The Family ENCYCLOPEDIA OF MEDICINE AND HEALTH

Consultant medical practitioner: Dr Maxine Long

Robinson
LONDON

Robinson Publishing Ltd
7 Kensington Church Court
London W8 4SP

Previously published as *Medi-Quest* partworks by
Marshall Cavendish Partworks Ltd 1987, 1988

**This revised, paperback edition first published in the UK
by Robinson Publishing Ltd 1996
Reprinted 1997, 1998, 1999 (Three Times)**

A copy of the British Library Cataloguing in Publication Data
for this title is available from the British Library.

ISBN 1-85487-359-8

Note
This book is not a substitute for your doctor's or health
professional's advice, and the publishers and authors cannot
accept liability for any injury or loss to any person acting or
refraining from action as a result of the material in this book.
Before commencing any health treatment, always consult your
own doctor.

Printed and bound in the E.C.

Introduction

Welcome to *The Family Encyclopedia of Medicine and Health*. It will, I am sure, be useful in several different ways – in providing simple explanations for technical terms, in offering a guide to the cause and treatment of common conditions, and especially in supplying the sort of background information that will allow you, the reader, to understand medical matters that may affect you and your family.

It is true to say that no medical reference work, however good and comprehensive, can be a substitute for a professional medical diagnosis, or offer the advice that comes from a fully considered assessment of symptoms in individual cases. Turning to the entry on headache, for example, there is a long list of possible causes – tension, migraine, sinus problems and so on – but also some potentially more worrying ones, such as brain tumour and meningitis. So it is important to try and distinguish between a simple, everyday ailment and something that is a symptom of a more serious problem, and in order to do this, and thus avoid unnecessary anxiety, it helps to bear in mind a few key points when consulting the book.

The first question, naturally enough, is 'Is it serious?' Every day millions of people with a multitude of complaints seek medical advice and the initial challenge for doctors is to decide whether the problem is relatively straightforward or requires further investigation or even referral for a specialist opinion. How do they do it?

The distinction between minor illnesses and the potentially more serious is made by assessing symptoms in three separate ways.

Is the symptom 'new'?

Consider a man in his mid forties who has woken with a pain in the chest. If he has had similar pains on and off over the years but which have not so far seemed to cause any harm then the probability must be that the pain is not serious – more likely to be due to muscle spasm than, for example, a heart attack. If, however, this is the first time it has happened there is a much greater likelihood the chest pain is, or at least must be presumed to be, potentially serious and appropriate tests are urgently required to clarify what that might be.

Have the symptoms persisted?
Most minor illnesses are 'self limiting', that is they get better of their own accord within a few days – often before a proper diagnosis has been reached. Thus, to return to the example of headaches again, if someone has had a headache for a few days (and he or she is not obviously unwell), it is usually permissible to treat with simple painkillers and see whether it does 'just get better'. If it does not, then clearly definitive steps need to be taken to sort out what is amiss.

Is the symptom getting worse?
This applies to symptoms that markedly deteriorate over a day or so, or more gradually over a fortnight. If an illness is noticeably becoming more serious over a relatively short period of time then it is urgently necessary to find out what is going on.

The rationale that emerges from these three criteria for distinguishing the minor from the potentially serious is easy enough to grasp. Doctors see a lot of patients with headaches and it would be completely wrong to investigate each and every one with expensive tests such as CT scans on the off chance that it might reveal a brain tumour or blood clot. If, however, the headache is 'new' – that is, the patient has not suffered from such a problem before, or if it has lasted for a week or more and is getting worse, then clearly urgent steps need to be taken to identify the cause. These three criteria of 'novelty' 'persistence' and 'deterioration', though not foolproof, act as a red alert system and if one or more are fulfilled, medical help should be sought.

There is one further important principle that can help the reader interpret the significance of the information in this book and thus avoid unnecessary anxiety. It is only natural to wonder – returning to the example of headache – how the doctor in the surgery can differentiate between head pain due to tension from that of migraine or sinusitis or indeed meningitis. The reason is simply that symptoms are highly specific, so the precise cause of a headache can be pinpointed by paying attention to its site, type, periodicity (frequency and length of duration) and exacerbating and mitigating factors. The bald statement 'I've got a headache' will not be of much use in identifying the cause unless it is also accompanied by these appropriate details. By contrast, 'I don't usually get headaches, but for the past month I have woken every morning with a real crasher. It usually gets better during the day, but is made worse by stooping or coughing,' should ring sufficient alarm bells for the doctor to conduct a thorough examination and arrange a prompt referral for a specialist opinion.

To sum up, knowledge (particularly 'a little knowledge') must be handled with care, so I hope that readers will find these brief notes useful when consulting what is a valuable and worthwhile family guide to medical information. It is certainly the case that the better informed people are about health matters, the greater their chance of staying healthy, and of getting any problems they do have sorted out quickly and efficiently.

Dr James Le Fanu

NOTE TO THE READER

This encyclopedia is intended for family use and has been written to offer clear, general information, with a minimum of technical terms. Entries are in alphabetical order, and within entries important references to other entries are made in small capitals – so for example, on looking up the entry for ALLERGY you will also be referred to ASTHMA. Italic is used for Latin names or necessary technical terms. While the limit of size means that the book cannot be absolutely comprehensive, we have tried to include some reference to all the common, and many not-so-common conditions, with descriptions of symptoms, variations, outlook and remedies. Illustrations have been included to show the appearance and function of many of the major organs and parts of the body.

Important: While every reasonable precaution has been taken to make sure that the information given here accords with current medical knowledge, personal circumstances vary so greatly that it is not possible to be sure that all advice given is right for everyone. So if you do experience health problems, you must consult your doctor.

A

A, vitamin, *see* **Vitamins**

Abdomen

The abdomen is the factory area of the body, containing most of the digestive system, the urinary system and, in women, the reproductive organs. It is also the biggest cavity in the body, extending from underneath the diaphragm, the sheet of muscle that forms the lower boundary of the chest, down to the groins. Bounded at the back of the body by the spine, and round its upper sides by the ribs, the front of the abdomen is covered by a thick sheet of muscle which can be felt just by 'pulling it in'.

Inside the abdomen

There are a great number of organs in the abdomen, often collectively called the *viscera*. Nearly all the ALIMENTARY CANAL lies inside the abdomen, starting with the STOMACH sited just under the diaphragm and ending with the RECTUM, which empties out via the anus. Associated with the alimentary canal are important abdominal organs such as the LIVER and PANCREAS, plus the SPLEEN, which is part of the defence system against disease. A huge network of blood vessels and nerves serves all the abdominal organs.

Behind the alimentary canal lie the KIDNEYS, each joined by a tube called a ureter to the BLADDER, which is in the lower part of the abdomen and in which urine is stored before it is released. Closely connected to the urinary system is the reproductive system. In women, nearly all the sex organs are inside the abdomen, but in men the testicles descend to a position outside the body before birth.

To keep everything in place, the abdomen is lined with a kind of tissue sac called the peritoneum and the organs are attached to it by sheets or strings of tissue known as the mesentery.

When something goes wrong

Because we cannot feel the abdominal organs working, we cannot actually detect when anything goes wrong, except 'by proxy' in some other part of the body. Thus the pain of a stomach ULCER, for example, is real enough but it is not in the stomach itself that the pain is felt but in nerve signals reaching the upper part of the abdomen.

Pains in the abdomen vary in position, type and intensity according to the cause of the trouble within and are in themselves good clues for the doctor's diagnosis. The pains are usually accompanied by other symptoms – nausea, vomiting and/or diarrhoea, as for instance in the case of food poisoning. And diseases of the abdominal organs can also be detected by pains in other parts of the body such as the back and shoulders.

Sex-linked symptoms

Many women become concerned about an uncomfortable, low abdominal pain which they get midway between periods. This is, in fact, perfectly normal, and it isn't worth bothering the doctor with unless the pain persists for more than 24 hours or is accompanied by bleeding. The pain is actually caused by release of an egg from an ovary (ovulation) halfway between each menstrual PERIOD.

Also connected with reproduction, but rather more unusual, is the set of symptoms known as *couvade*. Occasionally it is possible for a man whose wife is pregnant to suffer some of the same symptoms as a pregnant woman. In this condition, caused by extreme over-anxiety, the man suffers abdominal swelling and also sometimes morning sickness and food cravings. After the birth, the abdomen invariably returns to normal.

When to seek help

In obvious, everyday complaints, wait 48 hours before seeking medical help, but when severe, sudden abdominal pain strikes, never just 'grin and bear it' or take painkillers or laxatives. If an intense pain lasts more than a few hours, and particularly if it is accompanied by a swollen abdomen that feels tender to the touch and by blood or tarry substances in the motions, *see a doctor at once.*

Treating children's pains

All the same rules apply if children have pains in the abdomen, but if in doubt, always consult your doctor. In children, abdominal pain may also result from problems uncommon in adult life. Good examples are TONSILLITIS, middle-EAR infections and, rarely, lead poisoning from chewing lead-containing paint.

Anxiety is another common cause of tummy ache in both children and adults – and results from the natural tendency of the body to intensify the squeezing action of the intestine in times of stress. It is best to eat only small amounts or drink hot, soothing drinks to bring comfort and relief.

Examining the abdomen

If a doctor needs to investigate conditions affecting the digestive system, he makes an X-ray study. A barium enema is a study of the lower bowel in which radio-opaque barium sulphate is injected into the back passage and a series of radiographs is taken. A barium meal is an X-ray study of the upper parts of the gastro-intestinal tract and, in particular the stomach and DUODENUM. The patient is given barium sulphate to swallow, and a series of X-rays are taken.

Biopsy means removing a small piece of living tissue for examination as an aid to diagnosis. This procedure is carried out to investigate the digestive tract for a number of diseases including colonic cancer, colitis and peptic ulcers.

ENDOSCOPY is the name given to the technique of passing a flexible fibre-optic probe to view the inside of the stomach (gastroscopy), or colon (colonoscopy). Laparoscopy is a technique which is used to view the organs inside the abdomen or pelvis. Its most common use is in gynaecology.

Abortion

Doctors refer to any ending of pregnancy before the 24th week, even if it is due to natural causes, as abortion, but to most people abortion means the artificial termination of an unwanted pregnancy.

There are laws against indiscriminate abortions and abortion should never be regarded as a substitute for contraception. Generally, each case has to be judged on its merits, and two independent medical opinions are usually required before an abortion can be performed. Usually, this will be your GP or clinic doctor and a gynaecologist.

Reasons for an abortion

These can be roughly divided into the social and the medical. The most common non-medical reason is that the pregnancy was unplanned and unwanted. It may have resulted from contraceptive failure (or no contraception at all), from a casual affair, or even from rape. Other reasons include unfavourable circumstances, such as inadequate housing, a low income, or an unstable relationship between the couple.

In some cases, the pregnant woman may already have all the children she can cope with, or she may be in her 40s and view a late baby with alarm. On the other hand, a pregnant teenager may not be willing or able to bring up a child.

The main medical reasons for abortion concern the risk of mental or physical abnormality in the baby or the possibility of harm to the mother if the pregnancy continues. Abortion is generally recommended if RUBELLA (German measles) has been contracted in the first three months.

Abortion may also be suggested when SPINA BIFIDA (a serious defect of the spinal cord) or chromosome disorders, such as DOWN'S SYNDROME (which causes a mental defect), are detected.

The legal position

In the UK, according to the 1967 Abortion Act, an abortion can be performed provided two doctors agree that the continuation of the pregnancy involves greater risk to life or greater risk to the mental or physical health of the woman than if it were terminated. Existing children can also provide grounds for termination if it was felt that their mental or physical health might be adversely affected by an addition to the family. And, finally, an abortion can be granted if there is a risk that the baby will be born with a serious mental or physical handicap. In reaching their decision, doctors take into account both the woman's present situation and her possible future circumstances.

Abortions can be performed in Britain up to the 24th week of pregnancy. They are however much safer in the first 12 weeks. Only a very small minority of abortions are carried out at 21 weeks or more.

Counselling

Any woman who feels she should have an abortion will need to discuss the matter with someone. Counselling before any decision on a termination is taken is essential.

Sometimes the solution may be to have the baby adopted. This decision can be the right one for a woman who may feel that abortion is morally wrong. And sometimes the troubles and fears that a woman gives as her reasons for wanting an abortion can be alleviated by counselling. However, a woman who really wants and needs an abortion will always receive help.

How abortions are carried out

Early abortions, when the pregnancy is in its initial stages of development, are quicker, easier and much preferred by patients, doctors and nursing staff. After four to five months the foetus begins to move, and abortions at this stage may be followed by lactation (milk flow) which can be extremely distressing.

Two methods are currently used to carry out an early abortion. The first, D and E (dilation and evacuation), which is more commonly known as either vacuum suction or vacuum curettage, is carried out when the foetus is less than 12 weeks old.

The second abortion technique is a D and C (dilation and curettage), when the lining of the womb is scraped off. This is generally used for pregnancies of between eight and 12 weeks, but this can be extended to 15 weeks in some cases.

After the first three months of pregnancy, other methods have to be used. But whereas in the early stages the methods used are relatively safe, late abortion does have an element of risk.

Such late abortions (sometimes called a prostaglandin abortion) are carried out at about 16 to 24 weeks. Because the foetus is no longer small enough to be extracted by suction or curettage, an abortion-inducing solution is administered, usually vaginally but sometimes injected into the amniotic sac surrounding the foetus. This causes the patient to go into labour so that the abortion occurs through the natural process of delivery.

Before 16 weeks, the sac is not large enough to be located accurately, so this process of inducing labour by injections into the amniotic sac cannot be used safely before this time. A more recent method introduces a solution – usually in the form of prostaglandin pessaries – into the top of the vagina close to the womb, rather than the sac. This has proved effective in bringing on labour and has few side-effects.

There is a last method of carrying out a late abortion (16 to 24 weeks). Called a hysterotomy (not to be confused with hysterectomy), it is only used when induction methods have proved unsuccessful. As in a Caesarean section, the foetus is removed through a small incision in the abdomen, usually just below the pubic hairline. However, this technique has the highest risk of complications and it can sometimes limit a woman to Caesarean births in the future. It also involves several days' stay in hospital.

After-effects

There is very little danger attached to having an abortion in a hospital or clinic. The real danger is to the woman who goes to the back-street abortionist – where she could run the risk of infection, a punctured womb and even death.

But there are a few minor side-effects which can occur after even the most well-conducted abortion. A woman who is too energetic during the 48 hours following the operation may find she experiences heavy bleeding, and this will require bedrest. Blood loss following abortion varies from woman to woman: it may finish after a few days, like a period, or it may go on for two or three weeks. Some women get intermittent cramp pains for a few days afterwards.

Sudden pain, excessive bleeding, or a rise in temperature after abortion should always be reported to your doctor as soon as possible.

Because the cervix will remain open for a while after most types of abortion, there is a slight risk of infection. If an infection spreads to the Fallopian tubes, it could result in infertility. To reduce this risk, tampons or any other internal protection must not be used to staunch bleeding until after the first period has passed. Instead use sterile sanitary towels.

Some doctors also recommend not sitting or lying in a bath after the operation, though kneeling upright is all right.

Reassurance

After all abortions, final counselling should include contraceptive advice to avoid further need for terminations. In the case of the older woman who has completed her family, counselling should include discussion of sterilization for her or a vasectomy for her partner.

Occasionally, psychological effects are felt after abortion and these may be more likely after late abortion. Such emotional upsets may involve a sense of guilt and can lead to depression and a sense of loss or bereavement. This is not abnormal, and no woman should feel that, because abortions are relatively simple, she should just be able to breeze through it without any emotion. A great deal will depend on the circumstances that dictated the abortion, on the attitude of the partner, family and friends, and on the quality of the counselling before the decision was taken.

Abscess

Abscesses can occur anywhere in, or on, the body. They range from simple styes, PIMPLES and BOILS, which are abscesses in the skin's hair follicles, to serious tooth abscesses or other internal abscesses like an APPENDICITIS.

Causes
All abscesses are caused by INFECTION setting up inside a localized area of the body. Sometimes the entry point for infection is quite obvious: an abscess may occur, for example, as a result of a neglected injury to the skin or a large splinter. Often, however, there is no obvious site of entry for germs, but they can penetrate the skin through the microscopic pores in the skin surface. So if the skin is broken and dirty, abscesses are more likely.

Abscesses are also more common in moist areas of the body such as the armpit, groin and around the anus. Indeed, occasionally some people develop recurrent abscesses in these areas because the large glands which lie under the skin surface in time become deformed and persistently infected – a relatively rare condition called *Hydradenitis suppuritiva.*

Women who are breast-feeding sometimes develop a painful abscess in one segment of the breast, as a result of infection gaining entry through a cracked nipple.

Some people do, at times, seem to be more prone to skin abscesses. Occasionally this is an early sign of lowered resistance to infection. Diabetes may be one possible cause; another is the presence of virulent bacteria on the skin surface – *Staphylococcus aureus.*

Internal abscesses are usually secondary to some other problem – e.g. diverticular disease or a tumour. They may also occur after surgery.

Symptoms
The earliest sign of a skin abscess is a red, hot, painful swelling, which becomes filled with pus. If white blood cells are able to cope with the bacteria, the abscess clears up without any discharge, becoming a hard, painless lump which may disappear after some months.

Other symptoms, particularly of internal abscesses, are a fever and a feeling of being generally unwell. If the abscess is on the skin surface, glands nearby can become swollen and tender. So an abscess or boil on the arm can cause swollen glands in the armpit and one on the leg can cause swollen glands in the groin.

The great risk with an abscess is that, on bursting, it may release pus and dangerous live bacteria into the bloodstream, causing a serious type of blood-poisoning called septicaemia, or as in the case of an appendix abscess, into the abdominal cavity producing peritonitis (inflammation of the abdominal lining).

Treatment
Provided a skin abscess is treated at an early stage and the pus is drained safely away, it will cause little more than discomfort. A small superficial abscess will often discharge pus of its own accord.

Small abscesses can be drawn using a dry dressing covered with magnesium sulphate paste, which can be bought at any chemist; larger ones require medical attention. If the abscess is in an early stage of development, antibiotics taken by mouth, or given by injection may cure the infection. Once any large quantity of pus has formed, the abscess may need to be drained by an incision made under local or general anaesthetic. Often antibiotics are needed to ensure that there is no danger of the infection spreading.

Achillobursitis, *see* **Bursitis**

Acne

The mixture of blackheads, whiteheads and pink or reddish spots caused by *Acne vulgaris* occurs mostly on the face, the back of the neck, the upper back and chest, but can sometimes be found in the armpits and on the buttocks, too.

Causes

Acne affects young people of both sexes equally, but the lesions are evident at a younger age in girls and occur with earlier sexual maturation. The disease may be more severe in boys. It starts in adolescence because this is when there are great increases in the production of HORMONES from the sex organs and from the ADRENAL GLANDS.

Under their influence, and particularly that of the androgens, or 'masculinizing' hormones, the oil-releasing SEBACEOUS GLANDS in the SKIN, which normally produce just enough oil or sebum to keep the skin healthily supple, become over-active. They release too much sebum, causing a condition called *seborrhoea.*

The female hormones, particularly oestrogen, have the reverse effect, which explains – at least in part – why girls are generally less prone to acne than boys.

It was once thought that cutting out chocolate would help acne clear up more quickly and stop new spots forming. However, there is really no good evidence that acne is associated with particular items in the diet. Eating mostly fresh foods and plenty of fruit and vegetables will ensure a good supply of vitamins which should help to keep skin healthy.

Symptoms

Blackheads, accompanied by the pink or reddish inflammation which they cause, are the hallmark of acne. Bacteria that naturally thrive on sebum, particularly two called *Staphylococcus albus* and *Bacillus acnus,* are now known to be the cause of the inflammation, not the acne itself.

In response to the multiplying bacteria, the blood vessels expand to bring more infection-fighting cells to the site – this is the inflammatory reaction. As a secondary effect of acne, the bacterial infection may lead to the development of pimples, which are spots filled with pus.

This infection usually only becomes severe, involving the formation of larger BOILS OF ABSCESSES, if the deeper skin tissues become bruised and damaged as a result of squeezing the blackheads to release the sebum plugging the pore. Left undisturbed, each spot or blackhead usually clears up within about a week, but if secondary infection sets in it may take a month or more.

Dangers

Secondary infection is one of the chief physical dangers of acne, as it can lead to severe permanent scars and crater-like pits or pock-marks. Even more severe is the psychological danger, for acne can turn a happy extrovert into a morose introvert.

Treatment

The most important treatment is regular cleansing with a detergent solution. The use of abrasives is uncertain, but may help. An astringent cleansing lotion applied with clean cotton wool after thorough washing will help to remove any remaining oil.

A clean face will be of little help to the acne problem if it is then surrounded by lank, greasy hair. Unfortunately the overactivity of the sebaceous glands is not confined to the face but also affects the scalp, and the hair tends to become excessively greasy with the usual associated development of scurf or dandruff. The grease from the hair aggravates the acne, so hair should be washed regularly and kept reasonably short.

There are creams and lotions which can be used to treat acne. They usually contain antiseptics to reduce skin bacteria, and keratolytics which remove any plugs of sebum blocking the follicles. Preparations containing benzoyl peroxide are usually very successful in controlling milder forms of acne. The whole area should be treated regularly to keep the spots under control. Just treating individual spots will not help much.

Many acne sufferers find that spots clear up more quickly in summer. This is because the ultra-violet light in sunshine helps dry up grease on the skin and aids peeling of the top layer. For the same reason, ultra-violet ray lamps are occasionally advised for acne sufferers, but these should be used with care to prevent the skin burning.

It is always sensible for a teenager with bad acne to see a doctor, who may be able to prescribe treatment not available over the chemist's counter. Antibiotics in the form of creams may sometimes be recommended by the doctor for mild to moderately severe acne. Oral antibiotics are reserved to treat more severe pustular disease. For severe disease not responding to other treatments, an alternative drug called *oral isotretinoin* may be prescribed. Occasionally it may be appropriate for young women to take the oral contraceptive pill to counteract any hormonal changes worsening the acne.

Most acne eventually clears up on its own, although sometimes it may last from the teens into the late 20s or even the 30s.

Acrodermatis enteropathica, *see* **Trace elements**

Acromegaly, *see* **Pituitary**

 Actinomycosis, *see* **Fungal infections, Lungs and lung diseases**

Acupuncture

Acupuncture is an ancient healing art that has been used in China for several thousand years. It has its roots in the ancient Chinese philosophy of Daoism, where it was believed that each human is one with the universe and that all life is permeated with the life-giving energy of *chi*. Part of this belief is that all our experiences have opposites (hot/cold, day/night, masculine/feminine). *Yin* and *yang* are the names given to these opposite forces.

The theory is that *yin* and *yang* merge with and complement one another, creating a balance. When the forces are balanced we are in good health. However, when the flow is out of balance within ourselves, and with the universe, we feel unwell and disease may develop.

Acupuncture is used to restore the balance, the acupuncture points being the places where treatment is applied. These acupuncture points lie above lines under the skin called *meridians*, and the ancient theorists believed these lines acted as channels through which the *yin* and *yang* energies flowed. Whether one is sympathetic to this theory or not, acupuncture worked for the ancient Chinese.

Modern theory

Today, Western practitioners of acupuncture explain its effectiveness in more scientific terms, though still incorporating some of the Oriental beliefs. Their explanation is based on Western knowledge of the body's nervous system.

Beneath the skin is a widespread network of NERVES, the most important strands of which run along the meridians where most acupuncture points lie.

Among their functions, the nerves pass on messages that take the form of feelings which tell us what state our bodies are in. These messages come from all over the body, and when they arrive from a damaged organ, an 'alarm' sounds at the nerve endings in the skin. When this happens the alarm is felt as PAIN. The theory is that the pain may be referred – that is, it may be a signal of a problem located elsewhere in the body rather than where the pain is felt.

For instance, pain from the stomach is registered in the skin of the upper abdomen and the adjacent part of the back. The connection between the source of the problem and where the pain is felt is explained by the fact that both areas have interconnecting nerves.

There are 1000 or so acupuncture points in the body dotted along the meridian lines. There are 12 main meridians and each is associated with an organ of the body. The lines run along the major parts of the body (such as the arms and legs) and end at the tips of the fingers or the toes. For instance, the liver meridian runs down the inside of the left leg, from the midriff to the big toe.

How it works

Although the ancient Chinese believed that it was the rebalancing of *yin* and *yang* energies that brought relief, modern scientific studies have indicated that there are at least two alternative theories.

The 'gate theory' is that there are reflex mechanisms in the nerve pathways which can close off pain, rather as if a gate were being closed. This reduces the pain although the cause persists. Acupuncture works by closing these gates.

The other theory explains the success of acupuncture through the production of hormones called endorphins. These have a pain-killing effect, much like the drug morphine. There is now evidence that acupuncture causes the release of endorphins and these then travel to the brain, where they activate a mechanism which blocks the pain messages.

This theory helps to explain the pain-relieving effects of acupuncture and its ability to induce RELAXATION and a sense of well-being. However, no theory as yet manages to explain some of the claims of wonder cures.

The benefits of acupuncture

Acupuncture can be used to help with a wide range of specific problems, not just the relief of pain. These include HEADACHES, RHEUMATIC PAINS, digestive disorders, ASTHMA, high BLOOD PRESSURE, INSOMNIA, ANXIETY, and menstrual disorders. It is also used in CHILDBIRTH and even in operations.

The treatment also gives a feeling of well-being and relaxation. For this reason it is an appropriate treatment or preventive for the numerous ailments caused by STRESS in our high-speed society. But acupuncture is not a cure-all. It is not appropriate for anyone who is at risk from infection (i.e. severe diabetics or people taking steroids), nor for those who have bleeding disorders such as haemophilia.

Treatment

The patient is questioned about his complaint and asked whether diet, mood, personal habits, season and weather have any effect on the problem.

A thorough physical examination then takes place, with the acupuncturist taking particular note of any tender areas, various pulse rates at the wrist, signs of tension, and variations in body temperature. Further information is sometimes obtained from examining the tongue, iris, and soles of the feet.

On the basis of all this information a diagnosis can be made, either in terms of diseases or of the classical concepts of *chi* energy balance. The treatment then consists of applying needles, MASSAGE or heat to certain points on the body.

The heat treatment is called moxibustion because it involves placing rolled-up cones of the herb *moxa* on the correct meridian points and igniting them. A beneficial warmth is produced by their slow burning and the acupuncturist removes them before the skin is reached. Heat treatment can also be provided by electrical means.

The choice of the points depends on the condition of the patient; it will vary from person to person and from day to day as the condition changes. The number of needles used also changes; from one to 20 or more, and they may stay in for as long as the acupuncturist deems necessary.

The success of the treatment depends on many factors, among them diet and lifestyle.

One risk involved is that acupuncture applied thoughtlessly might hide a serious illness by taking away the symptoms. This is the reason for the very thorough examination and diagnosis.

A common response to the treatment is that the patients become so relaxed that they temporarily lose coordination after a session. For this reason, alcohol and sedatives should not be combined with acupuncture. Driving is also unwise, especially after the first session.

The virus that causes AIDS can be transmitted through contaminated needles. However, all properly qualified acupuncturists sterilize their needles and so there is no risk at all of transmission. It's up to you, however, to make sure you choose a fully qualified and reputable practitioner before accepting treatment.

Acupressure

Acupuncture can be used safely only by trained practitioners, but other forms of therapy are much better suited to being practised at home.

The most accessible and easy to learn is *shiatsu*, sometimes called acupressure or G-Jo. The person who gives shiatsu applies specific forms of pressure to localized points on the patient's body. However, the point at which pressure is applied is not necessarily the location of the part of the body that is being treated and may even be some considerable distance away. For example, pressure on the meridian that runs through the foot can be used to treat headaches.

Thus shiatsu is quite unlike Western massage, which most often involves the rubbing or manipulation of the affected limbs and muscles.

Shiatsu massage is used in the East for a very broad spectrum of complaints, some of which would be regarded in the West as serious illness. However, like many other complementary therapies, it would be unwise to regard shiatsu as a total replacement for Western medicine.

For minor problems, though, the beauty of shiatsu is that even a very superficial knowledge is sufficient for the treatment of specific disorders. You can relieve the pain of toothache by pressing hard on a *tsubo* (one of the 361 shiatsu pressure points) which lies at the corner of the mouth. Headaches and sinus problems can be relieved by applying gentle pressure around the eyes and forehead. Press the inside corner of the eye sockets, gently pinch along the eyebrows and then press the bony outer edge of the eyebrows.

Addison's disease, *see* **Adrenal glands, Endocrine system, Hormones, Melanin and melanoma, Salt, Steroids**

Adenoids

The adenoids are LYMPH GLANDS situated at the back of the NOSE just where the air passages join those of the back of the mouth or PHARYNX. The LYMPH SYSTEM is the body's defence against infection and the lymph glands, such as the adenoids, are full of infection-fighting cells. The adenoids are so placed that any INFECTION breathed in through the nose is filtered by them and – hopefully – killed. Sometimes, however, things can go wrong.

Adenoids are present from birth, but on the whole they disappear before puberty. They are most obvious from the age of one to four. This is because, between these ages, the child is continually exposed to new types of infection.

Not a great deal is known about how the adenoids become infected, but any respiratory germ can affect them. Once they become damaged, chronic infection may set in. If the adenoids are recurrently inflamed, they tend to swell and this can give rise to ill-effects.

Inflamed and swollen adenoids can block the eustachian tubes and lead to ear infection and even deafness.

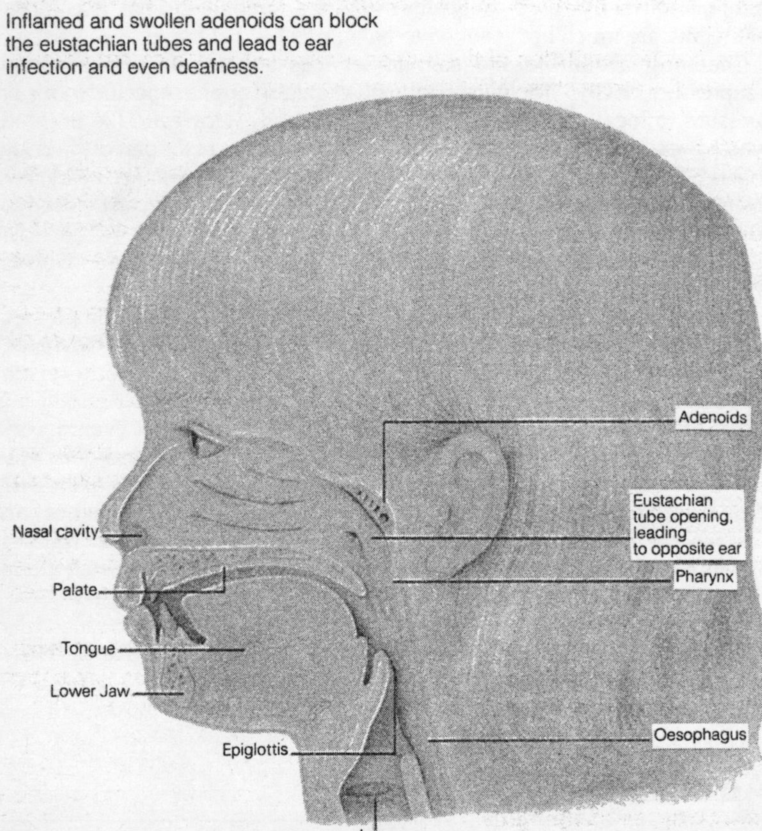

Symptoms
If the glands become swollen due to infection, they interfere with the flow of air through the nose so that the child has to breathe through the mouth. This may cause heavy snoring at night, and a nasal tone of speech. The child finds that his 'm' comes out as 'b' and 'n' sounds like 'd'. This is because when he closes his mouth to pronounce 'm' and 'n' through the nose, he cannot do so since his nose is blocked. BREATHING through the mouth also makes it very dry and the child may continually ask for something to drink.

As the adenoids fight infection, white blood cells – both dead and alive – are released in the form of pus. This pus will be seen as a discharge from the nose – quite different from the clear, watery discharge of a runny cold. The child sniffs to try to clear it but it then runs down the back of his throat and makes him cough. The cough is particularly obvious at night and is a typical sign of infected adenoids. In the morning, the swallowed pus may cause vomiting.

The normal ventilation of the sinuses is impaired which causes chronic sinusitis. Recurrent chest infections may also occur.

Dangers
Swollen adenoids can block the Eustachian tubes, which are a pair of tunnels running through the skull bones from inside each eardrum to the pharynx. Their function is to equalize the pressure in the middle EARS with that outside. If the tube is blocked by the enlarged adenoids, the pressure cannot be balanced.

But the main hazard is that natural secretions in the ear cannot drain from inside. This gives rise to a 'glue ear' in which the hearing apparatus is stuck up by secretions and hearing is impaired.

Treatment
Three types of medicines are helpful in treating adenoids. Decongestants and antihistamines are on sale at the chemist, but consult your doctor before using them. Antibiotics are available only on prescription.

As a last resort, when other methods have failed, the adenoids may be removed by an operation called an *adenoidectomy*. The operation is fairly simple and is carried out under a general anaesthetic in hospital. The TONSILS are often removed in the same operation.

The decline of infectious diseases and improvements in treatment mean that adenoids are not the problem they were 20 years ago. Often symptoms go away of their own accord when the child is six or so.

Adenomyosis, *see* **Hysterectomy, Uterus**

Adhesions, *see* **Salpingitis**

Adiposa dolorosa, *see* **Lipomas**

Adrenal glands

The adrenal glands sit, like caps, one on top of each KIDNEY. Each GLAND consists of two distinct parts: the inner medulla and the outer covering, called the cortex. These parts secrete different HORMONES, each of which has an entirely separate function.

The adrenal medulla

The medulla, or core, of the adrenals is the part of the gland which secretes adrenalin and its close relation, noradrenalin. Together these are known as the 'fight or flight' hormones because they prepare the body for the extra effort required to meet danger, cope with STRESS or carry out a difficult task.

The adrenal medulla is closely connected to the nervous system, which is exactly as you would expect of the gland responsible for priming the body to be ready for instant action.

Today, the dangers and stresses we face are as likely to be psychological as physical, but either way, the body has the same physical reaction. There is a surge in the production of adrenalin which makes the heart beat faster and more strongly. This raises the BLOOD PRESSURE, while at the same time constricting the blood vessels near the surface of the body, and in the gut, re-directing the flow of blood towards the heart – the reason we go 'white with fear'. It also turns glycogen stored in the liver and muscles into glucose required for extra energy.

When the danger is over or the stress removed, adrenalin production is reduced and the body returns to normal. However, if the danger or stress is constant, or if we are continually over-excited or under pressure, the body remains primed for action – and in time this can lead to stress-related conditions (e.g. high blood pressure).

The adrenal cortex

Wrapped around the adrenal core, the adrenal cortex secretes a series of hormones known as STEROIDS, the most important of which are aldosterone, cortisol and sex steroids.

Aldosterone: There are three types of steroids, each one performing a quite different function. The first, known as the 'salt and water' hormones, increases the water retention in the body. The principal hormone in this category is aldosterone, which acts as a chemical messenger and tells the kidney to reduce the amount of SALT being lost in the urine.

Salt determines the volume of BLOOD in CIRCULATION, which in turn affects the HEART's efficiency as a pump. Every molecule of salt in the body is accompanied by a large number of water molecules. This means that, in losing a lot of salt, the body loses even more water, and this reduces the volume and pressure of the circulating blood. As a result, the heart has difficulty in pumping enough blood around the body.

The secretion of aldosterone is controlled by the hormones renin and angiotensin. The system works rather like a see-saw: when aldosterone is low, the kidneys produce renin and the hormone level rises; when it is too high, the kidneys reduce their level of activity and the amount of hormone present in the blood returns to normal.

Cortisol: The sugar hormones, of which the most important is cortisol (hydrocortisone), are responsible for raising the level of glucose in the blood. Glucose is the body's principal fuel, and when extra amounts are needed, as in times of stress, cortisol triggers off the conversion of protein into glucose.

Many hormones act to push up the level of sugar in the blood, but cortisol is the most important. By contrast, there is only one hormone that keeps the level down, insulin. Relative insulin deficiency is quite common and results in DIABETES, where the level of blood sugar is high. Fortunately, diabetes can be treated with tablets or insulin injections.

As well as playing the key part in METABOLISM (the life-maintaining processes of the body), cortisol is also vital to the functioning of the IMMUNE SYSTEM, which is the body's defence against illness and injury. But if the normal level of cortisol is raised through medical treatment (for example, to prevent rejection after transplant surgery), the resistance to INFECTION is reduced.

Sex hormones: The final group of hormones produced by the adrenals are those known as the adrenal sex hormones. These are secreted by the adrenal cortex and they complement those produced in even larger quantities by the gonads, or sex glands.

The principal male sex hormone – also present in women to a lesser degree – is testosterone, which is responsible for increasing the size of muscles. Anabolic steroids are synthetic derivatives of male sex hormones. The main female hormone is oestrogen but the adrenals only make a little – most comes from the ovaries.

Control of cortisol

Cortisol is so crucial to body function that its secretion needs to be under strict control. The mechanism which regulates its production – and that of steroids – is another endocrine gland, the PITUITARY, situated at the base of the brain.

The pituitary secretes the hormone ACTH, which stimulates cortisol production and, as with the hormones renin and aldosterone, the two substances work in a see-saw action known as a feedback mechanism. When the cortisol is too low, the pituitary secretes ACTH and the level rises; when it is too high, the gland slows production and the level of cortisol falls.

Cortisol as a drug

Cortisol is used as a replacement drug in the treatment of the condition known as Addison's disease. When this occurs, either the adrenal cortex does not produce sufficient cortisol or the pituitary gland is defective.

As a drug, cortisol is also valuable for a number of other complaints – though it is best used as a short-term remedy. Because it reduces inflammation, it is used in rheumatoid arthritis as tablets, for skin complaints such as eczema as a cream to apply to the skin, and as an inhaler for conditions such as asthma.

It is also given to overcome the natural immune reaction so that the body will not reject 'foreign' tissue in TRANSPLANT operations, and, in combination with other drugs, to treat cancers.

Steroid therapy is not without its dangers, however. The most serious drawback is that the adrenal cortex is likely to stop producing its own cortisol when synthetic cortisol or a related drug is given for any length of time, and dosages must therefore be carefully controlled.

Steroids have more serious side-effects when taken regularly as tablets than in other forms. These include thinning of the skin to give easy bruising, thinning of the bones to give osteoporosis, and to cause an increased susceptibility to infection. Because of these reasons their use must be carefully monitored by a doctor.

Agammaglobulinaemia, *see* **Blood**

AIDS

Since the first case of AIDS – acquired immune deficiency syndrome – was recorded in 1981, confusion, misconceptions and recrimination have surrounded the disease. Meanwhile correct information is vital to prevent AIDS from spreading and to avoid unnecessary panic.

AIDS is caused by a VIRUS called human immunodeficiency virus, or HIV for short. To develop the illness, a person must carry the virus, and at present it is thought that not everyone who is infected with HIV (HIV positive) will eventually develop AIDS, although it is not known whether they may so do after many years, which at present has not been observed.

Cause

AIDS occurs after the IMMUNE SYSTEM – the body's natural defence against illness – has been destroyed by HIV. HIV attacks the immune system by killing off a special group of white cells in the BLOOD known as the T-helper cells. It is the T-helper cells which signal to the body's defence system when an invasion of BACTERIA or viruses has occurred. As a result, the body produces antibodies: chemical substances developed by the immune system which attack and, hopefully, destroy harmful bacteria and viruses.

Because they have fewer T-helper cells, people with AIDS are vulnerable to a whole range of INFECTIONS and CANCERS that other people do not normally get. It is the cancers and the infections, not the AIDS itself, that cause death. The most common causes of death in people who have AIDS are a type of pneumonia (*Pneumocystis carinii* pneumonia) and a rare form of skin cancer known as Kaposi's sarcoma.

Unlike most other viruses, HIV changes the structure of the cells it attacks.

It does this by incorporating its own genetic code into the genetic material of the cells it infects, becoming an integrated part of the cell and not leaving it again. After lying dormant, HIV then instructs the T-helper cells to make more viruses, which are then released. A person who has the virus will probably be infected – and be infectious – for life. HIV is a slow-working virus, and it can take years before someone develops AIDS.

Estimates suggest that 60 per cent of those infected are likely to get the disease, while others may develop less serious illnesses.

On the increase

Since the first cases of AIDS were reported, the disease has spread rapidly. By January 1990, 215,000 cases had been reported throughout the world. This may seriously underestimate the number of cases in Africa.

The number of new cases of AIDS continues to grow in the third world, but by 1995 had fallen slightly in Europe. The rate of increase has, in fact, declined since the AIDS epidemic began. Whereas in the US the number of cases was doubling every six months, in the past few years they have doubled only every 12 months. The first case of AIDS in the UK was reported in December 1981. By April 1990, adult cases in the UK totalled 3,223 (81 per cent of cases in homosexuals, 6 per cent in haemophiliacs, 6 per cent heterosexual contacts, 4 per cent IV drug abusers, 2 per cent blood transfusions, 1 per cent other).

It is difficult to know whether this rapid rate of increase in the number of people with AIDS will continue, in the absence of a preventive vaccine.

Transmission

Most people catch HIV through sexual intercourse with a person who is already infected with the virus.

In women, the virus might enter through ulcerations or erosions of the cervix or through the vaginal walls which become swollen with blood during sexual arousal. Cuts on a woman's genital area may also allow semen or blood containing the virus to enter her bloodstream. Similarly the virus may be passed more easily to a man if there are small cuts or sores on his penis.

Therefore, vaginal or anal intercourse carries a very high risk of infection. Other sexual practices, such as oral sex, are also risky if they allow body fluids – i.e. blood, semen and vaginal secretions – containing the virus to enter the body.

AIDS can also be spread through direct blood-to-blood contact, mainly with drug users who share needles or syringes. In the past, some people developed AIDS as a result of being given blood or blood products which had been infected with HIV. The risk of catching the virus this way has now been largely eliminated in Western countries.

Women who are infected with HIV can pass the virus on to their child during pregnancy or at birth, or possibly through their breast milk. It can also be transmitted via organ donation (kidneys, skin, bone marrow, corneas, semen, etc.).

There is no evidence that the virus which causes AIDS can be passed on through everyday, non-sexual contact with an infected person.

HIV is very fragile and is easily killed outside the body. You cannot get it from shaking hands. Nor will you catch HIV from toilet seats or towels, or from drinking out of the same cup as an infected person. If the virus could be contracted through normal daily contact there would by now be many reported cases of AIDS among health workers or family members and friends caring for people with AIDS. This has not happened.

Symptoms

Infection with HIV can produce a variety of symptoms. Initial infection may produce no symptoms or an acute 'seroconversion' illness with glandular-fever-like symptoms. This may occur up to six weeks after infection. More rarely it may affect the nerves of the brain, giving a reversible encephalitis or meningitis. Some people may develop persistent generalized lymphadenopathy with enlarged lymph nodes. The two main clinical signs of AIDS itself are tumours or 'opportunistic' infections, i.e. infections that do not usually infect a person whose immune system is intact. Tumours include Kaposi's sarcoma (flat, purplish, skin-cancer lesions). Infections include *Pneumocystis carinii* pneumonia, gastrointestinal infections caused by protozoa, fungi or viruses, tuberculosis, and toxoplasmosis infection of the brain.

Risk behaviour

More than three quarters of all people with AIDS in the UK are homosexual or bisexual men. This does not mean that AIDS is a homosexual disease; rather, certain behaviour – e.g. unprotected sex, anal intercourse, multiple sex partners – increase the risk of HIV infection. Anyone can get AIDS, men and women, homo- and heterosexuals. In Central Africa, where as many as one in ten people may be affected in certain areas, women and men are infected in equal numbers.

Drug-users who inject drugs carry a high risk of infection through sharing needles. If one of the previous users was HIV-positive, all the others could also become infected. It is now estimated that one in ten drug-users in the UK who inject drugs are infected with HIV. Over the next few years, a significant proportion of these will develop AIDS.

The best precaution against this risk is not to inject drugs. Those who do, should never share needles or other equipment for injecting drugs. In some parts of the UK, schemes to provide drug-users with free needles have been set up to prevent the spread of AIDS.

Prostitution is another high-risk behaviour, mainly because prostitutes have intercourse with a large number of partners. And as AIDS becomes more widespread within the heterosexual population, prostitutes will be at greater risk of catching the virus from their male customers, even though most insist that condoms are worn. Equally, there is the fear that prostitutes might spread AIDS to their customers.

AIDS and haemophiliacs

HAEMOPHILIA is a rare disease of the blood which mainly affects males. People who have haemophilia need treatment with blood products, Factor 8 or 9, to help their blood to clot, which are made from the blood of thousands of donors.

In the past, some haemophiliacs were treated with blood products which were contaminated with HIV. As a result, up to two thirds of haemophiliacs in the UK may now be infected with the virus. By April 1990 there had been 189 AIDS cases in this group.

Fortunately, the risk of people getting AIDS in future through treatment with blood products has been largely eliminated in the West as all Factor 8 and 9 is heat-treated to destroy the virus.

Blood transfusions

Before the HIV antibody test was developed in 1985 there was a risk of getting AIDS through blood transfusions.

Nowadays all donated blood in the UK is tested and any HIV-positive blood (i.e. blood that shows evidence of the presence of HIV) is rejected. People in high risk groups are not allowed to donate blood in the first place. So the risk of getting AIDS through a transfusion is negligible.

Unfortunately, this is not the case everywhere. In Africa, lack of money to test all would-be donors for infection with HIV means that the spread of AIDS through blood transfusion will continue.

Some people may be worried about getting AIDS through giving blood. Giving blood contains no risk. All the equipment at BLOOD DONATION centres in the UK is sterilized and used only once.

The risk of those handling donated blood and caring for people carrying the AIDS appears to be low. The most likely way in which HIV may be transmitted to health workers is through a needle that contains infected blood getting accidentally stuck into someone handling it and there seems to be little risk of infection from such accidents.

Other risks

ARTIFICIAL INSEMINATION is a possible way to catch HIV, if the semen of the donor has not been screened for antibodies. Most clinics now automatically test donors for infection with HIV, but women carrying out artificial insemination for themselves should choose their donor carefully.

Very few lesbians are known to have developed AIDS, but they are not immune to the disease. Although there is no evidence, so far, of the virus being passed on sexually from woman-to-woman, some lesbians may occasionally have sex with men who may be at risk.

Safer sex

'Safer sex' means performing sex in a responsible way to minimize the risks of either passing on or catching HIV from an infected partner. Any sexual act with an infected person that involves the exchange of body fluids is dangerous. The virus is carried in the fluids – that means blood, semen and vaginal secretions – and can enter the bloodstream through tiny cuts and grazes on the skin.

Safer sex means using a condom. But since condoms can break and tear, it is best to use them with a spermicide containing nonoxynol-9, which appears to be effective against the virus. If a lubricant is needed, this should be a water-soluble one such as KY jelly, not a petroleum or oil-based one as they will weaken the rubber.

Anal intercourse is particularly risky because the wall of the rectum is thin and easily damaged, allowing the virus to get into the bloodstream. It is safest not to have anal sex, but if you do, use a *strong* condom.

Oral sex is also dangerous since fluids can get into cuts and sores in the mouth. French kissing (where a lot of saliva is exchanged) may also be risky, although there is no evidence against it as yet.

The safest sex is that which does not involve the exchange of fluids. Hugging, massage, body kissing, using sex toys provided they are not shared are all perfectly safe and carry no risk of infection.

The antibody test

The HIV antibody test is a blood test which shows whether or not a person has antibodies to the virus which can cause AIDS. It is not a test for AIDS. What it shows is whether the person has been exposed to HIV.

In the UK, the test is used to screen donated blood and semen and also to test potential donors of organs. Opinions differ as to whether people should be screened for certain jobs, for insurance purposes, and so on, but the implications are far-reaching.

A positive result means that you have been infected with HIV at some time. It does not mean you have AIDS. However, anyone who is antibody positive is probably capable of passing the virus on to someone else and so needs to be aware of it for that reason. An HIV-positive person should take precautions during sexual intercourse, and should refrain from sharing tooth-brushes, razors or any other implements which could be contaminated with blood or other body fluids.

A negative result to the test usually means that a person is free from infection. However, it can take several months after infection for the body to produce antibodies to HIV. This means that, if someone were tested shortly after having been infected, the test would be negative. For this reason it is better to take a second test three to six months later. During this period, tested persons should not do anything that would put them at risk of infecting themselves or others with HIV.

If you think you might have been infected with the virus, it is worth having the test, which is available – free and with complete confidentiality – at hospital STD (sexually transmitted diseases) clinics, and also through your GP. Do not panic, however, if the test result turns out to be positive.

Not all HIV-positive persons contract AIDS, and even those who do are often symptom-free for years.

 Albinos, *see* **Enzymes, Hair, Melanin and melanoma**

Alcoholism

When people talk about 'alcohol', they are usually referring to drinks which contain varying amounts of pure alcohol. Alcoholic drinks have a restricted food value in the form of sugar (as in sweet wines, for example) and carbohydrate (in spirits and beers made from grain), but basically alcohol is a drug – that is, a substance which affects the workings of the mind and body.

Taken in moderation, alcohol can encourage the appetite and produce a feeling of well-being. This is because the alcohol stimulates the BLOOD flow to the skin which has the effect of making the drinker feel pleasantly warm. When it reaches the brain, ANXIETY is reduced and self-confidence increases. The effect is, of course, temporary.

Dependency

Heavy drinking, however, is quite another matter. If it is repeated over a period of time, subtle changes can occur in the personality – it is thought that these have a chemical basis – and this can lead to the need to carry on the drinking pattern. When every time a drink is delayed there is an urgent desire to have another, a state known as 'dependency' has been reached.

In the early stages of heavy drinking, this dependency tends to be psychological rather than physical. After all, it is anxiety and STRESS that usually lead people into drinking in the first place, but then they come to rely on the alcohol as a prop to keep them at their ease.

Unfortunately, if the drinking becomes increasingly heavier, psychological dependence can give way to a physical dependence. In the transitional period, this may not be noticeable, but as physical dependence grows, withdrawal will become more and more difficult and uncomfortable. Eventually, deprivation for any length of time will result in trembling, sweating and acute stress. The first drink will always relieve these feelings – until the next time.

Initial effects of alcohol

Alcohol tends to affect different people in different ways. The same amount can turn one person into the 'life and soul' of the party, bring out violent aggression in another, and send a third quietly to sleep.

Although it reduces tension, alcohol is not a stimulant, but a depressant. As soon as it enters the bloodstream, it begins to impair judgement, self-control and skill. Research has shown that workers with blood alcohol levels of between 30 mg/dL (the equivalent of one pint of beer) and 100 mg/dL have considerably more accidents than those with less than 30 mg/dL

With driving, the likelihood of having an accident increases when the blood alcohol reaches 30 mg/dL; at 80 mg/dL it is four times greater; and at 150 mg/dL (about five pints of beer) it is 25 times greater. This is because the coordination between hand and eye and the ability to judge distances deteriorates progressively.

The problems of alcohol

Once an excessive drinker begins to suffer harm as a result of drinking, he or she can be classified as an alcoholic.

Alcohol breaks up marriages, sets children against parents, and vice-versa, and costs individuals their jobs and their reputation in the community. Ultimately, of course, it can also kill.

When most people think of alcoholics, they visualize meths drinkers and down-and-out inebriates, but it is not just the deprived and inadequate members of our society that resort to the bottle as a means of escape – there are children too drunk to take in their school lessons after lunch, business executives incapable of working in the afternoons, and homemakers barely able to prepare a meal at the end of the day.

Alcoholism can strike irrespective of age, class, creed, colour or sex, and once afflicted, alcoholics will mix only with like-minded friends, neglect their families, break promises, lie and steal, and live only to drink.

A woman is more vulnerable to the effects of alcohol than a man; her liver and nervous system is likely to suffer damage with lower quantities of drink. Any woman who is pregnant should also drink as little as possible during pregnancy. Regular drinking, especially in the early months, may cause permanent damage to the baby, such as mental retardation or various physical deformities.

Reasons for heavy drinking

Drinking is an accepted and approved cultural activity. As such, it would appear that some people are more exposed to the risk of becoming alcoholics than others simply because of social pressures and conditioning. For example, studies of national groups reveal that the Irish have a high rate of alcoholism; in contrast, the Jews' is very low. Certain professions seem to encourage alcoholism – sales representatives, bar staff and company directors, among others, are particularly at risk. Presumably, extensive socializing and the availability of drink are responsible in these cases.

The housewife is increasingly a victim of this form of addiction. Often isolated, drinking can provide her with a welcome escape from an apparently humdrum existence. And the fact that most supermarkets today stock alcohol makes it only too easy for her to buy it as part of her routine shopping.

In most cases, drinking starts at an early age, with children, not surprisingly, copying the habits of their parents. It is statistically proven that the children of alcoholic parents have a higher than average risk of developing the problem themselves. Teenagers also tend to be strongly influenced by their friends.

However, studies of twins indicate some GENETIC influence, particularly in male alcoholics. Depression often occurs, as well as dependence on other sedative drugs.

Danger signals

The body develops a tolerance to alcohol and the danger lies in the fact that more drinks are soon needed to reproduce the original feeling of relaxation and well-being. The higher the daily intake becomes, the more difficult it is to give it up.

It can take between 10 and 15 years for someone to develop an addiction to the point where they can be classified as an alcoholic. But symptoms to watch for are: an obvious obsession with alcohol and the inability to give it up or even restrict drinking to a reasonable level; moral and physical deterioration; and obvious work, money and family problems. The typical alcoholic will probably need a drink early in the morning and may need continual boosters to keep going during the day.

Safe drinking

In a situation where an individual wants to drink, but not to excess, alcohol should be consumed as slowly as possible and some food should always be eaten beforehand so that the alcohol will be absorbed more slowly into the bloodstream. Consumption can also be kept down by interspersing alcoholic drinks with non-alcoholic ones. It is better not to drink alone, as it is all too easy to consume more than usual just in order to combat feelings of loneliness.

If you do not want to drink, you should not feel shy about saying no. And if you know how much you can drink, simply set a limit and stick to it.

Provided you keep your total intake over each week below certain limits there is virtually no risk of ill effects. For men this is 20 standard drinks in a week, and for women 14 drinks. Standard drinks all contain the same quantity of alcohol – one glass of wine or sherry, a single pub measure of spirits or a half pint of beer or cider. So for men the limit would be a total of 20 glasses of wine spread over a week *or* 10 pints of beer, *or* 10 double whiskies.

Finally, the combination of drinking and driving – or handling any type of machinery – is known to be lethal and is recognized as such by law. Those who have more than two-and-a-half pints or doubles prior to driving make themselves liable to prosecution.

People who know that they are going to drink should not travel by car; or, alternatively, they should take someone with them who does not drink to drive them home. Otherwise it is sensible for them to leave the car where it is and get a lift or take a cab. There are no half measures in this instance; the rule is clear and simple: *never drink and drive.*

The physical effects of alcoholism

- CIRRHOSIS of the liver – there is no cure for this most common disease associated with alcoholism
- Other diseases – alcoholics commonly develop PEPTIC ULCERS, KIDNEY trouble and HEART disease
- Pins and needles in hands and feet
- Loss of appetite and INSOMNIA make individual weak and tired
- Attacks of trembling and sweating when alcohol is withdrawn
- Delirium tremens – more serious form of attack after withdrawal, accompanied by frightening hallucinations

Aldosterone, *see* **Adrenal glands, Blood pressure**

Alexander technique, *see* **Relaxation**

Alimentary canal

Food is the fuel that powers the activities of the body. But before it can be of any use, it must be properly processed. The body's food-processing plant is the alimentary canal, a muscular tube about 33 ft (10 m) long. It comprises the mouth, the PHARYNX, the OESOPHAGUS, the STOMACH, the small and large INTESTINES and the anus. It is in the alimentary canal that the processes of DIGESTION and EXCRETION are carried out.

Allergy

An allergy is a sensitivity to a substance which does not normally cause people any discomfort or harm. HAY FEVER, which is caused by a sensitivity to pollen, is a well-known example. ASTHMA, ECZEMA, RASHES and a variety of other complaints can be caused partly or entirely by an allergy. In fact, allergies can affect almost any part of the body and be caused by a vast range of natural and artificial substances. The symptoms may be distressing but nowadays much can be done.

Allergies are a reaction to *allergens*, a name given to those substances (such as pollen) that spark off symptoms of an allergy in someone who is sensitive to it. Among the commonest allergens are foods (notably eggs, milk and fish), pollens, spores, insect bites (especially bee and wasp stings), animal fluff (such as cat's hair) and chemicals.

A common allergen in the home is the faeces of the house dust mite, a tiny creature, invisible to the naked eye, which lives in bedclothes, carpets and curtains. Some people are allergic to heat or cold so that their hands swell when plunged, for example, into hot or cold water.

Symptoms

As a general rule, the symptoms of an allergy tend to show up in those parts of the body which are exposed to the allergen. So an airborne allergen, like pollen, makes its severest impact in the eyes, nose and air passages. Food allergies reveal themselves through swollen lips, stomach upsets or diarrhoea.

An allergy to a metal would affect the skin, and an allergy to rubber would result in a rash on part of your body where, for example, the elastic of your underwear came into contact with your skin. But this is only a general rule, because, if an allergen gets into the bloodstream, it can cause reactions almost anywhere.

This is particularly true of food allergens, which are absorbed through the digestive tract into the blood. Because of this, food allergens can cause a wide range of reactions in sufferers, including eczema, nettlerash, asthma and even mental disorders.

Skin allergies: There are really three basic forms of allergic reaction affecting the skin. The most common, particularly among children, is eczema (*see* p. 270). Contact DERMATITIS is a particular type of eczema, often affecting adults, caused by direct skin contact with certain allergens. *Urticaria* is often called by its common names – nettlerash or hives. It appears as a red swelling which irritates intensely. The rash may appear suddenly, and there may be just a small area affected. But, if severe, it can cover the whole body with large, lumpy red wheals. Again, possible causes are many and varied. Certain foods, drugs, perfumes, flowers and plants may all be responsible. Some people even develop urticaria if their skin is exposed to intense heat or cold, or even because of severe stress.

Eye and ear allergies: Allergic reactions can also affect the eye, and these generally show up as irritation and redness in the white of the eye. Severe swellings can occur, but generally the symptoms are watering and soreness.

The ears, too, are sometimes the target of allergens; when this happens fluid will build up inside the ear and may temporarily affect your hearing.

Nasal allergies: Hay fever can affect the eyes and ears, though its principal target is the nose, which becomes stuffy, runny or sneezy. Unlike a common cold, which should clear up after four or five days in an otherwise healthy person, hay fever will last for as long as you are exposed to the particular pollen to which you are allergic.

Some people, however, suffer from symptoms very similar to those of hay fever all year round. They may have a stuffy, runny nose virtually all the time, although it will often be worse indoors and particularly at night and in the early morning. This condition is called *perennial rhinitis* and can be the result of an allergy to the house dust mite.

Food allergies and food intolerance: These have a wide variety of symptoms. The most obvious symptoms of an acute food allergy are a stomach upset followed quickly by nausea, vomiting or diarrhoea. People who are acutely sensitive to a food may also get a swollen tongue and lips. Sometimes the sufferer gets two kinds of symptoms; for instance, a child who is allergic to cow's milk may get diarrhoea and a skin rash. Apart from skin rashes, which may appear hours or even a few days after eating the food, these symptoms become apparent almost immediately after eating, usually within an hour. This makes it quite easy for the sufferer to identify the allergen.

Asthma attacks can also be brought on through an allergic reaction to foods and pollen, and this is characterized by wheezing, and difficulty in breathing.

Doctors now believe, however, that a variety of other physical and mental symptoms can be caused by food allergies though the cause can be difficult to identify. Recurrent tummy pains and hyperactivity in children have been attributed to food allergies. There have also been cases of bedwetting and CYSTITIS which have been blamed on food allergies.

The most severe – though fortunately, quite rare – symptom caused by allergy is *anaphylaxis*. In this instance, the patient's air passages swell and close and the blood pressure falls abruptly. This is an acute and life-threatening condition, though it can be reversed very quickly by an injection of adrenalin.

Causes

The basic difference between people who suffer from allergies and those who do not is still not known. Allergies do tend to run in families – and it is very common for people to develop hay fever, childhood eczema and asthma (a combined condition known as *atopy*). This may be due to an inherited characteristic in the cells which make up the IMMUNE SYSTEM, which is the body's defence system against disease. But this is theory rather than proven fact.

However, it is known that most allergies are the result of an error in the immune system. The body's defence forces react to the allergen as if it were a dangerous infectious organism.

White BLOOD cells called lymphocytes are one of the most important elements of the immune system. These cells are constantly on the look-out for foreign substances such as bacteria, viruses and proteins which are different from the body's own proteins and which may present a threat. When these white blood cells come across a potentially dangerous foreign protein they form a substance called an *antibody*, which combines with the foreign protein and neutralizes it.

A slightly different antibody is created to deal with each foreign protein, but once it has been formed the body is able to produce it again to deal with any future 'attack' by that protein. This explains why we usually get infectious diseases like measles only once in our lives: after the first attack the body has supplies of the antibody which can deal with the virus whenever it appears again.

By some highly complicated process, which is not yet understood by scientists, the immune system of a normal, healthy person knows how to tell the difference between a dangerous foreign protein (like a virus) and a harmless one, such as a food protein. But in an allergic person the immune system reacts to a harmless foreign protein as if it were a dangerous one, and starts forming an antibody. This antibody attaches itself to cells called mast cells. Mast cells contain a number of chemicals the most important of which is *histamine*.

When the body is exposed to the protein again, the antibody attached to the mast cells combines with the foreign proteins and tries to neutralise them. But in so doing it upsets the structure of the mast cell, which falls apart and releases its load of histamine. The surge of histamine produces an effect very much like the inflammation which follows a wound: it makes tiny blood vessels dilate, and as they dilate their walls become leaky, so that fluid from the blood escapes into the surrounding tissues. The dilation of the tiny blood vessels causes redness and itching, and the escaping fluid makes the surrounding tissues swell. In hay fever the mucous glands in the nose and sinuses are also stimulated to produce fluid, which causes stuffiness and a runny nose.

Diagnosis

The diagnosis of pollen allergies (and sometimes of food allergies, too) is performed with the help of a technique called the *prick test.* The doctor or nurse drops a watery solution containing a very small amount of one particular allergen onto your forearm. Then a fine needle is used to prick the skin through the drop before the solution is wiped off.

Up to 40 of these little prick tests may be performed at one session without much discomfort for an adult. If you are allergic to one of the allergens, a round, red weal will show up on the spot within about fifteen minutes.

Another type of skin test is used for people who have allergic eczema or dermatitis. Small patches of lint containing possible allergens are taped onto the skin and left in place for a day or so. If you are allergic to any of the substances, a small area of dermatitis will develop underneath the patch.

For people with perennial rhinitis a more complicated test may be needed. Possible allergens are sprayed into your nose, and then if symptoms appear shortly afterwards it is likely that you are allergic to that substance.

A special diet called the *elimination diet* is sometimes used to identify which food or foods are the cause of a food allergy. At first a very plain diet is provided, often consisting of little more than water and one vegetable such as potatoes with one meat such as lamb. All possible allergens are excluded.

If you get better after being on this diet for several days, it is likely that one or more of the foods which have been eliminated will be the cause of your problems. You may then be asked to try various foods again to see if your symptoms return. This process of elimination is how the identity of the allergenic food is discovered.

Another approach to an elimination diet is simply to remove those substances which are most likely to cause an allergy. Often the substances responsible are food dyes, such as tartrazine (E102), or other food additives. If food allergy is suspected, particularly in children, it may be worth feeding them nothing but fresh food without any additives for a while to see if the symptoms decrease. Similarly, small children with eczema may improve if cow's milk is removed entirely from their diet and substituted with goats' milk or soya-based milk substitute.

If there is great difficulty in isolating the substance causing an allergy then a provocation test is performed, in which the patient is given a small amount of a potential allergen to see if it provokes a reaction. This will need to be done under the close supervision of a doctor. This can be done to test for food allergies, and your reaction to chemicals which are commonly found in the home, as in cleaning agents, or used as flavouring, colouring or preservatives in food.

Treatment

If you have the acute kind of allergy which makes you sick whenever you eat say, strawberries or shellfish, you hardly need a doctor to diagnose your complaint. The cause and the effect are obvious, and the simplest way to deal with the allergy is to avoid the allergen.

If your doctor carries out prick tests, he will be able to tell you which substances you should avoid. So if, for example, the test shows you are allergic to wool, then you should avoid contact with it.

However, prick tests often show up an allergy to house dust mite faeces. It is very difficult to avoid exposure to dust but you may be able to keep dust down in your own house by avoiding too many loose furnishings such as heavy curtains, loose covers and deep carpets. Regular vacuuming of all carpets and curtains may help, and it is worth using pillows and duvets filled with artificial fibre rather than feathers as they will harbour less dust and fewer mites. They will also be easier to wash. Special mattress covers are now available and your doctor will be able to advise you about this.

Several kinds of drug are prescribed to deal with the symptoms of allergy. Antihistamines combat the inflammatory effects of histamine when it is released. They come as tablets, liquid medicine, nose drops or eye drops, and there are injectable antihistamines which can be used to deal with serious attacks. Antihistamines are particularly useful for hay fever, urticaria and perennial rhinitis. The one disadvantage of antihistamine tablets is that some of them may make you feel sleepy. If they do, do not drive or use any machinery, and ask your doctor or chemist for a different type.

Another drug, disodium cromoglycate (better known by its brand name Intal), works by preventing the mast cells from exploding. It therefore has to be taken before the symptoms occur; it can do nothing about histamine once it has been released. This drug can be given in the form of an inhalant (for asthma), eye drops (for allergic symptoms in the eye), tablets (for stomach allergies) or by a nose spray for hay fever or perennial rhinitis.

Corticosteroid drugs such as cortisone, which are very powerful and anti-inflammatory, are sometimes prescribed for skin allergies or, via an inhaler, to combat asthma. Asthma can also be controlled by a group of drugs known as bronchodilators, so called because they dilate (open up) the bronchi (the air passages around the lungs).

It should be stressed that these drugs are not cures; they simply relieve the symptoms. Nor are they without problems. Corticosteroids have to be used sparingly and if they are taken by mouth they should not be used for long periods.

Eczema often responds to quite simple measures, and it is important to ensure that the skin does not get too dry. So use of a simple moisturizing cream and oil in the bath will help.

Severe eczema can be brought under control with steroid creams but it is never advisable to use the stronger types of steroid creams over long periods. Hydrocortisone cream is the most widely prescribed type of steroid as it has few long-term side-effects. A weak version of this can be bought over the counter in a chemist's shop. Stronger creams need a doctor's prescription.

Food allergies can sometimes be relieved by drugs, but some doctors prefer to recommend diets which ensure that you eliminate all foods to which you have an allergic reaction. This can be quite difficult in the case of peanut allergy, which can be severe and most usually occurs in children – schools should be informed of the allergy. Peanut oil is a commonly used cooking ingredient of many foodstuffs.

Sufferers of the most severe type of allergy (anaphylaxis) may need to carry syringes of adrenaline with them to inject themselves immediately should symptoms occur before seeking help at the nearest hospital.

Self-help

There is quite a lot that sufferers can do to help themselves. Obviously, if you suffer from a food or chemical allergy you should make every effort to avoid your allergens. This means that you should read the labels on food packets carefully to see whether the product contains even small amounts of the substance causing your particular allergy.

Hay fever sufferers should be careful about going out in the open air during the pollen season, especially in mid-afternoon when the pollen count is highest. Dark glasses can protect your eyes against pollen or spores, and it might be worth thinking about buying a small air conditioner for your home or car which can extract pollen from the air. Some cars now have filters in their ventilation systems which are designed to catch pollen before it enters the car.

If you are going on holiday in the late spring or early summer, bear in mind that there is usually much less pollen in the seaside air than in the middle of the countryside.

Alopecia, *see* **Hair**

Alveoli, *see* **Breasts and breast cancer, Breathing, Emphysema, Lungs and lung diseases, Pneumonia**

Alveolitis, fibrosing, *see* **Lungs and lung diseases**

Alzheimer's disease, *see* **Amnesia, Mental illness**

Amnesia

The word *amnesia* literally means 'no memory', but medically it has come to mean a temporary loss of memory. Someone who is in a phase of amnesia may look confused and will often not know where they are, or perhaps who they are talking to. After the period of amnesia is over, the individual cannot recollect what happened during that time but often remembers clearly everything that happened before and after it.

The way in which memories are formed in the brain is complex and very poorly understood. But it seems clear that there is an early phase in the whole process during which a memory is processed so it can be stored in a retrievable form.

The processing of the memory may take hours or even days, but once it has been locked away in the memory system, it is not easily disturbed, although it can fade away over time.

When someone has amnesia, it seems that the processing mechanism is temporarily disrupted so that memories are not stored for a period of time.

Other more serious problems can permanently affect the processing of memories. For example, an elderly person suffering from Alzheimer's disease may be able to recall distant memories, but may remember very little of what happened since the disease started.

Head injury

Any severe blow to the head can cause *post-traumatic amnesia*, and the more severe the blow, the longer it lasts. A blow that causes memory loss is called 'concussion' and the distinguishing mark of concussion is that the person cannot recall the actual impact to the head. Immediately after the injury the person may seem confused and disorientated, but in time will usually recover and be able to recall events up to some time before the injury, and then for the whole period following full recovery.

Anyone with concussion should receive medical attention as soon as possible. It is not uncommon for someone playing team sports to receive blows to the head, but if there is any suggestion of amnesia, and if the person cannot remember the blow, they should stop playing and see a doctor.

Often a skull X-ray is taken to rule out skull fracture and then rest is needed until complete recovery occurs. The doctor may recommend observation in hospital because of the possibility of complications such as internal bleeding within the skull.

Physical problems

Many severe illnesses can interfere with the processing of memories and so cause spells of amnesia. For example, if someone is delirious with a very high temperature, they may not recall what happened during the time they were delirious. Serious kidney disease or other disorders which cause biochemical upsets in the bloodstream may also produce amnesia.

Similarly, a number of drugs may affect the memory. Perhaps the most well-known is alcohol. A heavy drinker may forget what happened during a bout of drunkenness. Longer periods of amnesia caused by alcoholism are a very serious sign of possible brain damage. Addiction to certain drugs such as heroin can have a similar effect.

Certain disorders of the brain itself can cause amnesia. For example, a temporary blockage of blood flow to the brain as a result of a blood clot in the arteries ('transient ischaemic attack') can produce temporary disruption of brain activity.

Amnesia caused by generalized illness will improve as soon as the illness is treated. If a brain disorder is suspected, the person may need to have a brain scan. When amnesia is due to drug addiction there may be some improvement if the person responds to the treatment given for addiction.

Hysterical amnesia

A sudden emotional shock or a period of unbearable stress can interfere with processing of memory in a way which is remarkably similar to the events of concussion. In the most severe cases, the individual may become totally disorientated, will not know where they are, or what caused the memory failure.

Sometimes he or she may go off on a journey, not knowing where they are going or where they have come from. With milder degrees of hysterical amnesia, there may simply be patches of memory loss which are hardly of any importance although the individual may feel other symptoms of distress. Some people believe that this type of memory loss may be a protective mechanism, in other words a process of blotting out an unpleasant memory. A more likely explanation is that sudden brain activity associated with the original stress somehow electrically disrupts the memory process.

With rest and reassurance – and possibly a mild sedative – the person is likely to recover. However, the treatment of someone who is still in a phase of amnesia may be quite difficult. Careful psychiatric assessment may be required to be followed up by long-term psychotherapy.

Amniocentesis, *see* **Pregnancy**

Anaemia

This is the name given to a disorder of the BLOOD, the composition of which is defective in some way. It is the red blood cells that are affected. These are produced in the bone marrow, and contain an essential ingredient, *haemoglobin*. This substance has the remarkable ability to carry oxygen, which it picks up in the lungs and then distributes to the tissues of the body where it is needed to provide energy.

The marrow produces two million red cells a second and these survive in the bloodstream for about 120 days. If the level of blood cells in circulation is reduced from normal levels for any reason, this results in a lack of oxygen reaching the tissues and produces the classic symptoms of anaemia: a lack of energy, fainting fits, and skin pallor.

Causes

In general, anaemia is a superficial symptom of something else that is wrong in the body, and because of this there are a number of causes. The main causes of anaemia can be divided into three main groups. First, there may be insufficient IRON or VITAMINS available for the bone marrow to make enough blood cells to keep pace with the rate at which they are lost from the circulation. Second, there may be some disease affecting the bone marrow itself so that it does not produce red cells quickly enough to keep up with the rate of loss. Third, the blood cells themselves may not last long enough to be replaced.

Lack of iron and vitamins

Every red blood cell is packed full of haemoglobin – a very complicated chemical molecule which contains iron atoms as part of its structure. The bone marrow must have a good supply of iron in order to produce haemoglobin, and certain B vitamins are essential too, particularly folic acid and vitamin B_{12}. There are some stores of iron in the body – particularly in the liver – so the body can make use of these if needed. But if these stores are depleted, red cells are produced without their usual quantity of haemoglobin, and the person becomes anaemic.

Iron is present in the diet in meat, particularly liver, fish and seafood, and certain vegetables such as beans, peas and cabbage. The most abundant form of iron is in meat, so vegetarians may become iron deficient unless they are careful to eat the right kind of vegetables. Children who have food fads and the elderly, making do without a proper mixed diet, can also become anaemic from lack of iron in the diet.

The other main cause of *iron-deficiency anaemia* is a total lack of stores of iron in the body. This will occur if there has been a high rate of loss of blood from the body and the iron stores have been unable to keep up with the demands of the bone marrow. Since iron is only absorbed from a diet fairly slowly, the stores can become depleted over time quite easily.

A woman who is pregnant may become iron deficient simply because her iron stores are used to supply the baby with iron (*see* PREGNANCY). Most commonly, however, iron deficiency occurs because of continued loss of blood from the circulation over a prolonged period of time.

Women who have regular heavy PERIODS may become iron deficient, or anyone who loses blood from PILES (haemorrhoids). More serious, however, is the possibility of internal bleeding giving rise to unnoticed loss of blood into the bowel. Someone with a stomach or duodenal ULCER may lose blood from the ulcer internally; growths or TUMOURS in the bowel may also bleed over a long period of time. Another, uncommon, cause of iron deficiency is the overuse of ASPIRIN for prolonged periods. Aspirin can cause small amounts of bleeding in the stomach lining.

Lack of folic acid and vitamin B_{12} in the diet also causes anaemia because the bone marrow cannot make the haemoglobin molecule properly without these two vitamins. Folic acid is present in green leafy vegetables, some nuts and fruits, and liver. People who do not eat many vegetables can become anaemic because of folic acid deficiency. Dietary deficiency of vitamin B_{12} is extremely rare because it is so widespread in foods and it is stored to a degree in the body.

However, the bone marrow may be deprived of vitamin B_{12} by a disease known as PERNICIOUS ANAEMIA. Vitamin B_{12} can only be absorbed from the diet if the stomach produces a chemical called 'intrinsic factor'. Some people develop antibodies to their intrinsic factor, and are no longer able to absorb vitamin B_{12}, thus becoming anaemic.

Bone marrow disorders

Anyone who has a chronic, serious disease, particularly LIVER disease or KIDNEY disease, risks becoming anaemic simply because the bone marrow does not function so well as it should as a result of the original illness. The bone marrow is also very sensitive to the toxic effects of certain drugs and indeed to the effects of RADIATION.

One of the most severe types of anaemia is called *aplastic anaemia*. On exposure to radiation, poisons and certain drugs, the bone marrow just stops making both red cells and white cells. A severe anaemia develops and the patient also becomes susceptible to infections because of the lack of white cells.

The bone marrow may also be affected by certain CANCERS, and LEUKAEMIA, which is a form of cancer affecting the bone marrow itself.

A few people suffer from hereditary disorders which cause the bone marrow to produce abnormally formed haemoglobin molecules. This haemoglobin does not work so well as it should, and sometimes the life of the red cells is reduced as well. SICKLE CELL ANAEMIA and THALASSAEMIA are such conditions. These hereditary blood disorders tend to run in families, from Africa and the Caribbean or from the Mediterranean region respectively.

Excess loss of blood cells

Occasionally, blood cells fail to last as long as they should and become damaged early. This condition is called *haemolytic anaemia*. It is rare, but is occasionally produced as a result of certain types of infection – including MALARIA.

Some people with enlarged SPLEENS may also have haemolytic anaemia because spleen damages the cells as they pass through, and it then traps too many cells in its tissues.

Symptoms

The most common symptoms of anaemia are lethargy, pallor and breathlessness, sometimes accompanied by palpitations depending on the severity and type of anaemia. Severe cases of anaemia – such as those resulting from rapid loss of blood – will cause fainting, dizziness and sweating. Symptoms of pernicious anaemia may also include 'pins and needles' in the hands and feet, nose-bleeds, and, in extremely severe cases, heart failure.

Aplastic anaemia can develop slowly, becoming obvious only weeks or months after exposure to a poison. It has all the normal symptoms of anaemia but is also accompanied by infections due to the deficiency of white blood cells.

Prevention

Most types of anaemia are impossible to guard against as they result from a malfunction of the blood-making system. But steps can be taken to prevent the onset of iron-deficiency anaemia. Eating a good balanced diet of milk, meat (especially liver), fresh fruit and vegetables, all of which contain an abundant supply of all those vitamins needed to make blood and which are also rich in iron, will contribute to good health and keep anaemia at bay.

Because of the demands made on their systems, pregnant mothers may be advised by their doctors to boost their iron intake with iron tablets, as well as folic acid. Vegans (i.e. vegetarians who also shun dairy products and eggs) should also take a vitamin B_{12} supplement.

Dangers

It is most important that the origin of the anaemia is diagnosed as soon as possible for a quick return to full health. With most forms of anaemia, the dangers are not immediate, but the condition can deteriorate progressively if left untreated.

However, in the case of acute blood loss, if the condition is not promptly controlled it may lead to a fall in blood pressure, and in extreme cases, the resultant reduction in oxygen supply may be a threat to the person's life.

It is very important that anyone suffering from severe iron-deficiency anaemia is carefully investigated. Apart from lack of iron in the diet, there may be other causes. If internal bleeding is suspected, special X-rays or ENDOSCOPY to check the lining of the stomach or bowel may be needed. The anaemia may be an early sign of an internal ulcer or growth which will need treating.

Chronic anaemia may often worsen an already existing disease, and this is particularly true of elderly patients.

Treatment

Treatments vary according to the anaemia, but invariably the patient will be treated to counteract the initial symptoms while undergoing tests to discover the underlying cause.

In addition to simple blood tests, other investigations may include a bone marrow biopsy. A needle is passed into the bone marrow under local anaesthetic in the breast bone or hip and a sample of bone marrow withdrawn into a syringe. Careful examination of this sample under the microscope will often provide the clue to the cause of the anaemia.

Simple iron-deficiency anaemia is normally treated with a course of iron tablets or injections.

With pernicious anaemia, the missing B_{12} vitamin has to be given by injection on a regular basis – usually once a month. And since the cause of the missing vitamin is the stomach's failure to secrete the intrinsic factor – a disorder that will never improve – the treatment lasts for life.

The treatment for aplastic anaemia is usually long term, the patient being treated in a special isolation unit designed to prevent infection. The treatment consists of giving antibiotics by drip to fight infection, and regular blood transfusions to keep fresh blood in circulation. The patient's bone marrow may be encouraged to recover with the use of certain drugs. In some cases, bone marrow transplants have been very successful as a treatment for this type of complaint.

Anaesthetics

These can be divided into several different groups, according to how and where they act to reduce pain. They can also be given to patients in a number of different ways.

General anaesthetics

These are used in treatments and surgery where the patient needs to be completely unconscious. They are always given by a qualified anaesthetist – a medical doctor who has taken special training in the types and administration of anaesthesia. It is the anaesthetist's job to control the exact length of time during which the patient is to remain UNCONSCIOUS and to keep a careful watch on his or her physical condition.

The anaesthetist keeps a regular check on pulse rate, BLOOD PRESSURE and a number of other signs throughout the anaesthetic. He or she may give intravenous drips and blood transfusions if they are required. The anaesthetist also has a variety of drugs available to correct any medical problems that may arise during the operation, such as changes in the heart rate or the circulation.

Anaesthetics are given in one of two ways – either intravenously (injection into a vein) or by the patient's inhalation of a gas. Whether the injection is used on its own or combined with a gas at a later stage depends on the type and length of the operation.

Loss of consciousness may seem to occur quickly, but it is, in fact, a gradual process which happens in three stages. In the first, the patient feels the pleasant sleep-like effects of the anaesthetic and starts to lose consciousness. This is the *induction* stage. With modern induction anaesthetics, the patient drifts off to sleep within seconds.

During the second stage, the patient is unconscious but still has some REFLEXES present and breathing is not quite regular. In the third and full stage, the patient is fully unconscious with quiet regular breathing and relaxed muscles. The anaesthetist is trained to recognize the physical signs shown by the patient at each stage and ensure that any necessary action is taken. This continual monitoring is helped by the use of extremely sophisticated equipment in the operating theatre.

Many anaesthetic gases have been developed over the past 15 years, all of which are pleasant-smelling and ensure a quick return to consciousness.

For most major operations that need a general anaesthetic, a muscle relaxant drug is given as soon as the anaesthetic has taken effect. This causes profound muscular relaxation and allows surgical procedures to take place much more easily. The drug also has the effect of paralysing the muscles used for breathing and this enables the anaesthetist to have much better control over breathing throughout the operation using a 'ventilator'.

This machine could be compared to a highly sophisticated set of bellows. When a ventilator is to be used, the anaesthetist inserts a small rubber tube called an 'endotracheal tube' into the patient's airway once the patient is asleep. There is an airtight seal between the tube and the windpipe. The tube is connected to the ventilator via a series of valves using flexible rubber tubing. Oxygen and anaesthetic gases are fed to the ventilator which then, in effect, breathes for the patient. The anaesthetist then has precise control over how quickly the patient breathes and the amount of oxygen given to the patient, and can control the amount of anaesthetic extremely precisely.

Provided patients remain in the deeper stages of general anaesthesia, there is no 'coming round', although it is possible that they may dream that this is happening. Where a very light general anaesthetic is used occasionally patients remember hearing voices during an operation, but this is very unusual, and they will always remain anaesthetized throughout the operation. Women who are having an anaesthetic for a CAESAREAN birth are given as little anaesthetic drug as possible to avoid it passing to the baby before it is born.

Once the operation is over, the effect of the muscle relaxant drug is reversed by the use of another drug given intravenously and the patient can once more breathe on his or her own.

Dental uses

Today, it is very uncommon for a dentist to administer a general anaesthetic. Any full general anaesthetic should be carried out in hospital – and many people now have their wisdom teeth removed under a general anaesthetic in hospital rather than in a dental surgery. A few dentists use brief general anaesthetics in their own surgeries to extract teeth, but it is still necessary for them to have an anaesthetist present and all the facilities necessary for a full anaesthetic.

Some dentists are now using tranquillizers, such as Valium, especially in the case of more nervous patients. These drugs, when given intravenously, produce deep sedation but they stop short of anaesthesia. Patients who are very nervous of dentistry may find such sedation very helpful.

Local anaesthetics

These are drugs which deaden a particular area of the body and so give local pain relief while the patient remains fully conscious; they are ideal for minor surgery, but can also be used for more complex operations if the patient cannot tolerate a general anaesthetic.

Most local anaesthetics are synthetic chemicals, although one of the oldest and best known is COCAINE, a derivative of the plant *Erythroxylon coca*. These drugs work by preventing the transfer of impulses along the nerves and so block information about pain to the brain. They have to be placed in direct contact with the nerves to do this, and so must be non-irritant, non-toxic – in other words, not poisonous – and very safe.

Most commonly used for the suturing (stitching) of wounds, the removal of splinters or small skin cysts, local anaesthetics actually have an extremely wide range of uses. Almost any part of the body can be rendered insensitive to pain by applying a local anaesthetic.

One method of giving a local anaesthetic is to inject it into the fat and soft tissue under the skin, so numbing the area into which the anaesthetic liquid has spread. This technique is also used before bigger needles are inserted –

for example, a BREAST BIOPSY (removal of a sample of breast tissue for analysis) is usually done in this way.

Injecting anaesthetic around the trunk of a sensory nerve will numb the whole area which the nerve usually supplies. In hospital, doctors use these 'nerve block' procedures to perform a number of different operations. Doctors may anaesthetize a finger to remove a nail, or inject under the armpit to deaden the nerves to one arm for special surgery. In obstetrics (medical procedures which may be carried out during CHILDBIRTH), the most common usage is the pudendal block: this injection deadens the whole pelvic outlet and allows forceps to be applied more conveniently to the baby.

When an epidural anaesthetic is used during childbirth, a local anaesthetic is injected into the lower back, just around the spinal nerves. This helps to give a relatively painless labour and also lowers the BLOOD PRESSURE at a time when high blood pressure could be dangerous.

Chemicals may also be injected into the spine in people who have severe and intractable pain, such as those suffering from bone CANCER. Such people obtain great relief from the use of special local anaesthetic placed in the SPINAL CORD.

In addition to deadening all the nerves in the spine below the point injected, spinal anaesthetics have the valuable side-effect of lowering the blood pressure. This can be extremely important in some difficult operations because it reduces the amount of bleeding.

After operations, epidural anaesthetics can be a good way of controlling pain. By leaving a very fine tube in the spine more local anaesthetics can be given at regular intervals and the patient kept pain-free for several days.

Local anaesthetics injected into the bloodstream can prevent and even stop irregularities of the heart. This can be life-saving in some circumstances.

When general anaesthetics can't be given to patients with severe heart or lung disease, even quite long and complicated operations can be performed on such patients using local anaesthetics. Similarly, elderly people may not be able to tolerate a full anaesthetic and so a local may be used.

A further benefit of local anaesthetics is that the surgeon can choose the type of anaesthetic to suit his or her purpose. Dentists can make use of a quick-acting, short-lasting anaesthetic, whereas a surgeon performing a protracted operation can choose a long-lasting drug.

Local anaesthetics are generally very safe drugs, but because they lower blood pressure, they have to be used with caution in a few patients.

After-effects

There are relatively few after-effects nowadays. With local and spinal anaesthetics, a little aching at the site of the injection may be felt for a few hours. In the case of general anaesthetics, the nausea and sickness that once occurred so frequently is now unusual. There may be some feeling of drowsiness, however, so that people who have had out-patient treatment or dental extraction should not drive a car immediately afterwards, and it is a wise precaution to see that there is someone to see them home.

If muscle-relaxant drugs have been used during general anaesthesia, muscular aches may occur for a few days after the anaesthetic.

Analgesics, *see* **Painkillers**

Anaphylaxis, *see* **Allergy**

Anastamoses, *see* **Circulation**

Aneurysm, *see* **Arteries and artery disease, Neurology and neuro-surgery, Smell, Stroke**

Angina, *see* **Arteries and artery disease, Coronary heart disease**

Angiogram, *see* **Ischaemia, Neurology and neurosurgery**

Angiotensin, *see* **Blood pressure, Circulation**

Ankylosing spondylitis, *see* **Arthritis, Spondylitis**

Anorexia and bulimia

'Anorexia' as a medical term has been around for centuries. It means loss of, or poor, appetite and is usually accompanied by loss of weight.

Anorexia nervosa

This is commonly known as the 'slimmer's disease', but despite this description, its cause is far more complex than any simple desire to lose weight. It is also far more compulsive in its effects than ordinary dieting.

It almost always strikes young people between the ages of 11 and 30, and it affects more girls than boys. Apparently those from better-off homes are more prone to it than those from less affluent ones. This tends to suggest that anorexia nervosa is very much more a problem of the Western world.

Dramatic loss of weight is the obvious sign that something is wrong, and the person may need hospital treatment if it has reached a really serious stage. But, in the long run, the underlying causes must be diagnosed and remedied if treatment is to work and any improvement in weight and health maintained.

Causes

Once rare, anorexia nervosa is now tragically on the increase. The parents of victims may find it difficult to understand its cause, but more often than not the problem lies within the family. A daughter who never rebels or gives trouble, who delights her parents in every way and seems part of a perfect family, may secretly be tortured by a basic lack of confidence, self-esteem and a true idea of herself as a person. She may be too submissive and anxious to please for her own good. Her parents may have unwittingly been the cause of this situation by being over-protective, thus deterring her normal adolescent drive towards independence and a separate identity.

Psychiatrists believe that such teenage girls may have a deep-seated fear of adult responsibilities and indeed a fear of sexuality. As their own bodies begin to show the signs of sexual maturity at puberty, they subconsciously yearn to escape from the adult world and revert to a neutral, asexual child-like figure.

The popular image of slimness and superficial prettiness that is promoted by films, advertising and television may give a girl exactly the justification for which she is looking to account for her rejection of food. In fact, she may not be overweight at all.

Other girls diet drastically to increase their sexual confidence. These girls can obstinately cling to the distorted idea that their extreme emaciation is beautiful, ignoring the harrowing evidence to the contrary which is only too obvious to everyone else.

When a normal person embarks on drastic dieting, they can stop when they so choose. Most find it so unpleasant to be hungry or deprived of favourite foods in the midst of plenty that the real problem is keeping to the diet. But anorexics, once set on a course of self-starvation, cannot go into reverse. It is as though they are the victims of a feeling not unlike that imposed by alcohol or drugs – and with something of the same light-headedness.

It has been suggested that anorexics may even have abnormal body chemistry, but this has never been proved. It seems far more likely that they simply have a different mental outlook and confused motives that can involve not only self-punishment but also punishment of their parents.

Dangers

Experience has shown that the more distorted an idea the victim has of herself, the more difficult the cure, and the longer the condition goes untreated, the more uncertain the outcome. In the past, death rates of between 5 and 25 per cent have been reported, but better understanding of the causes may improve the situation.

Anorexia nervosa must never be lightly dismissed as a passing fad or phase, which time and maturity will cure. The anorexic is *not* mature, nor is she suddenly likely to become so. Spontaneous cures rarely happen because the victim takes a positive pride in sustaining her hunger strike.

The longer the illness lasts and the more weight is lost, the greater the sense of achievement. This deepens in the anorexic the illusion that being thin is making her significant and outstanding as an individual. In more real terms, it is also succeeding in focusing attention and at last providing a form of personal rebellion against parental authority that should have been made much earlier – and in a less dangerous form – as part of growing up.

Symptoms

It is vital that the illness is recognized and that treatment is started as early as possible. This is not easy in the initial stages until the weight loss becomes so obvious that it is clear that something is severely wrong and a visit to the doctor really necessary. An unmistakable symptom in a girl, once weight has fallen about 2 stone (12 kg) below normal, is that her periods stop.

It may be discovered that she is making herself vomit, either to get rid of food she has been coaxed to eat or as part of a 'binge-and-vomit' pattern, enabling her to indulge in food without putting on the detested weight. In the end, the body becomes so accustomed to existing on a greatly reduced amount of food that it has difficulty in coping with a large meal.

In a few cases, anorexics use emetics, laxatives, diuretics and even enemas, and over a period of time they can badly disturb their body chemistry and greatly increase the risk of a fatal outcome. Obviously, prolonged starvation can mean a general weakening and a greater susceptibility to infection.

Other signs of anorexia include: bad school results, the committing of anti-social acts (e.g. stealing or deliberately breaking things), and withdrawal from friends.

Treatment

Alert families should call for medical help long before symptoms are acute. The first job is often to restore weight to at least above danger level, before psychiatric treatment can commence. American research suggests that there is a critical weight which must be achieved, between 90 and 95 lb (41 and 43 kg), before psychotherapy can penetrate the strange mental isolation that starvation imposes and allow real communication to take place.

Weight gain for the anorexic often requires a prolonged stay in hospital, with intravenous feeding in the early stages. To coax the patient gradually to eat normal food and gain a set amount of weight, a system of rewards and withdrawal of privileges has been widely used. The basis for rewards is often a list drawn up by the patient and includes such things as being allowed to get up to go to the toilet, having extra visitors, wearing day clothes, going home on leave or, finally, going home altogether.

Maintaining a successful weight increase at home is made difficult by the extreme cunning of anorexics, who will use fair means or foul to avoid eating. They will deceive parents into believing they are eating a main meal at school or at work, and at home will toy with food, pretending to eat while secretly smuggling it from the table in pockets or handkerchiefs. They have even been known to fake a weight gain on the scales by putting weights in their pockets.

In a hospital ward, of course, this type of deception is less easy; weight is monitored and bed rest imposed. Also, in the early stages, a tranquillizer may be given intravenously, if necessary, for those patients who know how to induce vomiting when given drugs or food by mouth.

Future action

Once enough weight has been gained for the patient to be out of immediate danger, the more difficult part of the treatment can begin. This will include some family counselling, so that parents can understand the nature of the illness and its causes and so learn to cope with it.

Initially, the victim has to be convinced that anorexia nervosa is not just a matter of weight loss. The girl, helped by the therapist, can then begin her own search and fight for identity, dealing with the inner doubts and fears that plagued her, accepting the challenges and appreciating the real promise of her own sexuality and maturity. She must be helped to realize that her old ideas about herself were distorted and to replace them gradually with a truer picture. With this will come the self-confidence to grow up.

Bulimia

Bulimia is the name given to another eating disorder which, this time, involves the compulsive eating of large quantities of food over a short space of time. These binges are usually followed by periods of strict dieting. Sufferers from bulimia may also indulge in strenuous exercise as well as inducing vomiting or taking large quantities of laxatives or diuretics in attempts to counteract the effects of the excessive eating and keep their weight under control.

Bulimia, which means 'insatiable hunger', has much in common with anorexia. Both involve an obsession with food and weight. But though many people with anorexia do binge eat from time to time, most of those who have bulimia as their main problem do not suffer from anorexia. Indeed they tend to be of normal weight or a little overweight. This means that if they are secretive about their compulsive eating, as is usually the case, it may take a long time for the problem to be detected.

However, we do know that bulimia affects mainly women and it generally begins between the ages of 15 and 24, often following a period of strict dieting. Researchers are not clear as to the causes. It does not seem to be associated with any particular personality type, but it may be precipitated by some very stressful event such as a bereavement or a broken relationship.

Most women report that they are tense before embarking on an episode of binge eating and that boredom or loneliness make it more likely they will succumb. Food eaten on a typical binge may vary from as much as three to 30 times the amount consumed in a normal day. It will probably include many sweet and fattening foods which are usually excluded from the diet. ANXIETY, it seems, tends to lift while food is being stuffed down, but is likely to return later once the binge is over.

It is estimated that over half those affected by bulimia induce vomiting either during or after the binge to avoid the food being absorbed by the body. Many do this secretly, using bags or other containers, which are later disposed of to avoid detection. Even more, it seems, use large quantities of laxatives in the mistaken belief that they will clear out the food from the body before it has the chance to be converted into energy. And a large number use diuretics, which have no real effect on weight but can cause POTASSIUM deficiency. Some bulimia sufferers are aware of this and eat oranges, which are rich in potassium, to make up the lack.

Treatment

Successful treatment of bulimia depends on the person concerned being aware they have an eating problem which may endanger their health and emotional well-being. They need to be motivated to change their eating habits and aware that there may be a difficult period of adjustment.

Treatment with a doctor or therapist should aim to help sufferers adopt new and more sensible attitudes to food and weight. They will need to cooperate in eating regular meals to maintain an agreed weight and to avoid excessive dieting and other inappropriate methods of trying to lose weight. They will need to recognize what precipitates their binge eating and find other ways of relieving their tension.

Bulimics may also require extensive dental work: the frequent exposure of the teeth to stomach acid brought up by vomiting can ruin the enamel.

Anoxia, *see* **Cerebral palsy**

Antenatal care, *see* **Pregnancy**

Anthracosis, *see* **Lungs and lung diseases**

Antibiotics

Being prescribed a course of antibiotics is such a common experience today that many people have forgotten that these drugs have made possible some of the most dramatic advances of modern medicine, and, of course, saved countless lives.

The first antibiotic, penicillin, was introduced in the 1940s. Since then the search for, and discovery of new types has continued, and the various antibiotics have, between them, dramatically reduced the mortality rates from several of the world's severe diseases.

Antibiotics are also used to combat infection in patients who have undergone surgery, or those with serious body wounds. Again, the number of lives saved is substantial.

And these drugs also cure many relatively minor problems such as THROAT infections, TONSILLITIS, CYSTITIS, ABSCESSES, carbuncles, and septic fingers.

What they can do

Most of the time, we are exposed to what doctors and scientists call micro-organisms – in other words, germs. They are in food, in the air we breathe, in plants, the soil and in our own bodies. Most are harmless to human beings, many are beneficial, but a few are not and these cause disease.

Micro-organisms which cause disease are divided into a number of different types. Perhaps the three most commonly encountered are BACTERIA, VIRUSES and protozoa. They all attack the body in different ways to cause different illnesses. Among the many conditions caused by bacteria are PNEUMONIA and TUBERCULOSIS. Viruses cause such ailments as the common COLD, FLU and CHICKEN-POX. Protozoa bring about among other things, amoebic dysentery and VAGINAL irritations.

Antibiotics are, quite simply, drugs which kill bacteria. They have no effect on viruses, are not prescribed for them and are used for only certain protozoal infections.

How they work

Antibiotics can be thought of as actually attacking micro-organisms, breaking them down and preventing their growth and multiplication within the body.

The most remarkable part of antibiotic action is that it is selective. This means that a given antibiotic drug only works on certain types of micro-organism, literally 'homing in' on the foreign bodies they are intended to kill, and leaving the other bacteria in the body unharmed.

To fully understand why antibiotics should be capable of this requires considerable specialist knowledge of chemistry. The basic theory, however, is fairly simple to understand. In nature, some micro-organisms just happen to attack and destroy others.

That this should be so was discovered by accident. Alexander Fleming, who discovered penicillin, noticed that certain bacteria stopped growing when placed close to a fungus called penicillium, most commonly found on mouldy bread. The most active part of the penicillium fungus had then to be isolated to produce an effective antibiotic drug. With this knowledge of the chemical substances which kill micro-organisms, researchers could then move on to the next stage: copying them to produce artificial antibiotics.

The fact that antibiotics occur naturally has meant that new ones have been discovered in what may seem to be extraordinary places. One, for example, was isolated from substances growing in dungheaps. But penicillin antibiotics remain to this day the most widely used.

Drawbacks

When antibiotics home in on bacteria, some will survive the attack and, remarkable though it may seem, 'learn' from the experience how to resist similar action in future.

The more an antibiotic is used, the greater the number of bacteria learn to survive attack – in other words, build up 'resistance'.

So antibiotics should be used as little as possible. If a bacteria becomes resistant to a certain antibiotic, as happened, for example, with the first penicillins, an alternative antibiotic has to be used. Luckily, the development of alternative and synthetic antibiotic types means that this is possible. This is one reason why researchers are continually developing new types.

Side-effects

Some people are allergic to penicillin, usually coming out in a rash when given it. They should always tell anyone who treats them medically if this is the case.

Many antibiotics can have side-effects, ranging from indigestion and diarrhoea to deafness and loss of balance. In most cases, it is a question of temporary discomfort to be tolerated for the sake of a permanent cure. However, you should always go back to your doctor without delay if an antibiotic is having a persistent, worrying side-effect.

Most antibiotics do not affect the action of the contraceptive pill, but one, rifampicin, destroys the contraceptive pill in the body, making it ineffective. Several others such as Amoxycillin, make the contraceptive pill less effective. So you should always remind your doctor that you are on the contraceptive pill.

Like all precision instruments, antibiotics need to be used properly. Medically, this means tailoring the drug to the patient's infection. Bronchitis or urinary problems may, for example, be caused by one bacteria in one attack, and a slightly different one the next. Each needs a particular antibiotic to treat it.

The side-effects of taking the wrong antibiotic can, in some cases, be very unpleasant, even dangerous. If you are being treated by a new doctor – especially abroad – tell him if you know of an antibiotic, or any other drug, that disagrees with you. Never take anyone else's antibiotics. Never take antibiotics given to you for a previous illness, or without being supervised by a doctor. Always complete the full course of antibiotics that a doctor has prescribed for you, in order to completely eradicate the infection: the doctor will have prescribed the shortest course possible to do this, and to take only part of the course will only partially treat the infection and encourage resistance to the antibiotic.

Antibody, *see* **Allergy, Blood, Blood groups and transfusions, Immune system, Immunization, Infection and infectious diseases, Lymphatic system**

Antigens, *see* **Blood, Blood groups and transfusions**

Antiseptics, *see* **Septic conditions**

Anxiety, *see* **Mental illness, Psychiatry, Psychology, Stress**

Aorta, *see* **Arteries and artery disease, Heart**

Aphthous ulcers, *see* **Ulcers, skin**

Apnoea, *see* **Cot death, Sleep and sleep problems, Snoring**

Appendicitis

The appendix is a narrow, tube-like piece of gut resembling a tail, which is located at one end of the large INTESTINE, attached to the part known as the caecum. The tip of the tube is closed; the other end joins on to the large intestine. It can measure up to 4 in (10 cm) long and about ⅖ in (1 cm) diameter. It is probably a relic of evolution.

If the appendix becomes inflamed, a condition called appendicitis results and the organ may have to be removed. This can occur at any time, from babyhood to old age. However, it is rare under the age of two, more common among teenagers, and then becomes increasingly rare again over the age of 30.

Causes

The history and incidence of the condition is extremely baffling. Up to the end of the 19th century, it was relatively unknown. This is still so in such places as Asia, Africa and Polynesia. But in Europe, North America and Australia, for example, appendicitis is now a very common complaint (recent emphasis on healthy eating may reverse the trend).

The reason for this is thought to be directly related to changes in our eating habits. The modern Western diet has become so refined that it now lacks sufficient fibre (roughage). This deficiency causes the food to slow down in its passage through the intestines. This sluggishness can lead to blockages, which may be a cause of appendicitis. Food residues can occasionally collect in the appendix and form an obstruction. Pips, fruit stones and other foreign bodies that may have been swallowed accidentally can also aggravate the appendix, but these are fortunately among the rarer causes of appendicitis.

Worms, the result of eating contaminated food, are another danger to the appendix. These intestinal parasites may lodge there and eventually cause an obstruction. Whatever their origin, blockages of any kind can lead to the onset of appendicitis.

The 'grumbling' appendix

Recurrent attacks of appendicitis, each lasting a day or two, can sometimes occur. As the appendix gets inflamed, the intestines nearby close round it to wall off the infection. If the inflammation clears up, the intestines may still be left stuck around the appendix. These 'adhesions' can restrain the normal movement of food around the system, resulting in colicky (griping) pains, which may then be felt in the appendix region during normal digestion. This gives rise to a 'grumbling' appendix, which will settle if it does not become inflamed again.

Serious symptoms

Fifty per cent of episodes may resolve spontaneously. However, for various reasons, a bout of appendicitis may not clear up on its own: the appendix is blocked and further action will be necessary.

The early symptoms of appendicitis are not easy to distinguish from any other form of tummy ache. Pain, which comes and goes in a colicky fashion is felt around the umbilicus (tummy button), as the appendix muscles contract while trying to drive any obstruction out. If there is no obstruction, there will just be a constant ache.

After 6 to 12 hours, the symptoms will change, as inflammation builds up around the appendix. The overlying PERITONEUM (lining of the abdomen) becomes irritated and, as this is well supplied with nerves, more pain is felt around the appendix. Usually, this is in the right lower abdomen. However, the site of the maximum pain is variable. The patient will feel more ill and may vomit as the infection progresses.

Diagnosis

Often the patient has to press his or her own stomach to establish where it hurts most. The most common site is two-thirds of the way along a line joining the top of the umbilicus to the top of the pelvic bone. This is called *McBurney's point*, after the American surgeon who first noted it. But the pain can move to the upper abdomen or down in the pelvis. In a woman, this is particularly confusing as it can be mimicked by gynaecological pains from the ovaries or womb. A rectal examination by the doctor may be needed to establish whether this pain is, in fact, caused by an inflamed, tender appendix.

The inflamed appendix often lies on the right leg muscle where it joins the back. Because this makes the leg stiff, the patient naturally bends the leg up to gain relief. Stretching it down then produces pain. The muscles in the front wall of the abdomen also go into spasm to protect the appendix from any painful movements the patient may make.

Although the appendix usually lies below the caecum, occasionally it tucks itself behind this part of the bowel and in this case there may be some difficulty in diagnosis. The pain may be felt further towards the back than the front and it may be higher up than is usual.

Mimicking other problems

When doctors see patients who may have appendicitis, they will first ask about the symptoms. They need to assess whether there may be other problems causing the pains. GASTRO-ENTERITIS may mimic appendicitis in its early stages, but there will often be some sign of bowel upset with gastro-enteritis, such as some DIARRHOEA. They will ask about urinary symptoms to rule out possible KIDNEY infection.

Women will also be asked detailed questions about periods and sexual activity. Do not be put off by this line of questioning. It is crucial for the doctor to know whether there is any possibility of PREGNANCY. Problems with a very early pregnancy lodged in the right Fallopian tube can mimic the pain of appendicitis. Also infection in the Fallopian tube itself may cause very similar symptoms. In this case, the woman may have noticed some irregular vaginal bleeding, possibly a vaginal discharge, and may have experienced deep-seated discomfort during sexual intercourse.

Having established the pattern of symptoms, doctors will check their patients' pulse. As infection sets in, the pulse rate rises, and the patients may also develop a temperature. Next, doctors will gently examine the patients' tummy. They will look to see how much the muscles of the abdomen move with breathing. If the area around the appendix has become inflamed, the stomach muscles will be tense and rigid. They will carefully feel for tenderness in the abdomen, which is usually most severe around the site of the inflamed appendix.

They may also suddenly remove their hand from the area; if the appendix has set up local inflammation, there may be 'rebound' tenderness, and patients will suddenly feel a twinge of pain as pressure is released. Doctors may carry out an internal examination – especially if the patient is a woman – to check on the internal organs.

In the early stages of appendicitis, it may be difficult for doctors to make a definite diagnosis. They may suggest that patients stay at home for a few hours, without taking any food, and then reassess the situation later. If the pains are caused by some other problem, then it is likely to become more obvious as time goes by. However, if appendicitis is a real possibility, doctors will advise hospital admission.

In children

The diagnosis of appendicitis in children is more difficult than in adults. Children may develop typical symptoms and signs of appendicitis and yet the signs are sometimes not caused by an inflamed appendix. They could result from a chest infection, and disappear as soon as the infection improves (appendicitis should always be suspected, however), or from swollen lymph glands in the abdomen. In these circumstances, the child is likely to have some other symptoms such as a sore throat and maybe a cough.

Even if a child seems to have obvious signs of chest trouble, it is very important to tell the doctor if he or she also has a tummy ache.

However, if the signs point to the possibility of appendicitis, the surgeon will carry out an appendicectomy because of the ever present risk of complications. Only when the operation has been done will the true situation be known. If the problem was caused by swollen glands, the illness – which is known as *mesenteric adenitis* – will resolve quite quickly.

When to see the doctor

If the pain has continued for a whole day or night and has become increasingly severe, and if the patient is vomiting and unable to get up, then it is clearly time to seek medical help. It may be quicker to take the patient to the doctor's surgery, rather than wait for him or her to call. Home treatments, such as painkillers or soothing drinks should not be tried at this stage. An operation may be urgently needed, and the stomach must be empty of food and drink before an anaesthetic can be given.

Dangers of appendicitis

If the problem is neglected, the situation can become dangerous. The tip of the appendix can become gangrenous, causing perforation.

The pus inside the appendix can build up to such an extent that it bursts through the wall of the appendix into the cavity of the abdomen. This then sets up PERITONITIS. An inflamed appendix is unlikely to perforate within the first 24 or 36 hours of the illness but if left much longer than this, the risk of perforation increases considerably.

Once the appendix has perforated, the patient's condition will deteriorate rapidly. He or she will have severe, generalized pain, may vomit more and there is a danger of collapse. When the doctor examines the abdomen, the muscles will be rigid, and on listening with a stethoscope, the doctor will discover that the bowel sounds have virtually disappeared. Operation is urgently required under these circumstances.

Another possible complication is the formation of an 'appendix ABSCESS'. In this condition, the appendix swells up considerably, swollen by pus, and there is intense local inflammation around the site of the appendix, but there is no sign of generalized peritonitis unless the abscess bursts.

Appendicectomy

Because the risks of neglecting appendicitis are greater than the risks of an unnecessary operation, the surgeon will operate, even if in doubt. But, if the symptoms are inconclusive, the patient may be put to bed and kept under observation. If things do not improve, an operation will be performed.

If the symptoms and signs are quite conclusive of a diagnosis of appendicitis and the patient is not too unwell, the surgeon will operate straight away. The operation is quite simple and takes less than an hour.

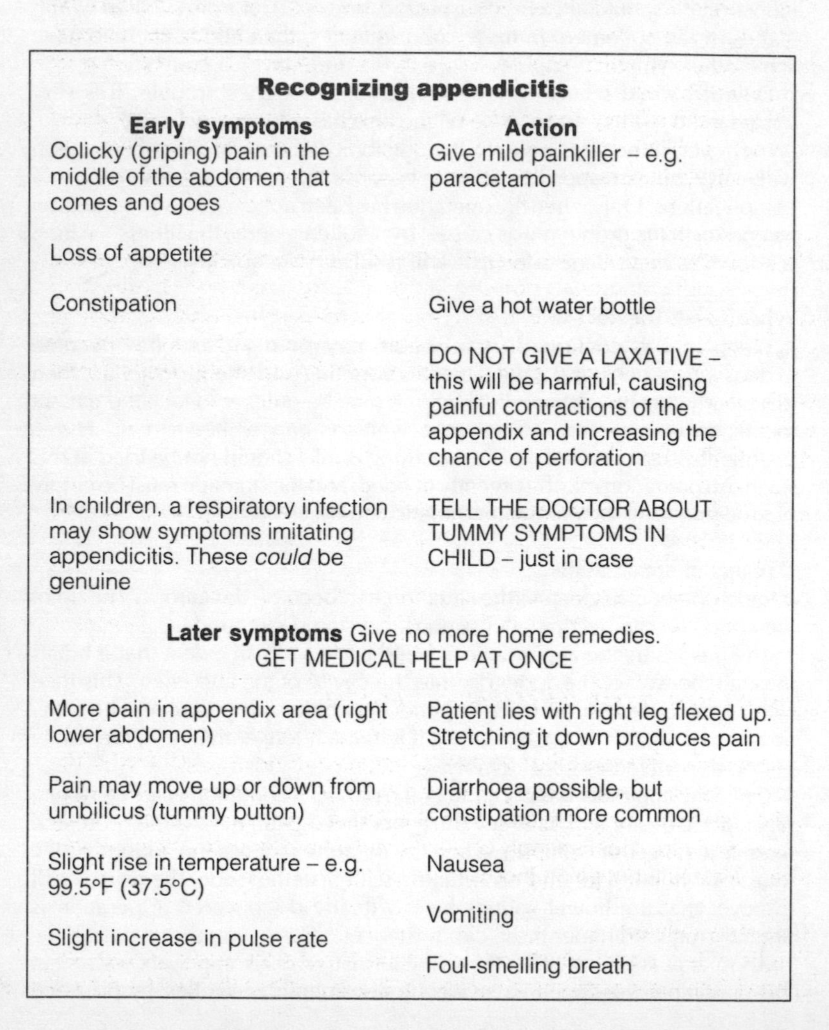

Recognizing appendicitis

Early symptoms	**Action**
Colicky (griping) pain in the middle of the abdomen that comes and goes	Give mild painkiller – e.g. paracetamol
Loss of appetite	
Constipation	Give a hot water bottle
	DO NOT GIVE A LAXATIVE – this will be harmful, causing painful contractions of the appendix and increasing the chance of perforation
In children, a respiratory infection may show symptoms imitating appendicitis. These *could* be genuine	TELL THE DOCTOR ABOUT TUMMY SYMPTOMS IN CHILD – just in case

Later symptoms Give no more home remedies.
GET MEDICAL HELP AT ONCE

More pain in appendix area (right lower abdomen)	Patient lies with right leg flexed up. Stretching it down produces pain
Pain may move up or down from umbilicus (tummy button)	Diarrhoea possible, but constipation more common
Slight rise in temperature – e.g. 99.5°F (37.5°C)	Nausea
	Vomiting
Slight increase in pulse rate	
	Foul-smelling breath

A small incision – usually about 2 in (5 cm) long – is made low down on the right side of the abdomen, following a crease in the skin. Through this small incision, the appendix is removed and the resulting hole in the intestine stitched. The layers of overlying muscle are stitched together and finally the skin is stitched or closed with clips. If the operation has been quite straightforward, tape alone may be used to close the incision.

If a surgeon discovers that the appendix has perforated, he or she will insert a plastic drain near to the incision to allow any infection to drain away. The patient will already have had signs of perforation of the appendix before arriving at hospital. If he or she is very ill by this time, the surgeon will give an intravenous drip to provide extra fluids straight away and then operate. Often, under these circumstances, a vertical incision is made near to the midline to allow the surgeon to clean out all the infection adequately. Intravenous antibiotics will be required if the appendix has ruptured or formed an abscess.

With expert surgery and modern drugs, even someone with a perforated appendix is likely to recover quite quickly from the operation. After an uncomplicated operation, the patient will be home within a few days.

The healing process

Once the stitches have been taken out, the scar still has to heal but the patient can soon lead a reasonably normal life again, though active sports are out of the question for several weeks. The patient is advised to undertake nothing more than light chores to begin with. A person with a desk job will probably be able to return to work after a few weeks but a manual worker needs at least 6–8 weeks to recuperate.

Areola, *see* **Breasts**

Arhythmia, *see* **Electrocardiogram, Heart disease, Pacemakers, Valves, heart**

Aromatherapy, *see* **Massage**

Arteries and artery disease

The arteries and VEINS are the two sorts of large blood vessels in the body. The arteries are like pipes, carrying BLOOD outwards from the HEART to the tissues, while the veins carry the blood on the return journey. The entire body depends on blood for its supply of OXYGEN and other vital substances without which life could not go on indefinitely.

The artery network

The heart is a pump which propels blood around the body through the arteries. The main pumping chamber on the left side of the heart – the left ventricle – ejects blood into the main artery of the body: the *aorta*. The aorta is a tube about 1 in (2.5 cm) across on the inside. The first of its branches arise as soon as the aorta leaves the heart. These are the *coronary arteries* which supply blood to the heart itself. The coronary arteries are particularly likely to be affected by disease. A blocked coronary artery – coronary thrombosis – causes a HEART ATTACK.

After giving rise to the coronary arteries, the aorta passes upward before doubling back on itself in an arch. Originating from this arch are the two main arteries to the head – the left and right *carotid arteries* – and one artery to each arm. The aorta then descends down the chest and into the abdomen.

In the abdomen, there are three main arteries to the intestines and the liver, and one to each kidney, before the aorta divides into the left and right *iliac arteries* which supply blood to the pelvis and the legs.

After passing through the *capillaries* – a network of tiny blood vessels linking the smallest arteries and veins – from which oxygen and nourishment enter the tissues, the blood returns to the heart in the veins. In general, the artery and vein supplying an area tend to run side by side. The veins empty into the right side of the heart, from where blood is pumped to the lungs and recharged with oxygen. From the lungs, oxygen-rich blood is drained by the pulmonary veins into the left side of the heart.

Here, it starts off round the body again by being pumped into the aorta by the left ventricle of the heart. The left ventricle generates a considerable pressure to force the blood through the arterial network. The tightness which the inflatable cuff used in taking BLOOD PRESSURE reaches around your arm is the same as the maximum squeeze in the left ventricle with each heartbeat.

The structure of arteries

Since the arteries are subjected to this force with each heartbeat, they have to be thick-walled to cope with the pressure. The outer wall of an artery is a loose, fibrous tissue sheath. Inside this there is a thick, elastic and muscular sheath which gives the artery its strength. There are also rings of muscle fibres encircling the artery in among the elastic tissue. The inner layer of the artery (the *endothelium*) is made of a smooth layer of cells which allows the blood to flow freely.

The thick elastic walls are most important to the system. Much of the force of each heartbeat is taken up in the elastic walls of the big arteries. They continue to push the blood forward in the pause between each heartbeat.

Artery disease

Arterial disease in any part of the body is dangerous because, if an artery is blocked or narrowed, it is possible that the part it supplies will die from oxygen starvation. There are two basic ways in which a blockage can happen.

Hardening of the arteries is the commonest serious illness in the Western world. Age is the most important cause, but many other factors affect the rate at which arterial disease progresses. One of these is SMOKING: for reasons that remain unclear, nicotine in the bloodstream causes arteries to narrow and, later, become rigid.

The changes in the walls of arteries which lead to hardening are called *arteriosclerosis* ('sclerosis' means hardening). These changes are caused by the development of an excessive amount of fibrous tissue. This can happen as a result of the straining of the artery walls caused by raised blood pressure.

The other type of disease is *atheroma*, which is the name given to fatty deposits which increasingly develop within the inner lining of arterial walls with advancing age. These fatty deposits look like porridge ('atheroma' is Greek for porridge).

Changes in the arterial network resulting from atheroma, as opposed to arteriosclerosis, are usually referred to as *atherosclerosis* – a word your doctor is more likely to use than arteriosclerosis. Arteriosclerosis and atherosclerosis can be used interchangeably.

Two types of abnormalities are seen in the artery wall. The first is the 'fatty' streak, a thin streak deposit of fat in the inner lining of the artery. These are seen in the main blood vessel, the aorta, of all children over 1 year old, and it is not known whether they develop to form the second type of problem, 'the atheromatous plaque'.

The atheromatous plaque develops in the inner lining of large and medium sized arteries such as the aorta and carotid arteries. It consists of a central mixture of cholesterol, a normal constituent of blood and one of the building blocks of normal cells. Patients with raised levels of cholesterol in the blood have a high chance of developing plaques, but they are also common in patients with high blood pressure or smokers.

Growth of the plaque results in a mixture of fibrous and fatty tissue blocking a proportion of the arterial lumen. The disease extends to a considerable depth in the wall of the vessel and encroaches on a large proportion of its circumference.

Once a large atheromatous plaque has formed, it may have a number of consequences. It may steadily enlarge, blocking the artery. Because of this, the flow of blood past the obstruction is reduced. This may activate the clotting system at the site of narrowing. The clot may well produce a complete obstruction known as a THROMBOSIS. Atheromatous plaques which are partly blocking an artery may also become displaced and swing across the lumen of the artery, like a lock gate, to block it completely. In addition, parts of an atheromatous plaque or parts of a blood clot that develops on top of a plaque may break off and travel towards a smaller artery which will then become blocked. This is a phenomenon known as *embolism*.

Atheroma develops most frequently at the points where arteries branch, where the flow of blood is less smooth and greater stress is placed on the arterial wall. This may injure the endothelium and allow plaques to develop.

Since arteries are necessary to supply oxygen to every part of the body, there is no organ which is completely immune to the effects of arterial disease. If an organ or a limb has its blood supply cut off by atheroma, it must eventually die. An area of tissue which has lost its oxygen supply is called an area of INFARCTION. When this process occurs in an arm or a leg, it is more usual to use the term *gangrene*.

There are obviously some areas where the effects of atheroma cause especially severe problems. The most important are the heart, the brain, the legs and, finally, the aorta itself.

Heart attacks and angina

Atheroma particularly affects the heart because the two coronary arteries (the arteries that supply blood to the heart) are under more mechanical stress than practically any others in the body. The heart is continuously contracting and relaxing with each heartbeat, and, in so doing, the coronary arteries, which lie on the outer surface of the heart, are alternately stretched and relaxed. This seems to give ideal conditions for atheromatous plaques to be formed. When a coronary artery becomes blocked as a result of atheroma, a heart attack results. Such an event may also be known as a coronary thrombosis, or a *myocardial infarction* (the 'myocardium' is the heart muscle and infarction is the formation of a dead area of muscle when it is deprived of blood).

But heart attacks are not the only problem which atheroma causes in the heart. Where there is a fixed obstruction which is not totally blocking the artery, the supply of blood to the heart may only be sufficient to meet the needs of the body when at rest. Exercise increases the need for blood in the heart and it becomes starved of oxygen. This causes pain arising in the heart which is known as *angina pectoris,* or simply angina. The two problems of angina and myocardial infarction are often lumped together under the title of *ischaemic heart disease,* ISCHAEMIA being a word which implies a lack of oxygen without total deprivation or infarction. *See also* CORONARY HEART DISEASE.

Strokes and aneurysms

In the brain, atherosclerosis may result in a STROKE. It may vary from the trivial to the fatal and may occur as a result of an artery becoming blocked through atheroma or embolism or through an artery leaking blood into the brain as a result of a weakened wall.

When the legs are severely affected by atheroma, they become painful and this pain is worse during exercise, just as with angina. If the disease is severe, gangrene results and the affected leg may have to be amputated.

Finally, the aorta itself is a very important area of atheromatous disease. Two different things can happen. The wall of the aorta may start to balloon out as a result of the weakening effect of the disease. This produces a sac-like swelling called an *aneurysm* instead of the regular tubular structure of the normal aorta. Aneurysms are usually found in the abdomen but may occur in the chest. An aneurysm may continue to expand and eventually start to leak, with disastrous results. Surgical treatment is the only hope, and the aneurysm is replaced with a tube made of artificial material. If the aneurysm has leaked or ruptured, and emergency surgery is required, then the results of the surgery are poor and many patients do not survive. When the operation is performed as a planned procedure then the results are good.

Another form of aneurysm which tends to occur in the chest rather than the abdomen, is called dissection of the aorta. This means that the layers of the aortic wall become split by escaping blood, the end result being much the same. Occasionally, patients survive dissection without surgery but, again, surgery is often necessary.

Those affected

There is now a well-established list of risk factors which indicate people who are more likely to suffer from 'accelerated' or 'early' atheroma. The most important of the factors is smoking, although also some diseases put people at greater risk. The two most important are high blood pressure and DIABETES.

People from a family in which atherosclerosis has occurred are at greater risk. Sometimes, members of such families may have high blood cholesterol levels (*familial hypercholesterolaemia*), which can trigger off the development of atherosclerosis. Even people from families who do not have a history of atherosclerosis may develop a high cholesterol level as a result of eating too much saturated FAT via meat and dairy produce. Moderation is the key here.

Prevention

What can we do to prevent or postpone the development of atheromatous disease? Both diabetes and high blood pressure must be treated. Otherwise the most potent risk factor is family history, over which there is no control, unless members of the family have high cholesterol levels which can be brought under control by a low-fat DIET. However, there is one controllable factor left – SMOKING. The most effective thing to prevent atheroma is to stop smoking immediately. Apart from significantly reducing the chances of your developing heart disease, giving up cigarettes will generally improve your health.

Arterioles, *see* **Blood pressure, Circulation**

Arteriosclerosis, *see* **Arteries and artery disease, Blood pressure**

Arteritis, temporal, *see* **Steroids**

Arthritis

This is an inflammation of the JOINTS and its causes are as varied and mysterious as the condition itself. It affects people of all ages and is a common complaint in temperate climates; it can be mild or severe, affecting one joint or several; and the different types include RHEUMATOID ARTHRITIS, OSTEOARTHRITIS, rigid spine disease (ankylosing SPONDYLITIS) and arthritis that has been brought on by an injury or other infection. Although its study is a well-established speciality called rheumatology, medical research cannot yet tell us all the answers.

Rheumatoid arthritis, osteoarthritis and spondylitis

These are discussed in full in the entries under these names.

Other causes of arthritis

An injury can trigger arthritis – this is called *traumatic arthritis*. The injury can either be direct – for example, from a blow to a joint – or indirect, as when you hurt your knee by falling heavily on it. Traumatic arthritis usually happens to men, although no one is immune.

The knee, ankle or wrist are the joints most commonly affected. A few hours after the injury, the joint becomes inflamed, painful and swollen. An X-ray is needed, in case a fracture has occurred, but rest, bandaging and painkillers may be all that is necessary.

Physiotherapy can also help restore mobility and muscle power to the affected limb. Occasionally the injury causes bleeding into the joint which becomes very tense and painful; this may have to be drawn out with a needle (aspirated) under a local anaesthetic. Any joint which has been injured in this way or has had a fracture of one of the bones on either side is always more susceptible to osteoarthritis later in life.

Germs can also cause conditions like *septic arthritis*, which is brought on by infection of the joint fluid. This happens either because of an injury or because the micro-organism is transmitted from the blood. Half of such cases involve the knee, but it can occur in any large joint. Both children and the elderly can be affected, but it is fortunately rare. A special type of septic arthritis is that caused by tuberculosis, but this is increasingly rare except in people from developing countries. It tends to affect the hip and spine.

Another rare form of arthritis can result from an attack of RUBELLA (German measles). This can happen to adults, who may experience swelling of their finger joints, knees and ankles which subsides after a few weeks.

In recent years, research has shown that a number of cases of *transient arthritis* (i.e. arthritis that is not long lasting) are associated with infections. This is probably much more common than had previously been recognized and may affect most people at some time in their lives.

The most well-known type of arthritis associated with infection is called REITER'S DISEASE, after the doctor who first described it. This type may affect the spine rather like ankylosing spondylitis, but also other joints including the knees and ankles. It seems to occur after certain types of infection. In some countries, it is mostly associated with particular germs which cause attacks of GASTRO-ENTERITIS, but it may also follow some types of sexually transmitted infection, particularly that caused by CHLAMYDIA which is sometimes known as NSU (NON-SPECIFIC URETHRITIS). When the original infection is properly treated, the arthritis gets better.

Another type of arthritis caused by infection is common in parts of the US and is found in the UK. Lyme disease is triggered off by infection with a 'spirochaete' germ transmitted by a tick. Again, treatment with the correct antibiotics prevents the development of arthritis. Apart from these more well-known types of arthritis caused by particular infections, it is clear that many virus illnesses may be followed by a period in which the joints ache and may become swollen, often for several months, although ultimately the condition will clear up.

People who have the skin disease PSORIASIS may also develop arthritis. This occurs in about one sufferer in ten, and tends to follow a similar pattern to that of rheumatoid arthritis.

Diagnosis and treatment

If you suspect that you have some form of arthritis, the worst thing you can do is to 'just put up with it'. Do not try to make the diagnosis yourself, but go and see your doctor. Any delay might mean the risk of permanent deformity, especially in the case of a child with Still's disease (the childhood form of rheumatoid arthritis), a condition which needs hospital care.

Your doctor will ask for a history of your illness and give you an examination. Often blood tests will be needed to test for the presence of infection, or to determine the cause of the arthritis. Special tests are available for rheumatoid arthritis and ankylosing spondylitis. X-rays may be required and can give an indication of both the type of arthritis and the degree of damage to the joints. He or she may prescribe simple painkillers such as paracetamol or distalgesic. More commonly a group of drugs called the non-steroidal anti-inflammatory drugs (NSAIDS) will be prescribed. These, along with aspirin, act by reducing joint inflammation and pain. They do, however, have side-effects on the gastro-intestinal system and should not be taken by anyone with gastric ulcers. If the patient is suffering from rheumatoid arthritis, certain treatments are available which may slow the progression of the disease.

You may have to rest the affected joints or wear an individually made splint to keep them in the best position and so prevent deformities from occurring. Swelling in joints can be treated by drawing off excess fluid under a local anaesthetic, or injecting an anti-inflammatory drug into the joint.

You may be feeling generally unwell and be advised to cut down some of your everyday activities and rest as much as possible. STEROID drugs (such as cortisone) may be prescribed to suppress the inflammation in the joints, but because they have side-effects, they will only be used when all other forms of treatment have been unsuccessful. Doses must always be kept at the lowest possible level at which they will control symptoms, and progress must be carefully monitored by a doctor.

If your symptoms persist, your doctor may recommend a visit to the rheumatology clinic or your local hospital for further investigation. An acute attack of arthritis with fever, swollen joints and a general feeling of being unwell may need immediate hospital treatment, including splinting.

Blood tests are made to check the amount of inflammation in the body at regular intervals.

Another technique, called arthroscopy (*see* ENDOSCOPY), involves a telescope-type instrument which is used to look inside the knee joint under local anaesthetic. Both the cartilage and lining tissue can be examined by this means, and small pieces of tissue can be removed for further microscopic examination to help establish the cause of the condition.

Exercise and physiotherapy

PHYSIOTHERAPY plays an important part in the treatment of all forms of arthritis.

For affected joints that are in a 'quiescent' phase – that is, free from inflammation – exercise is essential to prevent stiffness and loss of mobility and restore muscles around the joint that may have wasted. There is no evidence that exercising an arthritic joint in the quiescent phase causes it to flare up.

The physiotherapist at your local hospital will teach you exercises which can be continued at home. Heat can be used to ease painful joints. These treatments can include short-wave diathermy, when a heater pad is placed near the affected joint, or hydrotherapy (exercising in a small, very warm swimming pool). The effect of the heat is to relax tense muscles and, because the water supports the body, movement is increased.

If your doctor or physiotherapist advises it, an infra-red lamp can be used at home. Paraffin wax baths for hands and feet is another treatment that can be used very easily at home once the technique is learned. On the other hand, some therapists favour ice packs as a form of pain-relieving therapy.

The benefits of surgery

Great advances have been made in the replacement of badly damaged joints with artificial ones. In the first place, the decision that an arthritic joint needs surgery will be made by a specialist in the field, an ORTHOPAEDIC surgeon who has been consulted by either the patient's doctor or a rheumatologist.

One of the most successful forms of joint replacement is the replacement of the HIP joint. A 'cup' is implanted by the surgeon into the pelvis in place of the old joint, and then a stem is inserted into the femur with a metal ball attached to its upper end which fits precisely into the cup, so creating a new joint.

New materials such as ceramics are being used in the manufacture of these joints to extend their life, so that an artificial joint should last up to 15 or 20 years. Increasingly, other joints in the body can be replaced by artificial joints, although the success of the operation may not be so great as the replacement of the hip joint. Some joints in the hand, the shoulder joint, elbow and knee joints can all be replaced with metal or metal and plastic alternatives.

One of the most important results of replacement of arthritic joints is the relief of pain which can be dramatic and lift an intolerable burden from the patient's life. Deformity can be reduced and function improved. Benefits to the patient include restoring mobility, and in some cases, this may also mean restoring enjoyment of sexual activity which may have previously been very difficult.

Surgery can also relieve pressure around a joint, free gummed-up ligaments or remove the inflamed lining tissue of a joint (*synovectomy*) if it is excessively inflamed. An excruciatingly painful and useless joint such as may occur with osteoarthritis of the cervical spine (neck) or an arthritic knee is sometimes surgically fused (*arthrodesis*) to give relief, though this does involve loss of movement.

Arthrodesis, *see* **Arthritis**

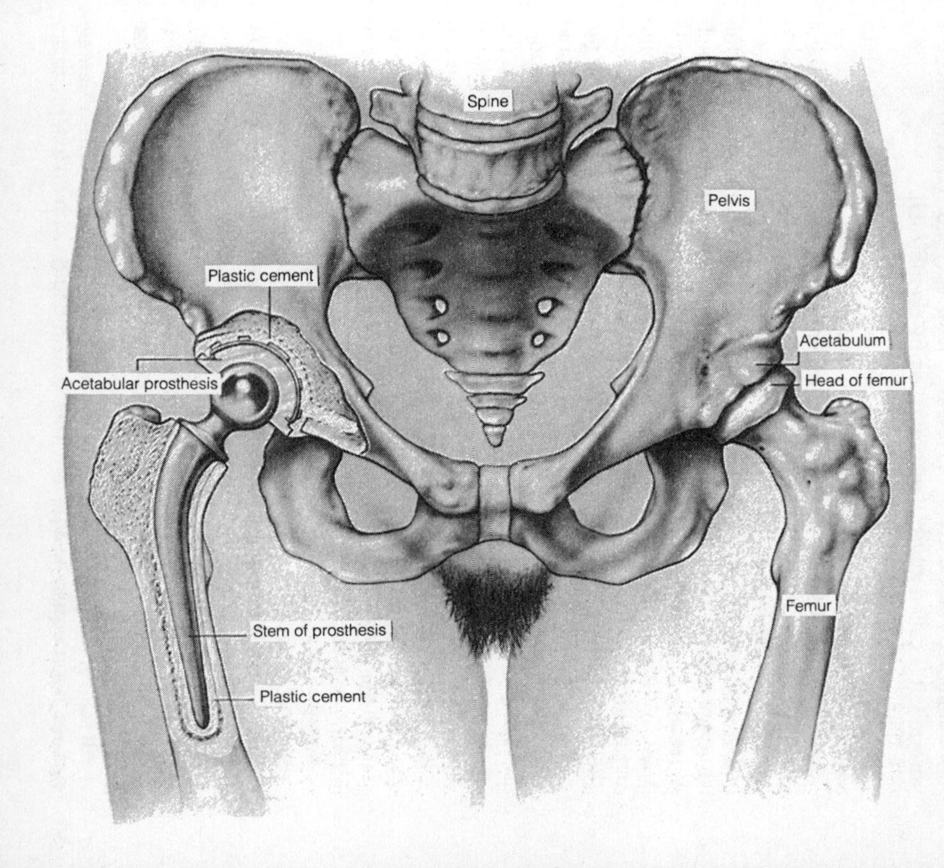

Hip replacement

The head of the femur is removed, holes are drilled and plastic cement is pushed in. A prosthetic ball and stem is inserted into the femur, and held in place by the cement. Stem and head are rejoined and traction is applied to maintain the position of the leg.

Artificial insemination

The term 'artificial insemination' refers to the process in which SPERM is inserted into the female reproductive tract by artificial means rather than through SEXUAL INTERCOURSE. The sperm is usually placed next to the woman's cervix (the opening to the UTERUS) using a syringe to which a long tube is attached.

Although increasingly used in cases of INFERTILITY, artificial insemination is one of several treatments available when couples fail to conceive. After carrying out tests, a couple's doctor will advise them on whether hormone treatment, surgery or artificial insemination will be the best treatment for them and will explain what is involved.

There are two forms of artificial insemination. If a woman has her husband's sperm inserted into her vagina, the process is called *artificial insemination by husband* (AIH). However, if the sperm of a different male is inserted, it is called *artificial insemination by donor* (AID).

Artificial insemination by husband

This method is used when there is some fault with the way the sperm is deposited in the VAGINA during normal intercourse. It may also be used to overcome some female reproductive problems.

For example, AIH might be used when there is some abnormality in the structure of the PENIS – a surprising number of men have the opening, which is usually found at the tip of the penis, situated elsewhere along the penile shaft. Most common of these conditions is where the opening is on the underside, back from the tip. So instead of the sperm being deposited next to the cervix, where they can easily swim up to meet the female eggs in the Fallopian tubes, they are deposited nearer the entrance of the vagina and conception does not take place. However, by using artificial insemination, the sperm can be placed directly next to the cervix and so increase the chances of conception.

Another case might be when a man is unable to achieve an erection or when he is unable to ejaculate within the vagina. These men may be able to maintain strong erections and have ejaculations when masturbating, or through manual manipulation by the partner or in oral sex, but they lose these abilities as soon as penetration is attempted.

For men who have low sperm counts, a technique called *split ejaculate insemination* is used, which also involves AIH. When the sperm count is low, the number of sperm in the semen that has been ejaculated may be too low for fertilization to occur. However, the first part of the ejaculate always contains more sperm than the rest, and if the first parts of several separate ejaculations are put together, the number of sperm increases. Using AIH, this collection of several ejaculates is introduced into the woman at the time when she is most likely to conceive.

AIH can also be used when the barrier to conception is found in the female partner. For sperm to be able to enter the womb and swim up to fertilize the egg (*ovum*), they must swim through the right quantity of watery mucus secreted by the cervix: some women produce too little mucus; others produce mucus so thick that the sperm cannot penetrate. AIH may solve this by attempting to put the sperm beyond the barrier.

Most parents tend not to tell the resulting child that he or she was conceived through the use of AIH. In fact, there is little to be gained by doing so.

Artificial insemination by donor

AID is used when the woman has no reproductive problems but either the man is sterile or the female is ALLERGIC to her partner's sperm. In this case, sperm is obtained from an unidentified male and introduced into the female in the same way that it is for AIH.

AID presents a good alternative, allowing a woman to have the experience of carrying and bearing a child which at least inherits *her* characteristics. And, since AID will be used only as a last resort to solve the problem of childlessness, most men feel quite happy about it. However, if there are already stresses in a marriage, AID should not be undertaken. A husband's disappointment that he cannot be the father of the child, or a wife's resentment at not being able to have a natural child, can be enough to destroy a marriage. So it is very important that any such conflicts are resolved first.

The greatest care is taken in matching the donor's physical characteristics, such as height, build and complexion, with those of the husband, so that the child has the greatest chance of looking like both parents. The donors are also matched for intellectual ability.

The donors' medical and family histories are also examined carefully to avoid passing on such conditions as DIABETES or other inherited ailments. Donors are also checked to make sure that they aren't carrying SEXUALLY TRANSMITTED DISEASES, including HIV. Furthermore, the characteristics of the female partner are also considered. If she does not have the RHESUS FACTOR in her blood, for example, then an Rh-negative donor is used to avoid future complications in pregnancy.

The matching procedures used are so effective that relatives, friends and the child itself do not generally suspect that AID has been used. But, in any case, genetic makeup of the offspring is far less important in the relationship between parents and child than genuine love.

Some doctors mix in some of the husband's sperm with that of the donor (except where the woman reacts against her partner's sperm). This provides a small chance that the one sperm to penetrate could, after all, have come from the husband.

Research has shown that the children conceived by artificial insemination show no difference in rates of abnormality than children conceived in any other way.

The treatment

Treatment is carried out at infertility clinics attached to gynaecological departments in some of the larger hospitals.

The first session in all cases of infertility consists of an interview with both partners. A medical examination is given to the woman, and a full medical and surgical history is obtained from both the man and the woman. Their attitudes towards one another, towards their infertility and towards children are also carefully discussed.

After this initial joint interview, the couple are usually examined separately: the woman has a gynaecological examination and a swab from her cervix is taken, and the man undergoes a full examination including his genitals.

Over successive sessions at the clinic, the doctors will establish the cause of the infertility. Once this has been discovered and artificial insemination considered, the insemination can be arranged to take place at the woman's time of ovulation to increase the chance of conception.

Artificial insemination is generally carried out on three consecutive days around the time of ovulation and may continue for a period of six months to a year. The sperm sample from either the husband or the donor is passed along a tube and inserted into the cervical canal. Where there is a cervical abnormality or a problem with the cervical mucus, the sample may be placed past the cervix within the uterus.

The success rate for artificial insemination varies, depending on the fertility of the woman, but, generally speaking, it is between 50 and 70 per cent.

The legal position

Once a child has been born using AID, it can run into legal controversy concerning its status. In Britain, for example, AID performed with a husband's consent does not constitute adultery or provide other grounds for divorce, but the child, in the eyes of the law, is regarded as illegitimate. By strict interpretation of the law, the birth certificate should state that the father of the child is 'unknown', but in practice they are rarely written out that way – the husband or partner instead being registered as the father.

The confused legal situation can lead to several problems which are not insurmountable but can cause irritation and distress. The first is that, when a birth certificate has been made out omitting the husband or partner's name, he will need to adopt the child legally to automatically guarantee inheritance where no will is made. Second, it is acknowledged that some husbands or partners feel a power differential between theirs and the mother's relationship with the child. Reinforcing the man's lack of physical contribution with a birth certificate that does not mention him hardly seems a way of correcting this imbalance.

The decision to tell children that they were conceived by AID must rest with their parents and will form part of the latter's early counselling. Donors remain totally anonymous, although there has been some debate as to whether superficial details should be released to parents so that they can provide their children with thumbnail sketches of their biological fathers. This would at least alleviate some of the stress should children discover themselves to have been AID babies but be unable to discover anything else.

Asbestos and asbestosis, ***see*** **Cells and chromosomes, Lungs and lung diseases, Phlegm, Sarcoma**

Ascariasis, ***see*** **Worms**

Ascites, ***see*** **Cirrhosis, Liver and liver diseases, Lymphatic system, Oedema, Peritoneum and peritonitis**

Aspergillosis, fungal, ***see*** **Fungal infections, Lungs and lung diseases**

Aspirin, ***see*** **Painkillers**

Asthma

About one child in ten develops asthma at some stage during childhood – it is one of the commonest LUNG problems in children and is becoming commoner, although experts are unsure why. This may be linked to the increase in atmospheric pollution in the Western world. Luckily, modern treatments are now very effective in relieving the condition. Some children grow out of asthma as they get older, but not all. About one adult in 20 has it, and, rarely, adults can develop the complaint later in life without any sign of it before.

What is asthma?

Asthma involves a severe narrowing of the bronchial tubes. These lead from the windpipe – trachea – into the lungs, carry the oxygen we breathe in to all parts of the lungs and provide a path for the carbon dioxide (a waste product of the body) to escape up the trachea when we breathe out.

The narrowing of the bronchial tubes – or bronchi – results from the contraction of the muscles lining them and causes difficulty in breathing that is most marked when breathing out. For this reason, asthmatics tend to inhale in short gasps and breathe out with a long wheeze – a result of the effort required to breathe against the obstruction.

The body's defences

Two different chemicals are responsible for causing the bronchial muscles to contract. One is histamine, which is released from mast cells (cells that store histamine) as part of an allergic reaction (*see* ALLERGY) and the other is acetylcholine which is a chemical released from the nerve endings which control the bronchial muscles.

These nerves are branches of the important vagus nerve which originates in the brain. The vagus keeps the bronchi in a constant state of contraction all the time and, as such, can be regarded as the main control over bronchial contraction, with additional control being provided by histamine.

To keep the balance between contraction and expansion (dilation), there are other substances that cause the bronchi to relax, thus working against the histamine and acetylcholine. These substances are called bronchodilators and a number of them are manufactured in the ADRENAL GLANDS situated above each kidney.

The most important bronchodilator is adrenalin, which acts as a stimulant during periods of stress and excitement; when we need more oxygen to provide energy during a dangerous situation, the adrenalin helps to open up the bronchi to allow more air through to the lungs during rapid breathing.

In addition to this, the bronchial muscles also contain enzymes – substances which are responsible for maintaining certain bodily functions on which life depends, including respiration (BREATHING). These help to protect the bronchial muscles from the action of histamine and acetylcholine.

Causes

Asthma is brought on by a number of different causes, ranging from breathing polluted air to emotional upset, which makes it a rather complex problem to treat. However, since all the causes of asthma trigger the release of either histamine or acetylcholine, it is important to understand these two chemical reactions in order to see why people are vulnerable to asthma.

Histamine release is the most common cause of asthma, and the process which brings it about is rather remarkable considering that the substances which trigger it – house dust containing the faeces of house dust mites, animal fur, pollen and fungal spores among others – are so varied.

Some people develop an excessive amount of an antibody (a protein made by the body as part of its defence system) to some substances breathed in – these substances (some of which are listed above) are known as allergens and they cause allergic reactions. It is this malfunction of the body's defences which starts the reaction leading to asthma.

What happens is that the antibody, which is known as immunoglobulin E, or IgE, attaches itself to the mast cells where the histamine is stored. The next time the allergen is inhaled, each molecule (particles which make up the whole antibody) of IgE pairs up with a neighbouring molecule and, as a result of this mating, the mast cell releases its store of histamine. The bronchi then begin to contract, making it increasingly difficult to breathe: the condition that we call asthma.

Acetylcholine release from the nerve endings in the bronchial tubes can be caused by a number of substances which irritate both the bronchial tubes and the nerve endings. These nerve endings then send messages to the vagus with the information that they have been irritated. In response, the vagus nerve then contracts the bronchial muscles and so starts asthmatic breathing difficulties. In addition, the lining of the bronchial tubes produces extra mucus which can lead to 'plugging' of the tubes, so exacerbating the breathing difficulty. The same sort of irritation is caused by viral or bacterial infections of the throat, which explains why asthma tends to get worse with chest infections and colds.

We also know that emotional upsets or anxiety may occasionally worsen an asthmatic condition, though how this happens is not clear. Other predisposing factors are some drugs (e.g. aspirin-like painkillers), occupational exposure to fumes (e.g. platinum salts in the electronic industry), atmospheric pollution and dusts. Asthma attacks may also be triggered by exposure to cold air, exercise or emotional upset.

Symptoms

The typical asthma attack is characterized by a sudden shortness of breath and wheezing, which is sometimes accompanied by coughing. Coughing and waking at night is a common symptom of asthma, and wheezing tends to be worse first thing in the morning. The bringing up of phlegm is not a prominent part of the attack and suggests that the patient may also have bronchitis. Generally speaking, asthmatics are more prone to chest infections, and this is caused by a failure to clear the lungs fully.

In many cases, the onset of asthma follows a seasonal pattern as the pollen count rises. This pattern is often accompanied by irritations to the nose and sneezing, which we usually refer to as hay fever.

Of course, allergies to house pets and the faeces of the house dust mite will occur all through the year as the allergen is constantly in the air. The mite is particularly keen on living in warm places, like beds, and for this reason asthma attacks often seem to happen at night. In fact, coughing at night in children may well be a result of this allergy and is often an early sign of the onset of asthma.

Treatment

The treatment given for asthma largely depends on the type of asthma and the severity of the attacks, but it is broadly divided into two: emergency treatment for severe attacks, requiring a visit from the doctor or admission to hospital; and everyday self-medication to prevent an attack occurring, which is known as prophylactic, or preventive, treatment and can be carried out at home.

The aim of emergency treatment is to bring relief as rapidly as possible. If someone has a severe acute attack, it is important to get drugs into the system as quickly as possible to relieve the 'bronchospasm'. These drugs are called bronchodilators. Those most commonly used are salbutamol and terbutaline. They can be given by injection but they are most effective given by a 'nebulizer'. This device is powered by electricity, and produces a fine mist or spray of the drug dissolved in sterile water. This mist can be inhaled through a mouthpiece, or a mask. Using a nebulizer, the bronchodilator usually works within five or ten minutes and will often relieve the spasm completely. If the attack has been severe enough to warrant medical attention, the doctor will often give a steroid drug to be taken by mouth for a few days as well. This reduces inflammation in the lungs and prevents further development of the attack.

If there is no nebulizer available, the doctor may use an injection of either a bronchodilator such as salbutamol, but he could use other drugs, such as adrenalin, or aminophylline. The disadvantage of adrenalin, however, is that it tends to cause palpitations; aminophylline given by injection can cause some nausea. A very severe attack may need to be treated with oxygen as well, and may need hospital treatment.

The aim of regular treatment for asthmatics is, however, to prevent any severe attacks from occurring and to allow the sufferer to follow as normal a pattern of life as possible. It may be possible to use skin tests to detect whether the sufferer has particular allergies. Many sufferers are found to be allergic to the faeces of the house dust mite and can be given advice on how to reduce exposure.

There are two main types of drug used in the maintenance treatment of asthma. First, the 'preventers' which are inhaled steroids (e.g. beclomethasone or fluticasone) and act by reducing the background inflammation in the airways causing asthmatic symptoms. Second are the 'relievers' which have a shorter action and act to relieve asthmatic symptoms (e.g. salbutamol or terbutaline). In addition, for more troublesome asthma there are other inhaled drugs or tablets (e.g. aminophylline) which can be added to the regular treatment. In general, a sign of deteriorating asthma is the need to use more of the 'reliever' medication during the day or night: this may indicate that an increased dose of the 'preventer' medication is needed on a regular basis.

Since these steroids are inhaled directly into the lungs, there is practically no absorption of the drug into the system and negligible risk of any side-effects.

For those who suffer from a more persistent and severe form of asthma, doctors may prescribe steroid drugs to be taken by mouth. Because of the side-effects of this type of drug, patients will be asked to stick rigidly to the doctor's recommended dosage, and to make sure that they always have the drug with them in case of an attack. The treatment should always be continued, as failure to do this may encourage a further attack.

Prevention

Most asthmatics will have their condition worsened or even triggered by everyday substances, and once the cause is identified, the only course is to avoid it by, for instance, keeping the house as clear of dust as possible, avoiding petrol fumes and tobacco smoke, certain 'reactive' foods, and also sudden exertion and emotional stress. But it is accepted that regular, controlled exercise (especially swimming) rather than sudden exertion does have a beneficial effect, and all asthmatics should be encouraged to take as much regular – but strictly controlled – exercise as they can manage.

Ataxia, *see* Cerebral palsy

Atherosclerosis, *see* Arteries and artery disease, Blood pressure, Heart attack, Stroke

Athetosis, *see* Cerebral palsy

Athlete's foot

This FUNGAL INFECTION is probably the most common foot complaint that doctors treat. It can affect almost everyone, though small children do appear to be immune.

The only real cause of athlete's foot is a failure to observe the necessary personal hygiene, along with carelessness in drying the feet after washing. People who suffer from sweaty feet are particularly prone to this complaint and the situation can be aggravated by wearing airless plastic shoes which prevent the feet from breathing.

It is the moist, sweaty areas between the toes that provide the soggy skin on which the fungus likes to settle. The fungus then lives on the skin, digesting the dead skin that the body sheds each day. Once the fungus starts eating the dead skin, it may then cause inflammation and damage to the living skin.

Symptoms and treatment

The first sign of athlete's foot is irritation and itching between the toes followed by the skin beginning to peel. This can be accompanied by bad foot odour.

In worse cases, painful red cracks, known as fissures, appear between the toes, and in the odd severe case, the toe-nails can be affected. These become either soft or more brittle as the fungus invades the nail substance.

Modern antifungal creams and powders are successful in the treatment of athlete's foot. Substances such as clotrimazole and tolnaftate are extremely effective as creams or ointments, and need to be applied daily while the condition lasts, and for two or three weeks after the symptoms have disappeared.

Where the infection is severe and the nails have been affected, a drug known as griseofulvin may be prescribed by the doctor to be taken orally. It is effective within a few weeks. It is then necessary to dust the feet, socks and shoes with antifungal powder to prevent re-infection.

Atopy, *see* **Allergy**

Autism

The word 'autism' is used to describe an extremely complex form of mental handicap. It is taken from the Greek word *autos,* meaning 'self', and means being turned in upon the self.

It has been a recognized – that is, medically classified – condition since 1943, when an American psychiatrist, Leo Kanner, first coined the word to describe the symptoms of a group of children whose common abnormalities of behaviour distinguished them sharply from the general mass of mentally handicapped children in his care. He identified what he considered to be the five most important symptoms common to them all, and from then on the condition became known as Kanner's syndrome, or 'infantile autism'.

Some years later, a working party of psychiatrists added four more symptoms to those selected by Kanner to make the 'nine points of autism' which for many years were used by doctors trying to diagnose the condition.

Symptoms

What most parents usually notice first in their young autistic child is the inability to look others in the eye – an autistic child tends to look past the shoulder of whoever is speaking to them in a way which, if he or she were older, might well be thought impolite.

In fact, this puzzling aloofness is only the tip of the iceberg. As the toddler develops, the parents slowly realize that he or she is unable to participate in *any* normal social behaviour.

An autistic child's fits of screaming and tantrums far outdo in length and volume those of even the most violent normal toddler. This is at least partly because autistic children, while seeing and hearing normally, appear to be unable to make sense of what they see and hear. Their everyday world becomes terrifying.

Nor is there any refuge in the world of the imagination. The autistic toddler does not develop 'pretend play' – a brick remains a brick, and can never be transformed into a garage or a fort.

Abnormalities of language vary from total muteness (inability to speak) to a literal, pedantic use of words. An autistic child, asked 'What do you do if you cut yourself?', might answer, 'I bleed!' Echolalia – repeating the question instead of answering it – is frequent.

Autistic children also exhibit strange fears – usually of totally harmless objects such as a bush or a box, but do not register fear when there is real danger. This is probably connected to their inability to make sense of the impressions they receive.

Then there is the fascination with bright lights, or with strange objects such as bits of broken plastic or elastic bands. And as if this were not enough, an autistic child may well show a disturbing indifference to heat and cold – being capable, for instance, of stewing in a hot bath without showing any reaction. Strangest of all, perhaps, are the odd body movements – grimaces, arm- or hand-flapping and jumping or springing from one foot to the other.

Many autistic children possess what are known as 'islands of normality'. These usually affect activities where the development of language and certain other skills are not necessary – such as music, maths, or art. A child who is incapable of uttering a single spontaneous word may be a near genius at mathematics, or have an extraordinary memory.

These islands of normality have even led parents of young autistic children to believe that they had an exceptionally gifted child, putting all other oddities of behaviour down to the quirks of genius, until the increasing number of 'quirks' eventually disillusion them.

A sheltered life

Other autistic children may develop a certain amount of useful speech and acquire many practical skills, but cannot tolerate the whirl of everyday modern life.

While they will always need to live in a sheltered environment, they are, however, capable of making important contributions to the success of that environment and of living full lives. Autistic people can earn a living as builders' labourers, accountancy clerks and piano tuners – all occupations demanding attention to detail without the burden of heavy responsibility.

At the other end of the scale, there are those who are so severely disturbed that their parents never had much doubt. At their worst, these children can turn a normal home to wreckage – tearing clothing, curtains, bedding, their own skin and hair.

We do not know the cause of autism. Over the years, many theories have been suggested, but none has been proved conclusively.

Without knowing the cause, it is, of course, impossible to find the cure. Most autistic children remain handicapped for life. Very rarely, a sudden easing of the symptoms' severity occurs, usually, oddly enough, when the child has been severely affected in the first instance.

Teaching autistic children

It has been proved that all autistic children do improve with special education, and parents should do everything to see that they receive it.

Much of the pioneering work which established that these children need a specialized type of education was done in the UK and there are now schools in many countries. There cannot be one single teaching method or technique to be applied to all the children (like Braille for the blind, or sign language for the mute). Different abilities have to be catered for in individual learning programmes.

To start with, long-established techniques for behaviour management are employed to cope with the autistic abnormalities. The worst ones – tantrums, screaming fits, hyperactivity and obsessions – usually have to be dealt with first.

Language problems present the most fundamental obstacles to teaching, since they are linked with the problems of behaving properly and learning to think. They are, therefore, given constant attention. Advice and help are sought from audiology (HEARING) clinics and SPEECH THERAPISTS.

Only after this is a language programme set up for the individual child. Language is concentrated on at all times – not just in the classroom. It is essential that all those engaged in teaching the child, at all levels, should themselves speak simply, using short sentences, and talk about things rather than abstract ideas.

Autistic children's lack of natural interest, motivation and concentration demand the teacher's careful organization of all daily situations in which the child finds itself. Normal children are taught to motivate themselves. Autistic children cannot – they have to be taught the *habit* of moving from one step to the next.

Autogenic training, *see* Relaxation

Auto-immune diseases, *see* AIDS, Blood, Immune system, Multiple sclerosis, Pernicious anaemia, Rheumatic fever, Rheumatoid arthritis, Steroids, Thyroid

Autonomic nervous system

As we go about our lives, many processes within the body, such as BREATHING and DIGESTION, keep us functioning smoothly. We usually take them for granted because they happen automatically. But all processes need some kind of controlling mechanism, and in the human body, two different systems provide this control.

'Automatic' control

One, the ENDOCRINE SYSTEM, affects much of the body's chemistry through the production of HORMONES, which regulate growth and reproduction, among other functions. But, on the whole, hormone-controlled systems do not have to work as quickly, or as spontaneously, as those controlled by the second system, the autonomic nervous system.

This system, which is part of the whole nervous system, is mainly concerned with keeping up the automatic functions, without deliberate mental or other effort on our part, of organs such as the HEART, LUNGS, STOMACH, INTESTINE, BLADDER, sex organs and blood vessels.

How it works

An understanding of how the autonomic nervous system operates is vital to medicine mainly because its workings – part chemical, part electrical – can be controlled or blocked by giving drugs. And this means, of course, that the organs it influences can be controlled too.

Think of the nervous system as the control system of the body. Thought and other conscious or 'deliberate' activities go on in the BRAIN hemispheres called the 'highest' part of the system. The ones dealt with here go on in the 'lower' parts of the brain and in the SPINAL CORD.

The actual process by which the nervous system works is truly complicated, but in simple terms, it can be thought of as electrical signals being transmitted down nerve fibres, each of which both end in and have nerve cells along their way.

Nerve cells are the tiny bodies which either transmit or receive messages or sensations. The fibres, known in medical science as axons, are the 'wires' along which the impulses, or stimuli, travel to and from the control centres of the brain and spinal cord.

Axons are not actually connected to nerve cells. There is a gap between the ending of an axon and the cell itself called a *synapse*, across which the 'message' is carried by means of a chemical. And this gap, with its chemical bridge, is what enables doctors to control the system. For, as will be seen, the action of these chemical transmitters can be imitated with similar, man-made chemicals.

Two types of control

The autonomic nervous system is divided into two parts, known as the *sympathetic* and *parasympathetic*. Each uses a different chemical transmitter where the nerve fibre reaches its target organ, each is built differently, and each has a different effect on the organ it serves.

Parasympathetic nerves serving, for example, the bronchial airways leading to and from the lungs, make them constrict, or grow narrow. The sympathetic nerves leading to the same area cause widening – that is, dilating – of the bronchial passages.

The chemical transmitter for parasympathetic nerves is called acetylcholine, and the one for sympathetic nerves is called noradrenalin – close relative of adrenalin, the main hormone released to get the body's processes moving fast in 'fight or flight' STRESS situations.

Manipulating the system

Armed with this knowledge, doctors have, for example, learned how to successfully treat ASTHMA. This is a drastic narrowing of the bronchial airways caused in the first place by ALLERGIC reaction to substances such as house dust. If the patient inhales a drug similar to noradrenalin, the sympathetic nervous system is assisted, the airways will dilate, and the attack will stop.

And when a chesty person is producing too much mucus, a drug which blocks the parasympathetic system, controlling the development of these substances, may help the patient too.

Belladonna

A drug commonly used to block the parasympathetic system is atropine. This used to be known as belladonna because beautiful ladies (in Italian *bella* means 'beautiful' and *donna* means 'lady') put drops of atropine in their eyes to widen the pupils in the hope of increasing their allure. The drug was extracted from, among other plants, deadly nightshade, which is also sometimes called belladonna.

However, if a patient is suffering from angina (poor delivery of oxygen to the heart; *see* ARTERIES), a drug to block the sympathetic nervous system and noradrenalin activity may be used. It is not surprising that this sort of drug, called a beta-blocker, sometimes causes asthma at the same time as relieving angina.

Surgery may even be used on the autonomic nervous system. The most usual of such operations is a vagotomy, or cutting of the vagus nerve, which is a large bundle of parasympathetic nerves in the chest. This reduces acid secretions which leads to relief of duodenal ulcers.

Diseases of the autonomic system

The autonomic system itself rarely gives serious trouble, but one minor problem to which it gives rise is relatively common – FAINTING.

Fainting attacks are technically called vaso-vagal attacks and the name gives a clue to the mechanism of the problem. *Vasa* are blood vessels and the vagus is the major nerve of the parasympathetic system. Relative over-activity of the parasympathetic system causes dilation, or widening of the blood vessels, particularly the smallest arteries (the arterioles). As a result, the BLOOD PRESSURE and flow of blood to the brain is reduced, causing loss of consciousness.

Occasionally, the autonomic nervous system may cease to work either wholly or in part. A disease of the autonomic nerves may occur on its own, and it is not simple to treat.

Palpitations (irregular heart action) can arise from a number of causes, but often are due to abnormal impulses from the autonomic nervous system. Drug therapy can, however, often control the condition.

B vitamins, *see* **Vitamins**

Babinski's sign, *see* **Head and head injury**

Back and backache

Ever since human beings stood upright they have been having trouble with their backs. This is why people gain such relief from getting down on all fours – we were just not designed to stand on two feet with our backs straight.

The natural position exaggerates the curvature of the spine at the waist, and this reduces pressure on the back. Standing, especially for long periods, provides little relief, and when combined with poor posture and uncoordinated or erratic movements, a considerable strain can be imposed on the back area and the main structure that supports it, the spine.

Apart from the neck, the spine is made up of 12 *thoracic* vertebrae at the back of the chest, five much larger bones in the *lumbar* region (in and below the curvature of the waist) and five fused vertebrae, called the *sacrum*, that form a triangular bone at the back of the pelvis. At the very base of the spine is the *coccyx*, five small vertebrae that are all that remains of our ancestral tail.

At each end of our spinal column is a ring or girdle of bones that provides support for the limbs. At the top, the pectoral girdle, to which our arms are attached, consists of the collar bone and shoulder blades, together with their various muscular attachments to the spine. At the base of the vertebrae is the pelvic girdle – the pubic bones, the iliac bones (that protect the small intestine) and the sacrum (*see* PELVIS).

The vertebrae that take the greatest strain of physical activity are those in the lumbar region; the thoracic vertebrae can also suffer.

Causes

Backache and back PAIN can be due to any number of reasons, relating either to a physical defect in the spinal column, or indirectly as the result of another disease or condition in some other part of the body. It can even be psychological.

The most common form of backache is LUMBAGO. It can occur quite suddenly or develop over hours – even days – and is caused by lifting or twisting, following injury or over-use, or it can happen for no apparent reason. The result is a tearing of the ligaments and inflammation of the JOINTS between the vertebrae.

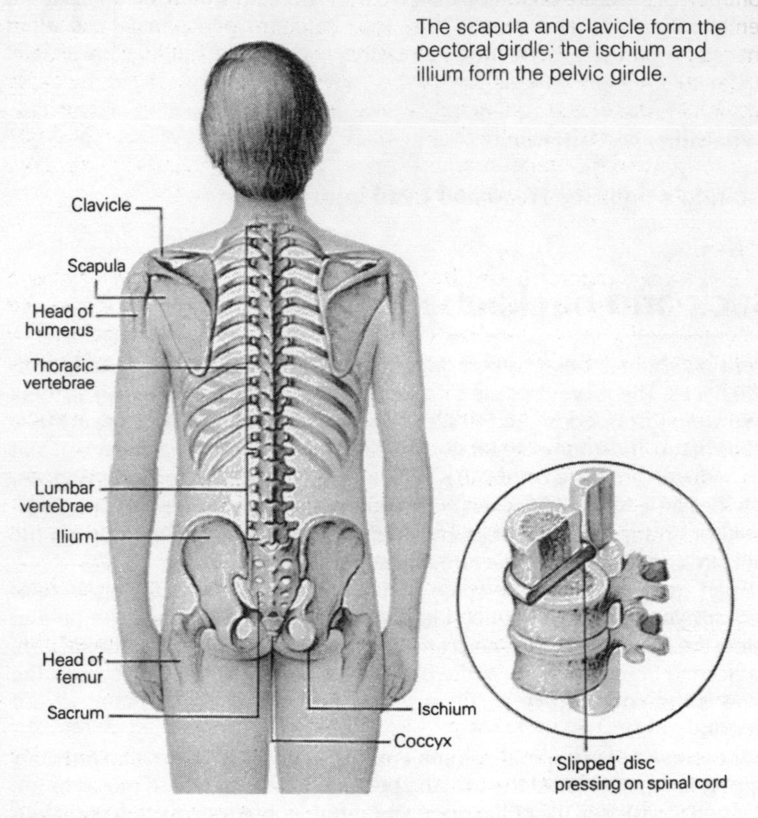

Bones in the back

The scapula and clavicle form the pectoral girdle; the ischium and illium form the pelvic girdle.

Slipped disc

This, and its treatment, is discussed fully in the entry on page 799.

Wear and tear

Spinal discs can be subject to a degenerative disease in later years. They can quite literally wear away, leading to great pain and disability. It rarely happens to anyone under 50, and is usually due to the general ageing process. Women tend to be the main sufferers, and the problem is caused by childbearing and housework, but men in physically arduous jobs are also potential victims.

The discs become progressively thinner, with those in the lumbar region being affected first. The condition places an increasing strain on the vertebrae and their supporting ligaments which often develop bony growths called osteophytes. These can cause a great deal of pain, and when the patient undergoes MANIPULATION, he or she will often hear sharp cracking sounds as they break up.

Problems with bones can also cause backache and back pain. The most common of these is a condition called OSTEOPOROSIS, in which the bones suffer demineralization. This means they lose calcium, phosphates and other important minerals, becoming increasingly weak and brittle. This usually occurs to a lesser extent as part of the ageing process, but it can suddenly accelerate. This leads to continual backache, the spine becomes increasingly bent, and very occasionally the vertebrae can even crumble. A bad fall, compression of the spine in an accident and bone TUMOURS will therefore cause bones affected by osteoporosis to fracture more easily.

Disease

Cancer of the vertebrae is rare, but it can spread to bones from other sites in the body. The disease makes a patient feel unwell, tired and run down and is confirmed by an X-ray or bone scan. Tumours usually respond well to radiotherapy, which will relieve the pain and arrest further growth of the tumour.

TUBERCULOSIS of the spine, which creates ABSCESSES on the muscles, is also a rare complaint, which can be quickly diagnosed by X-ray.

The pain from a GALLSTONE can lead to intense pain in the back. These stones cause no trouble until they block the tubes that intermittently empty the GALL BLADDER. Each time this happens, the patient will suffer pain that can last from two to three hours to several days. Pain from kidney stones can cause very severe pain on either side of the back. Central mid-back pain can be a presenting symptom of cancer of the pancreas.

SHINGLES can give rise to back pain that is often confused with a slipped disc.

Identifying the problem

The backache of worn discs and wear-and-tear arthritis can mimic the symptoms of a slipped disc, with characteristic intermittent bouts occurring every one or two weeks over several months.

The bone disease, osteoporosis, gives rise to various local symptoms which can be confirmed by X-ray or a bone scan. It causes a backache that leaves the patient feeling tender and sore. The bones are sensitive to pressure, there is constant pain and this can be made worse by any movement. Night pain is common and resting makes very little difference. Morning stiffness is also a symptom, just as it is of ankylosing SPONDYLITIS, a form of ARTHRITIS in which the vertebrae fuse to form a 'poker back'. The arthritic pain starts lower down, on both sides, with the spine becoming increasingly rigid as the condition worsens.

Any fracture of the vertebrae will result in a localized, unremitting pain that is intensified by movement. A low backache in the last three months of pregnancy is fairly normal, with the weight of the foetus placing a strain on the lumbar region.

Treatment

The main form of treatment for all types of moderate to severe back pain used to be bedrest in combination with painkilling drugs. Nowadays it is realized that a programme of regular exercises to keep the back muscles working is the most effective and quickest way to get better. Physiotherapists can give advice about exercises and postures. Sometimes an osteopath or chiropracter can help manipulate the back. The only circumstances when bedrest and painkillers are the best treatment is a slipped disc.

The sufferer should lie and sleep on as firm a surface as possible. A board can be placed over a mattress; an alternative is to lie on the floor. In some cases, such as lumbago, relief can be gained by bending the knees or lying on the side, with a cushion in the small of the back. Make the body comfortable and then keep still.

Persistent pain

If pain persists, take paracetamol, or something stronger if this does not work. Occasionally a muscle will go into spasm, resulting in a hot throbbing pain. This can be helped by administering a muscle relaxant, available on prescription only.

A doctor diagnoses the causes of back pain by a process of elimination. Strained muscles will improve within one or two days; torn muscles and ligaments take up to a week and a slipped disc at least two to get better. The only exception is the mild to intermittent pain of degenerative disease. In this case, shorter periods of rest are most helpful, with activity helping to maintain muscle tone and keep bones healthy.

Most people will seek advice on the onset of backpain, especially if it persists after a couple of days. If there is no improvement after two weeks, a doctor's help must be sought. Hospitalization will be advised so that tests can be run and bedrest monitored. The back may be manipulated, as in the case of osteoporosis, or the spine may be immobilized completely with traction. Alternatively, in the case of a fracture, a surgical corset or plaster cast is worn by the patient once he or she is back on their feet after two to six weeks. For severe pain radiating to the leg (SCIATICA), a spinal injection may be given to relieve pain.

Prevention

If you have to bend repeatedly, bend your knees to reduce strain on the spine. Then 'think tall'. Avoid slouching; ensure that all working surfaces are at a comfortable height; and only sit on chairs that have a good supporting back. A firm bed is best.

If you have to twist while lifting – even if it is your own body weight – make each movement in two separate stages. If you have to shovel sand, lift some on to the spade, then turn and deposit it elsewhere; and in getting out of a low car, first twist your body and place your feet on the curb, then stand up.

Keep your weight down; this will reduce strain on the back and aid posture. Finally, do not get overtired or unfit as this can also lead to bad posture.

If, despite all these measures, you still suffer back pain, take care once you have recovered. Always eat at a table; never slouch in a chair. Climb stairs with a straight back and avoid lifting or bending. Drive only short distances if possible.

It is not a good idea to embark on a heavy keep-fit programme; follow a series of exercises recommended by your doctor. Walking will do you good, as will swimming. And use the opportunity *not* to walk the dog, carry heavy shopping or push a pram.

Bacteria

These are minute, living things too small to be seen with the naked eye. At their largest, they measure only a hundredth of a millimetre across. Thought by biologists to be a very simple form of plant life, they are each made up of a single cell bounded by a tough wall.

Although they are so small, bacteria are one of the most successful groups of living things. They are found almost everywhere. Although bacteria have a bad reputation because they cause disease, on balance, they probably do more good than harm, for certain kinds help in the production of foods, and the manufacture of certain vitamins within the human intestine.

Different types

Microbiologists usually divide disease-causing bacteria into four main groups, based on their shape.

The *cocci* are spherical bacteria averaging about a thousandth of a millimetre in diameter. They arrange themselves in different ways: *Staphylococci,* responsible for infections such as BOILS and other ABSCESSES, are massed in bunch-like groups while the *Streptococci* that cause, for example, middle EAR infections and SCARLET FEVER are found in chains. *Gonococci,* the bacteria that cause GONORRHOEA, group themselves in pairs, as do those responsible for some types of MENINGITIS and PNEUMONIA.

Bacilli are rod-shaped bacteria averaging about three hundredths of a millimetre long by 1/5000 mm wide. They cause TYPHOID, CYSTITIS and TUBERCULOSIS.

The third group, called *Vibrio,* are comma-shaped and cause CHOLERA.

The fourth group, the *Spirochaetes,* are minute spirals. SYPHILIS, relapsing fever and trench mouth are three examples of disease caused by spirochaetes.

How they move and grow

Apart from the cocci, which are immobile, most bacteria can move, either by waving their whip-like projections or *flagella* or, in the case of spirochaetes, by twisting movements of their 'bodies'.

Bacteria multiply at great speed by splitting in two. At blood heat (37°C/98°F) and in places rich in things on which they can feed, they will divide in this way once every half an hour. In eight hours, one bacterium will have multiplied to produce over half a million offspring – remarkably, without having any form of sex.

When conditions are unfavourable, some bacteria – notably the ones that cause TETANUS – react by going into a kind of 'hibernation' state. They change into what is known as spores, with extra-tough outer walls. These spores are particularly dangerous because the toughened wall is extremely difficult to destroy.

Bacteria and the human body

The human body is able to cope with the presence of thousands of bacteria because over the centuries of human development, a situation of mutual tolerance has built up. It is also to the advantage of the bacteria not to kill the host that is providing them with a constant supply of nourishment. But there are some disease-causing, or pathogenic, bacteria to which the body is susceptible.

Methods of entry

To cause disease, these bacteria must first enter the body. They do this in contaminated food or water, through wounds in the skin via a cut or scratch or by being breathed in, especially in the minute droplets of water which are shot out at great pressure by coughs and sneezes. Some bacteria, particularly those that cause venereal diseases, are transmitted by direct person-to-person contact.

When bacteria have entered the blood or tissues, they do not show their effects immediately. They must first survive a growth or incubation period which may take from a few hours to more than a year.

They cause illness either by damaging body tissues, as in wound infections, typhoid, meningitis and WHOOPING COUGH, or by releasing powerful chemical poisons called toxins.

In food poisoning, the toxins irritate the intestine causing vomiting and diarrhoea, while in tetanus and DIPHTHERIA they damage the nervous system.

The body's defences

In response to infection, the body reacts by mobilizing its defence systems.

The first of these is inflammation, which means that the blood supply to the affected area is increased, and the white cells in the blood try to attack and engulf the invaders at the site of the infection. At the same time, the body starts making antibodies, which have the ability to attack the invaders.

Once bacterial infection has set in, of course, medicines can also come to the body's aid. The groups of drugs called ANTIBIOTICS and sulphonamides prescribed by doctors are the most effective.

Bacterial infection can be prevented by getting rid of breeding grounds, by killing them, or through IMMUNIZATION.

Balance

Humans are unique in the animal kingdom because we are the only creatures who always walk upright on two legs. To keep ourselves in this unusual stance, we rely heavily on a highly developed sense of balance.

Inside the ear

The body's balancing mechanism is intricate and is mostly contained inside our EARS. The ear is not just an organ of HEARING: it is also responsible for moment-by-moment monitoring of the position and movements of the head. And if the exact position of the head is correctly monitored, the body can adjust itself to stay balanced.

Well protected by the bones of the skull, the delicate organs of balance lie in the innermost part of the ear, appropriately called the inner ear. Here, there exists a maze of tubes filled with fluid, all at various levels and at differing angles. Of these tubes, the ones directly involved in balance are called the utricli, the sacculi and the semi-circular canals.

Detecting position

The utricle and the saccule are concerned with detecting the position of the head. Each of these two cavities contains a pad of cells overlaid with a jelly-like substance in which are embedded small granules of chalk.

When the body is upright, gravity causes these granules to press against sensitive hairs in the jelly. The hairs then send nerve signals to the brain that say 'upright'.

When the head leans forwards, backwards or sideways, the chalk granules push against the hairs, bending them in a different way. This fires off new messages to the brain, which can then, if necessary, send out instructions to the muscles to adjust the position of the body.

The utricle is also in action when the body starts to move forwards or backwards. If a child, for example, starts to run, the chalk granules are pushed back against the hairs as though the child were falling backwards. As soon as the brain receives this information it sends signals to the muscles, which make the body lean forwards, restoring its balance. All these reactions are reversed if the child tips backwards off his or her chair.

Starting and stopping

Jutting out just above the utricle of the ear are three fluid-filled semi-circular canals. At the base of each canal is an oval mass of jelly. Encased in this jelly are the tips of sensitive hairs, which become bent by movements of fluid in the canals as the head moves.

The semi-circular canals pick up information about when the head starts and stops moving – particularly important during quick, intricate movements.

As the head begins to move one way, the fluid in the canals tends to stay still, making it push against the sensitive hairs. The hairs then send messages to the brain, which can take action.

But when the head stops moving, particularly when it stops turning round and round, the fluid goes on moving inside the semi-circular canals for up to a minute or more making you feel dizzy.

Control centre

The part of the BRAIN most responsible for directing the action of the muscles in keeping the body balanced is called the cerebellum. As well as taking in messages from the balancing organs in the ears, this section of the brain receives a whole wealth of other information. Here messages from the eyes, the neck, spine and limbs – in fact from all over the body – are coordinated.

The EYES, too, have a very special part to play in balance, for they provide vital information about the body's relation to its surroundings. The eyes also have an important link-up with the semi-circular canals. When the head begins to move to the left, for example, the movement of fluid in the semi-circular canals makes the eyes move to the right. But the balance mechanism then makes them move to the left to adjust to the same position as the head.

This eye movement explains in part why people are more likely to be sick if they try to read while travelling during a journey in a moving vehicle, such as a car or bus. The reading tends to counteract these natural eye movements, which helps to trigger off those unpleasant attacks of nausea and vomiting which constitute TRAVEL SICKNESS.

What can go wrong

The most serious disease of balance is called MÉNIÈRE'S DISEASE, the cause of which is unknown. It causes sudden unprovoked attacks of VERTIGO with vomiting and loss of balance which lasts from minutes to hours. Ultimately it may lead to deafness. A similar set of symptoms (sometimes called Ménière's syndrome) can be caused by a wide range of conditions including certain drugs, strokes, tumours, multiple sclerosis or migraine.

Because the hearing and balancing mechanisms are so close together in the ear, problems concerning the hearing apparatus can also affect the balancing mechanism. This explains why a dizzy sensation often accompanies middle ear infections and bad colds.

An infection known as *vestibulitis* or labyrinthitis causes inflammation in the inner ear. The patient feels extremely dizzy and develops *vertigo* – a sensation of spinning round in space. When vertigo is severe, the patient may be unable to stand, and feels very sick; he or she may even start to vomit. If the cause of the vertigo is a viral infection, it may pass after a few days, although medical help should be sought; a drug to control the dizziness and sickness may be prescribed.

Doctors can perform several tests to find out whether the balancing mechanism is working properly. These include blindfolding patients to see how long they can balance without the help of their eyesight. Or patients may be put in a rotating chair to see if their eyes automatically start to move in the opposite direction. And another quite common test is putting iced water in one of a patient's ears, which should make the fluid in the semi-circular canals begin to move, causing the patient to feel dizzy.

Balanitis, *see* Penis, Thrush

Baldness, *see* Hair

Barium, *see* X-rays

Bartholin's glands, *see* **Vagina**

Basophils, *see* **Blood**

Becker's pseudohypertrophic dystrophy, *see* **Muscular dystrophy**

Bed sores, *see* **Ulcers, skin**

Bedwetting, *see* **Incontinence**

Behaviour therapy, *see* **Mental therapies**

Bell's palsy, *see* **Conjunctivitis, Taste**

Benign, *see* **Cancer, Tumours**

Benign breast disease, *see* **Mastitis**

Benzodiazepines, *see* **Tranquillizers**

Beri-beri, *see* **Vitamins**

Beta-blockers, *see* **Autonomic nervous system, Coronary heart disease, Tranquillizers**

Bile

This is a thick, bitter, yellow or greenish fluid (pigmented by *bilirubin* (orange-yellow) and *biliverdin* (green)) made in the LIVER and stored in the GALL BLADDER. Released from the gall bladder into the small intestine in response to the presence of food, it is essential to the DIGESTION of FATS.

It is also part of the body's excretory, or waste-disposal system, because it contains the breakdown products of worn-out BLOOD cells (*see also* JAUNDICE).

Bilharzia, *see* **Tropical diseases, Worms**

Bilirubin, *see* **Bile, Jaundice**

Billings method, *see* **Contraception**

Biopsy

This is the removal of a tiny piece of tissue from an organ or other part of a person's body for the purpose of microscopic examination. It is a relatively painless operation, often no more than the insertion of a special hollow needle into the organ in question to extract a sample from it. Biopsies are used in the diagnosis of various diseases, including cancer.

Birth, *see* **Childbirth**

Birthmarks

'Birthmark' is the word used to describe any noticeable abnormality, such as a swelling or any mark on the SKIN of a baby. It may be present at birth, or it may appear soon after.

Such marks can be thought of as defects in the development of part of the skin, and consist either of groups of abnormal blood vessels, collections of cells responsible for the production of pigment (colouring) or groups of cells responsible for the formation of the surface of the skin, properly called the epidermis. The usual word used by doctors to describe one of these marks is a *naevus.*

Birthmarks composed of abnormal blood vessels are called *vascular naevi*; those with pigmented cells are known as *melanocytic naevi*, or 'moles'; and those from the epidermis are described as *epidermal naevi.*

There are basically two types of birthmarks caused by groups of abnormal blood vessels. One, known as *naevus flammeus,* consists of a defect in the smallest blood vessels – the capillaries in the top layer of the skin. They dilate (widen) and this causes the redness of the overlying skin. Common names for some of these birthmarks are the salmon patch, the stork mark, the port wine stain.

The other main group of vascular birthmarks is derived from patches of primitive tissue from which blood vessels are formed. When they are present after birth, they are the blemishes known as strawberry marks or *cavernous naevi.* They rarely cause complications, and at least 90 per cent disappear by themselves.

Salmon patches and stork marks are visible at birth. They are pale pink, with fine blood vessels visible within them, and most commonly seen on the nape of the neck, the mid-forehead and the eyelids. The majority of them fade rapidly, and most have gone by the age of one year. They rarely, if ever, need treatment.

Port wine stains are less common than salmon patches, but are usually permanent. They occur on any part of the body, but are commonest on the face and upper part of the trunk. They range in colour from pale pink to deep red or purple and can vary in size from a few millimetres to several centimetres across.

Epidermal naevi are overgrowths of the skin surface, and are usually skin-coloured or yellow brown. They, too, are permanent.

Treatment

In the case of port wine stains, this has been generally most satisfactory. If the blemish is small enough to be completely cut out without the need for a skin graft, then a good result is assured. But if a skin graft is necessary, scarring usually occurs which can be as unsightly as the original birthmark. The best treatment in these cases is to hide the birthmark with make-up.

Occasionally, tattooing can be used to improve the colour match with surrounding normal skin, and freezing the skin and laser treatment have been used with some success.

Epidermal naevi can be cut out, but despite this, they sometimes return. Freezing is effective in some cases.

Pigmented birthmarks

Pigmented birthmarks can be divided into two basic types. There are the flat, uniformly pale brown marks 1–4 in (2–20 cm) across called café-au-lait patches; and there are the varieties of MOLES.

Café-au-lait patches, which occur in as many as 10 per cent of babies, are usually of no significance. Although they remain for good, they are usually on the trunk, and are not unsightly.

Moles are collections of pigment cells – those which give the skin colour. They are uncommon in babyhood, but become more and more common in childhood and especially during adolescence. When they are present at birth, they tend to be larger, and have a definite, though small risk of becoming malignant. Moles that develop later on in childhood have little risk of malignancy.

Blackouts, *see* **Unconsciousness**

Blackwater fever, *see* **Malaria**

Bladder and bladder control

The urinary bladder is a hollow, thick-walled, muscular organ which lies in the lower part of the PELVIC basin between the pubic bones and the RECTUM. It is a four-sided, funnel-shaped sac resembling an upside-down pyramid. The base of the pyramid provides a surface on which coils of the small INTESTINE or, in women, the UTERUS, rests.

How the bladder works

The walls of the bladder consist of a number of muscular layers which are capable of stretching while the bladder fills, and then contracting to empty it. The KIDNEYS pass a nearly continuous trickle of URINE down the ureters to its walls. However, rather than the bladder acting like a balloon, with the pressure constantly increasing as it is filled, the muscle fibres of the bladder allow considerable expansion by adapting to the volume of urine until the bladder is nearly full. When it begins to resist, the need to pass urine is felt.

The two ureters – the tubes through which urine passes from the kidneys to the bladder – enter near the rear corners at the upper surface. There are one-way valves in the openings where they join the bladder to prevent urine from flowing back towards the kidneys if the bladder becomes too full.

Urine is passed out of the body via the URETHRA, which opens from the lowest point of the bladder. Normally this opening is kept closed by a sphincter, a circular muscle which contracts to seal the passageway. While urinating, this sphincter relaxes simultaneously as the muscles of the bladder wall contract to expel the urine. In women, the urethra is only about 1 in (2.5 cm) long and is not a very efficient barrier against entry of BACTERIA from outside, especially if the sphincter is weakened by previous infection, old age or poor muscle tone. Men are better protected since their urethra has to pass through the PENIS and the PROSTATE GLAND to reach the bladder.

Bladder diseases and disorders

CYSTITIS is an inflammation of the bladder. It is commonly found in women, as

The urinary systems

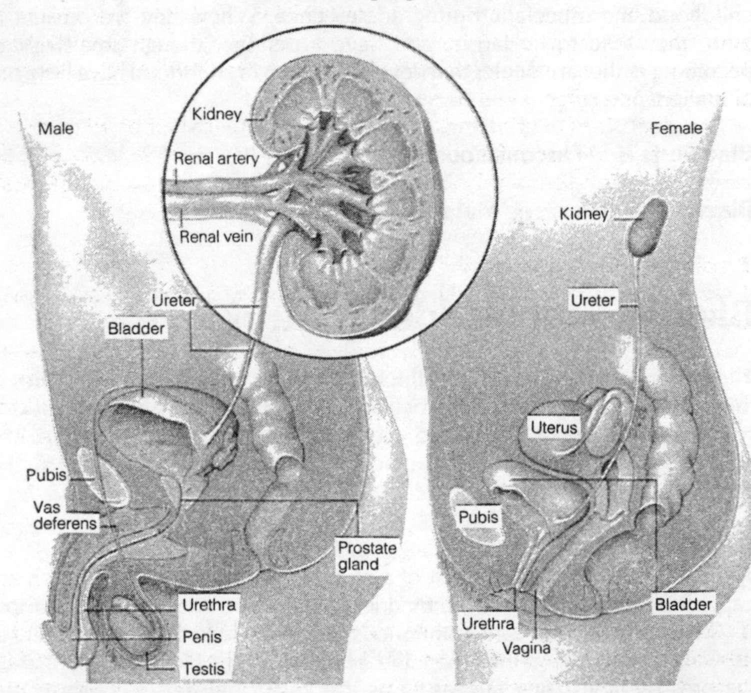

their shorter urethra affords less protection against bacteria. It may be caused by intestinal bacteria which have got into the bladder from the anus, from vaginal infections, or from an inflammation originating in an adjacent structure like the kidney. It can occur because of infections contracted through intercourse or childbirth, when there is damage to the urethra after nearby surgery, or when resistance is low.

KIDNEY stones (calculi), which are too large to pass through the urethra, can cause an obstruction, and result in an inability to empty the bladder freely. This condition brings acute distress with colicky pain and requires urgent medical attention. Smaller stones may pass through the urethra, but larger ones may need to be removed by surgery.

TUMOURS, usually benign, can also be present in the bladder, though sometimes they can become cancerous and will require medical attention. The main symptom is the sudden appearance of blood in the urine; there is no pain.

In men, enlargement of the prostate gland in the middle-aged and elderly can obstruct the flow of urine: straining and a decrease in the strength and force of the urinary stream are common symptoms. If medical attention is not sought, stones in the bladder or ureter and inflammation of the bladder may develop. A catheter may have to be passed up the urethra to release the urine which has collected in the bladder.

A decrease in the volume of urine passed daily may be due to a narrowing (stricture) or obstruction of the urethra, an inflammatory condition, drinking less fluid, or hot weather. If obstruction is the cause, the bladder becomes distended and surgery will be needed.

Any difficulties in urinating, or any change in the colour of urine, due to blood or pus, are cause for concern as they may be symptomatic of bladder disease, or some disorder elsewhere in the body. Seek medical advice as soon as possible.

Problems of bladder control

Congenital abnormalities of the bladder and urethra account for some cases of bedwetting, but an underdeveloped bladder is no cause for alarm.

The inability to control the reflex emptying of the bladder is usually a result of the loss of coordination in the NERVOUS SYSTEM due to possible injury or disease. The bladder may have to be emptied with the aid of a catheter, though sometimes it is possible to train the bladder to work at planned intervals. *See also* INCONTINENCE.

Blindness

Total blindness – that is, complete loss of vision in both eyes – affects only 5 per cent of the people who are termed 'blind'. The majority are, in fact, partially sighted, but with deteriorating vision. Such people may only be able to read the number plate of a car at a distance of just over 3 feet (about a metre) and most are even more handicapped. They can usually see little more than light or shade or count the number of fingers placed directly in front of them. They live in a dark, blurred and misty world or have 'tunnel' vision, which gives the effect of looking down a tube.

Why vision fails

There are many medical causes of blindness or failing vision. The EYE is a very complex sense organ and what you 'see' outside must be converted first into an image and then into nerve messages which are interpreted in the BRAIN. Loss of vision can be caused by any interruption of these nerve messages or from illness, accident, industrial or war injury, or disease that affects the eye or the nerve pathways within the brain.

CATARACT is one of the principal causes of blindness throughout the world. The clear transparent lens of the eye becomes opaque, preventing the passage of light and sight gradually fails. The majority of cataracts are caused by the process of ageing, but medical conditions or injury to the lens may also cause this problem.

Children who are born blind usually have congenital cataracts, or have a serious defect of the visual system. Cataracts can be surgically removed, but a condition called *nystagmus*, which is a fine involuntary tremor of the eye, often occurs and makes focusing extremely difficult.

Infections that cause blindness are rare in developed countries, but the commonest cause of blindness in the world is *trachoma*, a virus disease of the cornea, which causes scarring.

Should a pregnant woman contract RUBELLA (German measles), there is a possibility that the child will be born with cataracts. Similarly, should she develop *toxoplasmosis* – infection by a tiny parasite known as *Toxoplasma gondii*, which may be caught from domestic cats and raw meat, the child may be born blind.

Young children who are accidentally contaminated with dog excreta, while playing out of doors, also run a slight risk of contracting *toxocariasis*, from the WORM parasite *Toxocara canis*. This is known to affect the eye and cause a chronic inflammation of the retina.

The effects of ageing

People who are over 70 may suffer degeneration of the retina, for which there is no cure. The cells of the retina just age and die, particularly those in the area known as the macula, which is responsible for 'fine' vision. Although there is no cure for this condition, its effects can be lessened by magnifying the object.

Magnifying glasses are a practical aid for people with steady hands, but in the aged, this may present a problem. Closed-circuit television has been used to 'blow-up' the pages of books or magazines and project them on to a wide screen for easier and closer viewing.

Another common problem is when the retina becomes detached. This happens because it is, in fact, formed from several layers of cells which can be separated from the underlying eyeball. Should a tear also occur, fluid from the eye will leak behind the detachment, making it more difficult to replace.

The first symptom is blindness in the affected eye. This is quite painless and seems as if a curtain has descended on the view. Modern techniques have been devised to fix the retina back into position, either by surgery or by the use of laser beams. These fuse the retina and eyeball, so that they adhere normally and so save the person's sight. A detached retina may also happen to younger people, after a severe blow to the eye.

Older people are also prone to a condition known as GLAUCOMA, when the pressure of the fluid within the eye is raised.

Other causes of blindness

This can result from any condition that affects the optic nerve or the visual centre in the brain. Inflammation of the nerve can be brought about by a virus infection, poisons such as methyl alcohol (hence the expression 'blind' drunk), quinine, lead and arsenic, and even too much tobacco. When the inflammation is due to the nerve disease, *disseminated sclerosis*, it is often accompanied by a paralysis of the nerves that move the eyeball, which in turn produces double vision.

Vision can be partially lost if there is pressure on the optic nerve along its route to the visual centre. A tumour, haemorrhage or dilated blood vessel can produce complicated symptoms which need investigation and treatment by a specialist.

Sudden blindness, due to a blockage in the blood supply to the retina, usually occurs in one eye only. A clot in the artery that supplies the retina will cause instant blindness in the affected eye. It is not curable, but treatment of the medical condition causing it may prevent a similar episode occurring in the remaining 'good' eye.

A clot in the vein leading from the retina will also produce instant loss of sight, but this may return gradually over several weeks. Subsequent treatment with anticoagulants will be needed to prevent further occurrences.

DIABETES, KIDNEY failure and extremely high BLOOD PRESSURE are all conditions that can damage the retina, through ruptures of its tiny blood vessels and leakage of protein (exudates). Although there is no definite cure, sight can sometimes be improved by the use of laser beams to seal off the affected areas, so that the remainder of the retina can still function.

Retinitis pigmentosa, when patches of pigment form on the light-sensitive retina, is a condition that unfortunately runs in families. 'Tunnel' vision results, and because the periphery (outer area) of the retina is linked with night vision, people with this problem have difficulty in seeing in the dark. At the moment there is no successful treatment, and total blindness usually results by the age of 50.

Seeing spots in front of the eyes is a common experience, which doctors term *mucosae volitantes*. The little black spots are quite normal and tend to be seen when a person is young and a little anxious. It is not connected with failing vision or blindness in any way at all. This is also true of SQUINTS.

Blood

Blood is essential to body function. It is pumped by the HEART round the interior network of ARTERIES and VEINS, from before birth until death, delivering OXYGEN, food and other essential substances to the tissues and, in return, extracting carbon dioxide and other waste products that might otherwise poison the system. Blood also helps to destroy disease-producing micro-organisms, and through its ability to clot, it acts as an important part of the body's natural defence mechanism.

What the microscope reveals

Blood is not a simple fluid. Its proverbial 'thickness' is due to the presence of millions of cells whose activities make it as much a body tissue as bone or muscle. It consists of a colourless liquid called *plasma* in which float red cells (also known as *erythrocytes*), white cells (*leucocytes*) and very small cells called *platelets*.

To get an idea of the size of a single blood cell, you must first imagine the size of a micron – one thousandth of a millimetre. Each red blood cell is a flattened doughnut-shaped disc with a concave centre; it has a diameter of about 8 microns, and is 2 microns thick at its edge and 1 micron thick in the centre. In every cubic millimetre of blood, there are 5 million red cells, 10,000 white cells and 250,000 platelets.

Red blood cells

The red blood cells act as transporters, taking oxygen from the LUNGS to the tissues. Having done this, they do not return empty but pick up carbon dioxide, a waste product of cell function, and take it back to the lungs, from where it is breathed out. They are able to do this because they contain millions of molecules of a substance called *haemoglobin*.

In the lungs, oxygen combines very quickly with the haemoglobin to give the red cells the bright colour from which their name is derived. Carried in the arteries, this *oxygenated* blood arrives at the tissues. (A lack of red cells causes ANAEMIA.) With the help of ENZYMES in the red cells, carbon dioxide and water (another waste product of cell activity) are locked on to the red cells and taken back in the veins to the lungs.

White blood cells

The white cells in the blood are bigger than, and very different from, their red counterparts. Unlike red cells, white cells do not all look alike and are capable of moving with a creeping motion. Involved in the body's defence against disease, white cells are classified into three main groups known technically as *polymorphs*, *lymphocytes* and *monocytes*.

The polymorphs, which make up 50 to 75 per cent of the white cells, are also subdivided into three kinds. Most numerous are those called *neutrophils*.

When the body is invaded by disease-causing bacteria, these go to work. Attracted by chemicals released by the bacteria, they 'swim' to the site of infection and start to engulf the bacteria. As they do this, granules inside the neutrophils begin to make chemicals which destroy the trapped bacteria. The familiar pus that collects at the site of an infection is the result of the work of the polymorphs and is largely made up of dead white cells.

The second kind of polymorphs are known as *eosinophils* because their granules become stained pink when blood is mixed with the dye eosin. Composing only 1 to 4 per cent of the white cells, eosinophils combat bacterial attack but also have another vital role. When any foreign proteins (known as *antigens*) get into the blood, substances called *antibodies* are made to combine with the antigens and neutralize their effects. While this is going on, the chemical, *histamine*, is released. The eosinophils damp down the effects of histamine, for if too much is made, the result can be an ALLERGIC reaction. And once the antibodies and antigens have combined, the eosinophils remove the chemical remains.

The third type of polymorphs are the *basophils*. They make up less than 1 per cent of all the white cells, but are essential to life because their granules make and release the substance *heparin* which works to stop the blood from clotting inside the blood vessels.

Natural immunity

Lymphocytes form about one third of the white cells in our circulating blood and are entirely concerned with IMMUNITY. Lymphocytes are primarily derived from the bone marrow and then develop in two different groups. One group making antibodies which circulate in the blood are known as *B lymphocytes*. Another group, identical in appearance, are processed in the lymph glands where they become specialized in identifying and then REJECTING foreign (TRANSPLANTED) tissue and invading BACTERIA or VIRUSES. These are called *T lymphocytes*. Processing of the lymphocytes in the lymph glands is under the control of the THYMUS gland in the chest while we are still in the womb, and this controlling influence is maintained during childhood and continues even after the thymus gland shrivels up in our early teens.

B lymphocytes: The largest quantities of antibodies are made by an offshoot of the B lymphocytes known as plasma cells. The antibodies take the form of proteins called *immunoglobulin* (Ig) *receptors* which attack 'foreign' antigens. When this happens, the B lymphocyte is stimulated to produce antibodies and becomes a plasma cell. B lymphocytes can be distinguished from T lymphocytes by the use of a special fluorescent stain which shows up the presence of the Ig receptors on the cells' surface. T lymphocytes do not fluoresce.

T lymphocytes: These are made in the lymph glands by processing circulating lymphocytes originally from the bone marrow which makes B lymphocytes. How this takes place is not known. The T lymphocytes make chemicals which are released into the circulation and which are collectively known as *lymphokines*, more and more of which are being discovered, each with a different job to do.

T lymphocytes can be identified by their curious capacity to stick to the red blood cells of sheep. When mixed with lymphocytes, the sheep's red cells gather in clusters round the T cells but not the B cells, and look like a small rose with the T cell at the centre. For this reason the structure is known as a rosette.

There are several different types of T cell: *helper cells* which assist the B cells in the production of antibody to fight infection; *suppressor cells* which do exactly the reverse; and *killer cells* whose function is to destroy any invading tissue or infection.

These widely different functions of T lymphocytes are determined by the various lymphokines, or mediators, that they release. For instance, killer lymphocytes, or K cells, act with antibodies to attack and destroy particular target cells. They may play an important part in the body's mechanism for rejecting abnormal tumour cells.

Another mediator known as a helper cell or 'transfer factor' appears to be able to pass on sensitivity to specific antigens from one person to another. This means that it may find a use in therapy for difficult-to-treat disorders such as FUNGAL INFECTIONS and immune disorders.

In the main immune-deficiency diseases, many of which are inherited, B cells or T cells are absent, lacking or defective. For example, a lack of B lymphocytes, as in the disease known as *agammagloblulinaemia,* means that there is no mechanism for making antibodies to defend the body from disease. Children who inherit the disorder are normal for the first few months of life, but then begin to fall prey to various virulent infections such as PNEUMONIA. Infections can be treated with drugs, but IMMUNIZATION is usually ineffective. Replacement injections of gammaglobulin can now be given to combat infection.

Sometimes the mechanism by which lymphocytes produce antibodies breaks down and the body starts producing antibodies that attack its own tissues. Such auto-immune diseases include PERNICIOUS ANAEMIA, insulin-dependent diabetes mellitus, RHEUMATOID ARTHRITIS and various diseases of the THYROID gland. A decrease in the number of T helper cells, again because of a breakdown in the normal immune response, is characteristic of AIDS.

Monocytes: Last of the white cells are the monocytes, which form up to 8 per cent of the white cells. The largest monocytes contain large nuclei which engulf bacteria and remove the debris of cell remains, resulting from bacterial attack.

Platelets and clotting

The millions of minute platelets in the blood are similar to the red cells in having no nuclei. The platelets all have sticky surfaces and this is a clue to their function. If the minute blood vessels called *capillaries* are damaged, chemicals are released which make the platelets stick to the broken ends and plug them to stop the bleeding. The platelets are also instrumental in helping trigger off the process of blood clotting.

The ability of the blood to clot, or coagulate, and so prevent a person from bleeding to death if a blood vessel is severed, comes from the combined action of the platelets and a dozen biochemical substances called *clotting factors*, among which is the important substance called *prothrombin*. These factors are found in the fluid part of the blood – the plasma.

In the case of a wound, injured blood vessels bleed and platelets rush to the site to help seal it. Tissue-clotting factors are released and plasma factors enter the area. The reaction of the platelets, both types of factors and other agents convert *fibrinogen* into strands of fibrin. This becomes a jelly-like mesh across the break. Platelets and blood cells are trapped in this mesh, which now recedes, oozing out *serum* (the liquid part of blood without clotting factors) which helps form a scab. This will now prevent bacteria entering the body and so causing an infection.

Defects of the clotting process are of two kinds – failure of clots to form, and THROMBOSIS, in which blood clots form in the vessels.

Plasma

Although about 90 per cent of it is water, plasma is packed full of vital chemicals which it carries round the body. Among these are VITAMINS, MINERALS, sugars (GLUCOSE), FATS and PROTEINS – in fact, all the constituents needed for cell function and renewal. Other vital components are HORMONES, made by ENDOCRINE glands and carried to particular body organs to regulate functions as complex as reproduction. And just as the red blood cells carry away cell waste, so too does the plasma. The most concentrated chemical refuse in the plasma is urea which is ferried to the KIDNEYS for excretion in the URINE.

How red blood cells are made

The production of red blood cells begins in the first few weeks after conception, and for the first three months, manufacture takes place in the LIVER. Only after six months of foetal development is production transferred to the BONE MARROW, where it continues for the rest of life. Until adolescence, the marrow in all the bones makes red blood cells, but after the age of about 20, red cell production is confined to the spine, ribs and breastbone.

Red blood cells begin their life as irregular, roundish cells known as *haemocytoblasts*, with huge nuclei. These cells then go through a rapid series of divisions during which the nucleus becomes progressively smaller and is lost altogether. For red cell manufacture, the body needs IRON (the major constituent of the substance, haemoglobin), VITAMIN B_{12}, folic acid and proteins.

In their travels round the bloodstream, the red cells are subjected to enormous wear and tear and so need constant renewal. Each red cell has an average life of 120 days. After this, cells made in the bone marrow and SPLEEN attack those blood cells that are worn out. Some of the chemical remains are immediately returned to the plasma for re-use, while others, including haemoglobin are sent to the liver for further destruction.

The body has a remarkable ability to control the number of red cells in circulation, according to its needs. If a lot of blood is lost, if parts of the bone marrow are destroyed or if the amount of oxygen reaching the tissues is decreased through heart failure or because a person is at a high altitude, the bone marrow immediately begins to increase red blood cell production. And even strenuous daily exercise stimulates extra red cell output because the body has a regular need for more oxygen. Counts of blood cells show that athletes can have twice as many red blood corpuscles as people living sedentary lives.

Where white blood cells are made

The bone marrow is also the site of some white blood cell manufacture. All three types of polymorphs are made here, from cells called *myelocytes,* again by a series of divisions. The average polymorph lives only 12 hours and only two or three hours when the cells are involved in fighting bacterial invasion. In such circumstances, the output of all white cells is increased to meet the body's demands. As well as in the bone marrow, the lymphocytes, which live, on average, 200 days, are made in the spleen and in areas such as the TONSILS and the LYMPH glands scattered throughout the body. Both monocytes and platelets are made in the bone marrow. The length of monocyte life is still a mystery, for they seem to spend part of their time in the tissues, and part in the plasma. However, in a never-failing production line, the body manages to replace all its millions of platelets on average about once every four days.

Although bleeding, whether internal or external, is always a situation that should be taken seriously, the body's in-built survival mechanisms ensure that a person can lose as much as a quarter of all his or her blood without suffering any long-term ill effects, even if a blood transfusion is not given (see BLOOD GROUPS AND TRANSFUSIONS). And because blood is the supply line to and from the tissues, it is not surprising that body disorders and diseases show up via alterations in the blood. Apart from being a reflection of the body's state of health, the blood itself can be the site of a whole range of disorders affecting the red cells, white cells, platelets and plasma, each of which requires identification and treatment.

Blood groups and transfusions

BLOOD transfusions are not a new idea, but they have only become a safe, effective kind of medical treatment within the last 60 years, when the blood group system was fully understood and patients could therefore be given blood which was compatible with their own.

What are blood groups?

The major four blood groups are known as A, B, AB and O. What makes them different is the presence or absence of antigens on the red cells and of antibodies (which are part of the body's defence system) in the plasma, the colourless fluid part of the blood.

These proteins act rather like a badge or coat of arms: they enable cells to 'see' or judge whether other cells belong to the same clan as they do or whether they are potentially dangerous outsiders. If a cell wears a different protein from that of the native cells, it will be attacked and neutralized by the antibodies.

Group A and Group B red cells each have their own distinguishing protein on the surface.

Compatible groups

People with group O are 'universal donors': because their blood contains neither distinguishing proteins nor aggressive antibodies, it will be accepted by everyone. Group AB people are 'universal recipients', because they have no antibodies to destroy alien red cells. But although it may be relatively safe to mix blood groups in these circumstances, it is not done in practice. It is always safest only to transfuse blood of exactly the same group.

If someone is given a transfusion of the wrong kind of blood, the antibodies in their own blood will attack the red cells in the transfused blood, and the antibodies in the transfused blood will attack the patient's own red cells.

When an antibody attacks a red cell, they both clump together in a sticky mess which clogs up the blood vessels and KIDNEYS. A small transfusion would therefore cause JAUNDICE and fever, while a larger one might block the flow of healthy blood to major organs; the technical term for this 'clumping' is agglutination.

Heredity

Your blood is determined by heredity (*see* GENETICS). Broadly speaking, if parents have the same group as each other, their child will have the same group too. If one is A (or B) and the other O, the child will be A (or B). If one is A and the other B, the child will be AB.

If it were as simple as this, however, Group O would have disappeared by now, whereas it is, in fact, the most common group. It survives because anyone with a Group O parent retains what is called a recessive gene; if two people with this recessive gene have a child, it will as likely as not revert to Group O.

Certain blood groups are known to be more prone than others to particular diseases. For instance, people with Group O blood are more likely to develop duodenal ULCERS, gastric ulcers and PERNICIOUS ANAEMIA. Group A has a higher incidence of CANCER of the stomach, and both Group A and Group AB are susceptible to DIABETES. People with Group B are least susceptible to all these diseases.

The Rhesus factor

Apart from the ABO system, another very important aspect of blood grouping is the Rhesus factor, a protein found in the blood of the majority of the population. *See* p. 741.

Other ways of grouping blood

As well as A, B, AB and O groups and the Rhesus factor, there are more than a dozen other systems of grouping blood, all of which rely on identifying some kind of distinguishing protein in the blood cells. Two such blood types, known as M and N, were identified by the same Karl Landsteiner who discovered the A-B-O grouping and the Rhesus factor.

For the practising doctor worried about blood transfusions or the health of babies, these other groups are not of great practical importance. They are used principally in the study of heredity and in paternity tests and have little significance for health care on a day-to-day basis.

Some haematologists (blood specialists) now have such sophisticated techniques that blood-grouping will soon prove to be as positive a method of identifying individuals as finger-printing is well known to be.

Reasons for blood transfusions

The commonest reason for a blood transfusion is an acute loss of blood. Sudden bleeding of more than, say, about 2 pints (1 litre) can lead to shock, loss of blood pressure and ultimately heart failure. Serious accidents often cause hidden internal bleeding – injuries to the SPLEEN or LIVER, for example, can cause a loss of several pints into the abdominal cavity. And as many pints can be lost from a single fracture to the thigh. CHILDBIRTH may also be associated with abnormal haemorrhage either immediately before, or after the delivery of the baby.

To replace fluid needed to keep the blood flowing, a simple saline solution may be given initially, but then whole blood is used.

Major operations such as HIP replacement or removal of part of the BOWEL invariably need a transfusion, but even in some apparently straightforward operations, a transfusion may be needed if surgery proves more difficult than usual.

A patient with a bleeding duodenal ulcer, prolonged heavy PERIODS, or even infestation of hookworms (*see* WORMS) can lose up to 3.5 fl oz (100 cl) of blood a day. As this loss is chronic, it sometimes passes unnoticed until the patient becomes very ANAEMIC. Initially they may need a blood transfusion (before the cause is put right), but in this case, the transfusion is of concentrated red cells which are separated off from the blood plasma. This 'packed cell' transfusion lessens the risk of overloading the circulation with too much fluid.

In some diseases, such as LEUKAEMIA or APLASTIC ANAEMIA the patient may become deficient in white cells and platelets leading to increased risk of infection and excessive bleeding. White cells and platelets are removed from several pints of donor blood, suspended in plasma (the colourless part of blood in which red and white cells float), and given in a single transfusion.

Transfusions and disease

In parts of central Africa and other countries, where medical services are poor, collected blood may already be contaminated, but in the UK and most Western countries donors are initially screened for diseases such as MALARIA, HEPATITIS and HIV infection (the virus that causes AIDS). Then all blood is screened in the laboratory – for SYPHILIS, hepatitis and evidence of HIV infection. The one or two rare cases in the United Kingdom where AIDS has been transmitted by transfused blood were due to the fact that HIV can only be detected in the blood about 12 weeks after infection, so a recently infected person could donate blood which gives a negative test in the laboratory. Checking the donors for possible risks of exposure is thus crucially important, and now carried out most carefully by blood transfusion staff. The actual risk of transmission of AIDS in the UK is extremely small – less than one in a million. Blood is also screened for hepatitis B and C viruses, cytomegalovirus and syphilis.

To avoid any risk at all from infection, a technique has been developed in certain countries such as the United States for people who expect to have a major operation carried out on a routine basis. The individual donates his or her own blood – a pint each week over a period of a few weeks, while taking extra IRON to help make up the loss of red cells. This blood is then stored for use during the operation if it is required. This technique is useful where there is a high risk of blood-borne infection.

Blood pressure

When blood pressure is raised, a person is said to have 'high blood pressure', or *hypertension,* and if this is not treated, the chances of disease – or even death – are increased. In fact, the major causes of death in the Western world today are diseases of the HEART and blood vessels. Blood pressure is therefore not just a symptom but an urgent early warning signal.

Causes

The trouble starts within the ARTERIES themselves, thick-walled vessels that carry BLOOD from the heart to the tissues of the body. The blood is driven by the main pumping chamber of the heart, the left ventricle, and a great deal of force is required to send the blood out of the heart and into the arteries, through the tissues and then back into the heart again to be re-delivered to the arteries. Therefore, even under ideal conditions, the walls of the arteries are continually under considerable stress.

The level of arterial pressure is of great importance. If the pressure within the system is raised for any reason – a condition called hypertension – this stress is increased and paves the way for the development of arteriosclerosis, a narrowing of the arteries, due to the degeneration of the middle coat of the artery walls. The heart and the arteries can be severely strained and damaged by the blood pounding through.

On the other hand, seriously low blood pressure, or *hypotension,* is not a common problem and is usually the result of SHOCK from a HEART ATTACK, acute infection, or blood loss following an accident. Very occasionally it may occur in people suffering from Addison's disease – a failure of the ADRENAL GLANDS – which is extremely rare and can be corrected by drug treatment.

Because the maintenance of an adequate blood pressure is so important, very sophisticated mechanisms have evolved in the body to stabilize it. In the

West, the level of general STRESS has, however, led to many people developing a level of blood pressure that is far too high for the continuing good health of the arterial system. When this is not the result of disease elsewhere, it is called *essential hypertension*. The major long-term effect of high blood pressure is on the arteries of the brain, the heart and the KIDNEYS with the eventual likelihood of STROKES, heart attacks, or kidney failure.

Anyone who has had high blood pressure without any treatment over a period of years is several times more likely to suffer from a stroke or a heart attack than someone with normal blood pressure. If the individual also SMOKES, or has a high blood CHOLESTEROL level, the risks are many times greater.

What is normal?

The maximum pressure of each heartbeat, or *systole*, is called the *systolic pressure*, and the minimum pressure is called the *diastolic pressure*. It is these two pressures which are measured in order to determine a person's level of blood pressure. Obviously, some figure has to be adopted as 'normal'. For young and middle-aged adults, a pressure of 120 (systolic) over 80 (diastolic) – written as 120/80 – is considered normal, 140/90 is cause for concern, while one of 160/95 is definitely high and requires treatment.

Blood pressure starts to rise when people adopt a more 'developed' way of life. But why does the behaviour of blood pressure change in this way? Currently, the popular answer to this question is that it is caused by stress, and there is considerable evidence that it is involved. Genetic factors are important as hypertension can run in families.

The influence of diet

There is a significant difference in the type of food that is eaten by developed communities as compared to less developed ones. The amount of SALT consumed is particularly important, since it has been found that salt tends to increase the volume of blood in the circulation and put blood pressure up. It is now accepted that both salt intake and stress are among the factors that combine to produce essential hypertension.

Obesity is also associated with hypertension.

Control of hypertension

Whatever the causes may be, the tendency to essential hypertension is definitely connected with some kind of overactivity of the normal control mechanisms of the body.

There is an area in the lower part of the BRAIN, called the *vasomotor centre*, which controls blood circulation and hence the blood pressure. The blood vessels which are responsible for controlling the situation are called arterioles and lie between the small arteries and the capillaries in the blood circuit. The vasomotor centre receives information about the level of your blood pressure from pressure-sensitive nerves in the aorta (the main artery of the body) and the carotid arteries (to the head), and then sends out instructions to the arterioles through the sympathetic nervous system (*see* AUTONOMIC NERVOUS SYSTEM).

In addition to this fast-acting nervous control, there is also a slower-acting control operating from the kidneys, which are very sensitive to blood flow. When this fails, they release a HORMONE called *renin*, which in turn produces a substance called *angiotensin*. This has two effects: first, it constricts the arterioles and raises the blood pressure; second, it causes the adrenal gland to release a hormone called *aldosterone*, which makes the kidneys retain salt and causes the blood pressure to rise.

Diagnosis
Raised blood pressure may be the result of a number of conditions apart from essential hypertension. Many kidney diseases cause high blood pressure. Therefore, when a person is suspected of having this problem, their kidneys are usually checked. This is easily done in most cases with a single blood and urine test. Only occasionally is it necessary for the person to have a kidney X-ray.

Much information can be gained from the patient. The blood test measures the urea in the blood – this is likely to be raised if there are kidney defects. The blood level of various salts (sodium, potassium and bicarbonate) gives clues to other secondary causes of blood pressure. The urine is screened for the presence of protein, which also occurs in chronic kidney infection or disease.

The doctor will always check the EYES using an ophthalmoscope. This instrument allows the doctor to look directly at the blood vessels in the retina at the back of the eye. If blood pressure has been present for some time, these blood vessels tend to become damaged and there may also be damage to the retina itself – a condition called *hypertensive retinopathy*. The degree of damage to the retina is an indication of the likely effect on other organs of the body. These signs can also be useful to assess the urgency of treatment.

Many doctors will also perform a cardiogram and chest X-ray, to see if the raised blood pressure has affected the heart in any way.

If the kidneys are found to be functioning abnormally, it is possible that the raised blood pressure could be the result of renal (kidney) disease. On the other hand, the raised blood pressure can itself cause deterioration in the kidneys. This happens because continuing high blood pressure particularly affects the arterioles, causing their walls to thicken. This obstructs the flow of blood and has an adverse effect on kidney function.

Screening
The majority of people who have high blood pressure usually have no symptoms whatsoever. The early stages of hypertension may take several years to develop, and by the time symptoms have started to occur there may already be some damage to the arteries in the heart or the brain, which can cause an increased risk of strokes or heart attack later in life. For this reason it is now suggested that everyone over the age of 35 should have their blood pressure checked at least every two or three years. If there are early signs of hypertension, it will be much easier to treat and the extra risk of heart attacks or strokes can be reduced. This makes these regular checks worthwhile.

Symptoms
Occasionally, by the time that people feel it is necessary to see their doctor, their blood pressure is already very high indeed. They may already have BLACKOUTS, a minor stroke, and symptoms such as swollen ankles, or shortness of breath. This situation is particularly likely in *malignant or accelerated hypertension* and is fatal if left untreated.

The brain disturbances here are due to an increase in the pressures operating inside the skull and pressing on the brain. This can be detected by examining the eye with an ophthalmoscope. If there is undue pressure, the central nerve at the back of the eye will look inflamed. There are also likely to be signs of hypertensive retinopathy.

Apart from cases of malignant hypertension, symptoms of high blood pressure are not always definite. People may complain of headaches, but this does not necessarily mean you have hypertension. Dizziness (*see* VERTIGO) and NOSE bleeds are also common. Any middle-aged or elderly person who has a nose bleed – especially if they have several – should have their blood pressure checked as this may be an early sign of hypertension.

Treatment
Since treatment can dramatically increase the life expectancy of someone who has hypertension, it is clearly important that anyone who has significantly raised blood pressure should be carefully treated.

First, however, the doctor must check to see whether there is any specific cause for high blood pressure, such as Cushing's disease, or kidney problems. In these cases, the correct treatment is the treatment of the underlying condition. Cushing's disease may be treated by surgery to the adrenal glands; kidney disease also may need surgery to the arteries supplying the kidneys or to the kidneys themselves. Once the surgery has been completed, the blood pressure level will settle, and there will no longer be any excessive risk to the individual from hypertension.

Drugs and side-effects
However, in the vast majority of cases, there will be no obvious cause for hypertension, and then drug treatment may need to be considered.

Over the past few years, a number of drugs have become available for hypertension – each group works in a different way. However, many of these drugs have some side-effects, and any side-effects can become troublesome if patients have to take a drug every day for the rest of their lives – which is usually the case with the treatment of hypertension. So there have been many carefully conducted studies carried out to find out exactly which patients should be given treatment, and to find the best drugs.

Most doctors will now suggest that anyone with mildly raised blood pressure should first try to lose weight if they are overweight, avoid salt, reduce stress in their lives and perhaps exercise a little more. This alone may be quite enough to bring the blood pressure under control without the use of any drugs at all. Indeed, some doctors insist that a patient with high blood pressure and very high stress levels should immediately stop work, and take complete rest, often with sedatives.

If simple approaches like this do not work, or the level of blood pressure is very high or accompanied by significant retinopathy or heart trouble, then drug treatment will be needed.

The doctor will try to use the lowest possible dose of drugs to avoid side-effects, and may combine low doses of two or even three drugs rather than use very high doses of just one drug.

Initially the doctor will probably try a diuretic or a beta-blocker used alone. (Beta-blockers reduce the force of contraction of the heart muscle and decrease the production of renin.) Sometimes both will be used together. If the blood pressure is not controlled by this treatment a vasodilator drug may be used – either instead of one of the others or as well. Vasodilators decrease resistance to blood flow in the arterioles. More often drugs such as ACE inhibitors (which reduce the activity of angiotension in the circulation) may be tried as first line treatment in younger patients as they are often more acceptable to the patient than beta-blockers. Other drugs such as so-called 'alpha-blockers' and 'centrally-acting' drugs are reserved for the treatment of hypertension which has not responded well to other treatments.

Every individual responds differently to drugs for hypertension, so the doctor will have to keep a regular check on the level of the blood pressure and the possibility of side-effects. For those patients who have no symptoms whatsoever, it may prove very difficult to come to terms with taking drugs every day when they feel perfectly well, but it is vital for their future health that they do so.

Once the blood pressure has been brought under control, the long-term risks of a stroke, a heart attack, or kidney failure are much reduced.

Occasionally, an individual will develop seriously high blood pressure with symptoms. This may require urgent hospital treatment with drugs given initially by intravenous drip. The patient may then be given tablets to be taken regularly after the acute situation has resolved.

Blood sugar, *see* **Carbohydrates, Diabetes**

Blue baby

Babies born with congenital HEART defects – which are known collectively as 'hole in the heart' – can either have a healthy pink colour, or purplish blue lips and skin. The latter condition is known as *cyanosis*, and the characteristic colour of the blue baby occurs because there is insufficient OXYGEN in the BLOOD to change the colour to bright red.

Causes

In normal circulation, oxygen is extracted from the blood by the body's tissues, and so as the blood CIRCULATES around the body, it turns bluish in colour. The blood returns to the HEART and enters a collecting chamber called the right atrium, from which it travels to a second chamber called the right ventricle. It is then carried to the LUNGS, where it receives fresh oxygen, and is cleansed of carbon dioxide. This restores the red colour to the blood.

The blood then passes to the left atrium and into the left ventricle from where it is pumped into the body. The action of the blood moving through the lungs from the right side to the left is called *pulmonary circulation*; the movement of the blood from the left side of the heart, round the body and back to the right side of the heart is called *systemic circulation*.

A congenital heart defect allows bluish blood from the veins to pass through the heart and out to the body again without absorbing oxygen from the lungs. Any abnormality of the heart or blood vessels that allows one third or more of the systemic flow to consist of deoxygenated blue blood will cause a purplish-blue skin colour to appear in the baby from birth.

The abnormality can consist of a hole between the left and right atria or left and right ventricles, narrow openings to the chambers, or a mix-up between the great vessels that take blood to and from the heart. A child may have one or a combination of these abnormalities, each condition having a different medical name. The two that most commonly produce blueness as a symptom, however, are called *ventricular septal defect* and *tetralogy of Fallot*: together they account for a third of all congenital heart abnormalities.

Only about one out of every 1000 live babies born will have a congenital heart defect. It is not fully known why some children are born with defective hearts, but in some cases it is thought there may be a hereditary link. Exposure to RUBELLA during the first three months of pregnancy can affect a baby's heart, while other virus infections and certain drugs are other possible causes of abnormality. Congenital heart defects are also more common in babies with Down's syndrome.

Symptoms

Some babies with a heart defect may never look blue, while in others, the blueness may develop later if the defect has resulted in an abnormal heart function. Other symptoms of heart abnormality include difficulty during swallowing or crying, susceptibility to respiratory infections such as BRONCHITIS or PNEUMONIA, and less ability to recover afterwards.

To diagnose an abnormality, the chest is X-rayed to show the size of the heart. An ELECTROCARDIOGRAPH is then used to assess the size of the chambers and the thickness of the walls, and other painless, non-surgical tests such as an echocardiogram (which looks at the heart like an ultrasound scan) may be made to assess the amount and direction of blood flow.

A blue baby is likely to have one or many of these tests carried out within the first few days or weeks of life to determine whether surgery is necessary for the condition. Other babies with heart abnormalities whose colour is normal are often not so thoroughly investigated until they are at least three or four years old, or until doctors think they should be operated on.

If an operation is contemplated a final test called a *cardiac catheter test* is carried out. A fine tube is passed into the heart by the surgeon, under an anaesthetic, from a vein or artery in the leg. The pressures in the various chambers of the heart can be measured and special X-rays carried out. An exact diagnosis can then be made.

Treatment

The various abnormalities that cause blueness each have a different form of treatment, and the operations can be performed at different ages, from soon after birth to pre-school age or later.

The most common abnormality which requires surgery is ventricular septal defect, a hole between the left and right ventricles. The operation which carries a mortality rate of less than 5 per cent, consists of opening a ventricle, stitching up the hole or putting a plastic patch over it if it is too large to be closed.

Boils

Quite deep in the lower layer of human SKIN are hair follicles – a type of pore, or tiny 'pit' from which hairs grow. If a follicle becomes infected by invading BACTERIA, an ABSCESS, or swelling filled with pus, forms. This is a boil; the medical name is a *furuncle.*

A *carbuncle* is two or more boils occurring next to each other, and a boil occurring in one of the hair follicles along the eyelid is called a stye.

Boils can occur anywhere on the body, but they appear most often on the face, eyelids, back of the neck, upper back and buttocks. They specially favour places where clothing rubs, such as the area on the collar line.

The bacteria known as *staphylococci* are the most common cause of boils. They can be transmitted from person to person, and in fact, some live harmlessly on the skin all the time and in infected areas like cuts or pimples. They usually only cause trouble when excessive friction or rubbing buries them in a hair follicle.

Infection happens most easily when a person is overworked or ANAEMIC, or badly undernourished for some reason, as can happen with ALCOHOLISM.

DIABETICS can have a series of boils when their blood sugar concentration remains high. This is because the bacteria breed fast when there is sugar present in the tissues. And when the skin is broken, as in SCABIES OR ECZEMA, boils develop rather more easily.

A boil starts gradually with a tender area under the skin. It becomes hot and red and may be surrounded by swelling.

A centre of pus develops where the fight against the infection is fiercest. It is made up of the casualties on both sides – dead bacteria, dead white blood cells and destroyed body tissue.

On places such as the ear or nose, where the skin is tight and the surrounding tissue cannot stretch, the condition is very painful indeed.

As soon as the pus from a boil has been released and the central core of dead tissue is gone, the boil heals. This may take about a week. Occasionally the body's defences will get the best of a boil, and the inflammation will subside without bursting.

Scarring

A small boil will heal without leaving a noticeable scar, but large boils and carbuncles do form scar tissue which may shrink over the months, but never disappears altogether.

The best way to reduce the likelihood of a large boil or carbuncle scar is by early treatment. The sooner you see the doctor, the quicker he will be able to get the boil under control.

Many people believe that you can lessen the effects of scarring by rubbing vitamin E cream into the wound. In fact, there is little or no evidence to support this.

The main danger from a boil is if the infection enters the bloodstream and spreads round the body. Boils occurring round the eyes and nose are particularly dangerous because their poison could spread to the brain.

Treating boils

Boils usually clear up by themselves, but you can help them to form a head – and ease the pain at the same time – by bathing the area with hot water or by applying a hot flannel or poultice.

A kaolin poultice is the one normally used to treat boils. The kaolin paste is heated in a pan of boiling water until it is moderately hot, then spread liberally on some lint. This is covered with gauze and applied to the boil.

Although small boils can be gently squeezed without much danger, it is wiser to leave them alone. Large or painful boils must certainly never be squeezed, nor should you squeeze carbuncles or any boils, large or small, that are between the eye and nose.

Once a boil has burst and the pus begins to drain, a dressing should be applied daily. This prevents the bacteria in the pus from spreading the infection, and also stops rubbing by clothing.

Magnesium sulphate paste will help to draw the pus out once the boil is open. The paste should be applied liberally and covered with a dry dressing.

Medical attention

In rare circumstances, when the pus remains trapped, a doctor may have to lance a boil. If the inflammation appears to be spreading, or a carbuncle is forming, he or she may prescribe an antibiotic.

A series of recurring boils can occasionally be a sign of diabetes or other illness, and anyone suffering from these should be sure to seek medical advice. You should also seek medical attention if, in addition to one or more boils, you have a high temperature or general feeling of illness. In addition, anyone who is very young or old should consult a doctor if they have a boil.

Carbuncles are more serious than single boils and must have medical attention. Plenty of rest is necessary in the treatment of carbuncles, especially in the elderly.

Bone marrow and transplants

At birth, all the BONES in the body contain red bone marrow – that is, marrow producing BLOOD cells. However, at the age of about six or seven, the marrow in the outer areas of the body begins to stop producing cells and becomes yellow marrow. This process continues until, at the age of 20 or so, the red marrow is found only in the skull, ribs, vertebrae, sternum (breastbone) and pelvis, together with a small island in the head of the humerus (the long bone in the upper arm) and the head of the femur (the thigh bone). At the age of 70, the area of red marrow is about half that of a young adult. If demand for the manufacture of blood cells increases – as it does in a person with continuous blood loss, for example – the yellow marrow can turn back into red marrow, acting as a reserve site for the synthesis (composition) of blood cells.

Cell manufacture

Three types of cells are made in the bone marrow: the red blood cells responsible for carrying oxygen; the various types of white blood cells, whose main function is concerned with immunity or defence of the body against invaders; and lastly, the platelets, the tiny fragments of cells which are an essential part of the blood clotting and healing mechanism that follows an injury.

Bone marrow diseases

The bone marrow may be defective at birth, or it may become defective later on in life, as a result of acquired disease.

Congenital defects: A child may be born with the inability to manufacture one or more of the cells described above. Thus, he or she may be anaemic because of an inability to make red cells, or may succumb very easily to infections, because of a lack of white blood cells, or may bleed easily because of a lack of platelets, which form part of a blood clot.

Acquired diseases: Later in life, the bone marrow can be affected by various diseases. There can, for example, be a sudden failure of the bone marrow to produce the different types of cells. This can happen for no obvious reason or it can come about as a result of ALLERGY to certain substances, notably various drugs; the marrow usually recovers when the drug is withdrawn. Very large doses of X-RAYS can have the same effect, as can infiltration of the bone marrow with CANCER cells from a tumour elsewhere in the body. The cancer cells multiply in the marrow, preventing it from functioning.

The cells in the marrow can themselves become cancerous, leading to the production of vast numbers of unwanted cells. If the white cells are affected in this way, LEUKAEMIA can occur.

Bone marrow transplants

The success of a bone marrow transplant depends on various factors, the most important being the tissue type of the donor and of the recipient. If the tissue types match closely, the recipient's body does not try to reject the donor's marrow. Because marrow contains cells concerned with immunity, the reverse can happen: the donor marrow reacts against the recipient, in what is known as the *graft versus host* reaction (*see* REJECTION OF TISSUE).

There are about 100 different tissue types, and usually about ten of these in any one individual. There is about a one-in-four chance of two members of a family having the same tissue type; identical twins will, of course, have exactly the same type. The chance of two completely unrelated people having the same type is extremely remote, and so centres where bone marrow transplants are performed try to get thousands of people to be donors, to build up a 'tissue bank', with a computerized register of donors. In Britain, this task is undertaken by the Anthony Nolan Bone Marrow Trust.

Carrying out a transplant

The donor first has to have a blood test, from which the tissue type can be determined. Other tests can also be done at the same time, to exclude the presence of certain diseases which would make the person an unsuitable donor. He or she is anaesthetized, and about 17½ fl. oz (500 ml) of marrow is removed with a large needle from the bones of the pelvis and from the breast-bone.

The recipient is treated with large doses of X-rays to the bone marrow, and with drugs to remove any remaining cells, so that the transplanted marrow will not be rejected by the recipient's own marrow. The marrow transplant is then injected into the recipient and finds its way into the bones via the bloodstream. After the transplant, drugs have to be taken for the rest of the patient's life to prevent the graft versus host reaction.

Transplants are done for two main reasons: for patients born with defects in their own marrow; and for those with leukaemia. In the latter, the leukaemic cells are destroyed by X-rays and drugs, and the transplanted marrow takes over.

Bones and bone diseases

The primitive function of bones as armour-plating is still obvious today in certain parts of the human body. One needs to think only of the skull (*see* HEAD), forming a complete protective case around the brain, or the RIBS doing the same for the heart and lungs.

Bones also, of course, provide the support which keeps the many components of the body together and upright. It is interesting to reflect that when the body thinks support is no longer needed – such as in the prolonged weightlessness of space flight or just the experience of bedrest – the bones will lose their strength and will also break easily if put under strain.

Another vital, but not quite so obvious use of bones is as girders to which muscles may be attached. MUSCLES provide the power by which the various limbs and body parts are moved, and this is done in the first place by moving the bones relative to each other.

The insides of bones are hollow, and the body, with great economy of space, uses these cavities for the manufacture of BLOOD cells. They also manufacture another vital substance for the body – CALCIUM.

What bones are made of

Like everything else in the body, bones are made up of cells. They are of a type which creates what is technically called a fibrous tissue framework, a relatively soft and pliable 'base' material.

Within this framework, there is a network of harder material, which gives a result something like concrete, with lots of 'stones' (i.e. the hard material) providing strength to a 'cement' base of fibrous tissue. The end product is an extremely strong structure, with considerable flexibility.

The growth of bones

When bones begin growing, they are solid all through. Only at a secondary stage do they start to develop hollow centres.

Hollowing out a tube of material only very slightly reduces its strength, while very much reducing its weight. This is a basic law of structural engineering of which nature takes full advantage in the design of bones. The hollow centres are filled with a soft substance, known as BONE MARROW, in which the manufacture of blood cells takes place.

Bones start forming in a human baby during the first month of pregnancy, but they are at this stage made – just like the skeletons of primitive creatures – of cartilage, quite soft material with a rubbery flexibility. As the baby grows, this cartilage frame is replaced by the fibrous tissue, with little or none of the hardening agent. Hardening of the bones is a gradual process taking place throughout childhood and is only completed by the end of puberty.

Another important, and remarkable feature of bones is their ability to grow into the right shape. This is especially important for the long bones which support the limbs. They are wider at each end than at the middle, and this provides extra solidarity at the joint where it is most needed. This shaping – technically known as modelling – is specially engineered during growth and goes on all the time afterwards.

Different shapes and sizes

There are several different types of bone, designed to perform in varying ways.

Long bones, forming the limbs, are simply cylinders of hard bone with the soft, spongy, marrow interior.

Short bones – found, for example, at the wrist and ankle – have basically the same form as long bones, but are more squat to allow a great variety of movement without loss of strength.

Flat bones consist of a sandwich of hard bone with a spongy layer between. They are flat to provide protection (as in the skull) or a particularly large area for the attachment of certain muscles, as with the SHOULDER blades.

The final bone type, *irregular bones*, come in several different shapes designed specifically for the job they do. The bones of the spine (*see* BACK), for example, are box-shaped to give great strength and plenty of space inside for the marrow. And the bones that make up the structure of the face are hollowed out into air-filled cavities to create extra lightness.

The joints

Bones have to be joined securely, but some must be able to move very extensively in relation to each other. The way nature solves this problem is in the ball and socket and hinge type JOINTS.

The ends of the bones are lined with a pad of soft cartilage so that in movement and weight-bearing they do not damage each other. The joint is also lubricated by specially produced fluids. Tying the whole structure together are tough thongs known as ligaments.

Self-maintenance

Like many other parts of the body, bones have the extraordinary capacity to maintain themselves if infected or damaged. The most obvious example of this is the ability to repair themselves when broken – even completely in two.

People often find it hard to imagine how this can happen. The key to it, in the first place, is the fact that when a bone breaks, blood vessels running through the bone automatically break, too. Quite a large blood loss results (and needs to be replaced in many cases) but it is this blood, lying around the area of the break, which creates the scaffolding for the repair of the break by clotting (i.e. hardening) into a solid mass.

Next, cells from the broken ends of the bone spread into the clotted area and lay down fibrous tissue. This unites the two broken ends, but before the join is really complete, the hardening process must take place.

The finished join is actually rather large and unwieldy, forming a mass of new bone around the place of the break. But later on, the bone's ability to shape itself remodels the area into the original smooth shape.

This takes place over a period of years after the break is completely mended and the limb once again in use, so that eventually the place of the break – doctors call it a FRACTURE – is unrecognizable, except by X-rays, from original smooth bone.

Diseases of the bone

Bones are prone to four principal types of disease.

One of the most serious is known as *congenital bone disease* which is hereditary, or transmitted through families and is incurable.

The various forms of congenital bone disease are rare and they include such complaints as *brittle bones* – in other words, bones which are abnormally weak. Although the condition itself cannot be cured, it can be treated effectively, mostly by preventing situations where the bones are put under great strain.

Dwarfism can also be caused by bone disease. If a child does not grow to the normal height of an adult, but develops normally in other ways, this is caused either from failure of bone growth or a failure of control over the bone-growing process.

The final, least serious type of inherited bone problem is the misshapen bone – perhaps an in-curving little finger, or the existence of an extra finger or toe. Such deformities, if they can be called that, are often present in several generations of a family and practically never cause serious problems.

Chemical problems

Then there are what are known as the *biochemically caused bone diseases*. This means a failure of the body's chemistry to supervise bone formation properly.

One of the best known is now virtually a disease of the past – RICKETS. It used to be caused by a lack of VITAMIN D due, in turn, to bad or insufficient diet experienced in poor living conditions. Weakening of the bones occurs, giving the legs especially a characteristic, bowed look. Although rare, it is sometimes seen in strict vegetarians and treatment is by vitamin D supplements.

Another disease in this category is called *osteomalacia*, and again gives rise to abnormally weak bones. Its underlying cause is actually a disease of certain parts of the stomach causing malabsorption of calcium, and it can be treated.

Rickets and osteomalacia may also occur in association with KIDNEY disease. This is probably due to failure of the kidney to activate vitamin D. Treatment is aimed primarily at the kidney failure itself, along with supplements of specially 'activated' vitamin D.

Infection

Bones can become infected by invading bacteria just like any other part of the body. Probably the best known such infection of the bones is called osteomyelitis. This can usually be cured by treatment with high doses of antibiotics. Tuberculous osteomyelitis can also occur, producing a much slower development of symptoms. It is very rarely encountered nowadays.

Polio (POLIOMYELITIS) is often classed as a bone infection, though it is not, strictly speaking, one. It is actually an infection of the nervous tissue which in turn means that the nerves and muscles controlling the bones in the affected area do not work in a way they would normally do.

Bone tumours

Bone lumps, or TUMOURS, may be a more serious cause for concern. Quite often they have been present for years – for example, as a hard lump (*exostosis*) on the skull – and cause no trouble at all. But some lumps are malignant (i.e. cancerous), and these grow quite quickly and invade other tissues.

Bone cancer, occurring of its own accord, is rare. However, cancer occurring from the spread of a tumour elsewhere is more common.

Bone cancer is always a serious matter, but these days it is controllable to a very considerable extent. The types of treatment available are extremely effective, totally eliminating the pain of the swelling caused by the growth in the bone.

The spread of cancer to the bones does not mean the patient has to retire to bed. On the contrary, there are likely to be many pain-free, active years ahead.

Other types of bone diseases

Further types of bone diseases are OSTEOPOROSIS and *hyperparathyroidism*. The first means 'thinning and weakening' of bone and occurs mostly in the elderly. It can be helped by treatment. The second is a problem caused by excess production of a certain type of hormone – the body's chemical controlling agents. It may be diagnosed by X-ray and testing for high blood calcium levels. Again, it causes weakness of the bones, but can be effectively cured by removing, in an operation, the parathyroid gland (*see* THYROID AND PARATHYROID), or part of it, which is responsible for producing the hormone in these excessive amounts.

One type of bone disease, PAGET'S DISEASE, seems to be on the increase. It affects the elderly, its cause is unknown and it causes haphazard growth of the bones. Treatment with a hormone that stimulates the production of bone-hardening substances seems to be successful.

OSTEOARTHRITIS and RHEUMATOID ARTHRITIS – which affect the lining of joints and the cartilage space between bones – eventually attack the bones themselves. Osteoporosis is a generalized thinning of the bones. It is commoner in post-menopausal women and a common cause of fractured hips in later life.

See also SKELETON.

Bornholm disease, *see* **Diaphragm**

Botulism, *see* **Diarrhoea, Food poisoning**

Bowel, *see* **Colon and colitis, Intestines and intestinal disorders**

Brain and brain disease

The brain is at the centre of the complex network of nerves that runs through the body, and together with the spinal cord it makes up what is known as the central NERVOUS SYSTEM. This controls the whole body by means of messages which are continually passing up and down its nerve pathways.

All the information we receive about our surroundings comes from our five senses. The nerves carrying this sensory information up to the brain are known as *sensory nerves*. Once the brain makes a decision, it sends its instructions for action down other nerve cells called *motor nerves*.

All nerve impulses going to and from the brain have to go up or down the SPINAL CORD. But now and then, such speedy action is needed that there is no time for the message to go all the way to the brain. So the message goes only as far as the spinal cord, which processes the message and responds to it on a relatively simple level. The result is known as a REFLEX.

When a doctor taps your knee and makes it jerk, he is looking for possible damage to the spinal cord by testing how fast your reflexes are. Other examples of reflexes are blinking, reactions to PAIN, and sexual responses.

All the messages flashing to and from the brain are transmitted by minute electrical impulses. They travel through special nerve tissue cells called neurones. The electrical activity in the brain creates waves which can be picked up on a machine (ELECTROENCEPHALOGRAM or EEG) and studied for abnormal patterns.

Together the brain cells form a mass of soft, jelly-like tissue, surrounded by three layers of protective membrane known as the *meninges* and some fluid called *cerebrospinal fluid.* Four arteries in the neck supply the brain with blood, without which it cannot survive.

Major divisions of the brain

The brain consists of the brainstem, cerebellum and cerebrum which has four lobes. Speech, taste, touch, hearing, smell, vision and areas controlling body movement are controlled by specific areas.

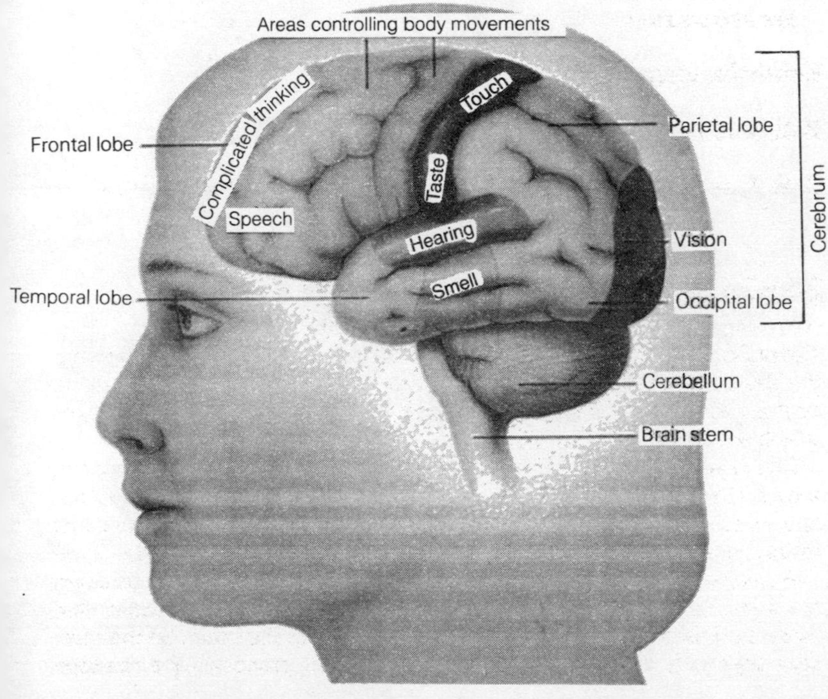

Mapping the brain

Basically the brain can be divided into three different regions: *hindbrain*, *midbrain* and *forebrain*. Each of these regions is in turn divided into separate areas responsible for quite distinct functions, all intricately connected to other parts of the brain.

The largest structure in the hindbrain is the *cerebellum*. This is the area that is in charge of BALANCE and coordination, and it works very closely with the organs of balance in the inner EAR.

Also part of the hindbrain is the *brain-stem*, which links the brain with the spinal cord. This is the part of the brain that was the first to evolve in primitive human beings. It is here that all incoming and outgoing messages come together and cross over, for the left side of the body is governed by the right-hand side of the brain, and vice versa. The various structures in the brain-stem

Internal structures of the brain

This cross-section highlights the major structures of the brain. The limbic system (inset) located within the thalamus is chiefly concerned with memory, learning, deep-seated emotions, and sociability.

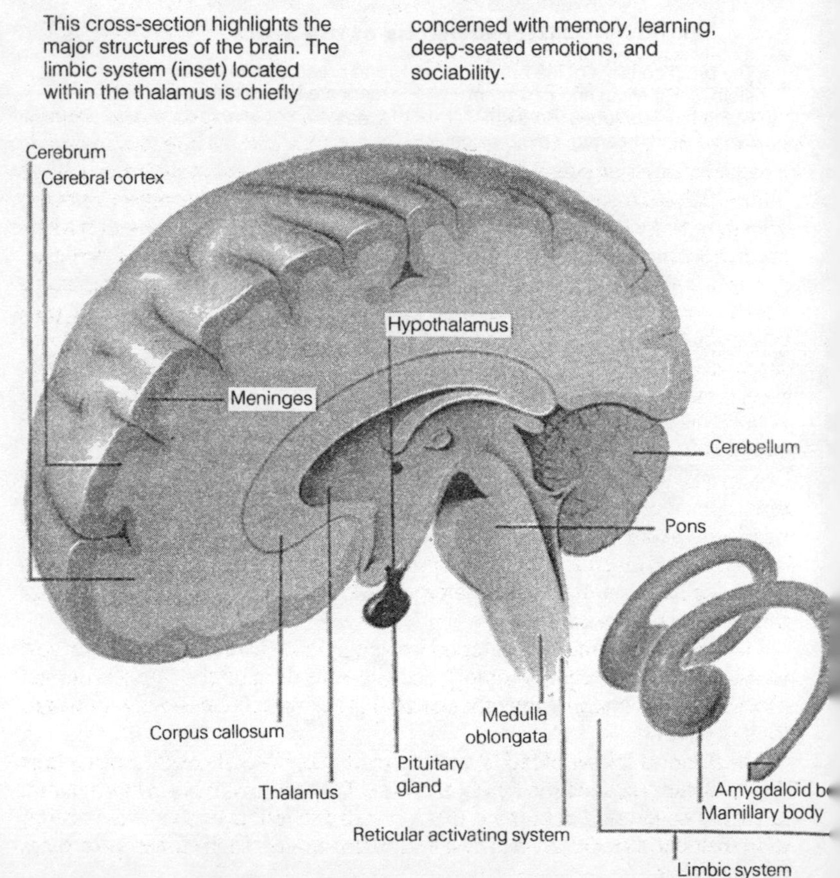

– including those known as the *medulla, pons* and *reticular activating system* – are in charge of life itself, for they control HEART rate, BREATHING, BLOOD PRESSURE, swallowing, COUGHING, hiccuping, VOMITING and consciousness.

Controlling the level of consciousness is one of the brain's most crucial functions. It is this mechanism, in the brain-stem's reticular activating system, that sifts through the mass of incoming information and decides which is important enough to alert the brain. It does this by controlling the amount of electrical activity each part of the brain receives. In turn, the reticular activating system is affected by the brain's decisions. It is this interplay that determines alertness and consciousness.

Central structures

Just beyond the brain-stem, in the midbrain, is an area devoted to controlling eye movements and pupil size. Beyond this, the forebrain begins. Here the *thalamus* is located, acting as a sort of relay station for incoming information.

Just below the thalamus is the *hypothalamus.* This is involved in such bodily functions as hunger and THIRST, body TEMPERATURE, SEX and SLEEP, and it works closely with the PITUITARY gland.

Nearby is another important system: the *limbic system,* comprised of a number of structures including the *hippocampus, amygdala* and *septum pellucidum.* This is the second most primitive part of the brain and is concerned with deep-seated emotions like rage, excitement, fear, sexual interest, pleasure, even relaxation and sociability. It is also closely connected with the smell centres of the brain, and there are rich connections with areas involved with other senses, behaviour and the organization of memories.

As well as information from our sense organs, we also receive messages from our internal organs, and these are relayed to the decision-making part of the brain by the limbic system. This accounts for the fact that these sensations are usually tinged with emotions – and that they can affect digestion.

Divided in two

The largest part of the entire brain is the *cerebrum,* which is located in the forebrain. It is divided right down the middle into two halves known as hemispheres, which are joined at the bottom by a thick bundle of nerve fibres called the *corpus callosum.* Although the two hemispheres are mirror images of each other, they have completely different functions, and work together through the corpus callosum.

The cerebrum is more developed in humans than in any other animal, and is essential to thought, memory, consciousness and the higher mental processes. This is where the other parts of the brain send incoming messages for a decision.

The 3 mm-thick wrinkled layer of 'grey matter' folded over the outside of the cerebrum is called the *cerebral cortex.* This part of the brain has become so highly developed in humans that it has had to fold over and over in order to fit inside the skull. Unfolded, it would cover an area 30 times as large as when folded.

Among all the folds there are certain especially deep grooves which divide each of the two hemispheres of the cortex into four areas called lobes.

The *temporal* lobes are involved with hearing and also smell; the *parietal* lobes with touch; the *occipital* lobes with vision; and the *frontal* lobes with movement and complicated thinking.

Within each of these lobes, there are specific portions devoted to receiving the sensory messages from one area. The sense of touch, for example, has a tiny area in the parietal lobe devoted to nothing but sensation from the knee, and a large area for the thumb. This is why areas like the thumb are more sensitive than areas like the knee. And the same principle applies to the other sensory parts of the cortex and to the motor, or movement, parts as well.

Of course, none of these areas of the brain can work by itself. Every instruction is in effect a joint decision, resulting from the different areas comparing and pooling their information, then coordinating the resulting action.

Personality

Most of our behaviour consists of movements. In addition, we go over possible behaviour in our heads, and we can use language to think as well as act. This gives us a sense of our relation to the outside world, which we feel as our consciousness or personality.

While the whole of the brain takes part in this process, it is the frontal lobes which act as the organizing and coordinating areas. They are concerned with directing our behaviour in accordance with the plans they formulate, and also ensuring that our behaviour is socially acceptable.

Brain damage

The skills and technology of modern medicine have changed our attitude to brain damage and disorders and brought new hope to patients. Although many parts of the brain are completely uncharted, specialists can still make a diagnosis. They know enough about the brain to work out what may be wrong – usually by a process of elimination. Then they perform tests, generally with electronic machinery such as the CT scan (which gives an X-ray picture of sections of the brain) to narrow down to a final diagnosis.

It is very important for those who have the misfortune to see friends or family suffer brain damage not to assume automatically that it is untreatable.

It is tempting to take this view, simply because brain damage *sounds* so serious. In the past, it usually was, and brain damage can cause major and worrying changes in the person concerned, such as UNCONSCIOUSNESS, PARALYSIS or loss of SPEECH.

In fact, it is amazing how much recovery is possible after, for example, a severe blow to the head in a car crash. The patient *may* seem deeply unconscious; he or she *may* spend days without showing a sign of life. But this can be the result simply of extensive but temporary paralysis of the neurones – the nerve cells – and, if so, large areas of the brain will eventually recover and work normally, just as before the blow.

In addition, the brain has what doctors call a large 'reserve of function', which means that it contains 'spare areas' which can take over the work which the damaged areas can no longer manage. Children, in particular, can make astonishing recoveries from brain damage because their brains are not so rigidly organized as those of adults, and their reserve areas can adapt more flexibly to what is required of them.

There is, however, a limit to what can be hoped for in terms of recovery, and the key factor in this is how much damage there has been to the brain-stem. Through this, all the brain's messages to the various regions of the body must pass. It also contains centres which keep up such vital processes as breathing and blood circulation, and without these, of course, life soon slips away.

When a patient with severe brain damage is first brought into hospital, these functions may well not be working anyway. It will be important to get them to do so artificially – by means of special machinery called life support systems – until the brain recovers enough to take over again. The introduction of these machines has meant the possibility of recovery where before there was no hope. But they also bring their problems.

In a few days, it may become clear that, however long support is given, recovery is impossible because so much nerve tissue has been lost following brain damage. The patient is then said to be in a persistent vegetative state.

Such situations will, of course, be hard to accept, but occasionally some people, and some doctors, have to face them. So the only realistic approach when someone is put on a life support machine is to remember that this does not mean there will be recovery, only the possibility of it.

Blows to the head

One of the most common HEAD INJURIES is caused by some sort of blow. The effect of a blow to the head is determined by the severity and the location, as well as the angle of the blow. The brain does not fit inside the skull tightly; when the head receives a blow, the brain is thrown against the inner surface of the skull and some of its cells are damaged.

Even slight blows can sometimes cause *concussion*, which is the medical name for the loss of consciousness caused by such an injury. Concussion itself is the mildest form of brain injury, and it may cause no real permanent damage. If the blow is severe, there may be headaches, giddiness and lowered concentration for some weeks after.

Sometimes the brain may actually be bruised as a result of a blow. In this case, there will be some permanent damage to the nerve cells and fibres, but how this affects the person depends on how much bruising there is.

A blow that is hard enough to FRACTURE or break the skull will usually also cause concussion. The fracture itself causes little trouble unless the broken part of the skull is pushed inwards, tearing the brain tissue and causing bleeding.

Penetrating injuries

An injury to the head from falling on to a sharp object like a pencil, or other item that actually penetrates the skull, exposes the surface of the brain to infection. In addition, the object itself may carry infection into the brain. The amount of damage that is done in any injury of this type depends on where the object enters.

Bullet wounds to the head carry these risks, and additional dangers as well. Their explosive entry into the skull sends shock waves through the brain which can disrupt quite distant nerve cells and also cause tearing of the blood vessels.

Brain damage at birth

If, during birth, the blood supply to a baby's brain is for some reason inadequate, some of its brain cells will die. If a lot of cells are damaged, a condition known as CEREBRAL PALSY results. Similar brain damage can occur after birth if an infant is starved of oxygen because of a lung disorder.

The term 'spastic' is used to describe the movements such children make. Their muscles tend to be stiff – especially those in the legs. The number of limbs affected and the severity of the condition varies from child to child. The level of intelligence also varies – some children with cerebral palsy may have learning difficulties, while others are of average or even above average intelligence.

Abnormal growths

Abnormal growths in the tissue of the brain are called brain tumours. The most common cause is CANCER somewhere else in the body, in which case the growth in the brain is known as a secondary tumour.

Like other tumours, brain tumours can be either malignant (cancerous) or benign (non-cancerous). Malignant tumours are those that grow quickly and tend to invade the surrounding tissues. Benign tumours do not invade, but they can create trouble as they grow, pushing against the rest of the brain. The pressure of a growing tumour causes such symptoms as persistent headaches, nausea and eventually drowsiness leading to *coma* (very deep unconsciousness) if not discovered in time.

Symptoms of brain disease

As well as the symptoms caused by the increasing pressure from a tumour, there are also other symptoms which indicate something is wrong. When a particular area of the brain becomes diseased, it will stop performing its own specific function properly.

A doctor will recognize these symptoms as a possible indication of some sort of disease in that area of the brain. A tumour is one possibility, but there are also other diseases that can cause a portion of the brain not to work properly (*see* DEMENTIA, EPILEPSY, MENINGITIS, MULTIPLE SCLEROSIS, PARKINSON'S DISEASE, STROKE).

The symptoms that appear as a result of a disease depend on the area of the brain that is affected. For example, symptoms of disease in the left side of the brain might include: halting or jumbled speech; difficulty in reading or writing; loss of feeling or vision or a general weakness on the right side; or a change in personality. These are all serious symptoms that need immediate investigation.

Symptoms of disease in the right side of the brain could include weakness, numbness or visual loss on the left side, or difficulty in dressing or even in finding one's way about.

Disease in the area of the thalamus, cerebellum, midbrain or brain-stem can be indicated by a dramatic change of mood or strange appetites, double vision, unsteadiness, severe giddiness, or a reduction in the ability to control breathing.

Of course, none of these symptoms is a definite indication of brain disease, and not necessarily a cause for alarm. The best thing to do is to see your doctor, who will discuss any worrying symptoms with you and arrange all the appropriate investigations.

Today's delicate brain surgery can be used to treat a range of conditions causing brain damage. Operations can now be successfully performed where previously they would never have been attempted.

Treatment of bleeding and blood clots

If you have a severe blow to the head, the blood vessels in the meninges – the membranes covering the brain and the spinal cord – or in the brain itself are torn and bleeding. This is called a *traumatic brain haemorrhage.* A blood clot may form on the membrane lining the brain, putting pressure on the brain itself. Surgery is often required to remove the clot.

Sometimes bleeding shows as a slow ooze and pressure gradually builds up. This is called *chronic subdural haematoma.* Here again surgery is called for. A general anaesthetic is always given and the patient is carefully monitored afterwards. The stay in hospital should be a matter of weeks.

More serious is a 'depressed fracture', where the broken part of the bone has pushed into the underlying brain and torn it. Surgery is needed.

A blood clot in the brain (thrombosis) occurs spontaneously. It builds up gradually and is often associated with high BLOOD PRESSURE. A clot can occur in any part of the brain. When it is sited in a suitable position, it may be possible to treat it by surgery; or its effects may be limited by anti-coagulant drugs.

Leaking may occur from a group of blood vessels near the base of the brain with bleeding into the subarachnoid space which will cause increasingly severe headache or blackout.

This condition – called a *subarachnoid haemorrhage* – is due to a weakness in the vessels present since birth. The haemorrhage may happen spontaneously or it may be triggered off by a rugby injury, for example. An operation is necessary to tie up these blood vessels.

Treatment of brain tumours

Tumours do not usually arise in the actual nerve cells but in the tissues which surround them – the neuroglia cells – or in the cells of the meninges. Sometimes tumours develop in the PITUITARY gland and press upwards into the brain.

Once a tumour has been detected, it is essential to find out whether it is malignant or benign in order to arrange treatment. An operation called a BIOPSY may be necessary to obtain a piece of the lump for examination under the microscope to determine the nature of the cells.

Depending on where the tumour is sited in the brain, surgery may be possible. Where it is difficult to get to, RADIOTHERAPY or steroid drugs may effect a cure instead.

Breasts and breast cancer

Most people think of the budding of the female breasts, which begins before the start of the menstrual PERIODS, as the first sign that a girl is on the road from childhood into womanhood. In fact, the breasts appear in rudimentary form in both boys and girls long before birth, and when only a few days old, a baby of either sex may produce a few drops of *colostrum* (a clear but nutritious fluid that used to be called 'witch milk') from the nipples as a result of the action of the mother's hormones.

Development

At the start of sexual development, and stimulated by the PITUITARY gland at the base of the brain, a girl's OVARIES begin to release large amounts of the HORMONE oestrogen. This hormone travels in the bloodstream and triggers the enlargement of the nipples, the growth of the milk ducts and the depositing of fat.

The completion of breast development, which takes about 18 months from the first appearance of small swellings on the chest, depends on another sex hormone, progesterone; this is produced monthly during the menstrual cycle. Under its influence, the ends of the ducts swell out into lobes, each composed of many smaller lobes (called lobules) containing glands that *lactate*; this means they can produce milk. Meanwhile the continued release of oestrogen by the ovaries results in more fat developing between the lobules.

The mature breast is roughly hemispherical in shape with a tail-like extension towards the armpit. The slightly upward-pointing nipple contains 15 to 20 minute openings from the ducts, too small to be seen with the naked eye. They are surrounded by a ring of rosy-coloured tissue, called the *areola*.

Apart from the tissues directly involved in the production and release of milk, each breast contains nerves and fibrous supporting tissue that gives it its firmness and shape. The nipple is particularly well supplied with nerves. These are important in breastfeeding because it is their stimulation that causes the nipple to become erect.

What happens in pregnancy

Whether the breasts are large or small, they increase in size when a woman is pregnant and may feel more tender than normal. During the course of PREGNANCY, the placenta makes enormous amounts of oestrogen which, together with other hormones from the placenta and secretions from the pituitary and other glands, causes the ducts to grow in size and form more branches. At the same time, the hormone progesterone, which is secreted by the placenta, stimulates the glandular tissue to enlarge. The sacs (*alveoli*) lined with true milk-producing cells produce the colostrum which flows into the ducts and out through the nipples even before birth.

Large amounts of fat are also deposited in the breasts during pregnancy so that the total breast weight increases by about 1 kg (2 lb). Through the effects of hormones, the areola round the nipple takes on a brownish hue.

Although they stimulate breast enlargement during pregnancy, the hormones oestrogen and progesterone, created by the placenta, are thought to suppress the secretion of milk until after the baby is born. But immediately following birth – and the loss of the placenta and its hormones – the hormone *prolactin*, which is secreted by the pituitary gland, has an unopposed action on the breast and stimulates the milk-producing cells. For the first two or three days, the cells, prior to releasing true milk, secrete colostrum – the thin, milky fluid that contains the protein, minerals and nutrients necessary for the baby.

Breast cancer

The idea of breast cancer is so frightening to some women that they do not even dare check for abnormalities, and may ignore a lump in their breast or any other unusual symptoms until it is too late, rather than face the doctor. But if breast cancer is diagnosed early, treatment will most likely be successful, so it is vital not to incur greater risks by unnecessary delay.

Breast cancer is the commonest form of cancer in women, affecting about one woman in 12, more usually over the age of 50 though, of course, it does occur in younger women. But although prompt action is essential, should a possible symptom occur, there is no need to be too anxious at this stage. Only about one in ten women consulting their doctor with worries about a lump in their breast turn out to have breast cancer, though many more will need to undergo tests to make absolutely sure.

Causes of breast cancer

It is not yet known what causes breast cancer so we are not able to take preventive action. That is why early detection is so important. What is known, however, is that a tendency to breast cancer does seem to run in families. So a woman whose mother has had breast cancer, for example, does have a slightly increased risk, particularly if another close relative has also developed it.

It is not yet clear whether taking the contraceptive pill, particularly the new lower-dose contraceptive pill, puts women at any greater risk of developing breast cancer. Research studies should make this clearer in the future. Nor is there, as yet, any clear evidence that women with a particular type of personality are more prone to breast cancer, or that breast cancer is a reaction to STRESS, although some research has suggested this. Finally, although there is also no conclusive proof for the theory that breast cancer is linked to a low-fibre, high-fat DIET, it does make sense for us all to switch to a diet with plenty of fresh food, less fat and more fibre, for our general health.

Symptoms

To detect any changes that might possibly be an early sign of breast cancer, all women should do a monthly examination of their breasts. It is only by becoming familiar with their normal shape and feel that anything unusual can be discovered and treated in its early stages.

The main signs you are looking for are a lump which does not change in size or consistency during the menstrual cycle, unusually tender areas, discharge from, or involution of, a nipple (one that is pointing inwards), puckering or dimpling of the breast, or a change in the size or shape of a breast and swelling of the upper arm or in the armpit. There are likely to be perfectly harmless reasons for the appearance of any of these symptoms but do check with your doctor immediately.

Apart from a natural lumpiness in the breast prior to menstruation, due to changes in hormone levels, the most commonly found breast lumps are cysts, due to milk sacs which become distended with fluid following a blockage in part of the duct system of the breast. The next most common lump is known as a *fibroadenoma.* This is simply a collection of fibrous glandular tissue which has become knotted together to form a solid lump. Both these conditions, though harmless, feel very similar to lumps due to cancer so special tests are usually required before an accurate diagnosis can be made.

In many women, nipples are retracted from puberty onwards and this is nothing to worry about. But if a nipple which has previously pointed outwards becomes retracted over the course of a few weeks or months or there is any discharge, see your doctor.

Investigation

The doctor may be able to give a reassuring diagnosis, but is more likely to refer you to a hospital specialist who can, if necessary, arrange for special tests. These may include:

Mammography: This is a method of taking breast X-RAYS which shows up very early abnormalities in the breast, often before they can be detected by manual examination.

Needle aspiration/needle biopsy: A needle is inserted into the lump and a few cells removed for laboratory inspection (*see* BIOPSY). If the lump proves to be a cyst, the fluid may be withdrawn then and there and the lump will disappear.

Surgical biopsy: The whole lump will be removed in a surgical operation under general anaesthetic. Some surgeons prefer to have the lump examined while the patient is still under the general anaesthetic and to operate immediately if it is found to be malignant (cancerous). While this may be very sensible in some cases, it is important that it is discussed carefully with the surgeon first so that it is quite clear what may happen. If patients need more time to think, they may give the surgeon permission only to do a biopsy at this stage. The operation can then be performed a few days later when they have had time to fully prepare themselves.

Treatment

There are now a variety of treatments for breast cancer, used on their own or in combination with others. These treatments are surgery, RADIOTHERAPY, hormone therapy and chemotherapy (treatment with cytotoxic or anti-cancer drugs). Treatment is selected on an individual basis depending on factors such as age, general health, the type and size of cancer and how far it has spread.

If breast cancer is diagnosed, it is important to talk things over very carefully with the doctor to understand why a particular treatment is being recommended, and what will be involved. If the patient is still worried, they should ask their doctor to refer them for a second opinion.

Surgery: A number of different operations are performed for breast cancer. A *lumpectomy* involves the removal of the affected lump and surrounding tissue. More surgeons are now performing lumpectomies where possible, as this is a simple operation and less upsetting than the removal of the whole breast, and, in many cases, appears to be just as effective. Where larger amounts of breast tissue are removed, the operation is known as a *segmentectomy*.

Sometimes surgeons will recommend the removal of the whole breast in an operation called a MASTECTOMY. They should explain in detail why the mastectomy is necessary, to help their patients come to terms with it. Very occasionally a radical mastectomy is performed. As well as the breast, some of the muscles of the chest wall, and possibly the LYMPH glands under the arm have to be removed to arrest the spread of cancer.

It is now often possible for women who have had a mastectomy to have their breast reconstructed either through surgery or by means of an implant. These possibilities should be explained at the beginning of your treatment.

On leaving hospital after a mastectomy, the patient is given a soft, temporary prosthesis to slip inside the bra so that the breasts match. Once the scar has healed she can select a more permanent prosthesis. She need not feel restricted in her style of dressing and can wear low-cut dresses and specially designed swimwear.

Radiotherapy: This is a treatment which uses specially directed high energy rays to kill cancer cells, while doing as little harm as possible to normal cells. It is often used as a back-up some weeks after surgery, though it may be a treatment on its own. Depending on the individual, a course of radiotherapy may last between three and six weeks, and sessions may be daily or several times a week. Radiotherapy itself is painless, but the patient may experience some side-effects such as nausea and tiredness, and will need as much support from family and friends as possible. The skin over the area treated by radiotherapy, may become red with dilated blood vessels.

Hormone therapy: Some cancers are very sensitive to hormone levels. Sometimes the ovaries are removed to reduce hormone levels in a younger woman when tumours have recurred or are likely to recur, though it is obviously distressing as it brings on an early menopause. However, treatment is often successful through hormone therapy, usually in the form of tablets or injections. *Tamoxifen,* one of the most common hormone treatments, helps reduce particular hormone levels, and has few side-effects. It is often given after surgery or radiotherapy as an extra precaution where there is thought to be a higher risk of the disease recurring.

Chemotherapy: This involves the use of drugs, given by mouth or injection,

How to examine your breasts

Every woman whatever her age should regularly examine her breasts for unusual lumps to help detect the early signs of cancer. It is important to do this at the same time during the menstrual cycle. The best time is the week after your period as the breasts are naturally lumpy before menstruation. Examination is equally important after the menopause.

(1) With arms by your sides study your naked breasts in the mirror for any changes in size or position, any puckering, and discharge or involution of the nipples. Do the same with arms raised above your head.

(2) Put your hands on your hips and push firmly forward with your elbows so that the muscles which support your breasts are tightened and lifted. Now look carefully for the same changes, such as swellings, or skin puckering.

(3) Lie down and put a pillow under your left shoulder. Put your left hand behind your head and with fingers straight out and close together, examine your right breast for lumps or tenderness.

(4) Starting with the upper outside of the breast, press gently with flattened fingers, rotating in small circles round the whole breast. Lumps often occur between nipple and armpit.

(5) Then use gentle pressure only to carefully probe the tissues under the nipple and the nipple itself. Never squeeze the nipple when checking for any changes in size or shape.

(6) To complete the examination, feel for lumps in and around the armpit and along the top of the collarbone. Repeat the individual breast examination on the left breast.

(7) Large breasts can be examined with both hands – one underneath to support the breast, and the other to examine the upper surface. Then support the breast with the upper hand to examine the under surface.

to destroy cancer cells. Each treatment usually lasts a few days. There is then a gap of several weeks to enable the body to recover from the side-effects. As the drugs temporarily decrease the number of normal white blood cells in the body, the patient is more likely to contract an infection. They are also likely to tire more easily. Other possible side-effects include nausea, vomiting and diarrhoea and possibly hair loss, but these disappear once treatment finishes. Hair will grow quickly again.

The fact that breast cancer is so common, that we do not know what causes it and that it can be successfully treated in its early stages means that women have to take responsibility for checking their breasts for abnormalities. This means asking your GP or family planning clinic for check-ups and doing regular and relatively effortless self-examination.

Breathing

Awake or asleep we breathe an average of 12 times a minute, and in 24 hours we breathe in and breathe out more than 8,000 litres (282 cu. ft) of air. During heavy physical exercise, the breathing rate will increase considerably: up to 80 times a minute.

The purpose of moving so much air in and out of the body is to enable the LUNGS to do two things: to extract the OXYGEN needed to sustain life and to rid the body of carbon dioxide – that is, the waste product of internal chemical processes.

Development of the respiratory system

The respiratory system begins to develop early on in the growth of the foetus in the womb, the branching pattern of the airways and arteries being complete by the 16th week after conception. At 28 weeks, cells which secrete surfactant, a fluid, start to develop in the lungs, preventing them from sticking together. The vital gas-exchanging parts of the lungs, where oxygen is absorbed into the bloodstream and waste carbon dioxide removed, then remain filled with fluid until the baby is born.

This fluid can be a problem in premature babies who are often not strong enough to breathe deeply, which would inflate the lungs, allowing the fluid to disperse. Artificial surfactant can now be given to help the breathing of premature babies.

In full-term babies, all the parts of the respiratory system are fully developed. However, it is not until the age of eight that the gas-exchanging part of the lung in children, whether premature or full-term, is fully formed.

Inhaling

Inhaled and exhaled air goes through the NOSE and mouth. As air enters the nose, dust particles and other foreign bodies are trapped by coarse hairs. The air continues its passage into the nasal cavity where the moist membrane that lines the walls warms the air and produces mucus to collect even more

How the body breathes

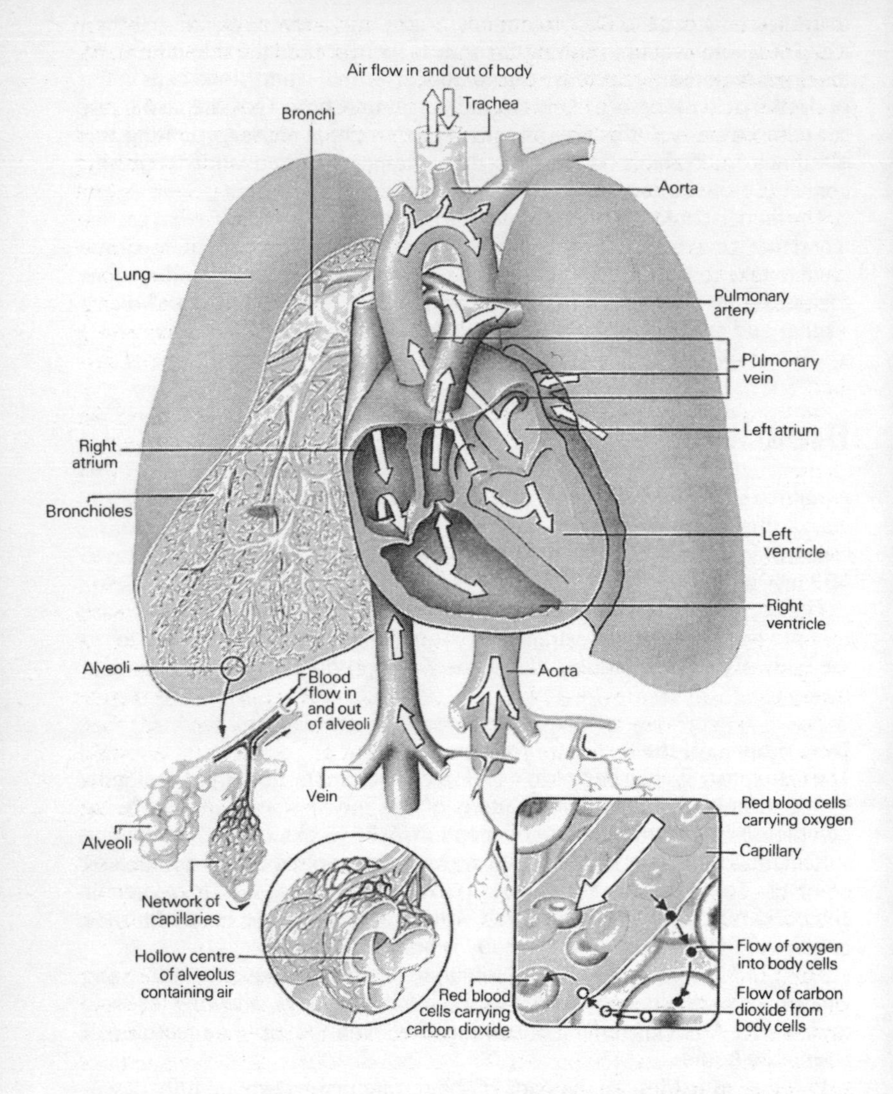

Air inhaled via the trachea, bronchi and bronchioles reaches the alveoli where oxygen from the air is transferred to the capillaries surrounding each alveolus. The oxygenated blood is carried to the pulmonary vein and into the left side of the heart and pushed into the aorta. Blood then proceeds around the body, through arteries to the capillaries. The oxygen carried by the red blood cells is given to the tissue cells which transfer their waste product, carbon dioxide, to the red cells. This is carried back through the veins into the right side of the heart and finally the blood flows out through the pulmonary artery and into the lungs. At the site of the alveoli, the circulating blood gives up its carbon dioxide, and takes in oxygen.

particles of dirt. Hairlike projections on the membrane, called *cilia*, are continually in motion, pushing the film of mucus and its trapped contents back towards the throat to be swallowed.

At the back of the nasal cavity and above the mouth lie two bodies of lymph glands, the TONSILS and the ADENOIDS. Because their role is to pick up and destroy invading bacteria, they often become infected and swollen, causing tonsillitis. A sustained build-up of invading bacteria also creates the swelling and irritation of the throat that causes colds and flu.

From the THROAT, the filtered, moistened and warmed air passes into the windpipe (*trachea*) where, as in the nasal cavity, cilia waft the mucous layer and its contents towards the throat for disposal by swallowing. Once past the trachea, the inhaled air has received all the screening it will receive before passing into the lungs where oxygen from it is absorbed.

At its lower end, the windpipe divides into two smaller tubes called the *bronchi*, one leading to each lung. It is here that infections such as those that cause BRONCHITIS and PNEUMONIA can build up and cause severe breathing problems.

In the lungs

Within the lungs, each bronchus divides into smaller tubes, the *bronchioles*; these, in turn, branch and form millions of tiny air sacs, the *alveoli* – each surrounded by a meshwork of fine capillaries – where the exchange of oxygen and carbon dioxide takes place. The branches of the pulmonary artery carry carbon dioxide-rich blood, and this gas is given up in return for the oxygen in the new air which has entered the alveolar sacs. The lungs then exhale the carbon dioxide in the de-oxygenated air, along with a certain amount of water vapour, which comes from the moist membranes of the alveoli. On cold days, this water vapour condenses and becomes steaming breath.

The lungs fill most of the chest cavity and are inflated and deflated by muscular movements of the chest, and the rise and fall of a sheet of muscle, the DIAPHRAGM, that lies under the ribs and divides the chest cavity from the abdomen.

Each lung is surrounded by a double membrane, the *pleura*. The outer pleura is attached to the chest walls and the diaphragm; the inner pleura attaches itself to each lung. Between the two membranes is a cavity: a thin film of fluid on its surface protects the delicate tissues as they move against each other as the lungs inflate and deflate.

Exhaling

When breathing is normal, the diaphragm does most of the work. The muscle contracts and the volume of the chest cavity increases. The ribs are pulled upwards and outwards by muscles, called *intercostals*, that lie between them, and as the pressure within the lungs drops, air is sucked in. Breathing out is a passive process: the diaphragm and the intercostal muscles relax and the natural elasticity of the lung tissue forces air out.

Breathing rates

Breathing is controlled by the respiratory centre of the BRAIN, the *medulla oblongata,* and is regulated according to the levels of carbon dioxide in the blood, rather than the amount of oxygen present. The brain will respond to an increased production of carbon dioxide, such as when the body undergoes physical exercise, and adjust the breathing rate accordingly. Breathing will become deeper and faster so that more oxygen is inhaled, stimulating the heartbeat; blood flow will increase and the carbon dioxide will be burned off. Once the exercise ceases, the carbon dioxide level falls and breathing will return to normal.

Voluntary alterations in breathing rates occur during talking, singing and eating. Yawning, sighing, COUGHING and hiccupping involve still other kinds of respiration. Laughing and crying, both long breaths followed by short bursts of exhalation, are respiratory changes due to emotional stimuli.

Holding your breath, either deliberately (when swimming under water), or unwittingly (as a result of an attack of nerves) also alters the breathing pattern. The carbon dioxide level falls after the first few deep breaths, which are then held, and the brain ceases to be stimulated. This can lead to a blackout and, when swimming underwater, death by drowning if the person cannot return to the surface. On the other hand, high-altitude sickness may occur when the unacclimatized person climbs to high altitudes. The body tissues may become unoxygenated, and the person feels giddy, nauseous, and as he or she goes higher, there will be a feeling of sublime indifference (euphoria), a loss of muscular coordination and, eventually, UNCONSCIOUSNESS if the person does not either receive oxygen or make a rapid descent at the onset of these symptoms.

Breech birth

Babies are usually born head first. When one arrives feet, knees or bottom first, this is known as a 'breech birth'. Approximately 3 to 4 per cent of babies enter the world bottom first; knee and foot presentation are rarer still. As a result of modern screening tests during PREGNANCY, women today usually know in advance whether a breech birth is expected, so any risks can be minimized.

Causes

There are certain circumstances in which a breech birth is more likely to occur. For example, when a MULTIPLE BIRTH is expected, it is more than likely that at least one of the babies will be 'breech'; twins will often present themselves as one head first (*cephalic*) and the other 'breech'.

A breech birth can also be the result of an abnormality in the pregnancy, but this is usually picked up early. Such a problem is the retention of excessive fluid around the baby, a condition known as *hydramnios.* This fluid – called *liquor* – permits ease of movement, but the more there is around the baby, the greater the likelihood of a breech birth.

It is normal for a woman to notice changes in the position of her baby from mid-pregnancy onwards. At this stage, there is more fluid in relation to the size of the baby; therefore, many premature babies are born 'breech'. But at about 36 weeks, the presenting part of the foetus normally sinks into the pelvis, a position known as 'engagement'; once this occurs there is no further movement. At this stage, doctors can tell the position the baby will be in at birth.

Symptoms

Many women who have a breech birth are able to feel their baby's head pressing under their lower ribs towards the end of their pregnancy. This can be very uncomfortable, particularly when sitting down. Once the bottom slips into the pelvis, however, this discomfort will ease. However, engagement does not always occur at 36 weeks, especially if the mother has had one child already.

On the whole, a pregnancy that results in a breech birth will progress like any other. But when the bottom engages into the pelvis, the doctor and midwife will take special precautions to ensure the safe delivery of a breech baby. They will check the dates to make sure the baby does not have any extra time for growth beyond the calculated date of delivery; this avoids the head being too large to pass easily through the pelvis.

On the whole, because breech births are now so much safer, many obstetricians prefer not to take the risk of turning a breech baby around. In rare cases, the waters can break, inducing a premature birth; the umbilical cord can also be pulled accidentally, and any decrease in the supply of oxygen could have serious consequences.

Special tests

Most pregnant women these days are examined under an ULTRASOUND scanner as part of their normal antenatal care. This machine measures the size of the baby, and can prove particularly useful in estimating the size of a breech baby's head to ensure a safe and easy journey through the pelvis. For this reason, the pelvis is usually measured too.

Labour

Labour will vary when a baby is breech, and the length depends on how efficiently the presenting part – the bottom, knee or feet – can press on the CERVIX (neck of the womb) to open it up. If there is no progress at all – as can easily happen in either of the last two cases – a CAESAREAN section may have to be performed.

A great deal of skill is required in dealing with a breech birth. The correct time of the birth must be gauged and the baby carefully guided into the world, the obstetrician usually delivering the head with forceps to prevent accidental injury.

When the cervix is finally fully dilated, the doctor will be able to see the presenting part of the baby's body: the bottom, an arm or leg. To allow easy passage for the baby and control of the delivery of the head, a small cut, called an *episiotomy*, is made in the perineum, the area between the vagina entrance and the anus.

As the buttocks descend, the legs will ease out gently. If they are extended, the knees can be gently eased and flexed.

The cord is checked to ensure it is not compressed at this stage and watched carefully for the rest of the labour.

The weight of the baby's body will draw down the shoulders which will naturally rotate. With luck, it may well not be necessary to touch the baby. Then, as the woman pushes, the shoulders and head should follow.

If a breech birth goes well, the body of the baby will emerge in its own time – slowly and safely. The one danger is at the end, when the head might be born too fast. The woman may give an unexpected push and the head suffers too sudden a pressure, causing possible damage and internal bleeding. The medical staff will watch carefully, and if there is any danger, forceps will be used to hold back the head.

After the birth, the baby will be checked thoroughly by the paediatrician who is always on hand during a breech birth. As there is a slight risk of internal bleeding in the baby if its head is delivered too fast, it may be given an injection of VITAMIN K to help the blood to clot.

Brittle bones, *see* Bones and bone diseases

Bronchiectasis *see* Lungs and lung diseases, Phlegm, Pneumonia

Bronchitis

Bronchitis is an inflammation of the main bronchial tubes of the LUNGS – the bronchi – caused by a bacterial or viral infection. It may develop suddenly, following a head COLD (acute bronchitis), or it may persist or return regularly for many years, causing progressive degeneration of the bronchi and lungs (chronic bronchitis).

Certain people are more susceptible than others; men are more so than women, outnumbering them ten to one – the reasons why are unclear. Smokers are 50 times more likely to get chronic bronchitis than non-smokers.

Causes

Generally, bronchitis occurs with greater frequency in winter, in damp, cold climates, and in heavily polluted environments. Chilling, overcrowding, fatigue and excessive SMOKING are contributory factors.

Most cases of acute bronchitis arise from a viral infection, which spreads to the chest. Chronic bronchitis causes irritation and COUGHING, which leads to the lining of the bronchi being damaged and narrowed by scarring. The lungs lose their elasticity, and the exchange of vital oxygen, which is breathed in, and waste carbon dioxide, which is breathed out, is impaired (*see* BREATHING). The bronchial tubes become permanently inflamed, and this results in an increased production of mucus from specialized cells in the walls of the bronchi, called *goblet cells.* The mucus coughed up is called *sputum* (PHLEGM).

Because it is difficult to look at the bronchi directly, doctors rely on the chief symptom, sputum production, to make a diagnosis. The colour of the sputum shows how serious the bronchitis is.

Symptoms

In acute bronchitis, the initial symptoms are often a head cold, running nose, fever and chills, aching muscles and possibly back pain. This is soon followed by the most obvious feature: a persistent cough. At first, it is dry and racking, but later it becomes phlegmy. It is worse at night, and when the person breathes in smoke and fumes.

Chronic bronchitis is defined as a cough productive of sputum on most days of the week, for three months of the year, for more than two years. Its main characteristic – a cough with sputum – often occurs in paroxysms. Other symptoms depend on how much, or how little, EMPHYSEMA is present. This means that the tiny air sacs in the lungs become inflated, and so the lungs become overstretched, making breathing out more difficult.

The chronic bronchitic with no emphysema tends to be overweight and have a bluish tinge to his lips due to *cyanosis* (a bluish colour in the blood caused by lack of oxygen). Shortness of breath only occurs during exercise. The bronchitic with a great deal of emphysema, who has lost a lot of his or her oxygen-exchanging ability due to the condition, is short of breath at all times. Bronchitics with emphysema tend to be underweight and, as the disease worsens, develop a barrel chest. The chronic bronchitic also wheezes because of the obstruction.

Treatment

The best treatment for acute bronchitis is bedrest in a warm room. Aspirin or paracetamol will reduce the fever, and cough medicines will relieve the cough. ANTIBIOTICS are usually needed to eliminate bacterial infection.

Treatment of chronic bronchitis is more difficult. The patient's lungs are already damaged, and the obstruction of the airways is not easily reversible.

Bronchodilator drugs may be given to relieve any such obstruction, while PHYSIOTHERAPY will help the patient get rid of any sputum. Postural drainage can also be tried: the patient lies on a bed, a large cushion raising the groin, and smaller pillows supporting the chest. Tapping the chest in this position causes the patient to cough up sputum. Yoga, and breathing exercises generally, may assist shortness of breath. In severe cases, urgent hospital treatment may be required. Oxygen might have to be given through the course of the illness. For severe cases oxygen may be required for 16 hours a day at home from an oxygen concentrator or cylinders.

However, the best form of relief is to try to remove as many bronchial irritants as possible. The patient should stop smoking immediately – although chronic bronchitis cannot be reversed, it can be arrested. Chronic bronchitics should try to avoid environments where there are irritants as these can bring on attacks.

Prompt treatment of chest infections is important. Sufferers should have a flu jab each winter.

Outlook

With acute bronchitis, the fever may last as long as five days, and the coughing for weeks afterwards, but if the patient receives treatment and takes sensible precautions, the illness will simply run its course and outlook is good.

Chronic bronchitis is far more serious. It is a degenerative disease, particularly when combined with emphysema, and can result in death due to respiratory failure when there is insufficient oxygen in the blood. One of the most important complications due to this problem is *carbon-dioxide narcosis* (stupor), together with increasing breathlessness, ankle swelling, and even HEART failure.

Brucellosis, *see* Occupational hazards

Bruising, *see* Purpura

Buerger's disease, *see* Ischaemia

Bulimia, *see* Anorexia and bulimia

Bunions

A bunion is an abnormal enlargement at the joint between the foot (*see* FEET) and the beginning of the big toe, which arises as a result of pressure.

Any JOINT is surrounded by a special capsule of fibrous tissue and there may also be a bag of fluid, called a *bursa*, which cushions the movements of the various parts of the joint. When the big toe joint gets swollen and inflamed, more fluid collects there and the end of the bones may actually enlarge. Instead of the joint lying in a straight line, it is forced outwards at a sharp angle. This puts pressure on the tissues between the bones and the shoe – the result is the formation of a bunion.

The overlying skin may also become thickened and inflamed, and matters can be made worse by the fact that all this happens just where most shoes rub.

How bunions develop

This distortion of the big toe joint is caused by wearing shoes which are too tight for your toes. Women's shoes have traditionally been made narrower at the front than men's (although the anatomy of male and female feet is exactly the same), so consequently women have always tended to develop bunions more frequently than men.

The trouble is increased by women's shoes having higher heels. These force the foot deep into the tight front of the shoe and put maximum pressure on the side of the big toe. If this sideways pressure continues, day after day, the big toe joint is pushed out of place and becomes deformed, leading to a condition that is called *hallux valgus*.

When this arises, the big toe points across to the other toes, while the foot bone under the skin leading to the big toe points outwards. Once this state of affairs is established, any further pressure from shoes will particularly fall on the big toe joint and cause a bunion to form there. At the other side of the foot, a similar deformity can arise, forming a smaller bunion at the little toe joint.

Some people are born with a tendency to *hallux valgus* and therefore are more likely to develop bunions. This may be because they have feet that are unusually broad in front, so that 'off the rack' shoes never fit properly. More rarely, the foot bone leading to the big toe may have started life abnormally and already be pointing outwards.

Whatever the cause, once it is started, this deformity will tend to progress and not right itself, even if no shoes at all are worn. This is because the TENDONS running to the toe bones become displaced. Instead of lying directly over the joint, they pull across to the inside. Then, every time the muscles contract to flex or extend the big toe – which happens at every stride when you are walking – the pull of the tendons makes the condition a lot worse.

Prevention and treatment

Shoes with very high heels and pointed toes that are worn regularly are bound to lead to problems, even in those fortunate enough to have narrow feet. Anyone who feels pain or notices redness of the skin on the outside of the big toe, when taking off their shoes, should discard them immediately.

To see just how much room your feet take up, stand barefoot on a piece of paper and draw around your feet with a pencil. Compare the outline with the space allowed by your shoes, and check particularly to see that there is enough space in your shoes for your toes to spread naturally.

Due to the 'bowstring' effect which is suffered by the tendons, treatment tends to be unsatisfactory. Wide-fronted shoes are a first essential. A special pad may be worn between the big and index toes, to try and correct the alignment of the big toe and reduce pressure on the bunion. In the end, many women feel they have no alternative but to ask for an operation – but, it is wise to remember that, basically, prevention is better than cure.

Complications

By itself, a bunion is not a serious condition. Occasionally, however, it can become infected, and this needs immediate treatment. The trouble may be caused by attempting to pare down the thickened skin as if it were a corn – this should never be done. Nor should you open any blister which may form over a bunion. Once the skin is broken, infection is easily introduced and quickly spreads to the fluid of the bunion and then to the big toe joint. The joint will become even more swollen, red and painful and eventually pus may be discharged from it.

Treatment with ANTIBIOTICS is then urgent to prevent any further spread of the infection and avoid septic destruction of the joint. If the sufferer's health in general is also in a run-down condition, the infection may take a long time to clear up completely.

As a long-term result of *hallux valgus,* the abnormal alignment of the big toe joint causes excessive wear and tear – and consequently ARTHRITIS. If the pain of the bunion has made you walk in an abnormal way to compensate for the pain, it is possible that arthritis in other joints could also develop; this is a further complication which could have been avoided.

Surgery

Surgeons are reluctant to operate on bunions just for cosmetic reasons. And merely cutting out the bunion is never sufficient, as the trouble will only recur. To correct the deformity, a full operation must be performed, which actually removes the offending joint by cutting away the bone. Eventually, this is replaced by strong bands of fibrous tissue which grow in its place – this will allow some degree of movement but it will never be able to function like a joint.

After the operation, it takes some time before the patient can walk without pain. For about three months, any type of shoe will hurt, and most people do not feel they have had any benefit from the operation until a period of about six months has elapsed.

Bursitis

More commonly known as 'housemaid's knee', this condition tends to afflict people in specific trades or activities. A *bursa* is a fluid-filled pouch formed in soft tissue, usually overlying a BONE OF JOINT. Bursitis is the inflammation of one of these sacs, and is a common and occasionally painful condition requiring prompt treatment to prevent the inflammation becoming acute or chronic.

There are two types of bursa. The most common type, known as *anatomical bursae,* occur on specific sites where TENDONS cross BONES OF JOINTS. There are 15 such bursae around the KNEE joint alone. These usually pass unnoticed until they enlarge, and bursitis develops.

The second kind of bursa is one which arises purely as a result of repeated friction or injury to soft tissue overlying a bony surface. These are known as *adventitious bursae,* and may develop, for example, over the pelvic bone in the buttock from sitting on too hard a seat for several hours a day.

Both types of bursa act as shock absorbers and pressure pads, reducing the friction where tendons or ligaments move over bones. Only when the bursa becomes chronically enlarged or acutely inflamed will bursitis develop. Housemaid's knee, anatomically known as *prepatellar bursitis,* is caused by repeated pressure to the knee; any friction or injury causes the bursa to secrete fluid, resulting in the swelling.

A type of bursitis that appears in children is called *semimembranosus bursitis,* and involves swelling behind the knee. The cause is unknown. Usually the condition disappears without treatment in a couple of weeks; during that time, strenuous or prolonged exercise involving the knee is best avoided.

Causes

Not all the causes of bursitis are always clear. Although it can affect both children and adults, some people are more prone to it than others.

Where friction causes the development of the bursa, the condition may be due to the way certain occupations or activities are carried out. *Bursitis of the elbow,* for instance, is common among students leaning on desks, and miners crawling along tunnels. Porters sometimes develop *bursitis at the neck* from the pressure caused by humping heavy boxes or baskets, as do hod carriers from balancing loads of bricks. Weavers, who sit for long periods on hard loom seats, can develop *bursitis on the buttock;* gardeners who work from a kneeling position are often likely to develop *bursitis on the knees.* However, the rubbing effect is not the complete explanation as some people develop bursitis much more quickly than others.

In rarer cases, bursitis can be caused by bacterial inflammation in the bursa or in a connecting joint. TUBERCULOSIS was a common cause in the past. In some cases of RHEUMATOID ARTHRITIS, the bursa around a joint becomes inflamed; in rare cases, GOUT may develop in a bursa.

In bursitis of the elbow, which commonly occurs in older men, there rarely appears an identifiable cause at all and yet within a matter of hours a swelling the size of a hen's egg can appear.

The heel – or, more precisely, the Achilles tendon of the ankle – is also rather prone to become inflamed with bursitis. This is called *achillobursitis.*

Symptoms

In acute bursitis a swelling appears over a joint or bone. The swollen area is painful, tender to touch, and may feel hot and appear red; in severe cases, movement is very painful. The fluid in acute bursitis is produced by the cells that line the wall of the sac. They produce straw-coloured fluid which is often tinged with blood as inflammation causes the minute blood vessels to leak. Where there is bacterial infection, this fluid becomes filled with bacteria and white blood cells to form pus which may occasionally discharge.

Chronic bursitis is caused by repeated attacks of acute bursitis or repeated injury causing swelling of a bursa. Slightly painful or even painless swelling may follow exercise or injury.

Treatment

The treatment for acute bursitis should be supervised by a doctor in case the cause is bacterial infection, or another rarer cause.

If the cause is unknown, or if it is due to rubbing or friction or excess use, resting the affected joint or area, and only passively exercising the surrounding muscles is the cure. If there is pain, PAINKILLERS may be necessary. Anti-inflammatory drugs, such as those which are used in arthritis, may reduce the amount of fluid secreted by the cells lining the bursa. Antibiotics will only be necessary if there is a bacterial infection. A cold compress, or ice pack, may help reduce the inflammation. Cool a polythene bag full of glycerine or crushed ice in the fridge. Mould the cold bag to the skin, checking it is not so cold as to burn the affected area. Then bandage lightly, with an elastic bandage, keeping this on for half an hour before removing. If this provides relief, repeat the treatment as often as possible, up to every four hours until the condition improves.

If it does not improve within two or three days, the doctor may drain or aspirate the bursa using a hypodermic needle; this usually gives the patient some relief. First, a little local anaesthetic is applied and then the needle is inserted deep into the bursa and some of the fluid is then sent to a hospital laboratory to check for bacteria.

The doctor might also inject hydrocortisone, a steroid drug which has an anti-inflammatory effect, into the bursa. This drug helps to prevent the accumulation of more fluid in the bursa. Once drained, the bursa is bandaged firmly. This treatment may have to be repeated a number of times.

When a chronic bursa is removed surgically, one of the interesting characteristic findings is the presence of the clumps of clotted protein, known to doctors as 'melon seeds' because of their size and colour. These have no significance. The surgeon clears these out and cuts away as much of the fluid-forming sac as is possible. This surgical removal of the bursa is usually successful, although in a small minority of cases, the bursa will form again in a few weeks.

Outlook

Pain and difficulty on movement is to be expected in acute bursitis and with treatment this condition usually clears completely within a week or 10 days. If the cause is bacterial inflammation, the likelihood of recurrence is very rare indeed.

With chronic bursitis, the condition usually only recurs if the stimulus of rubbing or friction is repeated. For this reason, taking preventive measures is very important.

Bypass surgery, *see* Coronary heart disease

C

C, vitamin, *see* Vitamins

Caesarean birth

A Caesarean birth (often called a Caesarean section) means that the baby is born through a surgical incision made in the mother's abdominal wall and UTERUS (womb). It is performed either as an emergency when the life and health of the mother or baby are at stake, or it is planned in advance because the doctors know that natural birth is impossible or unsafe in the particular circumstances.

A planned Caesarean

A Caesarean operation may be planned in advance by the obstetrician because of problems which could make a normal delivery difficult if not impossible. The bones of the pelvis may be small, or the baby large or in a difficult position – for example, lying across the abdomen rather than vertically (*see also* BREECH BIRTH). The mother may have medical problems which could cause problems in labour – or she may have had previous Caesarean operations. Sometimes a Caesarean is planned because the placenta is very low in the uterus (*placenta praevia*) and may obstruct the labour or cause bleeding during a normal delivery.

Most women who are having a Caesarean section come in to hospital at 38 weeks of pregnancy or before. Tests will make sure the baby is mature enough to be delivered without being harmed.

The night before the operation a routine examination and pubic shave will be carried out, and the mother will be given an enema to clear her back passage. Blood samples will be taken in advance for grouping and cross-matching in case a blood transfusion should be needed (*see* BLOOD GROUPS AND TRANSFUSIONS).

If a general ANAESTHETIC is to be used, the mother will be given nothing to eat or drink from midnight the night before the operation. However, some hospitals do a Caesarean section under epidural anaesthesia (an anaesthetic inserted into the epidural space just in front of the spinal cord, which numbs the area below). With an epidural, the mother can hold her baby immediately after birth and her partner may be allowed to watch the birth – so if you know you are to have a Caesarean section, it is worth asking about an epidural if you want to be aware of what is happening.

An emergency Caesarean

Although this sounds like a life or death situation, it very rarely is. An emergency Caesarean section may be necessary because of sudden bleeding from the placenta at any time before labour actually starts. During labour, the baby may not be getting enough oxygen from the placenta, or labour may just be too slow for safety. In either case, an emergency Caesarean may then be required.

Preparations for the operation will be performed quickly. An intravenous infusion (drip) will be set up. Fluids are essential for the prevention of SHOCK and extra blood through a blood transfusion may be required. The abdomen and pubic area are quickly prepared by shaving prior to the anaesthetic.

With a general anaesthetic, the mother will now be unconscious. A rubber tube (catheter) is placed in your bladder to empty it before the operation. The midwife checks the foetal heart on the monitor at regular intervals before surgery. The father may not be permitted in the operating theatre in an emergency in case it upsets him, but he is usually allowed to wait close by.

The operation

Most obstetricians – doctors who specialize in birth – make the incision in the lower part of the abdomen on the 'bikini line' where a scar will not show.

After the incision is made, forceps are inserted to hold back the layers of tissue. The lower segment of the womb (UTERUS) is exposed and the internal incision is widened. The doctor puts his or her right hand into the womb to lift out the baby's head. The assistant presses the top of the womb to push the baby out. Forceps may be used to deliver the head. The afterbirth (placenta) is delivered and a drug (ergometrine) is given to the mother to contract the womb. The abdomen is then sewn up.

The baby, meanwhile, is given immediately to the paediatrician (baby doctor) who is always present to check the delivery. The suddenness of the birth can cause babies some shock and it can take a few minutes for them to respond normally. For example, it may take a little time for their breathing to become regular and for their heart rate to steady. This is normal, and nothing to worry about. Sometimes babies can be a little floppy because of the anaesthetic given to their mothers and may need drugs to counteract this.

Most babies are put into incubators to warm up and to be observed while the mother comes round from her anaesthetic. If all is well, mother and baby can go back to the ward and both parents may hold and cuddle the baby. This is an important moment between parents and baby.

Mother and child will usually be able to go home after about one week or so after the birth.

Calcium

Ninety-nine per cent of body calcium is in the SKELETON and TEETH. Calcium crystals form solid building blocks which are held together by a fibrous network: the result is a strong, resilient material for supporting your body – the bones. However, calcium is not permanently sited in the bones for it can be mobilized to help maintain the correct levels in the body tissues elsewhere.

Small amounts of calcium also regulate the impulses from the nerves in the BRAIN. Similarly, they influence MUSCLE contraction. BLOOD clotting also relies on a set amount of calcium in the blood.

Calcium balance

We absorb calcium from our food – foods rich in this MINERAL include milk, cheese, eggs, meat and most dark green vegetables. Calcium then passes, via the INTESTINE, into the bloodstream. Some is lost in the URINE, but some is stored in the bones or reabsorbed into the bloodstream.

To maintain a balanced level of calcium in our blood, our bodies have an elaborate control system involving several substances, the most important of which are parathyroid hormone (PTH) and VITAMIN D. PTH is secreted by the PARATHYROID glands situated in the neck, and acts on the bones and kidneys to release more calcium, and also to decrease loss in the urine.

When our calcium levels are low, more PTH is passed into the bloodstream. When our levels are high, less PTH is put out, and so a constant balance is maintained.

VITAMIN D is also essential for maintaining our calcium balance. Without it, we cannot absorb calcium from our food. It also acts with PTH to release calcium from our bones.

Excessive calcium

If we have too much calcium in our bodies, symptoms develop such as vomiting and stomach pains. More seriously, excess calcium may be deposited in the KIDNEYS and form renal stones. (Renal stones are usually excreted naturally without an operation.)

The causes of too much calcium could be a parathyroid TUMOUR secreting uncontrolled amounts of PTH. Or it could simply mean that the sufferer had taken too many vitamin D pills. In addition, in the later stages of cancer, too much calcium may be found in the bloodstream.

To reduce calcium levels, an increase in fluid intake is essential. In an emergency, they can be reduced by an injection of one of a group of drugs known as the *biphosphonates*. A parathyroid tumour will usually require surgery. If the cause is too many vitamin pills, the person must stop taking them.

A lack of calcium

If there is too little calcium, a condition known as *tetany* occurs. The term describes cramp-like spasms of the muscles, especially of the hands and feet. Later, the LARYNX may be affected, producing *stridor* (a harsh, high-pitched noise). A common cause of tetany is hysterical over-breathing (*hyperventilation*) triggered off by fear or emotion, which results in a chemical change which temporarily reduces the available blood calcium. As the hysteria passes away naturally, the body returns to normal.

If the parathyroid glands have to be removed – to treat a parathyroid tumour for example – PTH levels can suddenly drop and cause tetany. This can be successfully treated by giving calcium through a vein and oral vitamin D. Kidney failure is the commonest cause of a low calcium level. Sufferers are prescribed a drug to take regularly, which acts like vitamin D and increases the calcium levels.

As well as tetany, a low calcium level can produce abnormal blood clotting and unbalanced heart rhythms. In fact, the muscle spasms always reveal themselves first and treatment prevents the other problems developing. *See also* CATARACTS.

If low levels of calcium are left untreated for months, the body may mobilize calcium from the bones to compensate, leaving them weak and without adequate minerals. This condition is called *osteomalacia* in adults and RICKETS in children. It is usually caused by a lack of vitamin D, either due to a poor diet or a disease affecting the gut where the vitamin D is poorly absorbed. Treatment is with a drug such as vitamin D. (This condition should not be confused with OSTEOPOROSIS, in which there is thinning of the bone substance itself, leading to reduced strength and an increased risk of fracture.)

Calluses, *see* **Corns and calluses**

Campylobacter, *see* **Diarrhoea**

Cancer

Cancer is the result of disordered and disorganized CELL growth. This can only be fully understood by looking at what happens in normal cells.

The human body is made up of many different tissues – skin, lung, liver, etc. – each of which is made up of millions of cells. These are all arranged in an orderly manner, each individual tissue having its own particular cellular structure. In addition, the appearance and shape of the cells of one organ differ from those of another. For example, a liver cell and a skin cell look completely different.

In all tissues, cells are constantly being lost through general wear and tear, and these are replaced by a process of cell division. Occurring under strict control in normal tissues, so that exactly the right number of cells are produced to replace those that are lost, a cell will divide in half to create two new cells, each identical to the original. If the body is injured, the rate of cell production speeds up automatically until the injury is healed, and then slows down again.

The cells of a cancer, however, divide and grow at their own speed and in an uncontrolled manner – and they will continue to do so indefinitely unless treatment is given. In time, they increase in numbers until enough are present for the cancer to become visible as a GROWTH or TUMOUR.

In addition to growing too rapidly, cancer cells are unable to organize themselves properly, so that the mass of tissue that forms does not resemble normal tissue. A cancer obtains its nourishment parasitically from its bearer, and will serve no useful purpose for that person whatsoever.

Cancers are classified according to the cell from which they originated. Those that arise from cells in the surface membranes of the body, like the skin and the gut, are called *carcinomas*; those arising from structures deep inside the body, such as bone cartilage and muscle, are called SARCOMAS.

Carcinomas are much more common than sarcomas. This may be because the cells of the surface membranes need to divide more often in order to keep these membranes intact.

Not all tumours are cancerous. Although tumour cells will grow at their own speed, tumours can be *benign* or *malignant*. Benign tumours tend to push aside normal tissues, but do not grow into them. Cells of a malignant tumour (a cancer), however, grow into the surrounding normal tissue, a process called *invasion*.

It is these claw-like processes of abnormal cells, permeating the normal tissues, that are responsible for the name cancer – which is Latin for 'crab'. They enable the cancer to spread, if unchecked, through the body and ultimately cause death.

The word 'malignant' means 'bad': this can be contrasted with 'benign' meaning 'harmless'. Both accurately describe the outcome of the two types of tumour without treatment.

Origin and spread of cancer

Cancer cells develop from the body's own normal cells, and a single cancer cell is enough to start the growth of a tumour. However, the change from normal cell to cancer cell is a gradual one, taking place in a number of stages over several years. With each stage, the cell becomes slightly more abnormal in appearance, and slightly less responsive to the body's normal control mechanisms.

This process is usually unseen, until a cancer develops, but in a few situations, pre-cancer can be recognized and treated. The best known of these is seen in the uterine CERVIX (neck of the womb) and this can be detected by a cervical smear.

It is the ability of cancer cells to spread inside the body that makes the disease so serious. Fortunately, the stages by which it does so tend to be orderly, with the cancer initially spreading into the surrounding tissues. This produces local damage, which in time creates symptoms.

Next, cells begin to break off from the cancer and float in tissue fluid. In time, this fluid finds its way out of the tissues into a system of channels called LYMPHATICS, which ultimately return the fluid (now called lymph) to the bloodstream. On its journey, the lymph passes through a number of glands called lymph nodes, which filter out dead cells and infection. Cancer cells are usually trapped in the lymph nodes nearest to the cancer where most of them die. Sooner or later, however, one will survive and start to grow in the gland, forming a secondary growth.

Later, cancer cells are carried through the lymph nodes to reach the bloodstream; from here they are carried to the various organs of the body, such as the lung, liver, bone and brain. Most of these cells die but a few may survive to form secondary growths called *metasteses*.

Causes

Cancer is commonest in late middle and old age. Thanks to sanitation and modern medicine, people are living longer, and it is this rather than any defect in lifestyle, that is responsible for the increasing frequency of cancer in the Western world.

Of course, some cancers are associated with the Western way of life. Cancers due to SMOKING are still rare in the Third World, but are becoming commoner as industrial development takes place and more people start to smoke.

The commonest forms of the disease are LUNG, bowel (*see* COLON and RECTUM), STOMACH, PANCREAS and BREAST cancer. Despite modern medicine, cancer is still responsible for 20 per cent of all deaths in England and Wales each year. The commonest cancers in children and young adults are LEUKAEMIAS, SARCOMAS and KIDNEY cancer. Fortunately, these cancers are rare, and their treatment has improved greatly in recent years.

The cause of cancer is unknown, but two fundamental abnormalities are recognized. First, cancers are not subject to the normal influences that control cell growth; second, the body will tolerate the presence of the cancer without rejecting it as a foreign invader – the fate of parasites. This makes them difficult to deal with.

Environmental factors, such as chemical POLLUTION and exposure to RADIATION, are thought to lead to some cancers, but there are several other possibilities. The *viral theory* states that a cancer cell is infected by a VIRUS and that it is this that causes the cell to grow. The *immunological theory* considers that abnormal cells are constantly being produced by the body, but that these are destroyed by the body's defences – i.e. its IMMUNE SYSTEM. For some unknown reason, this defence system breaks down and an abnormal cell survives to form a cancer.

The *chemical theory* relies on the knowledge that certain chemicals – tar, for example – will cause cancer when painted on the skin of laboratory animals. These chemicals are irritants that may alter a cell's genetic structure and turn it into a cancer cell. Large numbers of experiments have identified chemicals that will cause cancer in animals; these are called *carcinogens*. A certain number have been identified, the best known being tobacco smoke. However, despite research, it has not yet been possible to identify carcinogens responsible for many of the common cancers.

Radiation is known to alter the genetic material of a cell – radiation from the atomic bombs dropped in Japan in 1945 is known to be the cause of many cancers, some occurring 10 or 20 years after the exposure to radiation.

As no single theory explains all the facts about cancer, it seems probable that it has many causes, some unknown.

Diagnosis

It is no longer true that cancer is invariably fatal. There has been a vast improvement in treatment in recent years and many people are cured of the disease. However, a small cancer is much easier to cure than a large one, so early diagnosis is vital and is helped by the prompt reporting of significant symptoms to the doctor. If he or she suspects cancer, this is usually followed by referral to the local hospital out-patients department: from here the specialists will take over.

The diagnosis will first be confirmed. This may initially involve X-RAYS and scanning tests to show the presence of a lump inside the body. A part of the cancer will then be examined under the microscope. This can be done either by BIOPSY or by cytological examination.

A biopsy involves the removal, by a surgeon, of a small piece of the tumour which is then sent for examination by a pathologist. This will determine whether the tissue is cancerous or not. Cytological examination is where body fluids, such as sputum (PHLEGM) or mucus from the cervix, are studied specifically for cancer cells.

A thorough clinical examination is made, taking particular care to check the lymph nodes adjacent to the tumour. Simple blood tests are run to check liver and bone function and a chest X-ray looks for evidence of spread to these sites. If the doctor is suspicious of spread to a particular part of the body, this area may also be scanned. Various techniques are used. In isotope scanning, a very small amount of radioactive substance is injected into the body and the blood carries it to the suspected organ or area of tissue. If it does contain a cancer, this will take up a different amount of the isotope compared to the rest of the healthy tissue. The patient is then scanned with a special instrument which detects the radiation and the cancer can be seen. Many organs of the body can be examined in this way, especially bone, the liver and the thyroid.

The doctor will now have a detailed knowledge of the type of cancer involved and the stage of its development and progress. Using this information, the form of treatment that is most likely to be effective will be decided upon.

The aim of all cancer treatment is to kill or remove every cancer cell from the patient. With skilled use of the available treatments, this is often possible.

Surgery

Effective cancer surgery aims at removing all of the cancer from the patient. It usually involves removing the visible growth with a wide margin of surrounding normal tissue, to make sure every cell has been removed. In addition, the surgeon will remove the draining lymph nodes. During the operation a thorough examination of any adjacent structures is made (e.g. the liver during an abdominal operation).

After removing the tumour, the surgeon will, where possible, reconstruct the patient's anatomy. In some circumstances this is not possible – following the removal of a cancer in the rectum, for example. Here the surgeon creates a new opening for the bowel on the abdominal wall, called a COLOSTOMY.

There are some circumstances in which surgery is carried out without investigating the patient first. Obviously when the patient is presented as an emergency, surgery is performed both to diagnose and treat the patient. There are also some situations when a biopsy and a cancer operation are carried out under the same anaesthetic. For example, it was once common practice to biopsy a breast lump, examine the tissue and to then perform a MASTECTOMY if the lump was found to be malignant. This had the advantage of speeding up treatment, but nowadays, the two procedures are kept separate to allow the woman to come to terms with the operation.

Radiotherapy

The aim of RADIOTHERAPY is to destroy the cancer with irradiation. Radiation damages the genetic material of cancer cells, so that they are unable to divide. Unfortunately it also damages normal cells, but thanks to the body's remarkable ability to repair itself, quite large doses of radiation can be safely given – provided that it is given slowly enough.

Cytotoxic chemotherapy

If a cancer is too widespread or secondaries are present, it may not be possible to irradiate it completely or effectively. In this situation, drug treatment is now available. The drugs used combine with and damage the genetic material of cells so that they cannot divide properly. They were originally developed from mustard gas, when soldiers recovering from this form of poisoning were noticed to have low BLOOD counts. It was quickly realized that the gas was interfering with the division of cells in the BONE MARROW, where blood is made.

Nitrogen mustard (the active drug in mustard gas) was therefore tried in cancer patients in an attempt to poison the cancer cells and this proved successful. Treatment has now been greatly refined; many new and safer drugs have been discovered and effective combinations of drugs developed. Unfortunately, these drugs poison *all* dividing cells, hence the term cytotoxic ('cell poison').

The best way to minimize the damage to normal cells is to give larger doses of these drugs in single doses all together. There is then a gap of a few weeks (usually three) before the next treatment to allow normal cells to recover.

The cells in the body that divide the fastest are the cells of the skin, gut, and bone marrow. It follows that the side-effects of cytotoxic drugs are hair loss, nausea and lowering of the blood count.

Hair loss occurs with a few of the cytotoxic drugs but the hair regrows when treatment stops. The patient will be warned if hair loss is likely to be serious and a wig may be provided.

Nausea sometimes follows the injection of some cytotoxic drugs, but usually lasts only a few hours. Drugs that combat nausea can be prescribed.

Alternatively, when it is expected to be severe, the patient is admitted to hospital and the treatment given under sedation. However, this is rarely necessary.

The safe dose for the various cytotoxic drugs is now known and allowed for by the doctor, so serious depression of the blood count is now much rarer than it was. However, the blood must be regularly tested both before and during such treatment.

Chemotherapy is not solely used for extensive cancer. It is also used to treat blood cancers, such as leukaemia, as it has proved effective on bone marrow. Other cancers, such as HODGKIN'S DISEASE, may respond better to carefully monitored chemotherapy than to extensive radiotherapy.

In some cases where there is an inclination to relapse after surgery and/or radiotherapy, chemotherapy is given even when there is no sign of cancer present. This is called 'adjuvant chemotherapy' and there have been encouraging results with breast cancer and childhood cancer.

Hormone therapy

HORMONES are chemical messengers that circulate in the blood to control the growth and metabolism of tissue. If a cancer cell arises in a hormone-sensitive organ such as the womb, it may continue to recognize and respond to hormonal messages. If the patient is then given an inhibitory hormone – one that tells the cells to stop dividing, the cancer will stop growing. This type of treatment is particularly useful in breast, uterine and prostate cancers. Its great advantage is its freedom from unpleasant side-effects.

Combined treatment

Where more than one treatment is effective in treating a cancer, it is logical to consider combining them in a planned sequence of treatment. In some childhood tumours, surgery is followed by local radiotherapy and then one year of chemotherapy; the results are very encouraging. In head and neck cancer, chemotherapy is followed by local radiotherapy, and then any part of the tumour remaining is removed surgically.

Whole body irradiation and bone marrow transplantation

In recent years, it has been possible to transplant bone marrow from one person to another. This very specialized procedure requires large doses of radiation to be given to the recipient of the graft beforehand – called 'whole body irradiation'. At present, this treatment is only used in rare anaemias and leukaemia. In the future, however, it may be possible to treat other forms of cancer in this way.

Candida, *see* Fungal infections, Myalgic encephalomyelitis, Thrush

Cannabis, *see* Marijuana

Capillaries, *see* Arteries and artery disease, Blood, Circulation, Lungs and lung diseases

Carbohydrates

The major part of our food intake consists of carbohydrates, or, put more simply *sugars, starches* and *dietary fibre.* All carbohydrates contain atoms of carbon, hydrogen and oxygen in varying configurations. It is the arrangements of these atoms that give the different carbohydrates their specific properties and names. The basic units are called *simple sugars,* monosaccharides, such as glucose, and these consist of a single molecule; the next up the ladder are the *disaccharides* or double sugars, such as sucrose, lactose and maltose, which are the sugars we normally encounter in food; *starches* are polysaccharides such as glycogen and amylopectin, which are made from long chains of glucose molecules. *Dietary fibre* is made out of non-starch polysaccharides and is largely removed in the processing of food.

During digestion, almost all carbohydrates are broken down into simple sugars – especially glucose – which can be absorbed into our bodies where they are used as fuel to provide energy for all our metabolic processes.

The glucose absorbed into the body does not just pour into the bloodstream after being digested. A certain amount is diverted to the LIVER. Here it is 'captured' and turned into glycogen, or animal starch. In effect, the liver acts as an energy store for the body. When extra glucose is required, the liver converts some glycogen into glucose and releases it into the bloodstream. Thus, strangely, a high-glucose meal has no special energy-giving properties. In fact, extra glucose is like topping up the petrol tank of a car – you may have more fuel, but the car does not go any faster. Even if there is a temporary lack of carbohydrate, the liver is able to synthesize glucose from fats and proteins.

Blood sugar: About 0.1 per cent of the blood consists of glucose, and this is continuously supplying the energy needs of our various body tissues. It is particularly vital to the BRAIN which has no means of storing fuel. It is therefore important that the body monitors and regulates the concentration of sugar in the blood. Several HORMONES are involved in the fine control necessary to strike the correct balance between the ready availability and storage of glucose – the most important of these is insulin (*see* DIABETES). When the level of sugar in the blood rises, the PANCREAS releases insulin into the bloodstream and this enables glucose to be stored or used by the tissues. Too little insulin, or a total lack of it, leads to high concentrations of blood sugar; this is *diabetes mellitus,* or sugar diabetes.

On the other hand, too much insulin in the bloodstream leads to a condition called *hypoglycaemia,* which results from too little sugar in the blood. This condition quickly impairs brain function, and leads to such symptoms as hunger, uneasiness and sweating; it may even lead to EPILEPTIC fits or UNCONSCIOUSNESS. Diabetics may develop hypoglycaemia if they take more insulin than they need or if they miss a meal. They learn to recognize the symptoms and eat a sugar-rich food to arrest the problem.

Glucose

Every cell in our body needs energy just to stay alive, and glucose provides the basic fuel which the body burns. Glucose and fructose are the two most important examples of a group of sugar compounds found in various foods such as fruit (fructose) and milk (lactose). They are all changed to glucose when they are absorbed into the body. The ordinary white sugar that we buy is actually a substance called sucrose, which is glucose combined with fructose. This provides the 'sweetness' that we associate with sugar. It is energy-producing, but is now blamed for all kinds of physical ills.

All the various sugars are made of the same three chemical elements – carbon, hydrogen and oxygen, so this change to glucose is not as complicated as it seems. The only difference between them is that the hydrogen and oxygen atoms are 'hung' on to a carbon backbone in slightly different arrangements. This simple chemical structure gives the name *carbohydrates* to all the foods that are based on sugar molecules.

How glucose works: The body has many mechanisms which make sure there is an adequate level of glucose in the bloodstream to supply its needs. These depend on switching on or off the release of glucose that is stored in the liver. Glucose is stored as a compound called glycogen, which is a loose-knit mesh of glucose molecules. Glycogen is also stored in the muscles.

Once glucose is released into the blood, it is taken up by the cells. To do this, a hormone called insulin is essential. Insulin, like amylase, also comes from the pancreas, from special islands of tissue called islets of Langerhans. But, unlike amylase, it is secreted into the blood, not into the intestine.

When the glucose is inside the cells, it is broken down to produce energy. Carbon dioxide gas and water are the waste products of this process. The carbon dioxide is carried in the blood to the lungs, where it is excreted back into the air, whilst the water simply joins the pool making up 70 per cent of the body weight.

Just as the liver stores glucose, in the form of glycogen, so the energy made from burning glucose has itself to be stored in each cell, to be used little by little to provide power for the chemical reactions on which the cell depends. The cells do this by creating high-energy phosphate compounds that are easily broken down to release the energy. These phosphate compounds (adenosine triphosphate or ATP is the chemical name for the commonest) are like a battery that can be used and recharged at will, to supply small amounts of energy as they are needed.

Emergency sources of energy: The stores of glucose-producing glycogen in the body are not very large and if they run down as a result of fasting, for instance, other sources of energy are necessary. The body has two solutions to this problem. First, it may start to convert protein – the main structural compound of the body – into glucose. Secondly, it may start to burn fat in the tissues instead of glucose. The fat provides just as good a source of energy as glucose, but in doing so produces extra waste products called ketones.

Starch

Starchy foods have in the past had a bad reputation as fattening foods, but they are mostly good healthy nutritious foods with plenty of fibre and vitamins.

We tend to eat a large amount of starch in our DIETS purely because foods rich in it are usually cheaper and more readily available than proteins. In itself, starch has no special properties that make us fat – it is simply a ready supply of glucose that the body requires for its metabolism to have the energy it needs in order to work.

Many slimming diets claim that you should cut down on starchy foods. But this is based on old-fashioned nutritional ideas. Current medical evidence shows that starch is the best thing you can eat – if you need to lose weight you should cut down on fat in your diet.

Sources of carbohydrates: Plants manufacture carbohydrates by the process of photosynthesis, whereby they convert carbon dioxide gas from the atmosphere and water from the soil into a simple sugar, utilizing the energy from sunlight in the presence of the green pigment chlorophyll. The sugar is soluble in water and is transported to the parts of the plant that need energy for growth or repair. The excess sugar is converted into insoluble starch and stored, ready to be converted back into sugar when the plant needs it. Plants such as potatoes that have large storage capacity, therefore, contain a large quantity of starch.

The digestion of carbohydrates: When we eat starchy foods, the process of DIGESTION begins in the mouth. Food is first broken into manageable pieces by the teeth and then mixed with the saliva produced by the salivary glands in the mouth. The saliva contains a starch-digesting enzyme called *ptyalin*, or amylase, which is capable of breaking down the starch into simple sugars. There is, however, little time for it to act before the ball of food is swallowed and passed into the stomach. In the stomach, there is no digestion of carbohydrates.

When the stomach contents are passed into the DUODENUM (the beginning of the small INTESTINE), usually after about an hour, enzymes from the pancreas continue to break down all carbohydrates into simple sugars such as glucose. This end-product of digestion is absorbed into the body, enters the hepatic portal vein and is transported to the liver before entering the bloodstream.

The liver and glycogen: In the same way that plants store starch for use when sugar supplies are low, so the body also stores a form of starch called glycogen or animal starch. Glucose absorbed in the small intestine can be converted to glycogen in the liver which usually holds about 100 grams. The muscles also contain substantial quantities. As glucose is used up in the body to provide energy, so the equivalent amount of stored glycogen is broken down by enzymes to glucose. In this way, the concentrations of glucose in the blood and body fluids can be kept within limits.

The deposition of glycogen and its re-conversion to sugar is controlled by hormones – most importantly, insulin from the pancreas. When we eat meals that contain a lot of starch and sugar, the amount of sugar in our blood can double within a matter of minutes. This rapid increase triggers off the pancreas to pour out insulin, which acts on the muscles and the liver and instructs them to withdraw sugar from the blood before it is lost in the urine, and to store it as glycogen. However, the muscles and liver can only store a limited amount of starch and the excess is either converted to fat and laid down in fatty tissue or burned off by the body.

Several other hormones are also related to glycogen breakdown and storage. Adrenalin (*see* ADRENAL GLANDS) and THYROID hormones accelerate the conversion of glycogen to glucose and tend to act when the body is very active, or is prepared for action. Corticosteroids (*see* STEROIDS) increase its manufacture from proteins, while a hormone called glucagon (from the pancreas, like insulin) inhibits the storage of glycogen and helps break it down to glucose.

Sugars and health

Although sugar contributes to providing energy for the body, an excess of sugar can include being overweight and having TOOTH decay. In addition, sugar may be a contributory factor in hardening of the ARTERIES (*arteriosclerosis*).

There is a certain amount of evidence that an excess of sugar in the diet, along with smoking and a high fat intake – especially animal fats – can contribute to fatty deposits in arteries (*atherosclerosis*). Also, sugar is a very potent source of calories, and although we all vary in the amount of calories that we eat before we start putting on weight, people with a tendency to OBESITY should avoid pure sugar. Although all the starchy food we eat is converted to simple sugar in the body, it seems that the healthy way to eat is to take starchy foods in their 'highly complex' forms – as in brown rice, pulses and other 'whole' foods. By doing this, we may alter the body's way of handling FATS, the other main source of calories. This helps to guard against atherosclerosis. In all, a healthy diet contains more starch and less fat and, if possible, little refined sugar.

It is also thought that sugar and sweet things cause bad teeth. This is quite correct, but not the whole truth. All sugars can have an effect on dental health but their action is indirect.

Our mouths are a natural breeding ground for all sorts of BACTERIA, and these bacteria find the sugars just as good for them as we do. A bacteria in the mouth will feed off any sugars or starches left clinging to the teeth and produce waste products that, being acid, attack and etch the teeth until a cavity is produced.

Dietary fibre

Dietary fibre is largely non-starch polysaccharide of which several types exist. The main types of fibre are cellulose, the hemicelluloses, lignins, pectins and gums. None of these are digested by gut enzymes. However, fibre can be partially broken down in the lower part of the gut called the colon by the bacteria that colonize it.

Sources of fibre: All plant food when in its natural form (unprocessed) contains fibre. Good sources of fibre are fruit, vegetables, potatoes and wholemeal bread. Wholemeal foods are those foods with the fibre still present. Fibre can also be taken in the form of bran which comes from wheat and can easily be added to food to increase its fibre content.

Importance of fibre in the diet: Dietary fibre has recently been recognized to have a very important role in our diet. Having a high fibre intake reduces the chance of constipation occurring, and reduces the symptoms of diverticular disease and irritable bowel syndrome. It is also thought to reduce the risk of colonic cancer, the incidence of which is particularly low in countries where the intake of dietary fibre is high. The recommended intake of dietary fibre is 25–30 g a day. Food that is highly refined and consequently contains very little fibre can lead to obesity if eaten regularly in the diet.

Carbuncle, ***see*** **Boils**

Carcinoma, ***see*** **Cancer**

Cardiomyopathy, ***see*** **Heart disease, Ventricular fibrillation**

Caries, dental, ***see*** **Dental care**

Carpal tunnel syndrome, ***see*** **Neuritis, Pins and needles, Raynaud's disease, Wrist**

Caruncles, ***see*** **Urethra**

Cataracts

The lens is situated behind the pupil of the EYE, and is involved in focusing. It has no blood supply of its own; therefore, when it is damaged in any way, it cannot form new cells and responds by becoming opaque, forming what is called a 'cataract'. The cataract causes a gradual, painless loss of vision.

Eventually the cataract reaches a 'mature' state and, if not surgically treated, vision can be permanently lost (*see* BLINDNESS).

Causes

The most common cause of cataracts is ageing, in which case they mostly affect the centre of the lens first, and blindness is delayed for many years until eventually the whole lens is affected. Many patients therefore outlive their eye problem, but regular eye tests are recommended for the elderly, so that cataracts can be diagnosed and treated.

Some cataracts are congenital – that is, people are born with them. Within the first few months of development of the human embryo, the cells of many organs, including the eye, can undergo injury from infections (e.g. RUBELLA) or drugs that are in the mother's blood system during PREGNANCY. Other less severe congenital cataracts consist only of a light filming of the eye that resembles powder throughout the substance of the lens. Such cataracts rarely require any treatment at all, and vision is likely to remain good.

A low level of CALCIUM in the blood (*hypocalcaemia*) – for any reason – can cause cataracts. Patients with poorly controlled DIABETES mellitus can also form cataracts. Sudden increases in blood sugar levels in young people can result in rapid clouding of the lens, but this can be reversed by early treatment of the underlying cause.

Cataracts can form for other reasons too. A high concentration of drugs in the blood can have a toxic (poisonous) effect on the lens, while STEROID drugs, taken either by mouth, in the eye (in the form of eye drops), or by injection, may induce cataracts if given over a long period. Exposure to electromagnetic, cosmic, microwave or infra-red RADIATION can have a similar effect.

Cataracts can be formed as a result of accidents, and industrial and play injuries. A blow to the eye will sometimes cause a cataract to develop several years later. A minute injury from a needle, thorn or metal foreign body, if it involves the capsule or lens of the eye, can lead to a similar problem long after the accident has occurred.

Symptoms

The most obvious symptom is a loss of distinct vision, and sometimes the inability to see in bright light. As the cataract matures, near vision is lost and finally only light and dark can be distinguished. Usually one eye is affected before the other, but nearly always both will show signs of developing cataracts, and if treatment is not given, blindness may occur. Eyes affected by cataracts have a distinctive milky film over the surface.

Treatment

When cataracts affect only the centre (nucleus) of the lens, drops containing drugs which dilate the pupil are helpful; they enable light to enter the eye at the outer edges of the lens. However, the majority of cataracts affect the entire lens, and for this reason, the only effective treatment is surgery.

There are three basic methods, depending upon a person's age and the type of cataract present.

The first method, which is mostly used for children and young people, consists of the removal of the lens fibres of which the cataract is formed. If these lens fibres are soft and likely to be easily washed out by water solutions, simple procedures are followed. The cataract fibres are broken up by piercing the front capsule of the eye and the lens. Some that are left will slowly become absorbed and removed via the channels of the inner eyes.

The second method of removal is by ULTRASOUND (Phako-emulsification). This advanced procedure combines the opening of the eye capsule and washing out the cataract, and can be used for any age group.

The advantage of this method is that only small incisions into the eye are necessary. The disadvantage is that a second operation is sometimes necessary at a later date to produce better vision.

The third type of operation, used in patients over the age of 20, is the removal of the complete lens. In this method, the eye is opened and the lens removed by forceps or a cryoprobe (a probe with a frozen tip). Often a substance is used to dissolve the ligaments that hold the lens in position. A return of good vision is usual and a second operation rarely needs to be performed.

Correction of vision

After the cataract has been removed, the vision must be corrected. Since the lens of the eye accounts for a third of its total optical power, after successful surgery the sight can only be corrected by the use of strong optical lenses, either in the form of spectacles, or contact lenses. The only exception is when a cataract is removed from a very short-sighted person, and then the eye requires no correction, as his or her normal spectacles will be adequate to give improved vision.

Spectacles can only be prescribed if both eyes have been operated on for cataracts or if one eye only has been treated and the other is not used. Unfortunately the lenses of spectacles tend to limit part of the field of vision and they also magnify objects, sometimes resulting in difficulty in getting about.

Alternatively, contact lenses can be worn. If there is also astigmatism (a condition which causes distorted vision), and soft lenses are worn, additional spectacles will have to be prescribed. Hard contact lenses will correct all the vision.

Intra-ocular implants (plastic lenses) are the last option, and are useful for patients when one eye has undergone surgery. It is a complicated operation, with the implant being placed in the eye after the cataract has been removed. Contact lenses or spectacles might have to be worn once the eye has recovered.

Generally speaking, once a cataract has been operated upon and vision corrected, the patient will be able to see quite satisfactorily again.

Can cataracts be prevented?

There is some evidence that cataracts in the elderly can be prevented if ultraviolet light is avoided. Therefore, people should wear sunglasses on sunny days and when on holiday, or if they live at high altitudes or by the sea, to protect their eyes from sunlight.

Catarrh

Mucous membranes are the pliable, sheet-like connective tissues found throughout the body, lining, for example, the inside of the NOSE, the mouth, the THROAT, the windpipe, and air passages. They have a crucial function in producing a thick lubricating fluid for the body known as mucus. The membranes lining the nose and the windpipe help to warm and moisten the air flowing into the LUNGS, but they also help to trap dust and germs in the mucus.

It is, therefore, quite normal for the nose to have some mucus present at all times, but an excess of mucus in the nose is usually called 'catarrh'. Since the mucous membranes extend to the windpipe, excessive mucus may be produced in the chest, as 'sputum' or PHLEGM.

Causes of catarrh

The commonest causes of catarrh are an ALLERGY, infection or other irritation of the mucous membrane lining the nose. The response of the mucous membrane to irritation or infection is simply to produce more and more mucus which collects and forms catarrh.

Physical irritation of the lining of the nose can occur with dusts or cigarette SMOKE. Anyone who works in a very dusty atmosphere may be prone to catarrh (*see* POLLUTION).

Infection is perhaps the commonest cause of catarrh. The viruses which cause the common COLD affect the lining of the nose so that it produces copious quantities of catarrh in the early stages. INFLUENZA and a variety of other similar viruses may also produce catarrh in the same way.

Allergy is another possible cause. About one in ten people suffer from some form of HAY FEVER, which is a seasonal allergy to pollen grains. As they are filtered out of the air by the mucous membranes in the nose, they can set up an allergic reaction which triggers off irritation and catarrh.

Some people are allergic to other microscopic particles in the air. A few people are allergic to the faeces of the tiny house dust mite (*Dermatophagoides pteronyssinus*) that lives in house dust virtually everywhere. Such people may suffer from sneezing and catarrh the whole year round – so-called 'perennial RHINITIS' – although the symptoms are often worse after exposure to house dust caused by housework, or in the morning after exposure to the inevitable dust in a bedroom. Some people are allergic to the fur of cats or dogs or to feathers. Like other forms of allergic rhinitis, the result is a stinging nose and catarrh.

A small number of people suffer from more or less constant catarrh but without any clear allergic or infective cause. This is usually called 'vasomotor rhinitis' because it has been thought to be due to some unusual stimulus to the nerves supplying blood vessels in the nose – the vasomotor nerves. As yet the underlying cause has not been discovered, but it is thought to be as a result of an imbalance of the autonomic nervous system which supplies nerves to some of the nasal mucosa tissue.

Treatment of catarrh

The treatment must, to a large extent, depend on the cause. If catarrh is caused by dust or smoking, removal of the irritant is the first and most important step. If you smoke, stop smoking. If you work in dust, make sure that proper ventilation is supplied and use a face mask or respirator.

For a cold, you can help to relieve catarrh by using a steam inhalation. This will liquify the thick mucus and allow you to blow your nose more effectively. A decongestant nose spray from the chemist may help for a few days.

Hay fever and other types of allergic rhinitis do not usually respond very well to the decongestant sprays sold over the counter in the chemists' shop but are usually helped considerably by antihistamine tablets, which can be bought over the counter or may be prescribed by a doctor. Other treatments which a doctor may prescribe include special types of nasal spray containing either cromoglycate or a cortisone-like drug such as beclamethasone. These sprays may be used regularly and are effective only for allergic catarrh.

If catarrh is caused by an allergy to fur or feathers, relief can be obtained by avoiding animals, which may mean getting rid of pets. You should also avoid feather-filled pillows and cushions.

Decongestant sprays and nose drops should not be used for more than a few days except on medical advice. They often stop catarrh for a while, but this is frequently followed by worse catarrh than ever. They eventually act as irritants, damaging the lining of the nose and causing more catarrh.

Complications of catarrh

One of the commonest complications of a bad attack of catarrh is SINUSITIS. In this condition, the catarrh spreads from the nose into the sinuses, spaces lined with mucous membrane situated in the skull beside the nose and above and below the eyes. Bacterial infection can complicate matters and then pain in the face and thick yellow catarrh from the nose can indicate worsening infection. A doctor will prescribe antibiotics for a short-lived attack, but chronic sinusitis may need surgery to drain the sinuses.

Another complication of catarrh is middle EAR infection (*otitis media*). This is most common in small children, but can occur at any age. After a cold or measles, catarrh may travel up the Eustachian tube to the middle ear where secondary infection with bacteria may occur, leading to severe earache and often a fever as well; hearing may also be affected. Untreated, the ear membrane may rupture, but prompt treatment with antibiotics should halt the infection quickly. In severe cases, the eardrum may be punctured surgically, to prevent pus from seeping into the mastoid bone.

Catatonia, *see* Schizophrenia

Cells and chromosomes

The cells are the basic units of life, the microscopic building blocks from which the body is constructed. Within the cells are the chromosomes which contain the vast amount of information essential to the creation and maintenance of human life and personal characteristics.

Every adult body contains more than a hundred million cells, microscopic structures averaging only a hundredth of a millimetre in diameter. No one cell is capable of surviving on its own outside the body unless it is cultured (artificially bred) in special conditions, but when grouped together into tissues, organs and systems of the body they work together in harmony to sustain life.

Types

The body cells vary greatly in shape, size and detailed structure according to the jobs they have to do. MUSCLE cells, for example, are long and thin and contain fibres that can contract and relax, thus allowing the body to move. Many NERVE cells are also long and thin, but are designed to transmit electrical impulses which compose the nerve messages, while the hexagonal cells of the LIVER are equipped to carry out a multitude of vital chemical processes. Doughnut-shaped red BLOOD cells transport oxygen and carbon dioxide round the body, while spherical cells in the PANCREAS make and replace the HORMONE insulin.

Structure

Despite these variations, all body cells are constructed according to the same basic pattern. Around the outside of every cell is a boundary wall or cell membrane enclosing a jelly-like substance, the *cytoplasm*. Embedded in this is the nucleus which houses the genetic instruction in the form of *chromosomes*.

The cytoplasm, although between 70 and 85 per cent water, is far from inactive. Many chemical reactions take place between substances dissolved in this water, and the cytoplasm also contains many tiny structures called *organelles*, each with an important and specific task.

The cell membrane also has a definite structure: it is porous and is rather like a sandwich of protein and fat, with the fat as the filling. As substances pass into or out of the cell, they are either dissolved in the fat or passed through the porous, semi-permeable membrane.

Some cells have hair-like projections called cilia on their membranes. In the nose, for example, the cilia are used to trap dust particles. These hairs can also move in unison to waft substances along in a particular direction.

The cytoplasm of all cells contains microscopic sausage-shaped organs called *mitochondria*, which convert oxygen and nutrients into the energy needed for all the other actions of the cells. These 'powerhouses' work through the action of ENZYMES, complex proteins which speed up chemical reactions in the cell, and are most numerous in the muscle cells which need an enormous amount of energy to carry out their work.

Lysosymes – another type of microscopic organ in the cytoplasm – are tiny sacs filled with enzymes that make it possible for the cell to use the nutrients with which it is supplied. The liver cells contain the greatest number.

Substances made by a cell which are needed in other parts of the body, such as hormones, are first packaged and then stored in further minute organs called the *Golgi apparatus*.

Many cells possess a whole network of tiny tubes which are thought to act as a kind of internal cell 'skeleton'. All of them contain a system of channels called the *endoplasmic reticulum*.

Dotted along the reticulum are tiny spherical structures called *ribosomes*, responsible for controlling the construction of essential proteins needed by all cells. The proteins are required for structural repairs and, in the form of enzymes, for cell chemistry and the manufacture of complex molecules such as hormones.

What is a chromosome?

Each nucleus is packed with information coded in the form of a chemical called *deoxyribonucleic acid* (DNA) and organized into groups called genes (*see* GENETICS) which are arranged on thread-like structures, the *chromosomes*. Every chromosome contains thousands of genes, each with enough information for the production of one protein. This protein may have a small effect within the cell, and on the appearance of the body, but equally it may make all the difference between a person having, for example, brown or blue eyes, straight or curly hair, normal or albino skin. The genes are responsible for every physical characteristic.

Apart from mature red blood cells, which lose their chromosomes in the final stages of their formation, and the eggs (*see* OVARIES) and SPERM (the sex cells) which contain half the usual number of chromosomes, every body cell contains 46 chromosomes arranged in 23 pairs. One of each pair comes from the mother and one from the father. The eggs and sperm have only half that number so that when an egg is fertilized by a sperm, the new individual is assured of having the correct number.

At the moment of fertilization, the genes start issuing instructions for the moulding of a new human being. The father's chromosomes are responsible for sex determination. The chromosomes are called X or Y, depending on their shape. In women both the chromosomes in the pair are X, but in men there is one X and one Y. If an X-containing sperm fertilizes an X egg, the baby will be a girl, but if a Y sperm fertilizes the egg, then the baby will be a boy.

How a cell divides

As well as being packed with information, the DNA of the chromosomes also has the ability to reproduce itself. Without this, the cells could not duplicate themselves, nor could they pass on information from one generation to another.

The process of cell division in which the cell duplicates itself is called *mitosis*; this is the type of division that takes place when a fertilized egg grows first into a baby and then into an adult, and when worn out cells are replaced.

When the cell is not dividing, the chromosomes are not visible in the nucleus, but when the cell is about to divide the chromosomes become shorter and thicker and can be seen to split in half along their length. These double chromosomes then pull apart and move to opposite ends of the cell. Finally, the cytoplasm is halved and new walls form round the two new cells, each of which has the normal number of 46 chromosomes.

Every day a huge number of cells die and are replaced by mitosis; some cells are more efficient at this than others. Once formed, the cells of the brain and nerves are unable to replace themselves, but cells of the liver, skin and blood are completely replaced several times a year.

Making cells with half the usual chromosome number in order to determine inherited characteristics involves a different sort of cell division called *meiosis*. In this, the chromosomes first become shorter and thicker as in mitosis and divide in two, but then the chromosomes pair up so the one from the mother and the other from the father lie side by side.

Next, the chromosomes become very tightly intertwined so that when they eventually pull apart, each new chromosome contains some of the mother's genes and some of the father's. After this, the two new cells divide again so that each egg or sperm contains the 23 chromosomes it needs. The interchange of genetic material during this process of meiosis explains why children do not look exactly like their parents and why everyone except identical twins has a unique genetic make-up.

Identical twins are born when the egg from the mother splits in two after it has been fertilized by a sperm from the father; thus both members of the pair are always the same sex and carry exactly the same genetic instructions. It is for this reason that identical twins are so fascinating to scientists, for all the differences between them must, by inference, be due to differences in their environment.

Problems

Considering how many cells there are in the body, and the complexities of their structure and chemistry, it is surprising how little goes wrong with them during the average life, and how few badly affected babies are born.

Cells that receive some damage to their cell walls can often repair themselves, but if the cell is badly damaged it will die, to be removed by phagocytes which are specialized white blood cells which can 'reprocess' all the components of the cell so that proteins and other chemical constituents can be reused for other purposes.

Cells may also be damaged by disease, and by infections. The complicated chemical factory of the cell may be taken over by VIRUSES which use the reproductive system of the cell to replicate virus particles and in the process destroy the normal function of the cell. Cells can also be poisoned by toxins produced by BACTERIA. These can upset the chemical processes of a cell so that cells cannot carry out their usual functions.

Cancers and chromosomes

All CANCERS originally start with an abnormality within a cell. The affected cell starts dividing and forms daughter cells which continue to divide in an uncontrolled fashion. Sometimes the body seems to respond to slow down the abnormal division, but on other occasions, the divisions continue and cells split off to travel to distant parts of the body where they continue to divide forming further cancerous growths, often destroying other cells in the process.

The initial stimulus to this excessive growth does seem to be concerned with the chromosomes, although why the chromosomes give out false instructions to continue division when this is unnecessary still remains a mystery. In certain types of cancer, it appears that an abnormal gene which may have been inherited from one or other parent may be partly responsible; this problem can give rise to certain types of LEUKAEMIA. In other cases, the chromosomes or genes which control cell division may be damaged by a chemical irritant or may be affected by a virus. The chemicals in cigarette smoke are known to cause cancers by their effect on the cells in lung tissue, and a variety of other toxic chemicals have also been shown to produce cancers in a similar way. Certain types of asbestos fibre, particularly the fibres from 'blue' asbestos, are so tiny that they appear to be able to penetrate living cells without causing any obvious immediate damage to the cell. But in the long run, they can physically damage the chemical structure of genes in the cell, so that a cancer is eventually produced as a result of abnormal activity by the damaged gene.

Chromosome abnormalities

Since the chromosomes contain all the genetic instructions for creating a new individual, it follows that any abnormality in the chromosomes or in the genes which make up the chromosomes may cause a hereditary or congenital disease. (The word congenital means 'from birth'.) In 10,000 births, about 200 babies will have some congenital abnormality, although many of these abnormalities are minor deformities, such as an extra little finger, or webbed toes. Heart deformities (*see* BLUE BABY) and spinal deformities (*see* SPINA BIFIDA) are also among the more common abnormalities and may be associated with a genetic problem. Other genetic problems such as CYSTIC FIBROSIS or dwarfism are caused by an abnormality of a single gene. One of the commonest chromosome abnormalities is DOWN'S SYNDROME.

Chromosome abnormalities in new-born babies are not very common but can cause major disabilities. It is also likely that a proportion of foetuses which miscarry in the early months of pregnancy may also have chromosome abnormalities.

Cellulitis, *see* Rash

Cerebral Palsy

Cerebral palsy, sometimes called Little's disease, is a broad medical term which covers a range of conditions, all resulting in some form of PARALYSIS in early infancy because of imperfect development of, or damage to, the nerve centres in the BRAIN.

There is a widely held misconception that all people with cerebral palsy are mentally handicapped, but this is not true. Although some people with this condition may have brain damage that affects their intellectual development, many are of average or above average intelligence.

Approximately one in every 400 children born in the United Kingdom has this disorder in one of its three main forms, the damage having occurred during PREGNANCY or CHILDBIRTH or soon after. The most common form of cerebral palsy is *spasticity* or *spastic paralysis*. However the number of children with cerebral palsy is decreasing, a result of gradual improvements in obstetric care.

How the brain is affected

In each of the three main types of cerebral palsy, a different area of the brain has been affected.

Spasticity accounts for more than 80 per cent of all cases of cerebral palsy. In this condition the outer layer of the brain, the cortex, appears to have been damaged. The cortex deals with such functions as thought, movement and sensation – all vitally important.

In *athetosis*, damage is centred in the inner part of the brain, on a particular group of nerve cells known as the basal ganglia. These nerve cells are responsible for easy, graceful, flowing movement.

The third type, *ataxia*, results when the cerebellum (situated at the base of the brain) is affected. As the cerebellum is connected to the brain-stem, which links the main part of the brain with the SPINAL CORD, it controls balance, posture and coordination of bodily movements.

Causes

During pregnancy, certain illnesses and viruses can affect the foetal brain. RUBELLA (German measles) in the early weeks of pregnancy is known to cause damage to the foetus. Another virus called *cytomegalovirus* (CMV) is also known to cause brain damage to the foetus. Failure of the placenta to provide adequate nourishment can cause difficulties, but monitoring can detect any problems in the unborn baby.

Many doctors think that *anoxia* (prolonged oxygen starvation) at birth is probably the largest single cause of cerebral palsy. This may occur during a very difficult or prolonged labour, and the baby's delicate brain tissues, deprived of rich oxygenated blood, can rapidly deteriorate. Sometimes the position of the baby creates problems and the umbilical cord may be around the baby's neck. Very occasionally physical damage to the baby's head during delivery may result in brain damage, though this is now regarded as an increasingly rare cause of cerebral palsy.

Some newborn babies develop JAUNDICE and infections like MENINGITIS and encephalitis, which may cause brain damage. About a quarter of all children with cerebral palsy have been affected by a problem arising during pregnancy before the onset of labour, such as infection or a failure of the placenta, perhaps because of *toxaemia* (*see* ECLAMPSIA AND PRE-ECLAMPSIA). Just under half of all cases are caused by complications during labour, and about 6 per cent by brain damage occuring after delivery, usually from meningitis or other infections. However, in about 20 per cent of cases there is no obvious cause at all; the condition occurs after a seemingly normal pregnancy and delivery. In such cases, it can only be assumed that there was some period in which the supply of oxygen to the baby's brain was interrupted.

Symptoms

No two people who have cerebral palsy have precisely the same degree of handicap. In some, the results of the brain damage are so mild that there is no apparent disability; in others, the paralysis can affect all four limbs, speech, hearing and vision; it may also be accompanied by mental handicap and EPILEPSY. The majority of people with cerebral palsy are, however, only moderately affected, and their symptoms follow a common pattern.

A person with spasticity will have general muscular stiffness and weakness in one or more of his or her limbs. It will be difficult to use or control the affected limb or limbs and deformities can develop if treatment is not available.

The paralysis can affect either side of the body (*hemiplegia*), the legs only (*paraplegia*) or all the limbs (*diplegia* when the legs are mainly affected, and *quadriplegia* when the legs and arms are equally involved). The paralysis can either be spastic – that is, stiff and rigid – or flaccid, which is limp and relaxed.

People with ataxia walk in an awkward and uncoordinated manner and usually have very great difficulty in balancing. Those with athetosis have clumsy, awkward movements, with difficulty in controlling their limbs as well as muscles in their heads and bodies.

Additional parts of the brain can also be affected, and combinations of symptoms can mislead an onlooker. For example, the involuntary, writhing movements and awkward walk of some athetoid people, combined with an inability to control facial expression, have earned them the reputation of being mentally handicapped. This is particularly frustrating for those who are intelligent but unable to talk fluently.

Hearing, sight and speech may also be affected, because areas of the brain governing these functions have been damaged. If speech is badly slurred, the person may have difficulty in communicating, and where the hands are also affected learning can be very difficult and slow. Some people with cerebral palsy also have epilepsy, and problems with spatial reasoning are not uncommon.

Difficulties of early diagnosis

In some cases, the problem becomes obvious in the early days immediately after delivery. Doctors carry out a number of simple tests on newborn babies to establish whether the babies' movements are impaired and if the normal REFLEXES are absent or abnormal. However, even if a diagnosis of cerebral palsy is made at this stage, the doctors can rarely be certain about the nature of the outcome for the future. Even those children who are apparently quite severely affected as newborn babies can sometimes improve dramatically over the years.

On the other hand, some children who develop cerebral palsy may appear to be totally normal in the early weeks after birth. It is only later that the symptoms begin to appear. Often it is the parents who are first to notice something wrong – perhaps some clumsiness or difficulties in sitting, crawling or walking.

Because of the uncertainties which often surround the early diagnosis of cerebral palsy it is quite common for a team of doctors, nurses and physiotherapists to assess the child carefully in a special centre as soon as the diagnosis is suspected. A short period of admission to hospital may be recommended so that tests can be carried out – for example, blood tests, X-rays and also tests of nerve and muscle function.

Treatment

As it is not possible to reconstruct or regenerate cells of the brain, there is no cure for cerebral palsy. However, many of the symptoms can be lessened. Early diagnosis and appropriate therapy and counselling of parents are very important. PHYSIOTHERAPY helps to improve tone and develop movement in spastic muscles, and SPEECH THERAPY is essential in assisting communication and in helping with problems of feeding.

A few children need callipers or braces to help with walking, and others may need specially adapted feeding utensils so that they can be encouraged to feed themselves. There are now a vast array of different types of aids which may help such people. These range from simple items such as adapted articles of clothing with press fastenings instead of buttons, through to sophisticated aids run by a microcomputer.

Drugs are rarely of help for spasticity, but occasionally they may be prescribed to try to reduce tension in the muscles. In certain cases, surgery may be carried out to relieve excessive tension in one or two muscle groups so that movement is easier. However, neither drugs nor surgery can do anything to improve strength, whereas physiotherapy often can.

There are a number of paediatricians around the world who have taken a special interest in the treatment of cerebral palsy. Many have developed a particular approach and there are now several programmes in Europe and the United States which have been set up to provide intensive treatment for cerebral palsied children. One of the most famous is the Peto Conductive Education programme based in a world-famous institute in Budapest, Hungary. Undoubtedly some children make great progress in such institutes, but doctors are not sure whether there is any special merit in the individual approaches of each of these programmes. The benefit may simply be a result of intensive care of the child over a period of time. Nevertheless many parents are convinced of the benefits: if the child gets better with the treatment, theoretical discussions about the merits of the programmes are immaterial.

Cerebellum, *see* **Brain and brain disease**

Cerebrum, *see* **Brain and brain disease**

Cervical spondylosis, *see* **Osteoarthritis**

Cervix and cervical cancer

The cervix is the neck of the UTERUS (womb). It is shaped like a cylinder and its lower part projects into the vagina. The cervix is about 1 in (2.5 cm) long, and has a fine canal running through it which opens into the cavity of the uterus above, and the vagina below. If a finger is inserted into the vagina, the cervix can be felt as a small dimple.

In a woman who has not had children, this opening into the vagina is circular and quite small. During CHILDBIRTH, this stretches to allow the passage of the baby through it, and afterwards, it reshapes into a crosswise slit. If it has been badly damaged, it pouts open to form what is called a *cervical erosion*. Dilation, or stretching, of the cervix that occurs during one of the methods employed for the termination of pregnancy (*see* ABORTION), is another possible cause for this condition.

Sometimes, following damage or after a difficult childbirth, the cervix does not function properly. This leads to repeated MISCARRIAGES during the fourth to sixth months of pregnancy. When this condition is diagnosed early enough, however, a special stitch like a purse string can be put into the cervix.

Position of the cervix

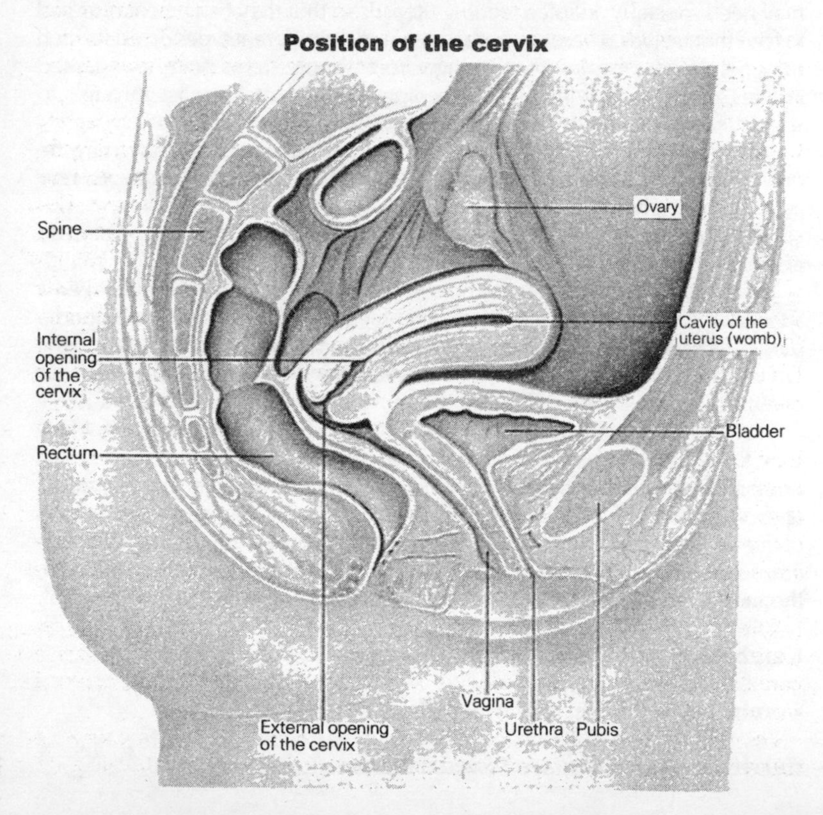

What is cervical cancer?
This form of CANCER develops at the neck of the womb or uterus (uterine cervix) where it projects into the vagina. Cancer is caused by the genetic abnormality of a single cell. This cell divides to form a 'clone' of potential cancer cells. The process of division gets out of control, so the cells continue dividing, developing into a lump. A malignant or cancerous tumour consists of cells which have the ability to spread beyond the original site, and if not treated, they invade and destroy the surrounding tissue, then spread through the bloodstream to other organs of the body.

In the case of cervical cancer, the early stages of cell abnormality do not produce any symptoms, but they can easily be detected by taking a *cervical smear.* Symptoms of more advanced cancer of the cervix may include discharge and bleeding between PERIODS.

In Britain, the incidence of positive cervical smears in 1984 was 8.4 per 1,000 smears taken, and is highest in women under 35 years of age.

The results of smear tests are categorized into groups according to the look of the cells. 'Normal' smears are, as the description suggests, entirely normal. 'Atypical' or 'inflammatory' smears are unusual and may indicate an infection, but are not pre-cancerous. Smears showing 'dysplasia' may be pre-cancerous. And smears showing 'severe dysplasia' are very likely to be pre-cancerous or to indicate a highly localized form of cancer called *carcinoma in situ.* Finally, smears may show obvious cancer cells.

A smear showing mild dysplasia is usually monitored by repeating the smear every few months, because the cells may return to normal without treatment. If mild dysplasia persists, or if there is a more severe type of abnormality in the smear, further investigations will be necessary. This means you will probably have to go to the out-patient department of your local hospital to have your cervix looked at under a special microscope. This procedure is called *colposcopy* and is usually done while you are awake. If the woman is showing severe dysplasia, affected areas can be frozen or cauterized under local anaesthetic. Laser treatment, where the cells are vaporized, is also used, and is becoming increasingly common.

The remaining women have carcinoma *in situ,* which is potentially malignant, and requires treatment of a relatively simple kind known as a cone BIOPSY. This entails the removal of the end of the cervix for further examination, and is carried out in hospital. In the majority of cases, all the premalignant cells can be removed by this method. Occasionally, a cone biopsy shows the spread of these cells into the cervix, and the uterus must also be removed (*see* HYSTERECTOMY).

Carcinoma *in situ* is about five times more common than invasive cancer (cancer of the cervix that has spread) so that the actual incidence of invasive cancer is less than one in every 1,000 of the women undergoing cervical smears.

For more advanced cancers, RADIOTHERAPY, chemotherapy or extensive SURGERY may be necessary. Repeat smears should always be taken on a regular basis, if there has been any abnormality in the past. Treatment for the early forms of pre-cancer are almost 100 per cent effective, but if left undiagnosed, the cure rates for later stages of cervical cancer drop dramatically.

Early investigations into the causes of cervical cancer implicated an infection transmitted sexually. Women who have never had SEXUAL INTERCOURSE almost never develop it. (The incidence among nuns is zero.) The rates are also low among women who use barrier methods of CONTRACEPTION, and among orthodox Jewish and Muslim women. Since the majority of Jewish and Muslim women have husbands who are circumcised, it has been suggested that the agent may be harboured under the foreskin of men. However, two studies have shown no difference in the incidence of the disease in Muslim and Jewish women who are married to circumcised or uncircumcised men.

There is now evidence that a virus, the human papilloma virus (HPV), is implicated in causing cervical cancer. Several different strains of HPV have been identified: HPV 6 and 11 are associated with genital warts and mild cervical dysplasia. HPV 16 and 18 are present in over 80 per cent of invasive carcinoma of the cervix and carcinoma *in situ*.

Additional factors in the development of the disease include SMOKING and taking the contraceptive pill. The younger the women's age at first pregnancy and having had any sexually transmitted disease are also risk factors.

Cervical cancer statistics

Deaths from cervical cancer make up approximately 3 per cent of all cancer deaths in British women. In 1985 there were 1,957 deaths from cervical cancer. It is the second most common gynaecological cancer – slightly less common than cancer of the OVARY, but more common than cancer of the uterus. However, the detectable, pre-cancer stage means that many of those 2,000 deaths could be avoided. Nevertheless, its incidence in younger women is increasing, despite screening.

In 1965, only 2 per cent of all women with cancer of the cervix were under 35, this increased to 11 per cent in 1980 and to nearly 20 per cent in 1983. The death rate among the under-40s has continued to increase.

Screening for cervical cancer

Screening is usually carried out by GPs and is also available at family planning clinics. A cervical smear should be taken within two years of the commencement of sexual activity or at the age of 25 years. After this it should be repeated at an interval of three years or more frequently if abnormal (this will be on the advice of the local hospital cytology service). This should continue until the age of 65 years and then stop if all smears have been normal, but should continue in women who have had abnormal smears. Cervical smears can also be taken more frequently if paid for privately.

Cervical smears

The taking of a cervical smear, or a Papanicolaou ('Pap') test, is a very simple matter and not at all painful. Some women feel embarrassed about having any form of intimate examination carried out, but it is more important to consider the consequences if a serious condition is later diagnosed. The best time to have a smear taken is 10–20 days after a period.

The procedure consists of a speculum being inserted into the vagina. Any discomfort that may arise is caused by the tightening of the muscles of the vagina during the examination, so it is important to relax. The cervix as well as the vaginal walls are inspected through the opened speculum with the aid of a bright light. The smear is then taken by lightly scraping off some of the cells of the outer lining of the cervix with a wooden spatula. The cells are treated with chemicals, which make it possible to see whether they are normal or show any changes that might indicate malignancy.

All women over the age of 35 should have cervical smears at intervals of at most, every five years.

Infections

A common condition affecting the cervix is that of infection (*cervicitis*). This may be due to one of the sexually transmitted diseases, such as GONORRHOEA or SYPHILIS, or to the less serious but more frequently seen non-specific genital infections, such as that due to a bacterium called CHLAMYDIA, responsible for some cases of NON-SPECIFIC URETHRITIS (NSU).

These conditions may produce an unpleasant vaginal discharge, but it is most important to remember that, in gonorrhoea – the commonest cause of cervicitis – there is often no discharge or, indeed, any other symptom at all. If gonorrhoea is a possibility, full examination by a doctor is an absolute necessity. Most vaginal discharges are, in fact, due to infection of the vagina rather than the cervix as for such conditions as THRUSH or TRICHOMONIASIS.

Syphilis does not cause a vaginal discharge, but rather a sore or an ulcer on the lips of the vagina or on the cervix, where there is the additional problem that it cannot be seen.

Syphilis or gonorrhoea of the cervix is treated with the appropriate antibiotic – most commonly penicillin – but both require very thorough follow-up to make quite sure that a permanent cure has been achieved.

Other causes for concern

Cervical erosions – in which cells from inside the cervix begin growing on the outside – may become infected and also give rise to discharge. They are treated by burning (cauterization) – either with some caustic chemical or electrically (diathermy) – or by being frozen (cryotherapy).

With a cervical POLYP, the vaginal discharge may be blood-stained, or actually consist of blood. Bleeding of this sort is due to a fleshy protuberance of the outer covering of the cervical canal. This might be 0.4 in (1 cm) in length and will continue to cause bleeding either spontaneously or during sexual intercourse until it is removed. Although it does not often happen, a polyp is capable of becoming malignant if left untreated.

Chemotherapy, *see* **Breasts and breast cancer, Cancer, Leukaemia**

Chickenpox

Chickenpox, whose medical name is *varicella,* is a highly infectious illness easily recognized by the RASH that it causes, which occurs mainly in children.

It is usually a childhood illness because although babies are born with a natural ability to resist the infection (passed on by their mother), by the age of two or three this wears off, leaving the child likely to catch the infection from other children.

The virus

The VIRUS (or germ) that causes chickenpox – *Herpes zoster* – is the same as that which causes SHINGLES in adults. For this reason, an adult with shingles can start a chickenpox outbreak in a child, and similarly, children who are infected can reactivate the virus in adults to cause shingles. This virus is so highly infectious that many outbreaks occur in children mainly between the ages of two and ten. The outbreaks are strongest in the autumn and winter and appear to occur in three- to four-year cycles as new groups of children lose their inborn resistance.

Although the virus is present, alive, in the spots which form on the child who catches chickenpox, it is chiefly transferred between people by *droplet infection.* Someone who already has the virus spreads clusters of the virus in the tiny droplets of water which are exhaled with every breath.

When a child breathes in an infected droplet, the virus starts to multiply and another case of chickenpox begins. Outbreaks cannot begin on their own – there has to be a source and this is almost always another child.

The course of the infection

Once the virus enters the body, it needs an incubation or breeding period of between ten days and three weeks in order to spread. The first a child will know of his or her illness will be a 24-hour period of vague headache, feeling unwell, occasional slight fever and sometimes a blotchy red rash which quickly fades. Parents may note that their child is 'off colour' or 'sickening for something'.

Within 24 hours the first spots will appear, and by the nature and position of these, the diagnosis is made. In very mild cases, it can be difficult to distinguish chickenpox from gnat bites, but in a full-blown case, with hundreds of spots, diagnosis is simple.

Spots first appear in the mouth and throat where they quickly burst, causing pain and soreness. They then appear on the trunk and face, only occasionally affecting the limbs.

A spot starts as a pink pimple which within five or six hours becomes raised to form a tiny blister, or *vesicle,* containing clear fluid which is full of viruses. These 'teardrop' spots gradually become milky in colour. Then they form a crust, and finally a scab. The time taken from the appearance of the blister to the formation of the crust is only about 24 hours. During this period the child may be fretful and run a temperature of 100 or 101°F (38°C). Some children only have 30 or 50 spots while others may have several hundred.

Immediately the crust forms, the spots begin to itch and this may last until the scabs drop off, leaving normal skin, after one or two weeks. Chickenpox spots come out in crops, which means that new ones will appear every day for three or four days. When examining the skin, an adult will notice that the spots will be at different stages even in the same area. This is typical of chickenpox and quite normal.

In the majority of cases the condition is very mild, but in others, the child is really quite unwell and needs careful and attentive home nursing.

Dangers

The dangerous complications of chickenpox are extremely rare. Most children feel well enough to play around the house during the illness.

Children who are taking STEROID drugs or those suffering from LEUKAEMIA are the only ones likely to be seriously affected and in whom the condition may be fatal. In a very small number of cases, a severe form of PNEUMONIA is caused by the virus. In other rare cases, there may be bleeding into the spots so that the patient becomes ill from loss of blood.

Children with chickenpox should, however, be isolated from old people in case they catch shingles.

Infection

The most common complications arise from infection of the skin at the spot, causing BOILS, or one or two other skin conditions. Similarly, spots near the eye may give rise to infective CONJUNCTIVITIS, commonly called 'pink eye'. In such cases, treatment with antibiotics is needed.

Cases have been known of ARTHRITIS and even inflammation of the heart or lungs following chickenpox, but they are extremely rare. The only other serious danger is when the virus attacks the nervous system to cause encephalitis (inflammation of the BRAIN), which it may do on the fourth or tenth day of the rash appearing. The patient becomes delirious and intensive hospital treatment is needed.

Treatment

Children with a high temperature who feel unwell may prefer to stay in bed or lie downstairs in front of the TV. Otherwise, there is no medical reason to enforce strict bedrest. The majority of children require no treatment at all.

Any pain from sore throat or headache is best relieved with a PAINKILLER such as paracetamol. As there is no medical cure for the virus, the condition is left to take its natural course.

Severe itching can be helped with application of calamine lotion, which has a cooling and an anti-itching effect. Alternatively, the itching can be reduced with an antihistamine drug. Should any of the spots become infected they may take longer to heal, and antibiotics will be necessary.

The majority of children with mild chickenpox start losing their scabs after about ten days and will then be completely clear of spots within two weeks.

Chickenpox infection produces life-long immunity to a widespread infection of chickenpox.

Childbirth

Having a baby usually means going into hospital, particularly if it is a first baby (*see also* CHILDBIRTH, NATURAL). It may seem strange that a hospital is where this unique and intimate event takes place as it almost always has nothing to do with ill health. But going into hospital is often advised just in case there is a problem during labour or some unexpected complication.

Of course, most women are unlikely to have problems and will enjoy a healthy PREGNANCY and normal labour. And a couple do have the right to choose where their baby will be born. So if you insist on having your baby at home, it can usually be arranged.

However, women giving birth in hospital, perhaps for the first time, will find it helpful and reassuring to know exactly what happens and what to expect – and so will their partners.

Labour: The first stage

No one really knows how labour begins, but there are a number of theories. The most recent is that the HORMONE levels in the baby change, triggering off labour.

Labour can begin in one of three ways. In the last months of pregnancy, the UTERUS (womb) prepares for birth with a tightening and relaxing of its muscles. When the tightenings become regular and strong, and last for more than just a few seconds, you can usually be certain that labour has begun.

Contractions occur every 10 to 15 minutes, and they remain constant: if they become irregular, it may be a 'false alarm'. This is why it is important not to rush into hospital.

When the baby is due, you may notice a small discharge of blood and mucus (a 'show') from your vagina when you go to the toilet, or you may simply find a slight discharge of mucus coming from your VAGINA. This can occur by itself, followed a little later by contractions. It is usually a sign that labour has begun, for the mucus acts as a plug over the CERVIX (neck of the womb). As the womb opens up, this plug is then released.

It is common for contractions to begin very soon after the discharge. If the contractions start first, the discharge often follows. Some women do not notice the discharge at all, especially if it is not bloodstained. (If there is any bleeding with contractions, this is not normal and you should call your doctor. With severe bleeding, an ambulance should be called to take you to hospital.)

The third way that labour may begin is with the 'breaking of the waters' (i.e. amniotic fluid) which protect the baby in the womb. In most cases, contractions will soon follow. Occasionally, the waters break and nothing happens. In this case, the baby is no longer protected from infection and you should contact your hospital at once.

Obstetricians may, for various reasons, decide to speed things up, in which case they prescribe a drug which stimulates the uterus and causes contractions. If this is done after labour has started, it is called an *accelerated labour.*

When it is done to start labour off, together with the 'artificial rupture of membranes' (breaking of the bag of amniotic fluid), it is called *induced labour* (*see* INDUCTION).

When should I go into hospital?

If there are no complications, home is the best place for you to be in early labour. It is extremely rare for a baby to be born within the first hour after the onset of labour.

If it is your first baby, labour may last about 12 hours; if it is your second, it is possible that labour will be quicker, lasting about seven hours, but this is not rigid and can vary enormously. A few women experience no contractions at all until the baby is about to be born.

If you feel able to relax at home between contractions, you can make your last-minute preparations at leisure. If possible, eat something but if you cannot face food, a hot, sweet drink will prevent your blood sugar from dropping as labour progresses and this will help prevent you from getting tired.

The labour ward staff can be kept informed by phone about the progress of your labour, and they will tell you when to come into hospital. If you are anxious, you may prefer to go in just in case, but there is usually no need to hurry.

On admission, the midwife will take particulars including a history of your labour up to date. She will normally carry out a vaginal examination (internal) to confirm the onset of labour by checking for the dilation of the cervix (opening up of the neck of the womb).

She will check the position of the baby, the baby's heartbeat, and carry out other routine observations which are designed to forestall any complications at an early stage and also to improve your personal comfort. These will include a check on BLOOD PRESSURE, pulse, temperature and the length of the contractions. She will also test your urine, as this will show her if the blood sugar level is satisfactory. Sometimes in labour the blood-sugar level drops and sugar water (glucose) is given to prevent exhaustion. Some hospitals do not allow you to eat while in labour, not just because some women may actually vomit, but because if there are problems which require a general anaesthetic, the stomach must be empty.

It was once common practice in hospitals for midwives to prepare women by giving a warm enema (to clear the back passage of faeces), and shaving the pubic hair, supposedly to reduce infection. These procedures are rarely carried out today.

Monitoring the birth

It is common in large maternity units for women to be electronically monitored in labour. This means wearing a rubber belt around the abdomen which has a large knob on the top attached by wires to a machine. The machine records when the contractions begin, when they peak and when they end. (The doctor or midwife will still feel for the contractions at certain intervals.) It also monitors the baby's heartbeat.

Monitoring does not mean there is something wrong. It is simply a way of saving work for the midwife by providing a constant check on what is happening to mother and baby. However, some experts claim that reliance on monitoring equipment (which can break down) has resulted in midwives and doctors losing their own diagnostic skills. In addition, many monitors require expectant mothers to lie down, rather than letting them walk about, which may be more comfortable for the women and healthier for the babies.

To check the progress of labour, the midwife will usually give you an internal examination every three or four hours, depending on your progress. On one of these occasions, she might fix a tiny clip to the baby's scalp which will be attached to the monitoring machine so that the heart rate can be recorded.

If labour progresses normally and there are no complications, routine observations and monitor recordings will continue with no other interferences. Occasionally, an intravenous drip-feed of glucose is used to keep up the blood-sugar level and prevent exhaustion. If you decide you would like an epidural to prevent pain, the obstetrician will ask the anaesthetist to give you one.

The progress of labour

If labour is progressing well – most hospitals have a graph which maps out what the normal progress should be – and the waters are still intact, they will not be broken artificially since this will eventually happen automatically. Occasionally, labour slows down and the midwife will break the waters to speed it up again. This is a quite painless procedure.

Towards the end of the first stage of labour, you will find that the contractions begin to get much closer together and that they can be very strong. Labour is now fully established and your baby is nearly ready to be born.

Midwives recognize this *transition* period as a sign that the cervix is more or less fully dilated. A positive sign that the cervix is ready is the gaping of the anus as the head of the baby arrives at the perineum – the area between the anus and the vagina. This area thins and bulges out as the head descends. There is a strong urge to push the baby out.

The second stage of labour

This is when all reserves of energy are required, and it is when partners or other birth attendants can be most useful in encouraging the mother-to-be. It is the end of labour, she is tired, and some really hard work is yet to come.

It seems unfair, but nature does provide compensations. Coping with those very strong contractions in the late stages of labour may seem almost unbearable, but when pushing begins, it may come as a relief – all one's energy goes into the pushing and the contractions do not seem too strong after all.

The urge to push is normally a natural reaction, but if you have had an epidural, you may not get this sensation and will need extra help. As the baby's head descends, the perineum will stretch. The midwife controls the head as it emerges to prevent the perineum from tearing. If the perineum is too thin, or if the baby is distressed and needs to be delivered quickly, then the midwife will cut the area with scissors. This is called an *episiotomy*. These used to be given routinely to all women in childbirth. However, most women will stretch adequately without any tearing, and it is now known that natural tears almost always heal faster and better than surgical cuts.

As the baby's shoulders emerge, the birth process is almost at an end. In an ideal situation, the baby should then be lifted on to the mother's tummy while clips or thread are used to block the flow of blood through the umbilical cord before it is cut by the midwife. Providing the room is warm and all is well, there is no reason for the baby to be whisked away – allowing for the beginning of the bonding between mother and child.

Holding the baby as soon as possible is very important. Research shows that mothers who cuddle and fondle their babies from birth are more likely to make the early, close relationships with them.

The third stage of labour

This means the delivery of the placenta, or afterbirth, and in hospital it is controlled by the midwife. She gives the mother a drug called *syntometrine*, which is injected as the shoulders of the baby are being born. This drug causes the uterus to contract and expel the placenta, and reduces the risk of serious bleeding after delivery.

Second, the midwife will gently pull on the cord to ease the placenta out. This process takes about three to ten minutes.

You may be unaware of this because the birth area is numb for a while after the delivery of the baby. When the placenta is left to be expelled without help, the process is usually a little longer, lasting from about 20 minutes to an hour.

If the baby is put to the breast immediately after birth, a hormone will be released which will cause the uterus to contract and expel the placenta. This was often done in the past before the use of drugs developed.

Shortly after the birth, Rhesus-negative mothers will be given an 'anti-D' injection (*see* RHESUS FACTOR). For a few weeks after childbirth, all mothers experience some vaginal bleeding and discharge known as lochia.

Forceps delivery

If the baby's head is slow to come down through the pelvis during the second stage of labour, or if there are signs that the baby is not getting enough oxygen from the placenta at this late stage, the obstetrician may assist the delivery with forceps. These instruments protect the baby's head and are used to help it through the birth canal. Occasionally, a different instrument is used, called the 'ventouse'. This is a metal cap which is attached to the baby's head while the baby is still in the birth canal, using suction. The obstetrician can then help the baby through the last stages.

Caesarean sections

The normal process of labour may be by-passed where necessary by a CAESAREAN section. This is an abdominal operation where the baby is born

Pain relief in labour

- Relaxation techniques (*psychoprophylaxis*) are very helpful. Ask at hospital if there are any classes you can attend.
- 'Gas and air' relief can be provided using Entonox, a mixture of nitrous oxide ('laughing gas') and oxygen. This is very effective and harmless to the baby. It is breathed in through a rubber mask. The only disadvantage is that it can make you feel sick (often because of the rubber mask).
- Transcutaneous electrical nerve stimulation (TENS) are sometimes helpful in early labour. The machine (a small box with electrodes attached) can be placed on the woman's back by herself, and can be used at home before going into hospital.
- Aromatherapy using lavender oils to help with relaxation is gaining in popularity in some maternity units.
- Pethidine was once the most commonly used pain-relief drug, injected into the leg muscles. It is not used as frequently now because it can cross the placenta into the baby's bloodstream and cause problems with the baby's breathing. Also, if given late in labour, it can make the baby very sleepy when born. A drug is now available, however, that can reverse these effects.
- Water baths can provide effective pain relief throughout labour; indeed the birth of the baby can occur in the bath. At the moment, however, their use is restricted to women who have had uncomplicated pregnancies and who are not expected to have difficulties during the birth.
- An epidural injection is a procedure whereby a local anaesthetic is injected into the epidural space (just in front of the spinal cord). A fine needle is placed in the middle of the back, which has a plastic tube inside. Once the tube is inserted, the drug is given.

  The area below will be numbed so that contractions are not felt. This drug is very effective and 'top-ups' can be given frequently as the drug wears off, without disturbing the mother.

  It may cause a drop of blood pressure or other minor reactions, such as shivering or faintness, but an intravenous drip may be used to counteract these symptoms. Sometimes the woman's ability to push the baby out is reduced because the pushing sensation is lost. A forceps delivery may be necessary.
- Local anaesthetics such as Lignocaine may be injected into the lower part of the vagina and around the nerves which supply this area to provide pain relief prior to a forceps delivery. These anaesthetics will not affect the baby, and the effect wears off fairly soon after delivery.

See also ANAESTHETICS.

through an incision either in an emergency when the life of the baby and/or mother are at risk, or as a planned procedure for those women who are known to have complications.

Possible complications

Having a baby today is considered an extremely safe experience. When all goes well, there is no need for interference and many hospitals will respect a couple's wishes for as natural a birth as possible.

However, there are times when things do go wrong, and what may have seemed a normal labour turns out not to be so simple. A midwife is trained to pick up the signs that show the labour is becoming complicated, and when she detects them, calls for a doctor. In hospital, he or she is immediately available: all obstetric units have obstetricians on call who check up on normal deliveries. (*See also* MULTIPLE BIRTHS.)

Childbirth, natural

There is really no such thing as completely natural CHILDBIRTH. Human beings are social animals and even the most primitive cultures have rituals, customs and taboos surrounding birth – and death. We all grow up strongly influenced by the ideas and expectations about birth which we receive from the community we live in. In Western society, there is an emphasis on the possible difficulties of childbirth, and the natural childbirth movement grew to counteract this.

A woman's right to choose

Over the past few decades or so, many women have questioned the need for some of the medical techniques used during childbirth. Obstetricians and midwives have also started to re-examine some of the standard routines adopted in both antenatal clinics and labour wards. While it is undoubtedly true that, in some circumstances, many of the advanced medical techniques can save the lives of both mothers and babies, it has also become apparent that some techniques have been applied as routine in many labour wards without any real justification. Women have felt that childbirth has become over-medicalized. The joyful, intimate nature of one of the greatest moments in a woman's life can be so easily destroyed by the use of inappropriate medical care.

A woman should have the right to make her own choices about the circumstances in which she would like to have her baby. Doctors and midwives have a duty to explain to women the reasons behind any proposed procedure, and a duty to justify to the woman what they wish to do.

In responding to public concern and women's desires for more natural childbirth, many hospitals now provide much improved facilities and have abandoned many routine procedures. Some hospitals provide 'birthing rooms', furnished with ordinary furniture, easy chairs and cushions where a mother may labour with her partner and other members of her family present, should she wish. A birthing stool may also be available, or the woman can give birth squatting rather than lying down, should she prefer this position. Routine shaving has generally been abandoned, as has the giving of enemas. Midwives now usually discuss whether or not the mother wishes to have pethidine during her labour should she be in pain.

In some areas, it is possible for a woman to be attended by her own midwife throughout pregnancy, and during labour. If the mother wishes to give birth in hospital, a 'domino' delivery might be possible. This term stands for Domiciliary-in-and-out. The scheme allows the woman to be cared for by her own midwife during labour in hospital and to come home again the same day that the baby is born, so that time in hospital is kept to a minimum.

Making a 'birth plan'

A woman who would prefer as natural a labour as possible should prepare herself during her pregnancy and attend classes to learn all about labour, and particularly to practise relaxation and breathing techniques.

A crucial part of the preparation for labour is a full discussion with a midwife about the procedures which may be carried out during labour. If the birth is to take place in hospital, the mother should see one of the senior midwives at the hospital's antenatal clinic to make a 'birth plan'. This lists the various points discussed, and should be signed by the mother and kept in her notes. Some clinics provide a simple form which can be filled in jointly by the mother and the midwife.

The birth plan should cover at least the following points:

Who may be present? Being alone in labour in a strange environment can be a frightening experience. Most women prefer the emotional support of their partner, or it may be possible for other children to be present during labour and delivery, so that the birth is truly a family affair. The woman's own mother or a friend can also be supporters. The woman may also have views about whether or not student midwives or medical students should attend her delivery. She has the right to refuse to allow students to be present.

Induction and amniotomy: The hospital policy about induction should be discussed. The mother must expect any proposal for induction to be fully justified to her before it is carried out. She may ask that an amniotomy is not performed unless it is essential. Once this procedure is performed, delivery must take place within a certain time as there is the added risk of infection as time passes following rupture of the membranes.

Shaving and enemas: The mother can ask not to be shaved, or given an enema, unless this is absolutely necessary for a specific reason.

Drugs: A preference for labour without drugs may be recorded in the birth plan. On the other hand, some women may wish to have an epidural anaesthetic instead of pethidine to relieve the pain of labour.

Posture during labour and delivery: Many hospitals are happy for a woman to walk about during labour, recognizing that gravity can actually speed things up. Moving about also helps to take the mind off the next contraction until it comes, and, left to their own devices, it seems that most women prefer to be as mobile as possible until the very end of labour. Doctors often prefer women to be lying down during labour so that they can easily see the baby's head being born, but many mothers prefer to give birth squatting, leaning against a wall or supported by their partner. A birthing stool is another popular alternative.

Episiotomy: For some years, episiotomy was routine, but it is now recognized that it is often unnecessary unless a forceps delivery is to be carried out. The mother's views should be stated in the birth plan.

Care of the baby: The mother may ask that the baby is born into a quiet room, with a low level of lighting, and is placed straight on to her abdomen so that she may instantly cuddle her baby following the birth. Research has shown that there is a sensitive period immediately following birth when mothers will accept and love their babies much more readily if they are allowed to hold and feed them. The mother may also wish to put the baby to the breast immediately after delivery. She can ask that the umbilical cord is not cut until it has stopped pulsating. It is only at this stage that the flow of blood through the cord has actually ceased. Cutting the cord too early is believed to cause some problems in the adjustment of the baby's circulation after delivery and is thought by some experts to have possible adverse psychological consequences for the baby. Some mothers may wish the baby to be placed in warm water soon after the birth – a technique which forms part of the Leboyer method.

Birth at home

Most doctors prefer babies to be born in hospital. Many women, however, want to retain the right to have their babies at home if they choose. Doctors on the whole feel that hospitals are much safer for both mother and baby if unexpected complications arise, whereas women often feel that birth is a natural, family event which should take place where the woman herself feels most relaxed, confident and in control of what is happening.

The advantages of having a home birth are that the woman is in a familiar place and therefore more relaxed. She will not be separated from her partner or children, she will have the sole attention of the community midwife who will probably also have been in charge of her antenatal care, and she will be much freer to have the kind of natural birth she wants in her own territory.

The disadvantages of a home birth are that the mother would not have all the hospital facilities on hand if anything did go wrong. In that situation, she would be dependent on the 'flying squad' from the local hospital, an emergency obstetric team who bring their skills and equipment from the hospital to the home. In addition to all this, she would also lack the range of pain-killing drugs available in hospital if she were to decide she wanted to use them. It may also be difficult for the mother to find a general practitioner who can provide obstetric care at home. In the past, when many women delivered at home, general practitioners were quite used to working alongside midwives in looking after women in labour and would assist if there were any minor problems or complications. However, since home deliveries are now

Methods of natural childbirth

• Psychoprophylaxis
The most widely used and popular method, it involves learning to use the mind to control the sensations of the body. (The word is formed from the prefix *psycho*, meaning 'mind', and *prophylaxia*, meaning 'preventive treatment'.) It consists of two main techniques:
Breathing: If a woman in labour synchronizes her breathing with her contractions, she feels more in control of what is happening, and in antenatal classes, she will learn four different levels of breathing for use during labour, from deep breathing for the weaker contractions, to very shallow breathing, when the lips blow rapidly against the index finger, for the strongest contractions.
Relaxation and dissociation: Exercises aim to teach the woman what a tight muscle feels like and how to relax it. This is easy in pregnancy because all the muscles can be relaxed, but during labour, a woman needs to relax all her other muscles while one of the most powerful, the uterus, is becoming very tense. The exercises need to be practised regularly until they become second nature. They include learning about the position and breathing which will help to push the baby out with the minimum of difficulty, and the massage which the woman's partner or other supporter can use to ease the pain.

• The psychosexual method
This is based on the view that birth is something which a woman should be free to experience with her entire personality. Its techniques, much the same as those of psychoprophylaxis but applied in a less mechanical way, emphasize the need for women to recognize and understand their feelings about birth and about their bodies.

• The crouching method
This is, in fact, a birth position. Women in most primitive societies give birth sitting, squatting or standing, simply because gravity makes the process quicker and easier. Tearing is less likely if a woman gives birth squatting, but anyone unused to the position should lean against a wall or have some other support.

• Birth in water
In this method, pioneered in the Soviet Union, the baby is born in water warmed to body temperature. There is greater relaxation during the first stage of labour, and because the mother's consciousness is relieved of the distraction of pain, she can help her child to come into the world more quickly and easily. And by recreating for the baby the conditions of the womb, it softens the shock of entering the world. Water birth is still quite rare (and not fully accepted) in Britain.

• Leboyer method
French doctor Frédérick Leboyer's 'gentle childbirth' method was developed to reduce the pain and shock of birth *for the baby*. The delivery room is very quiet and dimly lit, and there may be music playing softly in the background. The child is not held up in the air by the feet. Before the umbilical cord is cut, the baby rests on the mother's stomach for a few minutes and is gently massaged. When the cord is cut, the baby is put first into a basin of warm water, to recreate the atmosphere of the womb, and weighed later.

much less common, many general practitioners have lost the skills they once had in midwifery, and may not be prepared to look after a woman who opts for a home birth. It may, however, be possible for the woman to find a doctor other than her usual one who would be prepared to offer obstetric care at home.

Any woman who decides that she would like to have her baby at home, should first discuss the matter with her doctor. If she is under five feet tall, if it is her first or fourth baby, if she is over 30 years of age or has had any medical problems herself in the present or a previous pregnancy – such as DIABETES, KIDNEY or HEART DISEASE, or pre-eclampsia (*see* ECLAMPSIA AND PRE-ECLAMPSIA) – she will almost certainly be advised by her doctor not to have a home confinement on grounds of safety, but the final decision about whether or not to have a home birth is, of course, that of her and her partner.

Chiropody

Chiropody means the treatment of the feet and their ailments. It is carried out by chiropodists who are specially trained for this purpose. It is especially important in conditions where patients have diminished sensation in their feet: they are therefore more likely not to notice when they injure their feet, thus risking infection. This risk is even higher where the circulation to the feet is affected as well, as in DIABETES mellitus or peripheral arterial disease. People with these conditions may be advised to see a chiropodist regularly to prevent problems from occurring, as they are often more difficult to treat once the injury has already taken place.

Chlamydia

Chlamydiae are tiny BACTERIA that have been recognized since 1907, although their importance as a cause of disease has been realized only over the past 20 years or so. They are responsible for causing *trachoma* (which can cause BLINDNESS), certain types of SEXUALLY TRANSMITTED DISEASES and a lung disease called *psittacosis*. However, it has recently become clear that infection with *Chlamydiae* may be more widespread than previously thought. Research into the way they cause disease, and how they spread from person to person has been difficult because it has often been impossible to isolate or culture *Chlamydiae* in the laboratory. Techniques for doing this are now improving, however.

What are *Chlamydiae*?

Chlamydiae are an unusual type of bacteria. They are smaller than the majority of bacteria and consist of little more than some genetic material enclosed in a cell wall. Most types of bacteria can live and multiply on their own outside other living cells, making use of various chemicals in their environment so they can feed and grow. But *Chlamydiae* are different because they cannot feed, grow or multiply on their own. While they can exist in a dormant state outside other organisms, they need to enter a living animal or human cell in order to multiply. In this sense, they are more like VIRUSES than bacteria.

Once they have come into contact with the tissues of a 'host' organism, they are recognized as foreign particles and engulfed by the cells of the host in an attempt to destroy them. However, since *Chlamydiae* are parasites, instead of being destroyed they, in turn, take over the internal biochemical mechanisms of the cell and use the host cell to reproduce more chlamydial particles. These can break out of the cell and then infect other cells nearby. Each cycle of reproduction lasts between one and two days.

Types of *Chlamydiae*

It is now known that *Chlamydiae* are found in many warm-blooded animals, including humans. Domestic animals – cattle, sheep and many pets – as well as wild animals (both mammals and birds) have their own particular types of *Chlamydiae*, and most of these are unlikely to affect humans. However, certain types of *Chlamydiae* do appear to be able to affect humans and animals alike.

There are two main types of chlamydial organism which affect humans – *Chlamydia trachomatis* and *Chlamydia psittaci*. *Chlamydia psittaci* appears to occur naturally in some animals, particularly birds such as parrots, parakeets and pigeons.

There are a number of different subgroups of *Chlamydia trachomatis*; 14 types that affect humans have so far been discovered. Some of the subgroups (A, B and C) are responsible for causing trachoma; Groups D to K are responsible mostly for genital infections, and three other groups, numbered L1, L2 and L3, are responsible for a general infection called *lymphogranuloma venereum*, which is found mostly in tropical areas.

Chlamydial infections

Trachoma is the most serious type of Chlamydial infection in humans and is a common cause of blindness in developing countries. *Chlamydiae* can infect the EYE directly from contact with other sufferers, or it can be transmitted by flies. The infection causes redness and inflammation of the conjunctiva, which is the tissue over the white of the eye and under the eyelids. Pus is produced and gradually, as the eye becomes more heavily infected over the weeks or months, scarring of the cornea overlying the pupil can result. This may lead to complete blindness.

Chlamydia subgroups D to K may also cause a similar but milder eye infection, which can affect babies and also adults. These subgroups principally cause genital infections, but the disease can spread by contact or touch to the eyes. Newborn babies born to mothers who have a genital chlamydial infection may develop chlamydial CONJUNCTIVITIS of the eyes in the first two or three weeks after birth.

Genital infection can affect both men and women. In men, *Chlamydia trachomatis* causes an inflammation of the URETHRA. In women, it may cause inflammation of the CERVIX and possibly also the urethra, but it can also spread to cause chronic infection in the UTERUS. This may eventually lead to scarring of the Fallopian tubes and ultimately even to sterility. However, both men and women may carry genital *Chlamydia* without having any symptoms at all, but they will be infectious to a sexual partner.

Lymphogranuloma venereum is a rather more serious genital infection which is usually only found in the tropics. It causes chronic infection in the glands of the groin.

Psittacosis is the infection in humans caused by *Chlamydia psittaci.* These *Chlamydiae* are found quite commonly in over 100 different species of birds. Birds carrying the disease may seem quite healthy but can still be infectious, although some with psittacosis do become unwell. The infection can be transmitted through the air to people in close contact with infected birds. Once the organism is inhaled, it sets up an inflammation in the lungs. The sufferer feels ill, has a persistent cough and often a fever as well (*see* PNEUMONIA). A similar type of chest infection can occur in people infected by *Chlamydia trachomatis,* but this does not seem to be very common. In such cases, the organism spreads to the lungs from another part of the body, such as the eyes or genitals.

How *Chlamydiae* cause disease

Chlamydiae do not appear to be as infectious as some other diseases; close contact with a sufferer (such as sexual contact) or repeated contact seems to be necessary for the organisms to get into the body. They can only get into the system through certain points of entry, all of which are moist areas that are not protected by skin – such as the eye and the genitalia. They may also gain entry directly into the lungs from the air. Once established in the cells, *Chlamydiae* stimulate a local defensive response by the body which results in a type of chronic inflammation around the infected area. This is how symptoms are produced in trachoma, genital infections and psittacosis.

Chlamydial infections all tend to last a long time, but are not often fatal. Once established in the body, the infection can continue for many weeks, months or even years. The body produces antibodies to *Chlamydiae,* in the same way that it does to other germs, but the effectiveness of the antibodies in fighting off the infection depends on a number of factors. If the person suffering from a chlamydial infection, such as trachoma or genital infection, is poorly nourished and otherwise not particularly well, the infection tends to be more severe. Repeated exposure to infection or to re-infection from a number of different sources can also lead to more severe illness. So overcrowding in areas where there is trachoma will lead to more severe disease as the risk of re-infection is higher. Repeated exposure to genital infection through sexual intercourse with other infected individuals may also produce a more severe type of infection.

How common are chlamydial infections?
It has been estimated that there are some 500 million people with trachoma in the world, and about 5 to 10 million are blind as a result of it. It is the commonest cause of blindness in the world. Estimates for genital infection are more difficult because reliable diagnosis has only been possible for a relatively short time. It is clear, however, that the more sexual partners an individual has, the greater the chance of becoming infected with *Chlamydiae*. A study in London showed that nearly one in ten sexually active women were infected by genital *Chlamydiae*. An American study suggested that about 13 per cent of sexually active women were infected. A similar proportion of men are probably infected at some time in their lives; about a third of these men and women will develop chlamydial eye infection at some time or other as well. Genital *chlamydiae* are now one of the commonest causes of INFERTILITY in women; two or three attacks of severe genital chlamydial infection (*see* NON-SPECIFIC URETHRITIS) in a woman appear to reduce the chances of conceiving by up to 50 per cent.

Approximately one baby in 100 born in Britain develops neonatal chlamydial eye infection; numbers are greater in those areas where more women are infected with genital *Chlamydiae*.

Recently it has been shown that women who are pregnant and work with sheep during the lambing season are more likely to have a MISCARRIAGE if the sheep have chlamydial infections. It seems certain now that *Chlamydiae* can be transmitted to women farm workers and cause miscarriage. Women are now advised not to help with lambing (or calving) if they are themselves pregnant.

Diagnosis
One of the earliest forms of diagnosis was to use a swab to take samples of cells from an infected area and then to examine them under the microscope. Typical 'inclusion bodies' can be seen inside the cells. These represent areas where the *Chlamydiae* are multiplying. This method can be used to examine swabs from people with suspected trachoma, but direct examination is not very reliable for samples of other types of chlamydial infection. The most reliable test, which is now used routinely, involves treating the sample with special reagents in the laboratory so that any *Chlamydiae* present will fluoresce when the smear is examined under the microscope. Some laboratories are able to culture *Chlamydiae* in cells grown artificially in test-tubes, but this method of isolation is unreliable.

Psittacosis may occasionally be diagnosed by the typical appearance of an X-ray of the chest, but a blood test may also be used to detect antibodies to *Chlamydia psittaci*.

Treatment
Chlamydiae all respond to certain ANTIBIOTICS, particularly tetracycline and erythromycin. These may be applied locally for eye infection in drops or ointment but are usually more effective if they are taken by mouth (as tablets).

Depending on the site of infection, a course of between two and five weeks may be required to clear the infection completely. For pregnant women, erythromycin is preferred to tetracycline.

Once trachoma has caused blindness, however, antibiotics will not restore sight and surgical treatment using a corneal graft may then be the only remedy. Unfortunately the scale of the problem of trachoma worldwide means that this treatment can be available to only a very small percentage of those affected.

Prevention

There have been some experimental vaccines produced to try to prevent trachoma, but so far none has been successful in preventing it for more than a very short time. The main approach to prevention must be to improve hygiene and reduce overcrowding where trachoma is a problem.

The risk of genital infection can be reduced by avoiding indiscriminate sexual activity, particularly with many different partners. The use of a condom during sexual intercourse reduces the risk of transmission of many sexually transmitted diseases, and will reduce the risk of transmission of *Chlamydiae* to some extent. Thus using a condom reduces the risk of catching non-specific urethritis and *lymphogranuloma venereum.* But its effectiveness as a preventive measure against *Chlamydiae* seems to be less than its effectiveness in preventing other infections such as GONORRHOEA.

Cholesterol, *see* Arteries and artery disease, Coronary heart disease

Cholecystitis, *see* Gall bladder and stones

Cholera, *see* Holiday health, Tropical diseases

Chorea, *see* Rheumatic fever

Chromosomes, *see* Cells and chromosomes

Chronic fatigue syndrome, *see* Myalgic encephalomyelitis

Circulation

The body's circulation is a closed network of blood vessels – in other words, tubes which carry BLOOD around the body. At its centre is the HEART, a muscular pump with the job of keeping the blood in motion.

Arteries and arterioles

Blood starts its journey round the circulation by leaving the left side of the heart through the large artery known as the *aorta.*

At this stage, blood is rich in OXYGEN, food broken down into the microscopically small components known as molecules, and other important substances such as HORMONES, the body's chemical 'messengers'. On the early part of its journey blood flows through relatively large tubes called ARTERIES, and then it passes into smaller vessels known as *arterioles*. These lead

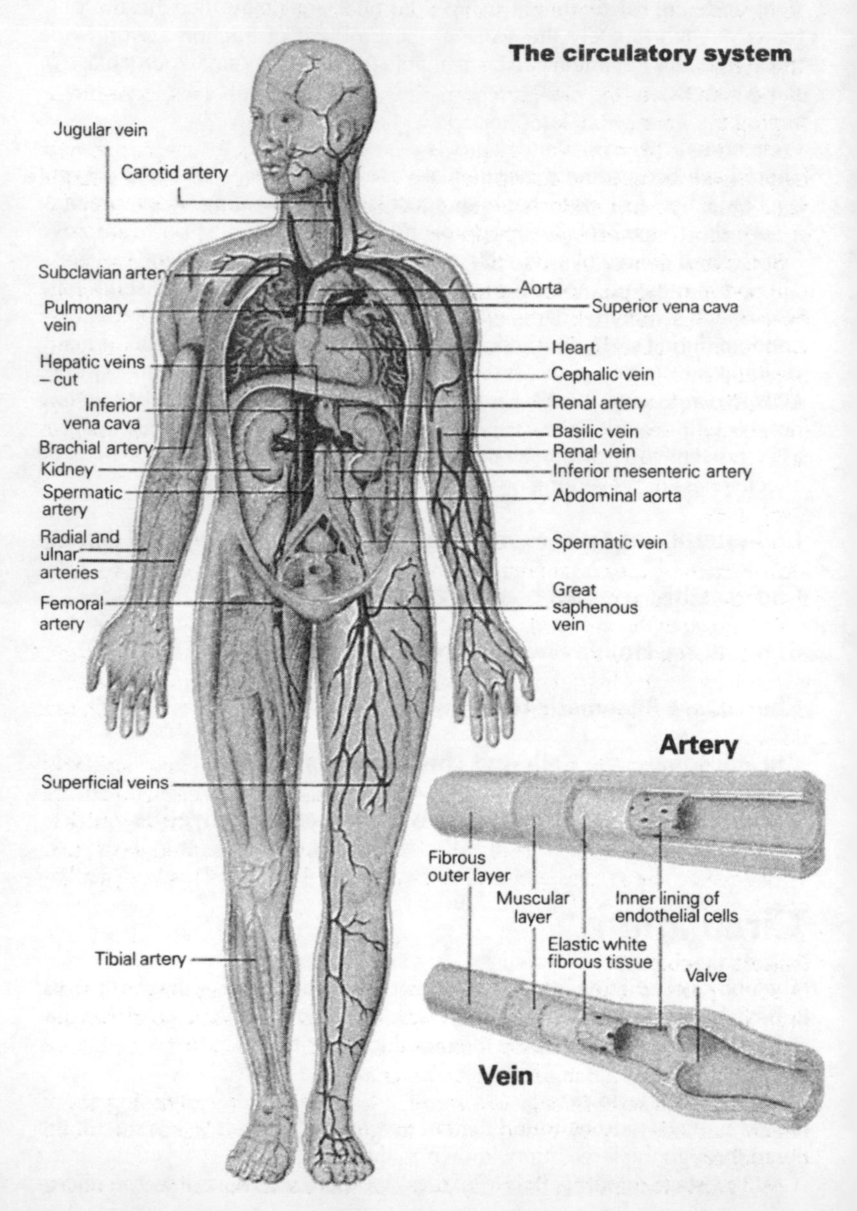

oxygenated blood to every organ and tissue in the body, including the heart itself.

From the arterioles, the blood enters a vast network of minute vessels called the *capillaries.* It is here that oxygen and life-maintaining molecules are given up in return for the waste products of the body's activities.

The veins

Blood then leaves the capillaries and flows into the small veins, or *venules,* starting the journey back to the heart.

All the VEINS from the various parts of the body eventually merge into two large blood vessels, one called the superior and the other called the inferior *vena cava.* The first collects blood from the head, arms and neck, and the second receives blood from the lower part of the body.

Both veins deliver blood to the right side of the heart, and from here, it is pumped into the pulmonary artery (the only artery to carry blood with no oxygen). This artery takes the blood to the LUNGS where oxygen from the air we breathe is absorbed into it and the waste carbon dioxide given up and breathed out.

The final stage of the journey is for the now oxygen-rich blood to flow through the pulmonary vein (the only vein to carry oxygenated blood) into the left side of the heart, where it starts its circuit again.

Short cuts

In general, the foregoing text describes what is meant by circulation. However, there are certain refinements of the circulation which help supply the body's special needs.

On leaving the INTESTINES, blood does not flow directly back to the heart but is taken to the LIVER by means of a special vessel called the hepatic portal vein. In the liver, some substances are sifted out for immediate use, others are put into storage, and poisonous or toxic substances are broken down.

And if the body is put under physical stress, such as when suddenly breaking into a run, blood vessels in the leg muscles increase in size and those in the intestine shut down so that the blood is directed to the site at which it is most needed. When you are resting after a meal, the reverse process occurs. This is assisted by a series of circulatory by-passes throughout the body called *anastamoses.*

Failsafe mechanism

In some parts of the body, such as the arms and legs, arteries and their branches are joined so that they can 'double up' on each other and form an alternative route for the blood if one is damaged: this is called a collateral circulation, and is a natural defence mechanism.

And when there is damage to an artery, the branch of the adjoining artery which has taken over grows wider to give a greater degree of blood circulation.

As it grows to maturity, the body develops more and more of these failsafe back-ups in its network of arteries, but they cannot cope with an extreme emergency such as the formation of a clot (*see* THROMBOSIS).

Distribution and rate of flow

The blood is not evenly spread throughout the system. At any given moment, about 12 per cent is in the arteries and veins which carry it to and from the lungs. About 59 per cent is in the veins, 15 per cent is in the arteries, 5 per cent in the capillaries and the remaining 9 per cent in the heart.

Nor does the blood flow at the same rate in all parts of the system. It spurts from the heart and through the aorta at a brisk 13 in (33 cm) per second, but by the time it has reached the capillaries, it has slowed down to a gentle one-tenth of an inch (0.3 cm) per second. The flow back through the veins gradually increases in speed so that blood is delivered back to the heart at 8 in (20 cm) per second.

Assessing the circulation

One of the main guides a doctor has to the condition of a patient's circulation is his or her PULSE, for it is a mirror of the heartbeat. Arteries have elastic walls which expand every time the heart pumps a wave of blood through them. You can actually feel this happening if you can find an artery near the surface of the body and press it against a bone. One such place, of course, is the wrist.

The normal pulse rate is between 60 and 80 beats a minute but varies widely, so a doctor taking your pulse is not only counting the beats but feeling for changes in their strength and regularity.

BLOOD PRESSURE is different from the pulse, being a measurement of the force with which the heart pumps blood out into the arteries.

If the blood pressure is higher than normal, the heart is probably having to work harder to push the blood through the circulation, and this may indicate that there is some disease of the system.

There might, for example, be *arteriosclerosis,* or a narrowing of the arteries. Clearly, the smaller the opening in a blood vessel, the harder the heart has to work to pump the blood through. If the heart works too hard over a long period, its life may be shortened, and this is one reason why doctors are on the lookout for high blood pressure.

Further controls

The width of the blood vessels is, in fact, a control on the circulation in its own right. Changes in the width of the blood vessels can be brought about by two means: the nerves and the HORMONES.

Overall direction of the behaviour of the arteries is provided by an area in the BRAIN known as the *vasomotor centre.* It receives messages from nerve endings, and in response to their signals, the centre issues instructions to the muscles of the arteries. If the blood pressure is too high, the muscles are 'told' to relax, so allowing the arteries to widen. And if it is too low, the opposite occurs.

As well as this central control, there are certain other factors which can cause changes in the width of blood vessels. A build-up of carbon dioxide in the body tissues from increased activity makes the arteries widen so that the cells receive more blood.

If, for some reason, the blood pressure drops, the KIDNEYS respond by secreting a hormone called *renin*: this acts on substances secreted by the liver to produce another hormone called *angiotensin*, which makes the arteries narrow, raising the blood pressure back to normal. In addition, angiotensin causes another substance called *aldosterone* to be released by the ADRENAL GLANDS: this also raises the blood pressure by causing salt and water to be retained by the kidneys.

TEMPERATURE is another local control. Heat makes the vessels expand so that more blood flows through them. As a result, more blood is available to be cooled by the outside air, and the overall body temperature drops. Cold makes the vessels contract, with the opposite result.

Taken together, these controls make it possible for the body to undertake amazingly varied and demanding roles in life.

If we need to sit still, the blood supply is automatically distributed to maximum advantage for digestive and other processes, with 14 per cent in the brain, 22 per cent in the kidneys, 28 per cent in the liver and 15 per cent in the muscles. But during hard exercise, this changes again with no conscious effort on our part, so that 14 per cent is in the brain, 22 per cent in the kidneys and more than 50 per cent in the muscles where it is most needed.

Capillary network

Measuring only about eight-thousandths of a millimetre, the capillaries are only just wider than one single blood cell. In them the blood cells jostle along in single file, giving up oxygen and other substances and taking in carbon dioxide and the cells' other waste products.

When the body is resting, blood tends to flow through so-called preferential, or preferred, channels. These are capillaries that have become larger than average. But if extra oxygen is needed by any particular part of the body – for example, by the muscles during exercise or by the heart – blood flows through nearly all the capillaries in that area. The capillaries in the skin also help to regulate body temperature (*see above*).

Each capillary consists of a very thin layer of tissue rolled up into a tube and surrounded by an equally thin membrane. All the capillary walls are thin enough to allow certain substances to pass in and out of the blood. Control of the capillaries is provided by muscles.

Being thin-walled, the capillaries can be easily damaged, and those which are most at risk are the capillaries in the skin. If the skin is cut or scratched, or receives a blow, the capillaries release their blood. A bruise is the after-effect of the capillary blood collecting in the skin. In old age, or as the result of excess alcohol over a long period, the capillaries may collapse, leaving purple patches or reddish lines on the skin.

Cirrhosis

This is a LIVER disease, characterized by a progressive destruction of liver cells (*hepatocytes*). These are then replaced with fibrous tissue, which gradually leads to hardening and less effectiveness of the organ. Clumps of small nodules give the cirrhotic liver a gnarled, knobbly appearance.

Causes

The commonest cause of cirrhosis is excessive ALCOHOL intake over a period of years. Although many people seem to believe that cirrhosis only occurs with certain types of alcoholic drinks, or that it only occurs with alcoholics who drink every day, neither of these beliefs is correct. The important factor is the average quantity of alcohol taken over the years. Any kind of alcoholic drink can eventually cause cirrhosis; it can occur in people who drink every day, or in people who just drink heavily over the weekends. It has been estimated that if a man drinks five pints of beer every day (or 35 pints each week) over a period of ten years, he is almost bound to get cirrhosis. Women are more susceptible to the effects of alcohol; about three pints of beer a day over ten years for a woman would have the same effect. Alcohol in excess acts as a chronic poison on the liver, causing gradually increasing damage to the liver cells. Small amounts of alcohol can be metabolized by the liver quite easily without causing damage, however, and two or three drinks every few days will not present a problem.

The second most common cause of cirrhosis is infection of the liver, known generally as HEPATITIS. This may be caused by several different types of hepatitis virus – in all five types have now been identified (A–E), but hepatitis viruses B and C are the major causes of cirrhosis. Viral hepatitis usually lasts between a few weeks and a few months. In some cases, the illness may linger, leading to a long-lasting inflammation called chronic active hepatitis, which in turn may develop into cirrhosis. A vaccine is now available against hepatitis B which is routinely given to all medical staff.

There are a number of other diseases which directly damage liver cells as a result of biochemical abnormalities, such as abnormal deposits of IRON or of copper in the liver cells. Such diseases may also lead to cirrhosis.

Primary biliary cirrhosis is an uncommon but serious form of cirrhosis which most often occurs in middle-aged women. The main symptom is skin itching. In the more serious cases liver transplantation may be required.

In 30 per cent of cirrhosis cases, no cause is found (cryptogenic cirrhosis).

Symptoms

In mild cases, there may be very few symptoms – maybe none at all. The onset of the disease tends to be gradual. Since the liver normally helps to excrete a number of waste chemicals from the bloodstream, early symptoms are caused by accumulation of these chemicals. The chest and upper body may develop small red marks called 'spider naevi'. Some of the body's HORMONES accumulate in excessive amounts – in particular, abnormal concentrations of female hormones which may cause, in men, atrophy of the testicles and growth of breasts. If BILE accumulates in the bloodstream, it causes JAUNDICE and itching of the skin. As cirrhosis develops, the liver gradually becomes harder, because the disease diverts blood flow to other parts of the circulation. Abnormally dilated veins may form on the abdominal wall, or in the gullet; these may burst, leading to internal bleeding. Other symptoms include swelling of the abdomen due to accumulation of fluid in the abdominal cavity; this condition is called *ascites.* Body muscles waste away and the hair becomes thinner. In the most severe cases, mental function deteriorates, leading eventually to coma, and possibly death. Sometimes internal bleeding from dilated blood vessels in the gullet (oesophageal varices) may be very severe, and the patient may die within minutes unless medical attention is immediately available.

Diagnosis

The first signs of cirrhosis may be picked up at a routine medical examination. The liver tends to be harder than normal, so the doctor may feel the edge of the liver just under the ribs on the upper right hand side of the abdomen. He may also notice spider naevi on the skin, or detect ascites in the abdomen.

Once suspicion is aroused, blood tests will demonstrate whether or not there is any sign of abnormality in the function of the liver. These tests do not usually determine the exact cause of cirrhosis, so a liver BIOPSY may then be carried out. A small piece of the liver is removed using a special needle inserted into the liver under local anaesthetic. This sample is examined carefully under the microscope, and usually the cause of cirrhosis will then be obvious.

Treatment

When the cause of the disease is alcohol abuse, abstinence is absolutely vital. It is not enough for the patient just to cut down on drinking, as the ability of the liver to metabolize even small quantities of alcohol will be impaired.

If cirrhosis is caused by blockage of the bile duct, it may be possible to unblock the duct surgically.

Sometimes, cirrhosis caused by chronic active hepatitis can be helped by certain anti-viral drugs. Cirrhosis caused by biochemical disorders can sometimes be helped by specific drug therapy to counter the biochemical defect. Treatment of biliary cirrhosis is with immuno-suppressive drugs.

If there is ascites, it may be controlled by diuretic drugs; abnormalities of blood clotting factors may be helped by certain VITAMIN injections.

Sometimes surgery is needed to deal with abnormally dilated internal blood vessels – for example, in the gullet – to prevent sudden haemorrhage.

Outlook

The liver does possess a remarkable ability to repair itself, so if the very earliest signs of cirrhosis are recognized, and the cause removed, recovery can occur and may be almost complete. If alcohol is the cause, complete abstinence can allow a virtually normal life expectation. However, once cirrhosis has progressed beyond the stage when destruction of liver cells outstrips repair, permanent damage will result, and the disease will tend to be progressive. In the most serious cases, death may occur within a year or two of diagnosis.

Within the past few years, some types of cirrhosis have been treated by liver TRANSPLANT. This procedure is now performed by several specialist centres and can lead to a dramatic improvement in the patient's well-being and life expectancy, with 70 per cent of patients being alive after five years.

Claudication, intermittent, *see* **Ischaemia**

Cleft palate and hare lip

A cleft palate and a hare lip are deformities which a few babies are born with and which sometimes occur together.

The palate is the roof of the mouth: the front part is hard and is called the *hard palate*; the back part is soft and is called the *soft palate*. Most of the hard palate is formed as part of the upper jaw bone, whereas the soft palate is made of muscle. The soft palate is lifted up to close the back of the nose in swallowing, and is lowered to let air escape through the nose to produce the sounds for *n*, *m* and *ng*.

Development of the palate

In normal development, the palate grows from two halves which meet in the middle: these initially create the floor of the mouth under the tongue and finally grow together in about the sixth week of life in the womb. In the eighth week, the halves grow up over the tongue and meet in the middle above it, in the front of what becomes the palate. The join slowly moves forward to the lip and back to the *uvula* (the dangling bit of tissue at the back of the throat). The fusing of the two halves is usually finished by the tenth week, and the nose is finally separated from the mouth.

Where the two halves of the palate do not unite, the palate is *cleft*, meaning it remains split open. Clefts vary in size and type, but wherever the palate is cleft, there is a hole between the internal parts of the nose and the mouth. Similarly, cleft lip (hare lip) occurs where the two halves of the lip fail to join.

Causes

No one knows exactly what causes cleft palate or hare lip. One of the most likely possibilities is that the condition is inherited. Clefts run in families, with relatives frequently showing the same type of cleft, but hare lip is more common in boys and cleft palate in girls. In a pair of identical twins, if one twin has a cleft, the chances are three to one that the other will have a normal palate and lip.

Another possible cause is a deficiency in tissue development within the first three months of foetal development.

Symptoms

Clefts are divided into types, depending on where they occur: lip only; in the ridge behind the teeth (alveolar); or in the palate. All three types can occur together, but because the palate joins in the front part first, and then closes forward towards the lip and back to the palate and uvula, clefts are more common in the lip and uvula than this front part of the palate.

The types of cleft can vary greatly: they range from a groove in the lip or uvula, to a complete separation of the two halves of the palate and lip. Clefts may be one sided; if they are two sided, they occur in alveolar clefts and lip clefts, with a cleft on either side of the two front teeth.

At birth, these clefts are clearly visible, but there is a condition called *submucous cleft* where the muscles of the two halves of the palate have not joined, although the skin covering the palate has. A submucous cleft may cause speech problems as the soft palate does not move normally and cannot close off the passage of air through the nose.

Problems

In babies with a cleft palate, swallowing is not usually badly affected, though there may be some regurgitation of food and drinks into the nostrils. Breastfeeding at first may prove difficult as the baby cannot press the nipple between his or her tongue and the roof of the mouth. Many babies adapt, but if they cannot specially designed teats and feeding bottles are available.

The most important effect, however, is on SPEECH. A baby with a normal palate making the usual babbling noises directs air either through his or her nose or mouth. Infants with cleft palates are unable to do this as air escapes from the nose and the mouth at the same time. The normal movements of the soft palate – down for the sounds 'n', 'm' and 'ng', and up for all other sounds – are very rapid, allowing air to escape through the nose when down and through the mouth when up. Specialist help from a speech therapist will be required.

Cosmetic problems may arise from defects of the palate or lip. With one-sided cleft palate, the bones of the face may be malformed or underdeveloped. With hare lip, the face may appear to grimace when speaking, as the muscles around the mouth are affected.

With the most severe types of cleft palate, defects may occur in the base of the skull and BRAIN: mental deficiency is eight times more likely with cleft palate. DEAFNESS is fairly common, even where the cleft palate child is not born deaf. This is because the nose cannot act as a filter to germs, and so there is a greater likelihood that the child will have ear infections which can lead to deafness. Regular assessments by an audiologist will be made.

Treatment

Hare lip is repaired by stitching the two edges of the lip together, using flaps of skin from other parts of the mouth if necessary. Where the palate is cleft, the two halves are sewn together, using bone and skin GRAFTS if the hole is large.

Cleft palate and hare lip are repaired as early as possible in order to prevent speech problems developing, and further surgery may be done when the child is older to correct any cosmetic damage.

The timing of surgery for cleft lip or palate can vary according to the surgical team involved and the level of abnormality involved: this can be as early as the first week or, more commonly, during the third month.

Sometimes it is considered more beneficial to wait until the second teeth are down before repairing the hard palate: the child can be fitted with a false hard palate called an *abturator* until surgery can be performed. This helps both speech and feeding.

If an operation needs to be postponed until the child is three or four years old, normal speech may develop by itself, but if not, SPEECH THERAPY can help the child learn how to control the direction of air and make the sounds of speech correctly. Other factors such as deafness that are sometimes associated with cleft palate may also prevent the child from speaking normally, but therapy will still be beneficial. When normal speech develops after surgery, the work of the speech therapist will often simply be a matter of assessment rather than treatment.

Dental work may also be necessary to encourage bone growth and development and improve facial appearance. An infant with a cleft palate may need a second operation later in childhood, adolescence or even adulthood to improve facial appearance if growth causes irregular nostrils or scarring of the lip.

Clitoris, *see* **Sex and sexual intercourse**

Clotting, blood, *see* **Haemophilia, Thrombosis**

Club foot, *see* **Feet**

Cocaine

Cocaine is found in the leaves of the plant *Erythroxylon coca* found principally in Peru and Bolivia. The drug is in the form of a hydrochloride salt, which is a white, crystalline solid. A newer form is 'crack cocaine' which is used in the practice of 'free-basing': this involves chemically separating the cocaine from its salt, so that it can pass to the brain more quickly. It can be smoked, sniffed or injected intravenously.

Effects

Cocaine is an addictive drug which causes nervous system stimulation, causing similar effects to amphetamines, such as agitation, dilated pupils, tachycardia, hypertension, hallucinations, hypertonia and hyperreflexia. Convulsions, coma and respiratory failure may develop in severe cases of overdose.

Medical uses
Cocaine is a controlled drug under the Misuse of Drugs Act, 1971, which strictly controls its medical uses. Medical uses of the drug are as a local anaesthetic: it quickly penetrates the mucous membranes and constricts blood vessels.

Dangers of addiction
There are many dangers of chronic cocaine abuse including hypertension, paranoid delusions, nasal ulceration, sleep disruption and, in pregnant women, spontaneous abortions and foetal abnormalities.

Coccidomycosis, *see* **Fungal infections**

Codeine, *see* **Painkillers**

Coeliac disease

Coeliac (pronounced 'see-lee-ack') disease means 'disease of the belly'. But the name is inaccurate because the complaint is a disorder of the lining of part of the small intestine called the jejunum, which prevents the body absorbing FATS, CALCIUM and other important nutrients from the diet. Sufferers have an intolerance, or a form of ALLERGY, to *gluten*, which is a natural protein found in wheat, rye, barley and possibly oats. Coeliac disease is not very common, affecting only one person in 500, but it is a permanent condition and sufferers need to follow carefully a gluten-free diet. It can present at any age, but most usually does so at the age of 30–40 years.

No one knows why gluten should damage the intestines of coeliac sufferers. It could be due to an allergy, to the lack of an enzyme which is supposed to break down gluten, to an abnormality in the intestinal membrane, or to a combination of all these possible causes. Coeliac disease also runs in families. There is a theory, though it is still controversial, that coeliac disease can be brought on by feeding infants gluten-containing foods at too early an age before their immune system knows how to cope with 'foreign' proteins.

Symptoms
The main symptom is loss of weight, due to food not being properly absorbed. Other symptoms include DIARRHOEA, a puffed-up painful stomach, and the passing of pulpy, foul-smelling STOOLS, which are full of undigested fat. Diagnosing the disease in babies is simple because the symptoms are obvious: they are sickly and bloated and fail to put on weight.

Coeliac disease is only dangerous when it is not diagnosed. Chronic diarrhoea, weight loss, ANAEMIA and MALNUTRITION can result.

Tests for the disease are carried out at gastro-enterology clinics. The patient swallows a small capsule attached to a polythene tube. An X-ray is made and a sample of the intestinal lining is then retrieved through the tube. In a healthy person, the lining is covered with little finger-like fronds, called villi. In coeliac sufferers, these are destroyed.

Treatment
The only effective treatment is a gluten-free diet. Once gluten is avoided, the villi grow back, but they will disappear again if gluten is eaten. Treatment is not a cure.

Gluten-free foods can be bought or prescribed by a doctor, though many of these are based on wheat and other gluten-rich cereals and still contain traces of gluten. Potato or soya flour can be bought from health food shops and these are genuinely gluten-free. Following a gluten-free diet outside the home may prove difficult. The best policy for eating out in other people's homes is to tell them in advance that you cannot eat floury foods, and in restaurants, you would be wise to avoid anything with pastry or a floury sauce, unless you can be sure it is gluten-free.

Coil, *see* **Contraception**

Coitus interruptus, *see* **Contraception, Penis**

Cold, common

The common cold is caused by infection by many different viruses. The symptoms that result are the same, and as an illness it is highly infectious. It can be transmitted to other people by droplets, e.g. by sneezing or by close personal contact (nasal mucus on hands).

There are at least 20 different types of viruses which are known to produce the common cold. Antibiotics are of no use in treatment, nor are there yet any effective anti-viral drugs.

Some people believe that taking large quantities of vitamin C, contained in citrus fruits, or in the form of ascorbic acid preparations, provides some protection. Hence, the old belief in honey and lemon mixture. However, experiments have not proved whether this helps.

The sick, the elderly or the under-nourished are not as good at fighting infection as healthy people, and so they are more susceptible to the ravages of the common cold. Young children, whose IMMUNE SYSTEM has not come in contact with so many viruses, can suffer 20 or more such infections each year – as is often seen with children starting school.

Symptoms and dangers
The first sign is a feeling of being 'under the weather', which lasts a few hours. This is usually characterized by aching of the joints and a cold, shivery feeling. The body temperature is commonly subnormal at this stage, but within the next few days – and sometimes hours – it goes up.

Usually the next symptom is a sore THROAT. The throat may feel dry and hurt when swallowing. Glands in the front of the neck may become swollen, and may be slightly sore as the infection takes hold. The sore throat – which can be quite severe and may be accompanied by HOARSENESS – usually lasts a day or two and then tends to clear up as the nose starts running. Large quantities of watery CATARRH often pour from the nose at first, with frequent sneezing. After a day or two, the catarrh tends to get thicker, and the nose becomes blocked. At this stage, most people also have a dry COUGH, particularly in the morning, when there may be a little PHLEGM with the cough. Gradually the nose clears, and the cough subsides after a few days.

SMOKERS tend to find that their colds linger rather longer than usual. This is partly because one effect of tobacco smoke is to reduce the ability of the tissues lining the nose and breathing passages to deal with infection.

HAY FEVER has symptoms that can often mimic those caused by cold viruses. Such ALLERGIC reactions are usually seasonal, and this is an important clue. However, if someone becomes allergic to material that is present in the air all the year round, like house dust, it can be quite difficult, without tests, to distinguish between an allergy and the common cold.

Treatment

Despite years of medical research, there is no cure yet for the common cold. All that can be done is to alleviate the symptoms. Unless you suspect some complication, there is no point in contacting your doctor because he or she will be able to do no more for your cold than you can do for yourself.

For the sore throat, simply sucking boiled sweets or medicated throat pastilles may help. Or you can gargle – with a proprietary antiseptic gargle from your chemist or a weak salt solution (spitting it out afterwards).

If you develop a temperature, or aches and pains, then take paracetamol or aspirin in the dosage recommended on the bottle. For children, use paracetamol tablets or medicine; ask your chemist for a suitable preparation, and ask advice about dosage.

Catarrh may be helped by a nasal decongestant spray from the chemist, but you should use such sprays for only a few days. Paradoxically, continual use may make the problem worse.

Cough medicines may help to loosen coughs, but again they are not curative and you should not expect too much from them. A soothing warm drink will probably help almost as much as a cough medicine.

If your nose is heavily blocked up with catarrh, it may help to use a steam inhalation. Boil some water in a kettle, fill a small basin with boiling water and add a few menthol crystals or some vapour-rub. Place the basin inside a washing-up bowl (for safety) on a table. Sit at the table and put your head over the steaming water. Drape a towel over your head to make a small 'steam tent', and breathe in the mentholated steam for ten minutes.

Complications

One of the commonest complications is a COLD SORE. This is a small blistering sore, caused by the HERPES virus, which tends to occur on the edge of the nose or upper lip. Sore, chapped lips usually precede the development of the sore, so if you are prone to cold sores it is sensible to use a lip-salve to keep your skin moist in order to prevent them developing.

A more serious complication of a cold is acute BRONCHITIS. This is particularly a problem for smokers, the elderly, or anybody who has a bad chest as a result of chronic bronchitis. The catarrh caused by the cold tends to pass down from the nose and throat and set up an infection in the lungs. Early symptoms of acute bronchitis are a severe cough, which is usually accompanied by some phlegm, wheezing or difficulty in breathing, and sometimes an ache or pains in the chest. The sufferer may develop a high temperature as the infection progresses. It is important to consult the doctor if you suspect bronchitis because the infection may progress to a more serious form of PNEUMONIA if neglected.

Another possible complication is SINUSITIS due to secondary infection with bacteria. Alongside the nose are a number of small cavities in the skull called sinuses, which can fill up with mucus when somebody has a cold. Sometimes the cavities then become infected, causing acute sinusitis.

A child with a cold may develop middle EAR infection (*otitis media*). Mucus from the back of the nasal cavity can travel up a Eustachian tube to the middle ear and infect it.

Cold sores

A 'cold sore' is the term used to describe the blisters that form around the mouth and inside the nose; they most often appear towards the end of a cold – hence their name.

These sores can be irritating and unsightly, and cause a lot of local discomfort, but they are not dangerous. They are produced by a virus called HERPES *simplex*, to which most people have been exposed by the time they are five years old; but the majority of us build up a natural immunity that is so effective that we never produce cold sores. Unfortunately, for the minority who suffer from them, they are a real nuisance.

The *Herpes simplex* virus is related to the one that attacks the genital area. That virus, however, is a SEXUALLY TRANSMITTED DISEASE and an immunity to the cold sore virus is not proof against genital herpes.

Causes

Once the herpes virus has infected the skin, it remains hidden there, lying dormant between attacks. The body produces a partial immunity that controls the virus for most of the time, until a certain 'trigger' causes it to flare up. This can be a cold, a bout of flu, a chest infection or a sore throat. Exposure to sunlight or harsh winds can also act as triggers. Some women have a tendency to produce the sores during menstruation.

It has not been proved that cold sores have a tendency to run in families, though it is possible that the inability to develop a sufficient immunity to the virus that causes it is hereditary.

Symptoms
People who suffer recurring attacks of cold sores soon learn to tell when one is starting: there is a sudden itchy tingling in the skin in the affected area, which can begin up to two days before the cold sore erupts.

When this has happened, an inflamed cluster of tiny blisters develops; these fill with a yellowish-white fluid and feel itchy and hot, a sensation which is followed by tenderness and some pain.

Occasionally these inflamed blisters will burst within two to four days of appearing, but in all cases, they start to heal by drying up. During this process, if the sore is left well alone, a crust forms which will eventually fall off. Most cold sores will heal naturally within a fortnight or so – three weeks at most.

Dangers
There is very little danger of scarring, except in severe cases. However, it is important to touch the sore as little as possible, or it will spread.

The crust should never be picked before the cold sore is fully healed and dried out, or it could become reinfected and the whole healing process would then be prolonged unnecessarily.

Treatment
There is no way in which the virus can be permanently removed from the skin once it is there, so if you suffer from recurrent cold sores, you cannot stop them from appearing when your lips get sore. But you can make sure that your lips do not get sore in situations that might trigger cold sores. Use lip salve or Vaseline when you have a COLD, barrier cream in very cold or windy weather, and a sunscreen cream in strong sunlight. Once a sore starts, dab it with surgical spirit.

Your doctor may prescribe an antiviral cream (Acycolvir), which to be effective needs to be applied within the first 24 hours of the cold sore appearing. If the ulceration is very severe, a course of antibiotic tablets may be necessary.

Once cold sore blisters have fully formed, there is no treatment that will stop them running their course.

Colic

Some babies are prone to attacks of colic for reasons that are not clear. It usually starts after the age of two weeks and rarely lasts longer than three months. The length of an attack is variable: anything from 15 minutes to several hours. During an attack the baby screams and is often hard to comfort, drawing its knees up over the stomach as though it had stomach ache. Babies with colic are usually perfectly healthy and the colic is thought to result from overactive bowel contractions instead of the smooth peristaltic movements that adults experience. Wind may exacerbate the problem by getting trapped in the intestine and distending the bowel. Weaning a baby too early – before two months – increases the chance of colic.

Treatment

Colic drops containing a drug called dimethicone or gripe water can be used, but trials have never shown them to be of definite benefit. The herb fennel is said to have a relaxing, calming effect and is available in drink form. Above all sucking is a comfort to colicky babies, and provides a distraction from the pain. Parents also find that rhythmic rocking or walking with the baby is soothing. A colicky baby can be very hard work and stressful for parents, and it is important for them to receive help and support from their health visitors.

Colles' fracture, *see* **Fractures, Wrist**

Colon and colitis

The function of the colon, or large INTESTINE, is to move solid material to the anus (the process of peristalsis) and to absorb salt and water delivered to it from the small intestine. *Colitis* is an inflammation of the colon's mucous membrane.

Colitis can occur as an 'acute' condition in which there is a sudden attack of colitis, or as a more long-standing or 'chronic' condition in which there is continued inflammation of the mucosa of the colon, which from time to time may flare up as an acute attack. Acute colitis may be caused by infections or as a result of poor blood supply (ischaemic colitis). Chronic colitis is usually the result of two diseases, ulcerative colitis or CROHN'S DISEASE.

Acute colitis

Most commonly, acute colitis occurs as a result of infection with bacteria such as *Shigella*, SALMONELLA or *Campylobacter*. These bacteria can be transmitted by touch from person to person, but most commonly are transmitted in food that has been contaminated as a result of poor hygiene. In tropical countries, amoebae may also be responsible for acute colitis.

Usually the onset is quite sudden. The patient will have DIARRHOEA, sometimes as often as once every half an hour. The diarrhoea will be very watery, but may also be accompanied by some mucus and, in more severe cases, blood as well. The diarrhoea may last between two days and several weeks. Recurrent abdominal pain will occur as long as the diarrhoea lasts, and often for several days after it has stopped.

The main danger of acute colitis is that the patient will become dehydrated as a result of fluid loss from the circulation into the bowel. This is particularly a problem if the patient is VOMITING as well, or has a fever. Another risk in severe cases of acute colitis is of perforation of the bowel.

For mild cases the only treatment required is to drink copious quantities of clear fluids. Small babies with acute colitis may need to be given special fluids made of a mixture of salts and sugar to maintain their fluid intake. You can buy these mixtures from the chemist, or your doctor may give you a prescription. In more severe cases, hospital treatment will be required. An intravenous drip will be used to replace fluid lost from the circulation. Specimens of diarrhoea will be examined in the laboratory to determine the exact cause of the colitis. If amoebae or *Campylobacter* are present, antibiotics may be prescribed, but they are not particularly helpful for other types of acute colitis. Perforation of the bowel requires emergency surgery.

Ulcerative colitis

Ulcerative colitis is one of two diseases which produce long-term inflammation of the bowel. The second is called CROHN'S DISEASE, and together the diseases are referred to as *inflammatory bowel disease*. It can be difficult to distinguish between the two, but a useful pointer for identification is that Crohn's disease may produce inflammation along the whole length of the gut, from mouth to anus, whereas ulcerative colitis is always confined to the colon, or the large intestine.

Ulcerative colitis is found all over the world, but it seems to occur more frequently in Western countries: about one person in every 1,000 suffers from the disease. CROHN'S DISEASE is only slightly less common.

Causes

What causes inflammatory bowel disease is unknown. Both conditions are found throughout the world, but are more common in the Western world and in Jewish people. They also tend to occur more commonly in certain families. CROHN'S DISEASE in particular is thought to be most likely due to an infection, but so far one has not been identified.

Symptoms

The symptoms arise from inflammation of the mucous membrane which lines the colon. The mucous membrane is the mucus-producing inner lining of the colon, and it is normally completely smooth. This inflammation starts in the rectum, and it may spread around the colon backwards from there. As a result, diarrhoea develops, varying in severity from one or two loose stools a day to repeated calls to pass stools – perhaps three or four times an hour. The other characteristic symptom is that blood and mucus may be passed as the smooth lining of the membrane is lost; and there may be extensive bleeding into the bowel.

Although in many cases, the diarrhoea will build up slowly, ulcerative colitis is characterized by acute, severe attacks as well as by chronic low-level bowel disturbance. An acute attack of the disease may be very serious. The bowel symptoms are severe and are accompanied by abdominal pains. The patient may appear toxic with a high fever.

Diagnosis and problems

The basis of diagnosing this disease lies in visual inspection of the lining of the bowel, and in BARIUM X-rays which outline the bowel from within. The bowel is inspected using a sigmoidoscope, which is a hollow metal tube passed into the RECTUM, or a flexible colonoscope (*see* ENDOSCOPY). If the disease is present, the mucous membrane will be raw and inflamed and will bleed easily on contact. Microscopic examination may also be necessary.

Although ulcerative colitis is primarily a disease which affects the colon, it may be associated with a number of problems outside the gut. For example, an odd skin rash called *pyoderma gangrenosum*, where the skin becomes inflamed in patches, is almost invariably linked with ulcerative colitis. Another skin rash, called *erythema nodosum*, where hard, red, coin-sized patches appear on the legs, may be associated.

ARTHRITIS, particularly affecting the spine, and inflammation of the eyes may also occur. These are the manifestations of ankylosing SPONDYLITIS, which has a strong association with ulcerative colitis.

Ulcerative colitis can be dangerous in an acute attack. The colon may blow up to an enormous size – a situation called *toxic dilatation*. The dilated colon may then burst, causing PERITONITIS, or there may be extensive bleeding from the bowel. If any of these complications occur surgical treatment may be advisable.

There is also a small risk of CANCEROUS changes occurring in the disease. This risk only applies to those patients who have had the problem for more than ten years; of them, 5–10 per cent develop cancer. Here, again, surgery is the answer, and it is often carried out simply to avoid the risk of cancer. Because of this risk, sufferers from ulcerative colitis are examined frequently by their doctors, and repeated sigmoidoscopies and colonoscopies are done as a routine part of the examination.

Treatment

A drug called sulphasalazine – a compound of aspirin and sulphonamide drugs – is very effective for many sufferers. If it fails, STEROID drugs are used. Mild attacks or those limited to the rectum only may be treated with steroid enemas. If the attack is moderately severe then oral steroid tablets may be required. In severe attacks intravenous steroids and fluids may be required.

Finally, if steroid drugs fail, there is always the possibility of surgery, which could, in fact, be said to constitute complete cure. In the removal of the colon, the end of the small intestine is brought out on to the abdominal wall – a procedure called an *ileostomy* (*see* STOMA CARE). Often after an interval another operation is performed to attach the ileum to the anus to form a pouch or artificial rectum, so that an ileostomy is not required long-term. Once the colon has been removed, the patient no longer suffers from ulcerative colitis.

Ischaemic colitis

This condition mainly affects middle-aged and elderly patients. It is caused by disease in the blood vessels which supply parts of the large bowel. The patient usually has signs of ARTERIOSCLEROSIS in other parts of the body as well, such as poor circulation to the legs, or possibly coronary HEART DISEASE.

It presents suddenly with pain in the abdomen, diarrhoea and the passage of bright red blood from the rectum. The patient's blood pressure may fall, and they look pale and sweaty. The abdomen will be tender to touch and may be swollen. Diagnosis is usually made as a result of a barium enema X-ray of the bowel.

The treatment is usually to rest the bowel, and to prescribe painkillers. In a few patients the blood supply to the colon is so impaired that gangrene forms and surgery is needed to remove that part of the bowel.

Colostomy, *see* **Stoma care**

Colostrum, *see* **Breasts, Immunization, Pregnancy**

Colposcopy, *see* **Cervix and cervical cancer**

Coma, *see* **Brain and brain disease, Diabetes, Unconsciousness**

Conception

This is a great deal more complicated than the simple joining of a SPERM and an egg. It is a complex process in which a variety of conditions have to be right to ensure that it is successful.

Menstrual cycle and ovulation

Every time a man ejaculates (*see* PENIS) he produces sperm, but a woman is physically ready to conceive only once during each menstrual cycle. Approximately 14 days before her PERIOD, she produces a single egg from one or her two OVARIES, which is then drawn into one of the Fallopian tubes. The egg lives for about 12 hours, and if it is not fertilized during that time, it dies and is absorbed into the cells that line the tube.

This is followed 14 days later by the menstrual period, and the cycle then begins again. The average menstrual cycle lasts 28 days, although some women find that their cycles are longer or shorter than that. Most women release approximately 12 eggs per year, assuming they have a regular 28-day cycle.

The sperm and ejaculation

If SEXUAL INTERCOURSE takes place around the time of ovulation, conception is very likely. A man produces around 400 million sperm in each ejaculation. These are surrounded by seminal fluid, which protects the sperm from the acidity of the VAGINA.

Once deposited in the vagina, the sperm immediately start their journey up the vagina through the CERVIX (neck of the womb) and into the UTERUS. They move by vigorously lashing their tiny 'tails'. Some of the sperm do not make this journey successfully, and will wither and die in the acid conditions of the vagina. This is nature's way of ensuring that damaged or unhealthy sperm do not manage to fertilize an egg.

How an egg is fertilized

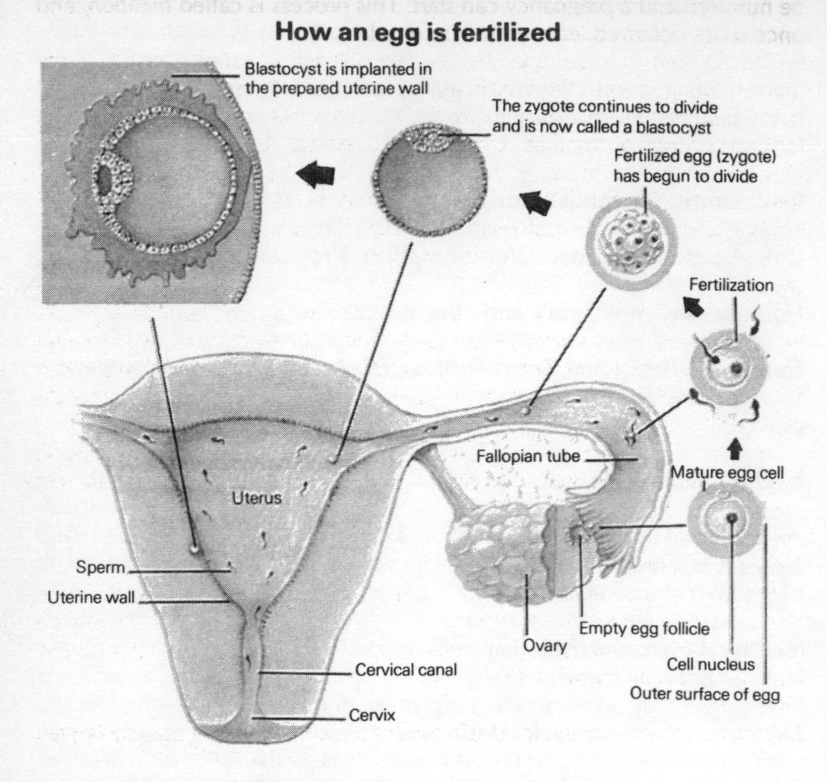

Fertilization

The millions of sperm that have reached the uterus are nourished by the alkali mucus of the cervical canal. They then travel up into the Fallopian tubes. This journey of about 8 in (20 cm) takes approximately 45 minutes – only about 2,000 sperm may actually survive. The sperm will stay alive within the Fallopian tubes for about three days, ready to fuse with an egg if ovulation takes place. If an egg is already present in the tube, fertilization may take place immediately.

Fertilization is accomplished when a sperm penetrates the surface of the egg. Each sperm carries an enzyme which helps liquefy the outer surface of the egg to make penetration of a single sperm easier. Once the egg is fertilized, the rest of the sperm die.

The egg and sperm (which has now discarded its tail) then fuse together to form a single nucleus, which then begins to divide into two cells. Within 72 hours the cells divide 32 times to produce a 64-celled egg.

The fertilized egg then travels down to the uterus within approximately seven days (day 21 of a 28-day cycle). During this time it grows tiny projections which help it to burrow into the lining of the uterus, where it can be nurtured and a pregnancy can start. This process is called *nidation*, and once it has occurred, conception is complete.

The egg can now be nourished by the rich blood supply present in the uterine lining. Soon after fertilization the egg produces a hormone called *human chorionic gonadatrophin* (HCG), which informs the ovary that fertilization has taken place (and ovulation ceases) and which maintains the blood flow to the lining of the uterus so that the egg can continue its development. The body therefore knows that the menstrual cycle must not continue, as a period would remove the fertilized egg.

Twins

Not every conception occurs in this way. If the egg divides into separate halves, instead of doubling the number of cells in a single egg, two separate embryos will be formed. They will be identical twins because they originated from the same egg and sperm. Non-identical twins occur when two separate eggs are released at ovulation, and are fertilized by two separate sperm.

MULTIPLE BIRTHS (three or more babies) occur for the same reasons. Though the use of fertility drugs has increased the number of such births, they are still rare.

Difficulties in conceiving

Although the majority of couples conceive within six months, it can take up to two years to become pregnant. But some still find great difficulty in conceiving. The cause of the problem may lie either with the man or the woman, or both. *See* INFERTILITY.

Concussion, *see* Amnesia, Brain and brain disease, Unconsciousness

Condom, *see* AIDS, Contraception

Conjunctivitis

The thin, delicate skin which covers the white of the EYE and the underneath of the eyelids is known as the *conjunctival membrane* or *conjunctiva*. Conjunctivitis is any inflammation of this membrane. The condition causes inflammation of underlying blood vessels, which become large and pink as a result – and also gives the condition its common name of 'pink eye'.

The type of conjunctivitis common among children is not serious, but there are other more severe types, including one called *trachoma* – found mainly in the East – which can cause BLINDNESS. Conjunctivitis therefore needs to be seen by a doctor so that he or she can diagnose the type and whether it is infectious.

Causes

The commonest cause of conjunctivitis is bacterial infection. Rubbing the eyes may transfer BACTERIA from the fingers to the eye surface. The bacteria may have originated in the nose – children with runny noses caused by a cold often develop conjunctivitis because they tend to rub their noses and faces a lot. Bacteria may also be transferred from towels or face flannels to the eye. Occasionally conjunctivitis occurs after a fly or other foreign body has landed in the eye. Even if the foreign object is quickly removed, it may leave germs behind.

A particular type of small bacteria, *Chlamydia trachomatis* (*see* CHLAMYDIA), is responsible for trachoma, which occurs in tropical countries. This type spreads by touch between people, especially if living conditions are difficult or overcrowded. Chlamydia may also cause conjunctivitis in Western countries, although the type of infection is not so severe.

The chlamydia bacterium is also responsible for the most common type of SEXUALLY TRANSMITTED DISEASE, called NON-SPECIFIC URETHRITIS, which may affect both men and women and sometimes causes very few symptoms. Somebody who is carrying chlamydia in his or her sexual secretions (semen or vaginal fluid) can transfer it to a partner by sexual contact, but the germ can be transmitted simply by touch to the eyes, and cause conjunctivitis.

Any woman who is pregnant and who carries chlamydia may pass the infection to her baby as it is born. The baby then develops chlamydia conjunctivitis within a few weeks of delivery. This type of infection is called *neonatal chlamydial opthalmia*. A severe conjunctivitis can also be contracted from the mother following birth; this is called *opthalmia neonatorum*.

ALLERGY may also be a cause of conjunctivitis. Anybody who suffers from HAY FEVER is likely to develop it during the hay-fever season. Pollen grains from the air get into the eyes, and set up an allergic reaction. Some people can become allergic to dusts in the air, particularly if they work in an environment where there are clouds of dust from, for example, wool or cotton. Chemical fumes may also trigger off conjunctivitis in susceptible individuals. Sometimes cosmetics such as mascara or eye-liner are responsible.

Occasionally, babies develop conjunctivitis in one eye, rather than both (which is usually the case with infective or allergic conjunctivitis). The cause is then likely to be blockage of a tear duct which leads from the eye to the nose and usually allows tears to pass down to the nose. In young babies, the duct may not be fully developed and partly blocked. The result is that the tears tend to run continually from the baby's eye, and the eye may become infected quite easily.

When contact lenses are first placed in the eye, they are like a foreign body, such as a speck of dust, and most people get an initial conjunctivitis. Usually it is not severe, but some people's eyes are particularly sensitive, and they find it is best to stick to spectacles. The softer lenses seem to cause less trouble.

Bell's palsy is paralysis of the nerves controlling the muscles of the face. The muscles which keep the eye tightly closed become weakened or paralysed and the eye cannot shut properly, even during sleep. It is thus easy for dust to blow into the unprotected eye and the chances of getting conjunctivitis are high. So to prevent this, special dust shields may be worn with spectacles.

Symptoms

The first symptom is usually a gritty feeling in the eye, with irritation just under the eyelids. The eye looks red as blood vessels in the conjunctiva become inflamed and enlarged. Pus forms under the eyelids and produces a discharge.

If the conjunctivitis is caused by bacterial or viral infection, large quantities of pus may be produced, which causes blurring of vision because it clouds the eye and causes a sticky feeling in it. The eyelids may even stick together when the sufferer wakes up in the morning, because the pus has dried on the eyelashes and eyelids.

Allergic conjunctivitis usually produces intense irritation and a watery discharge, but usually there is little pus. Sometimes it causes considerable swelling of the conjunctiva and eyelids, so that the lids become almost completely closed.

When the doctor examines the eyes, he or she is usually able to make a diagnosis of either infective or allergic conjunctivitis simply from this examination and by asking the patient about the type of symptoms. He or she may also use a swab to take a sample of pus from the eyes for examination in the laboratory. This examination can determine whether the infection is bacterial or viral, and help with the prescription of the most appropriate treatment.

Treatment

If the problem is an infective conjunctivitis, the doctor will probably prescribe antibiotics in the form of eyedrops or ointment. Chloramphenicol or gentamicin is often used. Drops may be prescribed for use by day, and ointment for night-time use because it is particularly helpful in preventing the eyelids from sticking together. If there is a lot of discharge, it is helpful to bathe the eyes or to wipe the surface of the eyelids carefully with cotton wool dipped in boiled water to which a little salt has been added – one level teaspoonful to a pint of boiled water.

Chlamydial conjunctivitis must be treated with an antibiotic that is suitable for this type of infection. Tetracycline eyedrops are usually prescribed, and often the patient is also given an antibiotic to be taken by mouth – either tetracycline or erythromycin – because the infection can be slow to clear with local treatment alone.

Allergic conjunctivitis is not treated with antibiotics, but with drops containing anti-allergy drugs. Antihistamine eyedrops, available on a doctor's prescription or over the counter at chemists, are useful for short-term treatment. For longer-term treatment, cromoglycate drops are usually prescribed, which counteract the allergic response in the eye and can be most effective.

It is most important that anybody who has conjunctivitis and is being treated for it keeps his or her towels and flannels separate from other people's, and is most careful about washing the hands after applying treatment to the eyes. This avoids transmitting the infection.

Constipation

The major sign of constipation is long, often irregular gaps of sometimes a week between BOWEL movements. These are accompanied by an enlarged, uncomfortable abdomen and often by flatulence (wind), bad breath, headaches and pain on defecation (the passing of motions or stools during a bowel movement).

Everyone has their own particular pattern of bowel movements, which can vary widely, from three times a day to once in every two or three days. So if you happen to be one of those who defecate at quite long intervals, do not automatically assume you are constipated. Worrying about constipation can actually cause it.

How it happens

Food is normally passed along the INTESTINES by rhythmic waves of muscle action called *peristalsis*. Constipation is simply some interference with this process. Among the several causes of such interference probably the most common is food itself.

The digestive system can break up and extract the goodness from most substances we eat as food, but there is one it cannot cope with. This is plant cellulose, which in its common forms occurs in the outer husk of grains (known as bran) and in fruit and vegetables. The everyday names for plant cellulose are *roughage* or *fibre* (*see* CARBOHYDRATES). Undigested cellulose in faeces stimulates peristalsis.

Some foods contain no fibre at all, and, as might be expected, if they are eaten alone, and in large quantities, they usually cause constipation. The most common are eggs, cheese and meat.

Simply a lack of food in the intestines is another cause of poor peristaltic movements, which is why some people on diets become constipated. For the same reason, people with illnesses that cause loss of appetite are also likely to suffer.

Three diseases of the intestines – IRRITABLE BOWEL SYNDROME, COLITIS and DIVERTICULITIS – may cause constipation. PREGNANCY can cause it, too, because the hormones produced at this time tend to interfere with the intestinal muscle movements, as does pressure exerted by the enlarged womb.

Weakness of the muscle in old age or after childbirth are also causes.

Constipation can be a side-effect of certain drugs – for example, some PAINKILLERS. It may also occur in some glandular conditions, such as an underactive THYROID (hypothyroidism) or high blood calcium (hypercalcaemia). In the elderly or after operations, immobility can lead to constipation.

If constipation is accompanied by pain on defecation, it tends to create a spiral of worsening problems. The pain, which is commonly due to damaged veins in the anus (PILES) or cracks (fissures) in the anus, causes reluctance to defecate.

This makes the faeces 'pile up' in the passage, which in turn causes water to be absorbed from them into the bloodstream. As a result, they become even harder and more painful than ever.

The psychological cause

Peristalsis, like breathing and the heartbeat, is controlled by the AUTONOMIC NERVOUS SYSTEM – that part of the nervous system which works without our direct control. However, we can, of course, control *when* we defecate. And this ability to hold back a bowel movement may cause trouble. If the brain can send commands for defecation, it can also 'overlook', as if absent-minded, signals from the intestine that the bowel is full and a visit to the lavatory is due. DEPRESSION, too, can often lead to constipation.

Treatment

Except when constipation is caused by a mental or physical illness, the best treatment is a common-sense one. Eat plenty of fibre. Drink plenty of fluids to soften the faeces. Take plenty of exercise to tone up the abdominal muscles, and give you relaxation from STRESS.

There are several different sorts of LAXATIVES. Bulk-forming laxatives (e.g. Fybogel) relieve constipation by increasing faecal mass, which stimulates peristalsis – thus acting in the same way as dietary fibre. Stimulant laxatives (e.g. senna) increase the speed of the intestines' movement and can often cause cramp. Osmotic laxatives (e.g. lactulose) retain fluid in the bowel and enable softer stools to be passed.

After the intestine has been cleared out in this way, it tends to hold the next supply of food longer than normal, so causing what seems like yet more constipation. The sufferer is likely to take another dose of laxative at this stage, and possibly several more when the process is repeated. This creates a real danger that the intestinal nerves may become so conditioned to the artificial stimulation that they will fail to work when it is withdrawn.

Children should never be given laxatives. Instead, increase the amount of fruit they eat and increase their intake of fibre.

If constipation occurs along with some obvious illness, such as APPENDICITIS or severe pain, consult your doctor – it could be dangerous to treat it yourself.

Should constipation remain after the common-sense treatments have been tried, also see your doctor. It might be a symptom of an underlying disease.

Consumption, *see* **Tuberculosis**

Contraception

Over thousands of years all kinds of ideas have been tried to prevent women getting pregnant – ranging from crocodile dung put into the vagina to standing up after intercourse, sneezing, drinking something cold, and jumping backwards seven times.

Fortunately, nowadays the reproductive system is better understood and far more reliable methods are available. The contraceptive pill is one of the best known, but not every woman can use it. However, there are other, very effective contraceptives available. Choosing which one to use can be totally confusing unless you know how they work and what they do to you. Only then can you decide which sort will best suit you and your partner.

See also PREGNANCY, SEX AND SEXUAL INTERCOURSE and CONCEPTION.

Spermicides

These create a barrier between the man's SPERM and the woman's egg (the ovum; *see* OVARIES). They contain chemicals which kill the sperm when they come into contact with them and they inhibit their movement up the VAGINA. They are not reliable used just on their own so they are generally used with either a condom or a cap. Spermicides take time to work, so a physical barrier such as a cap gives the chemical a chance to kill off sperm.

They are readily available from chemists without a prescription and come in a variety of forms – aerosol foams (which are the most reliable), tubes of cream and jelly, pessaries and foaming tablets, which break up in the moist environment of the vagina and release the chemicals. Some have been found to be almost totally ineffective, while others can cause rubber to deteriorate, so before you buy a spermicide, consult your local family planning clinic to see which brands they recommend. The creams, foams and jellies come with a syringe-like applicator with a plunger. The woman fills the applicator with spermicide and puts it in her vagina with the applicator tip as close to the CERVIX (the neck of the womb) as possible, to make sure that sperm which get this far will come into contact with the spermicide. The spermicide is released when the plunger is pushed.

Used with a cap, it can be applied up to an hour before intercourse. If you do use spermicide on its own, do not apply more than 15 minutes before full intercourse takes place. If you have intercourse a second time, you will have to apply more spermicide as there is only enough in one application to deal with sperm from one ejaculation (*see* PENIS). Sperm can live for six to eight hours in the vagina, so do not wash the spermicide away before that time.

Pessaries or tablets should only be put into place two to five minutes before intercourse takes place as they are not effective for long. Use your finger to place the pessaries as high up in the vagina as you possibly can.

Condoms

Known by a variety of names – including French letter, sheath, rubber, protective and prophylactic – a condom is a tube of fine rubber closed at one end. In its package, it is rolled up so it looks like a flat circle with a thick rim. It unrolls as it is pulled over the erect penis. It can then catch all the semen that the penis ejaculates and stop it reaching the woman's womb.

The tip of the condom should be held between the forefinger and thumb of one hand when it is put on as this keeps the air out and allows some space for the semen. It also reduces the risk of the condom bursting. Some condoms have a small teat on the tip for this purpose.

A condom should be put on not only before the penis enters the vagina but before it even touches the female genitals, because semen can leak out of the penis throughout loveplay. One of the common complaints against condoms is that the couple must stop love-making to put the condom on. However, many couples overcome this problem by making it part of their foreplay.

There are condoms available which have been lubricated to prevent them tearing when they enter the vagina. If this type is not being used, it is a good idea to use spermicide as a lubricant (*never* use Vaseline as it destroys rubber). Spermicide should be used in any case as an extra precaution as there is always a chance of a condom being faulty. Some condoms are treated with a lubricant containing a spermicide, and this increases their reliability.

When the penis is withdrawn from the vagina, either the man or his partner should hold the condom at the base of the penis so that the penis does not come out and allow sperm to escape.

Condoms are available in some countries in a choice of textures, sizes and colours, without prescription, from chemists and mail-order companies; they are also sold in dispensers in public lavatories. They are the only method of contraception – apart from withdrawal (*coitus interruptus*) and VASECTOMY (surgery which permanently prevents the presence of sperm in the ejaculation) – in which the man takes the total responsibility. Condoms of a reputable make are 96–97 per cent reliable if used properly with a spermicide. They also have the important added benefit of giving a good amount of (although not total) protection against SEXUALLY TRANSMITTED DISEASES, including AIDS and HEPATITIS.

Another way of combining the condom with a spermicide is for the woman to use a 'Today Sponge'. This is a small, round, disposable sponge with a depression at its centre designed to locate it over the cervix and a tape for its removal. It should be left in place 6 hours after intercourse. It is impregnated with spermicide and shaped so that it sits in the top of the vagina. It is designed to stay in place for 24 hours and has enough spermicide to last that long, no matter how many times intercourse takes place. It is not, however, very effective on its own and, for maximum contraceptive protection, should be used with the male partner wearing a condom.

Diaphragms and caps

These are round dome-shaped contraceptives made of rubber, which are inserted into the vagina and cover the cervix, preventing any sperm from entering the womb. There are three different types but they all work on the same principle. Used correctly – with spermicide – they are 96–97 per cent reliable.

The Dutch cap or diaphragm is the largest, varying from 2–4 in (5–10 cm) in diameter. It has a strong spring, and when it is in position, the front rim rests on a little ledge on the pubic bone and the back in a small crevice behind the neck of the womb. They are the easiest to use and, for this reason, the most popular. But they are not suitable for some women who have poor pelvic tone, which means their muscles are not strong enough to hold them in place. In these cases, one of the other types of cap can be used.

The cervical cap is much smaller than the Dutch cap; it looks like a thimble with a thickened rim. Some women find it is more difficult to handle, and men can sometimes feel it during intercourse as it is not as flat as the Dutch cap.

The vault cap is a cross between the other two types and, unlike the others, can be made of plastic, so women who are allergic to rubber can use this. Like the cervical cap, this can occasionally be felt by the man.

Using a cap: You cannot just go to the chemist and buy a cap. It must be fitted by a nurse or doctor to make sure it is the right size, as every woman is slightly different inside. A properly fitted cap should stay in place during intercourse without causing discomfort to either you or your partner. If it is uncomfortable or it moves, either it has not been fitted correctly or it simply is not the right type of cap for you.

A spermicide must always be used with a cap. The cap provides only a temporary barrier to sperm, so that the spermicide works during the 6–8 hours it stays in and prevents sperm getting to the cervix. Sperm could otherwise survive for up to two days in the vagina. Squeeze out about a spoonful of spermicidal jelly or cream on to both sides of the cap or diaphragm (note that Dutch caps can be used either way up). Smear more jelly or cream all around the rim and then squeeze the cap into a cigar shape, using your thum and finger to make it easier to insert. You may find it easier to insert if you squat down as this shortens the length of the vagina.

Check that it is in place by making sure you can feel the cervix through the cap. Your doctor or clinic will show you how to do this when you are fitted for a cap. If you do not have intercourse until more than an hour after you have inserted the cap, apply more spermicide without removing the cap. Leave the cap in place for at least six hours after the last ejaculation. To remove a Dutch cap or vault cap, hook a finger over the rim and pull. Cervical caps have a string on which you pull to remove them.

Wash the cap in warm water and check that there are no small holes or faults, especially around the rim. If there are any, see your doctor about replacing the cap and use additional contraceptive measures in the meantime. Dry the cap thoroughly and replace it in its box away from direct sunlight.

A cap can be used during a PERIOD. All that happens is that it will hold back the menstrual flow until it is removed. Keep the cap in for six hours after intercourse and then use a pad or tampon as usual. Intercourse during menstruation can be less messy and, therefore, more pleasant if you do use a cap.

A cap should be checked by your doctor to make sure it still fits at least once a year, especially if you have recently had a baby, gained or lost an excessive amount of weight or only just started having an active sex life.

Benefits: The most important benefit of the cap is that is has virtually no side-effects. Occasionally it causes a slight vaginal irritation and some women find it causes an attack of CYSTITIS (inflammation of the bladder). These conditions are, however, quite minor, and after a diagnosis by your doctor, they can be treated easily and effectively.

A few women find they cannot use any type of cap because their muscles are too relaxed for the cap to stay in place. Some young women may have a vaginal opening that is quite small and they have difficulty inserting it, and some just find it too distasteful. All contraceptives are not suitable for every woman. Doctors will help each one find one that is right for her.

Intra-uterine devices

Intra-uterine devices – commonly known as IUDs or coils – work in a different way from condoms and caps. They are inserted into the womb and, rather than forming a barrier between the sperm and the egg, they prevent a fertilized egg from implanting itself in the womb. Doctors are not sure why they work, but they are known to prevent the lining of the womb from thickening so the right environment for an egg to develop is not created. They are the only form of contraception available – apart from the contraceptive pill – that does not require any pre-intercourse preparation.

Coils come in many shapes and sizes and must be inserted by a medically qualified person under sterile conditions. The most commonly used are the Copper T-380S, Nova T and the Multiloads (especially Cu-375). They have a slightly higher reliability rate (98 per cent) than caps and condoms.

Coils are not a first choice method of contraception for women who have not had children. The womb and cervix have not been stretched by having a baby, and this makes it more difficult, and more painful, to insert a coil and there is more chance of the womb expelling it. There is also a higher chance of side-effects such as painful periods, bleeding and pelvic inflammatory disease.

Most coils come in sterilized packs with a fine plastic tube about 2 mm in diameter used for insertion. A coil is usually implanted just after or during menstruation because the cervix is more relaxed then.

The depth of the womb is checked by passing a small probe through the neck of the cervix. This shows the doctor how deep to insert the coil and also which type is more suitable, as the size of womb varies a great deal. The coil is straightened out inside the tube and the tube is inserted through the cervix. When the correct depth is reached the tube is detached and the coil springs back into shape inside the womb.

The insertion may be a little painful for some women, especially if they are nervous and tighten all their muscles. If the pain, however slight, continues for more than a couple of days, you should see your doctor. Each woman will react differently to having a coil fitted, but it is always a good idea to sit quietly for a while afterwards.

Some women may find they have heavier periods than usual for the first two or three months after having one fitted; sometimes there is a slight spotting between periods, backache or stomach cramp. These normally disappear within a couple of months, but if you are in a lot of pain, see your doctor.

Occasionally a coil may be expelled from the body for no apparent reason.

If this does happen, it is usually within the first three months and may be during menstruation so it can pass unnoticed. Coils all have a fine nylon string attached which hangs down into the vagina, and you should be able to feel this with your finger. If you cannot feel it or it seems longer than usual, you should go back to your doctor. Use some other method of contraception in the meantime.

You should check for the string once a week for the first three months. After this, check it once a month, preferably after menstruation as this is the time it is most likely to become dislodged.

Some men complain that they can feel the string during intercourse, and if this bothers them, it is possible for a doctor to shorten the string. Tampons rarely get caught up in the string, but if you feel a sharp pain when you remove a tampon check the string.

A coil can be left in place for several years, but you should have a medical check-up at least once a year. The copper IUDs have to be changed every three, four or five years according to the manufacturer's recommendations. They discharge small quantities of copper which seems to form part of the contraceptive process.

You are unlikely to get pregnant with a coil in place, but if you suspect you are, see your doctor immediately. It must be removed as it could cause a miscarriage. IUDs do not increase the chances of having an ectopic pregnancy: but if a woman does become pregnant with an IUD fitted, then it is more likely to be an ectopic pregnancy (10 per cent chance).

Morning-after coil: If a woman has had intercourse at the midpoint of her cycle – her most fertile time – without using any contraceptives, some doctors will fit a coil afterwards. It is usually the Copper T-380S, Nova T or Multiload and must be inserted not more than five days from the calculated date of ovulation. It is usually almost 100 per cent effective. It can be removed at the next menstruation and is considered more as a safety measure than a contraceptive.

Douching

It used to be thought that semen could be flushed out of the vagina with hot water or a mild solution hostile to sperm, but this is not so. Not only is it totally unreliable, it can be dangerous. A syringe with a rubber bulb at one end is inserted into the vagina and the contents squeezed out. A dirty syringe can cause infection.

Oral contraceptives

The contraceptive pill is made of synthetic hormones similar to those that occur naturally in a woman's body, and it prevents pregnancy. Some oral contraceptives work by stopping ovulation, others by making it difficult for sperm to reach the egg, or for implantation of a fertilized egg in the uterus' wall to take place.

The *combination pill* is made up of oestrogen and progestogen, and is taken daily for 21 days, followed by seven pill-free days in which a withdrawal bleed takes place. The *progestogen-only pill* (also known as the *mini-pill*) is taken every day. The *triphasic pill* is a type of combination pill, but contains a different amount of the two hormones for different times in the month.

Different types of pill work in different ways. The combined pill has hormones that are very much like those produced by the body when a pregnancy has occurred. This means that the PITUITARY gland, which normally sends a message to the OVARIES to produce their monthly egg, acts as if the body is already pregnant; it therefore does not send its egg-stimulating hormone and so no ovulation takes place.

The progestogen-only pill – the mini-pill – does not always stop ovulation from occurring. It makes fertilization by the sperm more difficult by thickening the mucus in the cervical channel leading from the vagina to the uterus, and inhibits the formation of uterine lining which is necessary for the fertilized egg if it is to implant itself. As a result, implantation (and pregnancy) do not take place.

The progestogen-only pills must be taken every day, and can cause changes in periods while they are being taken. Some women don't have any bleeding for several months; others have frequent breakthrough bleeds during the month. Many women have no problems of this sort at all. Bleeding does not mean that the pill isn't working properly, but if you find irregular bleeding troublesome, ask your doctor's advice. You are probably not pregnant, but if you are more than two weeks overdue, see your doctor. The progestogen-only pill is thought to involve less chance of circulatory problems, so is often a first-choice method for those who may be at risk from this kind of disease.

Effects on the body: The pill has many positive effects, not least the protection from unwanted pregnancy: 99 per cent or more reliability for the combined pill, 98 per cent for the progestogen-only pill. The pill can also actively protect a woman from certain kinds of disorders, such as the formation of benign BREAST lumps, can help to clear up ACNE, and reduce WAX IN THE EARS. Since the body is no longer going through the menstrual cycle, many of the problems associated with periods – PRE-MENSTRUAL SYNDROME, pain, or heavy bleeding – can be alleviated. Research also suggests that there may be some protection against THYROID and uterine disorders, but this has not yet been confirmed.

Troublesome side-effects may occur at the beginning of a course of pills. Some women find that, when they first start taking the pill, they feel slightly sick, or that their breasts become a little swollen and sore. Some women who suffer from MIGRAINES may find that their condition is made worse by the pill, although for others, the opposite is the case. The pill can also affect the ability to wear contact lenses, since the amount of fluid on the surface of the EYE may be reduced. It is also thought that the absorption of some VITAMINS may be slightly reduced, but this does not need to be a problem: the solution is a healthy diet providing more than enough vitamin intake.

DEPRESSION can also be caused by the pill, and in some cases so can loss of *libido* (sex drive). It you suffer from these symptoms, discuss them with your doctor, so that an alternative to the combination pill can be considered.

The most dangerous side-effect of the combination pill is the increased likelihood of BLOOD circulatory disorders, such as high BLOOD PRESSURE, THROMBOSIS, HEART ATTACKS and STROKES. These affect only a tiny minority of women on the pill, and the risk has been greatly reduced by the introduction of those pills containing a lower dose of hormones. However, because the pill does increase the likelihood of these disorders, prospective pill-users must be carefully screened to see if they are particularly at risk. Your own medical history, and that of your family, will need to be studied. SMOKING, being overweight, and being over 35 years of age all increase the risk of these disorders, so women who are in any of these categories are often advised not to use the combination pill. The progestogen-only pill does not seem to carry such risks, and is the one most often prescribed for them.

The progestogen-only pill is not quite so effective in preventing pregnancy as the combined pill. There is a tiny risk that, if an egg is fertilized, it will implant itself outside the womb. This is called an ECTOPIC PREGNANCY, and it can take place in one of the Fallopian tubes. The risk of it happening is very small indeed, but it is a dangerous condition, needing immediate treatment. Any pain in the lower abdomen should be reported to your doctor.

The return of the menstrual cycle may sometimes be delayed once a woman is off the pill, but it is now thought that it does not affect fertility in the long run.

Because of the relatively far-reaching effects of the pill, you should always inform any doctor you consult that you are taking it. A doctor knows what drugs might interfere with each other, and can avoid prescribing those that will reduce the effectiveness of the pill for you. He or she needs to be aware that you are taking it because this sometimes affects the results of laboratory tests. It is particularly important for a doctor to know what pill a woman is taking if she has to have an operation.

The choice of which pill is best for you to start off with will be made by your doctor. Most women start with a low-dose combination pill, and are given three months' supply. Any immediate side-effects should be discussed with your doctor on your next visit, or sooner if you feel that they are serious.

Your doctor will advise you to start taking the combination pill on the first day of your next period. You will be protected as soon as your period ends. The combination pill should be taken at whatever time of day is most convenient for you. Many women find that taking it last thing at night becomes part of a routine which is easy to remember. If a pill is forgotten, but you are not more than 12 hours late in remembering to take it, you will still be protected as long as you continue to take the rest of the packet normally. If you are more than 12 hours late, you will need to use additional contraceptive precautions for the next seven days. However, if those seven days extend beyond the end of your present pack of pills, you must start your next pack the day after you stop your present pack, without the usual seven-day break.

The progestogen-only pill will be taken first on day one of your period, and must be taken *at the same time every day*, since it is not quite so effective in protecting you against conception as the combination pill. You will need to take additional precautions for the first three days. Progestogen-only pills are at their most effective four hours after they are taken, so it is best to do this at a regular time early in the evening. If you are three or more hours late in remembering to take this pill, you should consider yourself unprotected for seven days.

The effectiveness of both sorts of pill may be affected by a stomach upset (either vomiting or diarrhoea), as it could mean that the pill has not been absorbed. If you have an attack of diarrhoea or sickness, follow the same procedure as you would for a missed pill, using additional protection for seven days. Other drugs, such as some ANTIBIOTICS, drugs for EPILEPSY, SEDATIVES and PAINKILLERS, can also reduce the effect of the pill.

You should see your doctor after the first three months on the pill, and thereafter have a check-up every six months. Your blood pressure should be checked, you should have a urine test, and you should be weighed.

Coming off the pill: How long a woman stays on the pill will depend on a number of factors, but doctors do recommend that the pill should not be used continuously for more than ten years without a break.

If you decide you want to get pregnant, it is worth going off the pill straight away to give your body time to get back into the menstrual cycle. You may find that there is a delay before regular periods return. Use other contraceptive methods until you have had two periods, after which time you can try to become pregnant. The delay that sometimes happens between going off the pill and the hoped-for pregnancy may not be due to the pill at all, or it may be that the body needs a little more time before ovulation begins again. If you have tried for a year or more to become pregnant without success, an INFERTILITY clinic may be able to help you.

Women who have to have any major surgery, or who are confined to bed for a time or have a leg in plaster, are advised to come off the pill until they are well again, since these conditions in themselves increase the risk of circulatory problems. Anyone who takes the combination pill would almost certainly have to come off it six weeks before an operation. A woman should, in fact, discuss this point with her doctor, whatever pill she is taking.

Depo-Provera injection

This is an injection of the female sex hormone progesterone given four times a year. It is 100 per cent reliable when given correctly. It is used mainly for women for whom other contraceptive methods are not suitable, and works by completely stopping the production of eggs. There are more side-effects with Depo-Provera than with the contraceptive pill, although they are not the same type of side-effects and serious problems are rare. Periods may become very irregular, and after the first injection, irregular bleeding is quite common, although after a few months, this tends to settle down. Many women then find that their periods stop altogether as long as they continue with the injections. A few women put on weight – often as much as a stone or two. Because Depo-

Provera is a long-acting contraceptive, it should be used only by women who definitely do not want a pregnancy for several years. When it is decided to stop the injections, it may take between six months and two years for the women to conceive. It usually takes about a year before normal ovulation starts again.

New and experimental methods

The Silastic ring is a flexible ring, impregnated with progesterone, which fits inside the vagina in the same way as a diaphragm. It releases the hormones into the body in the quantities normally present during pregnancy. The body is fooled into thinking it is pregnant and does not release any new eggs. The ring is worn for 90 days and then recommended for replacement. The ring moves freely within the vagina.

Another method that fools the body into thinking it is pregnant is a slow-releasing hormone rod the size of a grain of rice. Six of these are implanted under the skin of the arm and slowly dissolve, releasing hormones into the body. The device, called 'Norplant', releases hormones steadily, lasts for five years and is designed to be easily extracted. Since the device was launched, however, there have been many reports of severe side-effects, and the rods have often proved very difficult to remove.

New, more effective spermicides are being tested. The chief problem with present-day spermicides is that they do not affect the mucus in the cervix in any way. So once sperm have entered the cervix, they are beyond the reach of the spermicide. One approach is to develop spermicides that alter the cervical mucus or alter the sperm themselves. Disinfectants are attracting interest because they may also kill viruses, which has implications for sexually transmitted diseases.

Femidom

This is a new female condom which is designed to fit inside the vagina and has a ring to prevent it advancing beyond the vulva. The device is self-lubricating. Its advantage is that it can be inserted before intercourse when required and forms a complete barrier against STDs. Some women have found it unacceptable, but it seems to be less likely to rupture than the male condom.

The rhythm method

This involves a woman working out when she is likely to conceive and making sure that she does not have sexual intercourse during that part of her monthly menstrual cycle. Because it depends on determining which days are 'safe' from the risk of becoming pregnant it is often called the 'safe period' method. However the term is misleading because sexual intercourse, even with contraceptives, is never entirely free from risk of pregnancy. The terms 'natural family planning' or 'periodic abstinence' are much to be preferred.

How does it work?: The menstrual cycle is controlled by hormones. During the early part of the cycle following menstruation, the hormone oestrogen is produced by the ovary. Oestrogen ripens an egg in the ovary and prepares the lining of the uterus to receive it. When all is ready, the ovum is released from the ovary, a process called ovulation. After ovulation, the ovary produces a second hormone, progesterone. This prevents any more ova being released and causes the lining of the womb to secrete nourishment for the ovum should it be fertilized. Ovulation occurs about 14 days before the end of the cycle.

The ovum is available for fertilization for approximately 12 hours after it has been released from the ovary. How long sperm remain alive inside the woman is less certain, but they can lie in wait for up to five days. It is therefore possible to conceive following intercourse during the five days or so before ovulation and for a shorter time after.

So how do women work out the days on which they can have intercourse with less likelihood of becoming pregnant?

Calendar method: Ovulation occurs approximately 14 days before the next period. This formed the basis of the old calendar method. If a women kept a record of her cycles, she could (theoretically) predict the date of the next period and count back to the time of ovulation and the fertile time. It was usual to count back 11 and 18 days to cover the fertile time which occurred between these two dates. Because the date of the next period cannot be predicted with complete accuracy, the calendar method had a high failure rate and has been replaced by records of temperatures and mucus.

Temperature method: Ovulation is accompanied by a rise in body TEMPERATURE. By recording her temperature each day, a woman can know when she has ovulated.

During the early part of the cycle, the body temperature is at its lower level. At the time of ovulation, it shifts to a higher level and stays there until the next period begins, when it falls again. After she has recorded these consecutive daily temperatures at the higher level after the shift, a woman can have intercourse knowing that she has ovulated and that the ovum can no longer be fertilized. Intercourse can continue until the next period, which, on average, will be in 10 or 11 days.

Why must she wait until she has recorded the temperature at the higher level for three days when the ovum can only be fertilized for 12 hours? She needs to be sure her temperature is really on the higher level and has not gone up for a day for some other reason. Also a second ovulation may occur: this is how non-identical twins are conceived, so it must be allowed for. A second ovulation, when it happens, always follows shortly after the first because progesterone prevents the release of ova later.

To get a record from which it is easy to recognize the temperature shift (which is about half a degree Centigrade), the temperature must be taken immediately on waking, before getting out of bed, because the temperature is most stable at that time. It is best to use a 'fertility thermometer', obtainable from any chemist, as it is easier to read, but an ordinary clinical thermometer will do. The temperature must be marked on a specially designed chart. The shift is recognized by applying a simple rule – the first time in the cycle that the woman has three consecutive daily temperatures, all above the level of the previous six, she knows she has ovulated.

A feverish illness cannot be mistaken for ovulation as the temperature rise is much greater and the woman knows she is unwell. If the illness occurs before or after ovulation, it does not prevent the rise of temperature caused by ovulation from being recognized.

The temperature chart does not show when intercourse can take place before ovulation. This information is given by cervical mucus changes.

Mucus changes: In recent years, it has been observed that the appearance and amount of the mucus secreted from the cervix change during the menstrual cycle. Immediately after a period, mucus forms a thick plug at the cervix with the result that the vagina feels positively dry. As the time of ovulation approaches, the plug softens and mucus begins to flow from the vagina so that women usually become aware of a vaginal discharge. This starts as whitish, sticky mucus which gradually increases in amount and becomes clearer until a day or so before ovulation, when it is clear and slippery, rather like raw egg white. This gives a definite sensation of wetness in the vagina. The last day of slippery mucus is known as the 'peak'.

Intercourse in the early part of the cycle can take place only when the vagina is dry. As soon as mucus appears, there must be abstinence from intercourse until the fourth day after peak mucus or the third temperature after the shift. This way of ascertaining the time of ovulation through changes in cervical mucus is often called the Billings method, after the doctor who first described it.

Studies are continuing into the chemical changes which occur in the cervical mucus during the monthly cycle. Attempts are also being made to develop for home use special paper strips to test the level of these chemicals.

Advantages and disadvantages: The rhythm method is free from the risk of medical side-effects as may occur with the pill or intra-uterine device. In addition, there is nothing to interrupt love-making as there is with the condom or diaphragm. On the other hand, it makes considerable demands on a couple's mutual understanding and self-control. Abstinence may not be easy. In fact, in a large survey of couples using the rhythm method, the majority found abstinence difficult, although they considered the method had helped their relationship.

Charting temperatures and observing mucus changes give women an insight into the way their bodies work which many appreciate. The days when menstruation and all that goes with it were mysterious and not to be enquired into are gone. Women like to know what is going on inside their bodies; they also find it useful to know when to expect their periods, which they can if they know when they have ovulated.

Detecting ovulation may be more difficult at times of physical change, such as coming off the pill, after the birth of a baby or when approaching the

MENOPAUSE. Help from an experienced teacher is required and indeed should be sought by everyone learning the method.

It has been suggested that those who use the rhythm method run an increased risk of having an abnormal baby if conception accidentally occurs. If a couple do not wait quite long enough after ovulation, intercourse may result in fertilization of an ovum at the end of its short life span when it is beginning to deteriorate. Much work has been done on this, and while it remains a possibility, there is no conclusive evidence that this is the case.

Does the rhythm method work?: Couples use the rhythm method for a variety of reasons. Some women have been advised to come off the pill, or have become nervous about it and dislike using condoms or diaphragms. Still others are seeking to 'live better naturally' with the foods they eat, the exercise they take, and with family planning, natural childbirth and breastfeeding. Yet others have ethical or religious objections to the alternative contraceptive methods.

Whatever the reason, for the rhythm method to work a couple must be strongly motivated and properly instructed. Motivation is important in all types of family planning; in the rhythm method, it is vital. Mutual agreement about abstinence from intercourse, without at the same time allowing love to grow cold, is essential. Given that agreement and understanding, periods of abstinence can make the time of intercourse more satisfying – each month is a new honeymoon. But if mutual agreement is not there, natural family planning can be destructive to a relationship between a man and a woman.

Although the rhythm method is not as reliable as the pill, it can be as reliable as condoms or diaphragms. When motivation is good and couples have been properly instructed by an experienced teacher, it gives a reasonable degree of protection against pregnancy and provides a method of family planning which many people find more natural than the other available alternatives.

Convulsions

A convulsion is a term describing the seizures that can occur in EPILEPSY and is due to a paroxysmal discharge of neurones in the brain. Epilepsy is the continuing tendency to have such seizures, even if a long interval separates the attacks. Causes of convulsions are varied: a high fever in young children especially can cause 'febrile convulsions'. Other causes are MENINGITIS, brain TUMOURS, STROKES, head injuries, drugs and ALCOHOL withdrawal.

Copper, *see* **Minerals**

Cornea, *see* **Blindness, Eyes and eyesight**

Corns and calluses

A corn is a localized area of hard, horny SKIN, which has formed as a result of repeated rubbing or pressure. Dead skin cells build up and create a thickening of the *keratin* (protein) in the skin. As this piles up, the deeper skin cells underneath become inflamed, causing pain and discomfort. There is basically only one type of corn, although those that are very large are usually called *calluses*.

Causes

Corns are likely to occur whenever there is excessive wear on the skin. Manual labourers and barefoot walkers develop pads of hard skin, which are quite normal, never painful and therefore not true corns. In other people, such as violinists, who are continually rubbing their chin against wood, or those wearing a new pair of tight shoes, pads of skin may form at the site of the rubbing, causing considerable pain. These are true corns.

Although ill-fitting shoes and high heels do cause corns, the most common sites are on the ball of the foot, the side of the toes between the joints, and sometimes, on the heel (*see* FEET).

Corns frequently form over BUNIONS, although there is no special association between the two. The reason is simply that the bunion, being a prominent bone, presses against the side of footwear, causing pressure. Corns invariably appear over the bony prominences where the hard skin protects delicate structures underneath. Some people are more susceptible to corns than others; this is particularly true of the elderly.

Calluses can also develop where artificial limbs or appliances (prostheses) rub on the skin and, as such, are a normal response of the skin to excessive wear. In such cases, they can be useful, taking the brunt of pressure and impact and thus protecting the skin; but occasionally they may become uncomfortable and need trimming.

Symptoms

A corn can be recognized as an area of hardened, thickened skin, which often looks yellow in comparison to the surrounding skin. It can be conical in shape. Corns between the toes can be soft.

Corns may first be noticed because they cause aching at the end of the day or because they feel tender under pressure. When chronic or severe, the surrounding area may be slightly red and the corn extremely painful, even when the patient is at rest.

Symptoms vary considerably, and it is sometimes difficult to tell a corn from a VERRUCA (plantar wart). In general, verrucas are initially small and painful on pressure. When the top skin is rubbed off, tiny black roots will appear as dots; the area may then be seen as a WART.

Dangers

Corns are uncomfortable and painful, but only rarely dangerous. There is a more serious condition known as *hyperkeratosis*, in which the skin of the palms and soles thickens for no known reason, and soon spreads. Medical attention should be sought immediately.

The chief danger of corns is that as the skin is pared off as part of treatment, infection will occur due to the use of unclean instruments or too much skin being pared. For this reason it is important to pare a corn very carefully indeed.

DIABETICS are at special risk of complications from corns. Their blood circulation is likely to be poor, and the feet may also be less sensitive to pain.

Treatment

As corns are merely hard skin, they can be treated by removing the excess.

After a good soaking in the bath, a pumice stone should be rubbed over the corn. This is enough to keep some people's corns at bay. For more well-developed corns, scraping off the skin with a scraper or paring the corn with a safety knife is necessary. The tools used should be kept clean. The fine slivers of dead skin should be removed until soft pliable skin is felt beneath the corn. Care should be taken not to pare away too much skin; this could cause bleeding or introduce infection. Other tools may be used to remove corns, including a file or an emery board.

Corn plasters remove skin by softening it with chemicals: a 40 per cent salicylic acid is soaked on to a plaster. The plaster should be applied directly over the corn and left for 24 hours. The skin should then be lifted off with a pumice stone or corn grater. If the corn persists, further applications of plaster may be used.

Some older people become so accustomed to tolerating their corns that they cease to attend to them, simply padding them so that they are not painful. A variety of products for this purpose is available, the simplest being a ring of foam rubber on a sticky base with a hole in the middle.

Calluses can also be treated by applying a solution containing salicylic acid on a plaster and then paring them down.

Coronary heart disease

The HEART is a muscular bag which pumps BLOOD round the body. Like any muscle, it must be supplied with OXYGEN and food to continue working. This supply is carried in the right and left coronary ARTERIES, which are the first vessels to leave the *aorta* (the body's main artery) as it emerges from the heart.

Almost as soon as it branches off the aorta, the left coronary artery splits into two big branches. So there are, in effect, three coronary arteries: the right and the two branches of the left. They go on to completely encircle and penetrate the heart, supplying blood to every part of it.

A continuous supply of blood to the heart muscle is essential for the normal functioning of the heart. But unfortunately, all too often, the coronary arteries become diseased – a condition known as coronary heart disease. This in turn can lead to symptoms such as *angina*, or sometimes to a HEART ATTACK.

Coronary heart disease is one of the commonest and most serious diseases in the Western world. The earliest stage of disease that can be detected is the build-up of fatty material in the lining of the coronary arteries. This early stage may even begin in teenagers. Gradually this fatty deposit grows larger until it forms a *plaque,* or *atheroma,* which reduces the internal diameter of the coronary artery, so restricting the flow of blood through the artery. The process by which the fatty tissue clogs up the coronary artery is not completely understood, but it undoubtedly depends to some extent on the level of certain fats in the bloodstream. The plaques may also enlarge by microscopic blood clots becoming attached to their surface. However, it is now known that a number of factors are responsible for the development of coronary heart disease.

Risk factors

Research has been carried out comparing populations where there is very little coronary heart disease with those populations where there is a great deal, and the result of such studies have shown that certain factors – known as risk factors – are important in triggering the development of the disease. Somebody who has just one or two risk factors, has a small increase in risk. But somebody with several risk factors faces a much greater chance of developing coronary heart disease – often eight or ten times the risk for a 'normal' or average person.

Age and sex: There is a gradual increase in the risk of developing coronary heart disease with increasing age. The disease is rare in people less than 30 years old, but in men, the risk increases gradually beyond this age up to the 70s, when it is by far the commonest cause of death. In women, however, the increased risk of coronary heart disease starts slightly later. It begins to increase significantly only in the 40s, but then increases steadily in line with the increase in the rates for men, although it is always slightly less common in women.

Cigarette smoking: SMOKING is the most important cause of preventable death from coronary heart disease. Somebody who smokes up to 20 cigarettes a day has double the usual risk of developing the disease, and anybody who smokes up to 40 cigarettes a day has four times the usual risk. It appears that the various chemicals and toxins in cigarette smoke increase the likelihood of FATS being deposited in the walls of the coronary arteries, but smoking also increases the risk of a heart attack occurring by altering the way in which the blood clots.

High blood pressure: Abnormally high BLOOD PRESSURE is also a risk factor for coronary heart disease. Over the years, a high blood pressure level can lead to an increase in the amount of atheroma in the coronary arteries, and this may double the risk of coronary heart disease. In the early stages of high blood pressure – also called *hypertension* – there are no symptoms at all; it can be detected only when a doctor or nurse checks the blood pressure.

High cholesterol level in the blood: Cholesterol is a type of fat that is normally present in the bloodstream. Its level appears to be directly related to the risk of developing coronary heart disease – a very high level can treble the risk. The level of cholesterol in the bloodstream is related to some extent to the amount of 'saturated' fat in the diet. This type of fat is found in fatty meat and dairy produce, such as cream, full-cream milk, butter and cheese. Certain foods, such as egg yolks, do contain cholesterol, but the level in the bloodstream does not appear to be related so much to dietary cholesterol levels as to the amount of animal fat in the diet. The level of cholesterol is also determined to some extent by heredity.

Family history: Coronary heart disease can run in families, and a positive family history of coronary heart disease is an independent risk factor for an individual suffering similar illness.

Overweight and lack of exercise: Both of these are sometimes considered as risk factors, because there is no doubt that anyone who is very fat or unfit is at greater risk of developing coronary heart disease. However, it is probable that an overweight person is at more risk because he or she tends to have higher blood pressure and a higher cholesterol level. The same is true for people who are unfit. So becoming fitter or losing weight reduces the risk of coronary heart disease by reducing blood pressure and blood cholesterol levels.

Stress: Many people believe that STRESS is an important cause of coronary heart disease, but there is considerable controversy about this in the medical world. Certainly stress alone is much less of a risk factor than cigarette smoking or a high cholesterol level, but there is some evidence that continual stress can cause higher blood pressure than usual. In addition, a sudden stressful event can trigger off a heart attack in someone who already has coronary heart disease.

Multiple factors: In men aged between 45 and 60 years, the average risk of having a heart attack in any one year is about 1 per cent; in other words, one man in 100 in this age group has a heart attack. For a man with untreated high blood pressure, the odds go up to 1 in 50; for a heavy smoker the odds are about 1 in 25. But if a man has both untreated high blood pressure and is a heavy cigarette smoker, the risk in any one year is as high as 1 in 12 or 15.

Heart attack

See pages 352–3.

Angina

The other problem which coronary artery disease causes is angina. In this case, there is a partial block which allows the heart to function normally at rest but does not allow the extra blood flow necessary in response to exercise.

This relative lack of blood flow produces pain – the typical chest pain of angina which spreads to the arms, shoulders or neck. It is usually brought on by exertion or excitement and only lasts a few minutes. Patients who have angina may go on to develop a full-blown heart attack, and, conversely, patients who have had a heart attack may subsequently get attacks of angina.

Angina may, however, be a crippling disease even when the patient has not suffered a heart attack. At its worst, it may be impossible for the patient to move more than a few yards without pain. Fortunately, modern treatment has made a considerable impact on angina, in terms of preventing the symptoms.

There are three main groups of drugs that are used against the symptoms of angina: the nitrates, the beta-blockers and calcium-channel blockers. The nitrates have been used since the early part of the century. They act by widening the coronary arteries. Patients usually carry these pills about with them. When slipped under the tongue, they quickly stop attacks. They can also be used before any exercise that is likely to bring on an angina attack, to prevent the pain from occurring.

There has, however, been a treatment for angina since the development of the *beta-blockers* (*see* AUTONOMIC NERVOUS SYSTEM) in the mid-1960s – a great medical advance. These drugs block some of the effects (the so-called *beta effects*) of adrenalin (*see* ADRENAL GLANDS). In so doing, they also reduce the amount of work the heart has to do and therefore its need for oxygen. Taken regularly, not just when there is a pain, they not only reduce the number of attacks of angina but probably have some effect in preventing heart attacks. They can also reduce the mortality following a heart attack if prescribed within the first 24 hours. Unfortunately they are unsuitable for ASTHMA sufferers.

Calcium channel blockers also aim to widen the coronary arteries, and are safe to be taken by asthma sufferers.

Aspirin should also be taken by angina sufferers and immediately following a heart attack. It reduces the ability of the blood to form clots which can block off the coronary arteries.

Surgery

As an alternative to medical treatment, the last 20 or so years has seen a considerable advance in surgery for the treatment of coronary artery disease: *bypass surgery* and *angioplasty*.

Cortisol, *see* Adrenal glands

Cot death

There is nothing more tragic and disturbing for a family than the unexpected and unexplained death of a young baby. An apparently healthy baby is put to bed in a crib, cot or pram. When next looked at, it is dead, and for no obvious reason. This sad phenomenon, known as cot death, or *sudden infant death syndrome* (SIDS), is one of the most pressing and perplexing problems facing doctors. It is among the commonest causes of death among young babies – about 1 baby in every 500 dies from cot death.

Cot deaths are most common among babies aged between four weeks and one year, and occur particularly between the ages of two and four months. Apparently there are more cases among boys, twins and babies whose birth weight was low. They also happen more during the autumn and winter (often coinciding with local epidemics and influenza), and more often to bottle-fed babies.

There are no warning signs and death most often occurs when the baby has been left alone, often briefly in its pram or first thing in the morning in its cot.

Symptoms

Probably one of the most puzzling aspects of cot deaths is that there appear to be no warning signals of any kind. Yet recent research has shown that, in some cases, there may have been minor signs in the preceding few days. These may include a cold, the 'snuffles', listlessness, drowsiness or even a breathing difficulty. Some babies who die from cot death have shown a slight temperature.

In many cases, the baby was in its cot, and appeared to have a completely peaceful death – as if he or she just stopped breathing and died. Sometimes the baby simply dies in its mother's arms.

Possible causes of cot death

Whenever a child dies suddenly without obvious cause, it is a legal requirement in Britain that a pathologist examines the baby after death. In about a third of all cases of 'sudden infant death', the pathologist discovers a cause. It may be an infection, or a previously undiscovered internal abnormality such as congenital heart defect (in which the baby is born with an abnormality in the structure of the heart; *see* HEART DISEASE).

In at least two-thirds of all cases of cot death, however, a routine autopsy is quite unable to determine any apparent cause of death.

Infections

When a baby is born, it has quite a high resistance to infection because its bloodstream contains various antibodies transferred to it from the mother's circulation (while the foetus was in the womb). But over the first few weeks of life, these antibodies gradually disappear, and it takes several months for the baby to develop its own antibodies. For this reason, the level of antibodies in a baby's blood are at their lowest between the ages of two and four months. The baby is therefore most susceptible to infection during this time. It is thought that certain mild virus infections, or toxins from bacterial infections, could have a much more severe effect on a baby at this time than is normally the case with older children.

Abnormalities in temperature control

Once it was established that cot deaths are more common in winter than in summer, research has concentrated on possible explanations associated with changes in the baby's temperature. Paradoxically the evidence suggests that it may not be cold but an excessively high body temperature that should be associated with cot death. A baby is usually well wrapped up or kept in a vary warm room during winter. An ideal room temperature for the baby is 65°F (18°C). Thermometers are now widely available in children's shops to monitor the room temperature.

Heart problems

Some babies may die as a result of a previously unrecognized congenital abnormality of the heart.

Several researchers have investigated the hearts of babies who have died from cot death. The studies show that there may be minor abnormalities in the structure of the specialized parts of the heart that trigger the heart beat. Minor abnormalities in the function of parts of the heart may also occur as a feature of the normal development of these tissues, as the baby grows. The heart beat may then simply fail as a result of the type of electrical defect in the heart – possibly without any warning.

Allergy

More babies who are bottle fed appear to suffer cot death than those who are breast fed, but the reasons for this are unclear.

Breathing problems

Over the past few years, attention has been focused on the 'apnoea' theory. The word *apnoea* simply means cessation of breathing. Many people – adults, children and babies – have brief periods of apnoea lasting a few seconds in certain stages of deep sleep. Usually, this period of apnoea stops with a deep breath and then the normal rhythm of breathing continues. It is possible that, due to developmental defect, or simply immaturity in the brain centre that controls breathing, some babies are unable to switch from apnoea back into normal breathing rhythm.

Smoking

Deaths from cot death are much higher in families whose parents SMOKE (along with other respiratory illnesses). Cigarette smoke contains high levels of antimony, a substance which has possibly been implicated in causing cot death. It is therefore essential that parents do not smoke near young babies.

Posture

Most recent research has shown that babies should be put to sleep on their backs or sides – not on their fronts. Following this advice has dramatically reduced the number of cot deaths.

Mattresses

Much recent controversy has centred around concerns that substances used as fire retardants in mattresses (phosphorus and antimony) might be given off as a vapour if the baby became overheated and be involved in causing cot death. However, there is great debate about whether this is the case or not, though most manufacturers of mattresses have responded by no longer using these fire retardants.

Prevention of cot death

Since no one cause of cot death has been established, prevention is still very much a matter of commonsense care of the baby. It makes sense to try to breastfeed the baby – breast milk will provide additional antibodies to help the baby fight any infection, and reduce the risk of allergy. It is a good idea to keep a thermometer in the baby's room to check that the room temperature is right – not too hot or cold. It should be between 65°F (18°C) and 70°F (22°C). Light but warm bedclothes are also important. Babies should sleep only on their backs or sides until they are old enough to roll over on their own. Parents should not smoke near their babies.

If you suspect illness in a small baby, do not hesitate to ask for a doctor's advice – particularly if the baby has a very high temperature that you cannot bring down with cooling and paracetamol syrup.

Since the apnoea theory of cot death has received a great deal of attention, some parents who have already experienced a cot death or perhaps found their baby in an apnoeic attack, have used 'apnoea alarms' to monitor their baby's breathing at all times. These alarms are devices which consist of a small box of electronics, battery operated, connected to a sensor which is strapped to the baby's chest. The alarm gives an audible signal if the baby stops breathing, allowing the parents to check the baby and, if necessary, help the baby to start breathing again using artificial respiration.

However, it is far from clear whether or not the use of these alarms can actually save babies' lives. Normal children have apnoeic attacks, and there does not seem to be any clear relationship between the number of apnoeic attacks a child has and the possibility of cot death.

The alarm may, however, reassure parents of otherwise healthy babies to some extent, even though there may well be many false alarms. There are a very small number of clearly defined conditions when an apnoea alarm may be recommended by doctors.

Effects on the family

For the parents, profound shock is probably the first reaction, followed by feelings of guilt. Older children, who may have felt jealous or resentful of the baby, also suffer badly from guilt. It is essential for all the family to 'talk out' their feelings with an understanding outsider. Comfort and practical help can be sought from close friends, the family doctor, health visitor or a clergyman, and there are also self-help groups whose members have personal experience of cot deaths.

Coughs

A cough is the result of an explosive current of air being driven forcibly from the chest. It forms part of a protective reflex to ensure that the air passages remain free of any obstruction. As soon as the obstruction has been cleared, coughing stops. Irritation of the upper airways by noxious gases, or inflammation by infections, causes coughing by a similar mechanism, but in this case, the coughing is persistent.

A cough is a reflex action, triggered by foreign material in the windpipe or breathing passages. The cough is therefore a normal protective mechanism in that its function is to expel any foreign and potentially dangerous material and clear the BREATHING passages again. Dust from the air breathed in or cigarette SMOKE can cause coughing, but usually the commonest cause is the collection of mucus in the lungs and air passages. Coughing helps to clear this mucus, and so trying to suppress a cough with medicines may do more harm than good. Occasionally abnormal tissue or growths in the lungs can cause coughs because these tissues also irritate the lung lining and trigger the cough reflex.

Symptoms and treatment

Coughing, as such, is not a disease, though it may be indicative of some respiratory problem. The most important symptom is not the cough itself, but rather the material which is coughed up, the frequency of the coughing and whether there is any accompanying pain.

Most coughs, particularly those accompanying COLDS, are not dangerous and settle after a few days. A persistent cough of any type should however be investigated by a doctor. This is particularly important if there are other symptoms such as HOARSENESS, pains in the chest, breathlessness, fever or any coughing of blood.

One of the commonest types of cough is a dry, irritating cough. This can occur in the early stages of a cold as the lining of the breathing passages becomes inflamed. However, chronic inflammation of these passages may also be associated simply with smoking. Cigarette smoke destroys some of the natural protective mechanisms of the lung lining.

A tickling cough can often be caused by mucus dripping down the back of the nose ('post-nasal drip') and down the throat, thus irritating the vocal cords. This can be accompanied by the need to clear the throat repeatedly. In this case, treatment involves clearing up the nasal congestion leading to this problem.

A persistent dry cough associated with a fever may be the first signs of a lung infection such as PNEUMONIA. If there is hoarseness as well, there is a possibility of an infection in the LARYNX or voice-box (laryngitis). Any hoarseness in an adult that persists for more than a few weeks should be investigated by a specialist, because there is a possibility of a cancerous growth in the larynx, which can be treated successfully if discovered early, although more often the cause is a simple infection.

A 'productive cough' is one associated with some phlegm which comes up with the cough. A little clear white phlegm is common in the later stages of a cold, but thick yellow phlegm usually indicates the onset of infection, such as BRONCHITIS. Some smokers regularly bring up some thick phlegm, particularly in the mornings. This indicates the early stages of damage to the LUNGS by chronic bronchitis.

Sometimes a productive cough may occur with HEART problems even though there may be no lung disease or disorder. If the heart is not working as efficiently as it should, fluid can accumulate in the lungs as a result of back pressure building up in the veins leading from the lungs to the heart. This fluid can trigger off a productive cough; the phlegm is thin, frothy and often slightly pink because it is tinged with blood.

A cough associated with breathing difficulty tends to indicate a more serious problem. If the cough is caused by heart failure, it may be accompanied by quite severe shortness of breath. This may be so bad as to be a real medical emergency: anyone who is coughing and severely breathless should be seen as soon as possible by a doctor.

Bronchitis may be accompanied not only by a productive cough but some wheezing as well. The patient often complains that his or her chest feels 'rattly'.

ASTHMA can cause not only coughing, which is often worse at night, but also a characteristic type of wheezing in which it is harder for the sufferer to breathe out than it is to breathe in. Indeed, persistent coughing can be one of the early signs of asthma in children, and may occur long before the child develops any difficulty with breathing. Often such children also have chronic nasal CATARRH.

In children, if a cough is initially dry and then produces mucus and eventually turns into a barking, noisy cough with laboured breathing, *croup* is a possibility. Coughs that are violent and occur in spasms associated with vomiting and possibly a 'crowing' noise may indicate WHOOPING COUGH.

Coughing with pain is also an indicator of possibly serious conditions. PLEURISY is an infection of the lungs and the membrane covering them, which produces a sharp pain in the chest with deep breathing or coughing.

If the cough is accompanied by the production of blood, then medical attention is essential. Possible causes include viral or bacterial infections, TUBERCULOSIS, or heart failure; it may also be a symptom of some types of lung CANCER.

Treatment

Minor coughs usually get better on their own without any treatment at all. In fact, to suppress the cough with medicines may be harmful and, especially if it is a productive cough, may delay relief.

If you have a cough associated with a cold, you can get relief by using decongestant drops or a nose spray to relieve nasal CATARRH which might otherwise trickle down the back of the throat and cause more coughing. A warm soothing drink helps – honey and lemon is a good standby. Soothing fruit-based cough medicines can be tried, but are little better than an ordinary drink.

A dry cough can be treated with a cough suppressant such as pholocodeine linctus, but if it persists it is wise to consult a doctor.

Counselling, *see* **Mental therapies**

Couvade, *see* **Abdomen**

Coxsackie virus, *see* **Diaphragm, Motor neurone disease**

Cradle cap, *see* **Skin and skin diseases**

Cramps, *see* **Muscles, Periods and period pains**

Crepitus, *see* **Fractures, Osteoarthritis, Tendons**

Cretinism, *see* **Enzymes, Thyroid**

Creutzfeldt–Jakob disease

This is a slowly progressive dementia characterized pathologically by 'spongiform encephalopathy'. It is due to infection by a 'slow virus' which is resistant to usual sterilization processes. It has a long incubation period, up to several years. Symptoms are of increasing confusion and dementia. Infection has been found to be transmitted to children who were given growth hormone extracts (extracted from post-mortem pituitary specimens) to help them grow. Once the symptoms of dementia have begun, death is inevitable, usually within two years.

Treatment

At present there is no known cure. Concern has been raised because the disease in humans resembles that of 'mad cow disease' in cows, prompting the concern that it might be transmitted by eating infected meat. However, there is at present no definite evidence that this can occur.

Crohn's disease

Crohn's disease is a type of inflammatory bowel disease, the other main condition in this group being ulcerative colitis (*see* COLON AND COLITIS). Some of their features overlap. It occurs at any age, but particularly between the ages of 20 and 40 years, and affects both sexes equally.

Symptoms

Crohn's disease affects segments of the small and large bowel, causing intermittent fevers, weight loss, abdominal pain and distension, and diarrhoea. It can also present with right-sided abdominal pain and mimic appendicitis. Patients with extensive disease can have frequent relapses requiring hospital treatment. Occasionally, patients may have other parts of the body other than the bowel involved, such as joints, skin and eyes.

Investigations

Blood tests show ANAEMIA and abnormal liver function. X-RAYS of the bowel will be performed, especially a BARIUM X-ray of the small and large bowels. To confirm the diagnosis, biopsies of the bowel will need to be performed via an endoscope called a colonoscope.

Treatment

Patients with mild disease will just require symptomatic treatment, for example codeine phosphate to control their diarrhoea. Vitamins will be given to help correct deficiencies and anaemia. More serious disease will require treatment with STEROID tablets and other drugs to suppress the immune system such as azathioprine. Approximately 80 per cent of patients will require some form of operation at some stage to treat their Crohn's disease. The operation will remove part of the bowel, and it may be necessary for the patient to have a temporary or permanent colostomy.

Croup, *see* **Breathing, Coughs, Larynx and laryngitis**

Cryptococcosis, *see* **Fungal infections**

CT (computerized tomography) scan, *see* **Neurology and neurosurgery, X-rays**

Cushing's disease, *see* **Blood pressure, Hormones, Pituitary, Steroids**

Cyanosis, *see* **Blue baby, Bronchitis, Emphysema, Heart disease, Ischaemia**

Cystic fibrosis

This is an inherited condition in which there is abnormal mucus production by all the body's glands: it affects mostly the lungs and the pancreas. Cystic fibrosis is the result of a chromosome abnormality (on chromosome number 7) and is carried by 1 in 20 of the Caucasian population. It is unknown in the Afro-Caribbean population.

Symptoms

One of the first signs may be in a baby, when the small intestine becomes obstructed or blocked by very thick secretions called meconium, a condition called meconium ileus. In infancy and childhood the affected child develops recurrent chest infections requiring antibiotics and regular physiotherapy. Patients are taught to do their own physiotherapy called 'postural drainage' at home on a daily basis. For some reason the fingers develop a characteristically rounded appearance called clubbing. The pancreas can also be affected, causing malabsorption and DIABETES mellitus. Puberty may be delayed and children will be of short stature. Males are usually infertile, but females can conceive.

Diagnosis

This is by means of a skin test called a 'sweat test'. Genetic tests are now also available to reveal whether someone is a carrier.

Treatment

Regular antibiotic courses may be needed to treat chest infections. Dietary supplements are very important in maintaining body strength and general well-being. Diabetes may be treated with insulin injections. In end-stage disease, further treatments such as oxygen may be needed, and the patient may receive a heart-lung transplant.

Prognosis

The life-expectancy of sufferers has increased significantly over the last 10 years and now averages 30 years. This is due to better antibiotic and nutritional treatments. New treatments as the result of 'gene therapy' (i.e. replacing the abnormal gene) are now becoming available, as are drugs that are more efficient at breaking down the abnormally viscous secretions. Antenatal diagnosis can now also be performed on couples who have had a previously affected child or who are at high risk.

Cystitis

This is inflammation of the BLADDER. It is a common but distressing condition, which affects women much more than men; it is estimated that 80 per cent of women suffer an attack at some time in their lives.

The bladder is a stretchy muscular bag which collects and stores URINE until it is emptied. When the bladder becomes inflamed there are three basic symptoms: frequency of urination – the bladder signals 'full' much more often than usual, even though there is hardly any urine to pass; pain when urinating; and sometimes blood in the urine. These symptoms vary in intensity.

A woman's first sign of cystitis is a pricking pain, which can quickly become a burning, scalding sensation during urination. Gradually this develops into a sharp pain in the lower abdomen.

Causes

Cystitis is most commonly caused by BACTERIA called *E. coli* (*Escherichia coli*). *E. coli* live in the BOWEL and, like other bacteria which live in the body, are not harmful in this area, and sometimes even useful. The problems arise when

E. coli is transferred from the bowel and comes into contact with the urinary organs.

The design of the female body makes it all too easy for bacteria to be accidentally transferred from the bowel opening to the URETHRA (the tube leading out from the bladder). A woman's bowel opening, VAGINA, and urethra are all very close together. What's more, bacteria only have to travel about 1 in (2.5 cm) from the outside of a woman's body to the bladder, whereas to reach a man's bladder from the tip of the PENIS is 6 in (15 cm) or more.

E. coli flourishes in an acidic environment, and because normal urine is quite acidic, it thrives in the urinary passages. As it multiplies, which it does very rapidly, it causes an inflammation which, unless checked, can spread from the urethral opening and up into the bladder, ureters and, finally, the kidneys. If the infection reaches the kidneys, it is called *pyelitis* and, unless a cure is prompt, the infection can do lasting damage. The earlier the infection is checked, the better.

In some cases of recurrent pain on urination, the urethra becomes chronically inflamed – a condition known as *urethral syndrome*. This may be due to a deficiency in the female hormone oestrogen, and an oral supplement will usually cause the inflammation to subside. So urethral syndrome is not the same as cystitis.

Sex and cystitis

Cystitis used to sometimes be called 'honeymoon disease' because many women experience their first attack of cystitis when they first have SEXUAL INTERCOURSE. Because the urethral opening is so close to the vagina, frequent or very active sexual intercourse can lead to bruising of the tissue at the vaginal and urethral openings. Genital skin in both the male and the female is ten times more sensitive than any other skin on the body. The bruised tissues can easily harbour infection which then enters the bladder.

If the vagina is not moist and well-lubricated when a woman has sex, bruising can occur to the vaginal tissue. This becomes a breeding ground for bacteria and can result in infection. Some men inadvertently carry harmful bacteria under the foreskin of the penis. If you are prone to cystitis, the answer is not to give up sex, but matters may improve if both you and your partner take special care to keep this area very clean. This is even more important if your partner has not been circumcised.

Changes in the female HORMONAL cycle may make a woman more likely to suffer cystitis. If an attack occurs shortly after the onset of PERIODS, during PREGNANCY, after having had a baby, the MENOPAUSE or a total HYSTERECTOMY, it is worth mentioning this when you seek help from your doctor. Some experts believe that even when such dramatic hormonal changes have not taken place recently, hormone imbalance may be at the root of much unexplained recurrent cystitis.

Hormone imbalance can affect, among other things, the balance of acidity or alkalinity in the urine, or the level of moisture in the vagina – both of these may influence the likelihood of an attack of cystitis. The hormonal system itself is triggered by a variety of complex factors, and STRESS or DEPRESSION may disrupt the hormonal cycle.

If cystitis keeps recurring, it is worth considering what form of CONTRACEPTION is being used. A badly fitted diaphragm or cap may lead to bruising, and spermicidal foams or jellies may be causing irritation to the genital area.

The contraceptive pill, which works by 'tricking' the hormonal system, has been shown to make women using it more susceptible to common non-bacterial vaginal infections such as THRUSH and such infections can trigger cystitis symptoms. The germs which cause some SEXUALLY TRANSMITTED DISEASES, such as HERPES and TRICHOMONIASIS are also sometimes responsible for causing cystitis to flare up. Some women have found that cystitis occurs much less often when they stop using the pill.

Cystitis can also be related to blockage in the urinary system, such as KIDNEY stones, CYSTS or a thickening of the bladder walls, but these problems are less common and are usually corrected by surgery.

Cystitis tends to recur in some people. Many women get it three or four times a year and some have it once a month. This seems to be because the tissues situated in a previously infected area are weaker and more susceptible to re-infection, although some women seem especially prone to it.

Children and cystitis

Children, even babies, can get cystitis. As with adults, it is much more common in girls than in boys. It may not be all that easy to identify as they may show only the signs of general illness – fever, fretfulness, even vomiting – rather than bladder pain and a 'need to go'. Sometimes, however, the classic symptoms of pain and a need to pass urine every few minutes may be present in a young girl.

One reason may be that the child is not drinking enough liquid during the day. This can make the urine very concentrated so that, when it is passed, there is a burning feeling. This in itself does not constitute an attack but, if not remedied, can inflame the urethral tissues and result in cystitis. It is most important to check that a girl knows how to clean her bottom from front to back, so that germs from the bowel are less likely to come near the bladder opening. Luckily children respond very quickly to treatment for cystitis, but it is important to teach those who are old enough how they can prevent another attack.

Sometimes a minor internal abnormality of the kidneys or ureter may occur in children, which makes them more prone to cystitis. There is also a risk of infection travelling to the kidneys if a child has cystitis, so any attack should be reported to a doctor so that it can be properly investigated.

Treatment

It is most important to do something about an attack of cystitis straight away. By following the self-help tips here (*see box*) you can reduce the painful symptoms and prevent the infection spreading.

You should see your doctor within a day or two, particularly if you have seen blood in your urine: once the infection takes hold, it can be much more

Self-help for cystitis

Even the most unrelenting cystitis can be self-induced. The following hints can help to prevent it occurring, as well as bring some relief.

- Drink three to five pints of water-based drinks every day. Recent research has shown that cranberry juice can be effective in destroying *E. coli* bacteria.
- Urinate whenever you feel the need. 'Hanging on' can encourage an attack of cystitis.
- Bidets and bowls of water merely dilute bacteria. After defaecating, soap the anus only and pour warm water from a bottle down the area between the vagina and the anus from the front to the back. If away from home, use moistened paper tissues. Dry the area gently but thoroughly. Always wipe from front to back. Use only white tissues because the dye in coloured ones may contribute to soreness.
- Wash the vaginal area before and after making love and get your partner to do the same. Use a lubricant jelly if this helps to prevent soreness. Urinate as soon as possible afterwards to flush out any travelling bacteria.
- Your contraceptive may also be causing cystitis. Ask your doctor's advice.
- Wear cotton pants (never nylon), which should be boiled in plain water away from the family wash. Avoid tights and tight jeans or trousers.
- Do not use antiseptics, talcum powder, perfumed soap or deodorants near your genitals. If you must use soap, use an unperfumed brand. Do not use shampoo, bubble bath or bath oil in the bath, especially a product that contains hexachlorophene.
- Avoid certain foods, such as citrus fruits, soft fruits (strawberries, etc.), hot curries several times a week, and lots of black pepper on every meal – all can irritate the bladder. Try refusing foods with a high refined sugar or starch content.

When cystitis begins:

- Act at once, even if it is at night.
- Drink a pint of bland liquid (ideally cranberry juice) and keep drinking at the rate of half a pint every 20 minutes for three hours.
- Place a hot-water bottle, wrapped in a towel, between your legs. This helps to reduce the burning sensation when you urinate.
- Take one level teaspoonful of bicarbonate of soda in water every hour for at least three hours. (Note: if you have high blood pressure, ask your doctor before trying this remedy.)
- Take one or two mild painkillers if you need them.
- Make yourself as comfortable as possible, relax, and try to take your mind off the pain and anxiety. After three hours, most women find that cystitis begins to wear off.

If cystitis persists:

- Consult your doctor if, despite your self-help, cystitis persists after a day or two, if you are pregnant, or if you see blood in the urine. Ask yourself what might have triggered the attack. Be prepared to give a urine sample.
- Children should always be seen by a doctor.

difficult to treat. If you are pregnant, seeking early medical help is especially important because pregnant women are particularly at risk of kidney infection.

To prevent cystitis recurring, it is important to try to identify what caused it. Before you visit your doctor, drink some water as you may be asked for a sample of urine. The sample can be tested to find out whether your infection is bacterial or non-bacterial. If it is bacterial, you will be given an appropriate antibiotic.

If you are given a course of drugs by your doctor, especially if it is for a condition such as thrush or trichomonas, it's a good idea to check whether your partner should be treated as well. Your partner will not necessarily have any symptoms but might have an infection which is causing your cystitis.

Depending on how well your kidneys are functioning, the doctor may also prescribe potassium citrate, or a similar substance, aimed at reducing the acidity of the urine. Doing this will help stop the burning sensation which makes cystitis such a misery. However, some antibiotics actually work better if the urine remains quite acidic, so ask your doctor about this.

If the doctor decides that a hormone imbalance is causing the problem – for instance, during the menopause or after a total hysterectomy – you may be given medication in the form of creams or tablets, or referred to a specialist.

If cystitis attacks keep recurring, you may be sent for an X-ray to see whether there is any physical blockage or abnormality in the kidneys, bladder and tubes. The test – an *intravenous pyelogram* or *IVP* – involves injecting dye into a vein in your arm. After a while, allowing the dye to circulate through the blood system and through the kidneys, it is possible to X-ray the kidneys and the structure of the tubes that collect the urine coming out of the kidney. If a physical cause is found, simple surgery may cure it.

Some people have found that diet is an important way of reducing the risk of recurrent cystitis. Alcohol is almost certainly an irritant for a cystitis-prone bladder, and strong coffee or tea should also be avoided.

Cystocoele, *see* **Incontinence, Prolapse**

Cysts

A cyst is any abnormal sac within the body which contains fluid and sometimes solid matter. These sacs can occur in virtually any organ or tissue in the body and can be tiny or large enough to contain many pints of fluid.

Most cysts are *benign*, in that they expand but do not spread elsewhere or invade surrounding tissue. Others are *malignant* (CANCEROUS) and will eventually spread and invade other tissues.

There is no self-treatment for cysts. In virtually every case, the exact type and characteristic of the cyst must be determined by the doctor to see if it is cancerous. Usually the cyst is removed surgically and then sent to the laboratory for tests.

The common cysts occur in SKIN, BONES, BREASTS, eyelids, KIDNEYS, the LIVER, and, the tissues of women's OVARIES. They vary in structure.

Causes

In the majority of cases, a tissue will suddenly develop a cystic growth or swelling for no known reason. This accounts for the majority of cysts.

Some cysts form because of a small defect in the development of the body. A *dermoid cyst* is one that has arisen because some skin cells have been buried or closed beneath the skin. With time, they secrete fluid and the area swells to form a cyst.

In the case of a *polycystic kidney*, the tubules of the kidney had not joined completely into the drainage channels. Swelling takes place which becomes cystic as the urine is trapped and unable to discharge.

Blocked glands

For no known reason, some GLANDS have their exits obstructed, and as the secretion continues, the gland swells and a cyst forms. A common example of this is the sebaceous cyst under the skin where the sebaceous GLAND becomes blocked.

Cysts can also be caused by the formation of fluid in response to the presence of a parasite. Fortunately, these parasites are rare in countries with proper hygiene and veterinary procedures.

Very occasionally heavy blows can result in the formation of cysts within muscles. The blow ruptures a blood vessel, a clot is formed, and as it disperses, it attracts fluid from the blood. This forms a cyst.

Symptoms

The symptoms of a cyst will depend on its situation and type. The patient will probably notice a lump or bump if the cyst is under the skin. Where the cyst affects an internal organ such as the ovary, there may be some tenderness in the abdomen or just a generalized swelling, as the larger the cyst becomes, the less room is left for the normal organs.

In most cases, the doctor is able to feel the cyst or to see its presence either by X-ray or by scanning the area with thermography or a radioactive isotope. Some cysts are painful when pressed, especially if they are already swollen. A cyst near the skin will fluctuate with pressure like a soft ball.

Some cysts occurring in the scrotum – such as a *hydrocoele* – contain fluid, and light shines through them clearly as opposed to the dark shadow of the solid testes. This is known as *transillumination*, and indicates their precise position and size.

Complications

Any new lump which arises on the body could well be a cyst. Cysts are rarely dangerous unless they are cancerous, and this needs the opinion of your doctor. If there is any doubt, the earlier the cyst is removed the better the outlook.

Infection is also a danger. A sebaceous cyst that becomes infected turns into a sebaceous ABSCESS and may need to be opened. An ovarian cyst that becomes infected is a potential cause of PERITONITIS (inflammation of the membrane lining the abdominal cavity). This is serious. Like other large cysts lying free in the abdomen, it may twist on its stem, producing strangulation of its blood supply and subsequent degeneration. This may also occur if it bleeds into itself. In this case, the patient will feel intense abdominal pain and be very tender in the area of the cyst. It must be treated as an emergency and removed by surgery.

Outlook

Once removed, a benign cyst will not return. If new cysts develop in the same area, such as the breast (*see* MASTITIS), each one has to be evaluated by its behaviour.

Where a cyst is found to be cancerous, the outlook depends on the degree of malignancy and whether or not spread has already taken place. For this reason, surgeons removing cysts which are likely to be cancerous tend to remove surrounding tissue to prevent cancer cells coming into contact with other tissue and forming fresh growths.

Cytomegalovirus, *see* Cerebral palsy

D

D, vitamin, *see* **Vitamins**

D & C (dilation and curettage), *see* **Abortion, Miscarriage, Uterus**

Dandruff

This is an excessive scaling of the dead skin of the scalp. It forms part of what doctors call a *seborrhoeic tendency*: an overproduction of sebum, the natural oil secreted by sebaceous GLANDS in the skin. It affects all the areas where hair grows, especially the scalp; occasionally it appears on the eyebrows, chest and groin.

Causes

In the great majority of cases of dandruff, there is no known cause, but there are indications that heredity, diet or an upset in the body's hormonal balance may be contributory factors.

Stress and emotional upheaval can make dandruff worse; a good rest while on holiday may virtually abolish the condition altogether.

In addition, the excessive greasiness of an adolescent's skin is a well-known cause of the condition, while campers who are unable to wash their hair regularly may quite suddenly develop it, as will swimmers who bathe in salt water without wearing bathing caps.

Symptoms

Dandruff – scales of skin resembling tiny white flakes – occurs on the scalp and, in some cases, other hairy areas of the body. The scaling is sometimes, but not always, accompanied by intense itching.

In severe cases, there may be excessive greasiness of the skin and hair. Patches of scalp redden and tiny openings appear which ooze and form hard yellow crusts. The skin on the face, particularly on the forehead, cheeks and eyebrows, becomes reddened, and scaling occurs in the skin of the ears, and on the front of the chest, over the breast and collar bone.

The only serious complication occurs if any cracks in the affected skin open and crusted areas become infected, leading to the development of impetigo, a contagious skin infection. Occasionally the condition can turn into ECZEMA; the redness and inflammation worsen and the skin discharges a clear fluid. People with severe dandruff affecting the skin of the ears may develop *otitis externa,* an infection in the outer ear canal. This requires medical attention.

Similar problems
Dandruff should not be confused with ringworm, psoriasis (isolated tiny patches of skin) or exfoliative dermatitis (scaling all over the body), which is a serious condition that needs hospital treatment.

Treatment
The mainstay of the treatment for ordinary dandruff is regular – but not over-zealous – shampooing with one of the many anti-dandruff shampoos on the market. Doctors recommend coal-tar-based shampoos, which are safe and relatively inexpensive. Shampoos containing selenium sulphide or zinc pyrithione are also beneficial.

Only severe dandruff requires medical treatment, and this should be sought where there is scaling of the surrounding skin, severe itching and cracking of the scalp, or signs of spreading elsewhere on the body. Bouts of dandruff can be treated with steroid lotions or ointments to the scalp. Where there is a secondary infection in the scratched or cracked skin, antibiotics will help.

Deafness

This is the inability or reduced ability to hear. It can affect one or both EARS, the onset may be slow or sudden. It can result from a wide variety of causes, and many forms of treatment and devices are available to remove or alleviate the symptoms.

To understand deafness, it is necessary to know how the ear works. *See* HEARING and BALANCE.

Types of deafness
There are two main types: *conductive* deafness and *perceptive* deafness.

In conductive deafness, sound waves are prevented from reaching the inner ear. This can be because there is wax in the outer canal fluid inside, or the tiny ossicles (bones) in the ear have seized up (otosclerosis). In perceptive deafness, although the sound can reach the inner ear, there is a disease of the nerves leading to the brain or a condition affecting the function of the inner ear.

In the majority of cases, deafness falls within one of these two categories. In some instances, however, the causes may be confused. For example, an old person may have an excess of WAX causing conductive deafness, together with a hearing loss affecting the nerve that carries sound to the brain.

Mild or partial hearing loss is extremely common. In children, deafness can slow down the general ability to learn as well as speak. In adults, the deafness caused by gradual hearing loss or old age simply increases feelings of isolation and loneliness. Deaf people have to take special precautions in traffic or crowds and tend to be more accident prone because of their disability.

Diagnosis
Deafness is a symptom of malfunction of the ear. The earlier it can be identified, the sooner treatment can begin. A person with normal hearing can easily hear words or numbers whispered softly from about 1.5 m (5 ft) away. A slightly deaf person will miss most of the words whispered at this distance, and a very deaf person will be unable to hear a conversation 15 cm (6 in) from the ear.

There are various methods to test a person's hearing. Voice tests are the first, and the second is by means of a tuning fork. This produces a sound of constant pitch: the larger the fork, the lower the note. It is moved slowly away from the ear until the patient says he or she can no longer hear the sound and the distance is measured. The process is then repeated with the other ear. This makes it possible to plot hearing levels for different notes. Sometimes it is found that the patient hears best if the foot of the tuning fork is placed on the bone behind the ear. This test is used to identify hearing affected by conductive deafness.

The only scientific method of accurately assessing adult hearing is by the use of an audiometer. This machine emits standard notes at different volumes and the patient signals when a sound is heard. Not only does it measure the air conduction from the sound emitted which is heard in an earphone; it also tests what is known as bone conduction, when the sound is played directly into the bone of the skull.

Ears, like eyes, are precious. When deafness occurs, either suddenly or over a period of time, it is important, after its assessment, to start treatment quickly.

Coping with deafness
Where treatment is of no avail and deafness is permanent, a suitable hearing aid is likely to be necessary. If even this is of no help, the patient has to learn to lip read and to speak from memory. Small children have to be taught to speak and will receive special schooling; most deaf people also learn sign language.

Although deafness is a handicap, it is perfectly possible for deaf people to lead a normal and useful life. However, they must be additionally careful when driving. Total deafness may be considered a safety hazard to driving, but provided warning sounds can be converted into visual signals, most driving authorities allow deaf people to drive.

Defecation, *see* Excretory systems, Incontinence, Rectum

Deficiency diseases, *see* Malnutrition, Minerals, Rickets, Scurvy, Vitamins

Dehydration, *see* Water

Dementia, *see* Mental illness (esp. p. 522)

Dental care

Regular cleaning is vital for healthy TEETH and GUMS and for fresh-smelling breath. Without it, unpleasant substances develop in the mouth which cause tooth decay and gum disease. Of these, the most dangerous is PLAQUE. This spreads and clings to the teeth, breaking down sugar into acids, which attack the enamel surface of the tooth. This is the start of tooth decay, and once it is established, it slowly moves deeper into the tooth and holes – or *caries* – appear.

Apart from occasional bad breath (halitosis) caused by overindulgence in garlic, the usual reason for unpleasant smelling breath is dental problems. Badly brushed teeth, tooth decay, and gum disease can all cause bad breath. So anyone with persistent bad breath should take better care of their teeth, and if it doesn't go away, they should see a dentist for more advice.

Toothbrushing

Plaque re-forms within 24 to 48 hours, so the teeth should be brushed thoroughly at least once a day. Although many people have been brought up to brush their teeth three times a day after meals, this is not essential. It is most important to ensure that all plaque is removed completely once a day – it does not really matter when during the day you brush your teeth. A good tooth-brushing routine should take at least three minutes, and more likely five.

There is no 'correct' or 'incorrect' way to brush the teeth. The essential point is to brush both the inside and outside of every tooth thoroughly. It is useful to think of the teeth in sections and to concentrate on one section at a time. The upper teeth on each side can be divided into a rear section, a middle section and a front section, so there is a total of six sections, three on the left and three on the right. The inner parts of each section of teeth, nearer the tongue, should each be brushed with eight strokes of the brush. This makes 48 brush strokes. Then the outer part should be brushed with eight brush strokes – another 48 strokes. Repeat the same routine for the lower teeth and you should have made nearly 200 brush strokes.

There are several different brushing methods which may be used. The 'rolling' technique is quite popular, in which the brush is placed against the gum margin and swept down the teeth towards the biting surface. An alternative technique is the 'vibrating' method. The brush is held firmly against the side of the tooth and 'vibrated' backwards and forwards while trying to force the brush bristles into the gaps between the teeth.

Cleaning aids

Most dentists recommend a medium nylon bristle toothbrush with fairly fine bristles. The head of the brush should not be too large because this would make it difficult to reach the corners of the mouth. There is no need to wet the toothbrush before using it; a small amount of toothpaste will suffice.

Electric toothbrushes may seem a good idea, but there is little evidence that they are any better than careful brushing by hand, and they may encourage laziness! Water irrigation devices ('water piks') that squirt water at high pressure against and between the teeth are certainly much less effective than brushing. They do not remove plaque effectively and are *not* recommended by dentists.

It is just as important to remove plaque from the tooth surfaces in the less accessible regions – for example, between the teeth, as it is to polish up the front of the teeth which you can easily see in the mirror. An 'interdental' toothbrush which has just a single tuft of bristles may be used, but dental floss is more effective.

Floss is available either waxed or unwaxed – there is little to choose between the two, but many people find waxed floss easier to use. The floss should be inserted between two teeth then wrapped around the side of one tooth and pulled backwards and forwards while working the floss close that tooth. Once that side has been cleaned, the floss can be moved carefully to be wrapped around one side of the next tooth, without damaging the gums. If you are wary of using floss or if you have any crowns or bridges, it would be worth asking your dentist for advice on how to use dental floss.

Care of gums

Healthy gums are pink and firm. They should not be swollen or reddened around the edges and should never bleed, even if they are brushed hard. Careful daily brushing will keep them healthy. If your gums bleed or are inflamed, you should go to your dentist for advice. Gum disease starts when plaque accumulates around, and just under, the edge of the gums. Massage the gums with gentle brushing, but also see your dentist, as he or she can remove the plaque. The presence of plaque can be detected by using disclosing tablets, which can be supplied by your dentist or obtained from a chemist. They are particularly revealing if used immediately after you have brushed your teeth and think they are perfectly clean. If you then chew one of the tablets, the dye it contains will colour deposits of plaque a bright red colour.

It is particularly important to get into the habit of visiting your dentist regularly – every year or so – even if your teeth seem healthy. As well as carrying out any necessary treatment, he or she can also advise on how to clean your teeth properly, the planning of a diet that is kind to your teeth, how to detect plaque and brush it off.

Diet

It is now known that sugary foods of all kinds are the main cause of tooth decay, or caries. Within minutes of eating anything containing SUGAR, acid is formed by bacteria on the teeth, and this helps to rot them, causing decay. Any type of sugar can contribute to decay – including ordinary, brown or white sugar and those in sweets, honey and fruits.

Research has shown that it is not simply the amount of sugary foods that causes decay, but the number of times during the day on which they are eaten. Small, regular amounts of sugar are much worse than the same quantity eaten at once.

Children's teeth are most susceptible to the effects of sugar. Try to cut down on very sweet foods, and in particular avoid giving them sweet food or drink between meals, such as biscuits, cakes, pastries, ice cream, soft drinks, chocolates, toffees or other sweets. If a child is hungry between meals, give him or her a savoury snack.

Fluoride

Some dentists believe that the best method of preventing tooth decay, especially in children, is to brush teeth with fluoride toothpaste and take it in other forms. It is also thought to help repair enamel after it has been attacked and, in addition, to have an anti-bacterial effect.

In some parts of the country, fluoride occurs naturally in the water supply; in others, it is deliberately added. Ask your dentist if the water in your area is fluoridated. If it is not, you can use fluoride drops or tablets from your chemist, or your dentist can paint fluoride on to your child's teeth; fluoride mouthwashes are also available.

Opponents to fluoride claim that it can cause cancer, although most experts disagree and, so far, there has been no firm evidence to support the theory. However, it is true that fluoride in excess can cause bone disease and mottling of the teeth.

See also ORTHODONTICS.

Depo-Provera, *see* Contraception

Depression

Many people feel 'down' from time to time, but these are usually passing phases. In wondering where such moods end and proper depression begins, it should be remembered that this is not a simple condition. It can show itself in various ways and have a number of causes. Neither does it respect sex or occupation, and it strikes at any time from the teens to middle age, when it claims the greatest number of victims: for serious depression, the peak is about 60 years old for men and 55 for women; for milder cases, the peak age is about 50 for men and 45 for women.

Early warning signals

If you suspect that someone you live with is suffering from depression, what are the signs of serious trouble? Perhaps the most significant fact is that the victim loses interest and enjoyment in every aspect of life. Such a change is quickly noticeable to other people.

It can apply to work, the home, the family, food and drink, hobbies, sports and the desire for sex, and may extend to personal appearance and hygiene. Then the complaints begin about all kinds of physical problems – headaches, back pains, stomach troubles, 'tight' feelings in the chest, giddiness, constipation or blurred vision. And the depressed are also so apathetic that they are often unable to ask for professional help – it is up to others to seek medical or psychiatric advice for them.

The many faces of depression

Not all the symptoms of depression are shown by every patient – two people behaving in markedly different ways can both be classed as depressed. What makes the picture even more complicated is that the condition can be accompanied by acute anxiety (*see* STRESS) or PHOBIAS. Sometimes depression alternates with bouts of mania, a mood of almost forced gaiety, talkativeness and compulsive activity – hence the term 'MANIC DEPRESSIVE'.

In general depression, moods may vary from slight sadness to intense despair, and a feeling of utter worthlessness. Strangely, people with this condition seldom talk of these feelings to their doctor: instead they will grumble about aches and pains, tiredness or loss of weight. They may even find it difficult to speak at all; other people will seem to chatter constantly.

These variations in speech often occur as a result of thought difficulties. Patients often complain of not being able to think clearly, concentrate or make decisions – they *know* that something is amiss. This ability to realize their own unhappy state, without being able to do anything about it, affects depressives in another way. They tend to be preoccupied with themselves, and seem completely unable to count their blessings. Instead, they magnify the mishaps of the past and tend to blow them up into major disasters, always regarding themselves as totally to blame for these misfortunes.

This habit of distorting events to their own detriment affects their sleep, which may be already disturbed by the illness itself. On going to bed, they lie awake worrying about the past, their own state and the future. A vicious circle sets in.

As if all this was not enough, the depression itself can cause early morning wakening. Small wonder, therefore, that for many such people the beginning of the day is the most wretched time of all.

When depression is accompanied by anxiety, the sufferer is nearly always restless and has a nervous way of talking; this is in marked contrast to the apathy of other depressives who tend to hide their worries from others.

Heredity and environment

To some extent, depression is thought to run in families; but this influence is one of increased susceptibility to the condition rather than actually producing it. In fact, there is nearly always a definite stressful event or series of events that brings on the depressive state. Another way in which these symptoms can be 'transmitted' is that the parent who suffers from this condition invariably acts out their depression to others in the household. Seeing this demonstration in terms of behavioural patterns and actions, children inevitably tend to copy it themselves in later life, if they also feel depressed. This happens rather more easily than would be the case if they had no such model to copy.

When there is no family history of this condition, it is virtually always triggered by powerful patterns of outside events which affect the victim deeply. In such cases, the chance of recovery from the depression is somewhat better.

The effects of grief

A temporary, but still very real depression can be caused by bereavement. When you experience the death of a loved one, it is normal to express grief: indeed, to attempt to suppress grief reactions because they are painful, because you feel this is silly or because the deceased person 'wouldn't want me to be sad' is never helpful. In fact, it tends to prolong the period of grief.

Besides the usual reactions of distress, there are often feelings of guilt, irritability, lack of warmth towards others and sometimes an unnerving habit of taking on the personality traits or mannerisms of the dead person.

People in this state may also have problems with their relationships with other members of the family and with friends. They may show intense feelings of anger towards doctors, hospital authorities or 'uncaring' relatives. Alternatively, there may be a complete lack of apparent signs of grief, accompanied by periods of restlessness and virtually pointless activity, which are justified as 'keeping my mind busy', but which do no such thing. In any of these situations, the bereaved person should be encouraged to 'let out' their feelings and talk about their loss with friends, relatives or even with a doctor.

Treatment

Many people find it hard to appreciate the depths of despair which can affect the severely depressed person. In fact, about one in six cases of severe depression results in suicide. It is thought that this rate would be even higher were it not for the fact that the sufferer is often too apathetic to carry out a suicide attempt.

The use of drugs for the treatment of depression is less in favour than it used to be, possibly because psychological methods may better equip the patient for coping with the stresses or situations that contributed to their condition. However, drugs have their place, especially where inherited factors are concerned, because they are simpler to administer and do not involve extended visits to a specialist.

The most widely used group of anti-depressant drugs are known as the *'tricyclic' anti-depressants.* There are a dozen or more different drugs in this group – including imipramine, amitriptyline, nortriptyline, dothiepin, and mianserin. All have an effect on the level of certain chemicals in the brain, and it is thought that they work by improving the transmission of messages between various parts of the brain, although exactly how they work remains somewhat unclear. However, they all tend to improve the mood of the patient, and this seems to help lift the depression and allow the patient to begin to deal with the problems that may have caused the depression in the first place.

These drugs take several weeks to work, and they are effective in most, but not all, cases of depression. Where they do help, it may be necessary for the patient to continue to take them for at least three months and possibly much longer. Minor side-effects may be troublesome at first, particularly dryness of the mouth and slightly blurred vision, but these tend to fade away in time, or they can be reduced by the doctor adjusting the dose of the drug or switching to another one. Some tricyclic anti-depressants also act to relieve anxiety, whereas others are SEDATIVE. Still others, however, act as minor stimulants.

Another group of anti-depressant drugs are the *mono-amine oxidase (MAO) inhibitors.* These drugs, including phenelzine and tranylcypromine, are used less often than tricyclic anti-depressants because they may have more side-effects and the patient has to be careful about not eating certain foods while taking them. Nevertheless they can be very helpful for some patients with more severe types of depression who have not improved with other treatments. Side-effects may include dizziness, faintness, rashes and headaches. Some of the side-effects occur particularly if the patient consumes certain foods or drinks such as cheese, broad beans, yoghurt, beer and wine.

Another group of anti-depressant drugs – e.g. fluoxetine (Prozac) – inhibit the consumption of a chemical substance in the brain called *serotonin*, and are less sedative than the tricyclics.

Patients who have manic-depression may respond to the drug lithium carbonate. This is also used relatively rarely but, for certain individuals, can make a dramatic difference to their lives, releasing them from the severe mood swings which are so common in manic-depression. The use of lithium has to be very carefully monitored by a doctor because the dose varies considerably from patient to patient, and if the dose is too high, side-effects may occur, including heart or kidney problems.

When a patient with depression also shows signs of anxiety, a TRANQUILLIZER may be given as well as an anti-depressant. But tranquillizers, such as diazepam (Valium) or lorazepam (Ativan), cannot relieve the depression if used alone. Indeed, it is now known that patients who take such tranquillizers over a long period may actually become depressed as a side-effect of the drugs – and can become physically addicted – so they are now used carefully.

PSYCHOLOGICAL methods, such as a course in thought-examination or self-assertion (which can be obtained at certain clinics and therapy centres) as well as behavioural therapy techniques (*see* MENTAL THERAPIES) can work well in many cases. Even making this examination has in itself a certain power to lift depression.

Living with a depressive

Psychological treatment can do much to help sufferers to change their way of thinking about themselves. But if you have to live with someone in this condition, do not expect too much too soon, however infuriatingly negative their behaviour may be. What is needed is your continued friendliness, interest and support – even if it does not seem to be having much effect. Often, a positive approach is appreciated by the depressed person, even if they cannot respond, and will be remembered with gratitude later.

Curiously, the technique of not doing too much at once also applies to relaxation. Often someone will advise the depressive to 'get away from it all and take a holiday'. But not only will they fail to benefit from this, they may even become more anxious at not being on familiar ground. Holidays should be reserved for the time when the patient is well on the way to recovery, when everyone concerned will benefit more.

Hospital treatment

In severe cases, home care may become impossible. Then the patient may have to spend some time in hospital for continuous care and therapy. Hospital treatment provides a safe environment where the stress of home life can be relieved. The doctors and nurses in a psychiatric hospital are specially trained to give regular counselling and support to depressed patients, and to help them to reconstruct their lives and regain a sense of purpose. Not infrequently anti-depressants are prescribed as well, and their effects carefully monitored. Rarely, a treatment called *electroconvulsive therapy* (ECT) may be prescribed. For this, carefully controlled electric discharges are passed through certain parts of the BRAIN while the patient is anaesthetized. The current induces a CONVULSION in the patient's brain and body. This is not felt, but often produces considerable improvement in the patient's condition – as few as two or three treatments may be enough to produce a complete recovery. Although some temporary forgetfulness of recent events may result, many depressives believe that this is a small price to pay for the dramatic relief that ECT can provide. However, it is a technique which some doctors and psychiatrists question, as its results in some cases may be only very short-term.

See also POST-NATAL DEPRESSION.

Dercum's disease, *see* Lipomas

Dermatitis

This is a red, itching inflammation of the skin. The term actually covers a variety of skin complaints, many of which result from the skin's becoming oversensitive to some normally harmless substance. But, while the symptoms of each type are similar, the causes are quite different.

The commonest form – ECZEMA and contact dermatitis – are widespread, affecting people of all ages. But, though uncomfortable and unattractive, most types of dermatitis are temporary, not dangerous and not contagious.

Types of dermatitis

Allergic reaction: See ECZEMA and ALLERGY for a full discussion of this type of dermatitis.

Contact dermatitis: This is the other common type of dermatitis. Although its symptoms are similar to eczema – inflammation and irritation – the causes are rather different. This type of dermatitis is also an allergic complaint, but unlike eczema it is confined to those parts of the body that come into direct contact with the allergen.

Metals, especially nickel and chrome, are often to blame, though in fact the list of these contact allergens, as they are called, is almost endless. However, other common ones are: rubber, perfumes, certain drugs, synthetic resins (e.g. epoxy solvents), lubricating oils, chromate (found in cement), certain plants (e.g. primula and ragweed), wood oils and resins.

Contact dermatitis most often affects the hands because they are so frequently exposed to contact allergens. But a rubber allergy would be most likely to show up on the parts of the body exposed to the rubber elastic in underwear. Similarly, a perfume allergy would be likely to show up as dermatitis on the parts of the body where the perfume was applied.

Although allergies do tend to run in families, contact dermatitis is believed to be due more to regular and prolonged exposure to the substance.

Contact dermatitis has, in fact, been called a twentieth-century industrial disease, because modern industry – and its products – exposes workers, as well as consumers to so many potential allergens.

Dermatitis of the scalp: Another common type of dermatitis is seborrhoea, or seborrhoeic dermatitis. This is a condition that affects the hairy areas of the skin, particularly the scalp. It may become itchy and inflamed, with peeling of the skin and severe dandruff.

Seborrhoea is not caused by an allergy. It is thought that the condition is brought on by the over-activity of the skin's oil glands, or sebaceous glands.

Sensitivity to light: There is a type of dermatitis, called solar or photo-dermatitis, which is brought on by exposure to sunlight. In most cases the sun alone is not to blame, but sunlight can bring out some other allergy which has not been strong enough to produce symptoms by itself. Certain drugs, such as the antibiotic tetracycline, can increase the skin's sensitivity to light.

Treatment

Though there are no real cures for the various kinds of dermatitis, they can be relieved and controlled. The most important treatment is to keep the affected area clean and avoid scratching it. This allows the skin to heal naturally and reduces the risk of infections.

There is a wide range of ointments, creams, pastes and lotions which are prescribed by doctors or can be bought directly over the counter from a chemist.

Inflammations which are dry and flaking can be soothed and protected with oily preparations like lanolin or petroleum jelly, while wet, weepy inflammations are better treated with starch-based applications or an astringent.

Some of the more potent medicines are steroids. Anti-inflammatory, they are made into creams or ointments. The mildest type, hydrocortisone, can be bought at a chemist's shop, but stronger creams and ointments are available only on prescription.

The only permanent cure for dermatitis is to remove the cause. If an allergy is at the root of the trouble, the allergen should be identified and then avoided. This may not be easy, for sometimes the dermatitis shows up only days after the exposure to the allergen.

Barrier creams and sprays can protect the skin against irritating substances, and sun screens filter out some of sun's ultraviolet rays which can cause solar dermatitis.

Contact with some industrial allergens can be reduced by wearing gloves, a face mask or other protective clothing.

Dermatitis herpetiformis, *see* **Rash**

Dhobi itch, *see* **Fungal infections, Ringworm**

Diabetes

This is a condition where there is an abnormally high level of sugar in the blood. The disease, and its symptoms, have been recognized for hundreds of years. Affected people pass abnormally large quantities of URINE, as a result developing an abnormal thirst and losing a great deal of weight.

In the seventeenth century, when diabetes was known as 'the pissing evil', it was noticed that the urine of most sufferers was especially sweet. In a few cases, however, it was insipid – that is, it was not sweet.

The first type had *diabetes mellitus* (*mellitus* means 'like honey'), and is the disease we know today as plain diabetes. The second type, called *diabetes insipidus,* is extremely rare and results from a failure of the pituitary gland in the skull.

Millions of people all over the world suffer from *diabetes mellitus.* In the UK, for example, about 2 per cent of the population have it in varying degrees of seriousness, which amounts to about 560,000 diabetics. In some peoples – for example, the Pima Indians of Arizona in the US – nearly half the population have the disease.

Insulin

Diabetes results from a failure in the production of *insulin,* one of the body's HORMONES, or chemical 'messengers'. Its job is to keep the blood's SUGAR content in control.

Insulin is made by the 'islets of Langerhans', a cluster of hormone-producing cells in the PANCREAS. The purpose of the insulin is to keep the level of sugar in the blood down to normal levels. A lack of this hormone causes diabetes.

If the level of sugar in the blood begins to rise above certain limits, the islets of Langerhans respond by releasing insulin into the bloodstream. This then acts to oppose the effects of hormones such as cortisone and adrenalin (*see* ADRENAL GLANDS) – which raise the level of blood sugar.

The insulin exerts its effect by allowing sugar to pass from the bloodstream into the body's cells to be used as fuel. But if insulin is absent from the system, the mechanism for balancing the blood sugar level is removed, and because the sugar in the blood cannot be converted into fuel for the cells, diabetes results.

Treatment

The treatment for diabetes is to introduce insulin into the system. This will alleviate the problem by replacing the insufficiently produced hormone.

Most of the insulin prescribed for diabetics is now identical to the body's own insulin in chemical structure and is called 'human insulin'. In the past, insulin was extracted from the pancreases of cattle or pigs and therefore known as 'beef insulin' or 'pork insulin', but there was then the possibility of antibodies to the animal insulin being produced within the circulation. This would mean that, gradually, beef or pork insulin could become less and less effective. The problem has been overcome by the introduction of human insulin, because no antibodies are produced to it (since it is identical to the body's natural insulin).

Human insulin is produced artificially by GENETIC ENGINEERING. Special bacteria, bred in the laboratory, are given a gene which causes them to manufacture human insulin. This can then be extracted and purified, ready for injection by people suffering from diabetes.

There has been concern, however, that human insulin may not give as much warning of a hypoglycaemic attack (*see below*), thus making it more dangerous. Specialists are divided on this, but occasionally patients are recommended to return to pork or beef insulin if their symptoms are not well controlled.

Unfortunately, all types of insulin are destroyed by gastric juices if taken by mouth and so it is given by self-injection. In general, diabetics have two injections of insulin a day, one before breakfast and one before the evening meal.

How diabetes starts

In many diabetes sufferers, the lack of insulin is due to a failure of the part of the body responsible for producing insulin. This is the pancreas, and the failure is caused by the destruction of its insulin-producing cells. No one knows exactly how the destruction occurs, but it is the subject of much research. It seems that some people are more likely than others to develop diabetes, and that some event – possibly an infection – may trigger the onset.

The sort of diabetes which develops suddenly due to a complete or serious failure of insulin tends to afflict young people and children, and is often called 'juvenile diabetes' or 'insulin-dependent diabetes'.

The majority of diabetics, however, suffer from a different sort of diabetes. In this case, the pancreas does produce insulin, often in normal amounts, but the tissues of the body are not sensitive to its action and this produces a high blood sugar level.

The condition often goes hand in hand with being overweight, and the problem is treated by dieting so that the load of sugar is reduced. Dieting alone is often enough to keep this type of diabetes under control. If excess weight is reduced and sugary foods avoided, the body can manage with the insulin that is present in the circulation. Sometimes drugs to enhance the production of insulin may be prescribed, or another type of drug to increase the effectiveness of the body's own insulin.

This type of diabetes is often called 'maturity-onset diabetes' or 'non-insulin dependent diabetes', but despite the latter name, there may still be a need for insulin injections if the condition is severe and diet and tablets are insufficient to keep it under control.

How serious is diabetes?

The disease may be serious for two reasons. First, without insulin injections, the insulin-dependent diabetic simply continues to lose weight until he or she lapses into a coma and dies.

Second, diabetics can develop complications. Generally speaking, the better the level of blood sugar is controlled, the less likely complications are to occur.

The most serious concern the EYES and KIDNEYS and are caused by the disease's effect on the blood vessels. It is usually possible to see changes to the blood vessels in the back of the eye of any long-standing diabetic, and in a very few cases, this worsens to the extent that the patient eventually loses the sight of one or both eyes.

In addition, diabetics may also develop abnormalities in their nerves which, among other problems, can lead to a loss of feeling in the hands and feet.

Finally, the diabetic has, unfortunately, a tendency to develop ARTERY trouble, which in turn causes STROKES and HEART ATTACKS. For this reason, diabetics are particularly encouraged not to SMOKE, since this also increases the likelihood of arterial disease.

How insulin works

In general, it is the patient whose diabetes comes on early in life who needs insulin, although a fair proportion of those who start diabetes later in life will also eventually need it.

The hormone is given by injection, usually under the skin of the thigh. Diabetics learn to draw their own insulin up into a syringe and give themselves the injections. This usually has to be done twice-daily, and often different formulations of insulin are used to try and spread the total effect out during the course of the day. Some diabetics use a 'pen' device and give themselves several injections throughout the day as they need them.

Once diabetics have taken insulin, their blood sugar level will start to fall, but this is not, however, the end of their problems. Sometimes the sugar level falls too far as a result of taking too much insulin. Sugar is an essential food not only for the body's tissues in general, but particularly for the BRAIN. If the sugar falls too low, the brain ceases to function properly and the patient becomes UNCONSCIOUS.

Luckily, diabetics can learn the early symptoms of a falling blood sugar level. These are shakiness, sweating, tingling around the mouth and often a feeling of being rather muddled. The treatment for these symptoms, known as *hypoglycaemia* (which means 'low blood sugar'), is to take some form of sugar by mouth immediately. If a sugary drink or food is taken quickly, the symptoms of the 'hypo' will pass within minutes. Occasionally, in a severe hypoglycaemic attack, patients become so confused that they do not know what they are doing. It is then important that a relative or friend gives them a sugary drink: three of four teaspoons of sugar in a glass of water is usually enough. If the patient goes into a coma, however, medical help should be called straight away. The doctor can give a simple injection to bring the patient out of the coma.

Balancing the insulin

Because of the risk of 'hypo' attacks, it is important for diabetics to try and balance their food intake with their insulin injections so that the sugar level is kept somewhere near the normal range without too much soaring up and down.

This means regular meals containing similar amounts of CARBOHYDRATE (food that is broken down to sugar in the blood). All diabetics, whether insulin-treated or not, should avoid sugar itself or foods which contain sugar such as jam, sweets, cakes and squash. The sugar content of these is absorbed rapidly in the stomach to produce brisk increases in the blood sugar level. But clearly, the use of sugar to halt a 'hypo' is an exception to this rule.

Diabetics are encouraged to have a DIET high in fibre (including foods such as wholegrain cereals, vegetables and fruits) and low in fats. This diet encourages gradual absorption of sugars from the digestive system and, in the long run, probably also reduces the risk of the development of arterial disease.

Diabetics also need to balance the amount of EXERCISE they do with their food intake and insulin. If they do a lot of extra exercise, they will need more food and sometimes more insulin as well. But if they stop regular exercise, their food and insulin requirements may change too.

Measuring techniques

As well as carefully planned insulin injections and a regulated intake of carbohydrates, most diabetics use some form of measuring technique to keep a check on their blood sugar level.

The traditional way of doing this is to measure the amount of sugar in the urine, which gives an idea of the amount of sugar in the blood. This technique is now used only by diabetics who do not need insulin.

Diabetics who require insulin must keep a careful check on the level of sugar in the blood so that the dose of insulin can be adjusted according to the blood sugar level at any time. Special chemically impregnated strips may be used at home to measure the level of sugar in a drop of blood taken from a finger-prick. Most insulin-dependent diabetics check their blood sugar levels at various times in the day once every week, but some diabetics need to carry out tests every day, so that they can adjust their insulin dosage on a daily basis.

What causes a coma?

Diabetic coma is an unfortunate term, since it may refer to two completely different situations. One is hypoglycaemia (the 'hypo' attack) where a low blood sugar level causes fairly sudden loss of consciousness. The second is when the insulin-dependent diabetic starts to develop a high blood sugar level (*hyperglycaemia*).

Clearly, the two conditions are different, although some people may muddle them. A 'hypo' attack can develop in a matter of minutes, and is easily stopped by taking sugar. A high blood sugar level, on the other hand, takes hours or even days to develop, and may take hours to get back to normal.

As the sugar level rises due to lack of insulin, the cells are starved of 'fuel'. They have to burn something to keep alive, and so they start getting through fat instead. Used-up fat produces waste products called ketones, and it is the presence of excess ketones, which characterizes the sort of diabetes which requires treatment with insulin.

Diabetes inspidus, *see* **Hypothalamus, Kidneys and kidney diseases, Urine**

Dialysis

Dialysis is a form of renal replacement therapy for patients with end-stage kidney failure. There are two main types, haemodialysis and peritoneal dialysis. Nowadays, patients on dialysis are often using this form of treatment while they wait for a successful kidney transplant.

Haemodialysis

In this form of dialysis, blood from the patient is passed through a machine in which it comes into contact via a thin membrane with a specially designed solution. The waste products of metabolism that the kidney is unable to secrete are eliminated by diffusing into the solution, and salts that the body requires go in the opposite direction. Haemodialysis requires access to the patients' circulation, usually via a special 'fistula' created surgically in the forearm, into which special needles are inserted at the time of dialysis. A patient usually undergoes three or four hourly sessions a week of haemodialysis, and machines can sometimes be installed at a patient's home so that he or she does not need to come regularly to hospital.

Peritoneal dialysis

Continuous ambulatory peritoneal dialysis, or CAPD, is an easier and cheaper form of dialysis that can be performed on an out-patient basis. A small tube is inserted into the peritoneal cavity of the abdomen. Through this two litres of special dialysis fluid is passed into the abdomen where it stays for several hours in order that waste products of metabolism can be absorbed. The fluid is then run off and this process is then repeated four or five times a day.

Diaphragm

 When we BREATHE, most of the work is done by the diaphragm, a sheet of muscle and fibrous tissue that forms a complete wall between the chest and the ABDOMEN. The RIBS provide the upper part of the cage that encloses the HEART and LUNGS and the diaphragm forms the bottom.

If you were to look at the diaphragm from above, you would see a large central fibrous portion, connected by muscle fibres to the inside of the lower six ribs. This looks rather like the sun, with rays spreading out towards the rib cage to anchor it. From the front, the diaphragm appears as a dome, attached by muscular strings to the inside of the ribs.

How breathing works

The muscular fibres of the diaphragm contract when we breathe in, and flatten the 'dome' of the diaphragm, drawing the highest central part down into the abdomen. This increases the volume of the lungs and draws air into the chest through the trachea (windpipe). Breathing out happens by simple relaxation of the muscles, with the air being driven out in much the same way as when you let go of a balloon.

Like any other muscle, the diaphragm receives instructions to contract or relax from the NERVOUS SYSTEM. The nerves which supply the diaphragm are called the *left and right phrenic nerves.* Oddly enough, these nerves arise

The diaphragm and breathing

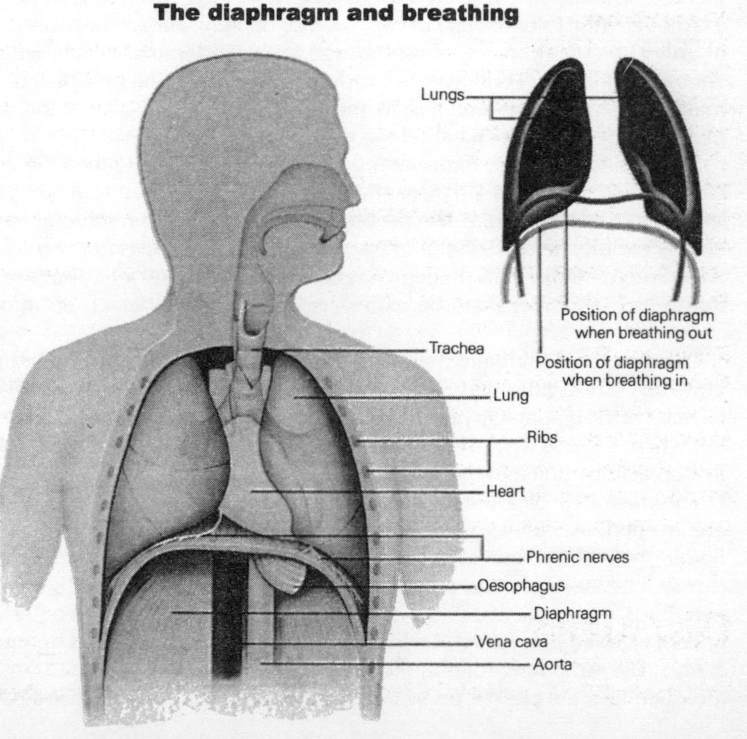

from high in the SPINAL CORD, and because of this have to make a fairly long journey from the neck down to the bottom of the chest. During early development of the embryo, the diaphragm actually starts as part of the neck structures, but as the foetus develops it moves downwards, taking its nerve supply with it.

The phrenic nerves can be damaged by injury or disease. However, despite the fact that the diaphragm appears to be an essential piece of anatomical equipment, people can breathe adequately if one side stops working. If both sides stop working, they can become short of breath when lying flat.

Developmental problems

Occasionally, when a baby is born, the diaphragm may not be fully formed. The result is that one of the lungs cannot expand properly and some of the organs that should be in the abdominal cavity may be in the chest. This condition is extremely rare but causes difficulty in breathing for the baby. Surgery may be needed at an early age to reconstruct the diaphragm.

Hiatus hernia

The diaphragm acts as a wall between the chest and the abdomen, but it is pierced centrally by two large blood vessels – a large artery (the *aorta*) and a large vein (the *inferior vena cava*). Another opening allows the OESOPHAGUS, or gullet, to cross from the chest through to the abdominal cavity, where it enters the stomach. Food from the mouth travels down the oesophagus and into the stomach. The opening in the diaphragm which allows the oesophagus through has been called the *oesophageal hiatus*.

Sometimes, however, this opening becomes too large and then the upper part of the stomach can slip through, up into the chest. This condition is then known as a *hiatus hernia*. The problem tends to occur in middle-aged and elderly people, because the diaphragmatic muscles get weaker with age. It is also more common in people who are overweight, because the pressure inside their abdomens can be excessive, forcing the stomach up into the chest.

The symptoms of a hiatus hernia can be unpleasant. Acid from the stomach flows up into the gullet very easily and causes severe heartburn. Normally the muscles of the diaphragm help to act as a one-way valve, stopping *acid reflux*, but where a hiatus hernia is present, there is no such valve and there is little to stop acid getting into the gullet.

The diagnosis of a hiatus hernia is complicated because special tests are needed. A patient with heartburn may be suffering from a hiatus hernia, but other conditions may cause similar symptoms – for example, stomach ULCERS. Even the symptoms of HEART DISEASE may be mistaken for heartburn. A BARIUM MEAL X-ray can show up a hiatus hernia readily. The patient is asked to swallow a white barium compound, which is opaque to X-rays. The radiologist follows the progress of the barium into the stomach, and then lays the patient on an X-ray table with the patient's head tipped down at a lower level than the feet to see whether the barium goes back into the oesophagus.

An alternative test involves the use of a flexible endoscope. This instrument is passed by the doctor down the oesophagus and allows a direct view of the oesophagus and stomach. The test is carried out with the patient under sedation. The doctor can inspect the lining of the oesophagus for signs of inflammation and can also see whether acid is coming up into it during the examination.

Drugs can be used for a patient with a hiatus hernia to reduce the amount of acid being produced by the stomach, but it also helps if the sufferer eats smaller meals and sleeps propped up in bed at night. In the most severe cases, surgery may be undertaken to try to reconstruct the oesophageal hiatus, but such surgery is not particularly successful in relieving the symptoms and the condition may recur because the diaphragm is weak.

Symptoms similar to those of a hiatus hernia may be experienced by a woman in the later months of PREGNANCY. Because the diaphragm is stretched, this reduces the effectiveness of the valve action which normally keeps the acid in the stomach. Fortunately the symptoms usually go away again once the baby has been delivered.

Pain in the diaphragm

Although the diaphragm is an unseen structure deep inside the body, it can occasionally be affected by disease and cause pain. Strangely, pain from the diaphragm may be felt not only around the lower ribs but also in the shoulder. This is because the nerves supplying the diaphragm also supply structures near the shoulder.

The diaphragm can become inflamed as a result of infection in the chest. PLEURISY affects the outer part of the lungs and the lining of the chest wall. If the diaphragm is involved, there may be pain on breathing, and this may be felt in the shoulder as well as in the chest.

ABSCESSES or inflammation under the diaphragm (e.g. when the GALL BLADDER is inflamed, as in cholecystitis) may also cause pain in the upper part of the abdomen, which radiates to the shoulder blades. These are very rare.

A slightly more common problem, which may occur without any warning, is a virus infection which can affect the diaphragm. A particular virus called the *Coxsackie virus* can cause generalized muscular aches and pains, headaches and feverishness but it particularly causes inflammation and pain in the diaphragm – to the extent that the infection may be confused with pleurisy. However, this infection, which is sometimes also known as *Bornholm disease*, invariably gets better on its own without treatment.

Hiccups start in the diaphragm, but why they occur remains a mystery. The diaphragm contracts, causing a sharp breath in. At the same time the larynx (voice box) suddenly closes off, causing the 'hic' and stopping air going into the chest. It is this breathing in with the diaphragm, while the upper part of the windpipe is closed, that makes hiccups so uncomfortable.

Diaphragms and caps, *see* **Contraception**

Diarrhoea

This is a symptom, not a disease. Usually it is caused by an INFECTION in the INTESTINES, though in some cases it may arise from a more serious problem. Diarrhoea can be dangerous in children, particularly in babies, and therefore medical attention should be sought if there is an abnormal change in a baby's stools.

Causes

Diarrhoea occurs because the lining of the intestine becomes irritated, either due to an infection, the presence of a toxic (poisonous) substance or some other cause. As a result, food and water pass through the length of the intestine much quicker than usual and fluid is not absorbed by the large intestine; this means that the stool remains very watery.

Not only may the walls of the intestine fail to absorb water, but they may also actually lose fluid as a result of inflammation, and this adds to the water lost in the diarrhoea. In severe cases, dehydration may occur, which may be fatal.

Diarrhoea may be due to a variety of causes. Food is one of the culprits. In food poisoning, BACTERIA grow on fly-blown food, producing toxins or poisons that give rise to diarrhoea and STOMACH upsets. This type of food poisoning may be caused by toxins from *staphylococcus* bacteria; a more severe type of illness called *botulism* may be caused by botulinum toxin, but this is very rare.

In other types of FOOD POISONING, it might be the bacteria itself which causes the infection. One bacterium called SALMONELLA causes diarrhoea, in addition to pain and, sometimes vomiting.

Diseases such as TYPHOID and dysentery are spread by bacteria being eaten with food. CHOLERA is spread by drinking water that has been infected by faeces. The difference between food poisoning and dysentery is that, in food poisoning, diarrhoea starts within a few hours of eating bad food, but dysentery may take up to 24 hours to produce diarrhoea, and will also last longer.

A bacterium called *Campylobacter* also causes diarrhoea, often with fairly severe stomach pains. This bacterium can spread between members of a household, or may be spread in contaminated food or water.

Much larger parasites can get into food and water and, once ingested, cause diarrhoea. This includes an amoeba, a single cell parasite, which can cause amoebic dysentery, a disease common to the tropics, and which, with its symptoms of diarrhoea alternating with CONSTIPATION, can go on for years.

Often diarrhoea is not due to bacteria or larger organisms, but to the smallest of germs, the viruses. In GASTRO-ENTERITIS, a virus infection causes diarrhoea, vomiting and abdominal pains. It can go under a variety of names: gastric flu, summer diarrhoea and so on.

Gastro-enteritis is a common affliction in babies, but loose stools should be distinguished from diarrhoea. Newborn babies do not pass normal stools, but instead pass greenish-brown sticky motions called *meconium*. Breastfed babies often have very loose motions, and they may pass several stools a day, whereas bottle-fed babies' stools are more like the consistency of adults' but the colour may vary greatly.

Despite the appearance of the stool, the baby who is breastfed is less likely to have gastro-enteritis as the breast milk protects the baby's intestines from any infection, and breastfeeding does not depend upon sterilizing bottles and teats for their safety.

Traveller's diarrhoea occurs when new strains of bacteria replace the bacteria which usually live in the large bowel, and are normally beneficial. It is a common experience for people to have this form of diarrhoea when they go abroad, and is not caused by a 'change of water' as is commonly supposed.

There are other causes of diarrhoea. If there is sustained nervousness, fear and anxiety (*see* STRESS), the intestine becomes overactive and diarrhoea occurs. Highly spiced foods can upset the bowels if a person is unused to eating them. Large quantities of fruit and shellfish can cause minor stomach upsets and loose bowels.

In children, diarrhoea can be caused by an infection which is completely unconnected with the bowels. Typically this happens in toddlers with EAR and THROAT infections.

Chronic problems

Chronic diarrhoea is not due to infections, but rather to other medical problems. One of the most common diseases is *ulcerative colitis*. The COLON (large intestine) becomes inflamed and the bacteria invade the mucous membranes which have already been damaged. No one cause has been found to contribute to ulcerative colitis, but theoretical causes range from ALLERGIC reactions to emotional upsets.

Diarrhoea occurs also when some other disease of the intestinal wall stops the proper absorption of foods. These MALABSORPTION problems – which include COELIAC DISEASE, in which the intestines have an intolerance or allergy to the gluten in wheat products – not only cause diarrhoea, but also leave patients badly undernourished.

A rather common symptom in the elderly is called 'spurious' or 'overflow' diarrhoea. What happens is that the lower bowel gets clogged up with faeces. However, some liquid matter manages to get past the blockage and gives rise to diarrhoea, which may cause the old person to lose control of the bowels and become incontinent. It is very important to recognize this as it is easily treated.

Dangers

Diarrhoea is not serious if it lasts a day or two in adults or older children. However, in babies and young children, diarrhoea can be dangerous, particularly if there is also vomiting, as the baby may not be able to take any fluid to replace the considerable amounts it is losing.

Persistent diarrhoea causes considerable loss of water and salt, which leads to dehydration. If untreated, it can be fatal. It takes much more to dehydrate an adult than a baby, but really serious infections, such as cholera, can cause death.

Treatment

The treatment for diarrhoea is dependent, in many instances, on finding out what the cause is, but basically the treatment is very simple. Follow the advice given under FOOD POISONING.

Diet, *see* Nutrition

Digestion

This is the process which breaks down food into substances that can be absorbed and used by the body for energy, growth and repair.

The digestive system depends on the action on the things we eat of substances called ENZYMES. These are produced by the organs attached to the ALIMENTARY CANAL and are responsible for many of the chemical reactions involved in digestion. These changes begin in the mouth. When food is chewed, the salivary glands beneath the tongue step up secretion of saliva, which contains the enzyme *ptyalin*. This starts breaking down some of the carbohydrates into smaller molecules known as *maltose* and *glucose*.

Food then travels down the OESOPHAGUS and into the STOMACH where the mixture of chemicals – mucus, *hydrochloric acid* and the enzyme *pepsin* – is poured on to it. Ptyalin stops working, but a new series of chemical reactions begins.

In the stomach

The amount of stomach juices is governed both here and in the intestine by nerve impulses, the presence of food itself and the secretion of HORMONES.

The hormone *gastrin* stimulates the stomach cells to release hydrochloric acid and pepsin after food is in the stomach, so that it can be broken down into *peptones*. Mucus secretion prevents the stomach lining from becoming damaged by acid. When the acidity reaches a certain point, gastrin production ceases.

In the small intestine

The food leaving the stomach – a thickish, acidic liquid called *chyme* – then enters the DUODENUM, the first part of the small INTESTINE. The duodenum makes and releases large quantities of mucus, which protects it from damage by the acid in the chyme and other enzymes. The duodenum also receives digestive juices from the PANCREAS, and considerable quantities of BILE, which is made in the LIVER and stored in the GALL BLADDER until needed to break down fat globules.

Two hormones trigger the release of pancreatic juices. The hormone *secretin* stimulates the production of large quantities of alkaline juices which neutralize the acidic, partially digested chyme. Pancreatic enzymes are produced in response to the release of a second hormone, *pancreozymin*.

Pancreatic enzymes help the digestion of carbohydrates and proteins, in addition to fats. These enzymes include *trypsin*, which breaks the peptones into smaller units called *peptides*; *lipase*, which breaks fat down into smaller molecules of *glycerol* and *fatty acids*; and *amylase*, which breaks down carbohydrates into *maltose*.

The digested food then enters the JEJUNUM and ILEUM, further down in the small intestine, where the final stages of chemical change take place. Enzymes are released from cells in small indentations in the walls of the jejunum and ileum which are known as the *crypts of Lieberkühn*.

Most food absorption takes place in the ileum which contains millions of minute projections called *villi* on its inner wall. Each villus contains a small blood vessel (capillary), and a tiny blind-end branch of the LYMPHATIC SYSTEM known as a *lacteal*. When digested food comes into contact with the villi, the glycerol, fatty acids and dissolved vitamins enter the lacteals, are carried through into the lymphatic system and they are then poured out into the bloodstream.

Amino acids from PROTEIN digestion and the sugars from CARBOHYDRATES, plus VITAMINS and important MINERALS such as CALCIUM, IRON and IODINE are absorbed directly into the capillaries in the villi. These capillaries lead into the *hepatic portal vein* which transports the food directly to the liver. This, in turn, filters out some substances for its own use and storage, and the remainder of these substances passes out into the body's general circulation.

Dilation and curettage, *see* **Abortion, Miscarriage, Uterus**

Diphtheria

This is an acute infection of the nose and throat which may prove fatal if it is not treated early. Although it is now rare in the Western world, it is still widespread in tropical countries, particularly those in Africa, where it kills thousands of children every year. It is only by widespread IMMUNIZATION that it has been largely eradicated from Western countries.

Causes

Diphtheria is caused by a bacterium called *Corynebacterium diphtheriae*. It tends to settle in the throat or nose where it grows on the tissues causing a 'membrane' to form. But the main threat from diphtheria comes not from the local growth of bacteria in the body but from a powerful toxin produced by them. The toxin is, in effect, a chemical poison that spreads into the bloodstream from the area where the bacteria are growing. It can then affect the function of the HEART or, later, the nerves (causing paralysis). Occasionally, diphtheria can cause SKIN infections, particularly in people who live in tropical countries.

DIPHTHERIA

There are several different types of *Corynebacterium diphtheria*, each with a different capability to produce toxin. The mildest form, called *mitis*, produces little toxin, and infection with it is unlikely to prove fatal but does give lifelong immunity to diphtheria. In some tropical countries, it has been found that up to half the population have been infected at some time in their lives. More serious types of diphtheria bacteria are called *intermedius* and *gravis*, and these produce more severe symptoms.

If an outbreak of diphtheria occurs, it is possible for the public health authorities to find out which people are already immune to the disease by using a special test called the *Schick test*. A tiny amount of toxin is injected into the forearm, and if the person is not immune to diphtheria (because of immunization or previous infection), a red reaction occurs. Anybody who is already immune gets no reaction to the injection and does not need to be immunized. All those who are 'Schick positive' need immunizing to ensure they do not get the disease and to control the spread and become a full-scale epidemic.

Symptoms

There are several forms of diphtheria, each with its own characteristic pattern of symptoms, although often the different types cannot be clearly distinguished from each other.

Nasal diphtheria: This is the mildest and commonest form. The patient – often a child – has a runny nose and there may also be some bloody discharge from the nose. There may be some white 'membrane' visible in the nostrils. The child is only slightly unwell, and as long as the infection does not spread, recovery is usually complete. The diphtheria toxin is not absorbed easily from the nose, so there is little risk of complications.

Tonsillar diphtheria: This type is more severe. A membrane forms on the tonsils, and the child can become quite unwell with a high temperature. He or she may have some difficulty in swallowing because the palate becomes paralysed. Recovery is usually complete after an illness of about a week, without long-term disability.

Naso-pharyngeal diphtheria: This type is a severe infection with a very real chance of the patient dying during the illness. The onset is rapid, with the child developing a fever, a severe sore throat and nasal discharge. A heavy whitish membrane builds up over the back of the throat, which can spread down the windpipe and, after a few days, may change colour to a dark greenish-grey. Glands in the neck can become enlarged to the extent that the child's appearance is described as 'bull-neck'. Large amounts of toxin are produced within the membrane, and this can affect the action of the heart. In the acute stage, within the first week or two, the PULSE may become poor or irregular, heart failure can set in, and the patient may then die. If the child survives the first few weeks, other late complications can occur as a result of the toxin's action on the nervous system. Apart from

PARALYSIS of the palate, which causes difficulty in swallowing, paralysis of the whole of the throat may occur, with consequent difficulty in breathing. This may then be made worse by paralysis of the chest muscles as well. Sometimes paralysis can affect the limbs, particularly the legs, and this may last for many weeks.

Laryngeal diphtheria: This is also a very serious type of diphtheria. The LARYNX (voice-box) is affected by the growth of the diphtheria membrane. Early symptoms include cough, croup and fever. The child can become rapidly unwell and may die either as a result of obstruction to breathing or as a result of the action of the toxins.

Skin diphtheria: The same diphtheria bacteria can also cause a quite different type of illness. It can produce small sores on the skin of the trunk or limbs, particularly the legs, which may take a long time to heal. Complications from toxins can occur, but are very rare. This type of diphtheria spreads readily by direct contact from person to person, and can give immunity to further attacks of diphtheria.

Treatment

Once diphtheria is diagnosed, early treatment can be lifesaving. Antibiotics, such as penicillin, are given to stop the growth of bacteria, but the most important treatment is injections of anti-toxin. This is a specially prepared serum which is an antidote to the diphtheria toxin. If it is given early enough, it can prevent heart complications and paralysis entirely. However, if the diagnosis is not made early enough and toxin has already been produced within the patient's body, the heart and nerves may already be affected and the anti-toxin may be of limited use.

A patient who has developed paralysis or difficulty in breathing as a result of laryngeal diphtheria needs intensive nursing care, and may also need a tracheostomy (*see* TRACHEOTOMY), a surgical opening in the windpipe to ease the breathing difficulty. Sometimes continuous artificial respiration is required as well.

Diplegia, *see* **Cerebral palsy**

Discharge, vaginal, *see* **Leucorrhoea**

Discoid lupus, *see* **Lupus erythematosis**

Disseminated sclerosis, *see* **Blindness**

Diverticulitis

This painful infection of the large intestine occurs as a complication of a very common condition called *diverticular disease* or *diverticulosis.* About a tenth of the population of Britain have diverticular disease by the time they are 50, a third by 60 and over half by 80. Often diverticular disease produces no symptoms at all until infection sets in, although there may be some disturbance of BOWEL action. However, about one in ten people with diverticular disease develop complications such as diverticulitis or more serious problems.

What is diverticular disease?

Diverticula are small pockets or pouches which form in the wall of the large intestine – the COLON – as a result of excessive pressure building up inside the bowel as it contracts. These pockets usually form in the lower, left side of the colon. For a long time, the cause of diverticula was unknown, but within the last few decades, it has become clear that this condition is one of the 'diseases of civilization'. It is virtually unknown in those parts of the world such as Africa and parts of Asia where a high-fibre diet (*see* CARBOHYDRATES) is usual. Even within Britain, it is twice as common in Scotland as it is in England and Wales. But the fibre content of a traditional Scottish diet is lower than that of an English diet.

It is now known that diverticula develop as a result of long-term CONSTIPATION. If the bowel is full of small, hard faeces, which result from a diet low in fibre, very high pressures build up inside the large intestine as it contracts to move the faeces along. The result is that the lining of the bowel is forced outwards and bursts through weak areas in the bowel wall – usually where blood vessels enter the bowel. Thus numerous little pockets are formed – diverticula. The number of these increase as time passes, but they are very rare among people who always eat a high-fibre diet – such as vegetarians.

Symptoms

Often there are no symptoms at all. However, the presence of diverticula does appear to upset the normal function of the muscles of the colon and there may be symptoms. Frequently, the patient has constipation, but this often alternates with periods when the motions are thin and slimy. There may be intermittent pain low down on the left side of the abdomen, but this tends to improve after a motion has been passed.

Diagnosis

If a patient consults a doctor about changes in bowel habits, the doctor usually orders either a *colonoscopy* of the bowel, in which the bowel is examined internally using a tubular instrument called a colonoscope, or a barium enema X-ray examination. In this examination, a barium solution is passed into the RECTUM through a small tube; the fluid outlines the bowel when X-rays are taken. The radiologist can diagnose diverticular disease from the characteristic pattern which shows up on the X-ray films.

Increasing fibre

The best way to deal with diverticular disease is to increase the amount of fibre in the diet. This helps to relieve the symptoms of pain and constipation, and may also reduce the risk of complications. The easiest way for most people to increase fibre intake is to switch from ordinary white bread to wholemeal bread, to increase vegetables and fruit in the diet, and eat a bowl of cereal – each day. Some doctors advise the use of raw bran in addition to these dietary changes, but initially this may produce a few griping pains if too much bran is taken too quickly. It may be necessary however, to take extra bran if dietary changes are insufficient to produce a regular bowel movement.

Complications and treatment

The commonest complication of diverticular disease is diverticulitis. Since the contents of the diverticula are stagnant, it is relatively easy for infection to set in. Each diverticulum then becomes full of pus and inflamed. The symptoms of the condition are increasingly severe lower left-sided abdominal pain (it is sometimes called 'left-sided APPENDICITIS'), with a fever and constipation. As the ABSCESSES build up, they can affect a larger and larger area of the colon. The patient may become severely ill and shocked. In some cases the abscesses spread beside the bowel, or the diverticula may burst, releasing pus into the cavity of the abdomen which then causes PERITONITIS – a dangerous condition needing emergency treatment.

Another complication is of bleeding from the diverticula. The mouth of a diverticulum may eat into a blood vessel and lead to quite severe haemorrhage into the bowel. The patient then passes large quantities of fresh blood from the rectum with a bowel motion.

If the patient is not too ill, it may be possible for treatment to be given at home. The doctor prescribes antibiotics and the patient needs to rest in bed until the inflammation and pain settle. However, often the patient is so ill that hospital treatment is required. An intravenous drip may be needed with high doses of antibiotics. If there is evidence that the bowel has perforated, surgery is required to remove the part of bowel affected by disease.

Bleeding from the rectum is always carefully investigated. Although diverticular disease is a common cause, other conditions may produce similar symptoms – for example, PILES or even CANCER of the bowel. However, if diverticular disease is present, the patient is likely to be advised to undergo surgery to remove the affected part of the bowel.

Mild diverticulitis is likely to settle easily with home treatment, but the patient may suffer recurrent attacks, although they should be less frequent if he or she takes a high-fibre diet. Sometimes anti-spasmodic drugs are helpful. A severe attack of diverticulitis is, however, a very serious, life-threatening illness.

DNA, *see* Cells and chromosomes, Genetics, Viruses

Douching, *see* Contraception

Down's syndrome

This used to go by the name of 'mongolism' because one of the characteristic features of children affected by it is rather small, almond-shaped eyes which slant down towards the nose. They are a little like the eyes of people of Mongoloid – or oriental – racial stock.

Down's syndrome describes a collection of abnormalities which develop during the baby's time in the womb and result from an inherited irregularity of the chromosomes (*see* GENETICS). The most distressing aspect of the problem is probably that all children born with Down's syndrome are mentally subnormal to varying degrees.

The abnormalities may not be too obvious just after birth, but a very striking and characteristic feature of the baby at this early age is its floppiness. The limbs feel disturbingly boneless.

In the first few days of life, other features become more obvious. The eyes are rather small, almond-shaped and slanting; the bridge of the nose is small, too, giving the nose an upward curve, and these abnormalities of the nose cause the baby to snuffle. The mouth is also small but the tongue is of normal size and so it tends to protrude.

As the baby grows, abnormalities of the hands and feet begin to show. The hands are short and broad, with a short little finger which curves towards the thumb. The gap between the big toe and the other toes is unusually large and the feet tend to be rather square.

There are also internal problems that may need corrective surgery. As many as 25 per cent of Down's syndrome children often suffer HEART defects. HERNIAS are common, too, and because of intestinal problems some children can be badly CONSTIPATED as a result.

But apart from these physical problems, the most obvious feature is mental subnormality. Generally the IQ ranges from 30 to 70 but it may go beyond 70 (the average for unaffected people is 100). However, with special care and tuition, the quotient can be raised up to 20 points.

Despite all these troubles, Down's syndrome children are usually easy-going, happy and friendly and, like all people, respond to love.

The causes

Down's syndrome is caused by an abnormality of the chromosomes – the particles which carry the hereditary elements that everyone gets from their parents. The syndrome occurs in one of every 660 births in Britain and is the most common type of mental handicap.

Normally people have a total of 46 chromosomes, in matched pairs of 23, which are numbered from the largest (number one) to the smallest (number 23). These pairs split for reproduction purposes, and one of each pair appears in the female egg and male sperm, so that the offspring has half its 46 from its mother and half from its father.

In Down's syndrome there are 47 chromosomes instead of 46. The abnormality always develops in the same chromosome – number 21. There are three main types of abnormality in this chromosome, but 92 per cent of Down's syndrome children suffer from what is called *trisomy 21*: three number 21s instead of the usual two.

Doctors do not know quite how this extra chromosome makes an appearance, but the most recent theory is that it happens when the egg or sperm is preparing for reproduction just before CONCEPTION, or at an earlier stage. So far, medical research has revealed little more than this.

Incidence of Down's syndrome

The condition is very much related to the age of the mother, but there is also some evidence to show that the age of the father is marginally relevant. When the mother is 20, the chance is one in 2300. This reduces to one in 290 at 30 years old and one in 46 over 45 years old. If a woman has once had a Down's syndrome baby, the chances of her having a second are doubled. If a Down's syndrome female has a baby (a rare occurrence), there is a one in two chance it will also have the syndrome. No male with Down's syndrome can father a child because his testicles will be underdeveloped and unable to function.

Why more older women have Down's syndrome children than younger women may be related to the age of the egg. By the time menstruation begins (*see* PERIODS), all the eggs are formed and ready in the OVARY. They are then produced at the rate of one every two months, each ovary taking it in turn to produce. It is possible, therefore, to have an egg resting in an ovary for 30 or 40 years before it is used. The same is not true of men, who produce SPERM at a constant rate. The long time during which the egg lies around could make it more prone to genetic damage from such things as virus infections. But as it is extremely difficult to test the make-up of the female egg in the ovary, scientists are not absolutely sure of this, and new theories often arise.

With expectant mothers over the age of 34, it is now routine to offer a test known as amniocentesis (*see* PREGNANCY), and women over 30 may request the test if they wish. It is a simple, quick and painless process. It involves removing a small amount of the amniotic fluid from inside the womb in order to study the cells shed by the baby, who floats in this fluid. The cells are examined under a microscope, where any abnormality can be seen. It is then a matter for the parents and physician to decide whether or not the pregnancy should be terminated (*see* ABORTION).

As an alternative to amniocentesis another test, called *chorionic villus sampling*, is being used in some centres. This test can be performed in the third month of pregnancy. An obstetrician removes a small piece of tissue from the inside of the uterus through the vagina. This tissue, from the lining of the uterus, contains cells with the same chromosomes as the baby, and so they can be studied in the laboratory in the same way as the cells removed by amniocentesis. This technique allows an earlier decision to be made about possible termination of pregnancy.

Blood tests can now be performed at an early stage in pregnancy to assess a couple's risk of having an affected baby: on the basis of the results, they will be advised whether amniocentesis is necessary. These tests are called the *triple test* (given at 12 weeks) and the *alpha-fetoprotein* test (16 weeks).

Action

It is essential that the parents are told as soon as possible of any abnormality so that they can prepare themselves to deal with the problem in whatever way best suits them.

They may choose to have the abnormal foetus aborted if they feel they cannot go ahead with having a mentally and physically handicapped child. On the other hand, if they choose to continue the pregnancy and feel they want help, they can contact an appropriate association or parents in a similar situation for help, advice and support. In Britain, the Down's Syndrome Association can provide help and practical advice for parents who want and need it. Organizations such as these also provide information on the development of the child and also give help to parents in adjusting to their own feelings. Guilt is a common reaction to having a handicapped child and can last for months, but discussion and counselling from other parents in the same situation can help new parents overcome this.

Development

On the whole, Down's syndrome children grow up to be happy, contented people. If they are given sufficient care and attention, some will develop well enough to earn their own living. Those who have found jobs are reported to be reliable, cheerful workers who rarely take days off for sickness.

The important factor in the development of Down's syndrome children is that they should be stimulated from the earliest possible age. Love and affection are, of course, very important from the very beginning of their lives. Also, parents should try to stimulate all their senses – by moving the child's limbs, playing different sounds to stimulate hearing, placing the child in contact with different textures and keeping the child visually interested. If this is not done, Down's syndrome children will not show a great deal of interest in anything and their condition will deteriorate.

Because of their low IQs, few Down's syndrome children will learn to read or write very well. However, some experts claim to have found that, with proper teaching, Down's children can achieve a remarkable improvement.

There is usually no difficulty in toilet training these children, or teaching them to dress and feed themselves. Those with higher IQs may also be able to handle simple tasks such as collecting items on a shopping list, but even so they may have some difficulty with money calculations.

Adolescence can sometimes be difficult for the child's parents as well as the child. It is often possible to arrange holidays away from home with groups of other children who are similarly handicapped through either a local authority or welfare group.

Down's syndrome children tend not to live as long as other people. The risk of severe pneumonia is much increased during childhood, and the inherited abnormalities of the heart may be so severe as to result in an early death. However, if there is no cardiac abnormality and the child passes his or her early years without trouble, there is no reason why a person with Down's syndrome should not live well into middle age.

It is important to remember that Down's syndrome children, like any others, vary enormously in their personalities. Each individual should be treated in a way that matches his or her state of emotional and intellectual achievements – just as any child.

Dropsy, *see* **Heart disease**

Duchenne's dystrophy, *see* **Muscular dystrophy**

Ductus arteriosus, *see* **Lungs and lung diseases**

Duodenum

Joined to the lower part of the STOMACH, the duodenum is the first part of the small INTESTINE and is important in the efficient DIGESTION of food. It is a horseshoe-shaped tube about 10 in (25 cm) long, curled round the head of the PANCREAS.

Structure and functions

Two layers of muscle in the wall of the duodenum alternately contract and relax (*peristalsis*) and so help to move food along the tube during digestion. Inside the muscle layers is the submucosa, containing many glands (called *Brunner's glands*) which secrete protective mucus. This helps to prevent the duodenum from digesting itself and from being eaten away by the acid mixture arriving from the stomach.

In the innermost layer of the duodenum, the mucosa are glands which secrete an alkaline juice containing some of the enzymes needed for digestion. The juice also works to neutralize stomach acid. The cells of the mucosa are in constant need of replacement, and they multiply faster than any others in the body: of every 100 cells, one is replaced every hour throughout life.

The partially digested, liquefied food coming from the stomach contains much hydrochloric acid. In the duodenum, this acidity is neutralized by the secretions of the duodenum itself, and by the actions of BILE and pancreatic juice which pour into the duodenum from the GALL BLADDER and pancreas through the common bile duct. These juices continue the process of digestion.

Duodenal problems

The most common duodenal trouble is the formation of peptic ULCERS – an eating away of small patches of the mucosa. In addition, the pancreas or gall bladder, whose secretions are essential to digestion, may not work properly, or the duodenum lining may become irritated by the poisons (toxins) produced by FOOD-POISONING bacteria. In such infections as these, vomiting and griping abdominal pains will be the usual symptoms.

When the duodenum is irritated in this way, its muscles contract while those of the stomach relax. As a result, partially digested food which has already passed through the stomach is pushed back again and this helps to trigger off the process of vomiting. As for all intestinal infections of this kind, the best treatment is to take nothing but fluids for 24 hours and to see a doctor if the condition has not improved within a couple of days.

CANCER of the duodenum is extremely rare.

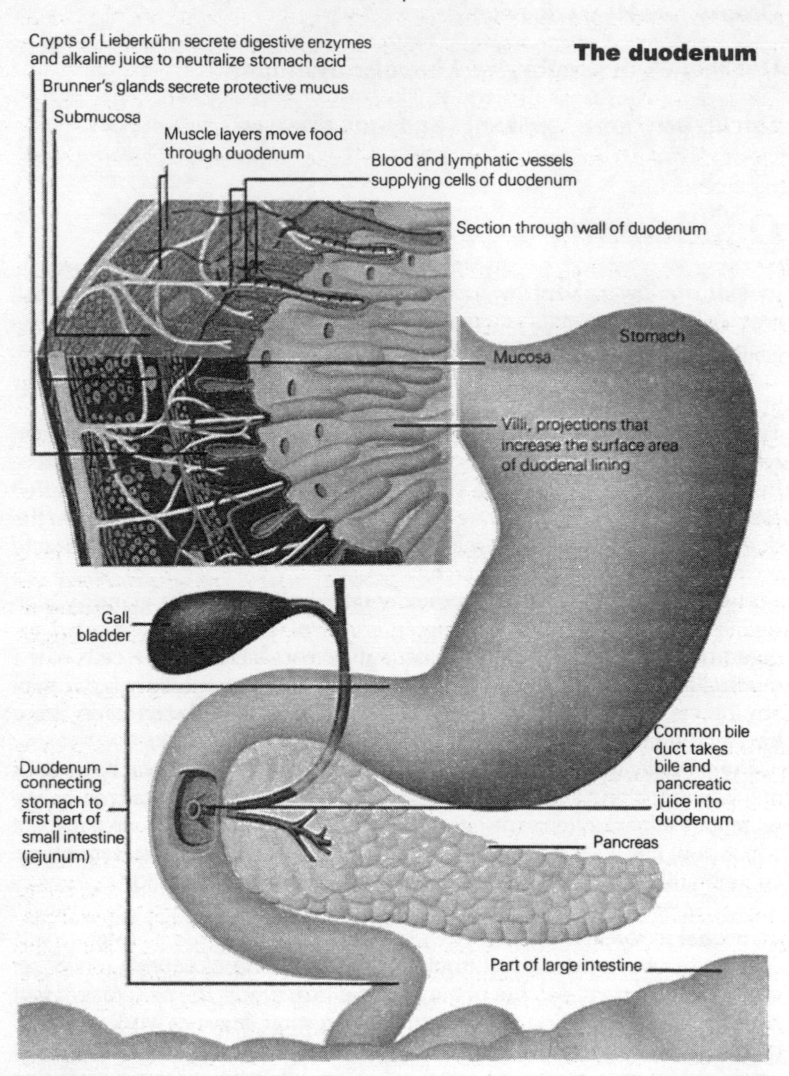

Dysarthia, *see* **Speech**

 Dyshormonogenesis, *see* **Thyroid**

Dyslexia

This is extreme difficulty with reading and writing – 'word blindness' is just one of the terms used to describe its many facets. It affects about one in ten children, is more prevalent among boys than girls and is caused by a small number of faulty cells in the brain, or by a delayed or incomplete development in one part of the brain.

Its consequences, if untreated, are serious as it will affect the child's progress in school, which in turn will create difficulties in adult life. Fortunately if it is recognized early, there is much that can be done to remedy the problem.

Causes

Dyslexia is caused by a localized BRAIN lesion, an area of scar tissue which can arise due to a brain injury, or by incomplete brain development. However, dyslexics should not be thought of as brain damaged as this implies that the whole brain is seriously affected, which it is not.

Dyslexia may be inherited: in about half the cases, it runs in families. It may strike both male and female members of the family, but it need not affect them all. It may produce different effects in different members of the same family, or affect them to very different degrees, from mild to severe.

Symptoms

In dyslexia, something goes wrong in the perception of words or letters. There is nothing wrong with the dyslexic's hearing or vision. The information goes into the brain satisfactorily, but something goes awry at the recording or playback stage, or at the stage at which the brain interprets marks on paper and converts them into sounds, or vice versa.

Being a symptom of a small and localized brain malfunction or incomplete development, dyslexia can take many forms. Sometimes it is confined to difficulty in reading and affects the person's ability to understand not only long or complex words but also words of one syllable. Often writing is affected, either because the child has difficulty in forming letter shapes or because the ability to learn to spell is affected.

Sometimes an inability to do arithmetic is involved, though the difficulty may largely be to do with problems of writing down figures correctly. Some children with this form of dyslexia perform fairly well with verbal questions, but if asked to write down the answers, they reverse the correct order of the numbers or even include a completely irrelevant number. Alternatively, there may be difficulties in touch recognition, where the child fails to recognize the shape of an object that he or she handles, or cannot tell the identity of a letter or number traced with the fingers. However, a dyslexic may have only one or a combination of these difficulties.

Dyslexics may be labelled as lazy, wilfully disobedient or 'thick', and typecast as not being worth worrying or bothering about. Consequently the child may be relegated to a slow learning group and, being often otherwise bright and intelligent, will become bored by school, come to dislike it and start playing truant. He or she will fail examinations, be left further behind and, if the dyslexia is untreated, not be able to catch up.

Treatment

Once the problem is recognized, there are remedial programmes for both children and adults, some of which may have to be tailored to the individual. This special tuition will not only help with the general difficulties of reading and writing, but also they will teach the speedy recognition of road signs and essential words such as 'danger', 'fire', 'no entry', 'caution' and so on.

Released from the pressure of achieving a 'normal' reading competence, the child may start to feel confident in other fields. Oral instruction, tape-recorded notes, films, pictures or video tapes are other alternative learning methods the child can use to minimize any reading difficulties.

Dyspareunia, *see* Sex and sexual intercourse

Dysplasia, *see* Cervix and cervical cancer

Dystrophy, *see* Muscular dystrophy

E

E, vitamin, *see* Vitamins

Ears

Each ear is divided into three parts: the *outer ear,* which gathers sound like a radar scanner; the *middle ear,* whose gear-like assembly of bones amplify the sounds they receive; and the *inner ear,* which converts sound vibrations into electrical impulses and works out the position the head is in – i.e. BALANCE.

The resulting messages are transmitted to the brain along a pair of nerves which lie side by side: the vestibular nerve for balance and the cochlear nerve for sound.

See also BALANCE and HEARING.

Problems

The lining of the ear canal is kept moist by WAX which is produced by the skin in the canal. It is quite normal for small amounts of wax to appear at the outside of the ear because the ear has a self-cleaning mechanism. Excess wax appearing at the outer part of the ear can simply be wiped away, but nothing should ever be used inside the ear canal, except under medical supervision, to attempt to clean wax away.

The most common problem with the outer ear is infection or *otitis externa.* This results in swelling, discharge and sometimes deafness if the ear becomes blocked by the discharge. It is particularly common and sometimes occurs repeatedly in people with very greasy skin and a tendency to dandruff. It also occurs as a result of swimming. Treatment is by ANTIBIOTICS, either taken by mouth or in the form of ear drops.

Middle ear inflammation (*otitis media*) occurs when VIRUSES or BACTERIA enter the Eustachian tube which connects the middle ear with the back of the throat. It is, therefore, usually preceded by a sore throat. These infections are very painful because the chamber is small and there is nowhere for the pus to go. The drum becomes reddened and bulges outwards, and when the infection is severe, the drum may actually rupture and the pus then drains straight from the outer ears.

In the majority of cases, the drum heals completely and hearing is not affected. Sometimes, however, the condition becomes chronic and DEAFNESS may result. Discharge from the ears, pain or any loss of hearing always warrant a visit to the doctor, this is especially important in children. Treatment of *otitis media* is always with antibiotics.

There are a number of different causes of deafness. Occasionally babies are

Structure of the ear

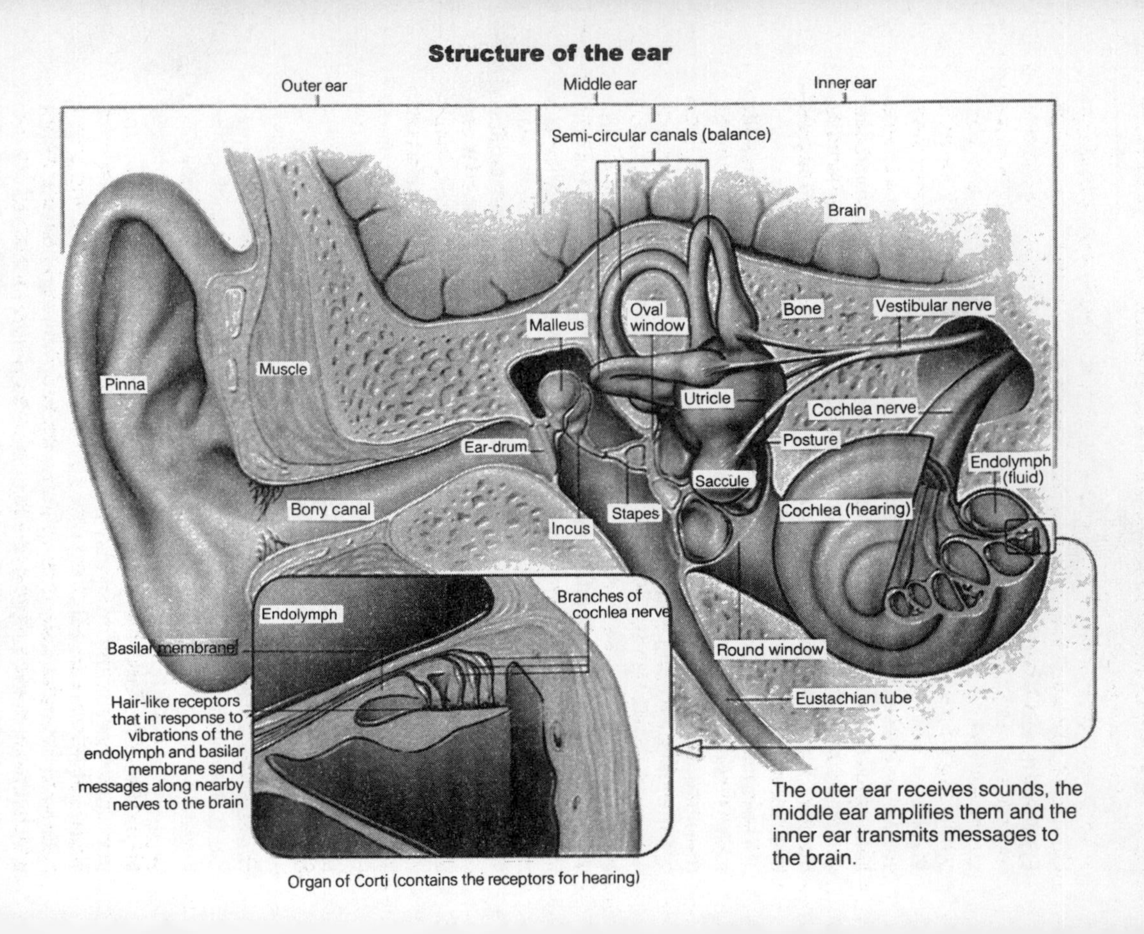

The outer ear receives sounds, the middle ear amplifies them and the inner ear transmits messages to the brain.

born deaf because of poor development of their inner ear, or this may result from maternal infection with RUBELLA during pregnancy. Any child born deaf needs very careful assessment and subsequently special education in order to help to develop speech.

Toddlers and older children may become deaf as a result of *otitis media* or chronic inflammation in the middle ear (called secretory *otitis media*, or 'glue ear'). Glue ear is a common problem, affecting up to one in ten children at some time in their lives. Thick fluid collects in the middle ear, effectively preventing normal movement of the small bones in the middle ear. This results in deafness. The cause of this condition is far from clear, although it may be that low-grade persistent infection or ALLERGY are possible causes. Any child who does not appear to be hearing well should see a doctor or have a hearing test, because deafness may seriously affect his or her education. Glue ear can be treated with decongestant medicines, or simple surgery to remove the gluey fluid if medicines do not work. Once treated, the child will be able to catch up with any education he or she has missed.

Adults may develop deafness simply as a result of the failure of hearing with increasing age. A hearing aid may then be needed. However, exposure to recurrent and repeated loud noise over the years can also damage hearing: surprisingly, this type of hearing damage is still common despite the provision of ear protectors by employers. One of the reasons may be the reluctance of some employees to use ear protectors properly. Another reason may be loud music at discos or in pubs. Even personal stereos can produce sufficiently loud sounds to cause damage to hearing, so the volume should not be turned up too high.

Otosclerosis is a relatively rare condition which affects younger adults, particularly women, and may run in families. The bones of the middle ear become stiffened and eventually stop conducting sound through to the inner ear. Hearing loss is gradual, but the hearing may be restored by an operation in which the stapes bone is replaced by a plastic substitute.

See also TINNITUS.

Ear-wax, *see* **Wax in the ear**

Echolalia, *see* **Autism**

Eclampsia and pre-eclampsia

These conditions can affect expectant mothers, particularly during a first PREGNANCY. Pre-eclampsia is the milder form of the condition eclampsia which, thanks to ever-improving antenatal care, is now increasingly rare.

Causes

None of the theories that have been put forward to explain these two forms of the condition has yet been proved to be true. They used to be called collectively 'the toxaemias of pregnancy', suggesting that a toxin (poison) was responsible, but this is not so.

A few things are known, however: the BLOOD flow to the pregnant woman's KIDNEYS slows down, partly explaining why she retains fluid; also the flow of blood from the mother to the placenta decreases, so reducing the amount of nutrient available to the growing foetus.

When pre-eclampsia becomes severe or continues for a long period of time, the baby's growth may be slowed down. This makes it vital that the development of the foetus is monitored in the womb by feeling the mother's abdomen or by ULTRASOUND the moment pre-eclampsia is diagnosed.

Pre-eclampsia is more common in women in a first pregnancy, in those expecting twins or triplets (*see* MULTIPLE BIRTH), and in those suffering from high BLOOD PRESSURE or DIABETES.

Symptoms and treatment

A woman with pre-eclampsia is seldom aware that anything is wrong: she may have gained weight excessively and have swollen fingers and ankles, but these are fairly common in a normal pregnancy.

Diagnosis is usually made at a routine antenatal clinic appointment by testing the urine for protein, and women are encouraged to step up their visits towards the end of a pregnancy so that symptoms can be monitored.

Severe fluid retention that results in a bloated appearance, very high blood pressure and large amounts of protein in the URINE indicate the imminence of eclampsia. This may be accompanied by nausea, vomiting, headaches, blurred vision or sensations of flashing lights. The patient may feel very ill and have a pain just below the ribs. These are all serious signs which, if left untreated, may lead to fits, kidney failure or coma.

Pre-eclampsia is not predictable. Usually the symptoms improve with strict rest, but sometimes they continue throughout the pregnancy.

The aims of trying to keep it under control are to deliver the baby before the mother is in danger of having an eclamptic fit, while ensuring that the baby is big enough to survive after birth. Observation and timing is, therefore, a very delicate matter.

In rare event of an eclamptic fit, the mother's blood pressure will first be lowered with drugs, labour will be induced and the baby delivered either normally or by CAESAREAN section.

After the birth, a woman's blood pressure usually returns to normal. She passes large amounts of urine and swelling is reduced. The majority of women who suffer pre-eclampsia in a first pregnancy deliver a normal baby. There is a chance that the condition will recur in the next pregnancy, but it is usually less severe.

The hormones in the CONTRACEPTIVE pill are similar to those released during pregnancy. Women who have had pre-eclampsia during pregnancy seem more likely to develop raised blood pressure while on the contraceptive pill, so a woman on the contraceptive pill who has suffered pre-eclampsia during pregnancy must have her blood pressure checked regularly. If it starts to go up, she should change to another form of contraception.

Ecstasy

Ecstasy is a hallucinogenic drug derived from amphetamine that is taken in the form of tablets, and has gained in popularity over recent years. Its proper chemical name is 3,4-methylenedioxymethamphetamine (MDMA).

Medical problems: The use of ecstasy is associated with several medical problems including excessively high body temperatures (hyperpyrexia), STROKES due to cerebral infarction and imbalance of body SALTS, particularly sodium, causing stupor and LIVER failure. In overdose it can cause effects similar to an overdose of amphetamines.

ECT (electroconvulsive therapy), *see* **Depression, Mental therapies, Schizophrenia**

Ectopic pregnancy

This is a PREGNANCY in which a fertilized egg implants itself outside the uterus (womb). There are four places where this might happen – in a Fallopian tube, an OVARY, the abdominal cavity or the CERVIX. However, the last three are extremely rare sites for implantation, and an ectopic pregnancy usually means that the egg has lodged in a Fallopian tube.

Normally, an egg is released from one of the ovaries and begins travelling down a Fallopian tube towards the womb. The egg is fertilized in the tube, and then continues down the remainder of the tube, embedding itself after about a week in the lining of the womb.

With an ectopic pregnancy, the fertilized egg is delayed on its journey to the womb and becomes embedded in the wall of the Fallopian tube. It then begins to develop just as if it were in the womb. A placenta starts to form, but it lacks the nutritious blood supply of the womb, and it has no room to grow. Ectopic pregnancies tend to be a little more common in women who have had previous infection in the Fallopian tubes, which damages the tubes and makes delayed passage of the fertilized egg more likely.

Symptoms and treatment

In the early stages of an ectopic pregnancy, there is rarely any reason to suspect that anything is wrong. The first signs of trouble usually occur between the 6th and the 12th weeks. Severe pain is felt in the lower part of the abdomen, often down one side, and is sometimes so intense that it makes the woman faint. There is no bleeding at first.

This pain may be mistaken for a MISCARRIAGE, but the difference between the two is that, in a miscarriage, pain always follows bleeding whereas in an ectopic pregnancy, pain comes first.

Any woman who experiences pain in early pregnancy should go to her doctor as soon as possible. If it is an ectopic pregnancy, the embryo may burst through the Fallopian tube, leading to severe internal bleeding.

If there is no doubt about the diagnosis on simple examination, an abdominal operation must be performed to remove the whole or part of the bleeding Fallopian tube, together with the pregnancy. If there is some doubt, laparoscopy (looking at the pelvic organs through an ENDOSCOPE) may be done.

Statistics do show that, in those women who have had an ectopic pregnancy, there is a 10 per cent risk of having a second one. So a woman who has had such a pregnancy should have an immediate check-up if she again becomes pregnant.

Eczema

This is a skin complaint that affects about one person in 12 at some point in life. It is an unpredictable and rather puzzling disease, often caused by ALLERGIES but just as frequently brought on by emotional upsets or by no obvious cause. It can be distressing, not only because it is irritating and itchy but also because it affects the skin in visible parts of the body.

The most familiar form of eczema – whose scientific name is *atopic dermatitis* – is closely related to ASTHMA and HAY FEVER, and it is quite common for people who have it to have one or both of these other complaints too.

Eczema usually makes its first appearance during infancy or early childhood, and tends to fade away as the child gets older. Sometimes, however, it appears in an adult who has not suffered from eczema as a child.

Most people who get it come from families with a history of eczema, asthma or hay fever, although it is common for one child in a family to be affected while the others escape it altogether. Babies may suffer from eczema because they are allergic to cow's milk, and recent research suggests that babies from 'at risk' families will have a better chance of avoiding eczema if they are breastfed.

Symptoms

The typical sign of eczema is an inflamed area of skin which becomes dry and cracked or covered with tiny red pimples or blisters. The most annoying symptom is an itch, and scratching the irritating area aggravates the condition, causing wet, bleeding sores and increasing the risk of infection spreading to other parts of the body. Eczema usually appears first on the face and scalp and then spreads to the hands and limbs, especially to places where the skin folds or is rubbed by clothing. Much of the discomfort is caused by scratching the patches of rash, rather than by the eczema itself.

Precautions

Eczema in itself is not dangerous or in any way a threat to life. The main problem for the parents of a child with eczema is to discourage him from making the condition worse by scratching the infected skin. Young babies with eczema often rub themselves on their bedclothes in a vain attempt to make the itch go away. Little children can be protected from hurting themselves if they wear cotton mittens (in bed as well as during the day), to prevent them from scratching. Eczema sometimes becomes worse as a result of exposure to certain substances or chemicals. Soap is a common culprit, so is soil. Occasionally even some house plants such as ivy or chrysanthemums may make a child's eczema worse, or even exposure to household pets – cats or dogs.

It is essential that sufferers from eczema should not come into direct contact with anyone who has COLD SORES (*herpes simplex*) because eczematous skin is very vulnerable to the herpes virus and is liable to widespread infection if it is exposed to it. Obviously, no one with a cold sore should kiss anyone with eczema.

People who suffer, or who have suffered from eczema are more sensitive than most to irritant chemicals, so it would be wise for them to avoid jobs which involve exposure to such substances. The risks are considerably reduced by taking such simple precautions as wearing gloves and a face mask, but young people with eczema should think twice before taking a job where it would be difficult to avoid well-known irritants such as cutting oils, resins and shampoos.

Treatment

If the eczema can be traced to an allergy, clearly the particular cause (the allergen) should be avoided. Breastfeeding disposes of the problem of an allergy to cow's milk in young babies, but if the mother cannot breastfeed, or if the child has to be weaned, there are alternatives: goat's milk does not cause allergic eczema as often as cow's milk, and there are also artificial milks based on soya which provide a nutritious diet for babies.

Dealing with an allergy is often only a part of the problem: other measures are necessary to relieve the eczema and prevent it from getting worse. First, materials such as wool, which can irritate sensitive areas, should be kept away from the skin. The child should wear cotton underclothes and cotton socks. If the skin is dry and cracked it should not be washed too often, because this tends to dry it even more. Obviously it should be kept clean to discourage infection, but in place of soap, people with eczema should use aqueous cream or emulsifying ointment, both available from chemists.

Alternatively, bath oils containing liquid paraffin added to the bath water prevent the skin from drying out – various proprietary brands can be bought from chemists or obtained on prescription. The most important part of the treatment is to keep the skin moist. Apart from bath oils, bland moisturising creams can be used liberally. Ask your chemist or doctor to recommend one.

There are a variety of medicines to control the inflammation and itching of the skin. Creams or ointments containing coal-tar extracts are well-tried remedies and may help, but they tend to smell rather strongly of tar. Creams containing small amounts of steroids such as 1 per cent hydrocortisone can reduce itching and inflammation very effectively. Stronger steroid creams can be used for more severe, localized disease, especially when the skin is very thickened. However, they should only be applied for limited periods and on doctor's advice: continual use of strong steroid creams could damage the skin.

Creams containing urea are sometimes prescribed to increase the water content of the skin to counteract the dryness of eczema, and an antihistamine drug can control the itching and burning. Bacterial infection can be treated with a steroid/antibiotic combination in cream form.

The chances are that children with eczema will 'grow out' of it after a time. Fifty per cent of them are, in fact, free of it by their sixth birthday, and only 10 per cent still have it by the time they reach their teens. However, like most allergic complaints, eczema has a habit of vanishing, only to make an unwelcome return in adolescence or adulthood.

Ejaculation, *see* Penis, Sex and sexual intercourse

Electrocardiogram

The HEART is a muscular bag which pumps blood by contracting and relaxing. Messages for the muscle to contract (shorten) are carried electrically from one part of the heart to another and it is this electrical current which is recorded on a machine called an *electrocardiograph*.

The reading it gives, called an ECG, is extremely useful in diagnosing heart complaints (*see* CORONARY HEART DISEASE, HEART ATTACK, HEART DISEASE, TACHYCARDIA). The process is totally painless and has no side-effects.

How it is done

Modern electrocardiographs basically consist of a sophisticated galvanometer, and the patient sits or lies on a couch, and electrodes (sticky patches to which small metal plates are clipped) are attached to each wrist and ankle. Another electrode is stuck to the front of the chest with a suction cup, and this is moved across the chest so that several readings can be taken from various points on the chest.

Inside the galvanometer there is voltage-sensitive needle with paper passing underneath it. Each time the heart beats, the flow of electricity makes the needle move and the heartbeats are traced on the paper as a series of humps and spikes.

ECG patterns

The heart has four chambers, two upper smaller ones known as the left and right atria (auricles) and the larger lower chambers, the left and right ventricles. The atria are receiving chambers and the ventricles are pumping chambers.

For the heart to beat at a regular rate of around 70 beats per minute, with a faster rate if exercising, it has to have a sophisticated timing system. The timing for the ventricles – the two main pumping chambers – comes from the atria, the thin-walled chambers that collect blood from the lungs and the rest of the body.

Each cardiac (heart) cycle starts with the two atria contracting (getting smaller); then, after a small pause, the ventricles contract together. Then they relax and begin a new cycle. This process shows up on the ECG as a small hump known as the P wave, which represents the atria contracting, followed by spikes which are the ventricles contracting. These spikes are known as the QR and S points.

Most of the electrical activity that the ECG picks up comes from the major thick-walled pumping chamber, the left ventricle, because this contains most of the heart muscle. The major spikes on the recording come from the voltage change as the left ventricle contracts. The ventricles then relax and recharge, shown as the T wave, before the cycle starts again.

The shape of the spikes and waves is different according to which part of the chest they are recorded from.

Diagnosing heart attacks

The most important use of the ECG is to show whether a person has suffered a heart attack or if there is lack of blood supply to the heart muscle which can be a cause of both angina and heart attacks.

The change in the pattern will be in the T wave part of the ECG. Subjects with an acute heart attack show an abnormal pattern between the QRS spikes and the T wave. As recovery takes place, the T wave turns upside down.

When no heart attack has taken place, but there is a lack of blood supply to the muscle, there are often minor changes which are picked up on the ECG while the patient is lying still. These changes may be accentuated if another ECG is recorded during or immediately after some form of exercise. Sometimes the changes are not present at all on the ECG taken at rest, but they become apparent when the ECG is taken during physical exercise. This is known as *exercise testing.*

Other faults

One of the most frequent heart problems is that the atria stop contracting properly and start uncoordinated activity, known as *atrial fibrillation.* Then the ECG shows no P waves, but instead a wavy line with irregular spikes.

Since the ventricles are working all right, this is not a serious problem, although patients may experience palpitations and the heart may beat too fast. The problem can be solved by giving drugs to slow down the rate. More serious is VENTRICULAR FIBRILLATION, when the ventricles do not contract and so stop pumping blood out of the heart. There are many other forms of disordered heart rhythm than can be seen from an ECG, some minor and some serious.

An ECG can also show if the left ventricle is having to do too much work – in the case of high BLOOD PRESSURE, for example. When this happens, its muscular wall becomes thicker, and this creates a greater flow of current, which in turn will make the spikes larger on the ECG reading.

Electroconvulsive therapy (ECT), *see* **Depression, Mental therapies, Schizophrenia**

Electroencephalogram

The amount of electricity produced by the BRAIN is very small and much is lost in conduction through the skull and scalp. Special amplifying equipment – the electroencephalogram (EEG) – records the brain's electrical activity by causing an ink pen to move over a roll of paper.

The electricity from the brain is picked up by special silver electrodes placed on the skin of the scalp. They are joined in pairs over adjacent parts of the brain so that, if the charge detected by one electrode is different from that detected by its partner, the pen is moved by this voltage difference.

If one electrode is over a negatively charged part of the brain and its partner is over a positive charge, the pen will move down; if the situation is reversed, then the pen will move up. If there is no charge, or if both parts of the brain under the two electrodes have the same charge, the pen does not move and the paper records a flat line.

Twenty or more leads are connected by their electrodes to the scalp to cover the whole of the top of the head. The highly trained technician who fixes the electrodes in place uses a special conducting jelly and a harmless – and removable – glue. The machine then records from pairs of electrodes in various combinations, so that the activity of the entire brain may be seen.

There are usually eight pens in a row, recording the reading simultaneously. The final set of lines measures both the strength of fluctuating voltage differences in microvolts (each one millionth of a volt), and their frequency.

The session – entirely harmless and painless – lasts between three-quarters of an hour and an hour and a half, and produces about 15 minutes' worth of brain waves on paper. Once the wires are in place, the person being tested relaxes on a couch. During the session, he will be asked to open and close his eyes and to breathe heavily, and 'strobe' lights may be flashed before his eyes. These are ways of showing up abnormalities in the EEG recording which might be missed in someone in a relaxed state.

What the EEG shows

Each strip of EEG recording shows eight fluctuating traces, one above the other. The operator marks the record to show the areas of the brain which are being tested by the individual tracings. The machine can be switched to test different areas at different times during the recording. Each electrode picks up brain activity from an area of brain a few centimetres across lying immediately under the electrode. Brain activity appears as different types of waves which can be analysed by the operator after the recording is over.

Alpha rhythms are waves that occur at about 8 to 13 times a second towards the back half of the head, and usually only when the eyes are closed and the brain is resting. *Beta rhythms* are faster – about 13 waves per second, or faster

– and usually occur towards the front of the head. *Delta waves* are slow, about 4 waves per second, and usually occur only when people are asleep, although they may be present in young children who are awake. *Theta waves* are of a rhythm between alpha waves and delta waves and are not often seen in perfectly healthy recordings – they tend to indicate some problem.

An EEG operator is familiar with all the normal variations in brain waves which show up on an EEG. The patterns produced in young children are quite different from those of an adult or elderly person.

The technician is first on the look-out for abnormal patterns of waves, which may indicate an area of the brain which is not functioning normally. There may be quite unusual types of waves, such as 'spike' discharges which can occur when the patient is EPILEPTIC. Such spike discharges may be triggered off by the stroboscopic light which is used during the recording, or may occur when the patient is asked to breathe very deeply.

Uses of the EEG

The most common reason for a doctor to request an EEG examination is the suspicion of epilepsy. While it is possible for an epileptic to have a virtually normal EEG, it is usual for some abnormality to be detected in the form of abnormal waves or spike discharges. The operator may even be able to localize the abnormal focus of activity to one particular area of the brain. This area may then be more fully investigated for an abnormality using other special investigations, such as an X-ray computer scan. The EEG recording usually clearly demonstrates the type of epilepsy.

An EEG may also be useful in diagnosing the severity of a HEAD INJURY and may be helpful to localize damage caused by a STROKE, or by an ABSCESS on the brain. It is sometimes used to help in diagnosis of unexplained coma (*see* UNCONSCIOUSNESS), or in patients whose mental ability has suddenly deteriorated.

Electromyography (EMG), *see* **Neurology and neurosurgery**

Elephantiasis, *see* **Lymphatic system, Parasites, Worms**

Elimination diet, *see* **Allergy**

Embolism, *see* **Arteries and artery disease, Infarction, Lungs and lung diseases, Phlebitis, Pleurisy, Stroke, Thrombosis**

EMG (electromyography), *see* **Neurology and neurosurgery**

Emphysema

Pulmonary emphysema is a serious and debilitating LUNG disease. The tiny air sacs in the lungs, called *alveoli,* and the narrow passages leading to the air sacs, called *bronchioles*, become permanently distended with air. The lung tissues lose their elasticity, and the number of blood vessels is reduced. As a result the lungs' ability to supply the blood with oxygen is progressively decreased, and the patient becomes breathless on the slightest exertion.

Pulmonary emphysema occurs less frequently in women. It rarely appears before the age of 40, but if it occurs in middle age, it causes disability and eventually death.

SMOKING is one of the greatest contributory factors, but continuous exposure to dust or high levels of air pollution may bring on various forms of emphysema. Many people with chronic BRONCHITIS also suffer from emphysema, which is also made worse by smoking.

Causes

Smoking is, therefore, a possible cause of emphysema, but not all smokers contract the disease, which may also occur among non-smokers. One theory is that a substance called elastase is produced by the white cells in the lungs. Smoke or dust particles may interfere with these cells, releasing elastase, which unless it is inactivated by a blood substance called $alpha_1$-antitrypsin, will attack the lung tissue. People who lack $alpha_1$-antitrypsin are particularly susceptible to pulmonary emphysema; if they smoke they are likely to develop a severe form of the disease.

Chronic bronchitis may also be a contributory factor. The airways of the lungs are blocked by mucus produced as a response to irritation by smoke or other pollutants. To breathe in, a person must make a great deal of effort to overcome the resistance of the mucus, and the inspiration of air may result in the distension of the alveoli. Bacterial infection, which is common in chronic bronchitis, may contribute to the process by weakening the lung's elastic tissue.

Symptoms

The most obvious symptom is breathlessness, followed by coughing, which can be brought on by the slightest exertion such as talking or laughing.

Chewing and swallowing may also be difficult, because of the breathlessness, and there may be discomfort after a meal because the lungs have expanded, pushing the DIAPHRAGM into the stomach. Loss of appetite might occur.

In severe forms of the disease, lung enlargement may cause the chest to expand into a barrel shape. Lack of oxygen in the blood may produce *cyanosis*, a blue coloration in the skin which is most noticeable on the lips and under the fingernails. As the disease is progressive, these symptoms will get worse with time.

Dangers

The loss of elasticity of the lungs and the presence of mucus in the airways may result in carbon dioxide no longer being efficiently eliminated from the lungs and insufficient oxygen being breathed in. The patient may have to make strenuous efforts to breathe, and may rapidly become out of breath.

In some patients, large holes may develop in the lung tissue and large air bubbles called *bullae* appear on the lung surface. Coughing may burst the bullae, causing the release of air into the chest (*pneumothorax*). In severe cases, the lungs collapse, and an operation is required to remove the air.

Emphysema can also affect the HEART. The loss of blood capillaries and thickening in the alveolar walls greatly increases the resistance of the lungs to the flow of blood. The heart has to pump much harder to force blood through the lungs, and it also has to pump a greater volume of blood when the patient exercises to deliver the amount of oxygen required. In time, this can cause the heart to become strained and begin to 'fail'.

Treatment

Although pulmonary emphysema cannot be cured, its progress may be slowed. The most important thing to do is to stop smoking. Some patients, particularly those who also have chronic bronchitis, may benefit from using bronchodilator drugs which help clear the airways, and which may be either taken by mouth or administered by aerosol spray. Breathing pure oxygen from a cylinder will allow enough of the gas to enter the blood. Portable cylinders can be used for short trips outside the home.

Operations to cut out the bullae can be performed. Weight loss can be combated by having small, frequent meals consisting of high-energy foods. Moderate or heavy exercise is inadvisable, but mild exercise may help maintain patients' muscle tone and prevent them from becoming house-bound.

If smokers give up their habit, and treatment is given, emphysema can be arrested. Replacement therapy with alpha$_1$-antitrypsin is now being given to selected patients with the deficiency who do not smoke. Also, if younger patients are severely affected, a lung transplant can be attempted.

Encephalitis, *see* **Brain and brain disease, Measles, Mumps, Rabies, Whooping cough**

Endocarditis, infective, *see* **Rheumatic fever, Valves, heart**

Endocrine system

Many of the most vital functions of our bodies are controlled by the endocrine system, which consists of GLANDS that secrete HORMONES, or 'chemical messengers', into the bloodstream. Since all the hormones are concerned with METABOLISM (the processes by which the body is maintained), they tend to interact.

Hormones are responsible for balancing the levels of basic chemicals such as salt, calcium and sugar in the blood. They are also essential to the reproductive system, controlling ovulation (*see* OVARIES), menstruation (*see* PERIODS), PREGNANCY and milk production in women, and SPERM production in men. They are of critical importance in the growth of children and their development during puberty.

There are many kinds of glands – the sweat glands (*see* PERSPIRATION) in the skin, for example. The PANCREAS, on the other hand, is a gland that has both endocrine and non-endocrine activity, since it secretes hormones into the blood, but also produces alkali and other digestive substances secreted directly into the intestine.

Overall control

A small gland in the base of the skull, the PITUITARY, is responsible for controlling much of the hormone system. It acts as a 'conductor', secreting hormones which turn the other glands on and off. The pituitary interacts with three important pairs of glands. The first is the THYROID, which is situated in the neck, just below the voice-box. Secondly, the pituitary directs the activities of the two ADRENAL GLANDS, which are found in the abdomen lying just on top of the kidneys, and thirdly, the sex glands – the two ovaries in a woman and the two TESTES in a man.

The control which the pituitary gland exerts acts in a very simple way, through what is known as 'feedback'. As an example of this, take the thyroid. When it is stimulated by TSH (thyroid-stimulating hormone) made by the pituitary, it produces the thyroid hormone. When this hormone's level in the blood rises, it turns off the secretion of TSH. But when the level of thyroid hormone starts to fall again, TSH is produced once more. In this way, a relatively constant level of thyroid hormone is kept in the body. This may be raised or lowered by the pituitary, which is itself controlled by the part of the BRAIN immediately above it, the HYPOTHALAMUS.

By the pituitary's control of the adrenal cortex (part of the adrenal gland), cortisone production is stimulated with ACTH (adrenocorticotropic hormone); also the action of the ovaries with FSH (follicle-stimulating hormone), or the testes with ICSH (interstitial cell-stimulating hormone). The balancing of the ovarian hormones, *oestrogen* and *progesterone* affects women's monthly periods.

Apart from its role in controlling other endocrine glands, the pituitary also secretes other important hormones including the *growth hormone,* which is essential for normal development in children, and *prolactin* which plays some role in the production of breast milk.

All these hormones come from the front part of the brain, or anterior pituitary. The back, or posterior pituitary, secretes only two hormones: *oxytocin,* which causes the womb to contract in labour, and *ADH* (anti-diuretic hormone), which is concerned with maintaining the amount of water in the body.

Acting independently

Various other glands and their hormones act more or less independently of the pituitary. Perhaps the most important is the pancreas, which secretes *insulin.* Insulin controls the sugar level in the blood; lack of insulin causes DIABETES.

Also important are the four tiny PARATHYROID glands, which are each about the size of a haricot bean, and lie behind the thyroid gland. These control the level of CALCIUM in the blood.

Finally, there are the hormones secreted by the walls of the gut and by the pancreas, which direct the processes of DIGESTION. These come from *exocrine* glands, in that they secrete their hormones directly on their targets, rather than via the bloodstream, as is the case with *endocrine* glands. Many of these gut hormones have only recently been discovered, and there is obviously a very complicated system of hormone-controlled mechanisms which affect such things as acid production by the STOMACH, alkali secretion into the INTESTINE by the pancreas and BILE from the GALL BLADDER.

The exact way in which the various gut hormones work is still being investigated. Perhaps one of the best known and understood is the hormone *gastrin*, which is secreted by the pancreas and causes acid production in the stomach.

Endometrium, *see* Uterus

Endorphins, *see* Pain, Pituitary

Endoscopy

This is a procedure where a doctor looks down a tube into a hollow part of the body to search for illness or disease. The instrument used to carry out an endoscopy is called an *endoscope*.

Types

Individual endoscopes have been developed for many parts of the body, including the ABDOMINAL cavity, OESOPHAGUS, RECTUM, BLADDER, LUNGS, STOMACH, INTESTINES, UTERUS, and KNEE joints. Each of these instruments has a different name in spite of their similarity of function. As long as there is space within an organ to manoeuvre the endoscope without causing damage, the instrument can be used. Notable exceptions are organs such as the LIVER and BRAIN because they are solid.

Early endoscopes (which are still used and are very effective for some diagnoses) consisted of a hollow tube made of metal often with a light bulb so doctors could see into organs.

More sophisticated endoscopes have since been developed, including the fibre-optic endoscope, which consists of hundreds of small bundles of glass fibres down which a light is shone. The image is reflected up inside the bundles which act like a tubular mirror so that the image appears at the eyepiece. As the glass rods are so thin, they can bend easily, making the endoscope flexible enough to wriggle around any organ.

For example, the fibre-optic *colonoscope* can be threaded along the bends in the COLON. By using a kind of pulley, the tip of the scope can be manoeuvred around the curves so that the whole length of the colon can be examined. The colonoscope has greatly improved on the straight *sigmoidoscope* which could only visualize as far as a straight rod could be placed without causing damage.

Other advanced endoscopes have steering mechanisms, clearing mechanisms, and surgical attachments to carry out minor operations, from BIOPSIES to STERILIZATION.

The only limitation to endoscopes is that they cannot see through the walls of organs or into solid organs, but as miniaturization continues, even more useful scopes will be developed.

Uses

Endoscopes are used primarily as diagnostic tools, allowing a doctor to look directly into an organ and see abnormalities and causes of disease.

Larger endoscopes have several channels in the bore: air can be blown in to distend the organ and improve viewing. Some endoscopes have attachments which can be used in carrying out minor operations. A biopsy attachment to an endoscope enables a piece of tissue to be removed, or an electric current can be passed to seal off a point of tissue that is bleeding. Other endoscopes, such as the *cystoscope* which is used for looking into the bladder, have refined attachments which can cut away a bladder tumour or remove small stones.

The most common endoscopies are carried out on the stomach (via the mouth) and large bowel (via the anus). In cases of severe injury or pain in the abdomen, a *laparoscope* can be passed through the wall of the abdomen to look for bleeding or damaged organs. Where a bladder abnormality is suspected, a cystoscope can be passed up the urethra. A *bronchoscope* can be used to look into a patient's lungs to diagnose the cause of a cough, or to look for a tumour.

In exceptional circumstances, it may be necessary to look into the uterus of a pregnant woman and check the development of the baby. This is known as *amnioscopy*. Alternatively, in cases of ECTOPIC PREGNANCY, where the foetus develops outside the uterus in one of the Fallopian tubes, a laparoscope can be used to look into the abdomen to confirm the diagnosis. Performing an endoscopy during pregnancy is often safer than X-ray examination which may harm the developing foetus.

Endoscopy is a harmless and painless procedure. It can save patients from complicated and often inexact investigations – its great advantage being that it gives a direct view of the part concerned – and from exploratory operations.

Treatment

The most common endoscopy that needs hospital admission is gastroscopy, where a fibre-optic endoscope is passed down the oesophagus into the stomach.

Having fasted for eight hours so that the stomach is empty of food, the patient is given some sedation, either by tablets three or four hours in advance, or by injection directly into a vein.

The endoscope is lubricated with jelly and placed in the patient's mouth. The patient then swallows it – retching is prevented because of the sedation – and the tube is fed down the oesophagus into the stomach. Some discomfort may be experienced, but no pain.

The surgeon then connects up the light source, the room is darkened, and he or she then begins viewing the oesophagus and stomach. The patient may be asked to lie in different positions to bring areas into view. In many cases, the procedure is so comfortable that the patient goes to sleep. When the investigation is completed, the surgeon slowly withdraws the instrument. The patient goes home when the sedation wears off.

Other endoscopies are more complex and lengthier procedures, especially the cystoscopy, and the laparoscopy, which is used to sterilize women. A general anaesthetic may be given. Providing the procedure is carried out by a skilled doctor, there is no danger of damage to an organ or tissue.

Enuresis, *see* **Incontinence**

Enzymes

These promote all the important chemical transformations that allow living organisms, including human beings, to function normally. Enzymes speed up some chemical reactions several thousandfold.

The role of enzymes

Enzymes are found throughout the body and come in hundreds of different varieties. Each variety promotes a different chemical transformation. These transformations are of two main types: those that involve the breakdown of large molecules to produce energy and smaller molecules, which are the building blocks of life; and those that use building blocks and energy for growth, reproduction and defences against infection.

Each cell in the body manufactures all the enzymes it needs to carry out its usual functions. Some enzymes are so important that they are produced by every cell; these enzymes are usually used within the cell itself. Others are produced only by certain specialized cells; these may be secreted and used outside the cell. An example of the latter are the enzymes involved in the digestive process (*see* DIGESTION) which act outside the cells in the gut itself.

Enzymes function by binding with a *substrate* (the substance involved in the reaction), which they convert into a specific product. In this way, they act as biochemical catalysts, and each is specific to one particular type of reaction. To work properly, they require the presence of other substances called *co-enzymes*, and must have the right conditions of temperature and acidity.

Enzymes are inherently unstable substances, and in the absence of the right conditions, they may become inactivated and fail to function. If they do, the biochemical processes they bring about also fail to happen, causing a wide range of disorders from albinism to serious life-threatening metabolic conditions (*see* METABOLISM). Many poisons act by blocking the action of essential enzymes, but the same effect can be turned to medical advantage. For example, sulphonamide drugs work by attaching themselves to enzymes essential for the growth of bacteria.

Problems

Certain substances can inactivate enzymes by occupying their working areas. Cyanide has this effect on an important enzyme called *cytochrome oxidase* and therefore small quantities of cyanide can rapidly cause death.

Many disorders are caused by enzyme deficiencies. For example, albinos lack an enzyme called *tyrosinase*, which is involved in making the SKIN pigment MELANIN. This is why their hair and skin are white. Other enzymes convert tyrosine to THYROID hormone: if one of these is missing at birth, the child will suffer a form of mental retardation which used to be known as 'cretinism'.

Enzyme deficiency disorders can be traced back to defects in genes (*see* GENETICS), which determine our inherited characteristics, and so cannot at present be cured. In many cases, they can be helped somewhat if the missing enzyme is replaced.

Many drugs prescribed by doctors work by altering the activity of enzymes. One of the effects of aspirin is to inhibit the activity of the enzyme *cyclo-oxygenase*, which is involved in producing substances called *prostaglandins*. Certain prostaglandins are thought to be connected with inflammation of the joints so aspirin is a useful treatment for disorders such as RHEUMATOID ARTHRITIS.

See also PHENYLKETONURIA.

Eosinophilia, *see* Blood

Epididymitis, *see* Testes

Epiglottis, *see* Larynx and laryngitis, Lungs and lung diseases

Epilepsy

This is a condition in which there are repeated periods of disordered electrical activity in the BRAIN, beyond voluntary control and resulting in a variety of symptoms, depending on the part of the brain involved. The most common are sudden UNCONSCIOUSNESS and twitching of the whole body – in other words, a generalized seizure or CONVULSION (commonly known as a 'fit').

The name 'epilepsy' comes from the Greek word *epilepsia*, meaning 'taking hold of, or seizing'. It was Hippocrates, the 'Father of Medicine', who first concluded in the 5th century BC, that epilepsy was due to a disorder of the brain, but it was not until 1929 that the coincidence between epileptic attacks and the occurrence of abnormal electrical discharges in the brain was confirmed.

Epilepsy affects about five people in every 1000 and is slightly more common in boys than girls. When it develops for the first time in children and young people, a cause is seldom found. When it happens for the first time in

Areas of the brain associated with epileptic attacks

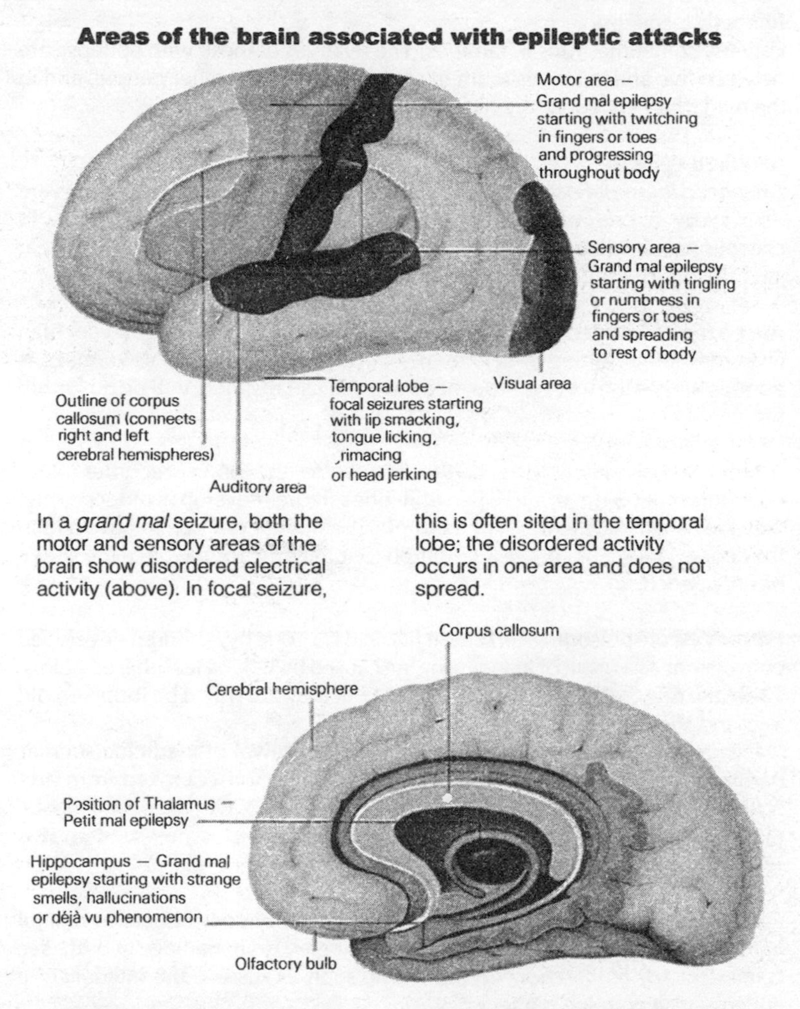

In a *grand mal* seizure, both the motor and sensory areas of the brain show disordered electrical activity (above). In focal seizure, this is often sited in the temporal lobe; the disordered activity occurs in one area and does not spread.

In *petit mal*, the thalamus, an area deep in the brain, is affected. Collections of cells in the thalamus act as pacemakers, synchronizing the pattern of electrical activity in the cortex, the outer part of the brain.

older people, it is more serious and may point to a disease of the brain such as arteriosclerosis (*see* ARTERIES AND ARTERY DISEASE) or TUMOUR.

Epilepsy is divided into two categories. The one in which there is no obvious underlying cause is known as *idiopathic* epilepsy; the other, in which the cause can be identified, is called *acquired* or *secondary* epilepsy. More than three-quarters of all cases of epilepsy belong to the first category.

Idiopathic epilepsy

Epilepsy sometimes runs in families. The relatives of those with epilepsy are between five and ten times more likely to have fits than other people, and in the twin of an epileptic, the likelihood is increased 20 fold.

Acquired epilepsy

After head injuries: Post-traumatic epilepsy can be a complication of a severe HEAD INJURY – one suffered in a road traffic accident, for example. In exceptional circumstances, the condition may develop months or even a year after the injury itself.

After a high fever: Seizures may be caused in normal children by a very high fever, and the resulting fit is known as a *febrile convulsion.* No damage is done as long as the fever is brought down, and usually there will be no further fits.

Arteriosclerosis: Narrowing of the arteries to the brain becomes more common as people age, and when epileptic seizures develop in older people, they are usually due to this. For example, it is not uncommon to have a fit in the course of a STROKE, but less common to suffer any trouble once the stroke has happened.

Poisons: Acute poisoning can cause fits. In days gone by, children developed convulsions as a result of lead poisoning caused by licking lead-based paints. These are now banned for household use but they are still to be found on old toys and Victorian furniture.

Fits may also be caused by too sudden withdrawal of medicine such as barbiturates. For this reason, doctors are nowadays discouraged from prescribing barbiturates for insomnia, although they have been one of the mainstays of treatment for epilepsy. It is important to remember that it is *withdrawal* of the drug that causes the fit.

Epilepsy in mental handicap: Epilepsy emphatically does not cause mental handicap. However, in people who have suffered brain damage at birth (*see* CEREBRAL PALSY), or infections in the womb such as RUBELLA, the incidence of epilepsy is very much higher.

What happens?

Normally, the brain controls the functions of the body, either by interpreting electrical messages from sensory nerves or by generating electrical impulses for transmission down the motor nerves to the muscles. The normal electrical activity can be measured by an ELECTROENCEPHALOGRAM (EEG).

During an epileptic attack, the electrical impulses recorded by the EEG increase in voltage and frequency so that what appeared to be a reasonably ordered pattern of electrical activity becomes a frenzy. The attack usually begins at one spot and then spreads as the fit develops to involve the whole brain. However, the EEG does not provide a sure diagnosis of epilepsy, since it records normal electrical activity in almost 25 per cent of cases, nor does it give much information about the cause of the fit. In a person whose EEG recording is normal, despite a history of recurrent fits, a doctor may try to induce a seizure by flashing lights in the patient's eyes. (This is known as 'photoic stimulation'.)

On occasion, abnormalities in electrical activity in the brain develop only during sleep. Sometimes EEGs are recorded during natural or artificially induced sleep in order to chart these abnormalities.

Types of epileptic attack

There are several forms of epileptic attack, depending on the part of the brain in which the abnormal electrical activity starts and also on how far the activity spreads.

Generalized seizure: This typical epileptic attack, better known by the name *grand mal* (French for 'great illness') follows a fixed pattern and is caused by disordered electrical activity over the whole brain. The attack, which seldom lasts more than a minute or two, may begin with the patient experiencing a strange sensation, or smelling an odd and unreal smell. Occasionally, there is also the feeling of having been in a particular place before (known by doctors as the *déjà vu* – 'already seen' – phenomenon).

This stage of the attack is known as the *aura* and it is followed immediately by the *tonic* seizure during which the muscles contract and remain contracted. The patient loses control and falls rigid to the ground, often sustaining some injury during the fall. (The tonic phase accounts for epilepsy being known in the past as the 'falling sickness'.)

The patient may shout out and will then pass into the *clonic* phase, when the arms and legs twitch and the breath is held. In both the tonic and clonic phases, the patient may become incontinent and bite his or her tongue. After the clonic phase, he or she will feel confused and drowsy and will tend to sleep. PARALYSIS may develop in one or more limbs and last for an hour or more.

Women sometimes have *grand mal* fits more often before a PERIOD, and during PREGNANCY fits may either increase or decrease in number.

Petit mal ('little illness'): This form of epilepsy develops in children only and rarely persists into adult life. The child with *petit mal* does not fall down but loses touch with the world for a couple of seconds. The fits may pass unnoticed at home, and at school, the child may be labelled as a slow learner or punished for inattention. Some children may have many attacks each day, which will cause them to be confused and forgetful.

A child with *petit mal* may be speaking at the time of the attack and suddenly stop for a second or two, only to continue after the break as if nothing had happened. In fact, he or she will be quite unaware of the attacks, and it will take an observant parent or teacher to spot them. The ECG recording is often abnormal in cases of *petit mal,* showing some typical changes in patterns of electrical activity of the brain which are considered to be constant.

Children may easily look vague and far away without having *petit mal.* A child in a daydream can be brought back to the real world without any difficulty; the child with *petit mal* is, for just a second or two, quite detached from it.

Focal seizure: This type of fit is caused by disordered electrical activity in one part of the brain which does not spread. The symptoms depend on the location of the activity and may show themselves as a twitching of an arm or a leg or of one side of the face.

A common site for the disordered activity is in the temporal lobe of the brain, and this gives rise to temporal lobe epilepsy. The outward signs of this include smacking the lips, making licking movements of the tongue, jerking the head and grimacing. The aura – the first stage of the attack – is strong: patients often complain that, during it, they experience unpleasant sensations, smell peculiar smells and have the feeling that their surroundings are familiar (the *déjà vu* phenomenon).

What to do if someone has an epileptic seizure

- It is not possible to stop an epileptic attack, but it is helpful to protect those having them from injury while they are thrashing about. Make sure that patients cannot bang their limbs against any hard furniture, and keep them well away from fire. A child having a convulsion should not be left at all until the attack is over.
- Do not attempt to push anything into the patient's mouth or to force open the jaws. They are clenched with immense power, and it is possible to cause an injury by trying to open them.
- When the fit is over, turn the patient gently on to one side and loosen the clothes at the neck, so that there is no difficulty in breathing.
- If the fit has happened in an unsafe place, such as the street, get the patient to safety quickly on a stretcher.
- If someone in your family has a fit for the first time, give the doctor a careful, detailed account of what happened during the attack and just before it: it will help towards the making of a correct diagnosis.
- A child who has a convulsion because of high fever should not be kept warm. Remove blankets and thick clothing, and if the temperature rises above 39.4°C (103°F), sponge the patient all over with tepid water until it comes down to at least 38.8°C (102°F).

Status epilepticus: When fits follow one another in rapid succession, persistent holding of the breath may cause brain damage through oxygen shortage. This form of epilepsy is a medical emergency and requires treatment in hospital as a matter of urgency. A single epileptic attack does not need hospital treatment, but it is wise to let the doctor know when one has happened, in case the particular medication needs adjustment.

Treatment of epilepsy

Grand mal seizures can be treated with a number of different drugs, such as phenytoin, sodium valproate, carbamazepine, primidone or phenobarbitone. *Status epilepticus* needs to be controlled quickly by the intravenous administration of a drug: the one often used in diazepam (e.g. Valium).

The anti-epileptic drugs are known collectively as *anti-convulsants* and their effect is to bring the abnormal electrical activity in the brain under control. If this is maintained for a long period of time, the fits may disappear entirely.

All medicines have unwanted side-effects, and this is especially true of the anti-convulsants. One common to most of them is drowsiness. Skill is needed to balance the benefits of the medicine in the form of fewer fits against the unwanted and uncomfortable effects of an unnecessarily large dose.

Episiotomy, *see* **Breech birth, Childbirth, Childbirth, natural**

Erysipelas, *see* **Rash**

Erythema, *see* **Colon and colitis, Rash, Rheumatic fever**

Erythrocytes, *see* **Blood**

Excretory systems

Excretion is the process by which the body rids itself of waste products. Different constituents of the body continuously produce their own by-products, and these must be eliminated if the body is not, in effect, to poison itself. Various organs – including the LUNGS, the KIDNEYS, the LIVER and the BOWEL – ensure that this does not happen.

The function of the lungs

Waste products are produced by the basic process of body cells burning up fuel with oxygen to produce energy. If GLUCOSE – the commonest body fuel – is being burned, the waste is the gas carbon dioxide. This dissolves in the bloodstream and is carried to the lungs and exhaled.

It may seem odd to think of the lungs as organs of excretion, but carbon dioxide is the most important waste product to be excreted by the body. If carbon dioxide starts dissolving in the blood in greater quantities than normal, then the blood becomes very acid. This, in turn, paralyses many chemical activities in the body and death can occur. This is known as respiratory failure and may be the final stage in chronic BRONCHITIS.

The kidneys

Most body cells use some protein in their chemical activities, and whenever protein is broken down, the waste products contain nitrogen. The kidneys are responsible for filtering this nitrogen-containing waste – the most common compound of which is urea – out of the bloodstream.

The kidneys also regulate the amount of water passed out of the body and keep the correct balance of salt in the body.

The action of the kidneys is complex. The kidneys receive about 1 litre (2 pints) of blood every minute. This eventually reaches a filter at the end of one of the kidney tubules – of which there are two million in each kidney – and is separated out so that the watery element of blood (the plasma) passes into the tubule while most of the rest stays in the bloodstream. As the filtered fluid passes down the long kidney tubule, most of the water, salt and other valuable substances are absorbed back into the bloodstream. Some water, urea, salt and other waste substances are passed in the form of urine down two tubes into the bladder.

The liver

The liver is a great chemical factory and storehouse with cells grouped in clusters around veins into which they pass their products. However, each cluster of liver cells is also very conveniently placed to excrete waste in the form of BILE into a bile duct. The bile ducts gather together and eventually form one large duct.

The gall bladder

Bile is stored in the GALL BLADDER which squeezes it out into the INTESTINES from the stomach. The reason for this is that bile contains substances that break down large droplets of fat into smaller droplets – a process called emulsification – and makes them easier to absorb. So the bile system not only provides a useful way of eliminating waste products from the liver but also plays an important role in the digestion of food.

The bowels

When food enters the STOMACH, it is churned around and broken down by acid until it is liquid. It then enters the small intestine (*see* DUODENUM) where the true process of DIGESTION takes place and all the desirable nutrients in the food are absorbed. Finally it enters the COLON or bowel. This is a long, wide tube which starts in the lower right-hand corner of the abdomen, then works up and round in a horseshoe shape before coming to an end at the anus.

It is during this passage through the large bowel that what remains of the original food gradually solidifies as water from it is absorbed into the bloodstream through the bowel wall. The final hardness of the food waste – the faeces – depends upon how much water is absorbed.

Most of the substance of the faeces is simply food residue after the nutrients have been removed. It is arguable whether this should be called excretion, but the bowel certainly does contain some true excretions, since it contains the waste products of cell chemistry in the form of bile.

The skin

On a hot day the body loses a large amount of salt and water in sweat (*see* PERSPIRATION). Sweat is the product of the sweat glands in the SKIN and its sole purpose is to regulate body heat since heat is lost as the sweat evaporates from the skin.

However, if someone were not to sweat at all for a day, any excess salt or water could easily be excreted by the kidneys. So sweat does not fulfil any essential function in the clearing of waste products.

Exercise

The amount of exercise needed to keep fit will vary considerably from one person to another, depending on factors such as diet (*see* NUTRITION), type of work, normal body weight (*see* OBESITY), METABOLIC rate and the ability to handle various forms of STRESS.

Walking, jogging, swimming, cycling and games such as tennis and squash are ideal forms of exercise for keeping the whole body in trim. Other types, such as yoga and callisthenics (from the Greek, meaning beauty and strength), exercise specific areas of the body or are used as part of an overall programme.

Additional exercise to that required to keep the body functioning properly usually involves increasing MUSCLE bulk and strength and developing the capacity of the LUNGS and HEART. This type of training is vital for any strenuous sport, but unnecessary for normal pursuits.

Why take it?

Being physically fit is not just a question of muscular strength. Someone who is badly out of shape may have an impaired digestion, a lowered mental alertness and shortness of breath, all of which will be improved by exercise. Our state of mind may also be affected by exercise – or the lack of it – because being fitter means being happier too.

The immediate effect of exercise is improved muscle tone. Even when the muscles are at rest, a certain amount of tension still remains; this exists to ensure the body is always ready to respond if demands are placed on it.

Occasional bouts of exercise are not the answer. In contrast, the cumulative effects of exercise on the heart and lungs are well known. Regular exercise will strengthen the muscles and increase the ability of the heart and lungs to supply oxygen to the tissues.

Exercise has been shown to reduce high BLOOD PRESSURE, and its importance in the prevention of some heart conditions is widely recognized. Many cardiovascular disorders are caused or aggravated by arteriosclerosis, in which deposits of fat accumulate in the ARTERIES, progressively reducing the blood supply. Exercise reduces the level of FATS in the bloodstream, making arteriosclerosis less likely.

Exercise is also a valuable part of any overall plan to lose weight. During increased muscular activity, the body's need for CARBOHYDRATES as a source of energy is increased dramatically. If the intake of food is reduced, the body has to rely on stores of fat to meet this, with a resulting loss of weight. If enough exercise is built in to a regular reducing programme, the need for dietary restriction will be less severe.

Who needs it?

As a general rule, planned exercise is good for everyone except very young children and people suffering from serious illness or a disability. However, the degree will vary according to age, sex and state of health. Children up to the age of six need no more exercise than their natural play; too much activity can wear them out.

For school-age children, a planned programme is often part of the curriculum. Some are naturally attracted to such a regime: those who are not are usually unfit to start with and embarrassed by their poor performance. But since exercise is essential for normal growth to ensure the proper development of muscles, BONES and ligaments, they should be encouraged to enjoy it for its own sake.

Statistically men are at far greater risk from stress-induced health problems than women. A period of vigorous exercise every day will reduce tension and increase mental clarity and alertness through the improved oxygen supply to the brain.

Excessive weekend exercise can be dangerous, especially to middle-

Before starting to exercise

- If you are over 30 and contemplating a vigorous exercise programme, consult your doctor first. He or she may suggest a medical check-up first, possibly including an ECG (ELECTROCARDIOGRAM) to make sure your heart is in good shape.
- Do not undertake exercise without consulting your doctor first if you suffer from DIABETES, high blood pressure, EMPHYSEMA, obesity or any heart condition or circulatory problem.
- ARTHRITICS, and anyone else with diseases of the joints, should start exercising only as part of a planned PHYSIOTHERAPY programme; otherwise the problem may be aggravated.
- Choose the right shoes and perhaps take some coaching in technique. The multiple small shocks of jogging, and many other sports, can cause backache and strained leg muscles.

aged and older men. The only way a body can be kept in good condition is through regular, steady training, at least every other day throughout the week.

Exocrine glands, *see* **Endocrine system, Glands, Hormones, Pancreas**

Exostosis, *see* **Bone and bone diseases**

Exposure, *see* **Hypothermia**

Eyes and eyesight

The eye is usually likened to a superbly designed camera when people want to explain how we can see. However, to understand fully how the outside world can be viewed inside the tiny chamber of the eye, one has to go back to basics.

Light

The fact that we can all see is, as most people instinctively realize, due to light.

The best way to think of light is as a transmitting medium. From whatever source – the sun or artificial light – it bounces off objects in countless directions, 'carrying' with it the possibility of the objects being seen.

The other important thing to understand about light is that although it usually travels in straight lines, it can be bent if it passes through certain substances, such as the specially shaped glass of a camera lens, or the lens made from tissues in a human eye.

Moreover, the degree of bending can be precisely controlled by the shape in which a lens is made. Light can, in fact, be bent inwards, or concentrated, to form tiny but perfect images of much larger objects.

The cornea

The cornea – the thin, transparent covering of the outer eye – forms the powerful, fixed-focus lens of the eye. The optical power of the cornea accounts for about two thirds of total eye power, yet the cornea is only 0.5 mm thick at the centre and 1 mm thick where it joins the white of the eye, called the *sclera*.

The cornea consists of five layers. On the outside is a five-cell layer called the *epithelium*, which corresponds to the surface skin. Underneath this is an elastic, fibre-like layer known as *Bowman's layer*. Next comes the tough *stromal layer* made up of a protein called collagen. This stromal layer, the thickest part, helps to keep the cornea free from infection, for in here are various infection-fighting antigens. The stroma is also thought to help control inflammation in the cornea.

After the stroma comes a layer called the *endothelium* which is only one cell thick. This thin layer keeps the cornea transparent and maintains a balance of water flow from the eye to the cornea. Once formed, the cells of this layer cannot regenerate and so injury or disease to the endothelium can cause permanent damage to sight. The final layer, which is called *Descemet's membrane*, is an elastic one.

A film of tears covers the epithelium. Without tears, the cornea would have no protection against micro-organisms, pollution and dust, and the epithelium would lose its transparency and become opaque, gradually leading to BLINDNESS.

The anterior chamber

After passing through the cornea, a ray of light enters the outer of two chambers within the eye, properly called the anterior chamber. This is filled

Structure of the eye

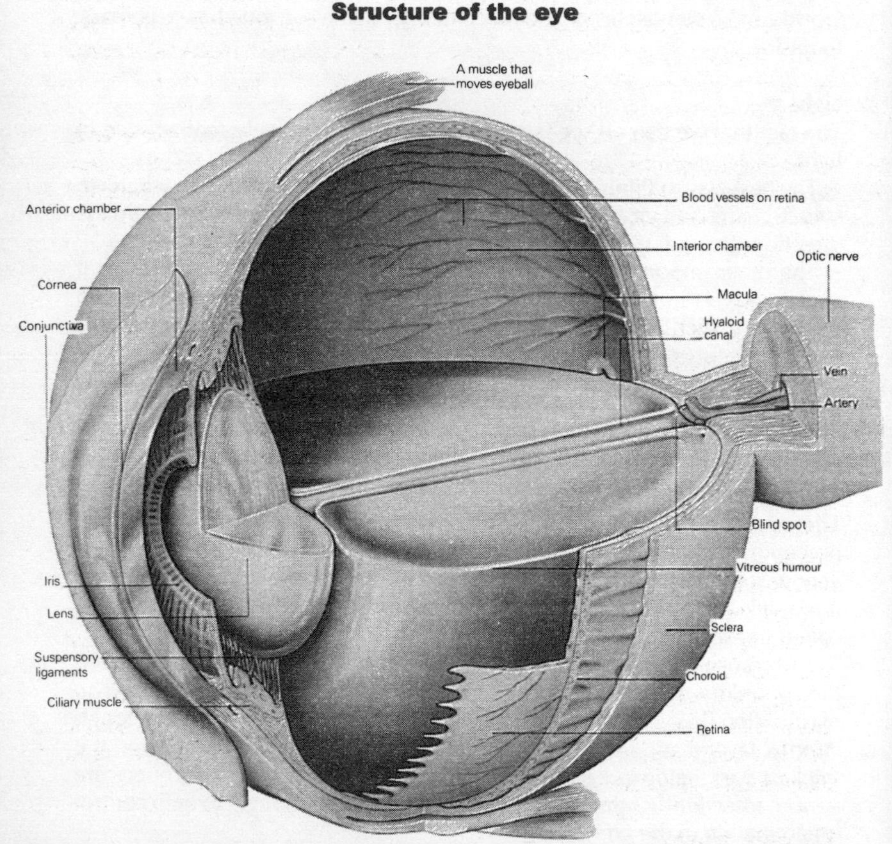

with a watery fluid called the *aqueous humour* that is constantly drained away and replaced.

The iris and the lens

Forming the back of this first chamber are the iris, and just behind it, the lens.

The iris is a circular, muscular diaphragm – in other words, a disc with an adjustable hole in the centre. In a human eye, this hole is called the pupil, and alteration of its size is done by two sets of muscles.

The iris is pigmented, or coloured, and it is this which gives the eye its colour when viewed from outside. (In fact, the word 'iris' itself is derived from the Greek word meaning 'rainbow'.)

The purpose of the iris is to control the brightness of the image entering the eye. If too strong a light falls on it, the pupil grows smaller, without our having to make any conscious effort. In dim light, it grows larger. Excitement, fear and the use of certain drugs also make the pupil widen or contract. *See also* UVEA.

Just behind the iris is the soft, elastic (and transparent) lens, whose job is the fine focusing of light rays. For this reason, the lens is adjustable. It is held round its edges by the ciliary muscle, which can change the shape of the lens.

The vitreous humour

Behind the lens is the main, interior chamber of the eye. This is filled with a substance called the vitreous humour which has a jelly-like texture, and makes the eye feel firm and rubbery. Running through its centre is the *hyaloid canal*, the remains of a channel which carried an artery during the eye's development in the foetus.

The retina

The curved inner surface of the eyeball is lined, all round the back chamber, with a light-sensitive layer called the retina. This is actually made up of two different types of light-sensitive cells, called rods and cones because of their shapes.

Rods are sensitive to light of low intensity and do not interpret colour, which is 'picked up' by the cones. There are three types of cones in the retina, specializing in seeing red, green or blue light. Colour blindness results from having too few of one of these types of cell. A person who is colour-blind does not actually see in black and white, but they will be unable to distinguish between certain colours, the most common being red and green.

The cones are also responsible for clarity and are most plentiful at the back of the eye in an area known as the *macula*. Here the lens also happens to focus its sharpest image, and this is where our vision is best.

Surrounding the macula, the retina still registers images with clarity, but out towards its edges is what is known as peripheral vision – all that area which we 'half see'. Together, this 'central' and peripheral vision make up a wonderfully complete view of the outside world.

The optic nerve

Every single cell of the retina is connected by a nerve to the visual cortex of the brain where information about pattern, colours and shapes is computed. All these nerve fibres collect together at the back of the eye to form one main cable known as the optic nerve. This runs back from the eyeball through a bony tunnel in the skull to emerge inside the skull bone just beneath the BRAIN in the region of the PITUITARY GLAND; here it is joined by its fellow optic nerve.

The nerves from each side then cross over so that some information from the left eye is passed to the right side of the brain and vice versa. Nerves from the outer part of each retina do not cross over and so stay on the same side of the brain, whereas those fibres from the inner part of the retina cross over to the opposite side of the brain.

Where the optic nerve leads away from the back of the eye, there is a small area where we are completely blind. We are not actually aware of this 'blind spot' because the eyes overlap their fields of vision.

At the centre of each optic nerve is a large artery which runs its entire length. This is known as the *central retinal artery*. This artery emerges at the back of the eye and the vessels from it spread over the surface of the retina. There is a corresponding vein which runs back down the optic nerve alongside the central retinal artery, and which drains the retina.

The vital job of these blood vessels is to 'service' the nerve cells of the retina: feeding with nutrients and draining waste products. They also enable a doctor, by means of an ophthalmoscope, to examine some of body's blood vessels without the hindrance of skin.

Common problems

Few eye disorders actually end in blindness. One of the most common, minor problems, especially among babies and young children, is CONJUNCTIVITIS, inflammation of the conjunctiva, the thin membrane covering the whites of the eyes.

The cornea is subject to various types of inflammation. Pain in the eyeball, redness, blurred vision and clouding of the cornea are all typical symptoms and anyone experiencing these needs immediate medical attention. Some people have an imperfectly curved cornea, and this throws a cock-eyed image on to the retina: this is *astigmatism*, which is corrected by glasses.

Glaucoma: Sometimes the normal circulation of the aqueous humour in the chamber behind the cornea is interrupted, and this causes a rise in pressure, which is painful and may lead to blindness. If treated early, chances of complete recovery are good.

Lens problems: About half the adult population of most Western countries wears glasses because of defects of the eyeball or of the lens or the muscle which changes its shape. If the eyeball is too long, or the lens lacks elasticity, there will be good close-up vision but poor distant vision: this is short sight. If, by contrast, there is difficulty in increasing the thickness of the lens, poor near vision but good distant vision results – which is long sight.

 Cataracts: These are a clouding of the lens which, for the person affected, is rather like looking through a window that is slowly frosting up. Most commonly caused by advancing age or DIABETES, they are painless and develop slowly.

Problems with the retina and optic nerve: Obstruction of the central retinal artery leads to sudden total blindness. Fortunately this is rare but may occur if the nerve becomes swollen in its bony tunnel and presses the artery as a result. The blood vessels running over the top of the retina may rupture and bleed over the surface, thereby cutting out the light. This is what often happens to diabetics.

Inflammation of the optic nerve itself is not uncommon during the course of MULTIPLE SCLEROSIS. This results in a special kind of visual loss resulting in a blind spot in another part of the retina; this is known as a *scotoma*. If the optic nerve is sufficiently inflamed, it turns pink and sticks out like the head of a drawing pin from the back of the eye, a condition known as *papilloedema*. Tumours of the pituitary gland may produce various visual abnormalities, depending on which nerve fibres pass beneath at that point. Perhaps the most common tumour to do this is the one causing the glandular condition known as acromegaly, an increase in the size of face, hands and feet.

It is common for a STROKE to interfere with the blood supply to the nerves passing through the internal capsule, the main telephone exchange of the brain. Damage here results in complete loss of movement and sensation on one side of the body and inability to see objects moving in from that side. Eyesight, movement and sensation is quite normal on the opposite side. This condition is known as a *hemiplegia*. Finally, damage to the visual cortex at the back of the brain may cause total blindness resulting from a blow to the back of the head.

Squinting: Squinting is an inability to focus both eyes on the same spot at the same time. This is caused by 'laziness' of one of the muscles which move the eyeball.

Nystagmus: This is the repeated, involuntary jerky movement of the eyes. It always affects both eyes and may be quite obvious in all positions of the eyeballs. However, in many cases, jerky movements may be noticed only with the eyeballs in one position, perhaps looking to the left or to the right. Nystagmus occurs even in people who are not normally affected when they are asked to look as far as possible out of one corner of the eye. The condition can be easily mimicked by asking a friend to look out of a train window: the eyes will jerk back and forth in an effort to focus on close objects as they flash by.

Movements of the eye are controlled by six muscles. Each muscle has a separate nerve supply from an area of the brain called the motor or 'action' area. As movements need to be extremely precise, these impulses are 'damped' by another set of muscles controlled by a part of the brain called the cerebellum.

The cerebellum, in turn, is connected with the organ of BALANCE in the EARS and is primarily concerned with this. Any damage or disease, either to the ears or the cerebellum, may thus result in an interruption of these 'damping' messages, and cause jerky eye movements. A good example of this can be brought on merely by turning round and round on the spot with your eyes closed: when the eyes are opened, the eyeballs continue to make jerky movements until the feeling of giddiness passes off. Sometimes a stroke involving the cerebellum will cause similar trouble. The same is true of inflammatory diseases of the ear.

A second cause of nystagmus is due to damage to the retina. The eye is moved about so that the image thrown on the retina is moved about too. This ensures that the damaged or blind part of the light receiving area is avoided. This type of nystagmus may also occur in albinos, and also in miners who spend a good deal of time working in the dark.

Corneal graft

This operation is done on diseased or injured corneas where the central portion is scarred or the curvature is deformed. In the latter, there is a thinning of the cornea, eventually forming an irregular cone shape.

The eye to be treated has a round disc cut out from the cornea, removing the diseased area or scar tissue. Most graft operations done to restore sight are 7–9 millimetres in diameter. There are two procedures. One is to cut the full thickness of the cornea and the other only part. The latter operation which is called a lamellar graft, is usually done to replace diseased surface tissues.

The donor eye (of a recently deceased person) has a similar-size disc cut from it, which is placed in position over the living eye. The graft is sewn into place using an operation microscope and very fine nylon or collagen thread mounted on a curved needle.

In most instances, the patient is allowed to leave hospital within a few days, and many notice an improvement in their sight even in this short time. If the graft starts to be rejected, anti-inflammatory drugs are used; in many cases, the graft survives.

The stitches will be removed several months later and then, providing the graft is clear, the sight is corrected by spectacles or contact lenses. At this point, if the operation has gone well, the patient should notice a great improvement in his or her sight. The graft will leave only a faint scar.

F

Faeces, *see* **Incontinence**

Fainting, *see* **Unconsciousness**

Fallot's tetralogy, *see* **Blue baby, Valves, heart**

Family planning, *see* **Contraception**

Fascioscapulohumeral dystrophy, *see* **Muscular dystrophy**

Fats

Together with PROTEINS and CARBOHYDRATES, fats complete a trio of substances that make up the bulk of the human diet (*see* NUTRITION).

They are important to us for other reasons. They make food more palatable – think of the difference between dry and buttered toast or salad with and without an oily dressing. And they are the most energy-rich of all foods. For instance, 3.5 oz (100 g) of bread supplies approximately 250 calories, while the same weight of butter, which is pure fat, provides 720 calories.

What are fats?

About 90 per cent of the fats we eat are known as neutral fats. They are made up of two chemicals – fatty acids and glycerol – which are formed from carbon, hydrogen and oxygen. The fatty acids and glycerol form chains called *triglycerides*.

These fats can be either *saturated* or *unsaturated* depending on the structure of the fatty acids. The more hydrogen atoms a fatty acid has, the more saturated it is. The degree of fatty acid saturation varies widely. Unsaturated fats are described as *polyunsaturated* if they have two or more hydrogen atoms below the full complement normally found in fat, making them especially unsaturated.

Most saturated fats are solid at room temperature, while unsaturated ones are liquid. One reason for this is that most saturated fats come from warm-blooded animals whose fat is only just liquid at their body temperature, which is above the temperature of the surroundings, while fish and plants containing unsaturated fats are adapted for life at much lower temperatures.

Which fat is best?

Research has shown that high levels of saturated fat in the diet can contribute to a higher risk of CORONARY HEART DISEASE, which can ultimately lead to HEART ATTACKS. A person who has a high level of CHOLESTEROL in the bloodstream is more likely to develop fatty deposits in the ARTERIES, particularly the coronary arteries, and this leads to coronary heart disease. The level of blood cholesterol depends on a number of factors such as heredity, and the level of physical activity a person takes, but also on the amount of saturated fat in the diet. The more saturated fat, the higher the level of cholesterol in the blood becomes and the greater the risk of HEART DISEASE. The body makes most of the cholesterol in the bloodstream from fats in the diet, and saturated fat intake is a more important factor in determining blood cholesterol level than the level of cholesterol in the diet. Although some foods do contain significant quantities of cholesterol (e.g. eggs), the cholesterol content of the diet is less important than the saturated fat content.

Nutritionists now advise that everyone should eat only moderate quantities of fat, and especially reduce the amount of unsaturated fat. So it is wise to use corn oil, olive oil or sunflower oil for cooking, rather than lard or coconut oil which are both saturated fats. It is worth choosing low-fat meat, or choosing fish more often (which has a higher proportion of polyunsaturated fat than red meat). Low-fat milks (skimmed or semi-skimmed) are lower in saturated fats, and it is also wise to reduce the quantity of other dairy fats such as cream, high-fat cheeses and butter.

It was once thought that polyunsaturated margarines were healthier than butter (highly saturated). However, it is now known that the manufacturing process that semi-solidifies the formerly liquid unsaturated vegetable oils to form margarine creates substances known as 'trans fats', which may actually be as harmful as saturated fats (or even more harmful).

How the body uses fats

Fats are part of the wall surrounding every body cell. The body uses fats to insulate it against cold, as a reserve store of energy, as shock-absorbers round bones and organs, to insulate nerve cables, lubricate the skin and help transport certain essential VITAMINS. It is because of this vitamin transport that it is not recommended that children under the age of two be given skimmed milk; when they are older, they will be able to get these 'fat-soluble' vitamins via a mixed diet.

Fats are broken down in the digestive system into their fatty acids and glycerol. The fatty acids are then broken down further to release energy for immediate use. Any excess is reconverted to triglycerides and stored in the cells under the skin and round the internal organs. The glycerol is converted into *glycogen*, which is either broken down at once to release energy or stored in the LIVER until it is needed. Once the liver's glycogen storage system is full, the excess glycogen is changed into fat and stored in the body cells, making you overweight if a lot is stored there. This is why it is important not to eat more than you need (*see* OBESITY).

Burning up fats

The rate at which the body burns up fats for energy is controlled by hormones from the THYROID, ADRENAL and PITUITARY glands (*see also* METABOLISM). At times of STRESS or during intense physical activity, the hormones adrenalin and noradrenalin have a very rapid effect on the rate of fat breakdown in the body, increasing the amounts of fatty acids in the blood as much as 15 times and pushing up the level of cholesterol. If these fatty acids are burned up in exercise, they seem to do the body no harm, but if they remain in the body, they can, with the cholesterol, contribute to a fatty build-up in the arteries. This is one reason why exercise helps to deal with stress.

Feet

Each of our feet is a mechanical masterpiece that consists of 26 BONES, 35 JOINTS and more than 100 ligaments. In many ways, the form of the bones, blood vessels and nerves of the foot resembles the structure of the HAND, but the proportions are different: for example, the *phalanges*, which are the bones making up the toes, correspond to the phalanges in the fingers of the hand.

It is not surprising that both the hand and the foot are similar in structure, as they have both developed, during the millennia of evolution, from the limbs of apes which were originally designed for climbing and grasping. In humans, the ability of the hand to make controlled movements was gradually refined, while the foot changed its function as people began to walk on two legs instead of four.

The foot has two important tasks – to support the weight of the body and to act as a lever to move the body forward when walking or running. However, it has been found that people who have lost the use of their hands are able to educate their feet to achieve almost the same dexterity and can even use them for writing and painting.

Walking

The foot is made up of many small parts and joints, so it is flexible and adapted to walking on uneven surfaces; most of its power is derived from the strong muscles in the LEG, with a series of smaller foot muscles to aid them in their task.

The weight of the body is supported on the largest bone in the foot, the *calcaneum* (or *calcaneus*), which forms the heel, and the heads of the *metatarsals* which make up the bones of the foot. The other bones are raised from the ground in the form of an arch, as this is the only way that a segmented structure (like the arch of a bridge) can hold up any weight.

The foot has three arches. Their anatomical names are the *medial longitudinal* arch, which runs along the outside of the foot; the *lateral longitudinal* arch, which runs along the inside of the foot; and the *transverse* arch, which crosses the foot. If you look at a wet footprint on the bathroom floor (and you are not flat-footed), you will see that it is narrower in the middle, because the inner arch is higher than that on the outside of the foot. All the arches are supported by an elaborate system consisting of ligaments and muscles.

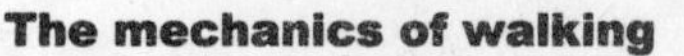

The mechanics of walking

The flexibility of the human foot is due to its intricate anatomy. Shown here are the many bones, ligaments and powerful muscles of the foot and leg that go into action with every step that we take.

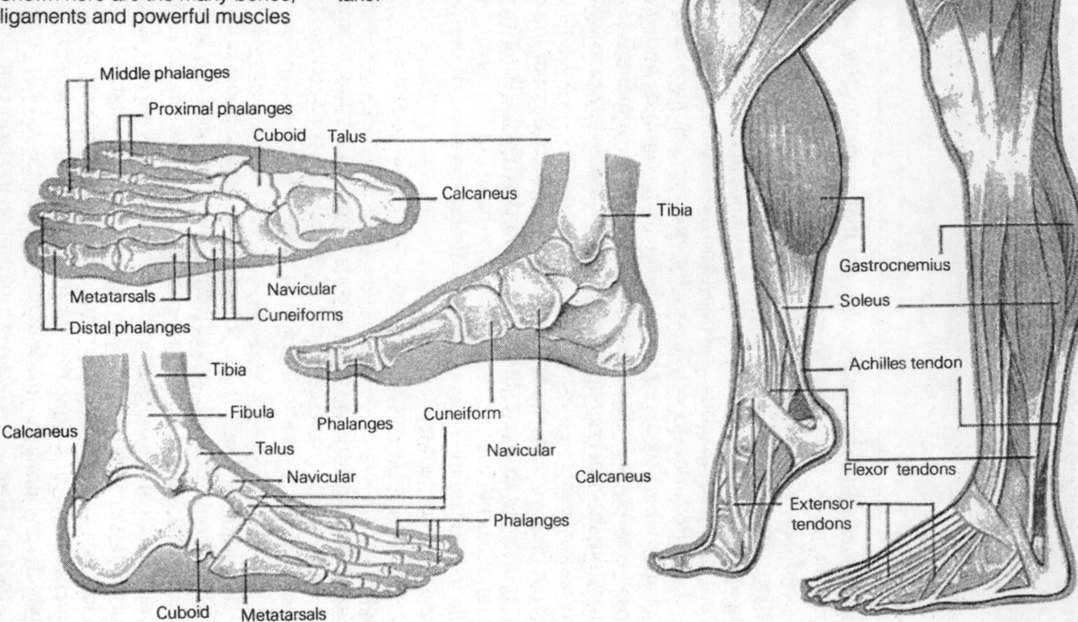

When you stand still, your body weight is supported on the heel and the metatarsals, but when you begin to walk, the load is borne first by the lateral margin (outside edge) of the foot and then heads of the metatarsals. The toes are extended as the heel rises and the contracting muscles shorten the longitudinal arch of the foot.

The body itself is thrown forward by the action of the powerful muscles in the leg – the *gastrocnemius* and *soleus* – which pull on the ankle joint, using the ankle as a lever, while the *flexor* tendons of the foot flex the toes for the final thrust forward. The toes are kept extended to prevent them folding underneath the foot. The big toe is the most important of all, but loss of the other toes does not affect your ability to walk.

Children's feet

Most babies are born with what appear to be flat feet and the arch only develops as tendons, muscles and ligaments strengthen with use. For this reason, it is most essential that young children should always wear well-fitting shoes, so that their feet can develop in the right way. In fact, it is not a good idea to give children shoes at too early an age. Let them run around barefoot as long as there is no danger from sharp objects.

Once your child has begun to wear shoes, make sure that his or her foot is measured for length and width about every two months. Most reputable shoe shops provide this service and will offer advice. As soon as shoes become too small, they should be discarded. Parents should keep an eye on this themselves because young children are unlikely to complain, even if their shoes are too tight. Cramped shoes are the cause of many deformities such as BUNIONS, ingrowing toe-nails and splayed toes which will be difficult to correct later in adult life.

Preventing foot problems

Adult shoes should be chosen with the same care as children's, despite the dictates of fashion. Unfortunately, most foot deformities are acquired as the result of wearing ill-fitting shoes, and problems can be accentuated by platform soles or high heels, because they tilt the body at an unnatural angle.

The same things that cause your feet to ache can also produce CORNS AND CALLUSES, which are hard areas of skin at the pressure points that also irritate the underlying nerves. Although it is tempting to try and treat corns yourself, it is always advisable to consult a CHIROPODIST.

Good foot hygiene is important in preventing infection. Because feet are mostly enclosed in socks or tights and shoes all day, they tend to sweat. Stale sweat not only smells unpleasant, but also creates a suitable environment in which infections may grow.

To some extent, the chances of contracting skin infections, such as ATHLETE'S FOOT, can be lessened by a careful choice of footwear. Socks made of cotton or wool absorb sweat better than synthetic materials such as nylon, and leather shoes allow the foot to 'breathe'.

Flat feet

The condition known as flat foot or *pesplano-valgus*, as the orthopaedic surgeons call it, can happen at any age. As the name suggests, the foot loses the arch on the inside, with the result that the entire sole is in contact with the floor. The 'bathroom test' will show you if your feet are flat – wet footprints made by normal feet are definitely narrower in the middle than those made by flat ones.

The inside arch of the foot acts as a spring that helps distribute your weight evenly through the heel and toes. If your feet are flat, it does not necessarily mean that this bracing is absent, merely that it is not shown by the presence of an arch. There are many athletes who have flat feet, and the only trouble they may suffer from is uneven wear of their shoes.

Perhaps the commonest cause of flat feet in adults is due to laxity of the ligaments holding the forefoot bones together. The forefoot splays and the arch drops – consequently there is often a generalized aching of the foot.

Many parents worry about their children's feet. The apparently flat feet of babies have, in fact, a large quantity of fatty tissue in the soles as well as a prominent pad of fat in the front of the heel which fills the arch and gives the flat appearance. By the age of three, when children are walking properly, their feet will no longer have such a flat look.

Unfortunately, surgery cannot correct flat feet, but the discomfort can be relieved by wearing well-supporting shoes or the sandals with instep supports which can be bought from chemists and some large stores.

See also VERRUCA.

Foot deformities

Common foot deformities that affect some people at the extremes of life are hammer toes and pigeon toes.

A hammer toe can be among the most painful conditions that may affect your feet. It usually affects only one toe, the one next to your big toe. The toe becomes bunched up so that the top of the toe may rub against the shoe. Hard skin develops where it rubs and this may become red and painful to the extent that you cannot bear to put your shoes on, and every shopping expedition becomes agony.

All the toes – apart from the big toe – contain three small bones with joints between them. If you take off your shoes and look at your toes, you will see that when you push the end of the toe next to your big toe in towards your foot, the toe concertinas at the joints and buckles up. This can happen if your shoes are too cramped at the front, or if the toe is too long. It can also happen if there is some imbalance of the small muscles of the foot which keep the toes straight.

This condition is not dangerous, and does not require treatment unless it is causing symptoms due to rubbing on the shoe. It may be sufficient just to stick a protective felt pad over the top of the joint to prevent it rubbing. A visit to the chiropodist may be helpful as he or she can remove any hard skin which may have developed on the toe.

If the pain is really severe, an operation may be necessary. It is a short one involving the straightening of the bent joint by cutting it out. Sometimes a stiff wire may be pushed through to keep it straight. After four to six weeks this is pulled out – painlessly – leaving the toe straighter and shorter than it was. The toe no longer rubs and is pain-free.

A similar condition is *curly toes*, where several toes are affected, often on both feet. They are like a whole series of hammer toes, and if they are causing painful symptoms, they can be treated in the same way as hammer toes. Obviously the best way to avoid trouble with your toes in the future is to wear shoes that have plenty of room at the front to stop them getting squashed, but many people seem to ignore this advice at the cost of painful feet in later life.

'Pigeon toes' is a term generally used when the toes of both feet turn inwards. Doctors use the medical term 'intoeing' to describe the same condition. The problem of intoeing can arise from several different causes. It can result because the forefeet are turned inwards (*metatarsus varus*). Usually, this will have been present from birth but becomes much more noticeable when the child is learning to walk. The other parts of the limb will be quite normal and the knees will face forward.

Intoeing can also result from walking with the whole leg turned inwards from the hip and this is the more common cause. The kneecaps tend to point towards each other instead of forwards. Fortunately, the exact cause of intoeing is not very important as in almost all children the problem corrects itself naturally with growth.

In the past, some of these children were given leg splints or special shoes to wear. However, these are no longer advised as they can be harmful if not applied correctly and the condition will usually disappear without treatment. In the few cases where it does not, walking or running is not normally impaired, and the concern is mainly because of the general appearance. The only effective method of correction in this case involves an operation to realign the bones of the upper leg so that the feet face forwards. However, this is very seldom necessary.

Club foot (*talipes equinovarus*) is usually a congenital defect (i.e. present from birth), but it can be caused by an injury that interferes with the foot's natural growth. The club foot is twisted out of the normal position, resulting in deformed muscles, tendons and bones. Some conditions can be cured by splinting and MANIPULATION if caught early. Special shoes may also be required. Severe cases may require surgery to rebuild the foot joints.

Fertility problems/treatments, *see* **Artificial insemination, Infertility, Test-tube babies**

Fever

This is not an illness: it is simply a raised body TEMPERATURE, and is usually a sign of some form of INFECTION. Everyone has 'had a temperature' at some point, and usually the cause is only too obvious – a cold, a cough or a sore throat. Most fevers are due to infections by BACTERIA or a VIRUS, but they can occur as a result of any sort of inflammation anywhere in the body.

Changes in body temperature

The body temperature is generally kept within fairly close limits by the HYPOTHALAMUS, the BRAIN region concerned with the control of many of the body's automatic functions (*see also* AUTONOMIC NERVOUS SYSTEM and HOMOEOSTASIS). When body temperature goes up, heat is lost by evaporation by blood being diverted to the SKIN.

When the temperature goes down, heat is made in the body by activity of the muscles, which burn glucose fuel and therefore create heat. This minor increase in muscular activity is not usually noticeable, but if a person becomes very cold, the activity increases greatly and he or she starts to shiver.

The normal body temperature – 98.4°F (37°C) – is only an average value: it is not uncommon for healthy people habitually to have temperatures anywhere between 96 and 99°F (35.6 and 37.2°C). In healthy people, body temperature rises through the day, starting at about 4 a.m. and reaching a peak about 6 p.m., and the variation may be as much as a degree or two Centigrade. The tendency of people with raised temperatures to sweat at night is nothing more than an exaggeration of normal heat loss during the day.

Very high temperatures can be fatal. A temperature over 106°F (41.4°C) can cause a CONVULSION in an adult, and permanent brain damage may occur if it rises to 108°F (42.4°C). However, temperatures as high as this are very rare. In most cases, a high temperature can be brought down by simply sponging the patient all over with tepid water.

Causes of fever

The reason why people develop a raised temperature with INFECTIONS and other causes of INFLAMMATION is not well understood. The white blood cells, which are an essential part of the body's IMMUNE SYSTEM, produce a substance called *pyrogen*. This acts on the hypothalamus, causing the body temperature to rise. Drugs such as paracetamol and aspirin bring about a reduction in high temperatures by blocking messages sent out by the hypothalamus.

The common causes of fever are, of course, virus infections such as INFLUENZA, which are usually associated with colds or sore throats. There is no specific treatment for viruses: the only thing to do is to rest until the fever passes.

Almost all other fevers in temperate parts of the world are brought about by bacteria, causing infections of the respiratory passages, the urinary tract, or the intestines and bowels. Bacteria also cause more serious infections, such as TUBERCULOSIS and TYPHOID fever, and collections of pus – ABSCESSES – which are accompanied by fever. Bacterial infections can be treated with ANTIBIOTICS.

In the tropics, there are many feverish diseases caused by parasites called protozoa, slightly larger than bacteria. The most obvious example is MALARIA.

Finally, there are rare fevers which may result from unusual forms of TUMOUR, or from drugs.

Children with fevers

A child can produce quite a high temperature with a very minor infection, and so temperature alone is not a particularly good guide to a child's health. A much better one is whether he or she seems generally ill. Symptoms such as loss of appetite, vomiting and miserable, lethargic behaviour are much more important signs than the degree of fever.

The common cause of feverish illness in children is a virus infection, usually accompanied by a cold, cough or sore throat. However, they are also likely (unless IMMUNIZED) to catch childhood illnesses such as MEASLES, RUBELLA, MUMPS, CHICKENPOX and WHOOPING COUGH.

Children who have a temperature do not necessarily have to be put to bed. They are often much happier taking things easy with the rest of the family for company, instead of being lonely and bored in a bedroom.

It is not necessary to force feverish children to eat solid food, but it is important for them to drink as much as possible: the danger of dehydration is particularly great in babies and very young children (*see* WATER).

Children tend to develop 'febrile convulsions' with very high temperatures – above 103°F (39.7°C). This happens mainly between the ages of one and three and rarely after the age of five. These usually respond to cooling the child and tepid sponging but, if they are prolonged, need to be treated by a doctor. A feverish child can be given paracetamol to bring the temperature down a little and avoid the risk of a convulsion.

Fibre, *see* **Carbohydrates, Constipation**

Fibrillation, atrial, *see* **Electrocardiogram, Hypothermia, Tachycardia**

Fibrillation, ventricular, *see* **Ventricular fibrillation**

Fibrinogen, *see* **Blood**

Fibroadenosis, *see* **Breasts and breast cancer**

Fibrocystic disease, *see* **Mastitis**

Fibroids

These are solid, whitish TUMOURS composed of muscle and fibrous tissue which grow on the UTERUS.

Their exact cause remains a mystery. However, they never appear in young girls who have not yet started their PERIODS, and they do not start growing after the MENOPAUSE, so it seems that their growth is dependent on the presence of the female reproductive HORMONES, particularly *oestrogen.* About one woman in five has some fibroids by the age of 40, although fibroids may start to appear in some women in the late teens or early 20s. They are more common among black women than among white or oriental women. Women who have never had a child, or had their first child late in life, are also more likely to develop fibroids.

Most fibroids grow in the muscle of the uterus and cause an enlargement of that area of it. Sometimes, however, they grow on the outside of the uterus. Occasionally they appear in the inside lining of the uterus, when they are called *submucous fibroids.* They may also grow within the CERVIX (neck of the womb).

The size of fibroids and their number is very variable. Sometimes just one or two may be present, or there may be several, or even as many as 10 or 20. Their size can also vary from that of a pea to that of a large melon. By the time they are diagnosed, there are often several fibroids present, each perhaps the size of a plum or larger.

Symptoms

The symptoms produced by fibroids vary according to their size and situation. One of the commonest symptoms is heavy periods which last much longer than usual. This is particularly the case with submucous fibroids, because the inner lining of the uterus is distorted by their presence, leading to a greater loss of blood during menstruation. Sometimes the periods may become so heavy that the patient becomes ANAEMIC, with symptoms of tiredness and possibly breathlessness.

Another common symptom is pain. Usually this is felt low down in the abdomen, although it may be felt as a dull, low backache. Pain during intercourse may also occur. Periods also tend to be more painful in a woman who suffers from fibroids.

Very large fibroids can enlarge the uterus so that it produces pressure on the BLADDER, causing a need to pass urine more frequently than usual.

Complications

Usually, fibroids are discovered when a woman consults a doctor because she is suffering from heavy periods or pain. Occasionally complications may arise which give rise to other, more acute symptoms. A fibroid may grow so fast that it loses its supply of blood, and then it can cause severe pain. Fibroids growing on the outside of the uterus can become twisted and also lose their blood supply – so-called *torsion* of a fibroid. Rarely, a fibroid can become infected, with the onset of severe pain and fever.

Another rare complication is the growth of cancerous cells in a fibroid, which can then grow rapidly. CANCER cells may then spread to other organs. When this occurs, the cancer is known as SARCOMA.

Fibroids and pregnancy

A woman with fibroids who is trying to become pregnant (*see* CONCEPTION) is less likely to achieve a pregnancy because the fibroids can distort the uterus and the Fallopian tubes that carry the egg from the ovary into the uterus. Thus it is more difficult for fertilization to occur, and it is also more difficult for a fertilized egg to become implanted in the lining of the uterus (*see* INFERTILITY).

If a pregnancy is achieved, any fibroids present tend to grow considerably. They may cause pain during pregnancy and occasionally complications during the delivery of the baby (*see* CHILDBIRTH). If the fibroids are very low down in the uterus, it may be necessary for the obstetrician to deliver the baby by Caesarean section.

Diagnosis

Often, the presence of fibroids can be detected by a doctor during a routine internal examination. An ULTRASOUND examination can then reveal the size and position of any fibroids. This test can easily be carried out in an out-patient clinic. If there is any doubt about the diagnosis, however, or if the gynaecologist suspects any other problem, the patient may be advised to have a D & C (dilatation and curettage) as a confirmatory examination, or possibly a laparoscopy. Both these examinations involve a general anaesthetic. A laparoscopy allows the gynaecologist to inspect the uterus through a small tube, rather like a telescope, inserted through a small incision near the umbilicus.

Treatment

If the patient is quite young and would still like to have children, the gynaecologist may advise that small fibroids are left alone until the woman's family is complete, or symptoms become severe. However, if the symptoms are troublesome, and the patient does not want more children, the gynaecologist may try to remove some of the fibroids from the uterus without removing the uterus itself. This operation is called a *myomectomy* and is most suitable when there are just one or two fibroids causing problems. The operation may also be recommended if the fibroids are thought to be the cause of infertility.

For older women, or if the patient's family is complete, the gynaecologist is likely to recommend a HYSTERECTOMY. The uterus is removed but, provided there is no other disease present, the ovaries are left in place, so there will be no risk of any premature menopausal symptoms.

Filariasis, *see* Tropical diseases

Flu, *see* Influenza

Fluoride, *see* Dental care

Folic acid, *see* Spina bifida, Vitamins

Fontanelles, *see* Skeleton, Water

Food allergy/intolerance, *see* Allergy

Food poisoning

This term groups together a number of different illnesses caused by eating food contaminated with BACTERIA, toxins or chemicals. It nearly always causes abdominal pain, VOMITING and DIARRHOEA which, in some circumstances, can be extremely serious because these can lead to dehydration.

Over the last decade or so, the number of reported cases of food poisoning in Britain has almost doubled. There are several possible reasons for this. The growth in popularity of chicken may be partly to blame, because raw chicken contains germs which cause food poisoning if the meat is not cooked properly. Another possible reason is the growth in numbers of 'fast food' outlets. To serve food quickly, some cafés or restaurants may keep partly cooked food at room temperature ready to reheat. This practice can encourage the growth of bacteria in the food while it is stored, and reheating may not kill off the bacteria completely. Finally, it may be that people have simply forgotten some of the basic rules of food hygiene that are essential if food poisoning is to be avoided.

Causes

There are three main causes of food poisoning.

Bacterial food poisoning: A germ, which may be present in raw food or may be introduced by contamination, grows in the food and multiplies before it is eaten. Once the food has been eaten, the bacteria continue to multiply in the stomach or bowel, and then produces typical symptoms of food poisoning. The commonest bacteria to cause food poisoning in this way are *Listeria* SALMONELLA (often from poultry or infected eggs, particularly duck eggs), *Clostridia* (usually from contamination of food with dirt or by flies), *Shigella* and *Escherichia coli* (from contamination of food or water by faecal material as a result of poor hygiene).

Toxin production: Certain germs that can grow in food kept in a warm place, or that has not been properly preserved, produce chemicals called toxins which can then cause severe symptoms when the food is eaten. *Staphylococci* are bacteria that are often present in BOILS or infected cuts; if someone with a boil on his or her hands prepares food, the *Staphylococci* can be transferred to the food, where they grow and produce 'staphylococci toxin'. Once the food has been eaten, the toxin rapidly causes symptoms.

Botulism is a very rare but dangerous form of toxic food poisoning produced by the bacterium *Clostridium botulinum.* This may occur in badly tinned or bottled food. Another form of toxic food poisoning is caused by *Bacillus cereus,* which grows easily in cooked rice. In the preparation of Chinese or other Eastern foods, it is quite common to keep cooked rice for some time before reheating or frying it. During this time, the *Bacillus cereus* can grow in the rice, producing a chemical toxin which is not destroyed, even by high temperatures. The toxin can survive cooking and can then cause symptoms when the food is eaten.

Chemical poisoning by food: Some foods contain natural chemical poisons. Certain fungi are very poisonous, even when eaten in small quantities. They contain chemicals which can cause coma, irregular heart action and even death in some cases.

A few foods which most people regard as harmless can, at times, cause problems. For example, some nuts contain small quantities of poisonous chemicals which may cause nausea and sickness if eaten in large quantities. Similarly the green areas on potatoes that have been exposed to the light contain poisonous chemicals. Uncooked kidney beans also contain a poison; the beans must be boiled in water for at least ten minutes to get rid of this.

Occasionally, food may be contaminated by pesticide sprays, although this is very rare. If foods containing pesticides are consumed regularly over prolonged periods, poisoning may result.

Symptoms

The earliest symptom of bacterial food poisoning is usually a fairly sudden onset of abdominal pain, which may be a severe cramping, followed soon afterwards by either sickness or diarrhoea – sometimes both. The pains can continue over a period of a few days and often worsen before a bout of vomiting or diarrhoea. Vomiting tends to settle after a few hours, although the diarrhoea may last longer, perhaps for several days.

The interval between eating the suspect food and the onset of symptoms is a clue to the type of food poisoning. If the cause is a bacterial infection, there may be an interval of 12 to 24 hours before symptoms start, which may involve abdominal pain as well as vomiting. If the cause is toxic food poisoning, the onset is much faster, often a matter of minutes. Staphylococcal food poisoning usually just causes vomiting and pain with no diarrhoea. Botulism usually begins after about 12 hours and causes vomiting, abdominal pain, paralysis and coma.

Dangers

The main danger of food poisoning, particularly in young children and the elderly, is dehydration. Diarrhoea and vomiting can lead to the loss of considerable quantities of fluids and salts from the circulation. This can upset the delicate chemical balance in the body and, if severe, may even lead to coma or death.

Death may also occur if botulism goes untreated. The toxin which causes it is thought to be the most potent poison ever known, and thus an anti-toxin must be administered swiftly, together with intensive nursing, to counteract its effects.

If contaminated food has been eaten by large numbers of people, such as in a school or hotel, an epidemic may occur. Usually the source is detected early, but where it is overlooked, goes on poisoning people and is undetected, or where it produces serious illness, such as botulism, the results could be fatal. Cases of food poisoning should always be notified to health officials.

Treatment

The most important treatment in most cases of food poisoning is to replace the fluid that is being lost as a result of vomiting or diarrhoea.

If the patient is a child over 12 years old, or an adult, he or she may be given small sips of boiled water which can be mixed with a little fresh fruit juice, even if the patient is still vomiting. Once the vomiting has stopped or if there is no vomiting, larger quantities may be taken. This is particularly important if there is diarrhoea because considerable quantities of fluid can be lost through diarrhoea. Do not give food for at least 24 hours, or until the patient is taking fluids well. Call the doctor immediately if the patient shows any signs of unusual drowsiness or confusion – these are the signs of dehydration. If sickness persists for more than 8 to 12 hours, or if there is severe pain, you should ask the doctor for advice.

Once the patient feels better, he or she can try a little food, but avoid fruit and green vegetables at first. Foods such as soups, milky drinks, jelly and ice cream are suitable.

Young children with food poisoning can become ill quite quickly. A small baby (under two years of age) who vomits for more than a couple of hours should be seen by a doctor, or if the diarrhoea is severe. Unusual drowsiness or confusion is again a possible sign of dehydration. If you suspect dehydration, you should call your doctor urgently or take your child for immediate treatment to the nearest hospital with a casualty department.

Babies and children with diarrhoea or vomiting should be given clear fluids. Boiled water can be used at first, but if sickness or diarrhoea continues, it becomes important to replace the salts the child will be losing. Ask your chemist or doctor for advice. A special 'electrolyte replacement fluid' should be used after a few hours. This can be made up with a special powder or tablets and contains a mixture of salts which is specially formulated to replace the fluids lost. In an emergency, if such special fluids are not available, a simple substitute can be made by adding two level teaspoonfuls of sugar and a generous pinch of salt to 200 ml of cooled boiled water.

If a baby who is being breastfed develops vomiting or diarrhoea, the feeds should continue, but additional clear fluids given by bottle or a spoon. If the baby is being bottle-fed, give extra clear fluids and half-strength feed (half as much powder or liquid for the normal amount of water).

Often food poisoning clears up in 24 or 48 hours, but if symptoms are persistent, or there is any chance of dehydration, your doctor may advise treatment in hospital. An intravenous drip may be used to replace fluids quickly: this treatment can be life-saving.

Depending on the cause of the food poisoning, treatment with ANTIBIOTICS may be given to clear up any infection. Often, however, antibiotics are not used because they may, on occasion, make the condition worse. Patients suspected of having botulism are admitted to hospital immediately. The patient's stomach is washed out, and he or she is given a botulism anti-toxin

Preventing specific types of poisoning

For general rules of hygiene, *see* GASTRO-ENTERITIS.

Salmonella
Strict personal hygiene must be maintained. Isolate infected individuals until three stool specimens are clear.

Staphylococcal
Treat all infected spots and infected areas on the body. Never touch infected areas when preparing food.

Botulism
Do not eat potted, tinned or bottled food that does not look or smell right, or that has a layer of fungus growing on top. When cooking outdoors, keep soil and earth away from food.

Chemicals
Fruits and vegetables may have been sprayed by insecticides and therefore must be washed thoroughly.

Mushrooms
Familiarize yourself with edible and poisonous mushrooms. If in doubt, do not eat them.

Mussels
Avoid mussels gathered near sewage outlets and those in rusty or red water. Mussels which cause food poisoning colour the water red. Never eat mussels that have remained closed after they have been boiled.

which may counteract the development of paralysis. Patients who are seriously ill have to be supported on a ventilator and need intensive care. Provided that the acute stage is survived, recovery can be complete and the outlook is excellent.

For fungal poisoning, an antidote may be given, depending on the type of fungus involved. The patient is usually admitted to hospital and rested in bed until the effects of the poison have worn off. In more serious cases, intensive care may be required.

Forceps delivery, *see* **Breech birth, Caesarean birth, Childbirth**

Fractures

The word 'fracture', when it refers to a BONE, means it is broken, but the severity of the injury can vary. The fracture may be a crack which runs only part way across the bone, when it is called a *greenstick* fracture; if it is bad enough for the bone to be separated into several small pieces, it is known as a *comminuted* fracture; if part of the bone is driven through the skin, it is a *compound* fracture, as opposed to a *simple* fracture where the skin is not damaged; and if the break occurs as a result of disease of the bone, the fracture is described as *pathological*.

The greenstick fracture gets its name from the way in which a willow sapling breaks along its outer edge if it is bent too far. Only the very young and supple bones sustain this type of injury, which is why it is usually found in infants and children.

Compound fractures are always more serious than those in which the skin is not broken (simple fractures), because of the greatly increased risk of infection. But both simple (closed) and compound (open) fractures may be comminuted.

When bones are excessively weak due to a condition known as OSTEOPOROSIS, found mainly in older people, or where there is a TUMOUR of the bone, pathological fractures may occur without any force being applied. This type of fracture which happens spontaneously, or as a result of minimal force, is always due to disease of the bone.

Causes

A great deal of force is needed to break a healthy bone, but its susceptibility to fracture also depends upon other factors – its anatomical location in the body, its thickness and the circumstances in which force was applied. The limbs, for example, are more prone to damage than the pelvis, so a footballer is more likely to break his leg than a snooker player.

The long bones of the limbs are very resistant to force applied along their length, but are much more likely to break if the same force is applied across the length. These long bones are not of uniform thickness, and tend to break at their narrowest point. This is known as the *surgical neck*. The three types of break that occur most frequently are fractures of the wrist, hip or ankle.

The commonest injury to the wrist is caused by a fall on an outstretched hand (which is used automatically to break the fall) and results in a break at the lower end of the large bone of the forearm (the radius). The broken lower end is displaced backwards, so that the forearm takes an upward bend before it reaches the hand. When viewed from the side, the resulting deformity looks like a dinner fork. This is known as *Colles' fracture* and can happen to people of all ages, but tends to be more common in the elderly.

Fractures of the HIP occur almost exclusively in old people. The injury results from a sideways fall and the fracture takes place across the upper part of the thigh bone (femur) at its narrowest point, just behind the joint with the pelvis. This is a medical emergency, because the unfortunate victim is unable to walk. Any elderly person who has suffered a fall at home and is then unable to get up needs to be taken to hospital by ambulance for an immediate X-ray.

The injury caused by a twisting motion of the ankle, with the full weight of the body above, is a mixture of a fracture of the bones of the lower end of the leg, combined with tearing of the ligament of the ankle. This is called *Potts' fracture*, after the man who first described it, and can happen to girls wearing very high heels or platform-soled shoes if their ankle 'turns over'.

Symptoms

Whatever the cause of the fracture, the symptoms are similar: the victim is in pain, the limb may be in an unnatural position and cannot be used, there may be signs of SHOCK (sweating and pallor) due to loss of blood from the broken ends of bone. If the bone is moved, the fractured ends may grind together (producing creaking called *crepitus*) which doctors feel by placing one hand over the fracture site. However, though pain is usually present, if the bones are not displaced at all, other signs may not be apparent. So an X-ray is necessary to check the diagnosis and exact position of the damage in the bone.

Fractures of weight-bearing bones, such as those of the leg, are more obvious, because the victim finds it difficult to walk, but a fracture elsewhere – for example, of the ribs or hand – may pass unnoticed. Fractures in very young children are also harder to spot, simply because they cannot explain where it hurts. And the very old may break fragile bones without much force being applied and without suffering much pain.

Dangers

The chief danger from a fracture is SHOCK, due to blood loss and pain. This can be a potentially life-threatening complication. Bone, like any other tissue of the body, is nourished by a rich BLOOD supply and the bigger the bone that breaks, the greater the loss of blood. For example, a motor accident victim who suffered a fracture of the pelvis and two fractures of the leg, could lose up to 7 pints (4 litres) of blood in a short space of time. This is why the immediate aim of medical treatment is to deal with shock and relieve pain before the fracture itself is repaired.

Fractures of certain bones must be treated very cautiously indeed because of the risk of damage to tissues underneath. Fractures of the skull (*see* HEAD AND HEAD INJURIES), for instance, may be complicated by damage to the BRAIN from increased pressure due to bleeding. Whenever a fractured skull is suspected, the patient is admitted to hospital as a routine precaution and is kept under observation for at least 12 hours. The best-known warning sign of brain damage is an increase in drowsiness after the injury.

A fracture of the lower part of the RIB on the right side could be complicated by rupture of the SPLEEN and on the left side by rupture of the LIVER. In each case, shock develops due to loss of blood, which must be dealt with urgently.

Fractures of the pelvis can lead to damage to the BLADDER or URETHRA. Fractures of the spine (*see* BACK) need particularly skilled handling to avoid damage to the SPINAL CORD and subsequent permanent paralysis.

Fractures of the limbs, although very painful, are not particularly dangerous, providing that loss of blood has been controlled. However, damage to blood supply to the bone sometimes occurs, with the result that the fracture does not heal. Examples of this are damage to one of the small bones of the hand or foot.

Young bone may stop growing if the line of the fracture runs across the 'growing' end. The result of this is that the affected limb does not reach the same size as the one on the other side. Obviously this problem will only affect children. The growing end of the bone is always close to the joint, so a fracture at the joint is more serious than a fracture through the shaft.

Treatment

Shock is corrected by giving the patient blood and pain is relieved with drugs.

Then the fracture is repaired. In cases where there has been no displacement of bones, the fractured ends need not be realigned: but in other cases, especially fractures of the leg, muscle spasm pulls the bone ends past one another and a pull needs to be applied in the opposite direction to correct this – this procedure is called *traction.*

The patient may be given a short-acting anaesthetic so that the bones can be realigned without causing discomfort. This process is called *reduction of the fracture*, and then the bones may be held in place by a plaster cast, applied while the patient is still asleep.

Badly comminuted fractures or spiral-shaped breaks may be impossible to bring together, and in these cases, the bone is joined with a metal plate screwed along the side. A good example of this type of 'unstable' fracture is through the neck of the thigh bone, which is held steady by a metal nail secured to a plate screwed along the side of the femur.

After realignment, the bone ends must be held in the correct position while healing takes place. This is usually done by means of a plaster cast, which is worn for a variable period of time, depending on the type and position of the fracture. Because of having to bear the body's weight, a fractured leg usually has to be kept in plaster for at least 12 weeks. But non-weight-bearing injuries, such as those of the arm, only need be immobilized for six weeks, or even less in children. Some fractures, for example fractures of the ribs, need no immobilization whatsoever.

Sometimes it is impossible to stabilize fractures using plaster, and then the bones may be kept in the right place by continuous traction. The patient is kept in bed, and a pin inserted through a bone near the fracture site, or some other type of appliance fixed to a nearby bone. Then continuous force is applied to the pin by connecting it to weights hung at the end of the bed, using a series of ropes and pulleys. This system is often used for fractures of the femur, pelvis or spine. The patient may need to stay 'in traction' for up to three months.

The speed at which healing takes place depends upon the blood supply at the fracture site. Age does not matter. We heal just as fast at 80 as we do at eight. If a screw has been inserted, a simple supporting plaster is all that is needed and weight-bearing can begin again as soon as the pain and swelling have subsided.

Freckles, ***see*** **Melanin and melanoma**

Frozen shoulder, ***see*** **Bursitis**

Fungal infections

The *mycoses* are a group of diseases and illnesses which are caused by a fungal infection. Fungi are plants which, because they cannot manufacture their own food, live by digesting other plant or animal tissue. Fungi live mainly in the air and soil, flourishing especially in warm damp places, but they are also found in food, in animal excrement and in water supplies.

There are hundreds of different types of fungi, but only a few of these can infect human beings and animals. The simplest of all fungi are the single-celled *yeasts* and *moulds*: these spread and reproduce by forming buds which then break off to form new cells.

More complex fungi consist of tube-like filaments of cells which are joined together; these are known as *hyphae*. The hyphae interweave in the tissues feeding from nearby cells to form a network of branched threads called a *mycelium*. These fungi spread either by producing spores (tiny seeds) which drift off to form new growths or by slowly extending the mycelium. Once settled, they digest the proteins of the host tissue.

Superficial fungal infections which only attack the keratin (outer layer of skin) are responsible for such common and easily treatable infections such as ATHLETE'S FOOT, RINGWORM and THRUSH. Other fungi can live deep in the body tissues, setting up infections in the lungs, heart and other organs. These infections are often difficult to diagnose and are sometimes resistant to treatment.

Fungi need a suitable environment and a susceptible host in order to start an infection of the skin. For this reason, the sweaty areas of the body are most easily infected. The deeper infecting fungi gain entry to the body through the lungs or as a result of a puncture wound of the skin. Warm, damp areas, and tropical climates, provide an excellent breeding ground for both types of fungi.

Superficial fungal infection

This type of fungal infection is extremely common and can be persistent unless treated properly. Most superficial infections are contagious so they can be passed on by direct contact, or by contact with towels or even contaminated surfaces such as bathroom floors. Some infections of this type can be caught from animals. In addition to athlete's foot, ringworm and thrush (which have entries of their own), the superficial fungal infections include:

Tinea infection in the groin: This infection has been described by a number of names, such as 'jock itch' and 'dhobi itch', although the medical term is *Tinea cruris*. The name 'dhobi itch' comes from an old belief that Indian laundrymen were the source of the infection in colonial times. The truth is probably that the condition is simply more common in warm climates such as that of India.

The infection involves a red, scaly rash which spreads outwards from the groin towards the top of the legs and on to the lower abdomen. It is caused by the fungus *Trichophyton rubrum* or *Trichophyton floccosum*. It is far more common among men than women.

Tinea versicolor (*Pityriasis versicolor*): This fungal infection, known by either of these names, is less common than ringworm and produces a quite different type of rash. It usually covers most of the trunk and results in slightly scaly areas, each 1–2 centimetres across. In dark-skinned people, the rash shows up as pale areas, but in people with pale skin, it appears as very light brown spots. If somebody with this condition becomes sun-tanned, however, the rash stands out as pale spots. It rarely itches or causes any other symptoms.

Treatment for superficial infections

Most fungal infections in the skin respond rapidly to a cream or ointment containing a drug such as clotrimazole or econazole. These preparations must be prescribed by a doctor, although effective creams for treating athlete's foot can be bought from a chemist.

If the nails or scalp are involved or the skin is heavily infected, treatment with griseofulvin may be required. This drug is taken by mouth and is very effective in clearing up skin infections. If the nails are affected, it must be taken for many months until the infection has completely grown out of the nail. For toe-nails, this may take more than a year.

Deeper mycoses

The deeper mycoses are more serious and can occasionally be fatal. They are caused by fungi which are found worldwide, but the infection only tends to occur in tropical areas with warm climates. Most of these fungi gain entry through the lungs, but others gain entry by penetrating injured skin. Once in the body, the deep fungi cause chronic infection in the lung or spread to other organs or body systems where they begin to destroy the tissue directly.

Deep fungal infections tend to occur most in tropical climates, but they may also affect people whose resistance to infection has been lowered. This can occur with certain types of CANCER, such as LEUKAEMIA, but it may also happen during treatment for cancer because the drugs used may reduce the body's response to infection. Patients with AIDS are also more prone to deep fungal infections.

The fungus which causes the condition *Madura foot*, although plentiful in local soil, is only contracted by walking barefoot with an open wound. From here it sets up an infection and forms an ABSCESS which can lead to crippling deformities.

Another fungus, the *Cryptococcus*, causes the condition *cryptococcosis*: abscesses form under the skin or in the lungs, or cause a type of MENINGITIS. A fungus known as *Actinomyces israeli* produces the serious and often fatal condition *actinomycosis*, where large abscesses may form in the region of the jaw, or more rarely in the abdomen, neck or lung, producing extensive destruction and scarring of tissue

The *Aspergillus fumigatus* fungus can cause several lung conditions, ranging from infected lung cavities (an *aspergilloma*) to an allergic-type reaction (*allergic bronchopulmonary aspergillosis*) with symptoms similar to asthma. The *Histoplasmosis* and *Coccidomycosis*, both of which are found in the southern states of the US, cause a chronic, slow lung infection which, in the former, may then spread to the spleen and the lymph glands. *Candida albicans*, the fungus that causes thrush, may also cause deep infections in the lungs or possibly other organs, including the kidneys and the brain. Often the patient is already ill from other infections, or with cancer, and the *Candida* infection takes hold because of lowered resistance.

The deeper varieties of fungi are slow growing in the beginning, and the symptoms the patient exhibits are often vague. This, plus the fact that the tests are not always reliable, makes these infections difficult to diagnose.

Deep fungal infections are often difficult to treat. There are very few antibiotics that are effective, and the few that are available cause considerable side-effects. The most widely used is amphotericin, which is usually given as an intravenous drip.

Furuncle, *see* Boils

G

Gall bladder and stones

BILE drains from the LIVER, where it is made, into a channel called the common bile duct and, from this, passes, during digestion, into the intestine through an opening in the side of the DUODENUM (the first part of the small intestine). Here it plays an important part in the DIGESTION of fatty foods before passing on to join the faeces.

Sprouting from the side of the bile duct, however, is a channel leading to a bag called the gall bladder, where ¼ pint (0.14 l) of bile can be stored. In the gall bladder, water is absorbed from the bile, so that it eventually becomes as much as ten times more concentrated than it was in its original form.

Exactly why our bodies store bile remains something of a mystery. If your gall bladder is removed by surgery, you can do perfectly well without it.

Formation of stones

Doctors also cannot agree exactly why some people have a tendency to form stones from the concentrated bile in the gall bladder. These are exactly as they sound – hard, 'stony' objects, varying in size from a pigeon's egg to a tiny bead. About one in ten people over the age of 50 probably has a stone or stones in their gall bladders which may cause trouble. The tendency to form stones runs in families.

Types

There are three different kinds of gallstones. The most common is known as *mixed stones* because these contain a mixture of the green pigment in bile and CHOLESTEROL, one of the chemicals produced in the body by the breakdown of FATS. They develop in clutches, up to 12 at a time, and have facets so that they fit together in the gall bladder.

Cholesterol stones, as their name implies, are formed largely from cholesterol. They seldom occur in more than ones or twos, and can grow up to ½ in (1.25 cm) in diameter, which makes them large enough to block the common bile duct.

Pigment stones are made largely of the green bile pigment, occur in large numbers, and are usually small. They tend to form as a result of illnesses affecting the composition of the blood.

Gall bladder problems

The main problem with the gall bladder itself is that it can become inflamed, a condition known as *cholecystitis.* The inflammation, in itself caused by bacteria, develops in many cases as a complication of gallstones already present in the gall bladder. Symptoms vary between individuals, but there is usually pain and vomiting.

Acute cholecystitis arises quite suddenly, with agonizing pain in the upper right side of the abdomen accompanied by fever and vomiting. Chronic cholecystitis is a long-standing inflammation causing an ache, nausea and flatulence.

Very occasionally, a large stone will find its way out of the gall bladder and become stuck in the common bile duct. The resulting complaint, called *biliary colic,* causes severe pain in the abdomen, high fever and sweating.

It also prevents bile from reaching the intestine, so that the faeces turn putty-coloured. This damming-up of bile also means that the pigment normally excreted in bile enters the bloodstream, and the patient turns a yellowish colour – in other words, becomes JAUNDICED. At the same time, the body tries to compensate by getting rid of the excess pigment in the urine, which turns dark brown or orange.

Diagnosis and treatment

Anyone suffering from cholecystitis, biliary colic or jaundice is examined for gallstones in order that the root cause of the problem may be found.

There are various techniques for this. Not all gallstones show up on X-ray pictures, and so the patient may be given drugs to take by mouth which are excreted in the bile and show up in the gall bladder on an X-ray. Alternatively, an ULTRASOUND scan may be carried out, which shows the gall bladder on a television screen.

Whether to leave gallstones well alone if they are not causing problems, or to remove them, is another point of disagreement between doctors. Some prefer to wait until the stone or stones actually cause trouble.

An operation for gallstones involves the removal of the gall bladder with the stones inside it. Nowadays, this is increasingly done by 'keyhole' surgery, using ENDOSCOPY, and involves only one night at most in hospital – traditional surgery requires hospitalization for 5–7 days and a number of weeks of recuperation. Sometimes there are stones in the common bile duct which need to be removed as well, but the duct is always repaired after stones are removed.

Very occasionally, stones may be dissolved by drugs taken over a long period of time, but this treatment is not always possible, or successful.

Gardnerella vaginalis, *see* **Leucorrhoea, Vagina**

Gastro-enteritis

'Enteritis' means inflammation of the large INTESTINE, and it occurs in various complaints – ranging from a short-lived bout of 'Spanish tummy' on holiday abroad to more serious infections such as dysentery and TYPHOID. Inflammation of the STOMACH lining is called 'gastritis'. When both are infected by a virus, the result is gastro-enteritis.

The causes of gastro-enteritis are complex. Microbes are by far the major source of the condition, especially those that cause FOOD POISONING. Bacteria contaminate food in one of two ways. They either produce toxins (poisons) which interfere with the absorption of food and the normal digestive processes of the bowel and result in inflammation, or they work more directly by attacking the lining of the stomach and the intestines. Here they cause minute ulcers, resulting in bleeding and loss of the fluids, salts and proteins that the body needs. Sometimes gastro-enteritis occurs as a result of infections that are passed from person to person in the same way that colds are spread. Some viruses may cause gastro-enteritis in this way. Mild attacks of dysentery – often caused by *Shigella* bacteria – may cause symptoms of gastro-enteritis. This infection is often spread from one child to another by direct contact, especially if hygiene is not completely scrupulous.

Poisonous mushrooms and berries can have serious ill-effects and large quantities of ALCOHOL, ASPIRIN, LAXATIVES or over-spiced food are also possible causes. A few people are ALLERGIC to certain foods, and these, too, can cause an attack.

Occasionally, symptoms of gastro-enteritis occur when people travel to an unfamiliar country, especially 'hot' countries – so-called traveller's DIARRHOEA. This is often not food poisoning but simply caused by a change in the type of bacteria present naturally in food, and particularly in fresh food such as salads, fish, and so on. If you travel to a new country, your system is not resistant to the local bacteria, which can then cause stomach upsets and diarrhoea (whereas local people are quite unaffected by the same bacteria).

Symptoms

An early symptom of gastro-enteritis is loss of appetite. NAUSEA and VOMITING may ensue, and there may also be considerable pain in the abdomen – usually of a 'griping' nature. Vomiting may be profuse, and include blood in severe cases.

If the patient suffers from diarrhoea and pain in the abdomen as well, the attack could be caused by infection. The stools (faeces) may be very liquid; sometimes they contain blood and slimy material called mucus; and these symptoms should be reported to a doctor.

Suspicion that harmful food has been responsible becomes stronger when there are a number of victims at the same time. Even so, to pinpoint the precise cause can be difficult. Symptoms may appear within a few hours of eating the food, but where there is infection by bacteria or viruses, this may take time to develop and the illness may not show itself until a day or two later.

Dangers

The diarrhoea and vomiting that occur in an attack of gastro-enteritis cause the rapid loss of a number of chemical elements such as sodium (*see* SALT) and

Prevention of gastro-enteritis

The majority of gastro-enteritis attacks are due to infection by bacteria or viruses entering the mouth and reaching the bowel. This is often due to inadequate care with food or poor hygiene in the lavatory.

Hygiene in the kitchen

- Follow manufacturers' recommendations about dates by which foods should be used. Many packed foods have date stamps to guide you.
- Wash hands and scrub fingernails before handling food.
- Keep work areas scrupulously clean.
- Do not allow pets near where food is being prepared. Prevent cats jumping on to tables.
- Keep food cool in summer. Use a refrigerator whenever possible.
- Avoid meats which have stood a day or more at room temperature after being cooked: recooking may not ensure safety.
- Eliminate flies.
- Keep all food covered.
- Dispose of food scraps, wrapped in plastic or paper. Keep waste bins covered and lined with a plastic bag. Do not allow children to play near waste bins.

Hygiene in the lavatory

- Wash hands thoroughly and scrub fingernails after using the lavatory. Remember that microbes could be transferred from the flush handle and the seat of a lavatory previously used by an infected person. Clean these with household disinfectant if there is an infected person in the house.

POTASSIUM. This deprivation can bring about biochemical changes in the body and may even lead to KIDNEY or LIVER damage.

The effect may also be serious if the patient is already unwell, elderly or very young. Babies, in particular, can become seriously ill. The sick child is very thirsty, but can suck only feebly and then be unable to retain what has been taken in. The result is dehydration (loss of water), a situation that needs immediate medical help.

Treatment

In gastro-enteritis, the first aim of treatment is restoring fluids to the body. Vomiting may be overcome by taking tepid drinks in very slow sips. This can be followed by well-diluted meat or yeast extracts, weak sweetened tea or citrus fruit juices. If the attack has been caused by a bacterial organism, an antibiotic may be necessary.

Rest in bed is important, and an easily digested diet with plain foods such as milk or strained broths, once the main symptoms have eased.

A seriously ill baby or small child, however, may need urgent hospital care to restore their fluid balance.

Genetics

Every feature of our bodies, from the size of our toes to the colour of our eyes, is determined from the moment of CONCEPTION by the chemical information supplied from each parent. This is contained in the twisted, thread-like structures called *chromosomes* (*see* CELLS AND CHROMOSOMES) which are sited in the nucleus of each cell.

Situated in a row along the length of each chromosome are the *genes* which carry the instructions for a particular characteristic. A single gene is constructed of the chemical *deoxyribonucleic acid* (DNA), formed like a twisted ladder – known as a double helix. Each ladder 'upright' consists of a chain of alternate sugar and phosphate units – the sugar is called deoxyribose.

Attached to each sugar unit in the chain is a biochemical compound called a base, of which there are only four: adenine, thymine, guanine and cytosine. The bases stick out sideways from the sugar–phosphate chains to form the rungs of the double helix ladder. The sequence of bases along the sugar–phosphate chains is called the *genetic code* and it tells all the other chemicals in the cell what to do.

When the gene goes to work in the cell, the two uprights of the DNA ladder break apart and the exposed bases 'read off' in groups of three – triplets – to form a carrier substance known as messenger ribonucleic acid (mRNA). This is also in the form of a double helix and is chemically very similar to DNA but it contains the base uracil in the place of thymine.

The vital function of mRNA is to organize the manufacture of *proteins*, the biochemical molecules essential to every bodily action, by directing the stringing together of smaller units which are called *amino acids*.

What can go wrong

Genetic mistakes may range from the inheritance of a gene which makes a single abnormal protein at one end of the scale to the loss of a whole block of genes – for instance, when a chromosome or piece of chromosome is missing – at the other end.

Mistakes are most commonly made at the time when the chromosomes divide into two, forming an egg (*see* OVARIES) or SPERM. Egg and sperm cells differ from every other cell in the body in that they contain only 23 chromosomes while all the rest contain 46. This halving in number is essential because, when the father's sperm and mother's egg come together, the recombination must then again make 46 chromosomes.

The halving in number is called *meiosis* and it is not difficult to imagine that, on occasions like this, chromosomes may get left behind, resulting in 24 chromosomes in one sperm and 22 in another, or that pieces of chromosomes may break off and get lost completely. Any resulting offspring may then be born with 47 or 45 chromosomes.

Sometimes a piece of chromosome may either be missing or an extra chromosome donated. The best known example of inheritance of an extra chromosome is the disease known as DOWN'S SYNDROME, the result of an additional chromosome number 21.

Nature usually deals with her mistakes by allowing a natural ABORTION, but if the child is born, then nothing can be done to treat the abnormality which is locked in the genetic code and which may be passed on to that person's children.

Where to turn for help

Genetic counsellors are specialists in both human genetics and statistics, and people are usually referred to them by their family doctor. Their job is to help people understand the way in which genetics is involved in certain disorders and to calculate the chances of disorders arising should a couple have children, or the risk of a second child being affected by a disorder that has occurred in an existing child.

Most of the couples who seek advice from a genetic counsellor are those with a child who has a serious disease or deformity, or who have a relative with a serious health problem. Other reasons are that one or both partners may have a family history of ill health, have an inherited disease themselves, or are worried because they are related.

In all cases, the first thing the genetic counsellor will do is to draw up a detailed family tree of both the man and the woman, if possible going back at least three generations.

To construct this 'pedigree', as it is called, the counsellor will depend heavily on the cooperation of the couple and of hospital and public record departments. Sometimes these pedigrees are very difficult to compile, either because a family has become very widely scattered or because records have been lost or never kept. It may also be difficult to make the pedigree totally accurate in medical terms because of the great advances in medical knowledge in the past century. But the counsellor will be able to make good use of what information he or she can find.

Having constructed the pedigree, the counsellor then has to work out the chances of the couple having a child with an inherited disease. The ease or difficulty of this part of the task depends very much on the type of disorder, the way in which it has been passed on in previous generations and the family relationship – if any – between the couple. He or she will also have to consider the frequency of a particular disease in the community as a whole, as this affects the statistical analysis. The counsellor may, in addition, want to obtain information from medical tests on any abnormal children already born to a couple to find out whether the abnormality fits into an hereditary pattern or is simply an accident of fate.

Dominant and recessive genes

For genetic counsellors, the easiest genetic diseases to asses in terms of risk are those which have a simple path of inheritance. Such diseases are called *dominant* or *recessive*, depending on the way the genes controlling them are expressed. (Of course, it is not only certain illnesses that result from dominant or recessive genes – hair and eye colour follow a similar if complicated pattern.) An inherited form of CATARACT is an example of a disease known to be caused by a dominant gene. This means that if a child inherits a normal gene from his mother but an abnormal one from his father (or vice versa), the abnormal one will show itself, even though it is present only in a single measure.

The disease PHENYLKETONURIA – a severe disorder of the METABOLISM in which the urine is a black colour, and which is associated with serious mental defects – is an example of a disease caused by a recessive gene. In this case, a child must inherit the gene for the condition from both parents.

Other examples of inherited disorders caused by dominant genes include one type of *dwarfism* in which the head and trunk are normal in size but the limbs are very short; brachydactyly, a disorder of the development of the fingers; Huntington's chorea, a disease of the nervous system in which the nerves gradually degenerate (*see* DEMENTIA); SPINA BIFIDA, a serious spinal abnormality; and some types of MUSCULAR DYSTROPHY.

These dominant traits are much fewer in number than those caused by recessive ones. In the case of recessive disorders, a person must inherit two abnormal recessive genes, one from each parent, for the disorder to become apparent. Both parents may, in fact, be perfectly normal but 'carriers' of a recessive gene each. Among the many diseases that have been found to be caused by inheritance of this type are albinism, in which there is a complete lack of pigment in the skin and hair (making them white) and in the eyes (causing them to be red); certain types of deafness and blindness; CYSTIC FIBROSIS, a disease of the mucous glands in the lungs and other organs; and many metabolic disorders, including galactosaemia, in which a baby cannot benefit from galactose, the sugar in breast milk.

Calculating the odds

If one partner is known to have a completely dominant disorder but the other does not, the genetic counsellor will assess the chance of the disorder being passed on as 50–50. With recessive disorders, the chances are one in four if both parents are carriers of the recessive gene.

Matters are complicated in the case of recessive traits by the facts that either or both parents may carry one recessive gene and that these may be combined in the children. This is something the genetic counsellor will be particularly keen to determine in the case of marriage between first and second cousins because the more closely two people are related, the greater the chance that they will both have inherited a recessive gene from the same grandparent or great-grandparent.

With some inherited diseases, the sex of the affected individual is also important. It is known that hereditary diseases such as HAEMOPHILIA (which affects the blood clotting process, and leads to excessive bleeding) only affects boys, while others, including CLEFT PALATE AND HARE LIP and some types of ALLERGY are much more common in boys than in girls. These so-called sex-linked diseases can involve dominant or recessive genes, and these are further factors the genetic counsellor will take into consideration. And there are many diseases that have a very complex method of transmission and expression because they depend on the simultaneous action of a whole group of genes – club foot is one example (*see* FEET). As a general rule, the more genes involved in the production of a defect, the less risk there is of parents passing it on.

See also HEREDITY.

Genitals

The word 'genital' is derived from 'generation', meaning 'bring into existence' and signifies the creation of life. The genital organs in men and women are those that nature designed for the purpose of sex and reproduction.

The male genitals

The male genital system is designed to produce sperm and deposit them in the female. It consists of the TESTES and the PENIS, which are situated outside the body, and the prostate gland, seminal vesicles and various tubes linking the genital system, which are found inside the abdominal cavity.

The testes are enclosed in a pouch of loose skin called the *scrotum* that consists of two compartments called *scrotal sacs,* one for each testis. Two functions are performed by the testes – the production of SPERM and of the male hormone *testosterone.* The latter is responsible for the development of the male genitals and has an important role in the secondary sexual changes of PUBERTY in boys, such as the growth of facial and body hair and the 'breaking' and deepening of the voice.

The female genitals

The woman's reproductive system must not only receive the sperm but also must produce ova (eggs) for fertilization and eventually nurture one or more eggs if fertilized, so that one baby or more can develop. Eggs are produced in the OVARIES and pass along the Fallopian tubes. However, it is only the parts of the female reproductive system below the CERVIX, or neck of the womb, that are usually understood to be included in the term 'genitals'.

Below the cervix is a muscular canal 4 in to 5 in (10 cm to 13 cm) in length called the VAGINA that encases the penis during SEXUAL INTERCOURSE, although normally the walls lie flat against each other. Its entrance is covered and protected by the external genitals known as the VULVA: two folds of flesh – the outer and inner *labia* (so-named after the Latin word for lips). The inner labia join together in front of the *clitoris,* a small fleshy organ that is covered by a flap of skin called the clitoral hood. The clitoris corresponds to the male penis and is made of erectile tissue that swells up during sexual excitement. *See also* UTERUS.

German measles, *see* **Rubella**

Giardiasis

This is an illness caused by a protozoa called *Giardia lambia*. It causes diarrhoea and the malabsorption of food. The commonest parts of the world in which it is found are the tropics, Russia and certain parts of Europe. The organism is transmitted as a cyst, which then colonizes the small intestine. It can either cause damage to the lining of the small intestine and lead to malabsorption, or, in carriers, can remain asymptomatic but risk transmitting the infection to others.

Symptoms

These include watery diarrhoea, nausea, poor appetite, abdominal pain and swelling. Stools become paler, as a result of the malabsorption of fats. If the illness lasts a long time, marked weight loss can occur.

Diagnosis

Examination of the stool can show cysts and parasites. Biopsies of the small intestine taken via an endoscope using a 'Crosby Capsule' can also reveal the parasite.

Treatment

Usually a short course of high-dose metronidazole will cure the infection, although sometimes this will need to be repeated. To prevent transmission when visiting endemic areas, personal hygiene and purified water are vital as no vaccine exists.

GIFT (gamete intrafallopian transfer), *see* **Infertility, Test-tube babies**

Gilbert's syndrome, *see* **Jaundice**

Glands

The body contains masses of different types of glands: organs which manufacture and secrete substances which have a wide variety of functions. They fall into two main categories, depending on where their secretions go.

Endocrine glands are ductless glands, scattered throughout the body, whose secretions pass directly into the bloodstream. The blood then carries them to the specific body organ that they stimulate. The endocrine glands secrete HORMONES and form the hormone system. They include, among others, the PITUITARY gland and the THYROID gland.

Exocrine glands include those glands which release their secretions to the surface of the body (for example, the sweat glands; *see* PERSPIRATION), or through large ducts (for example, the PANCREAS, which lies in the upper part of the abdomen, and secretes juices into the small intestine).

Finally, there are the glands of the LYMPHATIC SYSTEM. These are unusual glands in that they have no secretions, though they do produce the special type of blood cell called *lymphocytes,* and antibodies against particular infections.

Glandular fever

The cause of glandular fever is a micro-organism known as the *Epstein-Barr* VIRUS, which causes a generalized infection in the body. One of its most obvious effects is considerable enlargement and tenderness of the lymph glands (*see* LYMPHATIC SYSTEM) – hence the name glandular fever. The glands affected are often noticeable in the neck, armpits and groins. Another effect of the virus is to trigger a defensive mechanism in the patient's bloodstream (*see* IMMUNE SYSTEM) so that large numbers of unusual white blood cells – *mononuclear* cells – are produced. This gives rise to an alternative name for the illness: *infectious mononucleosis.*

The virus lives in the mouths and noses of people who have the disease, and can remain there for several months after the illness is finished. The virus is passed from person to person by close contact, probably in the tiny droplets that are exhaled normally with each breath, but possibly also by kissing. Outbreaks may occur in schools or colleges where young people spend a great deal of time in each other's company. But not all people who come into intimate contact with people who have glandular fever develop the illness because susceptibility to the Epstein-Barr virus seems to vary greatly from person to person.

Symptoms

After a symptomless incubation period of between four and seven weeks, the patient will begin to feel listless and fatigued. Headache and chills are followed by a high fever, an extremely sore throat, and swollen lymph glands in the neck and sometimes in the armpits and groin. The spleen may also become swollen.

Two sorts of rashes may appear. In about 15 per cent of cases, a redness appears under the skin of the trunk and inner surface of the arms and legs. This may develop into fine pimples which do not contain fluid. If a patient with glandular fever happens to be given certain antibiotics such as ampicillin or amoxycillin, a profuse red blotchy rash appears. This is not an allergy rash, but an abnormal reaction to the antibiotic which occurs only while the patient has glandular fever.

In many cases, the illness may be so mild as to be missed, or mistaken for another illness where the symptoms are a sore throat and swollen glands, such as TONSILLITIS. In severe cases, the symptoms are more obvious, and there may be complications. The LIVER may become inflamed, producing JAUNDICE. The SPLEEN may become so enlarged while it is forming white blood cells to fight the infection that it becomes painful and tender.

The virus may affect the NERVOUS SYSTEM, producing a form of MENINGITIS, or it may affect the LUNGS or HEART causing PNEUMONIA or PERICARDITIS, an inflammation of the pericardium, the fibrous sheath surrounding and enclosing the heart.

The two most helpful diagnostic tests are made from a blood sample. In one test, the blood cells are analysed under a microscope to see if the enlarged, abnormal lymphocytes, the glandular fever cells, are present. In the second test, known as the *Paul–Bunnel test,* a sample of serum is taken and tested against the red blood cells of sheep. In 90 per cent of infected cases, the sheep cells mass together and agglutinate; in non-infected cases, they do not. This test is often used to confirm the disease. A third test, called the *monospot test,* uses a specially treated latex suspension which is mixed with a sample of the patient's blood; it is easier to do than a Paul–Bunnel test.

Dangers

Glandular fever is not normally dangerous, but in very rare cases, some dramatic medical events may occur.

If pressed too hard or bumped in error, a very enlarged spleen may rupture. This condition would necessitate immediate blood transfusion and the surgical removal of the organ.

In very rare cases, meningitis may occur. This causes headache and photophobia (pain looking into bright light), but permanent damage is unlikely.

The danger of infecting other people is not great, but patients in hospital are barrier nursed to prevent other sick people from contracting the disease. This means they are kept in total isolation from the other patients. In normal circumstances, no such isolation is necessary.

Treatment

There is no curative treatment for glandular fever, only treatment for each of the separate symptoms. Because the illness is caused by a virus, antibiotics have no effect, although in certain circumstances, they are sometimes used, such as when the throat becomes ulcerated or the lungs become inflamed.

In mild cases, the patient should gargle frequently for the sore throat and take painkillers such as aspirin or paracetamol for headache. Bedrest is advisable, particularly in the early stages.

In severe cases, bedrest is absolutely necessary. The patient should have adequate fluids and a light diet, and take aspirin or paracetamol for fever and sore throat. Occasionally the sore throat is so bad that swallowing is difficult if not impossible. In some cases, STEROID drugs may be prescribed and they can be dramatically effective in reducing swelling in the throat, although they will not shorten the duration of the illness.

If a woman contracts glandular fever while she is taking the oral contraceptive pill, she is usually advised to stop taking the pill temporarily until the illness has settled. Glandular fever invariably causes some inflammation in the liver, and the pill can increase the possibility of more serious liver damage or jaundice.

Those patients who have a mild form of the disease may not need to take time off from school or work, but most patients will require a few weeks of resting and home treatment. The convalescent period is longer than with most infectious illnesses, and patients might not feel right in themselves for several months, even when the symptoms have gone. Most patients make a complete recovery over a period of about six to eight weeks; others may take longer, even up to six months.

Glaucoma

Although it usually develops late in life, glaucoma is a common cause of BLINDNESS, affecting one in 50 people who are over the age of 40.

Causes

The EYE is separated into front and rear portions (anterior and posterior chambers) by the lens, and the ciliary muscle supporting it. Just in front of the lens around the rim of the eyeball is a structure called the ciliary body which manufactures the fluid – the aqueous humour – which fills the anterior chamber. Since this fluid is constantly being produced, it needs to be continually drained away, and this is where the problem arises.

In glaucoma, there is an obstruction to the drainage of the fluid, and as a result, the pressure in the eyeball rises. No such trouble ever develops with the fluid in the posterior chamber, because it does not circulate.

Occasionally, babies are born with a defect in the drainage system in the eye, and can develop glaucoma very early in life. This is an extremely rare, although a potentially serious, condition.

In adults, there are three different possible causes for glaucoma. First, there may be a physical blockage to the drainage of fluid at the edge of the iris caused by the lens and the iris being pushed forward inside the eye. The angle between the iris and the front of the eye is reduced and this prevents proper drainage. This type – called *closed-angle glaucoma* – usually affects people who are long-sighted, and have relatively small eyeballs. It occurs in elderly people because the lens gradually enlarges throughout life, contributing to the changes that trigger this type of glaucoma.

A second type is *open-angle,* or *chronic simple, glaucoma.* In this condition, the anatomy of the eye is entirely normal and there is no simple physical explanation for the condition. The drainage of fluid from the front of the eye seems to become less efficient with increasing age, leading to a gradual increasing of pressure inside the eye.

Both closed-angle and open-angle glaucoma tend to run in families. Anyone who has an immediate relative with glaucoma has a one in 20 chance of developing the same condition.

A third type, which is very rare, is *secondary glaucoma.* In this, a disease of the iris leads to problems with drainage of fluid in the eye, and hence to a build-up of internal pressure and glaucoma.

Diagnosis

There are special examinations which may be carried out by an ophthalmic optician or by an eye specialist to detect the presence of glaucoma.

The first, and most important, is measurement within the eye. A drop of local anaesthetic is placed into the eye to remove sensation and then an instrument called a tonometer is applied to the front of the eye to measure the pressure. There are two or three different types of tonometers, although they all work on a similar principle. They measure the amount of distortion which can occur to the eyeball when a tiny force is applied to it by a probe on the instrument. Very accurate readings can be obtained with the most sophisticated type of tonometer.

Another test which may be carried out is careful 'mapping' of the visual field. Each eye is tested separately to find out the full extent of vision in all directions when the eye is focused constantly on one spot. This technique, sometimes known as 'perimetry', can detect 'tunnel' vision, which is an early sign of chronic glaucoma.

Finally, the doctor may examine the eye using a special lens called a gonioscope applied to the front of the eye, which enables the edge of the iris to be minutely examined with a special type of microscope focused on to the lens. This technique allows the doctor to decide which type of glaucoma is affecting the patient.

Symptoms

Closed-angle glaucoma usually begins suddenly, with inflammation and agonizing pain in the affected eye. There is severe blurring of vision. The patient may become so ill that he or she starts vomiting. Sometimes the patient may have had some warning pains in the eye previously. Often these occur in the evening, because the dilation of the pupil which occurs naturally in the dark can trigger off minor episodes of glaucoma. The patient may also notice 'haloes' round lights at night.

Chronic glaucoma, or open-angle glaucoma, is very different. There is usually no pain, but gradual deterioration in vision which can be so slow that the patient does not notice what is happening. The patient can slowly develop 'tunnel' vision, which, at first, makes getting about difficult but ultimately affects reading or watching television.

A doctor or optician may be able to spot the trouble early by looking into the eye with an ophthalmoscope. What he or she sees is the retina and the optic nerve supplying it, at the back of the eyeball. Normally the optic nerve has a pinkish colour and an edge which is continuous with the rest of the retina, but in chronic glaucoma the nerve looks pale and is pressed back.

An optician may also detect chronic glaucoma by using a tonometer routinely during an eye test.

Treatment

Acute closed-angle glaucoma must be treated in hospital. Drugs may be given by mouth or an intravenous drip to relieve the sudden rise in pressure in the eye. When inflammation is reduced, an operation called an iridectomy is usually necessary. A small hole is made at the edge of the iris using either a tiny surgical incision or a laser, so allowing the fluid to drain from the front chamber of the eye. This operation leaves a permanent new drainage channel, so preventing further attacks of glaucoma. It is necessary for both eyes to be operated on, but usually the operation in the second eye is delayed until the first eye has healed. Babies who are born with glaucoma also need emergency surgery to save their sight.

Chronic glaucoma usually responds to treatment with drugs. Pilocarpine eyedrops increase the rate of drainage of fluid from the eye; Timolol drops reduce the rate at which fluid is formed. If patients find it difficult to insert drops, a tiny piece of plastic film containing pilocarpine, called an Ocusert, can be placed under the eyelid. This needs to be changed only once a week – perhaps by a relative or a nurse if the patient cannot manage it. If treatment with drops is ineffective, an iridectomy may be necessary to relieve the pressure in the eye.

Prevention of glaucoma

It is advisable for everyone over the age of 40 to visit an optician at least every two years. Anyone who has a near relative with glaucoma should preferably be checked every year, whether or not they need glasses. If glaucoma is detected early, treatment can prevent deterioration of sight later in life.

Glucose, *see* Carbohydrates, Diabetes

Glue ear, *see* Deafness, Ears

Glue sniffing, *see* Solvent abuse

Goitre, *see* Thyroid

Gonorrhoea

Gonorrhoea – or 'the clap' – is one of the most common SEXUALLY TRANSMITTED DISEASES (STDs), and most often affects sexually active people between the ages of 16 and 25. The incubation period – the length of time between sexual contact with an infected person and the first signs of the disease – may be as short as 48 hours, and it is usually not longer than seven or eight days at the most.

Very few men have no symptoms. In them, urination usually becomes more frequent and painful. There may be a whitish discharge from the PENIS; in uncircumcised men, this can cause a reddening and irritation of the meatus (penis opening). Homosexual men may have an anal infection, resulting in soreness, redness and itching in a few cases. Untreated, gonorrhoea may spread to the glands leading off the urethra, causing the TESTES to swell.

Many women have no symptoms at all and are thus quite unaware that anything is wrong with them. In those women with symptoms, there may be a slight vaginal discharge and sometimes painful urination.

Gonorrhoea is rarely transmitted in any way other than by intimate sexual contact as the organisms quickly die once outside the body. Thus the toilet seat theory of transmission is a myth! It is possible, however, for an infected mother to give her daughter vulvo-vaginitis (vaginal infection) by cuddling her closely or by having her use her heavily infected towel.

Diagnosis

The symptoms of gonorrhoea can be very similar to those of another sexually transmitted disease – called NON-SPECIFIC URETHRITIS – caused by an organism called CHLAMYDIA. It is usually possible for tests to be carried out in an STD clinic on the spot to check the diagnosis. At most it will take a couple of days to get the result of the tests. These tests are essential to ensure that the right treatment is given. Tests for other diseases such as SYPHILIS or HIV infection (the cause of AIDS) can be carried out at the same time.

Dangers

The most obvious danger is the easy spread of the disease when the infected person has no symptoms.

The local dangers are confined to the male vas deferens and the female Fallopian tubes resulting in sterility (*see* INFERTILITY).

A more general danger is that sometimes 'silent' symptomless people, unaware that they have the disease, may continue to spread it to the community.

Treatment

Treatment with an ANTIBIOTIC is essential for all patients with gonorrhoea, whether or not they have symptoms. The recommended treatment is a single injection of penicillin, or a large dose of penicillin or ampicillin by mouth. If the patient is allergic to penicillin, other drugs may be substituted. Additional antibiotics may be given if there are other infections present.

Even though a single penicillin injection is all the treatment needed, repeat visits to a doctor are necessary to ensure that the cure is complete and that the patient was not incubating syphilis as well, as the two diseases may be caught simultaneously. The symptoms usually get better within 24 hours.

Unlike syphilis, gonorrhoea cannot be passed to a baby in the womb, but it may be transmitted during birth and the baby's eyes will become inflamed. Immediate penicillin treatment is given and is 100 per cent effective.

Sexual partners of gonorrhoea patients should also be treated and tested as a matter of routine, despite the fact that, under certain circumstances, there may be cause for some embarrassing questions to be asked. Doctors can refer patients to a local hospital where the trouble can be fully treated and freedom from relapse assured, or patients can refer themselves (with complete confidentiality) to any hospital's 'special' or GUM (genito-urinary medicine) clinic.

Patients should abstain from intercourse until tests show that they are free from infection. This takes at least three weeks from the start of antibiotic treatment.

Gout

Most people dismiss gout as just a painful inflammation of the big toe resulting from over-indulgence in food and drink. In fact, the causes are more complex, and if left untreated, gout can lead to serious BONE and KIDNEY damage.

Gout is caused by an abnormally high amount of uric acid in the tissue fluids. Uric acid is always present in the body as it is a product of certain foods when they are broken down and also of naturally worn out tissue cells. Normally the gut and the kidneys excrete uric acid so that the level in the body remains constant. In patients suffering from gout, either too much uric acid is formed or it is inadequately excreted.

Causes

There are various reasons for an increase in uric acid formation. In the past, the blame was put on over-indulgence in rich foods and alcohol, which produce uric acid after being digested. Certain foods rich in the chemicals known as *purines* will, after digestion, produce uric acid, an excess of which can lead to gout if the body does not excrete it efficiently. High-purine foods include sweetbreads, liver, kidney, brain, venison, heart, meat extracts, goose, duck, turkey, fish roe, whitebait, lobster, sardines, herring, bloater and sprats. These foods are best avoided in large amounts, but if eaten in moderation their contribution is relatively slight. Alcohol in moderation is all right, but an alcoholic 'binge' may temporarily decrease the power of the kidneys to pass out uric acid and so provoke attack. However, it is now known that the part played by diet is relatively small and other causes are far more likely.

The most common cause is the filtering process of the kidneys becoming inefficient at getting rid of uric acid. This can happen in some kidney troubles such as chronic NEPHRITIS (inflammation of the kidneys) or be due to the effect of certain drugs, such as *diuretics*.

Sometimes gout is caused by diseases of the blood and tissues which involve an excessive breakdown of their cells. There are also certain congenital (existing from birth) conditions in which the body chemistry creates more uric acid than is normal.

A person with a raised level of uric acid does not necessarily suffer from gout. However, in many cases the excess uric acid is deposited in the JOINTS, SKIN or kidneys. When this happens, the person may suffer either an acute (sudden) attack or a chronic (long-term) form.

Acute attacks

The first attack of gout is likely to be sudden and severe; it almost always involves the big toe. The condition used to be known as 'podagra' from the Greek words meaning 'a seizure of the foot'. Attacks may be precipitated by events such as surgical operation, dietary or alcoholic excess, diuretic drugs or starvation.

The patient may be woken in the middle of the night by intense pain. The toe is extremely tender and will hardly bear the weight of the bedclothes. Its base is swollen and the skin is dry, hot, red and shiny. The veins on the top of the foot may be distended. Sometimes the patient is feverish.

If an acute attack is not treated, the patient will suffer considerable pain for three to ten days and then the symptoms will subside.

However, treatment with anti-inflammatory drugs works successfully and quickly. The digestive systems of a few patients are sensitive to these drugs and they cause vomiting and diarrhoea. If this happens, they may be given as suppositories or injections.

They should be taken as soon as possible as delay makes them less effective. Aspirin should be avoided as it tends to lessen the kidneys' filtering out of uric acid.

Once the pain had gone, patients may think that that is the end of the matter. But the condition may be latent within patients, making them prone to further acute attacks at unpredictable intervals of weeks or months. Other joints may then be involved besides the big toe – usually extremities of limbs such as fingers or wrists. It is unusual for more central ones such as hips or shoulders, or several joints at the same time, to be affected.

Doctors will take blood tests and watch the patients' general condition to see whether further treatment is needed to try and prevent the gout developing into chronic gout. Patients who have had only a mild rise in their uric acid level, or have quite infrequent attacks, may not need further treatment.

Chronic gout

In chronic cases of gout, crystals of uric acid salts settle in joints, skin and kidneys, causing permanent damage.

At the joints, crystals of salts are deposited in the cartilage of the bone ends, roughening their smooth surfaces, causing swelling and stiffened movement similar to OSTEOARTHRITIS.

The skin may develop bumps at various points. These are formed of collections of salts and are known as *tophi*. Often they appear as small knobs on the rims of the ears but they may also form quite large swellings on the hands or the back of the elbows. Generally, they are more disfiguring than harmful, but occasionally a tophus becomes so large and inconvenient that it needs to be removed surgically.

Severe gout can cause kidney damage in two ways. Either deposits of uric acid can block the delicate filtering mechanism of the kidneys, leading to progressive damage, or the highly concentrated uric acid may crystallize and form kidney stones. About one fifth of patients who are not treated for gout develop kidney stones.

Long-term treatment

Patients who suffer frequent acute attacks, joint changes, the appearance of tophi, kidney damage or consistently show a very high level of uric acid in blood tests, need long-term treatment.

Under these circumstances, life-long treatment is very important to avoid long-term complications – particularly damage to the kidneys which could ultimately lead to kidney failure. Two different types of drugs may be prescribed. The one most commonly used, allopurinol, reduces the production of uric acid by the tissues in the body, so that the blood level is reduced. If, for any reason, this drug does not work for a particular patient, other drugs may be prescribed which increase the rate at which uric acid is excreted.

Patients who start on long-term treatment are likely to have to continue for the rest of their lives. Blood tests will be taken from time to time to show how they are getting on and whether the drugs or the dosage needs altering.

If the patient does not continue the treatment, the uric acid level may rise again and there may be further attacks. With long-term treatment, the attacks are likely to stop completely. If there are any, they will not be as severe as they would have been without treatment.

Graves' disease, *see* **Hormones, Thyroid**

Greenstick fracture, *see* **Fracture, Skeleton**

Growth hormone, *see* **Hormones, Pituitary**

Guillain–Barré syndrome, *see* **Neuritis**

Guinea worm disease, *see* **Ulcers, skin**

Gullet, *see* **Oesophagus**

Gut, *see* **Alimentary canal**

Guthrie test, *see* **Phenylketonuria**

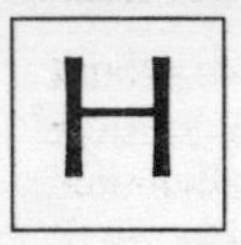

Haematocolpos, *see* **Vagina**

Haematoma, *see* **Brain and brain disease, Head and head injuries**

Haemoglobin, *see* **Anaemia, Blood, Oxygen**

Haemophilia

This is an inherited disease (*see* GENETICS and HEREDITY) affecting males almost exclusively, in which one of the essential factors required to make BLOOD coagulate, or clot, is missing. As a result, bleeding fails to stop when a blood vessel has been damaged, sometimes because of a slight injury or, with internal bleeding, without any obvious cause.

Cause

Haemophilia is due to an abnormal gene forming a part of the X-chromosome (the female sex chromosome; *see* CELLS AND CHROMOSOMES) which contains thousands of genes and which should ordinarily make a blood-clotting factor called Factor 8.

Blood clotting is a complicated series of chemical reactions which run in a chain using the 'knock-on effect'. The reaction starts with a special factor in the blood called the Hageman Factor, otherwise known as Factor 12. Factor 12 then knocks on to No. 11 and then to No. 10 and so on down to No. 1. The final step in the clotting process is the reaction of *thrombin* (an enzyme) with *fibrinogen* (a protein), Factor No. 1, to form *fibrin,* Factor No. 2. This forms a jelly-like mesh across any wound. Each factor in the chain is determined by a particular gene on a certain chromosome, so if one gene is missing the reaction fails to take place properly and the blood fails to clot.

How it is inherited

In order for males to develop haemophilia, the abnormal gene forming a part of the female sex chromosome must be inherited from a female carrier. A female has two X chromosomes and a male has an X and Y (male) chromosome – this means that, for a foetus to be a male, it must have inherited a Y chromosome from the father and an X from the mother. If the father has haemophilia, this would be carried on his X chromosome; this can never be transmitted to a son but it will always be inherited by a daughter, since a daughter inherits one X chromosome from her father and one from her mother. Therefore the son of a haemophiliac will be unaffected and will not transmit the disease, but all his daughters will certainly be carriers. On the other hand, there is a genetic possibility that female carriers will transmit the disease to half their sons, while half their daughters will be carriers.

For females to develop haemophilia, they must inherit an abnormal gene from a haemophiliac father and a carrier mother, but this is extremely rare since unions between two such people seldom take place and genetic counselling is now more widely available.

Symptoms

The symptoms of haemophilia often appear quite early in life. Babies affected by the disease bruise very easily. As they grow older, they develop more worrying symptoms, the most troublesome being bleeding into the joints (*haemarthrosis*). The result is severe pain and ultimately deformity of the affected joint itself. Repeated injuries of this type will result in the patient being crippled. Large weight-bearing joints are usually affected, most especially the knees and the ankles.

Mild haemophilia is often first discovered after a tooth extraction, when the dentist finds it difficult to stop the bleeding. The diagnosis is made for certain only by a measurement of the amount of Factor 8 in the patient's blood. The severity of the disease depends upon the level of Factor 8 present: in some instances, it may be only mildly lowered, but in others, there may be no Factor 8 at all and this can be serious.

Dangers

Bleeding may occur after what would normally be considered trivial injuries, even though there is no break or bruising over the skin. Bleeding into the abdomen can mimic other illnesses, including APPENDICITIS. In severe cases, the patient can become an invalid or have a massive fatal HAEMORRHAGE.

Treatment

If haemophiliacs are injured, they will require immediate supervision at hospital. The severity of their bleeding depends upon how much Factor 8 they have, and this will determine the amount of Factor 8 they will require. It is now possible to extract Factor 8 from donated blood and pool it all together. It can then be given in the form of an intravenous injection, or a transfusion to the patient.

Bleeding into the joints causes a lot of pain, but it can be rapidly controlled by the injection or transfusion. The injured joint must also be exercised passively (not by weight bearing) with the help of a PHYSIOTHERAPIST. Bleeding from soft tissues may take longer to staunch and treatment may need to continue for several days with repeated transfusions.

Haemophilia and AIDS

Factor 8, used for treating haemophilia, has to be extracted from human blood, which for this purpose is collected from a large number of donors.

Unfortunately, in the early and mid-1980s, some Factor 8 became contaminated with the HIV virus – the virus that is now known to cause AIDS. As a result, a large number of haemophiliacs were accidentally and, tragically, inoculated with the HIV virus.

Some of these people have already developed AIDS, although most are still quite well. Since the mid-1980s in Britain and the United States, and then in many other countries, all stocks of Factor 8 have been specially treated to kill any HIV virus that may be present. This action has eliminated the risk of transmitting AIDS to haemophiliacs.

Any haemophiliac already carrying the HIV virus from contaminated Factor 8 – and in some countries up to a third of all haemophiliacs are such carriers – must be careful to avoid spreading the virus to others, particularly their partners, through sexual intercourse.

Haemoptysis, *see* **Lungs and lung diseases**

Haemorrhage

Medically, haemorrhage simply means bleeding from any severed or damaged blood vessel in the body. Caused by accidents and diseases, or as the result of surgery, haemorrhage is described as *external* if the blood from the vessels is lost to the outside of the body, and *internal* if the blood is retained unseen within it.

Haemorrhoids, *see* **Anaemia, Piles**

Hair

Most of our bodies – except the palms of our hands and the soles of our feet – are covered by some sort of hair. It is most noticeable on the scalp, armpits, pubic area, arms, legs, eyebrows and eyelids and, in men, on the lower part of the face and on the chest.

The visible part of a hair is called the *shaft* : it is formed from a protein called *keratin* and is composed of dead tissue. The shaft is rooted in a tube-like depression in the skin called the *follicle.* The hair develops from a root, the *dermal papilla,* which is at the bottom of the follicle, and is nourished by the bloodstream. If the root is damaged, hair growth stops and it may never regrow.

The follicle also contains a sebaceous GLAND which secretes a greasy substance called *sebum.* This lubricates the hair shaft and surrounding skin and can give hair a greasy appearance. Lastly, the follicle contains *arrector pili muscles.* When a person is cold, afraid or alarmed, these muscles contract, making the hair stand on end and bunching the skin around the shaft to form what are known as 'goose pimples'.

Types

Adults have about 120,000 hairs on their head: redheads have fewer, blondes more. Hair type varies according to structure: there are fine, soft baby hairs which grow on portions of the body; long hairs which grow on the scalp; and short, stiff hairs which compose the eyebrows.

The type of hair shaft determines whether hair is straight or curly. A cylindrical hair shaft produces straight hair, and an oval shaft produces curly or wavy hair, and a flattened, or kidney shaped shaft produces the crinkly hair seen in many black people.

Growth and colour

The cells that make keratin for hair are among the most rapidly dividing of the body. Scalp hair grows an average of ½ in (1.25 cm) a month.

Hair growth is not continuous. Every five or six months, the hair goes into a resting phase, during which no growth takes place. The roots of resting hair become club-shaped – hence their name – *club hairs* – and lose their normal pigmentation. Up to 10 per cent of our scalp hairs are in the resting phase at any one time. It is the club hairs that seem to come out in handfuls when we wash our hair. No damage is done to the follicles, and when the root has finished its rest, normal hair growth begins again.

Lining the follicles and mixed in with the cells making keratin are other cells laden with a pigment called MELANIN. Melanin stains the keratin and gives hair its colour: red hair has an extra pigment. As we get older, the melanin-producing cells in each follicle gradually stop working, and as a result we go grey and ultimately completely white, though when this occurs tends to be determined by HEREDITY. Hair colour itself is also caused by heredity. Albinos lack the ability to form melanin and so their hair remains white throughout life, and they have very fair complexions and pink or red eyes.

Excessive hair

Hirsutism (excessive hairiness) is never due to an increase in the numbers of hairs, but rather to a change in the character of hair. Our bodies are covered with soft, downy hair called *vellus hairs*. In certain parts of the body, notably the scalp, the armpits and groin, these hairs become thicker, and are then called *terminal hairs*. At puberty, terminal hairs become more abundant on the face, in the armpits, the groin and pubic area and the legs. This change is brought about by male sex HORMONES called androgens. (Scalp hair, on the other hand, is not androgen dependent for growth.)

Certain types of people are hairier than others: for example, the hairiness of a European person would be considered abnormal in Chinese or Japanese people. Hairiness is either inherited from individual parents or it is part of a person's racial heritage.

Excessive hairiness is a sign of disease only in rare instances. It results from excessive production of androgen hormones, either from the ADRENAL GLANDS or from the OVARIES. This occurs as a result of a small TUMOUR, usually benign, which can usually be removed.

Development of hairiness in pre-pubescent children needs hospital investigation.

Male-pattern baldness

This hereditary condition is the most common cause of baldness in men. It tends to be inherited from the mother's side of the family and involves the presence of an active form of testosterone (one of the androgens) to set off the gene-programmed balding process. The growing time of hair is shortened, making all hairs increasingly thin and short until the roots produce nothing but fine down.

Most men who become bald first start losing their hair at the temples, as the hair line begins to recede on each side. By the age of 70, more than 80 per cent of men show this pattern of baldness, although it often starts quite early in life – in their 20s or 30s. Some men find that their hair becomes thin at the crown of the head first, but the hair may then gradually become thinner over the whole of the top of the head, leading eventually to a 'bald pate'. Men whose mother's fathers became bald early in life are very likely to follow a similar pattern: even the type of baldness tends to be the same.

Treatments for baldness

The most effective disguises until recently have been wigs, hair-pieces or toupees. These can be made to measure and fitted very carefully so that they are hardly noticeable. Some can even be carefully sewn on to the existing hair so that they will not come loose, and it is even possible for a man to go swimming with such a hair-piece in place.

Hair transplantation offers another possible solution, although often the end result is not particularly natural. One of the techniques used is that of 'punch' grafting. Using a local anaesthetic, a plastic surgeon takes small pieces of skin from the back of the scalp and transplants them to the balding areas on the top of the head. The hair follicles in the transplanted skin continue to produce hair. If this procedure is carried out carefully, a reasonable growth of hair may be expected. The result is often very patchy, however, and unless the surgeon is particularly careful in siting the transplanted hair, it often does not grow naturally in the right direction. Another disadvantage is that several operations may be required – at considerable expense.

Recently a drug has become available which has been found to promote hair growth on previously bald areas. This drug is the only one so far that appears to be successful in promoting hair growth. It is called *minoxidil*, and is sold under the trade name Regaine, only on private prescription. The drug was originally developed to be taken in a tablet form for the treatment of high blood pressure, but it was soon found that it caused hair to regrow in some bald men. The drug manufacturers then developed the drug in a lotion formulation for application to the head. It is still not clear why this drug makes hair regrow and there is doubt that it will do so in all cases, but tests have shown it to be safe. The major disadvantage with this treatment, however, is that it must be used every day to maintain the growth of hair. It is also very expensive, and medical supervision is also necessary.

Causes within your control

Mistreating hair can cause temporary baldness. Wearing a ponytail, plaits or other styles which pull hair tightly, or even just frequent tugging, can cause a hair loss in men, women and children. The medical term for this is *traction alopecia*. Sometimes temporary baldness also results from over-bleaching or perming the hair. PROTEIN and VITAMIN deficiencies can damage the hair.

These types of hair loss are generally not permanent, with the hair growing back to normal strength and thickness once the cause is removed.

Alopecia areata

This curious form of hair loss can affect men and women. A patch of normally hairy skin suddenly loses all its hair. The patch can be as small as ⅖ in (1 cm) across, or it can be 4–6 in (10–15 cm) in diameter. It may affect the scalp, or the hair on the beard area in men, or the body hair in either men or women. Despite research, there is no clear indication as to how this condition arises. Apparently a stressful event – such as sudden bereavement – can trigger off *alopecia areata* (*see* STRESS). It also appears to be slightly more common in people with certain disorders, such as DIABETES and PERNICIOUS ANAEMIA.

The most usual pattern of alopecia areata is for a few small bald areas – perhaps up to ⅘–1⅕ in (2–3 cm) across – to appear on the scalp. The person may wake up to find a handful of hair lying on the pillow – or the loss can be more gradual. Often the hair regrows after a few weeks or months, although in some cases there is no regrowth at all.

Occasionally large areas are involved. All the hair of the head may be lost – this is called *alopecia totalis*. Very occasionally the person may lose all his or her body hair, which is called *alopecia universalis*. In both of these conditions, regrowth is not likely.

There is no very satisfactory treatment for *alopecia areata*. If the areas are small, a doctor may try injecting the areas with steroid drugs to try to trigger regrowth, but this is seldom successful.

Halitosis, *see* **Dental care**

Hare lip, *see* **Cleft palate and hare lip**

Hashimoto's disease, *see* **Thyroid**

Hay fever

This condition results from an ALLERGY to inhaled dusts, the most common of which is grass pollen. The parts of the body affected are those most commonly exposed to allergy-causing dusts – the eyes, the nose, the sinuses and the upper part of the throat. There is a watery discharge from the nose and eyes, as well as irritation and sneezing.

HAY FEVER

Causes

While the most common cause is an allergy to grass or tree pollens, identical symptoms may result from inhaling other dusts such as fungal spores, animal hair and scurf, and the faeces of house dust mites.

The symptoms are usually seasonal and the precise timing of their appearance depends upon the sort of dust to which the patient is allergic.

The first pollens to appear each year are tree pollens and, depending upon the severity of the winter, these can cause hay fever in the UK as early as mid-March. Pollen from plane trees and silver birch are powerful allergens (substances that cause allergic reactions) and frequently cause hay fever. Later in the season, typically in mid-summer, grass pollens appear and have a short season, and are then followed by nettle pollen. From mid-summer until late autumn, fungal spores are abundant in the air and are the most likely to cause trouble in autumn.

Symptoms

The blood vessels increase in diameter (dilate), and the mucous cells in both the nose and the sinuses begin to generate more mucus. As a result, the eyes itch and stream, the nose and sinuses become blocked and cause feelings of stuffiness and heaviness in the head. The throat becomes sore and the patient feels generally unwell.

Sneezing is common first thing in the morning; the patient may sneeze repeatedly between rising and eating breakfast. If asthma is associated with hay fever, the patient usually suffers his worst symptoms at night.

Treatment

By far the best treatment is to avoid the cause of the allergy. If the cause is the family cat or the rabbit at the bottom of the garden, this is usually a fairly simple matter. However, there is no way of avoiding exposure to dusts like tree and grass pollens, although if you take your holidays by the sea you are less likely to be affected.

Local treatment: Medicines are placed in the nose by means of a spray or puffer, or in the eyes by means of drops. A solution of sodium cromoglycate is made up to treat both the eyes and the nose. This prevents the release of histamine. It usually has to be administered three times a day throughout the hay fever season. An alternative preparation, for use in the nose only, is a puffer containing a steroid which is given in very low doses three times a day. Both these medicines stop the symptoms from developing but are of little relief once they have developed.

General treatment: Antihistamines may be of some help in hay fever, but many cause sleepiness which some people find intolerable. Steroid injections bring dramatic relief, but because they can have undesirable side-effects, they are not used unless the patient's symptoms are really incapacitating.

Head and head injuries

The head comprises the skull, a rigid bony structure which houses the BRAIN and the organs of sensation for hearing, balance, sight, smell and taste.

The skull consists of two parts: the cranium which encloses the brain; and the face which provides a bony framework for the eyes, nose and mouth. The eight bones of the skull are joined together by *cartilage* before a baby is born. This permits the bones to move over one another if necessary to allow the head to pass down the mother's birth canal. The cartilage is gradually replaced by bone during the first 18–24 months of life – after that the skull becomes rigid.

The brain and spinal cord

The brain fills the cranial cavity. It comprises a soft, jelly-like substance which is easily compressed, torn or crushed. It is wrapped in an extremely tough layer of tissue called the *dura mater* and it is this, and the bony part of the skull, which protect the brain. But if the brain is damaged and swells, its tissue can be further damaged by being crushed against the bony outer layer.

At the base of the skull are several openings, enabling arteries, nerves and veins to pass through. The largest of these spaces, called the *foramen magnum,* is the outlet for the SPINAL CORD. This passes down through the vertebral (spinal) bones in a channel called the *spinal canal* which is widest at the top end and narrowest at the bottom. The skull rests on the first cervical vertebra, the *atlas,* which articulates with the second cervical vertebra, the *axis.* These are the vertebrae that allow the head to move backwards and forwards and to rotate. If the spinal cord is cut across or damaged at this level, death results almost instantaneously.

Injuries

Almost two thirds of people who die under the age of 35 do so because of head injuries, not necessarily from skull fractures, but from serious damage to the soft tissues of the brain which results from a violent blow on the head.

Injuries result from two causes: *deceleration,* when a head that is moving is brought suddenly to rest – for instance, by striking the windscreen of a car or hitting the pavement in a fall; and *acceleration,* when a head that is stationary is violently struck, as from a blow with a cosh. The result of these shocks is that the soft tissue of the brain is violently shaken. Two typical injuries result: one immediately beneath the point where the head has come into contact with something solid, the *coup injury*; and another inside the part of the head furthest away from the blow, when the brain is either pushed against the skull or pulled away from it by the force of the blow – called the *contrecoup injury.*

The most critical factor in every case is whether damage has been done to the blood vessels. If bleeding begins, blood is spilled into the brain substance, spreading through it with relative ease and occupying a great deal of space. Because the brain is contained within the bony skull, the pressure rises rapidly and some of the brain substance is crushed. Much of this damage can be prevented if the bleeding can be stopped or the rise in pressure relieved.

There is evidence to suggest that repeated blows to the head over a prolonged period of time will cause small haemorrhages throughout the brain, resulting in diminished mental ability, slurring of speech and general slowness; this is called being 'punch drunk'.

Diagnosis of head injuries

Doctors divide head-injury cases into three groups: those who are fully conscious at the time they are seen; those who have been UNCONSCIOUS since the time of the accident; and those who have been conscious for a period of time following the accident, but are slipping into unconsciousness again.

The major concern for doctors is to distinguish between *concussion*, from which the patient recovers, usually without brain damage, and bleeding inside the skull which may cause further damage and eventual death. One of the problems with brain tissue is that, once it has been destroyed, it never regenerates.

Minor injuries

These are most often the result of an accident in the playground or on the football field, or of a fall at home when the head is knocked against a solid object. The usual symptoms are those of concussion: unconsciousness seldom lasts for more than a few seconds; the victim often sees 'stars' and feels dizzy; sometimes he or she has a HEADACHE which is made worse by exertion, stooping or by emotional excitement; and the events which happened in the minutes immediately following the injury may be forgotten (a state known as *post-traumatic* AMNESIA), but it is most unusual for the events leading up to it to be forgotten. These symptoms seldom last more than a few hours. You should see your doctor after such an accident, especially if the period of unconsciousness has lasted much more than five seconds.

Serious injuries

A more serious state of affairs exists when the victim has been unconscious since the time of the accident. As with any unconscious patient, the first priority is to ensure that he or she is able to breathe. The person must be placed on one side to lessen the risk of inhaling any vomit and therefore suffocating.

This is the type of injury that can be complicated by bleeding inside the brain and there are certain warning signs for which the doctor is always on the lookout. One of these is an increase in size in one or both pupils of the eye, caused by stretching and paralysis of the nerve that supplies the muscles of the iris. At the same time, when a bright light is shone into the eye, the pupil does not constrict. These symptoms occur because the brain swells from the increase in pressure caused by internal bleeding.

Another well-known warning sign is the direction in which the big toe points when the sole of the foot is stroked. In a healthy person, the big toe usually points downwards when a blunt object is rubbed along the sole of the foot. But in the case of a serious brain injury, the direction is reversed and the toe may point upwards. This is known as *Babinski's sign*, after the man who first described it. Patients with this kind of head injury need to be taken to hospital as soon as possible for urgent treatment.

Sometimes, after a brief period of consciousness, perhaps less than an hour, the patient lapses into unconsciousness again. Typically, this is the result of a blow in the region of the temples, beneath which there is a vulnerable artery inside the skull called the *middle meningeal artery*. This condition is usually caused by bleeding between the tough covering of the brain and the skull, which is called an *haematoma*. The trouble begins when the bleeding occupies enough space to compress the brain beneath it. This pressure can be relieved almost at once if a surgeon drills a small hole in the skull over the site of the haematoma.

Problems

Doctors encounter a rather more difficult problem when bleeding occurs between the tough covering of the brain and the brain tissue itself – this is known as a *subdural haematoma*. In this case, the skull injury causing the trouble may be so trivial that the patient may not remember it happening. What can complicate matters further is that the period of unconsciousness may occur several weeks after the original injury. Both extradural and subdural haematomas may occur on both sides of the skull, just like coup and contrecoup injuries. Again, drilling holes in the skull to remove the blood clot rapidly relieves pressure.

Treatment

In many cases of minor head injury, only first aid measures will be needed although sometimes observation in hospital for 24 hours is needed as a precaution. In more serious cases the patient will need hospital care.

As described, subdural and extradural haematomas may be removed by a relatively simple operation, but there is not much that can be done for bleeding deep within the brain, although everything possible will be tried. To ensure normal breathing, a tube may be placed in the patient's windpipe and a mechanical ventilator used. There then follows a period of waiting to see whether the brain recovers from the injury. This may sometimes last for months, but full recovery has occurred after very long periods of unconsciousness, during which time the patient's life is supported on a respirator machine and the electrical activity of the brain monitored.

An after-effect that occurs in 20 per cent of cases following serious head injury is EPILEPSY, which is usually the result of damage to the brain tissue. The interval between the head injury and the first attack is usually about five months, but it may be much longer, even years, particularly in children. Concussion itself seldom leads to epileptic seizures.

Patients may also suffer from troubles such as headaches, giddiness, depression or excessive nervousness – which may have a psychological basis. In spite of such possibilities, it is important to remember that complete recovery is possible in many cases.

Headache

Everyone experiences headaches at some time or other, and all home medicine chests contain mild PAINKILLERS.

Simple factors such as excessive noise – in a disco, for instance – or a chronic COUGH, lack of sleep or STRESS can cause a headache in an otherwise healthy person. But a headache is also an extremely common symptom of more serious conditions such as NOSE, THROAT and EAR INFECTIONS, high BLOOD PRESSURE, and damaged blood vessels in the BRAIN.

If you have a headache that persists, recurs or is particularly severe, or a headache accompanied by other symptoms, you should go to your doctor as it may need treatment.

The exact site and nature of the pain helps to trace the cause, and it is important to tell the doctor as much as possible about when and how the headache started.

The doctor will usually examine the eyes and take the patient's blood pressure. If the diagnosis is still in doubt, the patient may see a neurologist and have skull X-RAYS taken, or possibly a CT scan, a series of X-rays which produce a computerized picture of the brain.

Common causes

The brain itself cannot feel pain but the tiny nerve endings within the arteries and veins that supply the brain are very sensitive to changes of pressure. A few very rare conditions, such as growths inside the head, can affect the pressure and result in persistent headaches.

The sensation of pain may also be transmitted to the brain by substances called *prostaglandins* from nerve endings in the skin, the eyes, and nose.

The most common headaches are ones that develop with a mild VIRUS infection like a cold, or with tension from intense concentration or worry. *Tension headaches* seem to be caused by an increase in the tension in the muscles of the scalp. These are usually mild and clear up quickly with the help of simple painkillers such as aspirin.

Migraine: This is an intense type of headache, thought to be caused by the blood vessels on the one side of the brain first contracting and then dilating. Some people seem to be more susceptible than others, and all sorts of things can trigger an attack. The headache is usually preceded by a feeling of sickness and there may be blurring of vision or flashing lights in front of the eyes. *See* MIGRAINE.

Sinuses and teeth: Inflammation will cause headache as well as producing tender areas at the site of the trouble. *See* SINUSITIS and TEETH.

Faulty eyesight: This is a common cause of headaches which occur in the region of the brow especially after close-up work such as sewing. They may be accompanied by a feeling of grittiness in the eye or sometimes blurred vision. *See* EYES AND EYESIGHT.

Poisons: Headache with a high temperature is usually caused by the toxic (poisonous) products made by viruses. Other toxic substances can also cause a headache. Alcohol and tobacco, if taken in excess, may result in a headache. Foul air from lack of ventilation, lead poisoning, carbon monoxide poisoning, and petrol fumes all cause chronic, mild headache. Even stomach upset can result in one.

High blood pressure: Severe high BLOOD PRESSURE in arteries supplying the brain stretches the tissues and may result in a recurrent throbbing headache. However, high blood pressure usually produces no symptoms.

Neuralgia: If a pain actually arises in nerves supplying the head or face, headache is acute and may be set off merely by the touch of a brush or comb. *See* NEURALGIA.

Pre-menstrual syndrome: PREMENSTRUAL headaches are common but their cause is not really fully understood. Some doctors believe they are caused by excess fluid that is stored in the body before a period starts, others believe they are the effect of hormone levels. Sometimes a *diuretic* drug which removes the excess fluid from the body will help to relieve this type of headache.

More serious causes

Brain TUMOURS, although not common, can cause persistent headache, usually accompanied by other symptoms such as vomiting. Careful investigation is needed to plot the exact site and plan treatment.

MENINGITIS is an inflammation of the meninges, the tissue layers covering the brain and SPINAL CORD and separating them from their bony casing. The patient develops a severe headache, a stiff neck and a dislike of light (photophobia). Treatment is usually by means of drugs and rest.

If blood vessels supplying the brain are damaged in an accident (*see* HEAD AND HEAD INJURIES), it can lead to blood leaking in the space between the skull and the brain tissue, or may even cause a blood clot. A severe headache may be the first sign that something is wrong. The condition may be self-correcting or surgery may be required.

Because the symptom of headache has so many causes, the information given by a patient is very important and may give the diagnosis before examination and tests confirm it. Remember when the headache started and if there were warnings. Note the frequency of the attacks and how long they last.

Hearing

What we hear are sound waves which are produced by the vibrations of air molecules. The size and energy of these waves determine loudness, which is measured in decibels (db). The number of vibrations or cycles per second make up frequency; the more vibrations, the higher the pitch of the sound. Sound frequency is expressed in terms of cycles per second, or hertz (Hz).

In young people, the range of audible frequencies is approximately 20 to 20,000 Hz per second, though the ear is most sensitive to sounds in the middle range of 500 to 4,000 Hz. As we get older, or if we are exposed to excessively loud noise over a period of time, our hearing becomes less acute in the higher frequencies. In order to measure the extent of hearing loss, normal hearing levels are defined by an international standard. The patient's level of hearing is the difference in decibels between the faintest pure note perceived, and the standard note generated by a special machine.

How we hear

Sound waves transmitted through the air are collected by the pinna, the outer ear, and are funnelled through the ear canal (*see* EARS). When they reach the eardrum, they cause it to vibrate. This vibration is passed on to the three bones of the middle ear – the malleus, incus and stapes – which are arranged in a chain and which transmit this vibration to the inner ear.

Diseases which affect the middle ear, resulting in this bony chain seizing up, will cause conductive hearing loss (*see* DEAFNESS). If the normal pathway to hearing is obstructed, transmission of sounds across the bone of the skull is also possible, but there is nevertheless a considerable hearing loss of about 25 to 30 db. This type of hearing loss may occur in otosclerosis, where the stapes becomes rigidly attached to the inner wall of the middle ear.

Sound vibrations are then transmitted to the inner ear which is filled with a fluid called endolymph. This transmits sound waves to the cochlea, which is shaped like a snail. Cells bristling with specialized hairs, which are sensitive to movement, are distributed along the length of the cochlea. As the waves pass, they are 'sensed' as pressure and transmitted along the cochleal nerve to the auditory area of the brain where they are interpreted. High frequency tones are sensed only by the specialized cells in the first part of the cochlea, whereas medium and low tones are sensed further along.

The way in which waves are turned into electrical energy and interpreted by the brain is not understood. One theory is that cells of the cochlea measure pressure waves in the endolymph and turn them into electrical impulses. It is also not clear how the ear distinguishes between loudness and pitch.

Diseases of the inner ear result in the disordered interpretation of sound.

Hearing tests

The simplest hearing test consists of whispering standard phrases at varying distances from the patient's ear. Next come tests with a tuning fork which the doctor taps and holds against the patient's ear. The doctor then moves the fork an inch or so away from the patient's ear until he or she can no longer hear any sound.

More sophisticated tests are done with a machine called an audiometer. These are conducted in a soundproof room, with the patient wearing earphones. A machine emits notes at different volumes, beginning with sounds beyond the hearing range and gradually bringing down the sounds until they are just audible. The patient signals that he or she can hear the sounds by pressing a button. Not only does the audiometer measure the air conduction from the sound emitted and heard in the earphone, but it also tests what is known as bone conduction, when the sound is played directly into the bone of the skull.

The results can be presented graphically, with frequency and hearing loss plotted on a scale. This shows the number of decibels required to be generated above those considered to be just audible in order for the patient to hear the tone.

Heart

The heart is a large muscular organ in the middle of the chest. Although it is often thought of as being in the left-hand side of the body, it actually straddles the mid-line with more of it on the left than the right. It weighs about 12 oz (340 g) in men and a little less in women.

The right-hand border of the heart lies more or less behind the right-hand border of the breastbone. On the left side of the breastbone, the heart projects out as a sort of rounded triangle with its point lying just below the left nipple. This point can be felt pulsating with each heartbeat. It is called the *apex beat.*

What the heart does

The job of the heart is to pump BLOOD around two separate CIRCULATIONS. First, it pumps blood out into the ARTERIES via the *aorta,* the central artery of the body. This blood circulates through the organs and tissues delivering food and OXYGEN to them. The blood then returns to the heart in the VEINS, having had all the oxygen absorbed from it.

The heart then pumps the blood on its second circuit, this time to the LUNGS to replace the oxygen. It is then returned to the heart with its oxygen renewed.

The circulation to the lungs is called the *pulmonary circulation* and the one to the rest of the body is called the *systemic circulation.* There are pulmonary and systemic arteries which carry the blood outwards from the heart and pulmonary and systemic veins which return it.

Structure of the heart

There are four main chambers in the heart operating the pumping arrangement. Each chamber is a muscular bag with walls which contract to push blood onwards. The thickness of the muscular wall depends on the amount of work the chamber has to do. The left ventricle has the thickest walls as it does the largest share of the pumping.

The chambers are arranged in pairs, each having a thin-walled atrium which receives blood from the veins. Each atrium pumps the blood through a VALVE into a thicker-walled ventricle which pumps the blood into a main artery.

The two atria lie behind and above the two ventricles. Both the atria and

Structure of the heart

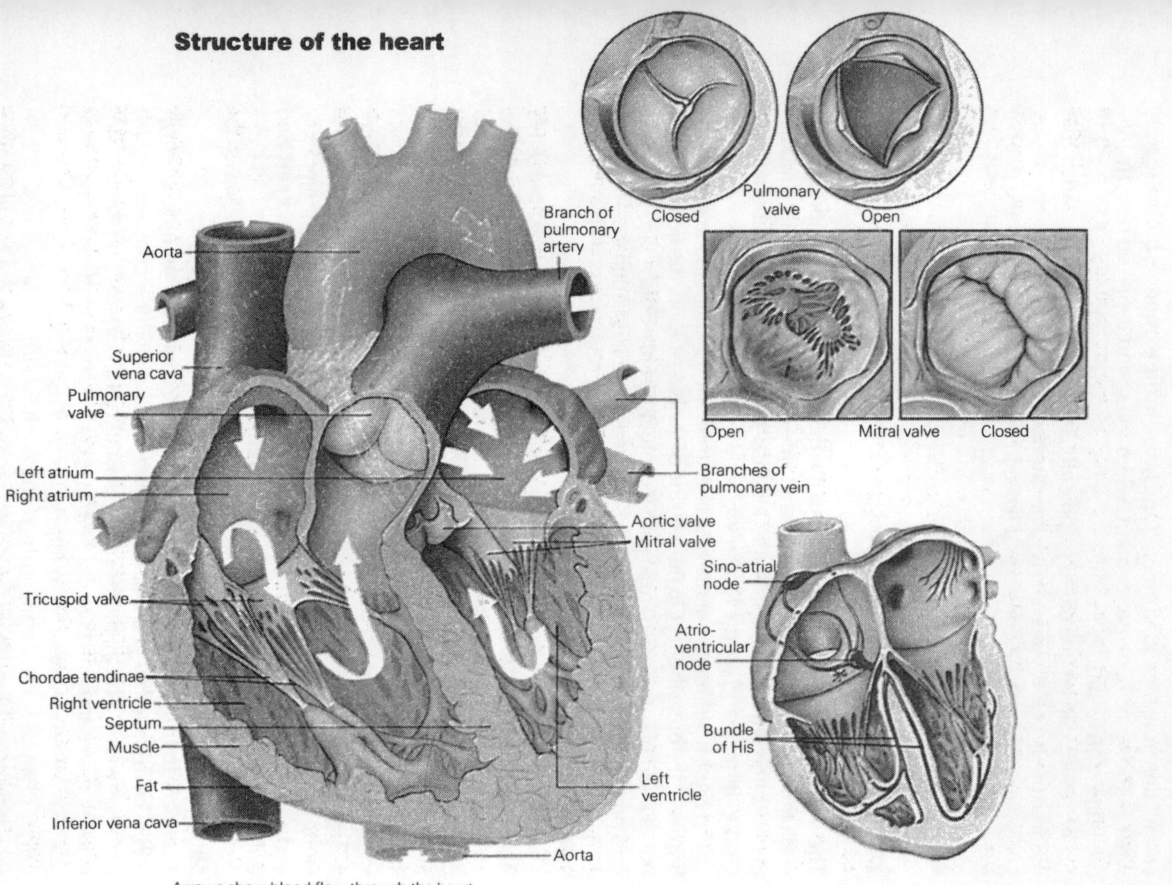

Arrows show blood flow through the heart

both the ventricles lie side by side. The portions of their walls which separate them are called the *interatrial* and *interventricular septums.*

How it works

Blood returns to the heart from the lungs in the pulmonary veins with its oxygen store renewed. It goes into the left atrium which contracts and pushes the blood through the *mitral valve* into the left ventricle.

The left ventricle then contracts and as it does so the mitral valve shuts so the blood can only go out through the open *aortic valve* into the aorta. It then goes on into the tissues where it gives up its oxygen.

The blood returns to the heart from the body in a large vein, the *inferior vena cava,* and from the head in the *superior vena cava.* It goes into the right atrium. This contracts and the blood passes through the *tricuspid valve* into the right ventricle.

A right ventricular contraction sends it out into the pulmonary artery, through the *pulmonary valve,* and through the lungs, where it has its oxygen renewed. It then returns to the heart in the pulmonary veins ready to start all over again. This process is repeated 50–60 times every minute.

The valves

The pulmonary and aortic valves have very similar structures. They have three leaf-like cusps, or leaflets, of yellowish-white membrane which open upwards to allow blood to flow forwards but fall back into place to stop any backward flow.

The mitral and tricuspid valves are more complicated, although they are similar to each other in structure. They also have leaflets – two for the mitral and three for the tricuspid.

The bases of the leaflets are planted in the ring which forms a border between the atrium and the ventricle. Cords called *chordae teninae* go from the leaflets to part of the ventricle wall called the *papillary muscles.*

By pulling down on the chordae tendinae during each ventricular contraction, the papillary muscles make sure no blood flows backwards into either atrium. The blood can only go forwards into the right and left ventricles.

Timing system

With each heartbeat, the two atria contract together and charge up the ventricles with blood. Then the ventricles both contract.

This orderly series of contractions depends upon a sophisticated electrical timing system.

The basic control comes from the *sinu-atrial node* which is in the right atrium. Impulses pass from it through both atria and make them contract. There is another node, the *atrioventricular,* at the junction of the atria and ventricles.

This delays the impulse to contract and then passes it down through a bundle of conducting fibres in the intraventricular septum called the *Bundle of His.* After passing through the bundle, the impulse spreads out into the ventricles causing them to contract after the two atria.

Heart attack

The heart depends on its own blood supply to provide it with the oxygen that is essential for it to function properly. If the oxygen supply to an area of heart muscle is interrupted, that area of muscle cannot function.

Over a period of months or years, *atheroma* (fatty deposits) can attach themselves to the wall of a coronary ARTERY – one of the two arteries which supply the heart with blood (*see* CORONARY HEART DISEASE). In time, this impedes the blood flow passing through that artery. A total blockage occurs when a blood clot forms in the middle of the artery at the point of maximum narrowing. It is not known exactly why this clot (THROMBOSIS) should occur, but the fact that the wall of the artery is heavily coated with atheroma is obviously a contributing factor.

A heart attack is a continuous process. Interruption of the blood supply is the first stage. As the blood supply to the heart muscle (*myocardial cells*) is stopped, the patient feels pain. The affected cells die, and if the blood supply remains obstructed, that area of muscle will die and be replaced over a period of weeks with fibrous tissue scar, which could weaken the heart if a very large area of muscle has been affected.

The people most at risk from a heart attack are SMOKERS, people who eat a lot of FAT, people with a history of high BLOOD PRESSURE, DIABETICS and those with a family history of heart attacks. They are most likely to occur in middle-aged men. They are unusual in women before the MENOPAUSE and in men under 35.

Warning signs

In some people, the first 'coronary' will be totally unexpected, but in many, there is a warning sign – the development of angina. This is a central chest pain which happens during exertion or excitement and lasts a few minutes. Often the pain spreads to the neck and shoulders, and may shoot down the arms.

Anyone who develops angina, or has angina which is increasing in frequency or in the length of each attack, should see their doctor to have a check-up.

Symptoms of an attack

The main symptom of a heart attack is a dull or heavy pain, usually in the centre of the chest. There may be sweating, nausea or vomiting, and breathlessness as well. The patient may look ill and grey. The severity of the symptoms varies from a severe pain and collapse to very trivial discomfort. It is even possible to suffer a heart attack without noticing any symptoms at all.

If you do suffer from an attack of pain which you think might be a heart attack, you should call your doctor, but do not get too alarmed; there are other conditions with similar symptoms, such as INDIGESTION, a chest infection, GALL BLADDER problems or the washing back of the acid contents of the stomach into the gullet (OESOPHAGUS).

Diagnosis and treatment

The first priority for any doctor treating a patient with a heart attack is to relieve the pain. This is usually done with an injection of morphine or a similar drug.

Then it is important to confirm the diagnosis and this may be done with an ELECTROCARDIOGRAM (ECG) which traces out the pattern of the heartbeats. Usually it will show characteristic abnormalities on the trace which confirm that the pain is due to a heart attack. Having confirmed the diagnosis, the next stage is to try and prevent any complications or to deal with them if they occur.

Modern treatment also involves the use of drugs to dissolve the clot in the coronary arteries. This is called *thrombolysis* and should be given as quickly as possible once the diagnosis of a heart attack has been made. In addition, if the attack victim is still conscious, an aspirin should be given as this helps to prevent platelets in the blood from sticking together. Soon after the heart attack, a drug called a *beta-blocker* will be given regularly for at least the first year; this helps to prevent any serious complications.

Coronary care units in hospitals provide special care to both prevent and treat the disorders of heart rhythm which may occur after heart attacks (*see* PACEMAKER). Modern treatment of rhythm disturbances is with drugs and electric shock treatment where necessary.

Rehabilitation

Patients who are admitted to a coronary care unit will probably spend a day or two there receiving treatment and then be transferred to a general ward. They are not usually kept in bed for longer than a few days, and if there are no complications, they will be discharged in 10–14 days.

Patients should aim to build up to their normal level of activity gradually.

In a few cases, there may be severe damage to the heart muscle and these patients usually take a little longer to recover full physical activity.

What to do if someone has a heart attack

- Phone the patient's doctor and he or she will either come to the patient or tell you to phone for an ambulance. If you cannot contact the doctor, phone for an ambulance.
- If the patient regularly suffers from indigestion, it is worth them taking indigestion tablets to see if they bring any relief.
- The patient should rest, either sitting in a chair or lying down with the head and shoulders raised. He or she should not get up and walk about.
- Stay with the patient until the doctor or ambulance arrives. If the patient becomes UNCONSCIOUS with loss of breathing and loss of pulse, mouth-to-mouth resuscitation and heart massage should be given. Continue this until medical help arrives.

Heartburn, *see* **Diaphragm, Indigestion, Oesophagus, Pregnancy, Stomach**

Heart disease

Because the heart is vital to life and has to work continuously, it is very prone to disease. The majority of people with heart problems suffer from CORONARY HEART DISEASE, but there are also other types of heart disease.

Valve disease

The heart depends on four VALVES to keep blood flowing in the right direction. Diseases of these valves used to be very common – often as a result of RHEUMATIC FEVER in childhood – but it has become much less so in the West because of a general increase in the standard of nutrition and hygiene.

Most valve problems today arise from abnormalities in structure which have been present since birth (congenital problems). The inlet and outlet valves (mitral and aortic valves) of the left ventricle, the main pumping chamber of the heart, cause the most trouble.

There are two things that may go wrong with a valve. It may become blocked and impede the forward flow of the blood – a condition called *stenosis* – or it may leak and allow backward flow, which is called *regurgitation* or *incompetence*. Stenosis and incompetence often occur together. Usually people with minor abnormalities of the heart valves have no problems.

Congenital heart disease

The reason the heart is so prone to abnormalities is that its development in the womb is very complicated. During the early weeks of PREGNANCY, it evolves in the embryo and foetus from a single straight tube into a four-chambered pump with two separate circulation systems. This is a complex process which can occasionally go wrong.

Sometimes a baby is born with holes in the partition between the two atria or the two ventricles. These two conditions are called *atrial* and *ventricular septal defects*, respectively. If the blood flow to the lungs is insufficient, the blood never becomes enriched with oxygen, and the result is a BLUE BABY (a condition known as *cyanosis*).

Modern heart surgery has advanced so much in recent years that it is now standard practice to operate on tiny babies.

Inadequate pumping

Sometimes there are problems if the force of the pumping is inadequate because the power of the muscular walls of the heart starts to fail. This condition is called *cardiac failure*. If the left side of the heart is failing to work properly, the condition is termed *left ventricular failure*. The patient feels weak and breathless and finds it difficult to carry out even the slightest exertion. Back-pressure builds up in the LUNGS and excess fluid accumulates in its spaces. A cough with white frothy sputum then develops. Sometimes this condition worsens at night, especially if the patient is lying flat in bed. He or she may wake up fighting for breath, although there is often relief when the patient sits up straight.

If the right side of the heart fails as well as the left, then the term *congestive cardiac failure* is used. Back pressure builds up in the veins all over the body, and OEDEMA (fluid) accumulates in the lowest parts of the body – the ankles and shins if the patient is upright, or the back if the patient is lying in bed. In the past, this was known as 'dropsy'. Although congestive heart failure is one of the commonest causes of oedema, swollen ankles can occur as a result of a number of other conditions that have nothing to do with the heart.

Cardiomyopathy

Congestive *cardiomyopathy* is a heart muscle disease which makes the muscle become weak and flabby so that the heart gets bigger and bigger as the muscle wall dilates under the strain. In most cases, the cause is not known.

Occasionally the muscle thickens and obstructs the flow of blood out of the left ventricle. This condition is known as *hypertrophic cardiomyopathy* and is one of the very few heart diseases that runs in families.

Viral myocarditis

Certain viruses may occasionally affect the heart muscle, causing inflammation in the muscular tissues. The patient can develop chest pains, similar to those of ANGINA, and may even have heart failure. This condition can affect people of any age – children included – but young adults seem to be more at risk. Usually patients recover completely after a few weeks without any long-term damage to the heart.

Heart rhythm disorders

The electrical conducting system of the heart is responsible for making sure that each part contracts in its proper sequence. There are two disorders that can happen – either the heart beats too quickly or too slowly.

Either of these may cause dizziness and even UNCONSCIOUSNESS because of an inadequate supply of blood to the brain. With a slow heartbeat – known as a *heart block* or *arrhythmia* – the heart beats so slowly that not much blood flows forwards. On the other hand, when the heart is going very fast, it does not have time to fill properly between each beat with the result that again very little blood moves forward.

When the dizziness and fainting are due to fast rather than slow beating there are often *palpitations* – an uncomfortable sensation of the heart beating. Heart rhythm disorders can happen as a result of other heart diseases or they may occur on their own.

To diagnose the cause of symptoms, an ECG (ELECTROCARDIOGRAM) will be done. A great advance in this field is the 24-hour ECG recording using a small tape recorder which the patient wears for a whole day. The results are then analysed on a machine which speeds up the recording by about 60 times.

Slow heart rates are treated with PACEMAKERS and fast ones with drugs.

Symptoms and diagnosis

Despite the fact that there are so many causes, the symptoms of heart disease are remarkably few.

There is pain (angina) when the heart is starved of oxygen. However, other conditions, such as indigestion, can give angina-like pain. The other main symptom of heart disease is heart (cardiac) failure. Treatment is by means of *diuretics* which will cause much excess fluid to be excreted through the kidneys with the result that the swelling is greatly reduced and breathlessness improves.

The presence of heart failure is easy to discover. Fluid on the lungs can be heard through a stethoscope as 'crackling' with each breath, and fluid around the ankles is quite obvious by the uncomfortable swelling it causes. The doctor will also check the patient's BLOOD PRESSURE. High blood pressure may eventually cause enlargement of the heart, or coronary heart disease.

The key to diagnosis is examination of the heart itself. The doctor will feel the patient's pulse for irregularities and to measure its rate, and the chest wall where the heart can be felt. The heart becomes enlarged with heart failure, and its beat becomes unduly forceful if the wall of the ventricle is thicker than normal, and the doctor can feel this.

The doctor also listens to the sounds of the valve closing during different phases of the heartbeat and listens for *murmurs.* Murmurs are sounds caused by the turbulent flow of blood through the heart. When a valve is obstructed or leaking, it will cause a murmur.

Having examined the heart, a doctor may decide that there should be further investigation. An ECG is often carried out. The test picks up the electrical impulses generated by the beating of the heart. The doctor can use the test to analyse the rhythm of the heart, and it will also indicate whether there is enlargement of the heart, or areas that are not working properly, perhaps because of coronary artery disease. If the first test is normal, a further ECG may be carried out while the patient is exercising. This is called an *exercise stress test,* and can reveal abnormalities as the heart speeds up. A chest X-ray may also be performed to check on the size of the heart, and the condition of the lungs.

Further examination may also be done with a *cardiac catheterization.* This is an X-ray procedure where tubes (catheters) are passed into the heart through the arteries or veins. Patients have to go into hospital for a few days to have this test done. The tubes measure the pressure in the various chambers of the heart. Special X-ray dye may be injected into the tube to outline the heart's chambers and show up abnormalities, and to reveal any blockages or narrowings in the coronary arteries, which may be corrected by surgery. Catheterization is usually done on patients who are being examined before a heart operation because while basic diagnosis is easy, more technical matters have to be investigated before open-heart surgery.

Heart transplants

Transplanting a HEART is a skilled, but from the point of view of surgical technique (rather than medical back-up), not an excessively difficult operation. The first heart transplants were, in fact, being pioneered as long ago as the 1930s. The early heart transplant surgeons had, however, one major problem – how to overcome the process known as REJECTION. This simply means the body's tendency to fight off foreign tissue in the same way as it fights off infection from invading germs. However, as medicines to damp down rejection (or, in medical terminology, suppress immunity) gradually improved, it became clear that the human body could be helped to accept foreign tissue, such as a transplanted heart.

Because the operation is so expensive, it cannot be offered to everyone who needs it. So, those with an established, general disease, such as DIABETES or CANCER, in addition to heart trouble, are usually excluded, as these other conditions could impair recovery.

Of course, patients who *are* selected are all extremely ill with heart disease, probably near to death because the heart muscle has been weakened by successive HEART ATTACKS.

Before the operation

For the transplant operation to happen at all, there must first be a suitable donor. Unless the new heart matches the recipient as far as possible in certain important respects, it will be rejected, however efficiently the reaction is suppressed with drugs.

This matching is achieved by tissue-typing. Samples of blood and other cells from the recipient's body are analysed, and the internal organization that holds a computer file of all available transplant organs is alerted for a donor with suitable tissue.

Potential donors carry cards on them at all times, giving doctors permission to remove various organs from their body in the event of their sudden death.

Also vital is the state of the donor's heart. It needs to be about the same size as the recipient's in order to fit the chest cavity. So, for this reason, both donor and recipient need to have similar overall physiques.

Of course, the donor heart has to be free of disease, and therefore hearts from people above the age of 35 are generally unsuitable.

Transporting the donor heart

The length of time taken to transport the donor heart to the recipient is also critical. Clearly, it cannot usually be arranged for the donor to die conveniently near the recipient, so painstaking organization is almost always needed.

Light aircraft, helicopters and police escorts are routine requirements, and the general rule is that the 'cold ischaemic time', which is the technical term for the period when the heart is between bodies, should not be longer than three hours. On its journey, the heart is packed in sterile polythene bags and stored in a special container designed to preserve it at a low temperature – 39.2°F (4°C).

Meanwhile, the recipient is prepared for surgery (among other precautions, a bath in sterile solution is taken by the patient to cut down the chance of infection, a particular risk in this type of operation). In the operating theatre, surgeons open the chest, methodically tying off or clamping blood vessels and finally exposing the heart cavity by levering the breastbone apart with a spreader.

This is routine surgery but it can take as long as two hours. If all goes smoothly, the recipient is ready for the new heart when it arrives.

The transplant

Essentially, this involves sewing the muscular part of the donor heart – that is, the left and right ventricles, together with their 'plumbing' (the blood supply vessels) – beneath the atria (the low-pressure pumping chambers) of the recipient's heart.

While the recipient is without a heart at all, blood is diverted through a heart–lung machine which pumps and oxygenates the blood. In this way, every part of the body is kept serviced with the oxygen and nutrients on which it depends.

Once connected, and receiving its new blood supply, the donor heart usually begins to beat straight away. Sometimes support is required in the form of a tiny electronic PACEMAKER which gives electrical impulses similar to the heart's own timing system.

In the first few days following the operation, the new heart is likely to be a little sluggish, so a perfect, regular beat may have to be established by boosting with a stimulant drug.

After the operation

The patient is usually conscious within about six hours, able to talk and take food. As early as three days later, the patient's new-found fitness can be tested on an exercise bike.

However, the critical period is not over. Between one and three days after the operation, the body always tries to reject the heart, however well tissue-typed.

A clue as to when the process will start in earnest is given by the machine (called an ELECTROCARDIOGRAM) which monitors the new heart's rhythm. A slight irregularity shows up on the screen, and the diagnosis is then confirmed by a BIOPSY of the heart muscle.

Controlling rejection

The heart specialist can then step up the doses of immunosuppressant drugs, choosing from the variety now available.

The most vigorous rejection continues for two or three months after the operation, after which the IMMUNE SYSTEM usually adapts to the new organ. However, taking immunosuppressants in moderate doses has to continue as long as the patient lives.

Suppressing the body's immune system also means suppressing its ability to fight infection in the form of germs. So during the critical period after the operation, the patient has to be guarded against infection to an astonishing degree: letters and cards are sterilized, and visitors must shower and change into sterile gowns.

Given the ambitious nature of the operation, together with its risks of rejection and infection, survival rates are impressive. Of those who survive the first year after the operation, 90 per cent return to a full life. The majority live over five years after the operation.

See also TRANSPLANTS.

Heatstroke, *see* **Sunstroke**

Helminths, *see* **Worms**

Heparin, *see* **Blood, Phlebitis**

Hepatitis

This is a highly infectious VIRUS disease, involving inflammation of the LIVER. The virus is transmitted in BLOOD, in faeces or saliva. It is a disease affecting people of all ages, but tends to occur more in the young or among those whose work entails handling contaminated material.

Causes

There are three viruses that are chiefly responsible, known as hepatitis A (formerly called infectious hepatitis), hepatitis B (formerly known as serum hepatitis) and the recently identified hepatitis C (formerly called non-A non-B hepatitis).

Hepatitis A is usually transmitted by food or water that has been contaminated, although this virus can also be transmitted in infected blood. The disease is only infectious in the incubation stage, and it is not transmitted by carriers. Outbreaks happen from time to time in areas with overcrowded housing and poor sanitation. This is the type of illness that can be caught on a trip abroad, for example, after eating contaminated food. Epidemics can also break out in schools and other institutions if hygiene is poor.

Hepatitis B takes longer to incubate, probably many months. It is transmitted in infected blood, either from hypodermic needles or as a result of a transfusion of infected blood or plasma, though stringent precautions against these forms of transmission are taken in hospitals. It has also been known to result from use of unsterile tattoo needles or razor blades. About 40 per cent of addicts who inject drugs are carriers of the B virus.

This virus also has the ability to infect an unborn child, by crossing through the placenta and so getting into the foetal bloodstream. Hepatitis B may also be transmitted sexually, either between heterosexual couples, or between homosexuals who appear to be especially at risk from this infection.

Hepatitis C is transmitted in the same manner as hepatitis B, and can cause disease following transfusion of blood or blood products. Since 1991, it has been routinely screened for in donated blood.

A group of people especially at risk are hospital personnel, particularly those whose work involves handling blood regularly in operating theatres or renal dialysis units (where sick patients are treated on kidney machines).

Symptoms

It is known that the majority of infections with either the A or B virus are mild and may even pass unnoticed, although both viruses leave chemical evidence in blood after an infection and signs of this can be found in blood tests.

When the disease is severe enough to cause sufficient inflammation of the liver to block the drainage of BILE, the sufferer becomes JAUNDICED. When this happens, the skin and the whites of the eyes develop a yellowish tinge. This is caused by bile pigments made by the liver entering the circulation instead of being eliminated through the intestine.

Jaundice may occur fairly rapidly after an infection by hepatitis A, but is usually slower if the illness is due to hepatitis B.

Very often the victim feels unwell for some time beforehand, going off food and losing any desire to smoke. Pain is felt high in the abdomen, on the right side. There may also be arthritic-type pains in the joints as well as a RASH. While the jaundice is most marked, the patient feels sick and frequently vomits. The jaundice does not usually last for more than a fortnight and recovery takes place within six weeks or so.

Unfortunately, in a few cases, the infection does not clear up and chronic inflammation of the liver develops, ultimately resulting in CIRRHOSIS. (The liver cells are progressively destroyed and replaced with fibrous tissue, which gradually makes the liver less effective.)

Doctors have little difficulty in diagnosing hepatitis when typical symptoms are present, which can be confirmed by blood tests. Tests can show which virus (A, B or C) has caused the disease. If the diagnosis is in doubt, a liver biopsy is performed, in which a tiny sample is taken from the liver for examination. This is neither risky nor particularly painful and is performed under local anaesthetic.

Dangers

Until the recent increase in liver disease produced by ALCOHOLISM, viral hepatitis was without question the most common cause of cirrhosis of the liver. If the infection was caused by hepatitis B, the virus may remain in the blood for months or years. Such patients then become sources of infection to others and cause problems if they have to be admitted to hospital for any reason at all. They may also be infectious to their sexual partners. But not all hepatitis sufferers are carriers; for reasons that are still unknown, some patients recover from the disease completely.

Treatment

It is not necessary to admit all hepatitis sufferers to hospital – only those who become extremely unwell or who are at risk – for example, expectant mothers, diabetics or the elderly.

While the liver is inflamed and also while it is recovering, its cells will be sensitive to all kinds of drugs and it is advisable not to take any medicines at this time, including the contraceptive pill. It is particularly important to avoid alcohol, which has a poisonous effect on the liver.

Whether the patient is being treated in hospital or at home, it is essential to try and reduce the chances of cross-infection by using separate cooking and eating utensils for the patient and being careful about personal hygiene.

There has been a good deal of medical argument as to the importance of complete bedrest. But it is felt by some doctors that the later complications (cirrhosis or chronic hepatitis) can be avoided provided the patient rests as much as possible while jaundiced.

It is best for the patient to avoid fatty foods, but to eat plenty of CARBOHYDRATES. Food should be made as tempting as possible to encourage the appetite.

Prevention

People who are exposed to infection by hepatitis, or who intend 'living rough' on walking or camping holidays in areas such as southern Europe, India or Africa, can be given temporary protection by an injection of gamma-globulin. This is especially effective against hepatitis A. People who are exposed to a high risk of hepatitis B – for example, homosexuals or hospital workers – can be given a vaccine to provide long-term protection.

Heredity

Every time we say 'it runs in the family' or 'she has her mother's eyes,' we are talking about heredity, or, in scientific language, GENETICS – the study of genes.

Genes are probably best described as biochemical codes. They are tiny, too small to be seen even under an electron microscope, but scientists know they are carried on the chromosomes, which are the tiny, thread-like structures that can be seen under a microscope within all human cells.

Everyone has 46 chromosomes, arranged in 23 pairs, one member of each pair coming from the SPERM of the father, the other from the mother's egg (*see* OVARIES). Together, these structures make a complete chemical blueprint for an entire person.

Simple forms of heredity

This pairing of chromosomes is most significant to the way heredity works because each pair contains similar genes, and the simplest forms of heredity can be traced to single pairs of genes.

Genes acting in this way can occur in two different forms, one the *dominant*, the other the *recessive*. Dominant genes are distinguished by the tendency to make their characteristics evident in the physical make-up of a person, even if they are only present in a single dose. A pair of similar recessive genes – one inherited from each parent – must be present if they are to make themselves obvious.

Geneticists have identified various dominant and recessive genes. For example, the gene for curly hair is dominant, so if a child inherits it from, say, the father, and also a gene for straight hair (which is recessive) from the mother, the curly hair gene will dominate, and the child will have curly hair.

In practical terms, this does not mean that you can predict whether your child will inherit your curly hair. The actual 'passing on' of genes is a random happening, the curly-hair dominant gene having slightly better than even chances of being transferred. But the principle does help us in a negative way – making it clear that we cannot count on a child having straight hair (if that is preferred) if one partner is curly- and the other straight-haired.

'Normality'

This form of heredity, known as *single-factor inheritance*, is relatively simple, and tells us some important and quite reassuring things about how our children will turn out in terms of their general health and make-up. This is because, fortunately, the majority of 'normal' characteristics are governed by dominant genes.

Just a few hereditary diseases are inherited on dominant genes, but recessive genes cause many more, including albinism (lack of pigment, or colouring) and some types of deafness.

Another important point to understand is that recessive genes, of their nature, can be 'carried' by a human all through life without the characteristics they convey actually showing up. Also, there is nothing to stop them being passed on to the next generation and, if the circumstances are right, showing up there.

So it cannot be precisely explained why, for example, musical talent tends to run in families to such an extent. No one knows how much of it is inherited, and how much occurs as a result of being brought up in an environment where music is part of family life. The same applies to acting ability, sporting skill, literary ability and many other talents.

Environment may also act as the trigger for an inherited physical characteristics. Two people, may, for example, be born with a tendency to go brown easily (which, in fact, involves the ability to make the pigment melanin in the skin). But if one of them stays indoors for most of the time, their skin is unlikely to go brown, while the other, doing an outdoor job, develops a healthy tan.

The question of heredity is further complicated by the fact that genes show their strength not only in terms of dominance over other genes, but by the degree to which they penetrate, which geneticists call *penetrance*.

Penetrance may be weak or strong. For example, the defect of the fingers known as camptodactyly is produced by a dominant gene, and can thus show up by being inherited in the single-factor method. However, the degree to which a person suffers from it will vary from severe stiffness of several fingers (full penetrance) to stiffness of just one finger (partial penetrance).

Hernia

This is a protrusion through a weakness in the abdominal wall. It can either be external – i.e. it shows as a lump on the surface of the ABDOMEN or in the groin – or it can be internal: for instance, a hiatus hernia, caused by a weakness in the diaphragm (*see* DIAPHRAGM for full details).

Types of external hernias

The commonest types of hernias occur in the groin, and are called *inguinal or femoral* hernias, depending on the exact site of the weakness. They can also occur near the navel (*umbical* hernia), in the upper part of the abdomen in the midline (*epigastric*), and through weakness in the posterior wall of the abdomen, when they are usually not visible as a lump. Hernias can also develop at the site of an operation, where the muscles have failed to heal strongly, and they are then called *incisional* hernias.

A hernia usually consists of a sac made of PERITONEUM, the thin membrane lining the abdominal cavity, which protrudes through the weakness in the muscular wall of the abdomen. If it is an external hernia, the sac will be covered with a layer of fat, over which will be the skin. The sac contains either part of an intra-abdominal organ, such as a loop of small INTESTINE, or of the *omentum*, the fatty membrane which covers the intestines. In fact, the omentum often fills the sac completely, preventing any other structures from entering it; as will be seen later, this helps to prevent the complications which may result from the presence of a hernia.

Causes

Hernias are very common and there are various causes for them. First of all, people may be born with a particular weakness which makes them prone to develop a hernia. This may mean that they develop a hernia in infancy, or later in life due to, for instance, heavy lifting.

Sometimes hernias occur as a result of a serious persistent COUGH. Children who have WHOOPING COUGH can develop hernias in the groin, as can adults with chronic BRONCHITIS. The cause is the excessively high pressures that occur in the abdomen during a bout of coughing. Any area in the abdominal wall where there is an existing weakness can then give way, producing a hernia. People who are overweight are also more prone to developing hernias (*see* OBESITY).

The commonest type of groin hernia – the inguinal hernia ('inguinal' means 'of the groin') – occurs more often in men than women, and in men is related to a weakness caused by the structures connecting the TESTIS to its blood supply passing through the muscular wall of the abdomen.

Symptoms

An inguinal hernia caused by heavy lifting will often come about suddenly: the patient may describe a feeling of something giving way, accompanied by some pain. This usually lasts only for a short time, and the patient then notices a lump in the groin. This lump is usually soft, bulges when he coughs, and goes away completely when he lies down. If it gets very large, it may extend down into the scrotum in a man or towards the vulva in a woman. However, hernias can get surprisingly large before they cause a number of symptoms. Of course, if the patent's job involves a lot of heavy lifting, the hernia may become uncomfortable all the time and prevent him from doing his job satisfactorily.

Femoral hernias also cause a lump in the groin, but instead of tracking down towards the genital area, they extend into the upper thigh. They are quite commonly painful, even if they are small.

Dangers

If strangulation occurs, a hernia becomes extremely serious and potentially lethal. Strangulation happens when the blood supply to the contents of the hernia is cut off by pressure on the blood vessels by the neck of the sac. First, the veins are obstructed, and this causes the contents to swell, causing further pressure on the arteries, eventually leading to gangrene of the contents if this includes part of the intestines.

The hernia, which had previously been soft, and perhaps only uncomfortable, becomes tense, tender and irreducible (i.e. it does not go away when the patient lies down). If the bowel is strangulated, the patient may develop symptoms of intestinal obstruction – vomiting, abdominal pain, distension and constipation. If this does happen, an emergency operation is needed to free the strangulated bowel and repair the hernia. If left more than a few hours, the bowel may become irreparably damaged, so that part of it will have to be removed and the two ends joined together again. Of course, if strangulation occurs in one of the rare internal hernias, there is no lump to feel and the patient becomes ill because of bowel obstruction.

The commonest hernia to strangulate is a femoral hernia, followed by inguinal and para-umbilical hernias.

Diagnosis

Most external hernias can be diagnosed by a doctor relatively easily simply by examination of the affected area. Often the doctor asks the patient to cough or strain to see if the hernia appears, and then asks the patient to lie down to check whether or not the hernia returns back into the abdomen.

It may not be easy, however, for the doctor to distinguish between an inguinal and femoral hernia if the hernia is fairly small. It is important that the site of it is identified because femoral hernias are more liable to complications.

Treatment

If there is a recognizable cause for a hernia, such as obesity, constipation, a cough or difficulty in passing water, this should, if possible, be treated.

Treatment for inguinal hernias involves either the wearing of a truss or surgical repair. A truss is a special belt, with an extra strap that passes between the legs to prevent it from riding up. It has a specially designed pad which presses on the area of the hernia, preventing it from bulging out. It may be uncomfortable to wear, and it can be dangerous in that it may allow the hernia, containing part of the bowel, to bulge out and then press on the neck of the sac, making strangulation more likely.

By far the best treatment for inguinal hernia is a surgical operation. This may be carried out to prevent strangulation in the future, or because the hernia is uncomfortable and is preventing the patient from working, or, finally, as an emergency because there is strangulation.

The operation is very simple, and can be performed under a local ANAESTHETIC if the patient is thin and the hernia is small, or if the patient is unfit for a general anaesthetic, although it is usually performed under the latter. The thin sac of peritoneum is carefully removed and tied off at the neck, after all its contents have been returned to the abdominal cavity. In a child, this is all that would be done, but in an adult the defect in the muscle wall of the abdomen is repaired. A strong, non-soluble stitch may be used, such as nylon, and the defect 'darned'. When the scar tissue has formed round the stitches (about three months after the operation), the area should be as strong as normal.

Nowadays the repair of the muscle wall is often performed with a piece of synthetic mesh, which is sewn in place over the defect. This type of repair often causes less pain in the early post-operative period than the conventional 'darn'.

Most incisional hernias have a very wide neck, so there is very little likelihood of their strangulating. In addition, they can be difficult to repair satisfactorily. A surgical belt is likely to control them very well.

Heroin

This drug is produced from morphine, which is made from raw opium. The major medical uses of heroin are to control severe pain that cannot be treated with morphine and ease the pain of certain terminal diseases.

If the drug is needed to ease the pain of serious injuries, it will be given in carefully controlled doses, tailored to the patient's exact needs, and there will be no danger of addiction.

Possibly the only circumstances in which morphine or heroin addiction could accidentally occur are if someone experiences injuries when they are days away from a hospital – for example, on an expedition to a remote area. If more than the stated dose is given for too long a period, physical dependence can occur.

Heroin addiction

It is not quite clear why heroin has become such a favoured drug of addicts – that is, people who began by taking the drug for pleasure rather than for medical reasons.

Its effect is no different in essence to that of morphine; indeed, it is changed by the body into morphine. However, there are a couple of probable reasons for its popularity.

First, heroin acts quickly, giving an instant, dramatic high, and also satisfies the addict's craving, once established, without any delay. Second, it is less bulky than morphine, and is therefore easier for those concerned in smuggling or trafficking in illegal supplies to store or carry. However, on the streets, where it is known by a variety of names such as 'H', 'smack' or 'horse', it is mixed with other substances such as dried milk or baking powder for bulk.

Heroin may be sniffed, but is usually injected with a syringe – first, into a muscle, but later, as tolerance builds up, into a major vein, often in the arm. Injecting makes the drug work more quickly and efficiently than sniffing, but has some considerable drawbacks.

With continual injections into the same vein, the skin becomes hardened and scarred, and the vein eventually collapses. If the needle is not properly sterilized, infectious diseases may develop.

So what does the addict get from heroin? After the injection (the 'fix'), he or she quickly experiences a strong feeling of well-being and contentment. The extent of this 'high' varies with the purity of the heroin and the emotional state of the addict before the fix. But generally, the more desperate the mood, the greater will be the 'high'.

In what by any standard is a short period, the heroin user will become physically addicted to the drug. In theory, the actual quantity needed to produce addiction is 60 milligrams (one grain) taken within a two-week period. In practice, this amount is different for every person (the larger your body size, the more you need to create the same effect), but essentially it boils down to the fact that remarkably few fixes during a two-week period will cause addiction.

With each successive 'fix', the duration of the effect becomes shorter and shorter. So the user starts taking more of the drug each time and also tries to get enough heroin to have several fixes a day – often as many as six or eight during a single 24-hour period.

The death rate among addicts is high, and average life expectancy has been estimated at 25 years, unless the addict started the habit at an early age. The actual causes of death are likely to be various – not only overdose of the drug itself, but also suicide and diseases caused by an infected needle.

Heroin and infections

A heroin addict becomes less resistant to infection as he or she takes more and more of the drug, even those addicts who only use the drug by sniffing. However, those who inject the drug are most at risk. Often addicts are so desperate for the next fix that they fail to clean their injecting equipment properly, so the needle and syringe are dirty and contaminated. This can lead to ABSCESSES in the skin, or blood poisoning which may prove fatal.

Some addicts, however, cannot obtain their own syringes and needles and so they share their 'works' with other addicts. This practice puts them at very considerable risk of developing those diseases that are most readily spread by direct blood transmission from one person to another. Infectious HEPATITIS B may be spread this way and can cause a serious liver infection with JAUNDICE and life-threatening LIVER failure. Those addicts who recover from hepatitis B may remain carriers of the virus so that they can pass it on to anyone else with whom they share needles or syringes.

Most worrying, however, is the possibility of the spread of AIDS by heroin addicts who share injecting equipment. In some parts of the US, one heroin addict in two is a carrier of the HIV virus that causes AIDS. Such people can pass on the virus to others through sharing injecting equipment, or through sexual intercourse. Both men and women can be infected in this way.

The cure

This is painful and lengthy. The only truly effective way of ceasing to be an addict is to be denied any supply of the drug whatsoever until the body learns not to need it any more.

Before reaching this stage, withdrawal symptoms have to be endured. This term describes the body's violent reaction to being deprived of the substance on which it has become so dependent.

Withdrawal symptoms begin between four and six hours after the last fix, and are at their most severe for about ten days. After that they begin to be less unpleasant, but a complete cure may take from three to six months. Even when the physical unpleasantness is over, the former addict is likely to need a period of adjustment to life without the drug.

Herpes

These are painful blisters which erupt on the skin in clusters or bands. They are caused by two distinct varieties of herpes virus. The first, and more serious, kind is called *Herpes zoster*, commonly known as shingles. The second kind, called *Herpes simplex*, is divided into two types: the type which affects the upper part of the body, particularly the nose and mouth, and genital herpes.

Herpes zoster (shingles)

Shingles is caused by exactly the same virus that produces CHICKENPOX, and only occurs in those people who have, at some time earlier in their lives, already had chickenpox. After an attack of chickenpox, the herpes zoster virus seems to lie dormant in the body, and then as a result of some trigger, suddenly becomes active again. The virus attacks a single nerve in the skin, often in the trunk, but sometimes on a limb or on the face. *See* SHINGLES for more information.

Herpes simplex

The two types of herpes simplex virus are known as type 1, which causes COLD SORES on the nose and mouth but can also be transferred to the genital area, and type 2 which causes nine out of ten genital herpes infections.

By the time children reach six years of age, about one in five has already become infected with type 1 herpes – usually contracted from a relative or playmate. By the age of 40, almost four out of five people have had the infection at some time or other. Once somebody has suffered an initial attack of herpes, the virus lies dormant in the skin and can produce further attacks at intervals.

Symptoms

The first attacks of herpes is usually the most severe. Type 1 herpes usually causes a 'primary' infection in the mouth and around the lips. Small painful blisters – cold sores – erupt on the tongue, inside the cheeks and on the lips. The affected area can become swollen and red. Often the pain is so severe that eating and drinking may be difficult. The blisters burst and heal after about five to seven days.

Subsequent attacks of type 1 herpes usually affect just small areas – perhaps $\frac{4}{5}$–$1\frac{2}{5}$ in (2–3 cm) across – on the edge of the lips or the nose. These attacks may be triggered off by a cold, a fever, or by exposure to bright sunlight or even cold winds.

Genital herpes is usually transmitted sexually from one partner who already has it to the other. It can be spread by oral sex to the genital area as well. The 'primary' infection can be very extensive. In a woman, irritating blisters can form all over the vulva and spread into the VAGINA, and occasionally even the inside of the BLADDER is affected as well. In a man, the whole genital area may also be affected. The sores heal within seven to ten days, but repeated attacks can then recur at intervals of a few weeks or a month, although the size of the affected area is usually only a few centimetres across. Each attack starts with tingling and itching in the affected area – the blisters appear a day or so later. Repeated attacks may be triggered by a FEVER, but also by emotional STRESS, and sometimes by soreness associated with sexual activity.

Dangers of *Herpes simplex*

Anyone who is suffering from a herpes infection can pass the infection on by contact. So somebody who has a cold sore should avoid kissing anybody else until the sore has completely healed. Similarly anyone who suffers from genital herpes should not have intercourse until the sores have healed completely. A woman with active genital herpes may pass the infection on to her baby during childbirth; in these cases, CAESAREAN sections are recommended.

Genital herpes in a woman has been suspected of being responsible for some cases of cancer of the CERVIX. It is certainly clear that there is a type of infectious agent associated with cancer of the cervix, but it is more likely that a type of genital WART caused by a virus is the linking factor. Nevertheless it is usually suggested by doctors that any woman who suffers from recurrent genital herpes should have a smear test carried out *at least* every three years.

Treatment

Primary herpes is occasionally so severe that hospital treatment is needed. A child with primary type 1 herpes may find it difficult to swallow and may need a drip feed to provide fluids. Anti-viral drugs can be given in hospital.

If a patient with primary type 1 or type 2 herpes is treated at home, acyclovir may be prescribed by the doctor in tablet form. Recurrent attacks can be treated with a cream containing acyclovir, which is very effective provided it is used early in the attack. Occasionally herpes sores become secondarily infected with bacteria, and then antibiotics such as penicillin may be required as well. Small cold sores usually heal without any specific treatment.

Hiatus hernia, *see* **Diaphragm, Ulcers, peptic**

Hidradenitis suppuritiva, *see* **Perspiration, Septic conditions**

Hip

This is the biggest JOINT in the body. It has two main functions, to carry the considerable weight of the upper part of the trunk and, with the help of the spine, to enable us to walk upright.

The description 'ball and socket' is particularly appropriate in the case of the hip joint, because it is here that a large hemispherical projection at the top of the thigh bone (the *femur*) fits into a cup-shaped socket, the *acetabulum*, in the *iliac bone* of the PELVIC girdle. This cavity faces outwards, so that the legs are kept far enough away from the mid-line of the body for effective balance and walking.

Smooth movement is ensured by the shiny cartilage that covers the head of the femur and lines the acetabulum, and lubrication is provided by the synovial fluid secreted by the synovial membranes. These membranes form the inner layer of the tough, fibrous capsule which makes a very strong hermetic seal around the joint. The capsule is thin at the back of the joint, but very thick at the sides and the front of the body, where the greatest pressure is exerted on the hip. Several accumulations of fatty tissue, which lie inside the tight seal provided by the capsule, serve as padding inside the joint and act as shock absorbers.

Added stability is provided by a set of ligaments which bind the head of the femur to the pelvic girdle, criss-crossing over one another to maximize their strength and to prevent the 'ball' from slipping out of its socket. Of these, the *iliofemoral ligament*, towards the outside of the joint, is thought to be the strongest in the body. It is essential for both walking and standing that the thigh does not move further back than an imaginary straight line drawn vertically down the side of the trunk. This constraint is provided by the ligaments. When the leg seems to be pulled back beyond this line – for example, before kicking a football – it is the whole pelvic girdle that moves, not the hip joint.

If you stand up and move your LEGS into several different positions, you will quickly see how many actions the hip joints allow. These movements are made possible by the muscles which lie over the ligaments. Take the action of pulling your knee up towards your head – this involves bending, or *flexion*, of the hip. Such a movement is brought about by two main muscles, the *psoas major*, which runs from the base of the spine across the front of the hip to the femur, and the *iliacus*, a flat triangular muscle which is attached to the pelvis at one end and to the femur at the other. These two muscles are assisted by others in the thigh.

Straightening your bent leg is called *extension*. To perform this action you use your outermost and biggest buttock muscle, the *gluteus maximus*, plus a group of muscles at the back of the thigh, known as *hamstrings*. It is these muscles that are actually at work when you are standing still.

Moving your leg out sideways is called *abduction*, and bringing it back again, *adduction*. The first of these movements involves several of the muscles that lie beneath the gluteus maximus; these are the *gluteus medius* and *gluteus minimus* which join the pelvis with the femur, and the *sartorius*, the longest muscle in the body, which runs from the pelvic girdle to the knee. The pulling power between the pelvis and the femur, needed for adduction, is provided by a group of muscles including the *adductor longus*, *adductor brevis* and *adductor magnus*. Many of these muscles are also used to allow the legs to rotate, although this movement is limited by the binding of the ligaments.

Congenital dislocation

Because of its complex structure, the hip is extremely stable compared to its counterpart, the shoulder. This stability means that, in adult life, dislocation of the hip is a very rare injury although, paradoxically, it is not only the most common hip problem of childhood, but also the most common at birth.

During the baby's development in the womb, the socket of the hip joint may not become deep enough so the hip can dislocate very easily in the early weeks of life. If this dislocation is not treated, permanent damage to the joints eventually occurs. Five times as many girl babies as boys are affected by congenital dislocation of the hip.

Examination of the hips is carried out immediately after the birth of every child, as a routine precaution. The baby is placed on its back, with its legs wide apart and held firmly by the feet. If the hips are dislocated, the doctor will hear a deep clicking sound as he or she bends the child's knees and hips. The sound is from the head of the femur as it goes into its socket. Another click will be heard as the femur disengages.

The doctor will also place his hand, so that his thumb is on the baby's groin and his middle finger is on the projection of the thigh bone. If the head of the femur is easily moved out of its socket, then he will suspect that the hip is potentially unstable, or 'irritable'. If this is the case, these tests are followed by X-ray examinations to check the diagnosis.

Nowadays, treatment for a congenital dislocation of the hip is extremely effective. Usually, the infant is put into a plaster splint, which keeps the legs wide apart, so that they are in a frog-like position. After a few months, the joint is X-rayed to check progress, and in most cases, the splint is then removed. Whether or not the baby has to stay in hospital during this period depends on domestic circumstances. The child can be looked after at home if this is possible.

If the hips are not actually dislocated, but 'irritable', the doctor may advise the mother to keep a double terry towelling nappy on the baby, so that the legs are kept wide apart until the ligaments and muscles around the joint have developed enough strength to overcome the problem naturally.

Diseases and injuries

Problems may arise in the hip joint later on in childhood, due to diseases which cause inflammation of the synovial membranes or, rarely these days, by TUBERCULOSIS. An unusual, but serious hip condition, which is very much more common in boys than girls, is PERTHES' DISEASE in which, for some unknown reason, the bony tissue in the head of the femur begins to disintegrate.

Children who start limping for no obvious reason may have had an unsuspected injury, but this symptom can be a warning sign of other hip problems. Apart from Perthes' disease, another common condition in children under ten is *synovitis.* The child starts limping and may complain of pain in the groin.

Infection in the hip – OSTEOMYELITIS – can start with similar symptoms, but if this problem is present, the child becomes quite ill and the pain gets worse rather than improving. Osteomyelitis always requires hospital treatment. High doses of antibiotics are given over several weeks to treat the infection.

Teenage children may develop pains in one or both hips as a result of a condition called *slipped femoral epiphysis.* The growing point at the end of any bone is called an epiphysis and is composed of an area of solid bone surrounded by softer cartilage. In teenagers, there is epiphysis at the head of the femur and it may simply slip out of place – sometimes as a result of an injury but occasionally without any obvious cause. The young person develops a limp and pain in the hip. An operation is required to return the epiphysis to its correct position.

Accidental injury to the joint is most common in old age (*see* OSTEOPOROSIS) and very often follows heavy falls. In such injuries, the most likely place at which a bone is broken is across the neck of the femur. First aid for a suspected hip FRACTURE is most effective if the victim's hips are immobilized by binding the legs together in several places, from the feet upwards, after which an ambulance should be called, because urgent hospital treatment is necessary.

Arthritis in the hip

The hip may be affected by a number of different types of ARTHRITIS. In younger adults, a condition called ankylosing SPONDYLITIS may affect the joints in the spine, but the hip joints may also become involved. RHEUMATOID ARTHRITIS usually affects small and medium-sized joints such as those in the hands, the elbows and knees. However, again the hips may also be involved and can become extremely stiff and painful.

The commonest form of arthritis in the hips is OSTEOARTHRITIS. This affects many middle-aged and elderly people: it is present in almost everyone who reaches the age of 70. Essentially, osteoarthritis is caused by excessive wear of the joint. People who are very overweight may develop severe osteoarthritis in their hips as early as their 40s. Anyone who has led an extremely active life or played a great deal of body-contact sports such as rugby football may also be prone to osteoarthritis in the hip.

Hirsutism, *see* **Hair**

Histamine, *see* **Allergy, Blood, Inflammation**

Histoplasmosis, *see* **Fungal infections**

HIV, *see* **AIDS**

Hives, *see* **Allergy**

Hoarseness, *see* **Larynx and laryngitis**

Hodgkin's disease

This is a form of CANCER which arises in the LYMPHATIC SYSTEM, the system responsible for defending the body against infection, which is itself part of the IMMUNE SYSTEM. Although the disease can occur at almost any age, it is most common between the ages of 15 and 30, although elderly people may develop a localized form of the disorder. About two people in every 1,000 develop Hodgkin's disease at some time in their lives.

Causes
Hodgkin's disease affects the lymph tissues, which are composed of lymph cells, or lymphocytes, a type of white blood cell. Lymphocytes are found in the BLOOD and BONE MARROW, and are grouped together in the lymph nodes in the neck, armpits, groin, chest, abdomen, and in the liver and spleen. In Hodgkin's disease, the lymph cells proliferate and the affected nodes become enlarged. One group of lymph nodes, usually in the groin or neck, is affected first, and then the disease gradually spreads from one group of nodes to the next until the whole lymphatic system is involved.

The cause of Hodgkin's disease is still not known, although at one time, it was thought that a virus could be involved in triggering off the illness. Twice as many men are affected as women in the younger age groups, although when the disease affects those over 65 years of age, the numbers of men and women affected are equal. The reason for this is also unknown.

Symptoms
Usually, the first symptom is a swelling in a group of lymph nodes. The patient may have suffered from a sore throat or some other trivial illness, then notices

that some of the glands which usually enlarge during illness have failed to go down again afterwards. Most often the glands affected are in the front of the neck or the armpit, but occasionally glands in the groin are enlarged.

About one in four people also have more general symptoms. There may be a fever, particularly at night, with sweating, some weight loss and considerable tiredness.

Diagnosis

Abnormally enlarged lymph nodes are quite common in response to local infection, but such infection is usually quite obvious to a doctor – for example, a SKIN infection or a BOIL. If an enlarged lymph node persists for more than three weeks without any obvious cause, the doctor may carry out some investigations. Blood tests may show another cause for the enlarged gland, but if the patient has Hodgkin's disease, the results may be quite normal.

The most commonly used test is a BIOPSY. Under a local or general anaesthetic, an enlarged gland is removed by a surgeon. It is then carefully examined by a pathologist using a microscope. Hodgkin's disease can be diagnosed with confidence using this technique.

Once the diagnosis has been made, further investigations are always carried out to try to assess the severity and extent of the disease. These tests are very important because the type of treatment depends on these results.

First, the patient is re-examined by the doctor, who checks every possible area where the glands could be enlarged – the neck and throat, armpits, abdomen and groins, and the back of the knee joints and elbow joints. Next, a chest X-RAY is taken to see whether internal glands in the chest are affected. The patient then usually has a CT scan (*see* NEUROLOGY), a special type of X-ray using a computerized X-ray machine which can produce detailed pictures of the soft tissues inside the body.

Another investigation that may be employed is a *lymphangiogram*. This is a type of X-ray in which the lymphatic system in the abdomen and chest is outlined by injecting a special dye into a lymph vessel in the foot.

Lastly, the doctors may decide to carry out a *laparotomy* as well. This is a major operation in which the abdomen is opened for inspection. All the possible sites of enlargement of lymph nodes inside the abdomen are carefully examined by the surgeon. Any enlarged glands may be biopsied for examination by the pathologist. The SPLEEN is removed for later examination, as well as a small piece of the LIVER. Laparotomy is less frequently used now that CT scanning is widely available.

Treatment

The treatment selected depends on the results of all the tests, and to some extent on the age and general condition of the patient.

Hodgkin's disease has been classified into different stages. Stage I is the earliest type of disease in which only one group of glands are affected; Stage II describes the next phase, where several groups of glands close together are involved; Stages III and IV are more severe types, with increasingly widespread involvement of glands.

Those patients with early disease (Stage I or II) are usually treated with deep X-ray therapy (*see* RADIOTHERAPY). Often it is necessary only to treat the neck, upper chest and armpits, or the abdomen and groins – depending on the site of the disease. Treatments are given daily over a period of several weeks. During treatment, there may be side-effects such as nausea and redness of the skin in the treated area, but these settle after the treatment. The aim of X-ray therapy is to kill off abnormal cells while leaving the healthy cells intact.

Patients with Stage III or IV disease are usually treated with a combination of several drugs. They are cytotoxic drugs, which kill cells that are dividing abnormally quickly such as the cancerous cells in Hodgkin's disease. Usually up to four different drugs are used at once for maximum effect. Side-effects can be very troublesome – nausea and vomiting and sometimes loss of hair – but are temporary. The drugs are given in a series of courses, a few days at a time, with three or four weeks between each course.

Forty years ago, most people with Hodgkin's disease died within two years of diagnosis. Today, treatment has advanced to the extent that Hodgkin's disease is one of the most successfully treated cancers, and most patients are eventually cured.

'Hole in the heart', *see* **Blue baby**

Holiday health

Becoming ill on holiday can be a serious matter. Everyone knows that foreign holidays can play havoc with the digestive system. If it is not DIARRHOEA, it is CONSTIPATION and then, of course, there are the unaccountable flu-type symptoms that some holiday-makers succumb to. You could run up high doctors' fees as well as a high temperature. Perfect health on holiday can never be guaranteed, but you can take precautions which will reduce the chances of illness.

For ambitious trips to remote areas, specialist advice on health protection can be obtained from such organizations as the London School of Hygiene and Tropical Medicine or the World Expeditionary Association. The Department of Health also publishes free information. (*See also* TROPICAL DISEASES.)

You should start enquiring about vaccinations at least two months before your departure, since some have to be given in two or more doses spaced several weeks apart. Your doctor should know which vaccinations you will need, but for the most up-to-date information, contact the embassies of the countries you are intending to visit.

Most vaccinations are recommended, not compulsory (unless there is an outbreak of disease), but you should still have them for your protection. They can nearly all be given by your own doctor, but YELLOW FEVER vaccination needs to be obtained at a special vaccinating centre – your doctor will have the address.

Vaccination checklist

Disease	How caught	Vaccination compulsory	Vaccination recommended	Other precautions
Typhoid	Contaminated food or water or milk		Everywhere except northern Europe, North America, Australia, New Zealand	Enquire about vaccination at least 6 weeks before departure. Take scrupulous care over food and drink on holiday
Polio	Direct contact with infected person; rarely by contaminated food or drink		Everywhere except northern Europe, North America, Australia, New Zealand	Everyone should receive this vaccine during childhood. 'Booster' dose if necessary
Tetanus	Entry of bacteria from soil into wound		Everywhere	Everyone should receive this vaccine during childhood. 'Booster' dose if necessary
Cholera	Contaminated food or water	Niger, Qatar	Most African, Asian, Middle Eastern countries; occasionally Mediterranean countries	Keep vaccination certificate in passport. Take scrupulous care over food and drink on holiday
Yellow fever	Bite from an infected mosquito	Most West African and some South American countries	Many other tropical African, South American and Central American countries	Keep vaccination certificate in passport. Avoid mosquito bites
Hepatitis A	Contaminated food or water or contact with an infected person		Countries where sanitation is primitive; most parts of Africa and Asia	Take scrupulous care over food, drink and hygiene
Smallpox	Disease now eradicated		No longer needed	
Rabies	Bite or scratch from rabid dog, cat or wild mammal		Only for explorers visiting remote areas of the world where rabies is endemic	Seek medical help immediately if bitten by dog, cat or wild mammal

Anti-malarial pills: For many areas of Africa, South and Central America, and Asia including Turkey and the Middle East, it is essential to be protected against malaria by taking anti-malarial tablets. You must take such tablets even if you are visiting a malarial area for only a brief stop-over. A single mosquito bite is enough to give you the disease.

Different strains of malaria occur in different parts of the world, and your doctor will select a suitable drug according to the area you are visiting. Your doctor will need to know exactly which countries you are visiting, and sometimes also which part of the country. He or she will then check with the latest information to find out which drugs are likely to be most effective against the strain of malaria present at the time. The tablets usually have to be taken once a week or once a day, before, during and for four to six weeks after you visit to the malarial area.

Tablets do not provide total protection, so for high-risk areas in the tropics, take extra precautions against mosquito bites. Minimize exposure to biting insects, and wear sensible clothing. Use insect repellents that contain diethyltoluamile (DET), and at night, use a mosquito net or burn pyrethrum 'mosquito coils'. (Electronic insect repellents do *not* work.)

Some medicines may be difficult to obtain abroad, so take a selection with you on holiday.

Taking your children on holiday

If you are taking small children, you need to apply a little forethought to your travel and accommodation arrangements. It is especially important to check up with your GP about vaccinations for your child if you are travelling abroad. Children are more susceptible to SUNBURN and SUNSTROKE than adults, so remember to take a sunscreen with a very high protection factor and also some hats for the children to wear in the sun. They may also suffer severely from insect bites, so make sure you have plenty of insect repellent cream and apply this liberally.

For babies who are bottle feeding, a supply of dried milk powder will be needed as well as the bottles. You will usually be able to get the bottles sterilized in a hotel, but if you are staying in a caravan, you should take your usual sterilizing equipment.

The risk of AIDS

AIDS is now present throughout the world, but it is far more common in some countries than in others – for example, in many African countries and some Asian ones. In certain central African countries, more than half the prostitutes are infected as well as up to 40 per cent of the rest of the population.

AIDS is transmitted in two main ways:

- By having sex with a man or woman who is infected with the virus.
- By allowing contaminated blood to get into your body.

Remember to take the following precautions whenever you are away from home:

- Do not have sexual intercourse with anybody other than your usual partner.

- If you do have a sexual contact with anybody, use a condom.
- Do not inject drugs.
- In some countries, blood used for transfusions is not tested for the HIV virus, which causes AIDS. A blood transfusion in these countries could be very risky. Try to avoid medical or surgical treatment in such circumstances. Make sure you have enough medical insurance to be flown to modern medical facilities urgently.

Travel sickness

Children are more vulnerable to TRAVEL SICKNESS than adults, the worst ages being between four and ten. Some people, of course, never grow out of it, and there is little they can do except buy travel sickness pills and take them before travelling, always following the instructions on the label carefully and keeping to the stated doses. Remember, if driving, that they cause drowsiness. Children need junior-strength travel pills.

Food and water precautions

Most places have healthy drinking water, but if you have any doubt, enquire at the hotel reception or ask the travel agent, if you are renting a cottage or villa. At camp sites you will be told which taps to use, but it is useful to take water-purifying tablets; these are available from chemists. If the water is impure, use the tablets even when rinsing your teeth.

Do not drink from local fountains or use the water to dilute fruit squash unless you know it is pure. Use bottled mineral water instead. Remember that ice-cubes are made from local tap water.

Wash any fruit and salad vegetables that you buy in pure water just before you eat them: or, alternatively, wash them when you bring them back from the shop and store them away from flies. Protect other food similarly and keep perishables in a cool place.

If you are reheating food, make sure it is done very thoroughly. Fresh cooked food is safer than reheated food. Keep cooked and uncooked meats separately and wash utensils and work tops thoroughly.

In places where the hygiene leaves something to be desired, the most dangerous foods are raw vegetables, salads, shellfish, cream, ice cream and underdone meat or fish.

Travellers' diarrhoea: It is impossible to say just how many travellers suffer from the short and usually self-limiting bouts of diarrhoea known simply as 'travellers' diarrhoea' – certainly a very large number. The symptoms consist of frequent passage of loose stools, abdominal cramps and colicky pains, persisting for anything from one to three days – there may also be nausea and vomiting. This syndrome is especially common in warm climates, where it may also lead to dehydration (*see* WATER).

Although travellers' diarrhoea has been studied extensively around the world, no uniform picture of how it is caused, and no clear policy of how it should be treated, has yet emerged. The micro-organisms thought to be responsible are usually non-pathogenic – that is, they do not normally cause disease. They may perhaps be different strains of the *E. coli* bacteria which normally inhabit the large intestine. It seems that travellers' diarrhoea may merely represent the body's response to a change in the balance of these bacteria within the intestines, following a change of diet and environment.

Travellers' diarrhoea rarely ever lasts more than three days. It never causes a fever, does not cause severe and persistent pain and is never associated with stools containing blood or mucus. Any severe bout of diarrhoea lasting longer than three days or associated with these symptoms should be taken seriously. Such symptoms are usually due to *dysentery*, an infection of the small or large intestine in which micro-organisms attack and damage the intestinal lining.

Minor diarrhoea can be treated with anti-diarrhoea tablets, which you should take with you on holiday, rather than rely on finding a local source of supply.

Homoeopathy

This is the name of the system of medicine which was established in Germany at the end of the 18th century by Dr Samuel Hahnemann. (It comes from two Greek words meaning 'similar to the disease'.) He based his theory on the principle that 'like is healed by like'. He reasoned that a very small dose of a drug could cure illness by stimulating the body's natural defence mechanisms against the illness. This is allied, in principle, to IMMUNIZATION in which a small dose of bacterial or viral substance is injected to promote the formation of antibodies – the elements in the body which defend it against further infection. Today, homoeopathy is practised by doctors who have completed extra studies in the subject after their regular training, and by some non-medically qualified people. In most Western countries there are long-established societies of homoeopaths.

The basis of homoeopathy

The theory of homoeopathy is based on the assumption that a healthy body has the resources to protect itself against illness, stress and all effects of the environment and to repair itself if it is temporarily overwhelmed. Ever since the time of the Greek physician Hippocrates, in the 5th century BC, some doctors have believed that the various functions of the body are controlled and maintained by a 'vital force' which exists independently of the cells, tissues and organs of the body.

In the last century, science and medicine have become increasingly materialistic, tending to discount anything which cannot be measured in a laboratory or discovered in a test tube. However, in recent years, research in physics and biology has demonstrated that there is no strict division between matter and energy. It takes energy to carry out all of the functions of life, and some of this energy forms solid structures, some provides the power for physical and chemical interactions, and some exists in the body as electricity.

Many scientists now believe that the 'vital force' is, in fact, a form of electromagnetic energy which organizes all the functions of life, and that as scientific equipment becomes more sensitive, we shall discover much more about it.

Homoeopathic practitioners believe that medicines gain effectiveness from an ability to influence and strengthen the patterns of electromagnetic energy which exist in and round the body. This, in turn, has a positive effect in reorganizing the response of electrical, chemical and physical processes and restoring health and vitality.

Purpose

Homoeopathy differs from orthodox medicine in that it doesn't regard a disease or an illness as a definable state which is exactly the same for any two people, since we all respond to the disorder in individual ways which are characteristic of physical type, personality, emotions and environmental circumstances. Therefore, there is no one homoeopathic medicine for influenza, for example, but rather a choice of remedies to suit the range of individual responses.

Homoeopathic prescribing is very precise: whether you have a tickle in your throat or not, dislike heat, enjoy sweet foods or cry easily will make a difference in the medicines you are given. Homoeopathic physicians claim to treat the whole person rather than the disease.

How homoeopathy works

Homoeopathic medicines are specially prepared from plant, animal and other biological sources. Each new remedy is arrived at by a process called 'proving', whereby healthy men and women volunteer to take the medicine to see what symptoms are produced, a process which is repeated several hundreds or thousands of times. The volunteers must describe in great detail all the symptoms produced by the substance. These are then collected in a book called a *Materia Medica*, which describes the symptoms associated with a particular remedy.

While he was testing his original remedies, Hahnemann made a remarkable discovery: the healing effect of a remedy *increases* if the amount of the substance present in the medicine is *decreased*. This discovery is incorporated in the preparation of doses of different strengths – a process called *potentizing*. It can be carried on almost indefinitely, and each successive potency contains less of the original substance. The most 'potent' dilutions used by homoeopaths can be shown to have no molecules left of the original substance. Yet the lactose powder or alcohol used for preparing the dilution retains the energy of the original substance in an enhanced and more potent form. This is very important, for many of the remedies would be poisonous if taken in large doses. Because there are no poisonous or toxic agents involved, there are no adverse side-effects. Consequently, homoeopathy – whether it is effective or not – is an intrinsically safe form of treatment.

Orthodox doctors do not accept that tiny doses of drugs can make any real difference to the health of the body or that they are sufficient to treat powerful diseases.

There are a number of other principles that guide the homoeopath. One important idea is that chronic disease may occur as a result of suppression of an acute one. Hahnemann pointed out, for example, that skin disease, if suppressed, may lead to some internal disease later on. In modern times it has been suggested by homoeopaths that using steroid preparations to suppress eczema may lead to a worsening of any accompanying asthma.

Homoeopaths also consider that signs and symptoms always progress in a particular direction: from within outwards, from above downwards, from important to less important organs, and in the reverse order to the way in which the disorder develops in the body.

A homoeopath always tries to choose a remedy that follows the 'natural' rules. So in the case of a child with ASTHMA and ECZEMA, he or she attempts to concentrate first on the asthma because it is internal and in a more important organ than the skin. Indeed, as the asthma is relieved, the eczema may worsen temporarily, only to improve later.

Types of homoeopathic remedies

Most homoeopathic remedies are based on natural salts and extracts of minerals or plants. Some remedies called 'nosodes' are based on extracts of diseased tissues or bacteria. Remedies can be prepared as tinctures, granules or powders.

A homoeopathic pharmacist begins the preparation of a remedy by obtaining the original substance in as pure a form as possible. If the substance can be dissolved, it may be prepared as a tincture. The chemist dissolves the substance in ten parts of pure 40 per cent alcohol. He then takes a tenth part of that solution and dilutes one part in ten parts of alcohol, shaking the mixture vigorously when the dilution is made – a process known as *succussion*. Further 1 in 10 dilutions are made until the required 'potency' is reached. A series of six 1 in 10 dilutions produces a '6D' or '6X' remedy. Often 1 in 100 dilutions are made, and then the remedies are referred to as 'C' potencies. A 6C remedy, which is a commonly used dilution for homoeopathic treatment, is diluted to 1 part in a billion.

Solids are diluted with pure lactose and sucrose powder, each successive dilution being made by grinding the powders together with a pestle and mortar. When the appropriate dilution has been made, the powder is made into pills or granules.

Illnesses that respond to homoeopathy

Undoubtedly many of the most successful cures described using homoeopathic remedies concern some of the illnesses that do not respond to traditional medicine. If viral infections such as INFLUENZA are treated early, resolution of the symptoms may be hastened. Chronic illness such as ARTHRITIS and chronic SKIN disease also seem to respond well. Physical problems that are associated with emotional or nervous symptoms, such as MIGRAINE or an IRRITABLE BOWEL, may also be helped.

Homoeopathic treatment

The homoeopathic doctor will want to take a detailed case history and will ask the patient questions which may, at first, seem unrelated to the illness. He will ask about reactions to the environment: to such things as heat and cold, whether sweet foods are preferred to savoury ones, and many other small details. He is trying to build up a composite image of the person as a whole, in characteristics and way of life. The object is to match symptoms and reactions to the effects created by the medicines in the *Materia Medica*, a reference book containing details of more than 2,000 different homoeopathic remedies.

In the course of the interview, or during subsequent treatment, the homoeopath may diagnose the 'constitutional remedy', one particular medicine to which the patient is particularly sensitive because it so well matches personality and physical type. A course of this remedy mobilizes various responses which improve general health and outlook. Many homoeopaths prescribe only one remedy at a time in order to assess the effect of each one in turn, although two or three remedies simultaneously is becoming more common. The potency of the medicine used will depend upon the age and health of the patient, how deep-seated the illness is, and whether it is acute or chronic. Usually, the dosage in acute cases is every half hour to hour until relief is obtained. In chronic illness it is not unusual for the homoeopath to choose a single remedy and to prescribe just one dose of a high-potency preparation.

Treatment is changed or suspended when there is improvement in the condition. However, it often happens that symptoms get worse for a short time before they get better; sometimes the symptoms of some previous illness may recur. Homoeopathic physicians claim that powerful modern drugs often suppress illness and drive the condition deeper into the system. As the defences are strengthened, old symptoms recur as the illness is eliminated. Although it may seem temporarily that the patient is getting worse, in fact, an overall improvement in health is taking place. After the first consultation, visits to the homoeopath are generally fortnightly or monthly and the time between them lengthens as improvements occur.

Homoeopathic preparations are dissolved on the tongue rather than swallowed whole, and stimulants such as cigarettes, coffee and alcohol should be avoided while taking the medicine, since they may diminish its effects. Homoeopathic medicines, at least in the lower potencies, are completely safe and no ill-effects will arise if the remedy chosen isn't quite right, but neither will there be an improvement. This makes many of the medicines suitable for use in a home first-aid kit. Many common afflictions, such as colds, sore throats and headaches can often be managed at home if care is taken to choose the right remedy. Tinctures can be used to make lotions and gargles for skin care and dental purposes. Homoeopathic chemists can supply a small kit at reasonable cost.

Homoeostasis

To remain healthy, our bodies must be regulated in a constant state of internal balance, under ever-changing conditions. The term used to describe this process is 'homoeostasis'. Many of the mechanisms involved in this interplay between ourselves and our environment can be thought of as separate and individual control systems, each with its own specific job to do, and which together form one overall system that is responsible for all our bodily functions.

Health and disease

The basic living unit of the body is the CELL and all our organs, muscles and bones are nothing but communities of cells, held together by supporting structures. Each type of cell is designed to perform some particular function, such as the red blood cells, which transport oxygen from the lungs to the rest of the body and carry carbon dioxide back to the lungs to be discharged. All the cells of the body are bathed in fluid which supplies their nourishment and carries away waste products. The characteristics of this 'extra-cellular' fluid must remain nearly constant to enable the cells to live and work properly. Homoeostasis is, therefore, a state of coordination which maintains the normal functions of the body until one or more of its systems gets out of balance. When this happens, all the cells of the body suffer, and disease or ill-health is the result.

A healthy body is able to resist disease and to repair and adapt itself to compensate for injury or stress, but in illness, this control is lost. Susceptibility to flu, for example, is largely determined in this way, which is why not everyone who is exposed to the illness will ultimately come down with it.

As we grow older, our capacity for adaptation lessens, increasing our liability to illness. Ageing can be seen as a narrowing of the range of circumstances with which the body can cope. Homoeostasis remains, but its effectiveness is reduced. A typical example is the older person who can no longer tolerate extremes of heat or cold in his or her environment. Similarly, the inability of the heart to adjust to sudden demands and emergencies can result in a HEART ATTACK, or homoeostatic breakdown.

Input/output

It is easy to imagine homoeostasis in engineering terms. All the control and regulating systems of the body act by a process of 'negative feedback', in which the 'output' of a given process is monitored by some other element. When the 'output' rises or falls beyond the desired limits, a part of it is diverted back to the source to act as a control.

A familiar domestic example is the thermostat which controls a central heating system. If the temperature of the room falls below the setting on the thermostat, an electrical circuit is completed which switches on the boiler and pump to circulate hot water through the system. When the desired temperature is reached the thermostat switches everything off again. However, unlike the central heating system, the body always has several different mechanisms available to perform similar tasks in different ways, thus providing 'fail-safe' back-up systems.

The regulators

There are several thousand control systems in the body which are coordinated to regulate virtually every function. The most vital regulators through the body are the NERVOUS SYSTEM and the ENDOCRINE (hormonal) SYSTEM. Because they are so closely interrelated, and each is necessary for the function of the other, they are sometimes referred to jointly as the 'neuro-endocrine system'.

Automatic regulation

The part of the nervous system primarily concerned in homoeostasis is known as the AUTONOMIC NERVOUS SYSTEM. This is involved with the 'automatic' regulation of the heart, lungs, stomach, intestines, bladder, sex organs and blood vessels.

The endocrine system consists of various GLANDS which release HORMONES into the bloodstream, so that they are carried to the necessary site of action. The hormonal system is much slower to react to a situation, but its effects last for some time, whereas the autonomic nervous system produces rapid responses, which are only sustained as long as necessary. Sometimes they work independently of each other, and often they work together, depending on the nature and severity of the problem. One example of homoeostasis which makes use of several possibilities is the regulation of BLOOD PRESSURE, which is a balance between the pressure output of the heart and the resistance offered by the arteries.

In the large carotid arteries of the neck, there are a number of specialized nerve cells, called *baroreceptors*, which react to pressure. If you were suddenly frightened, your heart would start beating faster, increasing your blood pressure. The baroreceptors sense this increased pressure and relay messages to the vasomotor centre in the brain stem, which immediately decreases the flow of nerve impulses to the arteries. The arterial walls thus relax and the blood pressure is lowered to keep it within its normal limits.

The buffer system

The baroreceptor cells are especially important for regulating blood pressure when you change the position of your body. If you have been kneeling or lying down for a time, and get up too quickly, dizziness or even a temporary blackout can occur. The sudden act of standing up causes gravity to reduce the blood pressure in the head and upper part of the body. The resulting lack of oxygen to the brain causes the dizziness. In this case, the baroreceptors sense the fall in blood pressure and immediately act to restore the balance – as a buffer system.

As well as the rapidly acting nervous control of blood pressure, there are at least three hormonal systems that also provide control by releasing hormones into the bloodstream. There is, besides, a slower-acting and more sustained control regulated by the KIDNEYS.

Numerous other vital functions such as BREATHING (respiration), body

TEMPERATURE and WATER balance are regulated in a similar way to blood pressure.

Hormone replacement therapy (HRT)

HORMONES given by mouth (or, in the case of insulin, by injection) are used to replace the body's normal hormones when one of the ENDOCRINE glands – the GLANDS responsible for secreting hormones – has stopped working properly. But there are glands whose secretions inevitably fail in all women, and these are the OVARIES. The decline and eventual cessation of oestrogen secretion by the ovaries or, to be more exact, the ovarian follicles, is responsible for the MENOPAUSE.

Oestrogen and the menopause

As the secretion of oestrogen by the ovaries fails – usually between the ages of 45 and 55 – there are a number of effects on the body, some of them obvious, others less so. First of all, the monthly PERIODS stop. Second, the well-known symptoms of 'hot flushes' and sweats may occur and be a disability.

In elderly women, falls tend to result in broken bones. This fragility seems to be related to the loss of oestrogen activity, but there are almost certainly other factors involved which have not yet been identified (*see* OSTEOPOROSIS).

The presence of oestrogen in the blood of women before the menopause seems to have the great advantage of protecting them from HEART ATTACKS which are, of course, a common cause of death in men in the same age range. This protection is lost after the menopause.

Without oestrogen, the skin of the VAGINA atrophies – that is, it becomes both dryer and thinner. The effect may be very uncomfortable and may cause older women to lose pleasure in their sex life.

Benefits of HRT

HRT unquestionably alleviates some of the symptoms of the menopause in women particularly troubled by them. It relieves hot flushes and helps to deal with vaginal atrophy, although this can also be done by the application of oestrogen-containing creams.

It is very difficult to determine whether or not HRT actually helps the psychological problems which may occur about the time of the menopause. However, there is a general impression that many women do find it helpful.

Post-menopausal osteoporosis is a major problem because FRACTURES, particularly of the HIP, can be dangerous in elderly women. There is evidence that HRT helps to reduce the severity of osteoporosis and therefore the number of fractures of the hip which result as a consequence.

Dangers

In the US, studies have suggested that there was an increased risk of cancer of the UTERUS with prolonged oestrogen therapy.

There are two major forms of this cancer. Cancer of the CERVIX (neck of the womb), which cervical smear tests aim to detect, tends to occur in younger women. Cancer of the main part of the womb is called cancer of the body of the uterus. It usually comes to light as a result of unexpected bleeding after the menopause, and its incidence was found to be increasing in patients taking HRT in the US. But these patients were taking quite high doses of oestrogen continuously and without proper checks. The risk of cancerous changes can be virtually eliminated by the use of lower doses of oestrogen combined with another hormone – progesterone – and leaving a week free of treatment after every three. This regime produces a 'withdrawal bleed' as the uterus sheds its lining, very much like a normal period. It is now generally accepted that oestrogen should always be combined with progesterone, although progesterone is often only given towards the end of each three-week course.

It seems reasonable to say that some women with troublesome menopausal symptoms should have them treated with cyclical oestrogen therapy for a year, during which time the problems will probably have diminished considerably. But the patient should not smoke, as the risk of complications involving THROMBOSIS (clotting of blood in arteries or veins) is increased when a woman takes oestrogen, either in the contraceptive pill or in HRT, and continues to smoke. Also, a doctor may advise against the treatment if there is a history of menstrual disorders, liver disease or a family history of cancer of the womb or breasts.

Hormones

These are the body's 'chemical messengers'. Unlike nerve impulses, which carry information round the body in the form of electrical charges, hormones are made and released in one part of the body, and are circulated (mainly in the blood) to other body cells – known as targets – where their effects are brought about. The organs largely responsible for making and releasing most of the body's hormones are the collection of ductless or ENDOCRINE glands, so-called because they discharge their products directly into the blood and not via a tube or duct. Those glands that do direct their secretions down a duct are called *exocrine* glands.

How hormones work

Compared with nerves, hormones tend to act more slowly and also to spin out their activity over a much longer time. Not all hormones act slowly, but many of those that do are involved in fundamental 'whole life' activities, such as growth and reproduction. In general, hormones tend to be concerned with controlling or influencing the chemistry of the target cells – for example, by determining the rate at which they use up food substances and release energy, or whether or not these cells should produce milk, hair or some other product of the body's METABOLIC processes.

Because they have the most widespread effects, the hormones made by the major endocrine GLANDS are known as general hormones; these include insulin (*see* DIABETES) and the sex hormones (*see* OVARIES and TESTES). The body makes many other hormones which act much nearer to their point of production.

One example of such a local hormone is *secretin*, which is made in the DUODENUM in response to the presence of food. The hormone then travels a short distance in the blood to the nearby PANCREAS and stimulates it to release a flood of watery juice containing ENZYMES (chemical transformers) essential to DIGESTION.

Other examples of local hormones, or transmitters, include the substance *acetylcholine*, which is made every time a nerve passes a message to a muscle cell, telling it to contract.

Proteins and steroid

All hormones are active in very small amounts. In some cases, less than a millionth of a gram is enough for a task to be carried out.

Chemically, hormones fall into two basic categories: those that are PROTEINS or protein derivatives; and those that have a ring, or STEROID structure. The sex hormones and the hormones made by the outer part or cortex of the ADRENAL GLAND are all steroid hormones.

Insulin is a protein and the thyroid hormones are manufactured from a protein base and are protein derivatives.

When each hormone reaches its target, it can only go to work if it finds itself in a correctly shaped site on the target cell membrane. Once it has become locked into this receptor site, the hormone does its work by stimulating the formation of a substance called *cyclic AMP* (adenosine monophosphate). The cyclic AMP is thought to work by activating a series of enzyme systems within the cell, so that particular reactions are stimulated and the required products are made.

The reaction of each target cell depends on its own chemistry. Thus, cyclic AMP produced by the presence of the hormone insulin triggers cells to take up and use glucose, while the hormone *glucagon*, also made by the pancreas, causes glucose to be released by cells and build up in the blood to be 'burned off' as energy-giving fuel for physical activity.

After they have done their work, the hormones are rendered inactive by the target cells themselves, or are carried to the LIVER for deactivation, then broken down and either excreted or used to make new hormone molecules.

Controlling the system

The whole system of hormone production and use in the body is very complex and is often likened to an orchestra whose 'conductor' is the PITUITARY gland. Lying at the base of the brain and connected to it by a short stalk, the pituitary gland is divided into two parts. The front portion, or anterior pituitary, secretes many hormones, which exert their influence by stimulating other endocrine glands to release their products. These are the *trophic*, or stimulating hormones, and include thyroid-stimulating hormone, which triggers the release of thyroid hormone, adrenocorticotrophic hormone, which stimulates the adrenal cortex to make *cortisol*, and follicle-stimulating hormone, which controls the release of hormones by the ovaries, and luteinizing hormone, which triggers the output of *testosterone* in a man and *progesterone* in a woman.

Other hormones made by the anterior pituitary exert their influence directly and include *growth hormone*, which acts on cells throughout the body to promote both growth in cell size and replacement. *Prolactin*, also produced by the anterior pituitary, stimulates milk and inhibits menstruation during breast-feeding.

The posterior part of the pituitary makes two important hormones – *anti-diuretic hormone* which travels to the KIDNEYS and helps to maintain a correct fluid balance within the body, and *oxytocin*, which triggers the 'let down' of milk from the breasts once a newborn baby starts to suckle. These posterior pituitary hormones are interesting in that their release is directly controlled by nerve impulses generated in the HYPOTHALAMUS, the part of the brain to which the pituitary is attached.

The only other hormones directly controlled by nerve impulses are *adrenalin* and *noradrenalin*, which are made and released by the inner medulla of the adrenal gland. It has been found, however, that there is an important, if less direct, link between the nerve cells of the hypothalamus and the secretions of the anterior part of the pituitary. What happens is that special nerve cells in the hypothalamus make so-called releasing factors, which must act on the cells of the anterior pituitary before they can send out their hormones.

Effects on emotions

The strong link between the brain and the pituitary goes a long way towards explaining why there is such a definite connection between the hormones and the emotions. Many women find, for example, that if they are anxious or upset, the timing of their PERIODS may be altered. And the levels of the same hormones – oestrogen and progesterone – that control the periods can also have profound effects on a woman's moods.

The sudden fall of hormone levels that happens just before menstruation is thought to play an important part in creating the symptoms of what has become known as PREMENSTRUAL SYNDROME, while the high hormone levels in mid-cycle are thought to give many women a sense of well-being. And it may not be an accident that this is the time at which women are both most fertile and most responsive sexually. But hormone levels can also be altered by emotional factors.

During sexual foreplay, for example, it is thought that levels of oestrogen and progesterone rise, as a direct result of pleasurable impulses on the brain, while the very thought of having sexual intercourse with someone who is physically repulsive is, quite literally, a 'turn off', because it inhibits the production of sex hormones.

At the end of her reproductive life – i.e. the time of the MENOPAUSE – a woman may experience great emotional ups and downs. This is partly because her ovaries stop responding to follicle-stimulating hormone, and so stop making oestrogen and progesterone. These changes of mood may also be due to psychological factors. But it is interesting to note that the sudden withdrawal of hormones from the system after a woman has given birth may have emotional effects similar to those of the menopause (*see* POST-NATAL DEPRESSION).

When we are under STRESS, our bodies prepare for 'fight or flight', a response that has evolved to help us cope with danger. Adrenalin is released by the adrenal glands, which increases the heart rate and sends more blood through the muscles, while less flows through the stomach and intestines. Extra cortisone is produced too. Psychological stress produces a similar response even when there is no physical danger. Panic attacks and abdominal discomfort can all be triggered by hormonal changes brought about by stress.

Hormones can be found in a huge range of preparations, from the CONTRACEPTIVE pill to the ointments used to treat ECZEMA. If your doctor recommends that these drugs can be useful to you, or a member of your family, it is important that he or she should point out the potential dangers to you; they must be used with care and, of course, exactly as prescribed.

Housemaid's knee, ***see*** **Bursitis**

HRT, ***see*** **Hormone replacement therapy**

Hunchback, ***see*** **Kyphosis**

Huntington's chorea, ***see*** **Genetics**

Hydramnios, ***see*** **Breech birth**

Hydrocephalus

This means, literally, 'water on the brain', and it refers to an excessive build-up of fluid in and around the BRAIN.

Cerebrospinal fluid is a clear, watery fluid that flows round the meninges, the membranes that cover the brain and SPINAL CORD, and through the brain's ventricles (cavities). The fluid has a cushioning effect and so helps to protect the vital brain tissue from injury.

The fluid is made continuously from the blood by specialized cells of the *choroid plexus* in the brain ventricles. Unlike the heart ventricles which have names, the brain ventricles have numbers. The numbering goes from the topmost to the bottom, and the first and second ventricles (known as the lateral ventricles) are the largest.

The fluid flows from the lateral ventricles through a narrow hole into the small third ventricle and then through an even narrower channel, the cerebral aqueduct, into the slightly wider fourth ventricle. From here it escapes through holes in the roof of the ventricle into the fluid-filled spaces (cisterns) which surround the brain stem at the base of the brain. Then the fluid flows up over the top of the brain (the cerebral hemispheres) and is reabsorbed by special outgrowths, called *arachnoid villi*, on the arachnoid membrane, one of three meninges covering the brain.

Hydrocephalus, which is a rare condition, occurs when something interferes with the circulation of the cerebrospinal fluid. The effect this has on children depends on whether the bones of the skull (*see* HEAD) have finally joined together before the pressure inside begins to rise.

In young children, whose skull bones have not joined together, the increased pressure forces the bones apart and the head increases in size. In older children and adults, the increased pressure cannot do this and the expanding fluid presses on the brain, causing progressive damage.

Causes

Various conditions can affect the circulation of cerebrospinal fluid. Some conditions are congenital (present at birth) though not necessarily inherited. But other causes may be acquired later in life.

Hydrocephalus is divided into obstructive hydrocephalus, where there is something which obstructs the circulation of the fluid, and communicating hydrocephalus where there is something wrong with the reabsorption of the fluid by the arachnoid membrane.

Obstructive hydrocephalus

This is the commoner type and it may occur in either adults or children for a variety of reasons.

An obstruction anywhere in the circulation of the cerebrospinal fluid means that the fluid will dam up behind the obstruction, gradually increasing the pressure in the brain and squeezing the delicate tissues inside the skull.

Children born with SPINA BIFIDA (a congenital defect of the spine) may also have an abnormality of the spinal cord in the neck or back (*meningomyelocoele*) and an abnormality of the structure of the lower brain stem and lower part of the cerebellum (area of brain in charge of balance and coordination). This is known as an *Arnold–Chiari malformation* and it has the effect of blocking off the exit hole at the bottom of the fourth ventricle, thus causing hydrocephalus.

In other congenital hydrocephalus cases, there may be obstruction, or failure, in the formation of the cerebral aqueduct, and this causes the third and lateral ventricles to swell up. If there is a collection of abnormal blood vessels or a swelling in one of the cerebral veins near the narrow cerebral aqueduct, these, too, may press on the channel and block it off.

Sometimes obstructive hydrocephalus is caused by an acquired condition, such as a TUMOUR growing within the brain pressing on the cerebral aqueduct or third ventricle enough to block the outflow of cerebrospinal fluid. Small tumours or benign CYSTS can cause hydrocephalus if they are in particular places and block aqueducts or exit holes.

Symptoms in children

The most noticeable change that occurs in children is an increase in head size. The bones of the skull normally join between the ages of six and ten years, so head expansion with hydrocephalus mainly occurs in younger children.

Children's heads vary enormously in size, and if a child's head is large, this doesn't necessarily mean that he or she has hydrocephalus. If hydrocephalus is the cause, the growth of the head size will be much faster and the shape of the skull quite distinctive, the forehead being prominent and the face being conspicuously small in relation to the rest of the head. Also, the eyes are pushed down so that a so-called 'setting-sun' face is seen with the whites of the eyes visible above the coloured irises.

If the condition is not treated, it can lead to double vision or even blindness. If the hydrocephalus is rapidly developing it may cause mental deterioration, paralysis and stiffness of limbs.

Diagnosis

Diagnosis is made using a CT scan (*see* NEUROLOGY) which is a form of X-RAY scan linked to a computer which enables the fluid-filled cavities of the brain to be clearly seen.

The scan will show up small tumours and cysts so the cause of the hydrocephalus may also be obvious. Further special X-ray investigations of the neck may be necessary if there are congenital abnormalities, such as the Arnold–Chiari malformation.

Occasionally special studies are done – using the CT scan and injected marker dyes – of the pattern of flow of the cerebrospinal fluid; these studies show those cases where the hydrocephalus is due to defective absorption of the fluid by the arachnoid membranes.

Treatment and outlook

In most types of hydrocephalus, surgical treatment is necessary. The ventricles can be drained by the insertion of a tube between the ventricles and the spaces at the base of the brain if there is an obstruction in the fourth ventricle or a narrowing of the aqueduct.

In other types of hydrocephalus – including most of the congenital sorts and normal pressure hydrocephalus – the cerobrospinal fluid is shunted from the ventricles to the bloodstream or the peritoneal cavity in the abdomen. A valve is necessary to prevent the flow going the wrong way. Common types are the Spitz–Holter, Pudenze and Heyer–Schulte valves.

A small hole is made in the skull and a tube is inserted which runs from the ventricles to either the right atrium of the heart or the abdomen. These 'shunts', as they are called, often have to stay in place for the rest of the patient's life.

The outcome of hydrocephalus after treatment varies considerably and is mainly dependent on what caused the hydrocephalus in the first place, whether damage to the brain occurred before the hydrocephalus was discovered, and whether there were any other congenital abnormalities. A child with a shunt in place has a good chance of developing normally in terms of mental ability if there has been no other brain damage. Children who have been treated for hydrocephalus have gone to university and have held down good jobs just like other people.

Hydrocoele, *see* **Cysts, Testes**

Hydrophobia, *see* **Rabies**

Hydrops foetalis, *see* **Rhesus factor**

Hydrosalpinx, *see* **Salpingitis**

Hypercholesterolaemia, familial, *see* **Arteries and artery disease**

Hyperhidrosis, *see* **Perspiration**

Hyperkalaemic paralysis, *see* **Muscles**

Hyperkeratosis, *see* **Corns and calluses**

Hyperparathyroidism, *see* **Bone and bone diseases**

Hypersensitivity, *see* **Allergy**

Hypertension, *see* **Blood pressure**

Hypochondria

People who suffer from an exaggerated concern about their health are described as hypochondriacs. A key factor in hypochondria is a family background in which the need to take care of one's health was overstressed. Early exposure to chronic illness in one or both parents or grandparents or deaths of near relatives can also have a profound effect on a developing child, who might grow up with a fear of illness or death. Excessive interest in keeping fit may be another subtle factor, for although it may be very important to EXERCISE regularly, there is a limit to the amount of time that needs to be taken up this way.

Anxiety and depression

There are a number of psychiatric disorders which are commonly found to be associated with hypochondria. The first is an anxiety state: the unpleasant apprehension that something awful has happened or is about to (*see* MENTAL ILLNESS). This is accompanied by a number of changes in the body's functions (*see* STRESS): increased heart and breathing rate and excessive sweating, especially of the palms of the hands and under the arms. Appetite may be lost or, in some people, it may increase dramatically. Either diarrhoea or constipation may occur. Sleep may be disturbed, dizzy feelings may be experienced and fainting might happen. In women, there may be changes in periods which can become infrequent or irregular. Hypochondriacs focus on any of these anxiety-produced symptoms, which are thought to be caused by any disease or condition that may be feared, such as CANCER or HEART DISEASE.

DEPRESSIVE states are a second contributing factor. Usually these arise following some unhappy event such as a serious illness in the sufferer or a loved one, or possibly a breakdown of an important relationship. Occasionally there may be some long-standing emotional conflict which has not been resolved, but which continues to smoulder deep in the mind. Again, bodily functions may be disturbed, usually slowed down in some way, and so lead to further feelings of depression or anxiety. In severe depressive states, delusional thoughts may develop, so that the person's fear of cancer becomes a belief that he or she actually has cancer.

Obsessions and hysteria

Obsessional states occur either through family environment, or the tendency may be inherited through genes. Persistent thoughts arise that something has gone wrong in our bodies, and we tend to ruminate over it. Often repetitive moments or habits develop: these are sometimes described as rituals, and may be related to numbers, such as touching the doorknob six times before turning it. Alternatively patients may become obsessed that they have a particular disease which may be related to deep guilt feelings related to past events.

The mental make-up of hysterical states may be inherited, which can become obvious when under stress. There is an exaggeration of ordinary bodily feelings, or symptoms of simple ailments. There may be a strong feeling that everything is out of control, so that the person develops an intense fear that his health or even life is threatened.

Psychotic disorders

Illnesses such as SCHIZOPHRENIA and MANIC DEPRESSION are well-known psychotic disorders in which hypochondria can appear. Symptoms may be bizarre or grotesque: the patient may imagine that his or her body is 'crawling with insects', 'filled with mould', 'shrinking' or 'swelling up'. Increasing interest in the body's functions may lead to severe introspection, even complete withdrawal from all outside activities.

Finally, some accident victims may develop a persistent belief that their injuries have left them with some permanent disability or handicap, even though their recovery has been complete. This is more common with patients with some pre-existing psychiatric illness.

Symptoms

There is a tendency to have many different symptoms, sometimes one after another, or even all at the same time. Alternatively, there may be one continuous single symptom which is the sole centre of attention. Usually the description is so graphic that a diagnosis of hypochondria is likely, particularly with complaints about the body's functions.

There can be difficulty in separating off symptoms that may be due to some other serious physical illness which is hidden by the marked anxiety about the symptoms complained of. A full examination must be made, and doctors must be continually on their guard in case the patient does actually develop a real illness.

Treatment

Simple reassurance by the doctor might help in the early stages, but it is generally only the doctor who feels reassured by negative clinical findings. Hypochondriacs are often unable to accept such findings and reassurance, and they remain convinced that they have some dreaded disease and that the doctor is not telling them the truth. The use of TRANQUILLIZERS and antidepressant tablets are usually of no real help.

In hypochondria, as in all illnesses, it is the cause and not the symptoms which must be treated. The family doctor is probably in the best position to help the patient, but it may be necessary to call in specialist help. A psychiatrist (*see* PSYCHIATRY) or psychotherapist (*see* MENTAL THERAPIES) could help reveal and deal with the underlying psychological or emotional disturbance.

Occasionally, however, severe hypochondria has to be accepted as a state of mind that has to be endured by the patients, by his or her relatives and friends and by the doctor. Fortunately, the passage of time often brings about changes in the patient's life situation, which reduce the intensity of hypochondriacal feelings and this brings relief.

Hypoglycaemia, *see* Carbohydrates, Diabetes, Unconsciousness

Hypokalaemic paralysis, *see* Muscles

Hypospadias, *see* Plastic surgery, Urethra

Hypotension, *see* Blood pressure

Hypothalamus

This lies at the base of the BRAIN, under the two cerebral hemispheres. It is immediately below another important structure in the NERVOUS SYSTEM, the *thalamus,* which acts as a 'telephone exchange' between the SPINAL CORD and the cerebral hemispheres.

The hypothalamus is actually a collection of specialized nerve centres, which connect up with other important areas of the brain, as well as the PITUITARY gland. This is the region of the brain concerned with the control of such vital functions as eating and sleeping. It is also closely linked with the endocrine (HORMONE) system.

How it exerts control

The hypothalamus has nervous pathways which connect with the *limbic system,* which is closely connected with the smell centres of the brain. This portion of the brain also deals with memory, and abnormalities here may cause the memory to be lost.

A vital function of the hypothalamus is temperature control (*see* FEVER). Fevers are caused by substances which act directly on the hypothalamus. In case of serious HEAD INJURY, when the hypothalamus is affected, high temperatures of over 105°F (40.5°C) may result for long periods.

Another connection is with the *reticular activating* pathways, which run up and down the central core of the brain and spinal cord. The reticular activating formation is concerned with SLEEP and waking and the condition that is called *narcolepsy* – when sudden sleep from which the person cannot be roused may occur at any time – is usually due to disease of the hypothalamus.

As if this were not enough, the hypothalamus is also the controlling centre for both appetite and THIRST. The two are controlled separately. Although problems in this area are rare, one of the commoner is gross obesity, due to massive overeating, which is usually associated with excessive sleeping. It is called the 'Pickwickian syndrome' after Dickens' fictional character.

The control of thirst and WATER balance is handled separately. The hormone which deals with loss of water from the kidney is called *antidiuretic hormone* (ADH). This is secreted from the posterior (back) part of the pituitary gland. This part is actually separate from the anterior (front) part of the gland, and is connected to the hypothalamus by the pituitary stalk. The 'receptors', which measure the concentration of the blood (and therefore help the hypothalamus decide how it should be organizing the body's water balance) are found in the hypothalamus itself. Disorders may result from abnormal retention of water by the kidney (excessive ADH activity) or from a loss of ADH secretion (this is called *diabetes insipidus*). This condition may result from head injuries, where the pituitary stalk has been damaged.

There is no doubt, too, that the hypothalamus is concerned with the control of behaviour and emotion. Withdrawn and confused behaviour with some aggressive outbursts may happen in cases of disease. Sexual over-activity may occur.

Links with hormones

Apart from its role in the nervous system, the hypothalamus is an integral part of the ENDOCRINE SYSTEM. The hormone ADH is actually formed in the hypothalamus and then passes down the specialized nerve cells of the pituitary stalk to be released from the posterior part of the pituitary gland.

However, the anterior part of the gland is anatomically separate and most of the important interactions occur between the hypothalamus and the anterior pituitary. It is really a little endocrine system of its own. Hormones – called *inhibitory or releasing factors* – are produced in the hypothalamus and carried to the pituitary in blood vessels which flow down the pituitary stalk.

The hormone TSH (*thyroid-stimulating hormone*) or *thyrotrophin*, which is produced by the pituitary stimulates the THYROID to release thyroid hormone. In turn, the production of TSH is stimulated by the *thyrotrophin-releasing hormone* (TRH) from the hypothalamus.

Similar systems exist to stimulate the release of *corticotrophin*, which controls ADRENAL activity, and FSH (*follicle-stimulating hormone*) and LH (*luteinizing hormone*), which stimulates the OVARIES or TESTES.

The anterior pituitary also produces two hormones which act directly upon the tissues. *Growth hormone* is one of these. It is essential for normal growth and is also involved in the control of blood sugar. Growth hormone seems to be controlled by two factors, one of which stimulates release, while the other inhibits it.

In contrast, the hormone *prolactin* – which stimulates lactation (the production of breastmilk) and inhibits menstruation – seems to be largely controlled by a substance called *prolactin inhibiting factor*, which restrains rather than stimulates secretion.

All these releasing and inhibiting factors are rather simple chemicals and the formulae for many of them have been worked out. Today, they can be made and used, not only to test pituitary function but occasionally for treating patients.

One of the most fascinating developments in this field has been the realization that some of these compounds, particularly TRH and *somatostatin* – the factor which inhibits growth hormone release – are actually widespread in the nervous system, acting as transmitters.

Disease of the hypothalamus is rare. TUMOURS may occur in that area, and infection of the nervous system in the form of encephalitis or MENINGITIS may also affect the function of the hypothalamus. Similarly, head injury or surgery may cause problems, which are difficult to treat. It is possible that some of the small, benign hormone-producing tumours which are known to occur in the pituitary actually result from overstimulation by the hypothalamus.

Hypothermia

The medical definition of hypothermia depends upon what is considered to be our normal body temperature. This is around 98.4°F (37°C), which is the temperature of the heart at the centre of the body, but the temperature of the skin or in the mouth can fall very much lower than this. Therefore, in the case of a subnormal temperature – that is, *hypothermia* – the routine method of measurement is very inaccurate. So doctors have to measure the temperature in the RECTUM. If this is below 95°F (35°C), the person is considered to have hypothermia.

What happens in the body

When the body loses heat, its automatic reaction is to try to generate more by shivering. At this stage, the person just feels uncomfortable and miserable, but as he or she gets colder, lethargy and drowsiness increase. Soon, all shivering stops. When this cooling-down process happens slowly, victims are less likely to shiver than when the cooling is rapid. But, whatever happens, their condition is potentially serious.

If cooling continues, mental confusion follows, then an overpowering desire to sleep and, finally coma. This usually happens when the body temperature approaches 89.6°F (32°C). When the temperature drops to around 86°F (30°C), the HYPOTHALAMUS (the organ situated below the brain) loses its temperature-regulating ability, cell activity and breathing rate slow, and the oxygen supply to the cells diminishes. The normal heartbeat is replaced by a condition called VENTRICULAR FIBRILLATION, when the heart muscles ripple, but do not pump blood.

The temperature at which ventricular fibrillation occurs is critical, because this marks the time when blood circulation stops, and unless something is done, the victim dies. Infants and children develop ventricular fibrillation at much lower temperatures than adults, sometimes as low as 69.8°F (21°C).

People at risk

There are two groups of people most at risk: those who are unable to defend themselves against heat loss with the normal protective reflexes of the body, and those who are exposed to a hostile environment.

Old people living alone sometimes find it difficult to look after themselves. During cold snaps, it is not unusual for them to sit in a chair and hope to keep warm because they are indoors, rather than to get up and switch on a fire; they may simply lack the will or motivation to do this, or, in some tragic cases, they may not be able to afford the cost of fuel. Their inactive state also prevents the body from shivering.

Very small babies are also at risk. Their bodies do not have a mature temperature-regulating mechanism, so they cannot shiver, and they have a large surface of skin in proportion to their body volume, and so their bodies act as very good radiators of heat.

The body's normal protective mechanism includes shivering and constriction of the blood vessels running to the skin, so that radiation of heat from the body is stopped. This constriction of blood vessels takes place over the entire surface of the body, with the exception of the head. The blood vessels running to the face and scalp cannot be constricted in response to cold, so however cold the victim, heat loss will continue from the head. When vigorous movement is not possible, because the victim is either very old or very young, shivering does not occur. As a result, heat loss is more rapid than normal. Matters are made worse when the victim is deeply unconscious.

This rapid heat loss also happens to people who are intoxicated with ALCOHOL or drugs, particularly barbiturates.

Exposure to the elements is another way in which people may develop hypothermia. This includes climbers and walkers, and divers in cold waters.

In divers, the rate at which heat is conducted away from the body by water is over 100 times greater than that of air of the same temperature. This heat loss is greatly increased if the wind is blowing, or if the water is rough. When boats capsize, death often results not from drowning but from exposure.

Treatment

If the patient is awake, with a temperature of greater than 32°C, rewarming can be achieved by placing the patient in a warm room, wrapping him or her in space blankets and giving warm fluids by mouth. This type of treatment is used for the patient who becomes hypothermic rapidly, as a result, for example, of exposure to the elements.

In old, frail or unconscious victims with severe hypothermia, warming should take place gradually, aiming at a rise of 1°C per hour and insulation with a space blanket and then warm woollen blankets is preferable. (A space blanket is made of heat-reflecting aluminium foil.) The patient is then left in a room which has a temperature of 95°F (35°C). It may take many hours, or even days for the rewarming process to be complete.

Hot food or drinks, although comforting, contribute very little and, in seriously ill patients, are better avoided because of the risk of them vomiting. Alcohol should never be given. It can contribute to heat loss by dilating (widening) the blood vessels too quickly.

Hysterectomy

This operation may be very advisable because of a serious TUMOUR in the UTERUS (womb) or associated tissues, or it may be suggested as a treatment for symptoms which are not always due to serious disease, such as heavy periods. In these cases, only the woman concerned knows how incapacitated she is by her symptoms and so she must decide.

The operation is becoming less common in Britain because many of the conditions for which it used to be performed are being treated in other ways: for example, abnormal bleeding from an otherwise healthy womb can often be successfully treated with HORMONE tablets, and CANCER of the CERVIX may be treated by RADIOTHERAPY.

Hysterectomy is, if possible, avoided in women who have not completed their families. Because of this and of the higher incidence of disease of the womb later in life, the operation is most commonly performed on women between the ages of 45 and 55.

During a woman's reproductive years the lining of the womb is shed at regular intervals and so she has a period. When she becomes pregnant, the foetus grows in the womb, so removal of this organ will put a stop to periods or pregnancies.

Reasons for hysterectomy

Dysfunctional uterine bleeding (DUB) is by far the most common reason why women require hysterectomies. DUB is a broad term covering abnormally heavy and/or frequent periods which do not seem to be caused by any identifiable condition, such as fibroids. Hormone imbalance is often to blame, for if a woman's ovaries are secreting too much oestrogen, the uterine lining (endometrium) thickens, resulting in lengthy and heavy bleeding which is often delayed.

A lack of progesterone also causes frequent menstruation – again, for longer than average – because the endometrium is too thin and expelled too soon. Before advising a hysterectomy, a course of synthetic hormones would be prescribed. Only if this approach fails will hysterectomy be advised.

Fibroids are estimated to affect about 25 per cent of women, and are another common reason for having a hysterectomy. They are non-cancerous bundles of fibrous tissue which may grow within the muscle of the womb, varying in size from a pea to a football. *Subserous* fibroids grow just beneath the skin on the outside of the uterus. Large ones may press against the bladder or bowel, causing pain. *Submucous* fibroids form beneath the endometrium, stretching the uterus and causing heavy, debilitating periods – and, because of excessive blood loss, sometimes ANAEMIA becomes an additional problem. The third type, *intramural* fibroids, grow inside the uterine wall and often go unnoticed unless their size causes the lower abdomen to swell out, creating a 'pot belly'.

Endometriosis and adenomyosis are both conditions affecting the endometrium. Normally, this lining is shed every month as a period. Endometriosis occurs when the cells which form the lining begin to appear elsewhere in the pelvic cavity. Tissue can grow outside the uterus, on the ovaries or Fallopian tubes, or even on the bladder or intestines.

Since these cells are programmed to grow in response to hormone levels, they continue to behave like this wherever they are. So when hormone levels drop, they automatically begin to break down and bleed – just as they do in the womb. But because they are misplaced, the blood has nowhere to go, and so can cause swelling, cysts, inflammation and pain. Adenomyosis is another kind of endometriosis which happens when, for some as yet undiscovered reason, the tissue invades the wall of the womb – causing painful expansion during menstruation, plus heavy blood loss.

Pelvic inflammatory disease (PID) affects many women at some time, and can usually be successfully treated with antibiotics. Infection may follow ABORTION, CHILDBIRTH or the use of an IUD (intrauterine contraceptive device.) SEXUALLY TRANSMITTED DISEASE or infections of other pelvic organs can also spread throughout the pelvis, especially if the disease has gone untreated for some time.

When PID is chronic – that is, long-term – and the patient is at risk, a hysterectomy may be the only final way to destroy the infection completely. However, antibiotics will certainly be tried for as long as two years before this option is taken. As a result, PID remains the least likely reason for hysterectomy.

Cancer of the cervix, uterus, or ovaries usually requires a hysterectomy – unless it is detected early enough when the cells are precancerous, and noninvasive. Cervical cancer is the most common form of gynaecological cancer, and through regular smear tests can be caught before it has developed and spread. Hysterectomy is then unnecessary, because the abnormal tissue can simply be removed from the cervix with laser or other treatment. Healthy tissue then grows back over the scarred area, and the problem may never recur. However, once cancer cells have invaded the body of the uterus, they are liable to spread, so they must be removed to prevent this happening.

See also PROLAPSE.

Different types of hysterectomy

There are four types of hysterectomy, which may be performed in one of two ways – depending upon which operation is appropriate. The four kinds are:

- **A subtotal, or partial, hysterectomy** – rarely performed nowadays because it leaves the cervix (neck of the womb) intact. Sometimes it is too difficult to remove the neck of the womb, which is attached to the bladder, because of extensive scar tissue from a condition such as ENDOMETRIOSIS. So to avoid damaging the bladder and bowel, or putting the patient at risk, a subtotal hysterectomy may be chosen.

  Because the cervix is a possible site for cancer, a woman who has had a subtotal hysterectomy still needs regular smear tests – and may continue to have very light periods.
- **A total hysterectomy** removes the uterus and cervix, but the ovaries and Fallopian tubes remain as functioning organs in the body. Oestrogen production and ovulation can, therefore, continue as before – although there will be no accompanying monthly period. When a hysterectomy is performed before a woman reaches the MENOPAUSE, the surgeon usually tries to leave one or both ovaries in place.
- **A total abdominal hysterectomy and bilateral salpingo-oophorectomy**, or TAH and BSO, removes the uterus, cervix, ovaries and Fallopian tubes, and is usually performed after the menopause – simply because a woman has no more use for her ovaries and tubes, and they may cause problems at a later date. It is also necessary if a serious condition has affected these organs, such as cancer, pelvic inflammatory disease, large FIBROIDS or extensive endometriosis.
- **A radical hysterectomy, or Wertheim's hysterectomy**, is an extensive operation which removes the pelvic lymph nodes and ligaments, two thirds of the upper part of the VAGINA, plus the uterus and cervix. It is performed when there is invasive cancer which could spread to these areas – but again, if the ovaries themselves are not affected, they may be left in women of menstruating age.

When the ovaries are removed before the natural menopause, menopausal symptoms often occur. These include: hot flushes; palpitations; formication (a kind of itching named after the Latin word for 'ants' which feels as if ants were crawling beneath the skin); and calcium loss in the bones (*see* OSTEOPOROSIS). In addition to these physical symptoms, there may be emotional problems such as depression, insomnia, forgetfulness and the onset of PHOBIAS. HORMONE REPLACEMENT THERAPY (HRT) may be given to counteract any menopausal symptoms that may occur. If HRT is inappropriate, because of the risk of deep-vein THROMBOSIS or pulmonary embolism (blood clot in the lung), other drugs will be prescribed – although nothing else is quite so effective.

Surgical procedure

The two possible routes a surgeon can choose when performing a hysterectomy are through the vagina, or through an incision in the lower abdominal wall. Abdominal hysterectomy gives the surgeon a view of all the pelvic organs and he or she can therefore check that they are healthy. If the APPENDIX looks unhealthy, it can be removed during a hysterectomy, freeing the patient from the need for an appendicectomy at a later date.

Two kinds of incision can be used. A vertical incision extends from the pubic bone towards the navel, and is used where the womb has become very enlarged by fibroids, or where a large ovarian CYST is present. It also allows the surgeon more room for manoeuvre than the other, more cosmetically acceptable, horizontal incision – popularly known as a 'bikini cut'. An incision of this kind curves across the abdomen just below the pubic hairline, ending beneath the hipbone on each side. Once healed, it is invisible under a bikini – hence its name.

One advantage of having a hysterectomy vaginally is that there are no visible scars afterwards – but it is difficult to perform unless the uterus has already dropped down, or prolapsed. The womb is normally supported in the abdominal cavity by a floor of muscle and ligaments which are attached to the region between the neck and body of the womb. These ligaments can become loose with age or child-bearing, and the womb tends to fall into the vagina. Sometimes this condition causes discomfort, and at other times, it also affects the bowel and bladder which push in on the vaginal walls – already weakened by the pressure of the prolapsed womb.

To perform a vaginal hysterectomy, the patient's position is the same as for an internal examination. An incision is then made close to the cervix at the top of the vagina, extending up through the uterus so that the ligaments which attach it to other pelvic structures may be cut away. The uterus and cervix are then removed through the vagina, and all incisions stitched back together closing the vagina at the top. A careful examination of the uterus takes place after either type of procedure, in order to check that there is nothing unexpected, or previously undiagnosed. It is then given to a pathologist for detailed laboratory analysis.

Although post-operative healing tends to be rapid (6 to 12 weeks), there is a 50 per cent higher risk of infection after a vaginal hysterectomy, plus technical difficulties during the operation itself. For these reasons, abdominal hysterectomy remains the more usual choice.

Hysteria, *see* Mental illness, Psychiatry

I

Ileostomy, *see* Colon and colitis, Stoma care

Ileum

This is the lower part of the small INTESTINE, and is the part which the food reaches last on its way from the STOMACH to the COLON, or large bowel. It is a 12 ft (3.5 m) long tube – leading on from the DUODENUM and the JEJUNUM and connecting with the large bowel – and accounts for just over half the total length of the small intestine.

The outer surface is protected by the PERITONEUM – the membrane which lines the abdominal cavity. Its interior consists mainly of muscular layers, responsible for moving the digested food along the intestines, layers of mucosa and, finally, an inner lining of cells which borders on the central cavity, or lumen.

It is the main purpose of the ileum to absorb food, and to do this efficiently, it requires a large surface in contact with the digested products in the lumen. This is brought about by the way in which the inner lining of epithelial cells is gathered into finger-like projections called *villi.* Each villus has an artery, a vein and a lymph vessel. The surface available for absorption is increased further still, because the cellular surface of the villus is also corrugated into what is known as the 'brush border'.

Food substances in the lumen pass through an epithelial cell, or in the case of fats, through the lymph vessel, and travel to the liver via the bloodstream.

Ileus

The most common problem of the ileum occurs when the lining of the abdominal cavity – the peritoneum – becomes disturbed or inflamed and the ileum, together with the rest of the intestines, stops working. This condition is known as *paralytic ileus* or simply 'ileus'. The muscular tube of the intestines becomes distended with stagnating food residue, secretions containing digesting ENZYMES, BILE, water and salts, and swallowed air.

Some degree of paralytic ileus occurs after every surgical operation on the abdomen where the peritoneum is opened, but the bowel usually returns to normal activity within 48 hours. However, if surgery is complicated by inflammation of the peritoneum from a burst peptic ULCER or APPENDIX, this causes the intestines to stop moving as if in an effort to prevent the spread of infection or toxic secretions inside the abdominal cavity.

Sometimes ileus is caused when the body chemistry of finely balanced chemicals, such as POTASSIUM, is upset by problems like DIABETIC coma and

KIDNEY failure. Lastly, the drugs used to prevent colic or intestinal spasms slow down *peristalsis* – the muscular contractions that move digested food through the intestines – and, if large doses are given, the ileum may stop working.

The distension of the intestines causes abdominal swelling, and although this is not necessarily painful, it may cause a lot of discomfort. As the intestinal contents are not moving, there are no bowel actions at all. The patient may also vomit fluids that have collected in the stomach.

If the cause of the ileus is recognized quickly and is successfully treated, the bowel action will soon return to normal. But, in the meantime, the ileus itself has to be treated. The body loses large amounts of fluids, body salts and protein into the gut lumen and in vomit. Distension of the gut by gases causes thinning and weakening of the intestinal wall, and the blood supply of the bowel is reduced.

Treatment consists of replacing lost fluid by means of an intravenous drip, and also sucking out the fluid and gaseous stomach contents to reduce bowel distension. A tube is passed, through the nose, down into the stomach, and is left there until the ileus clears up and the intestines start to work properly.

Other disorders

The ileum can be affected by other disorders, such as a protrusion of the gut through a weakness in the abdominal wall (a HERNIA), or having its blood supply interrupted due to ARTERY disease elsewhere. Fortunately, however, ileal disease is fairly uncommon.

From the surgeon's point of view, the two most important forms of ileal disease are *Meckel's diverticulum* and *intussusception*. A Meckel's diverticulum is a pouch, situated towards the end of the ileum, which is an abnormality of development which occurs while the child is in the womb. If left untreated, it may rupture like an appendix. Intussusception is a curious process where the ileum engulfs itself rather like a tuck in a sleeve. This condition affects children and babies rather than adults.

Immune system

This protects us from INFECTION and invasion by all sorts of BACTERIA, VIRUSES and other microbes. *Globulin*, made and released into the blood by plasma cells, circulates to attack all invaders, and specialized white cells (*see* BLOOD), *lymphocytes* on the attack, patrol the body and neutralize or engulf foreign material. Circulating globulins – *immunoglobulins* – are made by B cells in the BONE MARROW; white cells – called T cells – are manufactured by LYMPH nodes and, in our early life, are under the control of the THYMUS gland.

How immunity works

Immunity by B cells: The structure of a globulin molecule consists of two long chains of amino acids placed side by side and known as heavy chains because of their great size. On each cell of these chains and at one end of them are two small strings of amino acids known as light chains. Both heavy and light chains are manufactured separately and put together before the globulin leaves the plasma cell to join the blood.

Globulins differ in the sequence of amino acids at one end of the light chains and, according to these differences, can be divided into five groups: IgA, IgG, IgD, IgE and IgM (the Ig stands for 'immune globulin'). They are also known as *antibodies*.

IgA, the most important defence against bacteria and viruses in the blood, is made by plasma cells lining the intestine and the lungs and stops the entry of bacteria. IgE, which is responsible for ALLERGY, may be found attached to cells in the lung and elsewhere. What IgD does is not yet known, but IgM is known to be involved in the development of some auto-immune diseases.

Immunity by T cells: These cells attack viruses and foreign tissue (they are responsible for the REJECTION of transplanted organs, for example). They are made in the lymph nodes of the body, and when we are very young, they are under the influence of the thymus gland. If this gland is absent at birth, as it is in certain rare inherited diseases, the T cells do not work, and the patient usually dies before the age of about six months from a viral infection which the body, with no natural defences, cannot combat.

T cells destroy invaders of all types, and helper cells assist both them and the plasma cells. When they detect a foreign invader, they return to the lymph nodes and pass the message to developing lymphocytes. Like B cells, the T cells 'remember' the nature of an invader.

How immunoglobulins work

Plasma cells lining the lung and intestine make IgA antibody which is responsible for dealing with COLD viruses, INFLUENZA and the bacteria causing PNEUMONIA. It is also responsible for killing viruses that get into the intestine – for example, the ones that cause POLIO.

IgE antibody is responsible for ECZEMA, HAY FEVER and ASTHMA. IgE on the surface of 'mast cells' binds with antigens (e.g. pollens) to release substances such as histamines, so causing an allergic reaction.

What can go wrong?

Immunity depends on the ability of B and T cells to recognize an invading bacterium or virus. If they don't, they will not go into action against it. Once they remember an invader, they attack and repel it, sometimes with the help of vaccine injections (*see* IMMUNIZATION).

There is no immunity to the common cold because the cold virus keeps changing its appearance and so the body's immune system cannot recognize it.

There are a number of very rare INHERITED diseases, usually caused by abnormalities in the chromosomes (*see* CELLS AND CHROMOSOMES) that result in a deficiency in production of globulin antibodies or of T lymphocytes or both. In certain instances, one particular class of globulin is missing: for instance, the IgG antibody is the absent antibody in a disease called *agammaglobulinaemia*.

It is possible to survive severe deficiency of immunoglobulins because effective globulin from other people can be given to the person who needs it by injection, approximately every month. However, a complete deficiency of white cells is more difficult to treat and sufferers usually die young.

See also AIDS.

Immunization

The body's own immunity to certain forms of INFECTION is a very important protection against disease (*see* IMMUNE SYSTEM). This immunity may be acquired naturally through exposure to infection, or be provided through immunization, sometimes also termed *vaccination*.

Infections are caused by many different kinds of minute organisms, which can enter the body through many different routes. Some infections may be passed on through contaminated food or water, for example; through droplets in the air we breathe: through breaks in the skin, particularly wounds which are not cleaned and properly treated; through direct contact such as kissing or sexual intercourse; or as a result of animal or insect bites.

A large number of infectious diseases are transmitted by invisible micro-organisms known as VIRUSES. Infections caused by viruses – such as COLDS, INFLUENZA, CHICKENPOX, MUMPS and MEASLES – do not respond to treatment with ANTIBIOTICS. Patients may, however, need nursing care as the illness runs its course. Immunization offers protection against some infections caused by viruses.

Certain other infections, such as DIPHTHERIA, TUBERCULOSIS and TYPHOID, are caused by organisms known as BACTERIA. These do respond to the use of antibiotics, which in some cases can be lifesaving. However, with serious infections, such as those cited, prevention through immunization is a far more satisfactory procedure. Moreover, care is needed in administering antibiotics, because their too frequent use can result in some germs developing a resistance to treatment.

The body itself deals with infection by manufacturing specific *antibodies* to help overcome the particular germs it comes into contact with or by activating the immune system to respond in other ways. If the same germ then attacks the body at a later stage, the body has its defences prepared. This is why infections such as mumps and measles are usually encountered only once in life.

During PREGNANCY, the developing baby acquires some protective antibodies from the mother via the *placenta*. Protective antibodies are also contained in the *colostrum*, a sticky discharge produced by the breasts during the first few days after the birth before the milk comes in. Because colostrum helps to increase the baby's immunity to diseases during the vulnerable early weeks, it is important that he or she should be put to the breast for the first few days after the birth, whether or not the mother has decided to breastfeed her baby.

The fact that the body can acquire a natural immunity to infections may seem satisfactory as long as the course of the original illness is fairly mild. However, a severe attack of what was once a common childhood illness such as WHOOPING COUGH, diphtheria or measles can be dangerous or damaging to health. The aim of immunization is to prevent the occurrence of these infections by stimulating the body to produce the appropriate antibodies or other means of countering the disease. The number of infections for which immunization has been developed are relatively few, but because they include illnesses that are potentially serious, particularly in the case of young children, immunization programmes have resulted in vast improvements to health and to life expectancy in recent years.

There are two methods of immunization: active and passive. *Passive immunization* is a ready-made form of immunization which involves injecting the person with *immunoglobulin,* that part of the blood which is already rich in antibodies to a particular infection. This immunoglobulin may be derived from the pooled plasma of blood donors in the case of viruses such as mumps and measles, which are prevalent in the general population. In the case of rare infections such as HEPATITIS B, which are not prevalent, it is obtained from the pooled blood of convalescent patients or patients recently immunized with the vaccine.

Active immunization is the more usual form of immunization. It involves injecting either the inactivated (that is, dead) germ, or the live germ in a very weakened, attenuated form. The aim of the injection is to stimulate the body itself to produce the appropriate antibodies to protect it against that particular infection.

After passive immunization, protection against infection is immediate, although it gradually diminishes over the next three or four weeks. After active immunization, complete immunity may not develop for a month or so, but in some instances, it is lifelong.

Passive immunization

Passive immunization is used in certain cases where a person has been exposed to a serious infection and needs immediate protection. One common example is for the prevention of TETANUS (lockjaw) where someone runs the risk of developing the disease – for example, from a cut from a garden fork. The object of the treatment is to supply the patient with antibody which has been derived from another source. Horses have been used as reservoirs for this type of antibody since 1894, but more and more use is being made of human immunoglobulin (IgG). This has certain enormous advantages over horse globulin, the most important being that patients no longer have the allergic reaction to horse serum itself which was so common a few years ago. The disease caused by horse serum and known as *serum sickness* developed within 36 to 48 hours of an injection and was characterized by fever, aching joints, a rash and sometimes by the appearance of protein in the urine.

It is important to remember that passive immunization, although it provides protection immediately after the injection is given, does not last long and in no way protects the patient against the possibility of subsequent infection. For this reason, the anti-tetanus serum (passive immunization) is followed by an injection of tetanus toxoid (active immunization), unless the last injection of toxoid was given less than ten years previously. (A toxoid is a harmful substance treated to destroy its harmful qualities, but causes the body to make antibodies when injected.)

Passive immunization with a specific immunoglobulin may also be essential where people have been accidentally exposed to hepatitis B, either through intimate contact or through working with people suffering from the illness. Passive immunization is usually accompanied by active immunization with a hepatitis B vaccine or booster, unless the person is already known to have enough protective antibodies. In the case of hepatitis B, active immunization can take up to six months to confer adequate protection.

Active immunization

A safe form of inoculation by injection was introduced by a country doctor, Edward Jenner, in the late 18th century. He noticed that farm labourers who suffered a mild disease known as cowpox – for it was from cows that the disease was contracted – developed a surprising resistance to SMALLPOX. He reasoned that the cowpox germ was sufficiently similar in structure to the deadly smallpox germ for the antibody-producing system of the body to be fooled into making some sort of protective substance (now known to be globulins) which would kill both the smallpox and cowpox germs. The widespread use of smallpox vaccination has led to one of the great success stories of medicine; the last time smallpox was seen as a natural infection was in 1975.

The principles of immunization by vaccination are now widely applied to a variety of infectious diseases. The injected material used to raise the antibody response and provide protection may be living or dead. In certain instances, only a portion of it – for example, a protein derived from its cell wall – may be injected. The live vaccines are made less vigorous by growing them in the laboratory for generations or by growing them in animals. The process by which the vigour of the vaccine is blunted is known as *attenuation*. Live attenuated vaccines cause mild illnesses in the patient to whom they are given and are infectious.

The decision to make immunization against a particular infection widely available rests on balancing the risks of possible side-effects against the risks of having the disease or of passing it on to others who may be more vulnerable (*see* POLIOMYELITIS).

Controversy

The whooping cough (*pertussis*) vaccination programme has unfortunately proved more controversial. Whooping cough is a highly infectious and potentially serious disease which mainly affects young children. Severe complications and deaths occur most commonly in infants under six months. The best way to protect young babies is to ensure that their brothers and sisters and other children in close contact are immunized.

Timing of immunizations

Age	Vaccine	Interval
During first year of life	Triple vaccine (DPT=diphtheria/ tetanus/whooping cough) and oral polio vaccine (OPV). Hib (*Haemophilus influenzae* B).	1st dose: 2 months. 2nd dose: 3 months. 3rd dose: 4 months.
12–18 months	Measles/mumps/rubella (MMR) vaccine.	
School entry (4–5 years)	Diphtheria and tetanus booster; polio booster; measles/mumps/ rubella (MMR) for children not already vaccinated.	
10–14 years	Rubella vaccination for girls; BCG (tuberculosis vaccination) for boys and girls.	There should be a gap of at least 3 weeks between rubella and BCG.
5–18 years	Tetanus and polio boosters.	
Adults	Course of 3 doses of polio vaccine for previously unimmunized adults. Course of 3 doses of tetanus vaccine followed by booster 5 years later for previously unimmunized adults, subsequent booster doses every 10 years. Rubella vaccination for all women of childbearing age found not to be immune to rubella Hepatitis B vaccination for people in high-risk groups.	Interval of 4 weeks between each dose. Interval of 6–8 weeks between 1st and 2nd doses, and 4–6 months between 2nd and 3rd doses.

Before 1957, when the whooping cough vaccine was introduced, the average number of cases notified exceeded 100,000 a year, with approximately one death for each 1,000 cases. By 1973, with more than 80 per cent of children being vaccinated, the number of cases had fallen to around 2,500.

However, a certain amount of existing concern about the safety of the vaccine was intensified by a report in 1974 which stated that a number of children admitted to hospital with severe neurological illness had received the whooping cough vaccine in the previous week, although it could not be proved that the vaccine had caused the illness. The widespread publicity surrounding the report quite naturally gave rise to a great deal of parental anxiety, and the number of children receiving the vaccine fell dramatically to about 30 per cent in 1975. Unfortunately major epidemics of whooping cough occurred between 1977 and 1979, and again between 1981 and 1983, as a result of this fall in immunization. In 1978 alone, 66,000 cases occurred.

The Joint Committee on Vaccination and Immunization put the risk of side-effects at possibly one in 100,000 injections, but pointed out that, in the vast majority of cases, the effects are only temporary. Moreover, neurological complications are considerably more common after whooping dough disease. Public confidence in the whooping cough vaccine seemed to return with 67 per cent of children being immunized in 1986.

See also HOLIDAY HEALTH, MENINGITIS.

Immunoglobulin, *see* **Blood, Immune system**

Impetigo

This is a highly contagious SKIN infection which may arise in both apparently healthy skin, and in skin damaged by ECZEMA, insect bites, SCABIES or COLD SORES.

It is caused by the *staphylococcus* or *streptococcus* bacteria which are found in the nose. It may be transmitted by breathing or sneezing on to damaged skin, where it spreads rapidly, causing inflammation and weeping blisters. Unless hygienic precautions are taken and treatment given, impetigo may spread quickly to other members of the household or school, either by direct contact or contact with towels or face flannels used by the patient.

Symptoms

Impetigo first appears on the face, scalp, hands or knees as little red spots. These soon become blisters which quickly break, exuding a pale yellow, sticky liquid. They then dry to form large, irregularly shaped, brownish-yellow crusts.

If only a small area of skin is affected, there are usually no other symptoms, but if large areas are involved, or if the surrounding skin is also infected with another bacteria, the patient will feel unwell, with a temperature and swollen lymph nodes. Adults are usually less severely affected than children, except in hot climates where the spread of infection may be extensive.

Impetigo is, however, a life-threatening illness for newborn babies, who have very little immunity, and it is extremely important that no one with impetigo should be in contact with babies or their mothers.

Vary rarely, untreated impetigo may cause ABSCESSES elsewhere in the body, or NEPHRITIS (inflammation of the kidneys).

Treatment

Treatment must commence immediately. The area should be bathed with an antiseptic solution such as hexachloraphane or povidone-iodine. If the area is small, an ANTIBIOTIC cream should be applied three or four times a day until the crusts have healed. Larger areas will require additional antibiotics by mouth or occasionally by injection. Thick crusts may have to be soaked off with liquid paraffin.

Most importantly, spread must be prevented, both to patients, who may reinfect themselves, and to others. Always keep patients' face flannels and towels separate and boil these, and also clothing and bed-linen after use. Children with impetigo should be told not to scratch the crusts, as scars may form. They should be kept off school until the infection has cleared, usually after five days. If there is an underlying skin condition, such as eczema, both this and impetigo should be treated together.

Impotence

Sexual failure in men comes down, physically, to three things: non-production of SPERM in the TESTES; not being able to have or keep an erection (*see* PENIS); and finally, not being able to ejaculate. Strictly speaking, only the second factor is impotence. The first comes under the heading of INFERTILITY, and the third is distinguished as a problem of its own.

Premature ejaculation, meaning the problem of reaching orgasm too quickly, is also different from impotence, although it has similar causes and responds to broadly similar treatments.

All types of men, in all walks of life, are more likely than not to experience impotence at some stage of their lives. This is because impotence is most commonly caused by STRESS, relationship problems or lack of self-confidence.

Ageing is the other universal factor in impotence. Sexual functioning, just as other physical processes, naturally declines with age, so that, once again, all men are susceptible, though impotence caused this way is by no means inevitable.

Sexual arousal

The purpose of SEX is the penetration of the VAGINA by the penis so that fertilization (if CONTRACEPTION is not used) can take place. To do this, the penis has to be stiff and erect, rather than limp or flaccid as it usually is. The stiffness is caused by blood flowing into three spongy cavities within the penis, and being kept there by a muscular contraction at the base of the penis.

For the blood to flow to the penis, there must be a sexual response – in other words, a reaction to something which is sexually exciting. In humans, the 'trigger' for sexual excitement is mainly in the mind. Non-mental triggers for sex do exist, such as the cycle of HORMONE production, hormones being the body's chemical messengers. But unlike animals, we are not automatically 'turned on' sexually.

Once a man has an erection, physical stimulation does the rest. Friction of the walls of the vagina on the head of the penis, which is rich in nerve endings, stimulate various muscles until, at orgasm, they contract, pumping semen out through the penis.

Psychological causes

It should be no surprise, therefore, that a system so dependent on mental and nervous triggers should occasionally fail for mental or nervous – that is, psychological – reasons. By far the most common psychological reason for failure is the fear of failure. Society puts both men and women under great pressure to be sexually successful.

It can take something quite small to plant the seed of fear. Scornful words may do it – spoken, for instance, by a woman who, understandably enough, is disappointed when her partner is too tired to make love, perhaps because of overwork or stress.

Closely related to fear as a psychological reason for impotence is general lack of self-confidence. This is caused, typically, by redundancy, or failure to win promotion at work. Or there may be relationship problems – perhaps a lack of confidence in the relationship, or in the woman herself. But impotence is only a real problem if it persists.

Childhood events can make a man impotent in later life. Unhappy dealings with females – perhaps in his family – may give him an in-built resentment of women. Or he could have a naive tendency to idealize them.

Some men fear the consequences of sexual intercourse, not wanting the responsibility of children, or they may have a fear of hereditary disease.

Physical causes

In young, and not-so-young men, ALCOHOL is the most common (and joked about) physical cause of impotence. Anyone who has had too much to drink knows how it makes them willing but unable to make love. There may be an erection, but ejaculation either takes a long time, or does not happen at all.

Ageing is the physical cause of impotence to worry about least. At 60, a man is less able to perform sexually – in terms of frequency of erection, the length of time it can be 'held' and the time taken to reach orgasm. However, there is no set pattern, and some may find the rate of decline eases after 60.

As many elderly people know, this does not mean a deteriorating love life, just one with a different pace. Indeed, the length of time it takes a man to reach orgasm may mean greater pleasure for both partners, particularly the woman.

If you have a bout of flu, or even a cold, your sexual powers are likely to be weakened. Severe DIABETES can cause impotence, as can a few other serious degenerative diseases, such as CANCER of the COLON OR PROSTATE – although they may not always do so.

Besides diabetes, other endocrine disorders can cause impotence in which there are abnormal levels of testosterone or prolactin in the bloodstream. Disease of the arteries (atherosclerosis) can also affect the penile blood supply producing impotence. Many drugs, including diuretics, beta-blockers or cannabis, can also result in this.

Treatment

Temporary psychological impotence is almost always treated, at first occurrence, by the doctor. He or she will try to identify the cause and offer reassurance.

If the problem does not go away, it is likely to need treatment by a form of psychotherapy. Today, this offers great hope to couples who are prepared to cooperate with the therapist.

Sexual therapy entails a couple going to therapy sessions together to learn techniques which they then practise in their own home (*see* SEX AND SEXUAL INTERCOURSE).

For the most common physical cause of impotence – excess drinking – pointing out the cause is usually treatment enough. The same may well apply to young people who complain of impotence as a result of heavy use of cannabis (*see* MARIJUANA).

If impotence is caused by a short-term illness or over-tiredness, the treatment is equally simple: explanation, followed by reassurance that normal sexual functioning will return. More than 90 per cent of cases are psychological, and most respond to treatment.

When it is caused by disease – for example, diabetes – patients can often look for improved sexual ability in step with the progress of their treatment.

Decline due to ageing is not a medical problem, but the doctor or a sex therapist may offer advice on love-making positions which are easy and comfortable. Specialized urology clinics can offer help in the form of penile implants, or papaverine injections into the penis to produce temporary erections.

Incontinence

This is the inability to control the evacuation of URINE and faeces. It is a common problem, normally associated with the very young and the very old.

Incontinence of faeces is caused by a number of conditions, the most common being spurious DIARRHOEA in old age or during a weakening illness. Many old people have CONSTIPATION, due to a lack of bulk or fluid in the diet. They then take LAXATIVES causing liquid faeces to push past the constipation and cause spurious diarrhoea. The diarrhoea may have been caused by strong laxatives, or as a side-effect of ANTIBIOTIC treatment or IRON therapy. Patients with severe neurological diseases such as a SPINAL injury which affects control of the bowels or urinary BLADDER also develop incontinence, as do those with a serious abnormality of the RECTUM or anus such as a tumour or anal prolapse.

Faecal incontinence is often a sign of emotional problems in children; it is also common among severely handicapped, and patients with DEMENTIA.

Incontinence of urine also has a number of possible causes, resulting from problems with one or more of the mechanisms which hold urine in the bladder. These include the muscular sphincter at the base of the bladder, the muscular floor of the pelvis which consists of the *levator ani* muscle and the urogenital diaphragm, and the muscle wall of the bladder.

In women, some degree of urinary incontinence is very common indeed, especially in those who have a weak pelvic floor as a result of CHILDBIRTH. This is known as a prolapsed bladder (*cystocoele*). The weakness of the muscle allows the front part of the bladder to bulge down into the VAGINA making the sphincter less effective. This causes 'stress incontinence', where the urine leaks out whenever the patient coughs, strains or laughs.

A severe infection of the urinary tract will produce frequent urination, leaking and dribbling, with partial incontinence, especially in the elderly. The infection acts on the controlling muscles.

In men, an obstruction of the PROSTATE can lead to a retention of urine with a dribbling overflow. Alternatively, an operation for an enlargement of the prostate often makes some patients incontinent for a short time.

Incontinence in both sexes can occur where there is bladder CANCER, a *fistula* (wound or ulcer) or TUBERCULOSIS, or as a result of senility. Total lack of bladder control is very much more rare, and is usually caused by a neurological disease such as MULTIPLE SCLEROSIS.

In a small number of adult cases, there may be severe behaviour problems. However, when this occurs in children during the day, it is nearly always a result of such a cause. Incontinence during sleep is called *enuresis* and it is slightly different as the incontinence is involuntary. Bedwetting is a behaviour-linked condition, not true incontinence.

Treatment

Faecal incontinence can nearly always be cured and is only ever a permanent problem in a very small number of patients with neurological disease. Surgery to repair prolapse of the anus or to remove growths causing incontinence is usually very successful. Where the cause is impaction of faeces due to constipation, removal of the blocking faeces coupled with a very high-fibre diet is curative. Where patients have become incontinent following drug therapy from antibiotics or iron therapy, the condition will usually cure itself within a few days.

Children who are soiling in the daytime really need psychological help. They often have family problems or have become depressed, and they show their disturbance by soiling.

Most women suffering urinary incontinence can be helped by doing pelvic-floor exercises – squeezing the muscles between the legs as if trying to stop the flow of urine. If these are insufficient, the repair of a prolapsed bladder and weakened pelvic floor is a most effective operation. Where this is not suitable, an electronic implant, consisting of a coil and two electrodes, can be placed under the skin of the pelvic muscles, with another coil, powered by a battery, placed outside the skin. The device will stimulate and strengthen the pelvic muscles, reducing incontinence in many women. In other cases, a vaginal pessary that holds up the sagging pelvic wall, or even an ordinary tampon, will maintain continence.

For short-term bouts of incontinence, incontinence pads, changed immediately the patient is incontinent, should be used. However, they can be employed only in the short term as they may damage the skin.

In men, the length of the penis is a valuable aid to collecting urine. A sheath or open-ended condom can be placed over the penis, and linked directly to a specially adapted rubber tubing to collect urine in a sterile bag. This can be used where there is urinary incontinence due to spinal injuries. Women may need to have a catheter (tube) inserted, which collects urine in a bag.

Indigestion

Apart from the occasional rumble or belch, we do not usually notice the functioning of our DIGESTIVE systems. For most of us, the term 'indigestion' covers a wide variety of complaints, but most commonly it means pain after eating food, often accompanied by a bloated, sick feeling.

Indigestion is either a symptom of illness or, much more commonly, the result of eating unsuitable food. It may also result from the way food is eaten.

Depending on the individual, certain foods can cause indigestion. Cucumber and pickled onions are common culprits, as are spicy foods, such as curry or garlic, and rich foods loaded with cream or butter. Unripe fruit, undercooked meat and excesses of tea or coffee can also cause types of indigestion. It is not that these substances cannot be digested; it is only that the STOMACH takes longer to deal with them and is slow to pass them on into the remainder of the gut. The stomach contents and stomach acid lie in the stomach without being passed into the duodenum. Acid is poured out which causes heartburn and belching.

For some people, indigestion is brought on simply by hurried eating and failing to chew food properly. Drinking too much ALCOHOL can also bring on a bout of indigestion, and regular overindulgence can cause chronic indigestion. SMOKING too much can also be a cause.

Chronic indigestion is more persistent and severe, and is often a symptom of a medical condition which can usually be treated. In some people, the pattern of indigestion is indicative of a specific and usually treatable medical complaint, such as a peptic ULCER, a hiatus hernia (*see* DIAPHRAGM) or MIGRAINE.

There may also be psychological reasons behind bouts of indigestion. The nerve supply to the stomach is through the vagus nerve which controls acid production and the rate at which food leaves the stomach. Both anxiety (*see* STRESS) and DEPRESSION affect this part of the nervous system. Excess acid and slow emptying both cause indigestion and can lead to the formation of ulcers.

Symptoms

The degree of indigestion produces an individual combination of symptoms, from pain and flatulence (wind) to severe discomfort and regurgitation of acid food.

Symptoms vary depending on the cause. There is usually pain which is either colicky or constant and situated in the pit of the stomach or upper chest. Or there may be nausea, accompanied by a full and heavy sensation in the stomach; if the sufferer can be sick, the indigestion is relieved immediately.

Acid regurgitation from indigestion is also common. Acid comes up into the mouth to produce hoarseness of the voice and a pain in the chest, better known as heartburn. Sometimes a person with indigestion will experience a symptom known as *waterbrash* – where saliva flows like water – accompanied by excess belching, flatulence or hiccups.

In chronic indigestion, the tongue is dry and is coated with a brown fur-like substance, and the breath is stale.

Dangers

Isolated bouts of indigestion following heavy meals or drinking sprees are not dangerous. However, where the indigestion is chronic, or when the pain does not pass or becomes extremely severe, it is important to see a doctor, as some serious conditions have pains and symptoms which often mimic indigestion.

Inflammation of the GALL BLADDER, for instance, produces wind, sickness and central abdominal pain. Some rare cases of APPENDICITIS can produce the same symptoms. A HEART ATTACK or clot on the LUNG may also appear, at first, to be an acute bout of indigestion, but the pain remains fixed or worsens and is not relieved by taking an antacid. And where chronic indigestion is caused by a peptic ulcer, which is left undetected, the ulcer may perforate or bleed. Persistent indigestion may also be the first indication of stomach CANCER. Failure to diagnose any of these conditions is dangerous and could even be fatal.

Treatment and outlook

In the case of chronic indigestion where a medical condition, such as a hiatus hernia, cancer or an ulcer, is suspected, the sufferer will usually have a medical investigation, such as an X-RAY or an ENDOSCOPY, to establish the cause.

If the cause is a hurried way of life, stress or poor diet, this must be corrected or, in the case of isolated bouts of indigestion, treated with antacids – either bicarbonate of soda or magnesium trisilicate.

The outlook for people with a medical cause for their indigestion varies from case to case. Many people suffering from a hiatus hernia may have to control the condition by taking regular antacids and avoiding certain foods.

People with ulcers can normally be cured with drugs to cut down the amount of acid produced in the stomach, or antibiotics to control the bacteria that may cause them. However, if stress was the original cause of the ulcer, another may form if the way of life is not altered.

Induction

Some women will manage to have several children without needing an induction, which is the process of bringing on labour, but a woman who finds she needs an induction has no need to worry. On the contrary, without this technique many more women and their babies would die during CHILDBIRTH.

In a normal PREGNANCY, it is thought that hormone signals from the developing baby (the foetus) spark off labour, and this occurs at about the 40th week. The CERVIX (neck of the womb) softens (ripens) and the birth canal gets wider, the membranes covering the baby break, or rupture, and labour begins the process of birth. However, sometimes, it is necessary to bring the birth forward, but only for definite medical reasons.

The two most common situations where induction is needed are when the pregnant woman develops high BLOOD PRESSURE, or if the foetus is postmature (that is, over-ready).

High blood pressure

In this condition, known as PET (pre-eclamptic toxaemia) of pregnancy (*see* ECLAMPSIA AND PRE-ECLAMPSIA), the presence of the foetus induces high blood pressure in the mother. If it is untreated, the pressure will continue to rise and the mother's KIDNEYS will be affected. In serious cases, she can have epileptic-type fits and die. The mortality risk for the baby is also very high indeed, and it is for this reason that antenatal checks are so important.

Thankfully, this condition develops late in pregnancy, but if it does occur, bedrest and drug treatment are essential to control the blood pressure, followed by induction of labour. During labour, an epidural ANAESTHETIC is sometimes given; this not only numbs pain but also keeps blood pressure down. Provided the pressure continues to be kept down, the subsequent delivery of the baby should be completely normal. Rarely, a CAESAREAN section is necessary.

Postmaturity

This is a common situation, when the foetus remains in the uterus after the normal 40-week period. It is slow to send out signals to start labour and, at the same time, the placenta is becoming old. The essential function of the placenta is to supply nutrients and oxygen to the foetus, without which it would die. For this reason, when a baby is overdue, tests of placental function are performed to check that it is still working properly. These are done on specimens of the mother's blood and urine.

If it is found that the placenta is failing and the baby is no longer growing, the doctor will recommend induction of labour. In a case where a previous pregnancy has resulted in a foetal death, induction would be performed at 40 weeks. Otherwise, the doctor may recommend waiting for 10–14 days.

Other reasons

Other situations where induction may be necessary include serious illness of the mother – conditions such as DIABETES, HEART DISEASE or active TUBERCULOSIS; cases where the placenta has failed and the foetus has died and must be delivered quickly to avoid risk of infection; cases of RHESUS blood disease (where the mother develops antibodies that destroy the blood of the baby); the relatively rare condition where the placenta lies over the cervix and blocks birth (*placenta praevia*); and, lastly, when examination reveals that the head of the baby is larger than the outlet of the pelvis, when a Caesarean section will probably be required. In addition, if the expectant mother's 'waters' break – that is, the protective sac of amniotic fluid in which the baby lies ruptures – induction may be considered after some hours, to prevent infection reaching the baby.

Making the decision

In every case, the doctor has to weigh up the risks involved and decides on induction only when it is necessary. He or she will make a careful assessment of the risks and benefits of induction. Doctors do vary in their approach to the technique, and there is still a degree of controversy surrounding it. In many cases, the mother herself, or the midwife involved, may be given a choice, but the decision is based on the patient's previous obstetric history, the risks to the mother and baby and the facilities available where the baby is to be born. Unless the case is an emergency, the decision is made 24 hours beforehand. The patient knows and is ready, and so is spared any last-minute dash to the hospital. Induction is never recommended as a matter of convenience for the staff or doctors of the hospital.

Methods of induction

These are either medical, where drugs are used to bring on labour or surgical, where the membranes covering the baby are ruptured to release the amniotic fluid and start labour. The midwife explains to the patient the method that has been chosen for her; she is bathed and, in some hospitals, shaved of pubic hair if a Caesarean section is at all likely.

To establish how ready the womb is for labour, and how easy induction would be, the doctor performs a vaginal examination. If the cervix is very 'unripe', drugs called *prostaglandins* may be used. These may be given by mouth or inserted into the vagina.

The commonest method is to rupture the membranes surgically and, at the same time, to give a drug called *oxytocin* or *syntocinon* by means of an intravenous drip. The drug stimulates contractions. The amount given can be very accurately calculated in relation to its effect, so that contractions can be controlled, if necessary. A special electronic device is usually used to control the rate at which oxytocin is administered.

Once the membranes have been ruptured, it is essential to deliver the baby within 24 hours, as the uterus will no longer be sterile, but it is usually only a matter of ten minutes to half an hour, before contractions start.

The patient is usually connected to a *monitor* – an electronic machine that keeps track of the baby's heartbeat, the contractions and so on. This essential information about the condition of the baby and the progress of labour ensures that maximum precautions are taken to ensure a safe delivery.

Of course, progress depends on each individual case, but most will go on to have normal deliveries, some will need help from forceps and only a very small proportion will need a delivery by Caesarean section.

The greatest risk is of inducing a premature baby. This can occur if the induction has to be performed for medical reasons (e.g. pre-eclampsia).

Infarction

The life-line of every organ is the ARTERY which supplies it with fresh BLOOD and provides the OXYGEN and food on which its cells depend to remain alive. If an artery becomes blocked, the cells in the area are starved of blood and die. This cell death is known as *infarction*.

There isn't any real difference between infarction and gangrene. Both result from an artery becoming blocked and both refer to the cell death which results. It is normal to use the word 'infarction' to refer to this process occurring in an internal organ, while 'gangrene' usually refers to death of tissue in the arms and legs.

See also HEART ATTACK, HERNIA, STROKE, THROMBOSIS.

Infection and infectious diseases

'Infection' means the invasion of the body by an infecting organism such as a VIRUS or BACTERIUM. Infections can range from minor ailments such as COLDS and INFLUENZA to invariably fatal illnesses such as RABIES. Infections may be localized, affecting only a small area (an ABSCESS, for example), or one system (the way that PNEUMONIA affects the lung), or they may be generalized, affecting a greater part of the body, as in septicaemia (blood poisoning).

Strictly speaking, a contagious disease is one which is caught by touching an infectious person. However, many people use the word 'contagious' just to mean 'infectious'.

Causes

Infections are caused by tiny organisms (living creatures) which are too small to be seen by the naked eye: they are therefore called *micro-organisms*. Two sorts of micro-organism, the virus and the bacterium, cause the vast majority of important infections.

A third type of infective micro-organism is the *protozoa*: larger single-celled organisms and fungi (*see* FUNGAL INFECTIONS). MALARIA, probably the most important infectious disease in worldwide terms, is caused by a protozoa called plasmodium.

Once a micro-organism has entered the body, its object is to reproduce itself using the tissues as a food substance. Viruses go one stage further by using the chemical building apparatus of the cells to build new viruses. In contrast, bacteria reproduce simply by means of each individual bacterium splitting into two.

Micro-organisms cause disease in a number of different ways. Often the organism produces some poisonous substance, called a *toxin*, which causes symptoms. DIPHTHERIA is an example of such a disease. Organisms also cause disease by tissue destruction or by interfering with the normal functioning of an organ. Viral HEPATITIS, for example, causes JAUNDICE by interfering with the function of LIVER cells, while pneumonia may make large areas of the lung ineffective.

How the body defends itself

The body deals with infection by a remarkable and complex defence system called the IMMUNE SYSTEM.

Before an organism reaches the cells of the body, it must break through the SKIN: the skin acts as a primary barrier against infection. However, many infections enter the body through the respiratory tract or the ALIMENTARY (digestive) tract and so avoid having to cross the skin. Once inside the body, the organism may be consumed by a *phagocytic cell,* a cell which swallows up and destroys viruses and bacteria. These are the white cells of the BLOOD; there are similar cells in the tissues. In some cases, both the organism and the phagocyte will die, and this leads to the production of pus, which is no more than a collection of dead organisms and phagocytes. The activity and effectiveness of phagocytes depends on the immune system.

The immune system works through two major arms to combat invasion by foreign organisms. The first is the production of *antibodies*: these are protein molecules which travel in the bloodstream and among the tissues and bind on to the surface of specific micro-organisms. This makes it easier for the phagocytic cells to attack. Antibodies may also stop organisms from being effective: for example, they may stop viruses entering cells. Finally antibodies may trigger a system which actually leads to invading bacterial cells being broken down.

The other arm of the system is called *cell-mediated immunity*. The cells of this system, which are called *lymphocytes* because they come from the LYMPHATIC SYSTEM, may be specially primed to react with a particular organism and kill it. They may also produce substances which help phagocytes to attack infecting organisms.

The development of vaccines to protect against infectious diseases has been one of medical science's major contributions to health. Vaccination and IMMUNIZATION rely on the basic principle that the immune system in the body can be stimulated to produce antibodies by a substance or an organism which is very similar to that which causes the disease. If the person who has been immunized later comes into contact with that particular disease, the antibodies present in the body ward off the infection.

Incubation

When a person catches an illness, the bacteria or virus causing it must invade the body and become established some time before the symptoms begin. The time that elapses between contact with the disease and the actual onset or start of symptoms is known as the *incubation* period.

This can be as short as a few hours with diseases such as CHOLERA, or maybe weeks, as with rabies. However, for some diseases like TUBERCULOSIS, the organisms may lay dormant in the tissues for very long periods – sometimes even years. Such diseases do not have an incubation period in the normal sense of the word. The virus which causes COLD SORES – *Herpes simplex* – also remains in the tissues for some years, and only emerges occasionally, usually when some other infection is present.

Once a virus finds its way into the body, often through the lining of the nose or mouth, it invades the surrounding cells or is carried by the bloodstream to cells some distance away. Exceptions are the common cold and flu, which establish themselves in the nose and throat.

Once the virus is inside a cell, the virus cannot easily be reached by the body's defence system. Instead, it uses the cell's own building system to make more virus particles, and when these 'second generation' viruses are released into the bloodstream, symptoms begin.

With diseases due to bacterial infections, the bacteria must become established in the tissues, and the symptoms of the infection occur as soon as the organisms are present in large numbers. Bacterial infections become established quickly, so that incubation periods are usually shorter than those of viruses.

Diseases and their symptoms

Many organisms show a particular tendency to infect only one organ. For instance, the hepatitis virus lodges in the liver; the bacterium *pneumococcus* causes pneumonia in the lungs; and the pneumococcus' close relative, the *meningococcus* which causes MENINGITIS, results in an inflammation of the membranes lining the brain. Why organisms show this preference is unknown.

Other organisms, like the *staphylococcus*, may produce disease in any system. Once this organism has entered the bloodstream, it gets carried around the body and settles in organs far away from the point where it originally entered. Once settled, the staphylococcus can multiply and produce an abscess.

Finally, abscesses may produce toxic substances which poison particular areas of the body. TETANUS produces such a toxin which only affects the nervous system, while the cholera organism produces severe diarrhoea as a result of toxins.

However, in many cases much of the problem that a disease may cause results from the effect of interaction between the infecting organism and the body's defence mechanism. The production of large amounts of PHLEGM as a result of pneumonia is really a result of the immune response, and this phlegm is often the leading symptom of the disease. Similarly, the lung destruction that may follow from tuberculosis is primarily caused by the immune response rather than the disease itself.

Treatment

ANTIBIOTICS have made a great difference to the treatment of infection. These are drugs which are toxic to bacteria but not to human cells. Many of them actually act by interfering with the bacterial cell wall which has a different sort of structure to human cell walls.

Antibiotics are available to combat most bacterial diseases. Each is effective against a limited range of infections, so the doctor must choose the most appropriate one for the type of bacterium causing the illness. Occasionally, however, bacteria become resistant to antibiotics that would normally be used against them. If antibiotic resistance is suspected, samples can be taken from the patient and tested in a bacteriology laboratory to find out which antibiotics will still be effective.

Special antibiotics are also available for protozoal diseases and for fungal infections. However, there are as yet no antibiotics which can be used for most virus infections, such as colds, influenza or measles. Over the past ten years, one or two antiviral antibiotics have been developed but the range of infections which they can treat is very limited. There has been most success with the treatment of herpes virus infections.

No cure has yet been found for AIDS, and all those who develop symptoms eventually die of the disease or a secondary infection.

See also CHICKENPOX, GONORRHOEA, MEASLES, MUMPS, RINGWORM, SCARLET FEVER, SEPTIC CONDITIONS, SMALLPOX, SYPHILIS, THRUSH, TYPHOID AND PARATYPHOID, TYPHUS.

Infertility

It can come as a severe blow to a couple to find that they cannot have children. Many of the causes of infertility have no accompanying symptoms so it is only when the couple try to conceive that they realize they have a problem.

The indication of possible infertility is when a couple fail to achieve CONCEPTION after a year or more of intercourse without contraception. Some doctors prefer the couple to have been trying for two years before they begin tests and treatment, but this will depend to some extent on the age of the woman, since her childbearing years are limited.

About 17 per cent of couples are infertile and the numbers seem to be rising.

SEXUAL INTERCOURSE becomes a strain, focused as it is on the fertile time of the month, and many couples experience a loss of desire when they feel that each time they are trying (and failing) to make a baby rather than making love.

If the reason for infertility is not immediately obvious then tests are carried out to find the cause.

Causes

There are many different causes of infertility and it is a subject constantly under review with new discoveries of causes and treatments being made all the time. Infertility is just as likely to be caused by a problem in the man as in the woman, and in many cases, it is the result of combined factors.

The most common cause in women is failure to ovulate (release an egg from the OVARY each month) due to a HORMONE failure. Sometimes hormone imbalance can produce hostile mucus in the VAGINA that actually repels the male sperm or stops the fertilized egg from attaching itself to the UTERUS (womb).

In some women, the problem may be a physical one such as a hymen or vagina too tight for intercourse, or a malformation of the vulva (external genitalia), the vagina or any reproductive organ.

Other disorders that can lead to infertility may happen at any time – such as infection from BACTERIA or VIRUSES, SEXUALLY TRANSMITTED DISEASES (STDs), or the growth of FIBROIDS, POLYPS or CYSTS.

Emotional STRESS is another common cause. Psychological factors can stop ovulation or cause spasms in the Fallopian tubes which inhibit the passage of the egg to the uterus.

Infertility in men can be due to no SPERM or low sperm production, or sluggish sperm which do not swim as they should. High numbers of abnormally shaped sperm can cause infertility.

A blockage of one of the tubes that carries the sperm is another cause of male infertility. This may be the result of varicocele (VARICOSE VEINS inside the scrotum), a tuberculous infection of the PROSTATE GLAND or an untreated STD. Alcohol can reduce fertility.

IMPOTENCE and premature ejaculation (*see* PENIS) are other causes of male infertility, which may have a psychological basis.

Diagnosing the problem

An infertile couple will be referred by their doctor to their local hospital or infertility clinic. They should go together as it is just as likely for the man to be infertile as the woman, or for there to be a joint problem.

Diagnosing the trouble can be a lengthy affair. To start with, both partners will have a general physical examination and medical histories will be taken. The doctor will want to know when the woman's PERIODS started, whether she has a regular menstrual cycle (that is, regular periods), as well as details about both partners' past and present health and of their sex life.

The man will have a sperm count as there would be no point in carrying out tests on the woman if the man has a very low sperm count. He will be asked to produce a sperm sample at home by masturbating into a clean, preferably sterile, glass or plastic container. The sample is taken to the hospital laboratory. The couple should not have had intercourse for at least two days.

It is generally believed that the man has no fertility problem if the count is no lower than 20 million sperm per cubic centimetre of semen, that at least 40 per cent of the sperm are active and 60 per cent are of normal shape.

If no abnormality is found in the man, tests will continue on the woman. She will be shown how to prepare a basal temperature chart to show when she is ovulating. The basal body temperature (the temperature of the body at rest) rises when a woman ovulates, but as it varies with many factors – such as the time of day – it should be taken at the same time each morning before getting out of bed or having anything to drink.

Ovulation is indicated by a rise of about 0.4°F (0.2°C) or more. Sperm can live for 3–5 days in a woman's Fallopian tubes; the egg only lives for about 12 hours after it is released from the ovary. So the couple must make sure they have intercourse during those hours.

Doctors will usually recommend keeping a basal chart for several months so that they can establish the woman's ovulation pattern (*see* CONTRACEPTION).

But not all doctors consider this method of pinpointing ovulation reliable, so other tests may be used, among them the serum progesterone test. Using the woman's temperature chart as a guide or, alternatively, by giving her a blood test about six days before her next period, the rise in the level of the hormone *progesterone* – which happens immediately after ovulation – can be measured.

An endometrial biopsy is another test. By taking a sample of the endometrium (womb lining) and examining it under a microscope, the doctor can tell whether or not ovulation has occurred and approximately when. It is a reliable test and is usually done under general anaesthetic.

Other tests

An abnormality of the cervix or the mucus in the cervical canal can be diagnosed by a simple, painless test called the *post-coital test.* This involves taking some of the mucus from the cervix to see what is happening to sperm in the vagina after intercourse and whether the sperm are still active after several hours. The test is best carried out around the time of ovulation and the woman will be asked to have intercourse the night before or on the morning of the test. The mucus should be clear and still contain moving sperm.

Hysterosalpingography is a more accurate test which involves injecting dye through the cervix and up each Fallopian tube. Then X-rays are taken to reveal any blockage of the tubes, the shape of the womb and show whether the cervix is functioning properly. The test is usually carried out during the first ten days of the menstrual cycle. An anaesthetic is not usually necessary.

Laparoscopy allows a direct view of the uterus, Fallopian tubes and ovaries. It is done under a general anaesthetic as it involves piercing the abdominal wall with a slim needle through which gas is passed to distend the abdominal cavity. Then an optical instrument called a laparoscope is passed through a slightly larger incision just below the navel. The ovaries and uterus can then be biopsied if necessary. It is sometimes possible to carry out minor surgery through the laparoscope. *See also* ENDOSCOPY.

Male treatments

If infertility is a result of impotence or some other difficulty with intercourse, the first line of treatment involves simple counselling about sexual techniques – assuming that physical examination of both partners confirms that they are normal. Often the reassurance of a doctor is enough to solve the problem, but occasionally detailed psychological help may be needed. Physical causes for impotence are rare, but may be curable.

If impotence does not improve to the extent that intercourse becomes possible, then the doctor may recommend ARTIFICIAL INSEMINATION.

A common male factor is a low sperm count. If there is an obvious cause such as a varicocele (varicose vein in the scrotum), surgical treatment may help. If not, a number of simple general measures may be tried. Avoidance of both alcohol and smoking can improve the sperm count. Sperm grow best in the testicles when their temperature is lower than the normal body temperature. Because jeans and tight underpants raise the testicles nearer the body and keep them too warm for efficient production of sperm, the wearing of such clothing should be discouraged. Avoiding very hot baths can also bring about a worthwhile improvement in the sperm count.

Occasionally, drugs may be prescribed to improve the sperm count. In some cases, the female partner's secretions may reject the male's sperm so that they do not reach the egg and allow conception to occur. In such cases, the man may be treated with steroids or other drugs to reduce rejection.

In those instances where the sperm count is too low for natural conception to occur and fails to improve with treatment, there are a number of other options. One of the new techniques, such as *in vitro* fertilization (IVF), may be possible (*see below*).

If no sperm are present at all, however, another possible option is artificial insemination with sperm from a donor.

Female treatments

In at least a quarter of infertile couples, the main problem is a failure of regular ovulation. Often this is caused by an internal hormone imbalance. Treatment may involve the use of one or more different types of drug, depending on the exact cause. Blood tests and urine tests are usually needed to establish the cause, and sometimes further blood tests are made while treatment is progressing to assess the response to treatment. One of the most commonly used drugs is clomiphene, which is taken by mouth and helps to re-establish ovulation in many women. Hormonal preparations may also be needed, given by single injections at certain times during the monthly cycle. Occasionally, a continual injection of a drug called LHRH is used; a needle is placed under the skin and connected by a fine plastic tube to a special electronic control box which is worn in a holster under the clothes and which supplies the body with a regular dose of the drug.

Another common infertility problem in women is damage to the Fallopian tubes which blocks the passage of sperm and egg. This damage is often the result of a previous infection in the tubes, which may have been caused by a sexually transmitted disease. Any traces of infection are treated with antibiotics, and then sometimes surgery can be carried out to remove the blockage of the tube. However, such surgery is technically very difficult and not always successful.

The technique of IVF (*see* TEST-TUBE BABIES) is particularly valuable when a woman's Fallopian tubes are so badly damaged that surgery cannot restore them. However, IVF is not always successful, and often two or three attempts are needed to achieve pregnancy – each attempt requiring a stay in hospital. The success of the procedure is at most about 30 per cent (and can be much lower). Because the treatment is so expensive, it is often not available in state-financed health services, but can be provided in a few private clinics which have the appropriate specialist services.

Occasionally, IVF is useful as a treatment for a couple in whom the difficulty is a low sperm count – even when the woman has no other problem and normal Fallopian tubes. Ideal circumstances can be created in the laboratory for fertilization to occur, even when there are very few sperm present in the semen.

An alternative technique has been developed for this problem which is simpler than IVF. It is called GIFT (gamete intrafallopian transfer). The egg is removed from the ovary through a laparoscope in exactly the same way as in IVF, but is then injected directly into the Fallopian tube by the doctor, and a sample of semen is injected into the tube at the same time. Using this technique, a more natural process of fertilization can occur in the woman's Fallopian tubes. Complicated laboratory facilities are not needed, and the success rate, when used with semen which has a low sperm count, is as good as with in vitro fertilization.

Inflammation

Whenever tissues are damaged, cells at the site of the injury release a substance called *histamine*, which increases the BLOOD flow in that area and causes the blood vessels to leak large quantities of fluid into the tissues.

The fluid, known as an 'inflammatory exudate', can – like blood – form clots. The clots plug up broken blood vessels and join together, forming fibrous tissue to 'wall-off' foreign bodies and stop any infection spreading, while at the same time starting the healing process by binding the edges of torn or damaged tissues together (*see* IMMUNE SYSTEM).

Causes

There are three main causes of inflammation. Most commonly, the cause is an INFECTION by either a VIRUS or by BACTERIA. The infection damages cells in the area affected, and as they become damaged, they release histamine and other chemicals which trigger off inflammation. Sometimes bacteria themselves release chemicals or toxins which are responsible for setting off an inflammatory response.

Another cause of inflammation is a physical injury to the tissues of the body. This may take the form of a cut or abrasion, a bruise, or a burn. The inflammation of sunburn is also caused by physical damage to the cells of the skin by excessive ultraviolet light.

A more unusual form of inflammation occurs when the body produces antibodies to a foreign substance, and triggers off an allergic reaction (*see* ALLERGY). HAY FEVER is such an allergic response in which the body produces antibodies to grass pollens in the air. Inflammation can then occur in any of the mucous membranes in contact with air, so hay fever causes inflammation in the nose, eyes and sometimes lungs as well. Other types of allergic reactions can cause intensely irritating inflammation in the skin – a type of RASH called *urticaria*. Rarely, the body starts to produce antibodies against its own tissues, and this process may cause inflammation in various parts of the body. These conditions, called *auto-immune diseases*, are often painful and can cause deep-seated inflammation in internal organs. RHEUMATOID ARTHRITIS is such a condition, but certain types of inflammatory diseases of the bowel, kidney and liver are also thought to be due to auto-immune disease.

The process of inflammation

A number of changes take place in inflamed tissues which follow a similar sequence whatever the cause of the inflammation. Each stage can take only a few seconds in severe acute inflammation, but sometimes the process of inflammation develops over many days.

First, the blood vessels in the affected area widen to allow a greater flow of blood to the tissues. The walls of the blood vessels then become more permeable, so protein and white blood cells escape from the vessels and move into the tissues. Once this stage has been reached, blood flow in the vessels slows down again and the inflamed area becomes walled off from other tissues as the white cells build up around the inflamed area and the proteins in the tissues clot. In this way, other nearby tissues are protected from the cause of the inflammation. White cells can then set about dealing with the damaged tissues or with bacteria. They are able to engulf damaged tissues or whole bacteria and digest them by a process called *phagocytosis*. Once all damaged material has been removed by the white cells, healing can begin with new tissues growing into the previously damaged area.

The severity of inflammation depends on the severity of the original damage to the tissues – but also on the ability of the body to withstand damage. A person who is already weakened by illness, disease or malnutrition may have a poor inflammatory response to a new infection or injury, so the ultimate effects on that individual may be much more severe than would be the case with someone who was otherwise perfectly healthy.

Symptoms

The extra fluid in the inflamed area and the high blood flow cause swelling of the affected tissues. If the inflammation is on the surface of the skin, the area becomes red and hot. Release of chemicals in the area causes PAIN, which is more severe the greater the extent of inflammation. Some deep-seated organs, however, are not particularly sensitive to pain, so inflammation may be present in the LIVER, for example, without the patient feeling any pain at all. On the other hand, a small BOIL on a finger can be intensely painful.

Inflammation in the nose, throat or lungs may produce quantities of mucus which the patient coughs up. A boil on the skin may produce pus, which consists of white cells and inflammatory fluid. Other symptoms depend on the site of the inflammation. Inflammation of deep-seated organs will become apparent because the function of the organ is affected. So inflammation of the bowel may cause DIARRHOEA.

Inflammatory bowel disease, *see* Colon and colitis

Influenza

Known almost universally as 'flu', this usually occurs in epidemics when lots of people catch the illness at once. This usually happens in the winter, but it is also present somewhere in the population at all times, which is why people can get flu at any time of the year.

The cause

The VIRUS which causes influenza is special in that it is always changing its appearance, and these changes fool the body's defence mechanisms. Every year it changes by a process known as 'drift', resulting in outbreaks of flu. Every 30 to 40 years, a bigger change takes place, known as 'shift', during which a very different virus appears and causes a worldwide epidemic – a *pandemic*. Occasionally the flu virus changes to a form which resembles a previous virus, and people who were infected by that first virus are immune to the second one.

Influenza is transmitted from person to person by coughing and sneezing. This causes droplets of secretions containing the virus from the infected person to be breathed in by someone who is not infected, who starts to have the symptoms from one to three days later.

The part of animals in the spread of influenza is not well known. Certainly domestic pets do not carry the disease. There is some evidence, however, that farm animals – for example, horses, hens and pigs – do get a similar illness. In the pig, it is known that the virus is the same as the flu virus in human beings. In fact, the pig is thought to have acted as a potential carrier of swine influenza which caused a pandemic and killed about 25 million people in 1918–19.

Symptoms

The symptoms come on suddenly, with shivering and generalized aching in the arms, legs and back. The patient may have a HEADACHE, aching eyes, a sore or dry THROAT and sometimes a COUGH and a runny nose (*see* RHINITIS). Occasionally there may also be the symptoms of a stomach upset, with VOMITING and DIARRHOEA. If the temperature is taken at this point, it is above normal, usually over 101°F (38.5°C) and up to 102°F (39°C).

The symptoms and FEVER continue for two to five days and leave the patient feeling tired and weak. He or she may also feel depressed and washed out and should be reassured that a period of depression after flu is quite normal and may last a few weeks. The cough also may persist for one or two weeks After the other symptoms have gone.

If a patient with flu is examined by a doctor when he or she is ill, there is usually little to see, except a feverish person with an inflamed throat. These are the classic signs of flu. If a patient has some immunity, he or she may often have a milder illness, with fewer symptoms and only a small rise in temperature.

The difference in immunity explains why some people get the disease worse than others, and why people who have been in very close contact with an infected person may not feel ill at all. People become immune once they have had a certain type of influenza, because their bodies' defence mechanisms recognize the virus a second time and prevent it from multiplying and causing a real attack of flu. (This recognition does not happen if the flu virus has altered its appearance.)

Complications and treatment

Influenza can strike all age groups, but the old are particularly prone to the complications of flu.

The most common complication is a chest infection. This can vary from a mild cough to PNEUMONIA. Sometimes the virus itself causes this, but more commonly another germ enters the body which has been weakened by flu, and infects the chest. Old people and those who already have chest trouble are more likely to develop a chest infection after an attack of flu.

If the flu patient has a severe cough, is producing green or yellow sputum (PHLEGM), has chest pains, or feels breathless, it is advisable to call the doctor. People who have other things wrong with them – for example, chest trouble, heart disease or kidney problems – should let their doctor know if they catch flu because he may want to give them an antibiotic to prevent them from having complications.

If an attack of flu seems prolonged and is not progressing normally, it is wise to call the doctor without delay.

Very, very rarely the flu virus itself can cause severe pneumonia, or the disease can be caused by another germ, a *staphylococcus*, which gets into the body already undermined by flu. In very severe cases, the flu virus can also affect the heart or the brain, but fortunately this hardly ever happens.

Immunization

There is at present no cure for flu. The flu virus is always changing its appearance to fool the body's defences, and this explains why IMMUNIZATION sometimes does not work.

In spite of this difficulty, it is very useful, especially in communities such as schools, factories and old people's homes. It is also useful in attempts to prevent flu in people who are likely, because of some other illness such as chest trouble, or because of old age, to develop more serious complications.

The flu injection is given in a single dose in the autumn. It usually has no side-effects, but occasionally makes the arm sore or causes a slight rise in temperature for 24 hours. The injection will offer you 60 per cent protection against flu in the winter of the year when you have it, and even if you do get flu, it may make it a much milder attack than you would otherwise have had.

Inheritance, *see* **Heredity**

Insomnia, *see* **Sleep and sleep problems**

Intercourse, sexual, *see* **Sexual intercourse**

Intestines and intestinal disorders

The word 'intestine' is commonly used to mean the whole ALIMENTARY CANAL from the mouth to the anus, but strictly it applies to only two sections of the complete canal: the narrow, coiled small intestine, which leads from the lower exit of the STOMACH and comprises the U-shaped DUODENUM, the coiled JEJUNUM and the ILEUM, and the wider but shorter large intestine. The latter is made up of the caecum, the APPENDIX, the COLON, RECTUM and anus, from which the remains of digested food are eliminated.

It is in the intestines that the majority of the digestive processes take place, after food has been worked upon by a mixture of chemicals in the stomach, and here that the job of absorption takes place.

The workings of the intestines

The first part of the intestine, which takes food from the stomach, is the duodenum – so named because, in ancient times, its measurement in length was seen as 12 fingers' breadth (*duodecim* is Latin for 'twelve'). It curls round like a letter C at the upper right-hand side of the abdomen, quite near the backbone. In the centre of the curve of the C lies the PANCREAS, which produces

The small and large intestines

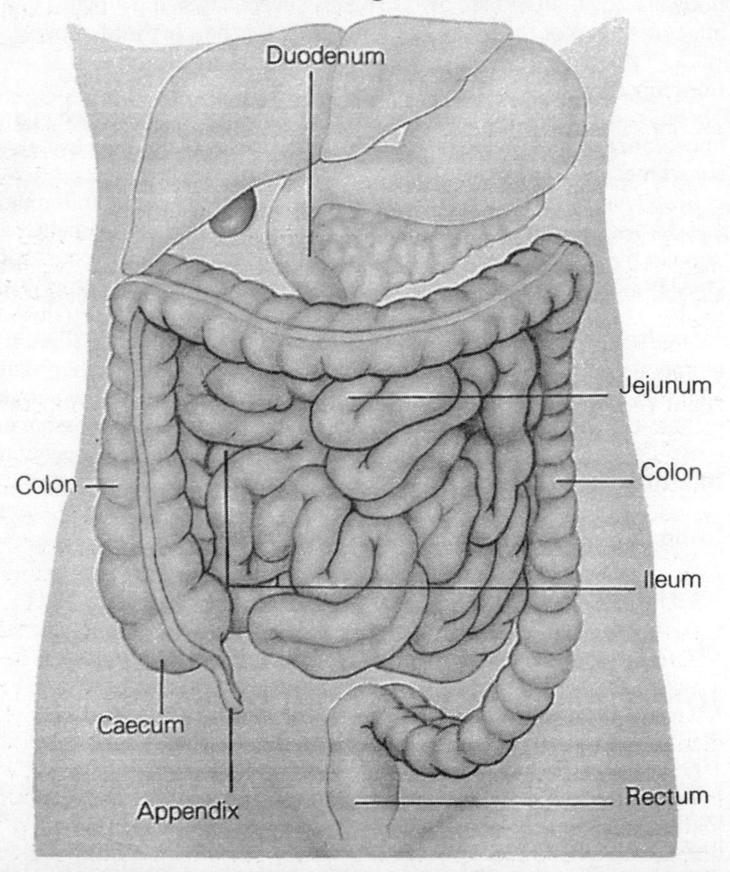

large quantities of ENZYMES that flow into the duodenum through a small duct. These are digestive enzymes which, in particular, help to digest fat and protein. In addition to the pancreatic juices, BILE from the LIVER also flows along the bile duct and into the duodenum to aid the process of digestion of fats.

The upper part of the small bowel is the jejunum, and the lower part is called the ileum. The lining of the jejunum produces some enzymes and extra fluid which lubricates the flow of the contents through the small bowel. By the time food gets to the jejunum, it is the consistency of watery paste. Muscles in the wall of the intestine contract rhythmically to push the contents through the bowel. Because the inner surface of the jejunum is folded upon itself many times, a large surface area is in contact with the food inside the bowel. Nutrients are absorbed into the wall of the jejunum and then pass into the bloodstream. Veins from the jejunum take the nutrients to the liver, where they may be changed into other chemicals which the body can use for repair of tissues or for energy. Most sugars are absorbed in the jejunum, along with some fats and proteins. Further absorption continues in the ileum until the contents reach the large bowel, or colon, by which time only indigestible fibrous material is left.

The lower part of the small intestine and the large bowel contain not only the remains of food but also large numbers of bacteria. These bacteria are useful to the body because they aid digestion, and do not cause any infection – unless they get into the wrong part of the body as a result of a disorder of the bowel.

The colon acts as a kind of filter to remove excess fluid from the solid waste matter, which is then stored as faeces in the descending colon on the left-hand side of the abdomen before passing to the rectum ready for the bowels to open.

Symptoms of intestinal disorders

Although there are a number of different types of disease that can affect the bowels, the range of symptoms they produce is quite limited.

Several different types of disease affect the ability of the small bowel to absorb nutrients, causing a condition known as MALABSORPTION. Sometimes malabsorption of only a few nutrients occurs, but more often it affects the complete process of digestion, so that the sufferer does not absorb sufficient food to satisfy the body's needs and loses weight – sometimes alarmingly quickly.

DIARRHOEA is another symptom of intestinal disorder. If the colon fails to absorb fluid from the contents that flow from the ileum, diarrhoea results. Many diseases of the large bowel, ranging from GASTRO-ENTERITIS to severe inflammatory disease of the bowel (*see* COLON AND COLITIS), can cause diarrhoea, but some diseases of the small bowel may also result in diarrhoea.

CONSTIPATION is often the result of a diet that has insufficient fibre, and it improves once the diet is corrected – with additional fibrous foods such as wholegrain cereals (*see* NUTRITION). But a change in bowel function from normal motions to constipation without any obvious change in diet should always be reported to a doctor.

Internal bleeding inside the bowel may occur without any obvious signs if the bleeding point is high up in the course of the intestines and the amount of bleeding is small. However, the patient may become ANAEMIC and the first sign of the problem may simply be tiredness and shortage of breath. If the bleeding is low down, in the large bowel, or if the bleeding is large in quantity, it will be obvious and may be mixed with the bowel motion. Such bleeding must always be reported to a doctor and investigated, because it may be a sign of serious bowel disease. Sometimes, however, the bleeding may come from haemorrhoids (PILES), which can be treated relatively easily, and are not a particularly serious problem.

Abdominal pain can occur as a result of abnormal stretching of the wall of the intestines, or as a result of excessive muscular activity in the wall of the bowel. Such pains are usually intermittent and griping or 'colicky'. If the intestines are inflamed, the pain is usually duller and constant, but can be severe.

Emotional stress

In both children and adults, emotional STRESS can upset the intestines. Some children react physically to emotional problems by VOMITING, diarrhoea and abdominal pains. Adults may have diarrhoea or colicky pains which occur at times of stress.

The answer to such problems is not to give medicine for the bowels but to sort out the cause of emotional stress. However, anyone with recurrent abdominal pain – particularly a child – needs a medical opinion just in case anything is physically wrong. There may also be a need for psychological help to resolve emotional difficulties.

Investigation of internal diseases

One of the most important parts of the investigation of any intestinal disease is the history of the condition, which the doctor records very carefully. The doctor notes the timing and frequency of symptoms such as pain, alteration in bowels or vomiting, and wants to know what the patient has been eating. The doctor also asks questions about general physical and psychological health.

Next, the doctor examines the patient's abdomen, often concluding with an internal examination of the rectum.

Further investigations depend on the suspected problem. Blood tests for anaemia, and for the function of the liver and KIDNEYS, are routine, as is a laboratory examination of the urine and often of the STOOLS. A plain X-ray of the abdomen may be useful to the doctor in an emergency, but it shows little detail of the bowel. Special X-rays using BARIUM to outline the intestines are more often carried out.

Sometimes the doctor wishes to examine the inside of the bowel directly. An instrument called a *sigmoidoscope* allows the doctor to see the rectum and lower part of the descending colon; a *colonoscope* is a flexible instrument which can be passed through the back passage to allow the doctor to look at most of the colon (*see* ENDOSCOPY). Small pieces of tissues can be removed for examination using either of these instruments.

Intra-uterine device (IUD), *see* **Contraception, Ectopic pregnancy, Salpingitis**

Intravenous pyelogram (IVP), *see* **Cystitis, X-rays**

Intussusception, *see* **Ileum**

In vitro fertilization (IVF), *see* **Test-tube babies**

Iodine

Iodine's vital role is in the production of THYROID hormone. This hormone, called *thyroxine,* is responsible for promoting normal growth and development and for maintaining the body's 'basal metabolic rate': its life-supporting systems. Too much thyroxine and the body's systems speed up; too little and they slow down.

Iodine is very readily absorbed from the small bowel and passes into the bloodstream. The thyroid gland – which is situated in the lower part of the front of the neck – extracts iodine from the blood passing through it and concentrates most of the iodine in the body into the cells of the gland. The gland then incorporates iodine into the two main hormones which it makes – thyroxine and tri-iodothyronine.

These two hormones are released by the thyroid gland when it is stimulated by a controlling hormone called *thyroid-stimulating hormone* (TSH), which is itself produced in the PITUITARY gland in the centre of the head just underneath the brain. If insufficient thyroid hormones are present in the bloodstream the pituitary releases more TSH, which causes extra thyroxine and tri-iodothyronine to be released and stimulates the production of more hormones.

If insufficient iodine reaches the thyroid gland to produce enough thyroid hormones for the body, the gland is stimulated by thyroid-stimulating hormone in an attempt to encourage it to produce more hormones. The gland then enlarges and becomes visible on the front of the neck as a *goitre.*

Sources of iodine

Seawater contains iodine and so the element is found in all seafood – fish and shellfish – and in seaweed. It is present in the soil in many areas, particularly low-lying farming land, so vegetables and other crops grown in these areas also contain appreciable quantities of iodine. However, it is not possible to list the iodine content of foods such as vegetables because it depends entirely on where they are grown. If seaweed or fish meal is used to fertilize the land, the crops will contain considerable amounts of iodine. Some natural water supplies contain iodine, but others have none.

The amount of iodine we need every day is about 140 micrograms (a microgram is one millionth of a gram). As there is plenty of iodine in any type of seafood, eating fish once a week will give more than enough iodine for everyone.

Antiseptic uses

A few years ago, it was thought that a dab of iodine was enough to kill all the germs in a cut. But now it has been shown that the antiseptic effect of iodine is neutralized by blood and thus it does nothing except dye the skin yellow. However, it quickly and efficiently kills germs on unbroken skin and surgeons use it on their hands and the patient's skin to prevent any risk of infection during operations.

More useful as an antiseptic is the iodine-containing compound iodoform (tri-iodomethane). Iodine is also a constituent of several drugs, such as that used to treat *Herpes simplex* (COLD SORE).

Iridectomy, *see* Glaucoma

Iritis, *see* Spondylitis

Iron

Iron is a MINERAL found in the body's red BLOOD cells. It cannot be produced in the body so, in order to maintain good health, it is essential to eat some foods that contain iron.

ANAEMIA, caused by iron deficiency, is one of the commonest deficiency disorders in women, but rarely occurs in men. This is because women lose blood with menstruation (*see* PERIODS) during the reproductive years of their lives and do not take enough iron in their diet to replace it. When iron-deficiency anaemia is found in children, men or post-menopausal women, however, it may suggest that there is a problem elsewhere. There may be a slow-bleeding duodenal ULCER or, particularly in children, there may be some disease causing abnormal iron absorption from food in the intestine (*see* MALABSORPTION).

Iron's role

The red blood cells contain haemoglobin, which is responsible for the vital activity of carrying oxygen from the lungs to the tissues, and which also gives blood its red colouring; iron is an essential ingredient of haemoglobin. A lack of iron, therefore, is by far the commonest, though not the only, cause of anaemia.

The body contains about $^1/_{10}$ oz (3–4 g) of iron. Seventy per cent of this is present in the red blood cells which circulate in the bloodstream, with a further small amount in the BONE MARROW. About 20 per cent of the iron is stored in the LIVER and the SPLEEN, much of it is in the form of *ferritin* – as iron-containing protein. A small amount of the body's iron is not concerned with the manufacture of haemoglobin, but is involved in equally important cellular functions. Many of the ENZYMES which regulate a normal cell's activity depend on iron for their activity.

Iron loss

The body has no way of excreting iron. However, since iron is widely distributed in the tissues the loss of cells from surfaces such as the skin and the lining of the intestine leads to iron loss.

The total amount lost in this way each day is about 1 milligram (mg). In women, although menstrual bleeding usually occurs only once a month, the average loss due to this amounts to a further 1 mg per day. Thus women normally lose about twice as much iron as men.

Female iron loss is also increased during PREGNANCY when the foetus and the placenta absorb much of the woman's iron stores. The total daily iron requirement during pregnancy is almost double that of a non-pregnant woman during her reproductive years. And, in particular, during the last four months of pregnancy a great deal of iron goes into building the blood volume of the baby. During these four months, up to 7.5 mg of iron are required per day. For this reason, iron supplements are frequently prescribed, but perhaps not until after the 14th week of pregnancy. This is because iron tablets can cause disturbance of the intestine and lead either to CONSTIPATION or DIARRHOEA, occasionally to NAUSEA and in some cases even to actual VOMITING.

Since the normal iron stores are quite large in an average man, it would take him about three years to develop iron-deficiency anaemia. However, it occurs much more quickly if there is blood loss, such as might occur if someone is suffering from slow bleeding from ulcers or PILES.

Severe anaemia is immediately obvious because the sufferer will become very pale. Less severe degrees can be detected by blood tests. If there is a low haemoglobin level in the blood, the fact that it is due to lack of iron is confirmed by looking at the red blood cells under a microscope. When iron-deficiency anaemia is present, the red blood cells become smaller, whereas in other causes of anaemia, they tend to enlarge or remain of normal size. To avoid confusion, a blood test can be carried out which measures the level of iron stored in the body – a 'serum ferritin' test. As iron deficiency may be caused by chronic internal bleeding – for example, from a stomach ulcer – further tests may be needed to find out why iron deficiency has occurred. If it is simply the result of a poor intake of iron, treatment is with iron pills, which are taken until the level of haemoglobin is back to normal. This will be confirmed by a blood test.

Iron absorption

Iron is absorbed from the small intestine. The normal absorption is in the region of 1 mg per day, which only just balances the normal losses. The fact that iron loss and iron absorption are set in this critical balance does explain why it is relatively easy to have an iron deficiency and, therefore, why it is quite a common complaint.

In fact, only about 10 per cent of the iron we actually eat ever gets absorbed, although this proportion may be higher when there is iron deficiency. Since the normal loss is about 1 mg, people should therefore eat about 10 mg of iron per day, though obviously menstruating women need more and should try and eat more of the foods which are rich in iron – such as liver, milk and eggs.

Iron is mainly found in red meat, particularly liver. There is also a considerable amount in pulses and in wheat flour which has not been refined. Purified white flour contains less iron, although iron is artificially added to flour and to breakfast cereals. Iron from vegetables is not as easily absorbed by the intestines as iron from meat.

Excess iron

Iron overload in the system causes a disease called *haemochromatosis*. This rare condition is known to be inherited as an autosomal recessive condition (*see* HEREDITY). Iron is absorbed in excessive amounts from the intestine. The disease may affect the liver, causing CIRRHOSIS, and may rarely accumulate in the PANCREAS, giving rise to DIABETES, or in a man in the TESTES, which may then cease to produce male hormones.

The treatment for iron overload is repeated removal of blood at intervals. This lowers the overall level of iron in the body. Once cirrhosis is established, repeated removal of iron will not make it disappear, but the treatment may help to slow down the progress of the disease and the effects of internal bleeding.

Irritable bowel syndrome

This is one of the commonest causes of abdominal pain and disturbance of bowel action. It has been estimated that about 40 per cent of patients referred to specialist gastro-enterologists for investigation have this condition. The precise cause remains unknown, although a link with STRESS is very common.

Over the years, a number of different names have been used to describe this condition including mucous colitis, spastic colon, irritable colon and nervous diarrhoea (*see also* COLON AND COLITIS). It is now usually known as irritable bowel syndrome (IBS) because doctors realize that most of the bowel is involved, even though the symptoms seem to be related largely to the colon, or large bowel (INTESTINE).

Irritable bowel is much more common among women than men – about five women have the condition to every two men. It can occur at almost any age, although symptoms usually start in early adult life. Most people with irritable bowel are in the age range 20 to 40. However, it can sometimes affect children as young as three or four.

Symptoms

Almost everyone with irritable bowel experiences pain. For any one patient, the pain tends to follow a particular pattern, but different patients experience different types of pain. Usually it is griping or colicky in nature and tends to occur in bouts lasting a few minutes or anything up to a few hours. Often the pain is worse after eating, and it may improve immediately after the patient has passed a bowel motion, although sometimes this makes the pain worse. The site of the pain is often on the left or right of the abdomen, although it can occur almost anywhere in the abdomen such as high up under the ribs or low down in the groin.

Most sufferers also have wind and distension; this may produce loud gurgling noises at regular intervals inside the abdomen, but can be passed by belching. Sometimes a large amount of gas is passed with bowel motions. The bowel habits are often disturbed. Sufferers may complain of DIARRHOEA or they may be CONSTIPATED. Loose watery diarrhoea is uncommon; it is more likely that the sufferer will pass frequent small-formed motions and often have the feeling that the bowel has not emptied properly. They keep going back to the toilet, but with little result. Sometimes slimy mucus is passed with the bowel motion – hence the old name for the condition, 'mucous colitis'.

Many sufferers also complain of various types of INDIGESTION. Nausea is not uncommon, nor is heartburn.

The symptoms may be worse first thing in the morning, but they can also occur at periods of stress. Some sufferers find that symptoms clear completely when they are free of worries.

Causes

A variety of possible explanations have been put forward to explain the symptoms of irritable bowel syndrome. It has been found that the symptoms experienced by individual patients can be reproduced by an experiment in which a small balloon is used to distend part of the bowel. However, this does not explain why symptoms arise in the first place.

Some patients seem to develop symptoms after eating particular foods, and it is possible that a type of food ALLERGY is responsible for a few cases.

In many patients, however, there is a very clear relationship to stress or DEPRESSION, and it appears that psychological factors are responsible for the syndrome in most cases. The activity of the intestines is governed by the AUTONOMIC NERVOUS SYSTEM which is linked to the subconscious part of the brain. Stress appears to upset the activity of the autonomic system in many people, and this can lead to a variety of symptoms – including the irritable bowel syndrome.

Some doctors have suggested that the syndrome is a direct result of a low-fibre diet, but this has not been proved – even though a high-fibre diet may help to relieve some of the symptoms.

Occasionally, the first attack of irritable bowel follows a bowel infection, such as GASTRO-ENTERITIS.

Investigation

Because the symptoms of irritable bowel may mimic those of a number of potentially serious physical conditions, doctors are very careful to exclude other possible causes. A thorough examination is carried out, and usually this includes an internal examination of the RECTUM. If the patient is a woman, the doctor may also carry out a vaginal examination. Often the pain experienced by women from an irritable bowel is indistinguishable from pains caused by abnormalities in the UTERUS or OVARIES. The pain of irritable bowel may even be triggered by sexual intercourse.

Once examination is complete, routine blood tests are usually performed to check for ANAEMIA. Other blood tests, such as a 'sedimentation rate', can help to exclude diseases such as ulcerative colitis. If the diagnosis remains in doubt, the doctor may suggest a sigmoidoscopy (visual examination of the rectum) or a BARIUM MEAL or barium enema. These tests can rule out other diseases such as CANCERS, and DIVERTICULITIS (bulges in the intestine caused by inflammation).

Treatment

Once the diagnosis has been established, the doctor usually discusses the significance of the illness with the patient in some detail. It is important for the sufferer to come to terms with the fact that the pains and upset bowel actions are mostly likely to be directly linked to some factor in his or her life-style. Over-ambition or stress at work or at home may be a potent factor in triggering the symptoms, and the remedy may lie in the patient's own hands. Sometimes it helps if the sufferer keeps a diary of daily events and of the symptoms experienced. This can help to pinpoint the trigger factors.

If there are obvious severe psychological factors, professional help may be needed from a PSYCHOLOGIST or PSYCHIATRIST. If the patient is depressed, he or she may be given anti-depressant medication. Otherwise the patient may be advised to relieve stress by regular EXERCISE and RELAXATION, or by taking a course in yoga or autogenic training.

If the bowel action is very irregular, it may help to increase the amount of fibre in the diet. Increasing fibre suddenly by taking large amounts of bran may trigger off distension and colic, so it is better to increase fibre gradually by eating wholemeal cereals or wholemeal bread and gradually increasing the amount of vegetables and fruit in the diet.

Drugs may be prescribed for irritable bowel, although their effect is unpredictable. Some people are helped by 'anti-spasmodic' drugs – others are not. Peppermint oil, given in a capsule, does help many sufferers. If the patient has diarrhoea, an anti-diarrhoea medicine may be needed whenever the symptoms are troublesome.

Ischaemia

This is the term used to describe an insufficient supply of BLOOD to any part of the body. All living cells require OXYGEN and nutrients, which are carried in the bloodstream via a network of ARTERIES and smaller blood vessels (arterioles). Ischaemia in the limb arteries (peripheral vascular disease) occurs when the vessels become furred up, either by blood cells (platelets) or fatty deposits, and the blood flow to the legs is reduced.

Causes

The commonest cause of ischaemia is atherosclerosis affecting the arteries to the lower limbs. In this condition, fatty deposits form inside the arteries, which can eventually lead to blockage of the affected artery. Usually, atherosclerosis affects most of the arteries once the condition is established, but some arteries may be more seriously affected than others. Atherosclerosis in the coronary arteries, which supply blood to the heart muscle, can lead to angina or HEART ATTACKS (*ischaemic heart disease*) and atherosclerosis in the arteries in the neck may cause STROKES.

There are a number of life-style factors which can predispose to atherosclerosis and actually lead to CORONARY HEART DISEASE, ischaemia in the legs or strokes. Cigarette SMOKING is the most important. A smoker is several times more likely than a non-smoker to develop atherosclerosis – heavier smokers are even more at risk. Indeed it is very unusual for anyone who is a non-smoker to develop ischaemia in the legs unless he or she is diabetic or has a family history of atherosclerosis.

Other risk-factors include high BLOOD PRESSURE and a high blood CHOLESTEROL level. OBESITY can contribute to both high blood pressure and a high cholesterol level, and a diet with large amounts of animal fat can contribute to high cholesterol.

Another, rarer, cause of ischaemia is a condition called *Buerger's disease*. The interior lining of the blood vessels becomes inflamed and thickened to such an extent that blood flow is reduced. This condition only affects smokers, and it can occur at a relatively young age – heavy smokers in their 20s may be affected whereas atherosclerosis is unlikely to cause ischaemia before 40 years of age. Chemicals in cigarette smoke appear to be responsible for this condition, although the exact cause has not been identified.

Symptoms

The earliest sign of ischaemia is usually a cramp-like pain which occurs in the calf and develops on walking. This pain is called *intermittent claudication*. At first the patient may be able to walk a considerable distance before the pain appears – say half a mile along the flat. But as the blockage to the artery worsens, the pain appears after only a few minutes' walking. Walking uphill brings on the pain much more quickly as does climbing stairs. In severe cases, the patient may be able to walk only a few yards before the pain appears. On stopping, the pain goes away after a minute or two. If the blockage from atherosclerosis is in the aorta (the main blood vessel in the chest and abdomen), pain may be felt in the buttocks and thighs; the patient may also experience IMPOTENCE.

In the most severe cases, pain may appear when the patient is at rest – either in bed at night, or simply sitting in a chair. The skin looks pale and white and hair growth over the affected area ceases. Once there is pain at rest, there is then a considerable risk of GANGRENE (tissue death). The feet may turn blue (*cyanosis*), and infection can set in easily if the skin of the foot is damaged.

Investigations

The doctor will first examine the limbs and check to feel the pulses in the feet and behind the knee. Once claudication has occurred, the pulses in the feet are usually absent. If pulses are absent behind the knee and in the groin, then this is a sign of a blockage in the arteries high up in the abdomen – for example, in the aorta or the iliac artery, which runs towards the groin from the aorta. The doctor will take particular note of the condition of the skin, looking for the earliest signs of possible gangrene.

The exact nature of the arterial damage can be assessed using a special type of X-ray called an *angiogram*. Contrast medium is injected into the arteries which allows them to show up on an X-ray, and then the size and extent of any blockages can be assessed.

Treatment

The first and most important part of treatment is for the patient to stop smoking – if he or she is a smoker. Whether the cause of ischaemia is atherosclerosis or Buerger's disease, stopping smoking will reduce any further damage. If the patient continues to smoke, the condition invariably worsens. The patient must pay careful attention to the care of the feet, keeping them clean and dry and avoiding damage to the skin of the feet at all costs.

Vasodilator drugs may be given which help open up alternative channels for blood to reach ischaemia tissues, and they may increase the distance the patient can walk before claudication appears, but they are not a cure for the condition.

Once a patient is disabled by claudication, or if there is any pain during rest, surgery will be considered. The surgeon may be able to bypass a blockage by grafting on an artificial artery made of special knitted plastic material (Dacron); a piece of vein taken from another part of the body is occasionally used. Sometimes it is possible for the surgeon to open the arteries which are affected, and remove the atheromatous deposits – a procedure called *endarterectomy*.

Itching, *see* Pruritis

IUD (intra-uterine device), *see* Contraception, Ectopic pregnancy, Salpingitis

IVF (in vitro fertilization), *see* Test-tube babies

IVP (intravenous pyelogram), *see* Cystitis

J

Jaundice

A person who looks yellow is described as 'being jaundiced', but jaundice is not a disease in itself but a symptom of disorder in the LIVER or elsewhere.

Red blood cells are constantly being broken down by the SPLEEN and replaced so that they can carry out their vital functions in the body efficiently. A substance called *bilirubin* is released during this process. It is carried to the liver where it is subjected to a process called conjugation. This makes the bilirubin dissolve so that it can be excreted in the BILE produced by the liver. The dark brown colour of faeces is due to bilirubin, which has been broken down into brownish-yellow pigments.

A raised level of bilirubin in the blood can result from a problem at any one of the stages in the release and elimination of bilirubin. It is this raised level that gives the yellow colour of jaundice.

Types of jaundice

Pre-hepatic: This type is rather uncommon, but there are certain congenital disorders of blood cell function which lead to increased breakdown of abnormal red blood cells. There are also other circumstances – known as haemolysis – in which too many red blood cells are broken down.

Hepatocellular: HEPATITIS, which is quite common, causes jaundice because it inflames the liver cells. Drugs such as the contraceptive pill, anti-diabetic drugs and some antibiotics may also cause inflammation of the liver cells or small bile ducts and produce jaundice but these are very rare cases.

ALCOHOL is a frequent cause of jaundice, either as a single attack after a prolonged drinking session, or else as a result of alcoholic CIRRHOSIS.

Obstructive jaundice: The commonest cause of obstructive jaundice is a gallstone lodged in the common bile duct (*see* GALL BLADDER AND STONES). The bile duct may also become blocked if there is a tumour pressing on it, and jaundice is a fairly common way for CANCER of the PANCREAS to come to light.

If a person's skin looks sallow and yellow when he or she is tired it is possible that there is a slightly higher level of bilirubin in the blood than is normal. This may be due to an extremely common congenital disorder called *Gilbert's syndrome,* where people suffer from a long-term, low-grade jaundice. It may be worsened by fasting or infection, but does not usually cause any trouble.

Symptoms

Yellowness is usually the first symptom, showing first in the whites of the eyes and then in the skin. Pain may occur as a result of the underlying disease.

In obstructive jaundice, patients often have pale stools and dark urine, as bilirubin is not making its way into the bowel. Conjugated bilirubin is being dammed up and is leaking from the liver cells back into the blood, and because it is dissoluble, it can pass through the kidneys and come out in the urine, making it darker.

Diagnosis

The cause of jaundice is particularly important. The hepatocellular sort may not always require specific treatment. In contrast, a gallstone blocking the common bile duct needs to be removed by surgery or an infection may start in the bile ducts behind the obstruction.

Blood tests may be used in the diagnosis; if necessary, an ULTRASOUND scan will show the bile ducts in the liver. If they are dilated, the cause is likely to be an obstruction, whereas if they are normal, a hepatocellular cause is more likely to be found.

When an obstruction is suspected, it may be diagnosed in one of two ways. The first is to insert a fine needle into the liver through the right side. This will enter one of the many small bile ducts and then dye can be injected to outline the obstruction. This is called a *per-cutaneous cholangiogram.*

Alternatively, a flexible gastroscope (*see* ENDOSCOPY) may be passed down to the bile duct, a tiny tube inserted and X-ray dye injected to show the site of any obstruction. Both these diagnostic techniques are carried out in hospital.

Jaundice in newborn babies

This is very common, resulting from the fact that the newborn liver is often not quite mature enough to cope with the normal breakdown of red blood cells.

Because the liver is immature, the bilirubin in a baby's bloodstream tends to be unconjugated. High levels of unconjugated bilirubin in the blood may lead to it being deposited in various parts of the brain, causing permanent damage. This means that severe jaundice in babies within the first few days of life has to be treated promptly. Treatment under a powerful ultraviolet light increases the breakdown of bilirubin in the skin, but in severe cases, a complete change of blood may be needed. This technique, called *exchange transfusion,* is only necessary in the first days of life. After this, the liver starts to conjugate the bilirubin.

Jejunostomy, *see* **Stoma care**

Jejunum

This is the part of the small INTESTINE, leading on from the DUODENUM and connecting with the ILEUM. The jejunum extends about 8 ft (2.5 m) before it merges with the ileum. There is no sudden break between them, more of a gradual change. The jejunum has a diameter of about 1½ in (3.8 cm), while that of the ileum is slightly smaller. The jejunum also has thicker walls than the ileum, although they both consist of two muscular layers on the outside, and inner layers of mucosa which line the inner diameter of intestines, or lumen.

Unlike the duodenum, which is more or less fixed firmly to the back of the abdominal wall, the jejunum and the ileum are supported on a membrane called the *mesentery*. This fan-like structure consists of two layers of PERITONEUM, and is attached to the back wall of the abdomen. The end which supports the intestine is about 6 yd (5.5 m) long. The depth of the mesentery, measured from its base all the way out to the intestines is about 8 in (20 cm) – this allows both the jejunum and ileum some room in which to float about quite freely within the abdominal cavity.

Role of the jejunum

The jejunum provides the site where the useful nutritional elements of food are absorbed, leaving mainly water and food waste behind. The absorption process is then completed in the ileum. To carry out this role, the jejunum has a very specialized interior designed to ensure that the greatest possible area is in contact with the food.

The interior of the jejunum consists of a series of circular folds. And if you were to look at this inner surface under a microscope, you would see that the whole surface is made up of delicate finger-like projections, called *villi*, each of which measures approximately 1 mm. The surface in contact with digested food is increased yet further because the cellular surface of each villus is gathered into what is known as the 'brush border'.

Absorption of food

Since the jejunum is designed to allow the passage of food from the intestine into the blood, it needs an efficient blood supply. The arteries and veins which carry the blood to and from the walls of the jejunum run in the mesentery. The veins which drain the jejunum, like the veins draining the rest of the intestine, do not go straight back to the heart, but are gathered together to form the portal vein which drains into the LIVER. This means that food absorbed into the blood is delivered to the liver for processing before it goes into the rest of the body.

As well as absorbing food into the blood, some of the fatty constituents of the food are absorbed into the LYMPHATIC SYSTEM instead. Each villus has a central lymph channel or *lacteal* which enables this to take place. This special fat-containing lymph fluid which drains from the intestine is called *chyle*.

Jejunal disorders

The jejunum can stop working as a result of problems, such as peritonitis – inflammation of the PERITONEUM – or major abdominal surgery. This condition is called *ileus* (*see* ILEUM) and soon rights itself once the cause is treated.

The jejunum can also present problems when its BLOOD supply is interrupted as a result of a loop of jejunum becoming stuck in a HERNIA, or because of arterial disease.

Although rare, jejunal disease usually gives rise to problems of MALABSORPTION. Most commonly, it is fat that is absorbed least well, and where this occurs, there is an excess of fat in the faeces, making them pale, bulky and more foul smelling than usual.

The usual cause of malabsorption is a disease called COELIAC DISEASE where the villi of the jejunum are lost, leaving a completely flat inner surface – and, of course, a far smaller area in contact with digested foodstuffs. This happens when people are sensitive to gluten, which is an integral part of wheat and other cereals. The treatment is a gluten-free diet.

Diagnosis of disorders of the jejunum is carried out by means of a technique called a jejunal BIOPSY, which is done with a device called a *Crosby capsule*. The capsule, which is attached to a long thin tube, is passed down into the jejunum, and suction is applied to the tube at the mouth. This sucks a little fold of jejunal lining into the capsule through a small hole in its side, which is then nipped off by a tiny knife. The capsule is withdrawn and the lining of the jejunum can be inspected in the laboratory to see if it is flat.

Joints

There are two main types of joints – *synovial* and *fibrous*. Synovial joints are designed to allow a large range of movements and are lined with a slippery coating called *synovium*. Fibrous joint movement is limited by fibrous tissue.

The synovial joints can be subdivided, again depending on the range of movement of which they are capable. *Hinge* joints, such as the ones at the elbow and KNEE, allow bending and straightening movements; *gliding* joints allow sliding movements in all directions because the opposing bone surfaces are flattened or slightly curved. Examples of these joints are found in the spinal bones (*see* BACK), the WRIST and the tarsal bones of the FEET. *Pivot* joints in the NECK at the base of the skull and at the elbow are special types of hinge joints which rotate around the pivot. The pivot joint in the neck allows the head to turn and the one in the elbow allows twisting of the lower arm to enable movements, such as turning a doorknob or a screwdriver. Joints which can be moved in any direction, such as the HIP and SHOULDER, are called *ball-and-socket* joints.

Synovial joints

The joints in the fingers are typical examples of hinged synovial joints. The bone ends are covered in a tough elastic material called cartilage and this is known as *articulating cartilage*. The entire joint is enclosed in a very strong coating of tough gristle, called the *joint capsule*. This holds the joint in place and so prevents any abnormal movement.

Lining the inside of the joint but not running over the articulating cartilage is the synovium. This is a layer of tissue sometimes only one cell thick which provides fluid which oils the joint and prevents it drying up.

Fibrous joints

The fibrous joints are those of the back, the sacrum (the triangular bone between the hip bones) and some of the joints in the ankle and the PELVIS. These joints have no synovium. The bones are joined by tough, fibrous tissue, permitting very little movement.

The joints of the spine are a special exception. Besides being jointed by fibrous tissue they are cushioned by a small bubble of jelly called a disc. This capsule of jelly acts as a shock absorber and there is one between each of the spinal bones (*see* SLIPPED DISC).

Cartilaginous joints

Some joints in the body are formed between bone and cartilage. Cartilage (or gristle) is a rubbery substance that is very flexible and this allows a good deal of movement without the need for synovium. The joints between the RIBS and breast-bones at the front of the chest are cartilaginous joints. Those attaching the ribs to the back are synovial joints. These allow the ribs to move up and down freely when we breathe.

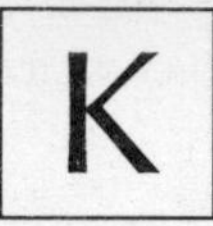

K, vitamin, *see* **Vitamins**

Kala-azar, *see* **Spleen**

Keratoderma blenorrhagia, *see* **Reiter's disease**

Kernicterus, *see* **Liver and liver diseases**

Keyhole surgery

Keyhole surgery is the popular term given to surgery performed using a laparoscope. This is a thin telescope that allows the surgeon to see and operate on organs within the abdominal cavity and the chest without having to make an incision through the skin. This has the advantage of reducing pain after the operation and usually allows the patient to leave hospital earlier. It also produces a far smaller scar.

The commonest operation performed using this technique is called laparoscopic cholecystectomy: this involves removal of the GALL BLADDER when it contains gallstones. Other operations that can be performed using the keyhole technique include HERNIA repair, appendicectomy, and operations on the stomach for HIATUS HERNIA and perforated ULCERS.

Kidneys and kidney diseases

The kidneys contain a complicated system of filters and tubes. Apart from their main function of filtering off impurities from the BLOOD, they enable many essential NUTRIENTS to be absorbed back into the bloodstream from the tubes. It is here that another important function of the kidneys is performed: balancing the SALT and WATER that is retained.

We have two kidneys, lying on the back wall of the abdomen. From the inner side of each kidney, a tube called the *ureter* runs down the back of the abdominal cavity and enters the BLADDER. The tube leading from the bladder is called the URETHRA. In women, its opening is in front of the VAGINA, and in men at the tip of the PENIS. The urethra in women is much shorter, and for this reason, they are more likely to suffer from various bladder infections than are men.

Functions

The kidneys contain thousands of tiny filtering units, or *nephrons*. Each nephron can be divided into two important parts – the filtering part, or *glomerulus*, and the *tubule*, where water and essential nutrients are extracted.

The glomerulus consists of a knot of tiny blood capillaries which have very thin walls. Water and the waste dissolved within it can pass freely across these walls into the collecting system of tubules on the other side. So large is this network of blood capillaries that it may contain – at any one moment – almost a quarter of the circulating blood and filters about 4.6 fl oz (130 ml) from the blood each minute.

The holes in the capillary wall form a biological sieve, and are so small that molecules beyond a certain size cannot pass through them. When the kidneys become infected, the glomeruli inflame and the 'sieve' fails to be so selective, allowing larger molecules to escape into the urine. One of the smallest protein molecules to find its way into the urine is *albumin*. This is why your doctor tests your urine for protein to see whether the kidneys are functioning properly.

The tubules run between the glomeruli to a collecting system which ultimately drains into the bladder. Each glomerulus is surrounded by a *Bowman's capsule*, which is the beginning of its tubule. It is here that almost all the filtered water and salt is reabsorbed, so that the URINE is concentrated. To reabsorb all this water, the body has a highly sophisticated system in which a HORMONE secreted into the blood from the PITUITARY gland in the brain changes the permeability of the tubule (its ability to reabsorb water).

While the hormone is in the blood, the tubule allows a great deal of water to be reabsorbed. When the hormone is 'turned off', however, the tubule becomes less permeable to water and more is lost in the urine – this is called *diuresis*, and the hormone concerned is known as *antidiuretic hormone* (ADH). In certain conditions, such as *diabetes insipidus* (not to be confused with 'sugar diabetes' or DIABETES mellitus), this hormone may be totally lacking. When this happens, the patient cannot conserve water, and so loses large quantities in the urine, which have to be replaced by drinking.

Another hormone, *aldosterone*, secreted by the ADRENAL GLANDS just above the kidneys, is responsible for exchanging sodium salt for potassium salt – so helping to control the balance of salt in the body. The kidney's production of an-other hormone, *renin*, is dependent on the level of salt. Renin activates yet another hormone, *angiotensin*, which is responsible for increases in BLOOD PRESSURE.

Parathormone, another hormone made by the four small PARATHYROID glands buried behind the thyroid gland, regulates the reabsorption of the essential mineral CALCIUM, from which our bones and teeth are made.

Kidney disorders

Once a nephron is destroyed, it seldom regrows. From birth onwards we gradually lose nephrons. Fortunately, we have so many that this seldom becomes a problem. Indeed, there are many more than are needed in the kidneys. In fact, about a third of all our nephrons do very little; they are gradually brought into use as wear and tear takes its toll.

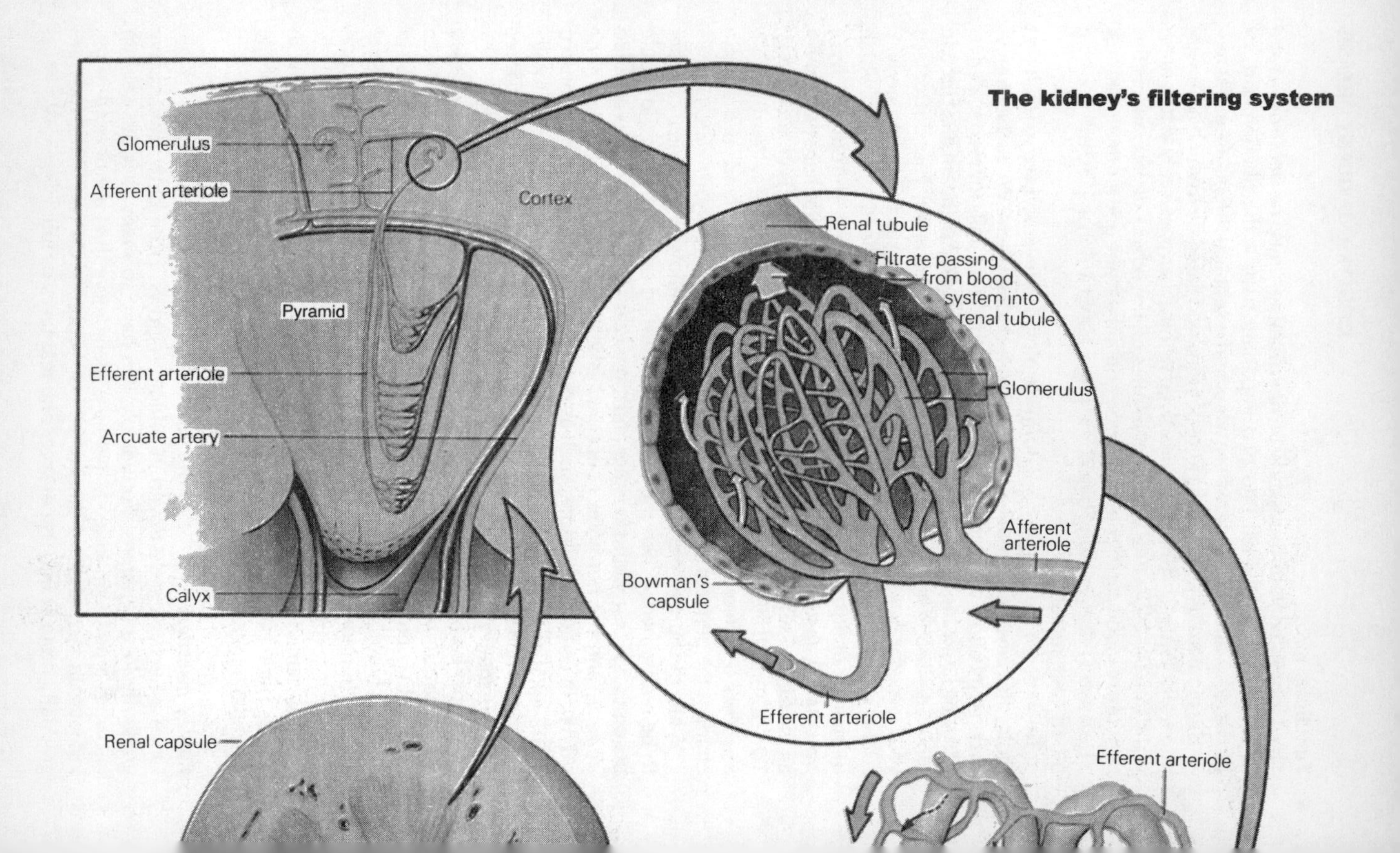
The kidney's filtering system
Glomerulus
Afferent arteriole
Cortex
Pyramid
Efferent arteriole
Arcuate artery
Calyx
Renal tubule
Filtrate passing from blood system into renal tubule
Glomerulus
Afferent arteriole
Bowman's capsule
Efferent arteriole
Renal capsule
Efferent arteriole

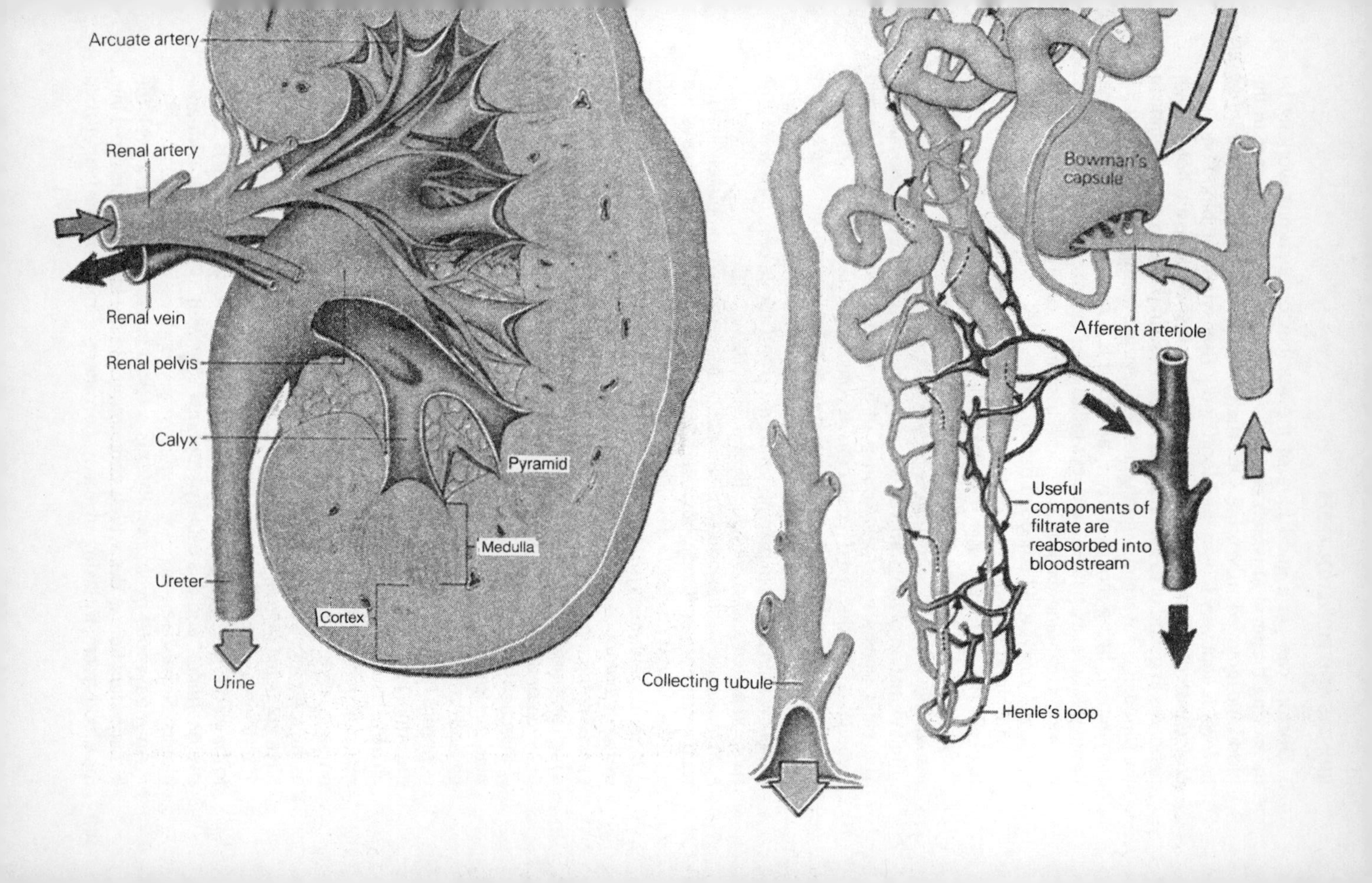

Arcuate artery
Renal artery
Renal vein
Renal pelvis
Calyx
Ureter
Urine
Pyramid
Medulla
Cortex
Collecting tubule
Bowman's capsule
Afferent arteriole
Useful components of filtrate are reabsorbed into bloodstream
Henle's loop

Doctors can get a good idea of the number of nephrons working by measuring the level at which certain waste substances are present in the blood and removed in the urine. One such waste product is called *creatinine.* Its level is kept very low in the blood and it rises when the blood becomes concentrated, as it does when we are thirsty, or when there are not enough nephrons to get rid of it. When doctors see a rise in the level of creatinine in the blood, it is a warning sign that the kidneys are failing. The rate at which creatinine is being removed from the blood is a better indication of renal (kidney) failure. If a patient's kidneys fail to clear more than 0.35 fl oz (10 ml) of blood creatinine each minute, the assistance of a DIALYSIS machine, or artificial kidney, will be needed before long.

High blood pressure causes the small blood vessels of the kidneys to thicken. This, in turn, causes damage to the nephrons and, as these are lost, the ability of the kidneys to remove waste products is hampered, ultimately resulting in kidney failure, unless the condition is treated.

Inflammation of the glomerulus can lead quite suddenly to kidney failure. The early signs are the appearance of albumin protein in the urine and sometimes particles of red blood cells. If your urine changes to a pink or rust colour, you should go and see your doctor as soon as possible. Excess water and salt cannot be excreted and so collect in parts of the body – which means either swollen ankles in patients who are up and about, or at the base of the spine in patients who are lying in bed (*see* OEDEMA).

In most cases, acute kidney inflammation settles down completely and full recovery is normal. Rarely, however, damage to the glomeruli is progressive, and the patient gradually develops renal failure. This is known as chronic *glomerulonephritis.* The most common cause of this condition is an ALLERGY to the *Streptococcus* bacteria. In the days before penicillin, streptococci caused epidemics of sore throat, followed by acute glomerulonephritis, and a high proportion of these victims developed chronic renal failure. However, this type of disease is seldom seen.

Infection of the kidneys, usually coming up the ureter from an infected bladder, is the most common cause of tubular disease. Repeated infections caused in this way can ultimately result in the destruction of sufficient nephrons to cause kidney failure. A tell-tale sign is the appearance of pus in the urine. In the early stages of disease, the patient's water may appear quite clear, and a microscopic examination is needed to spot the white cells which make up pus, but later the urine becomes cloudy. Of course, there are many other causes of cloudy urine, the most common being the first amount passed in the morning, which usually contains a deposit of undissolved salts which have collected overnight. Go and see your doctor if you are worried.

Kidney failure requires hospital treatment and usually the patient will have to have dialysis. Inflammation of the kidneys due to infection is called *pyelonephritis,* and this usually responds very well to treatment with antibiotics. *See also* NEPHRITIS.

An *intravenous pyelogram* (IVP) is a test done in hospital to check the kidney's function. A dye which concentrates in the kidneys is injected into the bloodstream. By taking an X-RAY, soon after the injection, the kidneys can be seen outlined by this dye, so giving doctors a good idea of their size. Later on, when the dye is excreted, the position of the ureters and the bladder can be seen. Patients suffering from an enlarged PROSTATE tend to be unable to empty their bladders completely, so any residual dye left in the bladder will show on the X-ray and confirm the diagnosis quite conclusively. This test is quite painless.

Called *calculi,* kidney stones are composed of the salts of calcium and phosphorus. The two main causes of kidney stones are infection and an excessive amount of calcium in the blood. Stones associated with infection are more common in women, and reach very large sizes so that they cannot pass down the ureter. They lie inside the kidney, and as they grow, they take up the shape of the collecting duct system in which they lie. When an X-ray picture is taken, they show up as a branched lump of chalk, looking rather like the antlers of a stag. Smaller stones may be passed down the ureter, causing colic and severe pain.

There is a dangerous form of kidney disease, which results in damage to the duct system, caused by certain drugs. *Phenacetin* has been particularly linked with this kind of kidney disease, but there is reason to believe that other anti-inflammatory drugs, such as *paracetamol* and *aspirin* may also cause trouble if large amounts are taken regularly. The people most at risk are those who take tablets of this kind habitually – especially if they live in hot climates, where the amount of the drug concentrated in the urine is likely to be high.

Klebsiella, *see* **Pneumonia**

Knee

This is the JOINT situated in the LEG between the thigh bone (the *femur*) and the shin bone (the *tibia*). It is designed in such a way as to allow great flexibility of movement, yet still be strong and stable enough to hold the body upright.

Structure and function

To allow easy movement, the knee joint is constructed like a hinge. The end of the femur is smoothly rounded off, and rests comfortably into the saucer-shaped top of the tibia. And the surfaces of the bones are covered with a layer of shiny, white and hard substance called *cartilage.*

To stabilize the joint further, yet still allow flexibility of movement, two leaves of cartilage lie in the joint space on either side of the knee. These are the bits of cartilage which get torn in sports injuries and may be removed in a cartilage operation on the knee. Without them, the knee can still function, but wear and tear seems to be increased so that ARTHRITIS may set in later in life.

To lubricate the joint, the surfaces are all bathed in a very slippery liquid known as *synovial fluid.* This is made and held in the joint by a capsule which surrounds the whole knee. There are also additional bags of fluid, called *bursae,* which lie in the joint and act as cushions against severe stresses.

Strength and stability are provided by fibrous bands called *ligaments.* Without hindering the hinge movement of the knee, these ligaments lie on both sides and in the middle of the joint, and hold it firmly in place.

The movements of the knee joint are governed by muscles in the thigh. Those at the front pull the knee straight and those at the back hinge it backwards. At the top these muscles are attached to the HIP and the top of the femur. Further down the leg, they condense into fibrous TENDONS which cross over the knee and are then attached to the tibia.

To prevent the tendon at the front from rubbing the joint as it moves, a bone has been built into the tendon. This bone is the kneecap, or *patella,* and lies in the tendon itself, unattached to the rest of the knee. It runs up and down the bottom of the femur in a cartilage-lined groove and is lubricated by synovial fluid. There are also two further bursae which act as the shock absorbers for the kneecap.

The knee joint is traversed by blood vessels which nourish the ligaments, cartilages, capsule and bones. And, as with all important structures, nerves run to the knee so that the BRAIN can know exactly the position of the joint, in order to coordinate balance and movement.

The knee is important principally for locomotion. At every stop, it bends to allow the leg to be brought forwards without striking the ground – otherwise the leg would have to be swung outwards by tilting the pelvis, as in the typical stiff leg walk. Once forwards, the knee is straightened and the foot brought back to the ground by movement at the hip.

Structure of the knee

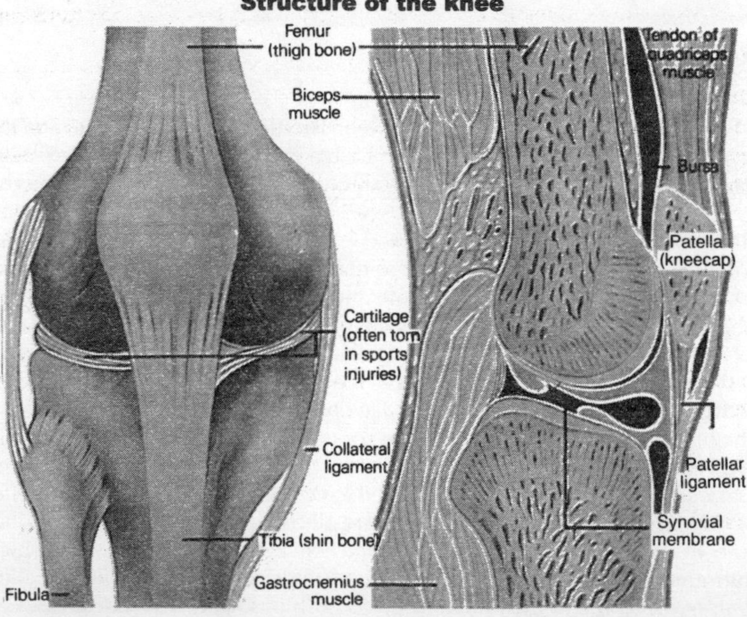

Treatment of injuries

Twists and sprains are common knee injuries caused by excessive forces stretching the knee joint ligaments. The knee swells, becomes stiff, and tenderness is felt over the injured ligament. On the whole, sprains get better by themselves with rest and gentle remobilization. A crêpe bandage, applied in a figure of eight, will give good support to the knee initially, and a walking stick can help take weight off the leg. In a severe ligament injury, the knee may need to be put in plaster.

Either of the two slices of cartilage in the joint space may get torn by a sudden twist of the knee; the knee locks and will not straighten, and also tends to give way. Nature often sorts this problem out, but if the symptoms persist, or recur, your doctor will refer you to an ORTHOPAEDIC specialist. In hospital, the diagnosis is usually confirmed by arthroscopy (*see* ENDOSCOPY). An arthroscope is a fine telescope which is actually put through a small cut into the joint. The torn cartilage can be seen through it and minor repairs performed by remote control. For more serious injuries, it may be necessary to remove the cartilage completely. However, the muscles will gradually strengthen to compensate for this loss.

DISLOCATION of the kneecap may result from a sideways knee injury. The kneecap is pulled out of its groove and the patient is unable to straighten the knee. Treatment consists of pushing the patella back into place, followed by a period of rest. Even so, the dislocation may recur with only minor stresses on the joint, in which case surgery may be necessary.

Severe injuries can break the bones at the knee with the result that the knee cannot bear weight and is very swollen and painful. The definite diagnosis is made by X-ray examination. Surgical correction may be necessary, followed by a prolonged spell in plaster.

Other problems

As opposed to the sudden loss of function following injury, many people find their joints getting stiff and painful with progressing age. Morning stiffness which improves as the day progresses is typical of arthritis. It may be caused by a previous injury or it may be RHEUMATOID ARTHRITIS, which is a disease, unrelated to a previous injury. Anti-inflammatory drugs will be given to relieve pain, but if the arthritis becomes crippling, the remedy may be for a knee replacement operation.

After persistent, unexpected activity, the bursae may become inflamed – a condition known as BURSITIS. The knee becomes tender and swells in the area of the affected bursa. Fortunately, bursitis settles with rest, but it does tend to recur from time to time.

Korsakoff's syndrome, *see* Vitamins

Kwashiorkor, *see* Malnutrition

Kyphosis

This is the excessive backward curvature of the spine (*see* BACK AND BACKACHE) which, in its advanced form, is known as 'hunchback'. It is often associated with lateral curvature (*scoliosis*). The two deformities, when combined, are called *kyphoscoliosis*. Sometimes the deformity is slight, but when it is severe, the patient cannot stand up straight and the upper part of the backbone sticks outwards.

Causes

One of the commonest causes of a kyphosis is simply poor, slouched posture. This may occur in children who develop a habit of dropping their heads and walking badly. If they continue like this into adolescence, they may still have a kyphosis in adult life. However, the bones remain perfectly mobile and the kyphosis disappears when the child stands properly.

Normal and kyphotic spine The backward curvature of the thoracic vertebrae (right) can result in varying degrees of hunchback.

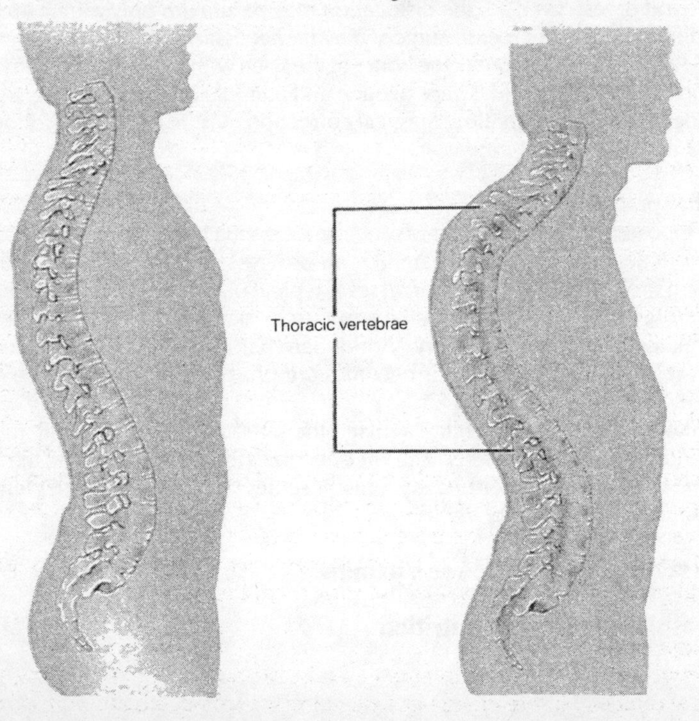

But the kyphosis can become 'fixed', which means that there is a constant deformity of the backbone whatever the patient tries to do to straighten up. In children, the cause of such deformity is usually unknown. Even children as young as three to four years of age can develop a kyphosis, which is often combined with a twist in the spine – a kyphoscoliosis. As the child grows, the deformity can worsen.

Adolescent children may develop a kyphosis as a result of a condition called *Scheuermann's disease*. The growing points in the child's vertebra become distorted, and growth in the vertebra is therefore uneven. Scheuermann's disease usually affects teenagers when their rate of growth is at its greatest – around PUBERTY. They become increasingly round-shouldered and may complain of pain in the back as well. Girls are affected twice as often as boys. The condition tends to burn itself out once growth finishes, and the kyphosis does not worsen after this time, but it does remain a permanent deformity.

Elderly people can develop a kyphosis as a result of OSTEOPOROSIS. It is much more common in women than men. About half of all women over 70 have osteoporosis, hence the name given to the kyphosis of elderly women: a 'dowager's hump'.

Osteoporosis is a condition in which a general thinning of the substance of the bones occurs throughout the body. Not only do the bones lose their calcium but the protein structure of the bones also becomes thin and weak. FRACTURES can easily occur as a result of minor injury – such as hip or wrist fractures. The vertebrae are affected early in the process of osteoporosis, and the bodies of the vertebrae simply collapse. This is usually a gradual process, but occasionally one or more vertebrae become crushed as a result of minor injury, or lifting a heavy weight. The elderly person becomes round-shouldered and diminishes in height, sometimes by as much as 6 in (15 cm).

A number of other bone disorders may cause a kyphosis if the bones of the vertebrae are involved in the disease process. Ankylosing SPONDYLITIS is a type of arthritis which tends to affect young adults, particularly men. The sacro-iliac joints in the pelvis are nearly always affected but the spine may become inflamed as well. Ultimately the joints between the vertebrae can become stiffened, and they may actually solidify, so that the patient has a fixed stoop.

TUBERCULOSIS may affect bones, and where it does, it usually affects one or more vertebrae. This condition is uncommon in Western countries but is still widespread in the Third World. A tuberculous ABSCESS develops in a vertebra – *Pott's disease* – destroying it so that it collapses, and the patient develops a sharp angulated kyphosis at the point where the tuberculosis is affecting the spine. Occasionally two or three vertebrae are involved; the patient may also be very ill as a result of the generalized effects of the infection.

Tumours or growths in the vertebrae may have a similar effect, causing a localized collapse of the spine, but such conditions are rare.

Complications

A very severe kyphosis, particularly if it is associated with a sclerosis, may cause difficulty in breathing because the LUNGS cannot expand fully. Occasionally even heart failure may result if the deformity is severe. More commonly, a long-standing kyphosis leads to ARTHRITIS in the bones of the back or in the PELVIS or HIP as excessive strain is placed on the joints because of the deformity.

Even if there is no immediate risk to health, a severe kyphosis in a young adult can be limiting for the individual simply because mobility is restricted. The impact on the individual's family and social life may also be severe.

Treatment

A postural kyphosis can readily be improved by spinal exercises. A PHYSIOTHERAPIST or remedial gymnast can prescribe a daily exercise routine to strengthen the back muscles, and in time this helps to straighten the spine.

Children who develop severe kyphosis or kyphoscoliosis at an early age need careful assessment, which includes special X-rays to measure the angle of the kyphosis and to rule out the possibility of a congenital deformity of the bones in the spine.

Early treatment in a brace may help to prevent the kyphosis or kyphoscoliosis from worsening. The most commonly used type is the 'Milwaukee brace' which is like a strongly boned corset, with a support resting on the hips and metal bars extending to pads under the chin and at the back of the head. The brace holds the spine straight and can be worn all day and night. Provided it is properly fitted and adjusted, the child can carry out virtually normal activities with little discomfort, even though the brace may look cumbersome.

Occasionally, even a brace does not fully correct a severe kyphosis or kyphoscoliosis in a teenager or young adult. An operation may then be carried out, although often this is delayed until late adolescence.

Ankylosing spondylitis is treated with anti-inflammatory drugs with the aim of reducing inflammation in the joints. The patient also has physiotherapy to ensure that the back stays as straight as possible. A patient with tuberculosis of the spine is given antibiotics over a period of many months to counter the infection, but may also need surgery to straighten the spine.

Once a patient has developed kyphosis as a result of osteosporosis, treatment may be difficult, and is unlikely to give much benefit. Calcium supplements may help to reduce pain from the bones. An osteosporotic fracture may be very painful and need painkillers. There is, however, considerable debate about how osteosporosis may be prevented (*see* HORMONE REPLACEMENT THERAPY).

See also LORDOSIS.

L

Labour, *see* **Childbirth**

Labyrinthitis, *see* **Vertigo**

Lactation, *see* **Breasts**

Laminectomy

This is an operation to take the pressure off nerves which are compressed by a SLIPPED DISC. A doctor always examines any patient with suspected slipped disc (more correctly called a PROLAPSED disc) very carefully, looking for certain danger signs. If there has been sudden onset of symptoms with weakness affecting the muscles in the legs, an acute disc rupture is likely. Often symptoms improve simply with bedrest, but if weakness in the muscles progresses and worsens, a slipped disc is very likely and needs urgent investigation. Another danger signal is any difficulty in control of urination or of the BOWEL. This can indicate a serious rupture of the disc pressing on the nerves in the spinal canal. Unless pressure is relieved quickly, permanent damage can be done and the patient could be left INCONTINENT.

Whenever a laminectomy is being considered, a special investigation called a *myelogram,* a type of X-RAY, may be carried out first. A dye is injected into the spinal canal and the patient tipped up and down to let the dye run around the SPINAL CORD. X-rays are taken which are then studied to see if there is any obstruction to the free flow of the dye, caused by the prolapsed disc. The radiologist can pinpoint the exact site of a slipped disc and guide the surgeon when planning the operation.

Nowadays, however, a more sophisticated scan is performed when possible. Called an MRI (magnetic resonance imaging) scan, this can accurately show the site of the disc protrusion without the need for injections.

How a laminectomy is performed

The name 'laminectomy' means 'removal of a lamina'. Each vertebra surrounds the spinal canal with an open tunnel. Overlying the canal are the *laminae* of the vertebrae – thin protective plates of bone which do not carry any weight but simply keep surrounding structures from pressing on the spinal cord. A small section of the laminae can be removed without causing any harm to the spinal cord, but once some laminae are removed, the surgeon can have access to the spinal canal. Usually the operation is carried out to remove a slipped disc, but occasionally a laminectomy is performed to operate on other obstructions such as small benign TUMOURS.

A laminectomy takes between one and two hours and is performed under a general ANAESTHETIC. The patient is usually placed on the operating table lying on one side, or sometimes kneeling face down so that the small of the back is easily accessible to the surgeon who works from above.

After cutting through the skin, the muscles are pushed apart from each side of the spine, exposing the laminae at the back of the spine. If the surgeon already knows precisely where the slipped disc is located, he or she may remove only the lamina on one side of the vertebra. He or she uses special instruments to nibble away the bone piece by piece until access is made to the spinal canal. Sometimes the whole of the laminae of one or more vertebrae are removed to give better access to the spinal canal. The spinal cord is then gently moved to one side to expose the prolapsed disc. The bulging disc is cut away and a small instrument passed into the space between the two vertebrae to scrape out the centre of the diseased disc. Rarely, two discs may be prolapsed, and both have to be removed.

Larynx and laryngitis

The larynx is the body's 'voice box', containing the vocal cords, which vibrate to produce SPEECH. As such, it is an extremely delicate instrument, but it also has a less complex function – a 'valve', guarding the entrance to the LUNGS.

When we eat or drink, it closes tightly, making food or liquids slide over it down into the OESOPHAGUS, which leads into the stomach. When we need to breathe in or out, it is, of course, open.

Position and structure

The larynx is placed at about the centre of the neck, at the top of the windpipe or trachea, out of sight round the 'corner' of the back of the THROAT.

The larynx is essentially a specialized section of the windpipe with an external sheath of *cartilage*. Positioned over it is the *epiglottis*, the flap-valve which comes down to cover the opening from the back of the throat into the larynx, known as the *glottis*.

The action of the epiglottis is automatically controlled by the brain, but sometimes it fails, and then liquids or food particles go down the 'wrong way'. Unless a lump of food is so large that it sticks in one of the passages below the larynx, it will be coughed up.

Within the larynx are the vocal cords, mounted on specially shaped pieces of cartilage. Air breathed out over them makes them vibrate, which produces sound. The cartilages can move in such a way as to tighten or relax the cords, producing high- or low-pitched sounds.

However, the quality of sound produced is also strongly influenced by the nature and action of the tongue, lips and jaw because the sound waves resonate or 'bounce around' the adjacent passages.

Position and structure of the larynx

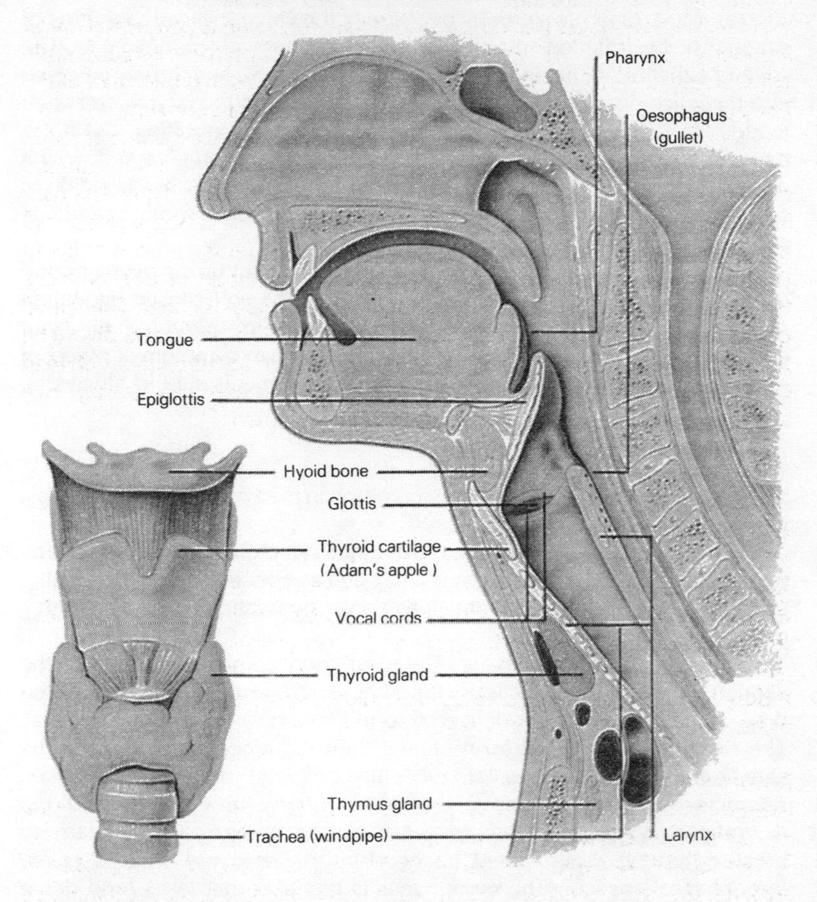

Injury to the larynx

If the larynx is damaged by injury, such as a blow or a knife wound, it may become blocked; equally, scalding vapours, liquids or poisons can burn and irritate its lining, which may in turn cause swelling and blockage. The difficulty in breathing and the pain of such injuries usually disable the patient severely.

Obviously the vital need is to restore the air flow to the lungs, and this is usually done in hospital. It may be possible for a tube to be passed down the trachea, creating a new, artificial passage; or it may be necessary to make a hole in the trachea below the larynx so that air can pass directly to the lungs. This is known as a *tracheostomy* (*see* STOMA CARE).

Laryngitis

Acute laryngitis means inflammation of the larynx caused by an infection, such as a COLD or INFLUENZA, or by over-use of the voice (typically shouting or singing) or by irritation, usually through too much cigarette smoke. The sufferer either has difficulty speaking, and has a hoarse and throaty voice, or else the voice disappears completely. There is pain in the larynx, and often tenderness is felt in the region of the larynx. It is an irritating, but not a dangerous condition, and passes if the voice is given a complete rest, which means exactly that – i.e. not speaking for as long as it takes the condition to cure, normally a day or two. Inhaling hot, steamy air with a soothing additive can help; antibiotics help only rarely.

As opposed to acute, chronic means a condition occurring over a period of time. Its cause is always irritation, mostly of the sort caused by violent shouting. Tobacco, smoke and dust and over-use of the voice are again common causes. Continued hoarseness may also be a symptom of CANCER of the larynx. But, whatever the cause, chronic laryngitis should always be reported to a doctor.

Cancer of the larynx

This type of cancer is ten times more common in men than women, and most common in heavy smokers.

It arises in the cells of the larynx and its initial symptom is hoarseness lasting several weeks. This is followed by a dry cough and occasionally by coughing up flecks of blood, followed some weeks later by swallowing and breathing difficulties.

Untreated, it can end fatally. Detected soon enough, it is one of the cancers which can be completely cured by RADIOTHERAPY alone. A controlled dose of radioactive rays is delivered to the area of the cancerous tumour. The malignant cells 'melt away' under their influence, and provided the cancer has not spread too far, this can completely cure the condition. There is no need to remove the whole larynx unless the condition is comparatively advanced. In these severe cases, patients learn to breathe through a permanent tracheostomy, and to use what is called 'oesophageal speech'. The oesophagus is the tube that takes food down to the stomach, and these people swallow air so that it passes down to the stomach, then belch it up, controlling the amount released, and the sounds produced, by means of the oesophagus. With practice, people who have had their larynxes removed become skilful at this type of speech, and can express themselves perfectly clearly, although they do have a rather unusual voice.

Polyps and nodes

Polyps are tiny lumps attached to tissue by a stalk – like a berry. If they develop on the vocal cords as a result of a long-term vocal abuse, they cause hoarseness and a 'breathy' quality of the voice. Vocal cord nodes (sometimes called singer's or teacher's nodes) are also lumps and develop from long-term abuse. They both need to be removed surgically.

Laryngotracheo-bronchitis

This is the technical name for *croup*, the dry, distinctive-sounding cough caused when inflammation narrows the larynx.

Such inflammation is frequently caused by a bacteria, but it may also be caused by a virus. The larynx, trachea and bronchi (the airways leading to the lungs) become so inflamed and swollen and such a sticky, heavy mucus is formed that the air supply is in considerable danger of being cut off.

If the case is severe, a tracheostomy is once again necessary. Milder cases respond to oxygen, antibiotics and ensuring that the atmosphere around the patient is warm and humid – which soothes the inflamed areas.

Laxatives

These are used in the treatment of CONSTIPATION. Usually they are completely unnecessary and, if taken over long periods, may even have serious and persistent side-effects.

Types

The first group of laxatives – the 'bulk laxatives' – are simply preparations designed to increase the amount of vegetable *fibre* (remnant of vegetable matter after nutrients have been absorbed) which passes through the bowel (*see* CARBOHYDRATES). The best example is bran, which is produced from the outer part of the wheat germ as it is milled into flour.

It is now accepted that bowel problems like constipation and diverticular disease (a type of bowel inflammation) are related to the fact that the Western diet does not contain enough fibre. Bulk laxatives are a way of increasing this fibre. They can be taken in tablet form or as granules, or, more simply, by eating wholemeal bread or bran breakfast cereals.

Bulk laxatives should be thought of as somewhere between a food and a drug. Their only drawback is that they are an expensive way of doing what [illegible] done by altering the diet.

The second group – the 'non-bulk laxatives' – fall into three types, each working in different ways. There are stimulants such as castor oil and senna, which act on the nerves in the bowel wall, increasing the power and frequency of peristalsis (rhythmic muscular contractions of the bowel wall which move food matter onwards). The next type, such as liquid paraffin, softens the STOOL and make it easier and less painful to pass. Finally, there are the osmotic laxatives. 'Osmotic' describes the process of drawing water from one place to another. As laxatives, they cause more water to be retained within the bowel, making the stool softer and bulkier.

All of the non-bulk laxatives ought to be thought of as drugs that should only be taken on a doctor's advice, for every drug has side-effects.

Dangers

Non-bulk laxatives which stimulate the large INTESTINE (bowel) and are taken over a number of years tend to poison the nerve fibres in the bowel. This means that people who have been in the habit of taking 'a little opening medicine' every day may end up with a bowel which is unable to produce muscular contractions at all and is therefore unable to move faeces onwards. When this happens, further stimulation is useless, and the change to bulk laxatives which work well in the normal bowel may only make matters worse. Osmotic laxatives may be some help, but because of the magnesium salts they contain, which can upset the body's chemical balance, they have to be used with care in the elderly and those with KIDNEY disease.

Uses

When a patient has a painful anal condition like PILES and fissures (ulcers), stool softening or osmotic laxatives can be of some use, though the object should be to increase fibre in the diet. Such non-bulk laxatives can also be used in angina and other forms of HEART DISEASE to prevent straining to pass a stool.

Many drugs make people constipated – for instance, the more powerful painkilling drugs such as opiates like codeine. Similarly, being ill and immobilized, particularly in hospital or confined to bed at home, may induce constipation. Laxatives may be useful to treat the condition in these circumstances.

Laxatives may also be used with safety to clear the bowel before investigations such as a BARIUM enema or a colonoscopy (inspecting the colon with a flexible instrument; *see* ENDOSCOPY) are carried out. More intensive preparations are used to prepare people for bowel surgery.

'Lazy' eye, *see* Squint

Leboyer method, *see* Childbirth, natural

Leg

Human legs have evolved as remarkable pieces of engineering, capable of supporting considerable weight and pressure. From your waist to your toes, there is an intercommunicating network of more than 60 different bones.

Bones

The *femur,* in the thigh, is the longest and heaviest bone in the body – a fact which is not surprising when you consider the amount of strain it has to take during standing, walking, running or jumping, or supporting the head and trunk.

At the lower end of the femur, it widens into the *lateral and medial condyles,* which articulate with the tibia below to form a hinged joint – the KNEE. The *patella,* or knee cap, a slightly teardrop-shaped bone, lies in front and protects the knee joint, but it is vulnerable to dislocation or FRACTURE.

The lower leg, like the forearm, is supported by two long bones, with shafts that are approximately parallel – the slender *fibula*, or calf-bone, and the heavier *tibia*, or shin-bone, which is the second longest bone in the body. The front of the tibia is only covered by a thin layer of flesh and is often painfully bruised when we bump our shins.

Another vulnerable spot is the bump at the lower end of the tibia, the *medial malleolus*, or outer ankle bone. A sudden sharp turn of the ankle can result in the break known as *Pott's fracture*. The fibula articulates with both the tibia and the *talus* bones. The remaining *tarsal* bones of the ankle correspond with the carpals of the wrists.

Muscles

Cloaking the bones of the leg are some of the body's largest muscles. Those of the thigh work in close conjunction with the HIP, to give us stability and balance when standing or walking. Important too, are the hamstring muscles.

The calf muscles are among the strongest in the body. As well as being involved in walking or jumping, they help to steady the legs in a standing position and control the movements of the feet. The muscles needed to straighten the leg include the *extensor digitorum longus*, the *extensor hallucis longus* and the *tibialis anterior*. The bulging calf at the back of the leg is formed by the *gastrocnemius*, the most prominent of the flexor muscles of the ankle. Together with the *soleus*, it is inserted into the heel bone by the most powerful tendon in the body, the *Achilles tendon*. To enable you to stand on your toes, it is the calf muscles at the back of the leg that have to contract.

Veins and arteries

Walking upright may have given humans immense advantages but it also provided the legs with their one, in-built drawback.

Like all other tissues, those of the legs, particularly their large bunches of muscle, need to be 'serviced' with oxygen and nutrients pumped to them in the bloodstream by the heart. Blood travels outwards to the legs in the ARTERIES, and then back to the heart in the VEINS.

Because it is such an uphill haul, it is this journey back in the veins which, as will be seen, tends to cause the problems if the leg veins tend to weakness.

Unlike arteries, the veins of the leg are not under direct pressure from the heart's pumping action. This is because all arteries become progressively smaller as they extend towards the body's extremities, finally ending in capillaries – the tiniest, thread-thin blood vessels. These then connect with tiny veins which grow progressively larger on the return to the heart. Blood can only travel through veins by a combination of squeezing pressure exerted by the muscle which surrounds them, by the effect of the palpitating arteries close by, and by certain other more or less outside influences, such as the action of walking, which has a helpful stimulating effect.

As a result, the walls of our veins are thinner than those of arteries – they just do not have to withstand so much pressure. If you stand upright, the weight of blood in the veins increases because in theory they are supporting a 'column' of blood reaching, in the end, to the heart.

This extra pressure would make the veins of the leg swell like balloons if it were not for a system of one-way valves within the veins which effectively reduce the columns of blood into small sections.

Some people, however, have veins whose walls tend to weakness. In time – often not until middle age – this will result in stretching of their walls, so that the non-return valves are made ineffective. This, in turn, means that the veins have to support a much longer and heavier column of blood; and not surprisingly, they react by swelling, knotting and twisting – the characteristic appearance of VARICOSE VEINS.

The legs are also high-risk areas for arterial problems. Arterial disease itself is a 'furring up' of the arteries by a build-up of fatty deposits. Some of its symptoms seem to overlap with those of poor circulation in the veins. If there is a complete blockage, blood flow out to the tissues is stopped and gangrene, or tissue death, can occur.

The body can, to a certain extent, compensate for arterial failure by developing what is known as *collateral flow*. This means that the arteries actually develop extensions which bypass areas becoming blocked. This remarkable ability takes a matter of weeks to develop fully. However, it should not be relied on as a cure-all for arterial problems, because obstruction can develop much more rapidly than that. The usual, and generally successful, treatment is with drugs to dilate the arteries, combined with a prescribed regime of diet and exercise and stopping smoking.

Clots can also be removed by surgery, and an operation exists to bypass an artery altogether (*see* THROMBOSIS).

See also PHLEBITIS and SCIATICA.

Legg–Calvé–Perthes' disease, *see* **Perthes' disease**

Leishmaniasis, *see* **Tropical diseases, Ulcers, skin**

Leucocytes, *see* **Blood**

Leucopenia, *see* **Blood**

Leucorrhoea

Vaginal secretions are the body's natural way of cleansing, lubricating and guarding the VAGINA against infections. Like the mouth and anus, the mucous membrane of the vagina constantly sheds and replaces its cells, passing them out of the body in a mucus secretion.

It is still quite rare for young girls to be told that, as well as starting periods, they may begin to notice a transparent, slightly milky fluid, which comes from the vagina and leaves a whitish-yellowish patch on their underwear. If a young girl does not know this, she may think it is abnormal; at the same time, if she does have an abnormal discharge, she may not be able to identify it. Leucorrhoea, more commonly known as 'the whites', is not a disease in itself, but it can be a symptom.

Normal discharges

The normal secretions of the vagina are related to the menstrual cycle (*see* PERIODS). They come from the CERVIX (neck of the womb), the walls of the vagina and the *Bartholin's glands* in the vaginal lips (*labia majora*). Vaginal and cervical secretions and mucus are present throughout the menstrual cycle in varying amounts.

Around the time of ovulation, these secretions become more profuse, wetter and thinner, and about 24 hours before they ovulate, many women notice that their vaginal mucus is clear and stringy. This change in the secretion makes it easier for sperm to survive in the vagina and also helps their upward movement towards the womb, increasing the chances of fertilization. Two or three days after ovulation the vaginal secretions usually become thicker and dryer, which make it more difficult for sperm to penetrate and fertilize the egg. These changes in vaginal mucus are used by some women in the 'rhythm method' of CONTRACEPTION.

Sexual arousal causes an increase in secretion from Bartholin's glands and an increase in secretions from the numerous tiny glands in the walls of the vagina. Together, these glands produce a clear, slippery fluid, which lubricates the vagina prior to intercourse. The increase in secretions caused by sexual arousal can be quite considerable.

An increase in the level of female hormones during PREGNANCY produces an associated increase in vaginal secretions. Women taking the contraceptive pill may also notice an increase, because the synthetic hormones of the pill imitate the state of pregnancy. This kind of increased discharge production is harmless.

The quantity of discharge can vary widely from one woman to another and may increase as a result of a number of factors, many of which are easy to diagnose and to remedy.

Abnormal discharges

Any discharge that is discoloured, causes soreness or irritation of the vagina or lips (vulva), or has an unpleasant smell is likely to be related to infection somewhere in the genital organs.

One of the commonest infections is THRUSH (also called monilia or candida), which causes a thick white discharge with intense irritation around the vaginal opening. Thrush can occur in young girls or women who have never had intercourse, and is more common if personal hygiene is inadequate, or if tight jeans or trousers are worn. It also occurs more frequently in women who are DIABETIC, because sugar in the urine tends to encourage the growth of the micro-organism (a type of fungus) that causes thrush. Occasionally, thrush is SEXUALLY TRANSMITTED because the infection can be carried by a male partner, particularly if he is not circumcised.

Another very common cause of leucorrhoea is infection in the vagina with a bacterium called *Gardnerella vaginalis*. Recent research has shown that this organism may be present in the vagina without causing any symptoms at all – possibly in as many as one woman in five. However, for reasons which are not yet entirely clear, some women do suffer symptoms from *Gardnerella* infection.

Typically, there is an increase in discharge, although this may not be very profuse, and there may be some irritation. The discharge tends to have a peculiar smell – a fishy odour is often described – which can be obvious to the sufferer or partner. Another typical symptom is discomfort during intercourse, with a dull pain in the vagina and an increase in discharge for a day or two after. Although *Gardnerella* infections can be sexually transmitted, this is not always so. It appears, however, that men carrying the infection usually have no discomfort: they have no symptoms whatsoever.

Trichomonas vaginalis infection tends to produce an intensely irritating greenish discharge which is quite profuse (*see* TRICHOMONIASIS). Again, men may carry this infection without it causing any symptoms to them but pass it on to their partners during sexual intercourse.

A number of diseases that are predominantly transmitted sexually may also produce an increase in vaginal discharge. Both GONORRHOEA and CHLAMYDIA may cause a discharge, but they are also likely to produce other symptoms, such as burning urination and pain in the lower abdomen.

Blood-stained discharge appearing between periods is a sign of some form of internal bleeding. If this occurs when taking the contraceptive pill, the pill is usually the reason for the irregular bleeding, but a check-up from your doctor is still advisable. Sometimes the cause is an infection, but occasionally the cause is something more serious, such as a CANCER of the womb or of the cervix. If such bleeding occurs, it should always be reported to a doctor, especially if the woman is over 40 years of age.

An 'erosion' of the cervix is a benign non-cancerous condition in which the surface of the cervix becomes slightly abnormal, and covered with an unusual, glandular type of tissue rather than the usual smooth covering. Often there are no symptoms at all from an erosion but it may cause leucorrhoea, which is usually non-irritating. Sometimes there may be a little bleeding from the cells in the surface of the erosion.

Vaginal lubrication decreases after the MENOPAUSE and becomes more alkaline. Sometimes this causes irritation and there is a greater likelihood of getting common fungal infections such as thrush. HORMONE REPLACEMENT THERAPY, sometimes used to treat various troublesome symptoms of the menopause, can also help minimize menopausal effects on vaginal secretions.

When to see your doctor

Any heavy vaginal discharge that happens before puberty is likely to be abnormal and should be investigated as soon as possible.

Women should not let an unpleasant discharge continue for more than a week before consulting a doctor about it. If you experience an unpleasant discharge, you should see a doctor without delay if it is accompanied by fever or abdominal pain, if there is a possibility of sexually transmitted disease, if it is blood-stained or brown and you are not close to an expected period, or if it is accompanied by pain or burning on passing urine, soreness, irritation or smells unpleasant.

Your doctor will first ask you a number of questions about the nature of the discharge, and he or she will also ask detailed questions about recent sexual activity and about your sexual partners. For example, your doctor will want to know if there is any risk of sexually transmitted infection. This is more likely if you have had a recent change in sexual partner, or if your partner has had any symptoms.

You should then expect an internal examination. Your doctor will take several samples of mucus on swabs to be sent to the laboratory for further investigation to see if there is an infection present and, if so, the type of infection.

You may be asked to wait for the results of these tests before treatment is given, but if the symptoms are severe, or if a simple problem is suspected – such as thrush – you may be given treatment straight away. Your doctor may decide to refer you to a hospital department of genito-urinary medicine if he or she does not have the full facilities available to carry out a complete range of tests. If you have an erosion or other internal problems, you may be referred to a gynaecologist for treatment.

If the cause is straightforward, the doctor will prescribe appropriate medication – tablets to take, pessaries to be inserted into the vagina or cream, these will quickly deal with the condition.

If the idea of talking to your family doctor about your sex life embarrasses you, it is not difficult nowadays to go to a 'special clinic' (sometimes called a genito-urinary medicine department) where you will be treated in confidence.

Leukaemia

This is a CANCER of the BLOOD which may start in the BONE MARROW or the LYMPH system. Bone marrow is one of the places where blood cells are made: red cells, which carry oxygen; white cells, which fight infection; and platelets, which form clots to seal injured blood vessels and prevent bleeding. The most immature white cells are called *myeloblasts,* which then become *myelocytes* and finally *granulocytes*. Leukaemia which starts in the bone marrow is called *myeloblastic or myelocytic leukaemia*. Sometimes these two types are referred to collectively as 'myeloid' leukaemia.

White blood cells called *lymphocytes* are made mainly in the lymph nodes and some in the bone marrow. Leukaemia of the lymph system is known as *lymphoblastic or lymphocytic leukaemia.*

However, in either case the leukaemic cells invade each other's territory so that, in lymphoblastic leukaemia, abnormal lymphocytes can be found in the bone marrow and vice versa.

Contrary to popular belief, leukaemia is not a disease which is more common in children. The incidence remains remarkably constant until the age of 75, at about 10 per 1,000,000 per year in the UK and thereafter it rises to a level of 50 per 1,000,000 per year.

However, lymphoblastic leukaemia is much commoner in children than in adults, reaching a peak incidence of 50 per 1,000,000 children per year between the ages of two and four years. Then it falls, only to rise to a second peak in adults after the age of 65.

Either type of leukaemia may be in acute or chronic form – this describes the speed with which the disease runs its course, 'acute' meaning rapid and severe and 'chronic' meaning longer-lasting and with less severe symptoms.

What happens in acute leukaemia

White blood cells cannot reproduce themselves, and after a life-span of a few days or weeks, they are replaced by new cells. With leukaemia, two things go wrong. In the first place, the leukaemic cells never seem to grow up into mature blood cells so they are unable to fight infection. Second, excessively large numbers of these immature cells are produced. This means that eventually they accumulate to such an extent that they clog up the bone marrow, then spill into the blood to invade the lymph system, the LIVER and the SPLEEN. Because the bone marrow is clogged with leukaemic cells, the production of normal red and white blood cells is considerably reduced.

Cause

The cause is unknown, but in the case of acute leukaemia, it is believed that it may be the result of a VIRUS. It is likely that infection with a virus changes the susceptibility of the patient or perhaps changes the structure of the surface of the immune cells which fight infection. This, in turn, may result in failure to recognize abnormal cancer cells which are normally killed the moment they develop.

Other factors are also important. One which is well known is atomic RADIATION, as was witnessed by the enormous increase in the incidence of acute leukaemia after the atomic bombs were dropped on Japan in 1945. More recently, it has been shown that the doctors who handle X-RAY equipment – radiologists – have a slightly increased risk of developing leukaemia.

The incidence of chronic leukaemia also increases following heavy exposure to atomic radiation, and chronic myeloid leukaemia is more common after prolonged exposure to the toxin benzene, a constituent of petroleum.

Both chronic types have a similar incidence, occurring in 15 new cases per 1,000,000 people per year in the UK. Both are relatively uncommon below the age of 20 years.

Chronic myelocytic leukaemia is also associated with an abnormality in the chromosomes (*see* CELLS AND CHROMOSOMES) in which a piece is missing from chromosome number 22. This was discovered by scientists in Philadelphia and has become known as the 'Philadelphia chromosome'. Because this chromosome is not present at birth and only appears in the leukaemic cells, it is thought to be the result and not the cause of the disease. Abnormalities of chromosome number 21, which are common in DOWN'S SYNDROME are also associated with an increased incidence of myelocytic leukaemia.

Research has identified abnormalities on chromosomes in other types of leukaemia. It is thought that this may be a link in the chain which leads to uncontrolled growth of leukaemia cells.

Symptoms

When the bone marrow becomes crowded out with the abnormal leukaemia cells, it cannot function properly and the patient becomes anaemic through lack of red blood cells, susceptible to infection because of lack of efficient white cells, and suffers from excessive bleeding because the blood cannot clot without platelets.

ANAEMIA may be one of the earliest signs and sometimes appears before any abnormal cells can be found in the blood. There may be bleeding in odd places like the gums. Easy bruising and repeated heavy nose bleeds are also warning signs. Infection occurs far more commonly, often resulting in dental ABSCESSES, SINUSITIS or PNEUMONIA. Liver, spleen and lymph nodes also enlarge as leukaemic cells grow in these organs. They are inside the rib cage and normally cannot be felt. In leukaemia, they may poke down below the level of the ribs so that they can be felt on examination.

Sometimes leukaemia tissue may grow in other places, such as the skin. If such tissue grows rapidly in the bones, there may be considerable pain.

Diagnosis

Doctors diagnose the disease by examining a blood sample under a microscope. Young leukaemic cells look quite different from mature blood cells.

The diagnosis may sometimes be made before such abnormal cells appear in the blood by taking a sample of bone marrow (*see* BIOPSY). This is done, under local ANAESTHETIC, by inserting a needle through the bone into the narrow cavity, often of the patient's breastbone.

Treatment

Treatment with modern drugs means that it is possible to cure lymphoblastic and lymphocytic leukaemia, and life expectancy can be greatly prolonged with myeloid leukaemia.

It is now clear that leukaemia should be treated by specialists in centres where the necessary facilities are available. The most important requirement in treatment is the need to control the patient's bone marrow function until this returns to normal. It has been found that the anti-cancer drugs which are so important can initially make the patient's bone marrow function worse, rather than better. Coping with such difficulties needs medical treatment and nursing of the utmost skill.

Two types of drug treatment (chemotherapy) are given. The first is vigorous treatment in hospital to kill all the white cells in order to get rid of the leukaemia cells.

Cells multiply by splitting into halves. When this happens, the genetic material DNA (deoxyribonucleic acid) in the nucleus of the cell is duplicated. The drug treatment interferes with this process so that new leukaemic cells cannot form. When treatment is finished, normal bone marrow cells are able to grow again and produce functioning white cells.

The second course of treatment is designed to keep the remission in check, and this can usually be taken at home.

Repeated treatment in hospital is usually necessary during the course of the disease. A patient is considered cured if he or she goes for five years without evidence of a recurrence of the disease.

Alternatively, RADIOTHERAPY may be used to suppress the reproduction of cells. An excessive dose of radiation stops the formation of all blood cells but a smaller dose only affects abnormal cells. This means that the leukaemic cells are more susceptible than the healthy ones, and the treatment can be adjusted to suppress their activity without destroying the healthy cells.

All children with acute lymphoblastic leukaemia are now routinely given X-ray therapy to the brain and spinal cord because leukaemia cells can grow in the NERVOUS SYSTEM at a later stage in the illness. Such treatment reduces the chances of this occurring.

With chronic leukaemia, the patient remains in remission for long periods and has no symptoms, but every now and again, the chronic leukaemia develops the features of the acute form and requires the same sort of vigorous treatment. Patients with chronic leukaemia have been known to survive for a number of years, and modern drugs have greatly improved the quality of life for them.

An exciting development in recent years in the treatment of myeloid leukaemia is the use of BONE MARROW transplantation.

Lice

Of the many types of louse, only two main groups – *Pediculus humanus*, which includes the head and body louse, and *Pediculus pubis*, pubic louse or 'crab' – live by infesting humans and sucking their blood. Fortunately, lice can be dealt with quite easily, but treatment varies as each type of louse – head, body and 'crab' – requires different conditions for survival.

Head lice

The eggs – 'nits' – of the head louse are laid in the hair close to the scalp, and are secured to it by a cement-like substance. Each egg is about one millimetre long, and can be seen by the naked eye. After eight days or so, the eggs hatch, and the lice begin to feed off the scalp by sucking blood.

Over a period of about nine days, the louse moults three times. At the end of this stage, the adult is fully formed and ready to reproduce. Each louse will then live for about two more weeks, during which time the female will lay as many as ten eggs every night.

The effects of head lice vary greatly from person to person. Some people experience only slight itching, while others may be driven to distraction by the itchiness of what may be a swollen and inflamed scalp. An itching scalp is the most obvious symptom of head lice, but on inspection, it is possible to see the discarded egg casing still cemented to the hair, which will indicate that treatment is necessary.

The safest way to deal with head lice is by using a special lotion which is sprinkled on the scalp and rubbed into the hair. The lotion has an alcoholic base and is inflammable, so it must be used with care and in a well ventilated room. The lotion must be allowed to dry naturally. Always ask your doctor's advice before buying a treatment for head lice because the lice and nits can become resistant to some treatments. Your doctor will know which treatment is being used in your area with success. Do not rely on medicated shampoos to treat head lice: these will kill off the lice but are not strong enough to kill nits. They can be used after treatment with lotion as a further prevention.

Head lice transfer easily from head to head. Children are more likely to be at risk, since they are often in close physical contact with each other when playing. School medical services are well aware that this is the case, and should inform parents if an epidemic of lice occurs. Keeping children's hair cut short may provide some protection and makes it more easy to use the lotion on the scalp, but there is little else that can be done to protect them from a possible infestation. Since lice are not killed by ordinary shampoo and water, cleanliness will provide no defence.

Since lice move so easily from one person to another, it is usually considered sensible for every member of the family to be treated if one is affected, including anyone with whom the child has been in contact. Do not forget parents and grandparents, who can carry lice just as easily as children.

Body lice

Body lice occur less frequently than head lice. They need to feed regularly and live in a constant temperature, so will thrive in any condition in which the host changes clothes infrequently. They have therefore been associated with groups such as troops in wartime or prisoners, where conditions exist in which they can develop undisturbed and easily transfer from person to person.

The adult female louse lays her eggs in clothing, preferring the safety of the seams where the eggs will be undisturbed. Even if the clothes are removed at night, this may not bring about a change in temperature sufficient to kill the louse and its eggs, so use of an insecticide is always advised. Lice will also be killed by extreme temperature, so washing clothes in hot water followed by careful ironing of all seams will ensure that the body lice are eliminated.

The adult female louse will lay up to 250 eggs. This reproductive rate makes it difficult to prevent the spread of body lice, and their numbers can reach epidemic proportions if the environment is suitable and they can reproduce unchecked. Their bites produce itchy inflammations which will alert the host to their presence.

There are a number of louse-borne diseases, the most dangerous of which is TYPHUS. The disease starts with flu-like symptoms, followed by a serious fever and rash on the body. It is, in fact, spread by excretions from the louse. Fortunately, however, the incidence of this disease is now far lower than it used to be.

Crab lice

The crab louse is usually found living in the pubic hair. It derives its name from its crab-like appearance. Once again, there is little that can be done to prevent them being caught. If there is close contact with a person who has crabs – and since they infest the pubic area, this contact is likely to be sexual – they may well transfer themselves. They thrive in warm conditions, and once a crab louse has made its way on to the pubic hair, it will lay eggs in a similar way to the head louse. The eggs are cemented on to individual hairs, and can be seen with the naked eye. A female louse lays up to 50 eggs in her lifetime.

After a month, the crab lice hatch from their eggs, and begin to feed off the human host. Symptoms vary from person to person, and are usually at their worst and most irritating at night. There may be inflammation of the pubic area, as well as an uncomfortable rash. Crab lice sometimes spread to the hair of the chest, armpits, eyebrows and eyelashes, but are never found on the hair of the head, as these hairs grow too close together.

Lichen planus, *see* **Rash**

Lipomas

These are benign TUMOURS of the connective tissue. They can grow anywhere on the body, and sometimes internally. Treatment is usually unnecessary unless they become large and are disfiguring.

Lipomas can arise wherever there are fat cells in the body. They are non-cancerous growths of fat cells, and can vary in size from a tiny pea-sized structure to large growths several inches across. Usually they have a fibrous outer capsule, although sometimes a great deal of tough fibrous tissue is present within the centre of the lipoma, and it may then be called a *fibrolipoma*.

Most lipomas occur singly, but in about one case in ten there are multiple lipomas. Sometimes the tendency to develop them runs in families.

Most commonly, lipomas occur in the fat layer under the skin. These subcutaneous lipomas range from 1 in (2.5 cm) or so up to 3 in (7.5 cm) across and can usually be felt easily as soft, rather jelly-like swellings under the skin. Most often, they appear in adults between the ages of 30 and 60, but they can appear at any time in life. The commonest sites are the neck, shoulders, upper arms, trunk and legs. They rarely hurt or cause pain.

Sometimes lipomas are found in muscle tissue. They become obvious only if they reach an appreciable size but can cause a swelling deep in the muscle – for example, in the thigh.

Rarely, lipomas occur inside joints. Even small ones in this location may cause minor problems with the use of the joint, although the cause may not be obvious until the joint is carefully investigated.

Internal organs of the body may also be affected by lipomas – for example, the intestines and various glands in the body, including the breasts. It is not uncommon for lipomas to appear around the kidneys, right at the back of the abdomen. These are called *retroperitoneal* lipomas, because they lie behind the peritoneal cavity which contains all the abdominal organs, including the intestines. In this location, lipomas may reach a considerable size and may weigh several kilograms.

Occasionally people who are overweight develop a number of subcutaneous lipomas which become tender and painful. This condition is called *Dercum's disease*, or *adiposa dolorosa*, which literally means 'painful fat'. Dercum's disease usually affects severely overweight middle-aged women, although men can be affected. Painful, firm lipomas tend to occur in the lower abdomen and on the outer surface of the thighs and buttocks. In this condition, the lipomas grow so fast that they cannot be supplied adequately with blood and there is some necrosis within the centre of each.

Treatment

The doctor first examines the lump to check that it is a lipoma because there are a number of other possible causes for SWELLINGS under the skin. However, lipomas have a very characteristic appearance, and there is seldom any doubt about the diagnosis. If a lipoma is small and causing no significant problems, it can be left alone. But a large lipoma is usually removed surgically. The surgeon will also remove any lump where the diagnosis could be in doubt, so that it can be examined carefully in a laboratory to exclude any cancerous condition.

Small lipomas are usually removed using a local ANAESTHETIC. The surgeon makes a single incision and, having removed the lipoma, sutures the skin. Healing should occur easily, leaving only a fine scar. If a lipoma is large or situated internally, a general anaesthetic is given.

If the patient suffers from Dercum's disease, it is vital that he or she loses weight before any surgery is undertaken. This also helps to relieve the symptoms. Only when the patient has reached a reasonable weight will the surgeon be prepared to operate to remove the lipomas.

Little's disease, *see* **Cerebral palsy**

Liver and liver diseases

The liver has two vital roles: making (or processing) new chemicals, and neutralizing poisons and wastes.

The organ stands four-square in the way of every drop of BLOOD coming away from our INTESTINES – blood which carries all the nutrients absorbed from the food we eat. In other words, blood can only get back to the HEART and LUNGS from the STOMACH by first passing through a system of veins into the liver, known as the portal system.

The liver is the largest organ in the body, weighing between 3 and 4 lb (1.36 and 1.81 kg). It is tucked underneath the DIAPHRAGM, protected from damage by the lower ribs. There are two projecting parts, or lobes, called the left and right lobes, the right being the largest, occupying the whole of the ABDOMEN's right side. The left is smaller, reaching the mid-point of our left side. It is not usually possible to feel the liver, but when it enlarges – as a result of disease – it protrudes from behind the rib cage, and can then be felt if the abdomen is pushed in.

Functions

Medical science calls the 'creative' cells of the liver *hepatocytes.* They are specialized to handle the basic substances that our bodies run on – PROTEINS, CARBOHYDRATES and FATS.

Protein processing: Proteins are essential for the renewal and creation of cells all over the body, for the formation of HORMONES (the body's chemical 'messengers') and for making ENZYMES, substances secreted by cells to bring about chemical change.

We eat protein in various forms, both vegetable and animal in origin. From these 'raw' proteins, the liver has to create proteins acceptable to the body by first breaking them down, and then actually rebuilding them.

Put simply, this process – or synthesis – means raw proteins being absorbed from the blood flowing through the portal veins into the surrounding hepatocytes, being synthesized by the liver's enzymes, and then being 'handed back' in their new form. Waste, however, does not return to the bloodstream.

Carbohydrate processing: These are the large class of chemical substances made of three atoms – basic building blocks of all physical matter: carbon, hydrogen and oxygen.

They occur most typically in sugary or starchy foods, and we need them for energy. Our muscles literally 'burn' sugar, or sugar-like substances, whenever they work – a process assisted by oxygen. The liver plays a vital role in organizing this 'fuel' into forms which can be used.

This it does by turning carbohydrates into two forms, closely akin to pure sugar. One is 'instant energy': *glucose.* The other is storable energy, a substance similar to glucose and called *glycogen.* Sugar shortage rapidly causes brain damage, and so the level of sugar in the blood must be precisely maintained, hence the need to store sugar for times of need, such as sudden exertion or starvation. Equally, if too much sugar is present in the blood, a hormone made by the liver can store the excess as glycogen.

Conversion of fats: Fats are essential to the body, too. They are turned by the liver into forms which can actually be built into or renew existing fatty tissue, typically the subcutaneous layer beneath the skin which acts as insulation and shock absorber. Fat, in addition, is a means of storing energy.

Waste disposal: Lining the veins of the liver are highly specialized cells called Kuppfer cells after the man who identified them – which 'vacuum clean' the blood of impurities, such as BACTERIA. These cells also 'weed out' excess red blood cells and 'hand them across' to the hepatocytes for processing.

From all the sources mentioned – blood itself, proteins, fats and, to a much lesser extent, carbohydrates – by-products are produced during the rebuilding that goes on in the hepatocytes. Some, such as ammonia (produced during the breakdown of protein), are poisonous, and the liver cells neutralize this, sending the harmless waste product urea, back into the main circulation. Fat and blood waste products pass out as BILE.

The same applies to actual poisons we consume – such as alcohol – and, indeed, medicines. If a drug is to be long-lasting in its effects, it needs either to be resistant to the liver's enzymes or to bypass the liver completely.

What can go wrong

The liver has a marvellous capacity to renew itself – a whole lobe cut away in an operation can be replaced in a few weeks. However, on rare occasions, destruction of liver cells outstrips the rate of replacement, and this leads to acute – meaning immediate – liver failure.

The most common form is viral HEPATITIS, or infection by a particular type of germ. Paracetamol poisoning, due to deliberate overdosage, is also a common cause.

The results of liver failure are easy to imagine by considering the jobs the liver performs. Blood sugar falls, and without a proper level, brain damage can result. Failure of protein production, including manufacture of those which cause clotting in the blood, make the patient bleed easily; it also leads, for various technical reasons, to complications such as accumulation of fluid in the abdomen, called *ascites.* Failure to eliminate waste causes JAUNDICE (the yellowish tinge given by too much bile pigment in the blood) and also COMA.

Certain inborn defects can cause long-term liver problems, notably failure of the liver enzymes to remove excess bile. Known as *kernicterus,* the condition is most common in premature babies. It is characterized by various degrees of jaundice that, if allowed to persist, may result in brain damage.

The enzymes which make and store glucose may also be deficient, causing rapid fall in the blood sugar level.

The liver sifts an enormous amount of blood, and this is why the liver is a common site for CANCER to settle in after spreading from the primary site through the bloodstream. Primary liver TUMOURS are relatively rare.

Poisons such as paracetamol and ALCOHOL, or infections such as hepatitis can cause such rapid destruction of liver cells that repair is not possible. This

How the liver works

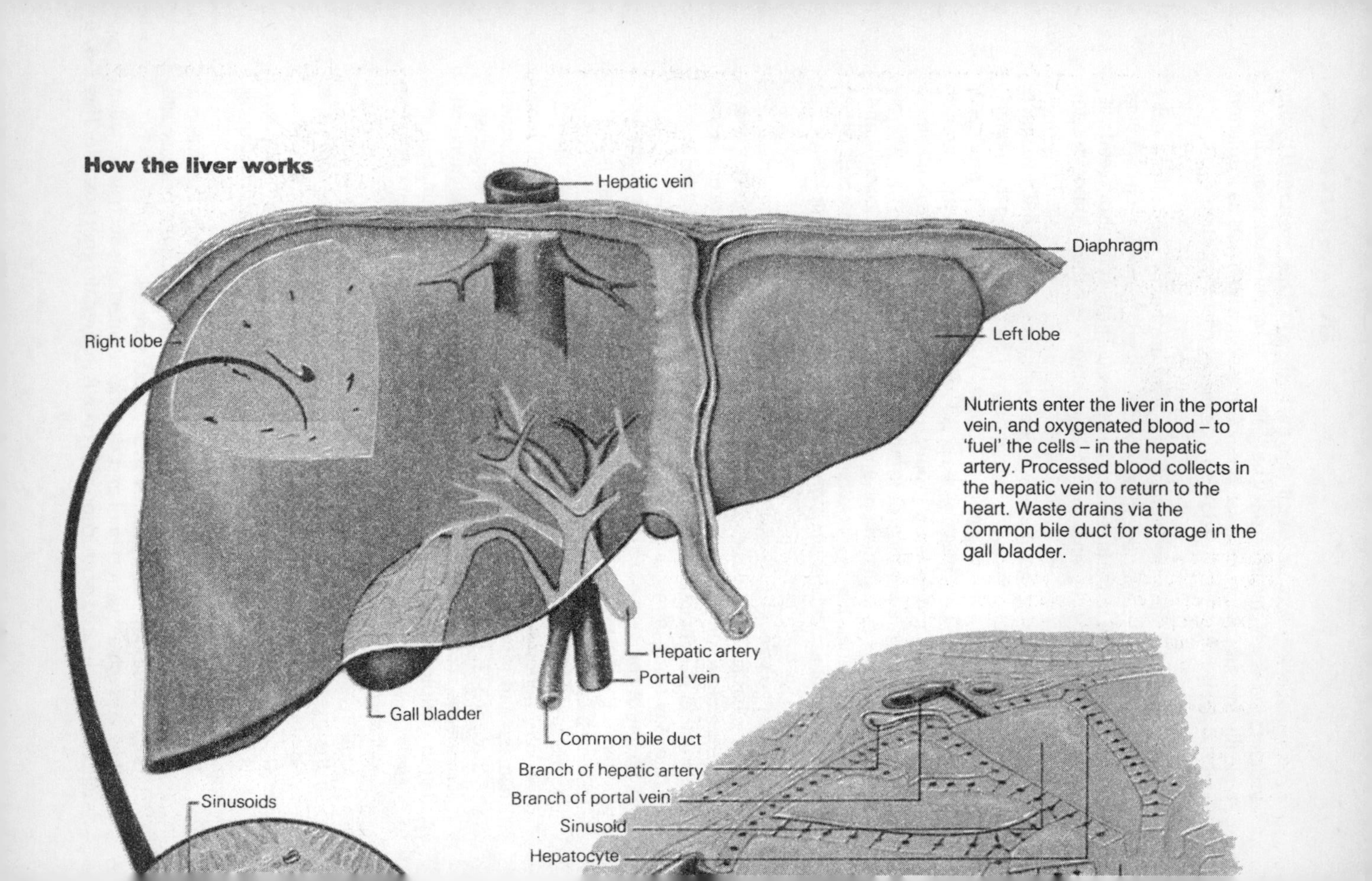

Nutrients enter the liver in the portal vein, and oxygenated blood – to 'fuel' the cells – in the hepatic artery. Processed blood collects in the hepatic vein to return to the heart. Waste drains via the common bile duct for storage in the gall bladder.

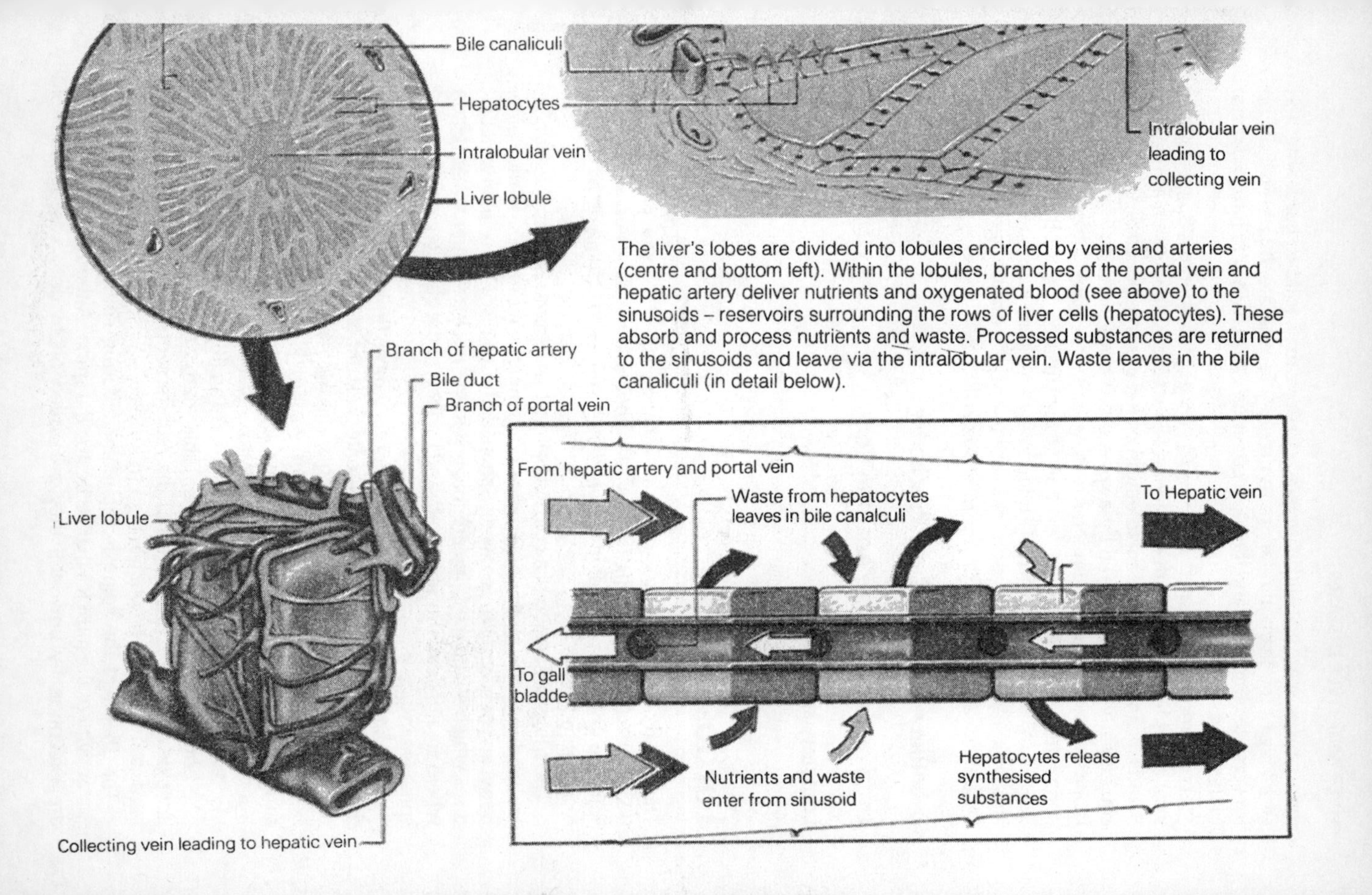

The liver's lobes are divided into lobules encircled by veins and arteries (centre and bottom left). Within the lobules, branches of the portal vein and hepatic artery deliver nutrients and oxygenated blood (see above) to the sinusoids – reservoirs surrounding the rows of liver cells (hepatocytes). These absorb and process nutrients and waste. Processed substances are returned to the sinusoids and leave via the intralobular vein. Waste leaves in the bile canaliculi (in detail below).

then causes scarring, and if severe, CIRRHOSIS may follow: hardening and shrinking of the liver, and failure to properly regenerate. It is eventually an irreversible condition, and the most common cause of liver failure and coma in the West.

Liver tumours are treated either by surgery or radiotherapy. Some forms of viral hepatitis clear up with rest after a few weeks. Others, such as hepatitis B and C, can cause persistent infection called *chronic hepatitis.* Cirrhosis, if caught early, can be slowed by a special diet and giving up alcohol. If the jaundice produced by kernicterus is severe, the baby's blood must be completely replaced, in an 'exchange transfusion'. Acute liver failure is treated by a low protein diet, injections of VITAMIN K, blood transfusion, antibiotics and the intravenous delivery of fructose (fruit sugar). In addition, in some cases a liver TRANSPLANT may be carried out.

Lobotomy, pre-frontal, *see* **Psychiatry**

Local anaesthetics, *see* **Anaesthetics**

Lockjaw, *see* **Tetanus**

Lordosis

The spine (*see* BACK AND BACKACHE) is a curving S shape, the lower part of which is the lumbar region (small of the back). Although the natural curvature of the spine in this area is called the *lordosis,* the term usually refers to an exaggerated curve.

The spine is made up of a column of vertebrae (jointed backbones) which are held together by the muscles and ligaments that lie beside the spine. Between each vertebra is a wedge-shaped fibrous disc. These intervertebral discs which shape the spine are thickest in the neck and the lumbar region where greater flexibility is needed, and thinnest in the chest region where the spine is rigid.

In the lumbar region, the spine is not only more flexible than the spine in the chest area, it also has to bear a greater amount of the body's weight, and it is the combination of these two factors which leads to pain in the lower back being such a common problem. There is an additional complication in the structure of the spine which increases the back's vulnerability – after the five lumbar vertebrae have made the bottom half of an S shape (the lumbar lordosis), the lowest one makes quite a sharp angle as it joins on to the sacrum (the bone at the base of the spine). This sharp angled joint has to carry a considerable burden; because of the requirements of CHILDBIRTH, the angle tends to be greater in women than men.

The shape of the spine is maintained during sitting and standing by the activity of the muscles that lie beside the spine. Although these muscles are exceptionally powerful, they are called on to do a vast amount of work. When they are overworked, low backache occurs; if they are simply not equal to some particular task and suddenly give way, the result may be a SLIPPED DISC.

Lordosis in pregnancy

In PREGNANCY, the weight of the growing womb in the pelvis puts an increased strain on the lower back. It also causes the lower stomach and pelvis to be tipped forward, increasing the strain by increasing the lordosis. In addition to this, all the ligaments that bind the various parts of the skeleton together relax during pregnancy, and although this is a valuable process because it allows the pelvis to become more flexible during childbirth, it has the disadvantage of placing yet more of a strain on the muscles of the back.

See also KYPHOSIS.

Lumbago

This is the old-fashioned name for the type of back pain which is felt in the lumbar region, or small of the back. *See* BACK AND BACKACHE.

Lumbar puncture

Cerebro-spinal fluid is the liquid which circulates around the BRAIN and SPINAL CORD and cushions them from injury. It is a clear, sterile liquid containing a small amount of PROTEIN and also SUGAR. Abnormalities in the spinal fluid can indicate the presence of certain illnesses; doctors can use a technique known as a lumbar puncture to take samples of it, in order to measure its pressure and sometimes to inject ANAESTHETICS or ANTIBIOTICS.

The sample of fluid can be analysed for the number of white BLOOD cells – leucocytes – it contains, and for the concentrations of proteins and sugar (glucose). With inflammatory conditions such as MULTIPLE SCLEROSIS, the amount of protein in the cerebrospinal fluid is increased; bacterial infections and tumours cause a reduction in the sugar concentration. Cerebrospinal fluid can also be examined using a microscope to determine the presence of specific micro-organisms or abnormal (cancerous) cells. In some cases, the disease organism in a sample of fluid can be 'grown' in a culture medium and then identified.

One of the commonest disorders usually diagnosed by means of a lumbar puncture is MENINGITIS, which involves inflammation of the meninges, the membranes within the skull which cover the outer surface of the brain. There are many forms of the disease, caused by bacteria (including TUBERCULOSIS and SYPHILIS) or viruses. Other disorders associated with abnormal spinal fluid include encephalitis, ABSCESSES or TUMOURS of the brain or spinal cord and various types of haemorrhage into the cerebrospinal space.

The technique of lumbar puncture

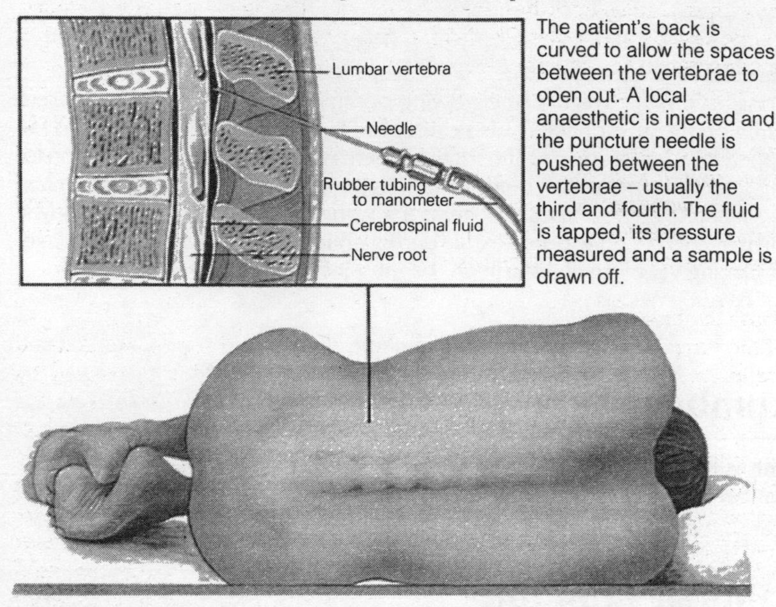

The patient's back is curved to allow the spaces between the vertebrae to open out. A local anaesthetic is injected and the puncture needle is pushed between the vertebrae – usually the third and fourth. The fluid is tapped, its pressure measured and a sample is drawn off.

How it is done

The patient is placed at the edge of the bed with his or her legs curled right up so that the spine is parallel to the bed. Alternatively, the patient may be sitting up. The small of the back is cleaned with antiseptic spirit.

Local anaesthetic is injected just under the skin to deaden the area. Then the hollow lumbar puncture needle is pushed through the skin until the doctor senses by its resistance that the spinal canal has been entered.

A stilette (probe) from the centre of the needle is removed and fluid flows up the hollow channel, to be collected for analysis. A manometer is connected so that the spinal fluid pressure can be measured. Afterwards, the patient must rest flat in bed for six hours, to avoid a headache.

Lungs and lung diseases

The lungs have an essential purpose – it is here that a vital exchange of gases takes place, when life-maintaining OXYGEN is absorbed into the bloodstream from the air we breathe and waste carbon dioxide is removed from the body.

The lungs themselves form little more than a dense latticework of tubes – those containing blood mingling with another system of tubes containing air; the structure is suspended on a framework of elastic strands and fibres.

Of the two lungs, the right is larger as the heart takes more room on the left side. Each lung is divided into lobes, which are fed by divisions of the bronchus, leading from the trachea (windpipe). The right lung has three lobes, upper, middle and lower. The left has only two, upper and lower. The lobes are separate from one another and are marked by grooves on the surface, known as fissures. These give important information to doctors, as they can be seen on a chest X-ray. By looking carefully at their position and observing, for instance, whether they have moved up or down, they can tell whether you have suffered a collapse of part of your lung.

The entrance to the trachea is guarded by a flap valve, the *epiglottis*. When we swallow, this shuts, preventing food from entering the lungs. Should this mechanism fail and food get into the trachea, violent coughing results.

How the lungs work

If the lungs were removed from the chest, they would shrink like deflated balloons. They are held open by surface tension, which is created by fluid produced by a thin lining around the lungs and the chest wall: the *pleural membrane* (sometimes referred to in the plural as the *pleura*). To picture this, think of two sheets of glass. If dry and laid on top of one another, they can be easily separated, but if wet the surface tension of the water sticks the glass sheets together. The only way in which they can be separated is by sliding them apart. In the same way, as long as a thin layer of fluid separates the lungs from the chest wall, the lungs are held open. When the chest expands, the lungs are pulled out and air is taken into the *alveoli* – millions of tiny air sacs in the lungs, each surrounded by fine capillaries (blood vessels) where the exchange of oxygen and carbon dioxide takes place. When we exhale, the rib muscles relax gradually. If we were to relax completely, the lungs would spring back rapidly. (*See also* BREATHING.) If air gets into the space between the lungs and the chest wall, the surface tension is broken and the lung collapses.

If the lining membrane becomes inflamed or irritated it may produce an excess of fluid which accumulates in the space between the lungs and the chest. Commonly called 'fluid on the lungs', its medical description is a *pleural effusion.*

In the alveoli, the exchange of oxygen and carbon dioxide takes place in less than one-tenth of a second. Oxygen is taken up by haemoglobin in the BLOOD and the red cells discharge their carbon dioxide, to be exhaled by the lungs.

Lung diseases

In adults, BRONCHITIS and EMPHYSEMA are by far the commonest chest conditions in Western countries. SMOKING is contributory to both and, to some extent, pollution. In bronchitis, the bronchial tubes become chronically inflamed and produce an excess of mucus, resulting in a COUGH that produces PHLEGM.

If suffering from emphysema, the patient becomes breathless, but does not usually cough or bring up phlegm. Both conditions can occur together.

Some impairment to breathing may also result due to obstruction in the

Cause and treatment of lung disorders

Disease	Cause	Symptoms	Treatment
Asbestosis	Inhalation of asbestos fibres	May give rise to tumours in the lung and in the pleura. 'Plaques' of chalky material in the pleura show up on the X-ray	Treatment of the tumours is very unsatisfactory. Prevention is all important
Asthma	Constriction of the bronchial tubes, often as an allergic reaction to something in the air (*see* ASTHMA)	Wheezing, and occasional cough	Drugs which have the effect of widening the tubes, usually given in an inhaler
Acute bronchitis	Inflammation of the lining of the bronchial tubes caused by infection (*see* BRONCHITIS)	Cough producing green or yellow sputum (phlegm)	Antibiotics
Chronic bronchitis	Inflammation of the bronchial tubes which persists even when there is no infection. Nearly always found in smokers (*see* BRONCHITIS)	Cough with sputum: coloured when the condition is due to infection, otherwise clear (white), produced for months at a time	Antibiotics help the acute flare-ups. The condition cannot really be cured although stopping smoking will help. Prevention: don't smoke!
Bronchiectasis	Inflammation with narrowing and widening of the bronchi. Follows a severe chest infection	Continuous production of large amounts of infected sputum	'Postural drainage' techniques are taught so that the affected part of the lung can drain its infected sputum. Surgical removal of the affected part may be required
Cancer	Various different types: all but a very few caused by smoking. Cancer of the lung actually arises in the lining of the bronchi (*see* CANCER)	May have no symptoms until widespread. Cough with blood (*haemoptysis*) or infection as a result of a bronchus being blocked by tumour; weight loss	Surgical removal is only possible in a few cases. Anti-cancer drugs and X-ray treatment are also helpful. To prevent: don't smoke!
Emphysema	Often occurs with chronic bronchitis. Caused by breakdown of the walls	Breathlessness. Other symptoms like a cough and wheeze indicate	Stopping smoking will help. Same sort of treatment as for asthma may

	between the small air spaces in the lung. Although the lungs may be larger, there is less area for oxygen to cross into the blood. Most sufferers smoke (*see* EMPHYSEMA)	that there is additional bronchitis or asthma	be of value in some cases. To avoid the disease: don't smoke!
Fibrosing alveolitis	Inflammation and eventual fibrosis of the alveoli (small air sacs). Can be a reaction to outside factors as in bird fancier's lung or farmer's lung	Shortness of breath and cough. Diagnosis confirmed through chest X-ray and special breathing tests	If there is an external cause, it must be removed. When not, steroid drugs can help
Pleurisy	Inflammation of the pleura. Usually due to a virus (*see* PLEURISY)	Pain on breathing	Rest and pain-killing drugs as for any other virus
Pneumonia	Infection and inflammation of the lung tissue as well as the bronchi (*see* PNEUMONIA)	Cough, fever, breathlessness. May bring on asthma or cause pleurisy	Antibiotics and sometimes physiotherapy
Pneumoconiosis	Inhalation of dust; usually associated with mining. Often occurs with emphysema	Breathlessness	Avoidance of dust. To prevent: keep dust levels down, and use masks at work
Pneumothorax	Air escapes from the lung into the pleural cavity (space around the lungs lined with the pleural membrane) causing the lung to collapse	Sudden breathlessness, often with pain in the chest	Air must be allowed out of the chest by inserting a tube through the chest wall
Pulmonary embolism	A clot of blood floating in the circulation (usually arising from thrombosis in the legs) breaks off and passes through the heart until it gets stuck in the pulmonary artery (the main blood-vessel to the lungs)	Collapse in severe cases. In less serious conditions, pleurisy-type pain and some breathlessness. Can cause haemoptysis	Blood-thinning tablets to prevent clots forming
Tuberculosis (TB)	Infection of the lungs by the TB bacterium. Other organs may be affected but the lung is the commonest site (*see* TUBERCULOSIS)	Cough, often with haemoptysis. Can cause a severe fever. Sometimes found with no symptoms	Treatment is with special anti-TB antibiotics

bronchial tubes. This may be persistent and difficult to treat in chronic bronchitis. Where the obstruction is easily reversed by medication or rapidly gets better by itself, the condition is called ASTHMA.

PNEUMONIA is an infection of the deepest parts of the lungs, beyond the main bronchi, and involves the alveoli, so that it can interfere with oxygen exchange. It caused many deaths in the days before ANTIBIOTICS. The infection may be confined to only one lobe of the lung. This is called *lobar pneumonia* and is caused by the pneumococcus bacterium which, mercifully, is sensitive to antibiotics.

Other bacteria may invade the whole lung, causing *bronchopneumonia*, when breathing may be severely affected. The organism responsible is the *Haemophilus influenzae*, which is not related to the influenza virus. Unfortunately it is resistant to penicillin but is treatable with other antibiotics.

Viruses can also cause pneumonia, and they can weaken the patient and make him or her more susceptible to bacterial infections. Serious bacterial pneumonia can complicate the viral diseases of childhood, such as MEASLES, WHOOPING COUGH, CHICKENPOX and INFLUENZA. Pneumonia typically affects the weak, the sick, the very old or the very young. Adolescent or middle-aged people who develop pneumonia are often smokers.

There are several types of lung CANCER, but in the last 40 years there has been an enormous increase in one type – known as a *squamous carcinoma*. This is certainly due to smoking, but may in part be caused by industrial pollution.

Shadow on the lung

An area of disease or infection in the lungs is more opaque to X-RAYS than healthy lung tissue. As a result the diseased area shows up as a shadow, which actually appears white on the X-ray film (because it is conventionally viewed as a negative image).

The most common types of shadow result from lung infections. Even relatively minor degrees of bronchopneumonia show up as patches of shadowing. TUBERCULOSIS, a bacillary infection, also commonly causes shadow in the lung fields. It usually attacks the upper parts of the lobes, often producing dense shadows.

Diseases of the HEART can produce abnormal shadowing in the lung fields because heart failure results in extra fluid accumulating in the lungs (pulmonary OEDEMA). When there is heart failure, the heart is also increased in size so that the normal heart shadow seen on an X-ray is greatly enlarged.

Various OCCUPATIONAL disorders can also cause shadows on the lungs, including *pneumoconiosis* (inhaling coal dust) and *silicosis* (inhaling sand dust). FUNGAL INFECTIONS can also show up – e.g. *aspergillosis*.

Lumpectomy, *see* Breasts and breast cancer

Lupus erythematosus

Lupus erythematosus, abbreviated to LE, is a term which may apply to two conditions. One is a generalized disorder which can affect several organs of the body. This is more precisely called *systemic lupus erythematosus*, or SLE.

The other involves only the SKIN, and is properly called *discoid lupus*. Neither condition is particularly rare.

Both forms are characterized by a RASH (most discoid lupus cases and about 50 per cent of SLE cases involve one), and it commonly occurs, sometimes with a 'butterfly' shape, on either side of the nose, making the face look wolf-like. (*Lupus* is the Latin for 'wolf', and *erythematosus* the Latin for 'redness'.)

Discoid lupus

This form of the disease generally occurs in people in their 20s and 30s and affects women more than men. The rash usually develops on the face, consisting of round, scaly, disc-like patches. As well as showing up on the cheeks, it can occur on the lips and nose. The rash is particularly sensitive to sunlight, and it is important for sufferers to keep their faces shaded. Blood tests on people with discoid lupus show the same sorts of abnormalities as those taken on SLE patients, but as it is uncommon for discoid lupus to progress to SLE, they are for practical purposes regarded as two separate diseases.

SLE

By any standard, this is an extraordinary disease. One of a group called the 'connective tissue diseases', it can affect almost any organ or system within the body, and gives rise to many symptoms in the same system.

The symptoms come and go, with patients having several trouble-free years followed by outbreaks of illness. SLE used to be considered serious; today it is generally not. Like discoid lupus, it is more common in women than in men, with about nine women affected for every one man. It also seems more common among black people.

Causes

Basically, the causes of either form of the disease are unknown. All that can be said for certain is that the disease is associated with abnormalities of the body's IMMUNE SYSTEM.

The immune system works by producing antibodies, or defence cells, which specialize in engulfing and destroying harmful invaders such as bacteria. In SLE patients, the immune system not only produces antibodies to fight 'outsiders', it also produces antibodies (anti-nuclear antibodies) which fight parts of the body itself. But none of this actually pinpoints the cause.

Symptoms and treatment

Discoid lupus has no symptoms other than the facial rash. SLE is characterized by bouts of recurring ill health, which may be associated with a higher than normal temperature. Then there are the more specific symptoms, varying from case to case.

Besides the skin rash, there may be pains in the joints reminiscent of ARTHRITIS, inflammation of the LUNGS (similar to PLEURISY) and involvement of the HEART. Most serious of all is the involvement of the KIDNEYS.

Discoid lupus can be effectively controlled by applying a STEROID cream to the affected skin area. Steroids are drugs which can 'damp down' the operation of the immune system, and they used to be the mainstay of treatment of SLE, too. But these days, doctors prefer not to use them if possible because of their tendency to produce side-effects if taken over a long period – which is likely to be necessary in an SLE patient.

The alternative is to use one of the immunosuppressive drugs (e.g. hydroxychloroquine) which have been developed to a considerable degree of refinement in recent years.

Lyme disease, *see* **Arthritis**

Lymphatic system

This forms a complicated network of very fine tubes which are designed to carry away surplus fluid from the BLOOD and tissues, and to make the white blood cells, or *lymphocytes,* which form part of the IMMUNE SYSTEM.

Structure

The lymphatic system is composed of tubes about the diameter of a needle which criss-cross the tissues to collect surplus fluid, known as *lymph,* from blood vessels and body tissues, and then return it to the bloodstream via a myriad of vessels known as *lymphatics.* Some lymphatics contain an involuntary muscle which contracts rhythmically in one direction, driving the lymph forward, with valves set at intervals of 1½ in (38 mm) to prevent the lymph from flowing backward.

Lymphatics are found in all parts of the body, except the central nervous system, and the constituents of the lymph they contain is dependent on their location. For instance, the vessels draining the limbs contain fluid surplus to body needs which is leaked from cells or blood vessels; the lymph therefore is rich in protein, especially albumin. On the other hand, the lymph in the intestines is full of fat, which it has absorbed from the intestines during digestion; this lymph has a distinctive milky-looking colour.

At various points, the lymphatics join together to form a knot of tissues known as a *lymph node,* or 'gland', where the lymphatic type of white blood cells, which act as part of the body's defence system, are made. (The term 'lymph gland' is inaccurate because glands make hormones and the lymph glands only process lymphocytes.) These lymph nodes collect around major arteries and can be felt at these points where the arteries run close to the skin – for example, they occur in the groin, in the armpits and in the neck.

All the lymph vessels join together to form two large ducts: the *thoracic duct* and the *right lymphatic duct*. The lymph enters and exits from these, then circulates to the rest of the body.

Functions

Lymphocytes are also made by BONE MARROW, but those processed by the lymph nodes are special and are called *T lymphocytes*. They receive chemical messages concerning the nature of foreign agents such as viruses and bacteria which invade the body, and then pass these messages on to the developing lymphocytes to help them make *antibodies* (a protein which inactivates the foreign agent).

Unless the infection is contained at the point of entry, the invading bacteria or viruses gather in the lymph and pass up to the nearest lymph node, resulting in a condition known as *lymphangitis*. The lymph channel becomes inflamed on the way, and this can be seen through the skin as a thin red line, which is tender to touch. Once the infection reaches the lymph nodes, these swell up. This is why a wound in the finger will produce a swollen lymph node in the armpit if not treated promptly.

Besides acting as a filter of bacteria and viruses which invade the body, the lymph nodes also trap CANCER cells which are carried away from the tumour in the lymph. Once in the lymph nodes, the cancer cells may lodge and begin to grow, forming a secondary deposit. Cancers of the breast, for example, will drain towards the lymph nodes of the armpit, and cancers of the lung may spread to the nodes in the neck. When the lymph node is invaded, it enlarges and hardens, but it is seldom painful as it is during viral or bacterial infections. The neighbouring lymph nodes often have to be removed during surgery for cancer.

Lymphatic obstruction

In certain instances, the lymphatic vessels can be blocked and the lymph dammed back. This seldom causes a problem in the chest or abdomen because the large network of vessels act as an alternative pathway for drainage, but if an obstruction arises in the limbs, this wide choice of routes is not available. Here the blockage of the lymphatics, which causes the fluid to collect outside the cells, usually results in a type of swelling known as *lymphoedema* (*see* OEDEMA).

Lymphatic obstruction can have various causes. Occasionally people may be born with deficient lymphatic channels. The deficiency may affect one limb or part of a limb or it may be generalized. However, this condition seldom causes a problem to the major organs of the body which receive lymph from such a massive network of vessels.

Obstruction of the lymphatic vessels in the legs may occasionally follow normal CHILDBIRTH, and although this is short-lived, swelling of the legs may persist in some instances. Some diseases are associated with lymphatic obstruction, the most well-known being a condition called *elephantiasis*, which is due to an infection caused by tiny parasitic worms known as filariae, which gain entry to the lymphatic system through the feet. The ensuing blockage of the lymph glands results in permanent damage and unsightly swelling. A similar condition may result in the arms.

When lymph channels have been damaged by surgery, lymphoedema also results and may be persistent. This may be seen in one or other arm following a MASTECTOMY operation for breast cancer. Sometimes, as a precautionary measure, the lymph glands are removed from the armpit on that side in case they too contain cancer deposits which may spread.

TUMOURS may also obstruct the lymphatic channels and this will result in lymphoedema. Because of the invasive nature of many tumours, the lymph vessels themselves may become perforated, leading to a leakage of lymph. Where there are large numbers of lymphatic channels such as in the abdomen and chest, leakage may be quite large and contain a great deal of fat. Lymph may then accumulate either between the lungs and the chest wall, forming an *effusion*, or in the abdomen, forming *ascites* (oedema in the membrane of the abdominal cavity). If a creamy white fluid is obtained when these accumulations are drained, the patient is likely to have a malignant disease.

Not only do the lymph channels and nodes form a means by which cancer is spread, they may also themselves be the site of primary cancers known as LYMPHOMAS or *lymphosarcomas*, the latter being of a more serious nature. Lymphomas can be cured if caught early.

Diagnosis

For less serious illnesses, the doctor can feel your armpits, groin, or round your neck to see if the lymph nodes are enlarged, but in other instances, special techniques may be required. If the disease involves the lymph nodes near the surface, a local anaesthetic is given, a small incision is made through the skin and a piece of node is removed for study under a microscope; this is a BIOPSY.

Biopsies of deeper nodes around the aorta (the major artery leaving the heart) are either done by an abdominal operation under a general anaesthetic, an inconvenient procedure, or by a *lymphangiogram*, where a special dye is injected, usually in the foot; this is then carried up to the lymph nodes, first in the groin and then in the abdomen, and will show up any abnormality on an X-ray.

See also ADENOIDS, AIDS, GLANDULAR FEVER, HODGKIN'S DISEASE, SPLEEN, TONSILS.

Lymphocytes, *see* **Blood, Rejection of tissue, Thymus**

Lymphogranuloma venerum, *see* **Chlamydia**

Lymphoma

This is a cancer of the lymph nodes (commonly called 'glands'), the islands of lymph tissue (*see* LYMPHATIC SYSTEM) which are found in the SPLEEN, LIVER and

INTESTINE, and around the large blood vessels of the HEART. *Non-Hodgkin's lymphoma* is rare below the age of two, whereas *Hodgkin's lymphomas* (*see* HODGKIN'S DISEASE) are more prevalent in people in their mid-30s to their mid-50s.

Hodgkin's lymphomas can develop into the more serious non-Hodgkin's lymphomas if treatment is not given, and these can, in turn, become *lymphosarcomas,* the most serious form of lymphoma, if left untreated.

Causes and symptoms

Viruses have long been suspected as a possible cause of lymphomas, but after much research, this theory has proved untenable and the cause of the condition remains unknown.

In the early stages, there may be no symptoms, but as the illness progresses, the most common symptoms are tiredness, loss of energy, loss of appetite and, particularly, weight loss. The patient may discover quite accidentally that his or her neck 'glands' are enlarged.

In Hodgkin's lymphoma, in the early stages, single lymph nodes or groups of nodes are involved, and it is only later that the disease spreads to involve nodes elsewhere in the body, and lymphoid tissue in the spleen and liver. The enlarged nodes have a curious, rather rubbery feel to them, though they are not painful, unlike other cancers or infected nodes.

Another symptom of lymphomas is fever, which has a curious pattern of rising in the evening, but this alternates with periods during which the temperature is normal, sometimes for days or even weeks. This fever pattern is known as *Pel–Ebstein* and, in rare cases, may be the only sign of lymphoma. One other curious symptom is a persistent skin itchiness and dull pain which develops in the neck nodes within a few minutes of drinking alcohol; no explanation for this has been found.

Late in the disease, blood abnormalities appear, the most striking being ANAEMIA. Though there is no increase in T lymphocytes (white blood cells created in the lymph nodes, which fight infection), those appearing in the blood under the microscope do not look normal, and there is a variation of cell appearance between the non-Hodgkin's and Hodgkin's lymphomas.

In some cases, where deeper nodes are involved, no obvious symptoms may be present, and the disease is only discovered during the course of a routine chest X-ray, where the lymphomas show up as lumps on either side of the heart.

Treatment

The earlier the treatment starts, the better the chance of cure.

First, an assessment is made as to how far the disease has spread: this is known as 'staging' the disease. This is done by feeling the nodes close to the skin, and in the liver and spleen to see if they are enlarged. For deeper nodes around the aorta, in the abdomen and thorax (chest), a CT scan is performed, or an abdominal operation to remove and inspect the glands may be needed. An X-ray called a *lymphangiogram* is rarely performed nowadays.

The staging system divides the disease into four groups, depending on the extent of spread. Choice of treatment is dependent on this.

In the early stages of the disease, radiation treatment is given, but in later stages, where the spleen is involved or there is evidence of spread both above and below the DIAPHRAGM, anti-cancer drugs, the same used in the treatment of LEUKAEMIA, are used in combination with RADIOTHERAPY. These powerful drugs are given in combinations of three or four at a time in periods, or 'pulses', since continuous treatment results in death of the BONE MARROW. On occasion, supportive treatment, known as maintenance treatment, with the STEROID prednisone, is given between pulses. Treatment for Hodgkin's lymphomas and non-Hodgkin's lymphomas is similar, but determining which stage lymphomas have reached is not always easy. If the bone marrow is extensively involved, a bone marrow transplant may be considered.

Outlook

Hodgkin's disease is now curable, depending on the stage the disease has reached, together with survival without recurring symptoms five years following the start of treatment. Survival from non-Hodgkin's lymphomas is not as good, but cure is possible.

McBurney's point, *see* **Appendicitis**

Macules, *see* **Moles, Rash**

Madura foot, *see* **Fungal infections**

Malabsorption

This happens when the STOMACH and INTESTINES become unable to digest and absorb food properly. It can affect both children and adults and can lead to MALNUTRITION, however full and varied the diet.

Malabsorption results from a variety of underlying diseases and conditions, but where wheat is a staple part of the diet, the most common is COELIAC DISEASE. This can appear from childhood onwards and results from sensitivity of the small intestine to gluten, a basic constituent of most cereals. The sensitivity vastly cuts down the intestine's ability to absorb digested food, as it decreases the surface area by flattening the millions of microscopic finger-like projections called villi. A similar disease, *tropical sprue,* causes many cases of malabsorption in the tropics.

Malabsorption can occur after surgery involving removal of part of the stomach for ULCERS. This is the most common cause of intestinal stagnation, when the waves of peristalsis which move food through the gut are temporarily interrupted, which, in turn, causes malabsorption.

If the flow of BILE from the GALL BLADDER and bile duct is interrupted, this will deprive the small intestine of vital bile salts and can trigger malabsorption. Alternatively, there may not be enough digestive juices to break down the contents of the small intestine if the PANCREAS becomes inflamed over a long period – a condition known as *chronic pancreatitis.*

CYSTIC FIBROSIS is a rare inherited disease where secretions of various sorts of glands do not work properly. This includes the digestive secretions of the pancreas, so poor absorption may result.

Symptoms

Malabsorption can be hard to recognize, as its symptoms are not specific, especially in the early stages. Later, there may be obvious malnutrition, but often blood tests are the only method of positive diagnosis.

There is nearly always some disturbance of the bowel with loose stools and sometimes DIARRHOEA. The stools often have distinctive features – they are abnormally pale, bulky, frothy, difficult to flush, and smell worse than usual.

Stomach aches, ranging from vague discomfort to acute pain, can result from excessive activity in the small intestine. If the condition is severe enough to cause ANAEMIA, symptoms of general ill-health, such as tiredness, weight loss and breathlessness are likely.

Symptoms of other blood disorders resulting from malabsorption can also appear. Pain in the bones and bowing of the legs, called RICKETS in children and *osteomalacia* in adults, indicates a low level of calcium in the blood caused by a lack of VITAMIN D. There is a slim chance of excessive bleeding from any wounds as poor absorption of vitamin K reduces the tendency of the blood to clot, but usually this is only obvious from blood tests.

Children with malabsorption may have additional symptoms of stunted growth, although it is sometimes difficult to judge if a child should have grown more or if a baby or toddler is thriving.

Malabsorption is a dangerous condition which can be fatal if left untreated. The patient can starve even though consuming food, as the body receives too few calories. IRON, folic acid and CALCIUM levels of the blood can drop below acceptable levels, too, involving serious illness related to blood deficiency.

Treatment

Treatment depends on the underlying cause. Coeliac disease is diagnosed by removing a tiny portion of the internal surface of the small intestine (BIOPSY) for examination under a microscope. An ingenious biopsy capsule is swallowed and triggered to remove the specimen when it has reached the right level. This disease is treated by restricting the patient to a gluten-free diet. Tropical sprue is treated with the antibiotic tetracycline and folic acid, but does not always respond well. Cystic fibrosis is greatly helped by the addition of extracts of pancreas to food, to aid digestion.

Intestinal stagnation has a variety of treatments, with surgery to reconnect the stagnant loop as a last resort.

Malaria

There are 1.5 billion people living in areas where they are at risk of catching malaria, but it is on the increase in many other parts of the world. For instance, it is now relatively common in Britain, since air travellers may catch the disease in malarial areas and not develop symptoms until they have returned home.

Malaria is commonest in the tropics (*see* TROPICAL DISEASES), but it may be found a good distance both north and south of them. It is particularly prevalent in Africa and is becoming more common in India and other parts of Asia. The only parts from which it has been successfully eliminated are Europe, Australia, the Asian areas of the former USSR, and North America. It is not found in very cold climates.

It should be remembered that the carrier of the disease is an insect, so air travellers who merely make a refuelling stop can be bitten and get malaria.

Causes

The parasite which causes the disease is called a *plasmodium*. Four different species of it cause malaria in human beings: *Plasmodium falciparum, P. malariae, P. vivax* and *P. ovale*. Of the four, the most important is *P. falciparum,* since it is the most commonly fatal form, and also causes the most serious complications: for this reason, falciparum malaria is known as 'malignant tertian malaria'. (The use of words such as tertian and quartan to describe the different sorts of malaria refer to the characteristic time courses of the bouts of fever accompanying the disease: in tertian malaria, the fever tends to come every third day, in quartan malaria every fourth day.)

The three other sorts of plasmodium cause less malignant malaria. ('Malignant' here does not mean cancerous; rather it implies that the disease is very virulent or infectious.) Their main feature is bouts of fever recurring at regular intervals, and with these forms of malaria, the parasites may remain dormant in the LIVER for long periods of time, and can occasionally cause the disease long after the original infection. (Serious complications, and even death, may occur with any form of malaria.)

Life-cycle

Malaria is spread by female *Anopheles* mosquitoes. They pick up parasites during a meal of blood taken from an infected human being, but for them to become carriers they have to take up both the male and female forms of the parasite, called *gametocytes*.

Once both are inside the mosquito's stomach, they fuse to form a fertilized egg cell inside the stomach wall. This eventually develops into something called a *sporozoite* which migrates to the mosquito's mouth parts, from where it can be injected into the next human being whom the mosquito bites.

Sporozoites entering the bloodstream as a result of an infected bite make their way to the liver where they remain for about a week without causing any symptoms. They then invade the red BLOOD cells where they start to multiply and to cause symptoms in the host.

Trophozoites – early stages in the plasmodium's life-cycle – increase in size inside the infected blood cell until they are large enough to divide into two *merozoites,* which are then available to infect other red blood cells. This process of division and release of merozoites results in the original blood cell being broken down and its contents being released into the bloodstream. When large numbers of red cells are infected, quite severe ANAEMIA can result.

Eventually, some merozoites develop into male or female gametocytes instead of fresh trophozoites when they enter a new red blood cell, and they can then infect a new mosquito if the human host should be bitten by one. No further development of the gametocyte takes place unless it finds it way into an *Anopheles* mosquito stomach.

In malignant falciparum malaria, the parasites continue to divide in the bloodstream once they have become established there. As there is no reservoir of infection elsewhere in the body, killing the parasites in the blood would eliminate the disease completely. In the other forms of malaria, there is the possibility of relapse if the disease is eliminated from the blood only, since parasites lying dormant in the liver can reinfect the blood.

Symptoms

People living in areas where malaria is common suffer from repeated attacks of the disease and so become partially immune to the local strains of the infecting parasites (*see also* SICKLE CELL ANAEMIA), whereas a visitor to the area may have a quite severe bout of the malarial disease.

The most important symptom is fever – in less severe attacks, it may be the only one. When the disease first develops, fevers may be fairly continuous, but as it progresses, the cycles of red blood cell breakdown and the reinfection of new cells tend to become synchronized, so that a whole lot of red cells are all breaking down at the same time. Fevers occur when this happens.

P. malariae produces fever every fourth day, usually in the evening. *P. vivax* and *P. ovale* tend to produce fevers every third day. Falciparum malaria may show very little regular swinging of the fever, but if it does, the swings occur about every second day.

A swing in fever often goes through three distinct stages: a 'cold stage', a 'hot stage' and finally a 'sweating stage', when the temperature returns towards normality. The other symptoms tend to be like those of flu: headache, a general feeling of illness and sickness. Vomiting and diarrhoea also may occur, giving the impression that the patient has a rather severe stomach upset.

The other common symptoms of all forms of malaria are anaemia (resulting from the recurrent breakdown of red blood cells), and enlargement of both the liver and the SPLEEN. In people with partial immunity, there may be a continuous low level of parasites in the blood with an occasional bout of fever.

Dangers

Infection with *P. falciparum* involves the most dangers, the gravest one being *cerebral malaria*. This affects the brain, causing mental disturbance, drowsiness, fits and, eventually, UNCONSCIOUSNESS, which is often fatal.

Malignant malaria may also cause quite bad infection of the liver and of the gut, giving rise to symptoms which can be mistaken for the liver disorder HEPATITIS or dysentery.

Failure of the KIDNEYS caused by malaria can be almost as dangerous as cerebral malaria. *Blackwater fever*, involving the kidneys, results from infections so heavy that large numbers of red blood cells are broken down, releasing considerable amounts of red blood cell pigment – haemoglobin – into the blood, whence it is passed out in the urine. Blackwater fever is not as common as it once was: it seems that the regular use of quinine to try and prevent malaria was frequently a factor in bringing it about. It appears to occur when people have lived in heavily infected malarial areas for a few months.

Treatment and prevention

Quinine is probably the best-known anti-malarial drug, but there are now many others as well. It is not wise to try to wipe out the infection completely in people living in malarial areas, since they would lose the immunity they have. Treatment for them consists of giving them just enough anti-malarial treatment to clear the blood and so avoid symptoms.

In contrast, people who get malaria and then return to live in a temperate part of the world should have what is called a 'radical cure': when they have been infected with one of the relapsing (recurring) forms of the disease, they should have one drug to clear the bloodstream and another to clear the liver.

It is important to build up blood levels of anti-malarial drugs by starting to take them a week or so before leaving for a malarial area, and it is even more important to continue taking them *for at least four weeks* on returning to a temperate country.

To prevent malaria: Mosquito netting secured in place over your bed at night reduces your chances of getting bitten. Burn a mosquito coil – a spring-shaped insecticide candle – in each room to discourage the mosquito.

Malignancy

In medicine, the term 'malignant' can be applied to any extremely serious or almost certainly fatal condition. In practice, it is used to describe cancerous TUMOURS which spread to other parts of the body and which would, if left, eventually kill the patient (*see also* CANCER).

In contrast, the term 'benign' suggests that the condition is harmless, with no serious consequences, and in practice, benign tumours are those which may grow larger but which never spread to other organs or parts of the body.

Malnutrition

This condition is any poor health or illness caused by an inadequate diet, so both semi-starvation and over-feeding can be to blame. While two thirds of the world's population have too little food, OBESITY is a major health hazard in the prosperous Western countries.

Food intake must be correct in both quantity and quality and in developing countries, both may be at fault. The average calorie intake for whole populations is often only half the minimum required to stay healthy, and whatever food is available lacks PROTEIN. This deficiency is so serious for children that, in many countries, half the population dies before the age of five.

However, malnutrition is by no means restricted to the developing world. Poor people everywhere go hungry or have to buy cheap, starchy food to feel full – which is why obesity is not the privilege of the very rich. Children, especially pre-school age, and old people are the most frequent victims of poverty-based malnutrition.

Causes

War, famine, drought and economic circumstances restricting food imports and availability are the major causes of malnutrition. The lack of a vital substance in the local food or water can cause VITAMIN deficiency for whole populations.

Poor eating habits are another serious cause, either from over-indulgence in the wrong foods, or through custom – in the Far East where beri-beri is widespread, causing general weakness and swelling of the limbs, the local diet is based on polished rice, and the nutritious husk is thrown away. Obesity is caused by taking in more calories than needed and storing them as fat.

Certain medical conditions either prevent proper absorption of food or, as with a baby with a CLEFT PALATE, restrict intake. PREGNANCY can render an adequate diet insufficient in protein and IRON for both mother and baby. Disease of the placenta can leave the baby severely malnourished.

Symptoms and treatment

Malnutrition has general effects and some specific conditions resulting from lack of essential vitamins or MINERALS.

A malnourished child appears pale from ANAEMIA, dull, small and thin. Lack of protein can cause *kwashiorkor*, a severe form of malnutrition in children, in which the skin and abdomen become distended from retained fluid, the liver swells, and there is loss of pigment in the skin and hair. Starvation brings children additional symptoms of dry, inelastic, cold skin and sparse hair.

An adult who is semi-starved can lose up to 70 per cent of body weight, some as water but much as protein shed from the muscles, liver, intestines, and heart. Lack of calories can cause ANAEMIA, low BLOOD PRESSURE, apathy, irritability and bouts of debilitating DIARRHOEA.

Skimmed milk is most frequently used to treat malnutrition as it provides excellent protein replacement and is easily transported. Vitamin supplements are necessary for severe cases, and where a medical problem is the cause, this must be controlled or corrected. However, in most cases, a balanced diet is such a rapid cure that, after two or three weeks, essential vitamins are replaced and resistance to disease is restored.

Unless puberty has been reached, a child can make up growth completely. Older people rapidly return to a lively, active state.

Mammography, *see* Breasts and breast cancer

Manganese, *see* Minerals

Manic depression

People whose moods swing wildly from intense elation to severe depression may be suffering from a condition known as manic depression. This is a severe mental disturbance. The condition is referred to as manic-depressive psychosis (*see* PSYCHIATRY), regardless of whether the full swing between mania and depression is shown.

Causes

Manic depression is an affective psychosis – that is, the patient becomes carried away by his or her emotions, either from habit, or in an effort to conceal anxiety and shyness. Manic depressives are often reserved, inward-looking, emotionally sensitive personalities, even though, during the manic phase, their behaviour takes on a very extrovert form.

A possible cause is a defect in the hormonal mechanisms that control the balance of our emotions. Two chemicals present in the brain influence mood: a low level of one, *serotonin*, may produce mood instabilities in general, while an imbalance of the second chemical, *norepinephrine*, determines the direction of the mood swing, a low level being associated with DEPRESSION and a high level producing mania.

Normally, manic depression arises without any causal stress, but it is possible that external factors such as outside tension, abnormal patterns of upbringing or unconventional attitudes may actually stimulate the brain to produce the chemicals which give rise to the mood swings.

Symptoms

The illness takes the form of mania (*hypomania* when not excessive, and *hypermania* when very intense) which is a highly over-excited and elated state. Patients in a manic phase work at high pressure at everything they do; they talk a great deal and at high speed, flitting from subject to subject; and usually get involved in doing several things at once because they are easily distracted.

In extreme cases, the patient behaves much like the popular notion of the raving maniac: continually pacing about, shouting, singing, screaming obscenities. Alternatively, they may be confused, disorientated, experiencing hallucinations and delusions (religious or non-religious) or act in a sexually unrestrained or unpredictably violent way. Patients seldom realize that anything is amiss, but they may change mood very suddenly and turn from being pleasant to being very aggressive if not tactfully handled.

Alternating with mania is the severe depressive state, with profound fatigue, despondency and sadness. In extreme cases, the patient becomes silent and motionless. Suicide can become a real risk during recovery from this phase, as before this, patients actually lack the determination to kill or seriously harm themselves. Manic and depressive moods often arise spontaneously, and last for some time – even weeks or months if no treatment is given.

Patients who are in the manic or depressive phase of the cycle are usually not dangerous to others, but living with them is not very easy. However, patients may become a danger to themselves if the condition is untreated: for instance, they can become undernourished through lack of time or will to eat. Many sufferers go on wild spending sprees and may get themselves into debt. But they have no idea that they are placing a financial burden on themselves and their families.

Treatment

The mania of manic depression will most certainly need psychiatric treatment, though hospitalization will only occur in extreme cases. Drugs will generally also be used, both to help lift any depression and to reduce the intensity of the manic episodes. In some cases, the moods are treated separately, using tricyclic antidepressants or monomine oxidase inhibitors to control the depressive swings, and SEDATIVES and TRANQUILLIZERS to control episodes of mania.

Lithium carbonate has been found to be a beneficial treatment for manic depression because it stabilizes the ups and downs of the manic-depressive cycle. The doctor introduces the drug gradually, checking its level in the blood every few days until the best dose is determined. Lithium is usually given for many months or even years and can be dramatically successful in improving the lives of sufferers. But it may have toxic effects on the THYROID gland and KIDNEYS unless the dose is very carefully controlled.

Manipulative therapies

Any treatment where parts of the body are manoeuvred to change their positions is called *manipulation.* It is used in many branches of medicine, usually by a highly skilled surgeon or PHYSIOTHERAPIST. Manipulation is most common in treatment for BONE and JOINT problems, but is occasionally used in obstetrics and in the treatment of HERNIAS.

Fractures

When a bone is broken, the two parts may become separated or misaligned. For instance, in a FRACTURE of the femur (thigh bone), there may be a clean break across the bone with the two ends overlapping considerably. Manipulation of a fracture requires considerable skill and practice as it is done by feel rather than sight.

This type of manipulation is usually performed under ANAESTHETIC but an experienced surgeon can perform the realignment very quickly with the minimum of injury to the soft tissues around the fracture. An X-ray is taken afterwards to check the alignment and then the fractured bone is held in place by plaster of Paris or traction (pulleys and weights) until the bone has mended.

Joints

When a joint is put out of place by an injury (dislocation), manipulation is needed to restore it to normal. The SHOULDER joint is frequently dislocated by a fall on an outstretched hand or by direct injury – for instance, during vigorous sports such as rugby. It is a ball-and-socket joint, and when dislocated, the ball comes out of the socket and lies beside it. At this stage, the pull of the muscles around the shoulder tends to hold the shoulder out of place.

An anaesthetic or sedation is needed to inhibit the pull of the muscles while the joint is manipulated to reposition its component parts. For the shoulder joint, a specific manoeuvre has to be carried out. The head of the humerus (the bone of the upper arm) is pulled away from the shoulder blade and the arm is twisted so the ball goes back into the socket.

Some joints, especially the small joints in the BACK, can become locked halfway through a movement. This is usually due to wear and tear in the joint and can sometimes be instantaneously cured by manipulation. This can be accomplished by a sudden quick movement which need not be painful and can be performed without anaesthetic. A skilled physiotherapist can perform this type of manipulation with immediate and dramatic results in certain cases of back and neck pain.

Joints become stiff from wear and tear or because the joint or surrounding LIGAMENTS have been involved in a fracture. This severely limits movement at the joint and causes pain. Manipulation under a general anaesthetic sometimes helps in these cases. The joint is put through its full range of movements, sometimes breaking tissues which have become bonded. This range of play should be preserved by regular exercises under the supervision of a physiotherapist.

The KNEE joint is most frequently affected by a fragment coming loose inside the joint. This can be either a small fragment of bone from the end of the tibia (the shin bone) or a cartilage, a piece of gristle at the side of the knee joint which can protrude between the joint surfaces if torn. In either case, there is a sudden locking of the joint so it is fixed in a bent position.

If the joint is not too painful, this can sometimes be remedied by twisting the joint so the loose bit flips out of the space between the two bones. Usually only an ORTHOPAEDIC surgeon or a physiotherapist can manage this, but some people with recurrent cartilage problems can be taught to manipulate their own knee joints when locking occurs. Persistent cases, however, may require surgery.

Pregnancy and hernias

Manipulation is sometimes used in PREGNANCY to turn a foetus so the head points towards the pelvis (*see* BREECH BIRTH). This is a difficult and sometimes hazardous procedure and can only be undertaken by an experienced obstetrician. Great skill is required to make the diagnosis, to turn the foetus very gradually round, and to time the procedure so that the head will stay in the pelvis until birth.

Manipulation is occasionally used to push a hernia back into the abdomen when it becomes slightly painful or will not go back on its own when the patient lies down. It can be extremely dangerous and should only be done by an experienced doctor or surgeon. This form of manipulation is only a temporary measure to make the patient more comfortable, and usually indicates that an operation will be needed to effect a complete cure: the hernia will be reduced by pushing its contents – that is, the protruding part of the bowel – back into the abdomen. After this is done, the empty sac of PERITONEUM is removed and the wound is stitched.

Manipulative treatments

Although manipulation may be used by doctors for certain specific conditions, such as fractures, practitioners of chiropractic and OSTEOPATHY have developed manipulative treatments for a whole range of medical problems. Both the therapies originated in North America and have certain similarities.

Marijuana

The Indian hemp plant, also known as *Cannabis sativa*, is the source of several different forms of the drug *cannabis*, of which marijuana is one. The plant, which reaches a height of several feet, can be grown almost anywhere in the world, although it grows naturally and is cultivated commercially in India, Pakistan, South America and Africa. Marijuana is the name given to the dried leaves and flowering tops of the cannabis plant. This form of cannabis may also be called herbal cannabis or 'grass' and is usually smoked in a cigarette called a 'joint' or 'splif'. The same leaves are sometimes used to make an infusion (tea) – this form is known as *bhang*. In India, the smallest leaves from the plant are known as *ganja*.

Cannabis may also be used in the form of *hashish*, which is the dried resin from the leaves of the Indian hemp plant. Usually this form is also smoked, mixed with ordinary tobacco in a 'joint'. *Cannabis oil* is prepared from hashish by a process of distillation.

It has been estimated that between 11 and 14 per cent of the population of the United Kingdom have tried cannabis in one form or other, and that between 2 and 5 per cent are regular users. However, estimating the usage of illicit drugs is very difficult, and it is possible that consumption is higher. Most cannabis used in the United Kingdom is in the form of hashish, whereas in the United States, marijuana is most common.

Effects of cannabis

A number of different chemical constituents have been isolated from the Indian hemp plant which are responsible for the effects of cannabis on the body. These drugs are called *cannabinoids*, and at least 25 different types have been isolated. One of the most potent is *tetrahydrocannabinol* (THC).

The effect of cannabis on the user depends on the source of the marijuana or hashish used, because different climates and growing conditions may affect the amount of cannabinoids in the plants. Hashish tends to be stronger than marijuana, but cannabis oil is the most potent. Smoking cannabis produces more rapid effects than eating the leaves of the plant or drinking an infusion made from the leaves.

After smoking marijuana (or hashish), the effects tend to come on after an hour or two and reach their peak at about three hours. At first, the user feels relaxed and has a sense of well-being. Often he or she starts talking a great deal. There may be heightened perception of taste, smell or touch, but some users can also have hallucinations. Often colours take on a vivid hue, or sounds develop special significance.

The effects of cannabis vary considerably from one person to another – some people become depressed or irritable after taking it. This may occur as an initial reaction to the drug, or a depressive mood may set in a few hours after an earlier euphoria. Usually the effects pass within 12 hours of a single dose.

Most worrying is the occasional case of severe MENTAL ILLNESS triggered off by cannabis. This is more common in very heavy users but can occur in certain individuals after one joint. The individual may become severely disturbed. Repeated hallucinations can occur and there may also be repeated bouts of confusion, emotional outbursts, and delusions. The illness may clear up within a few weeks with appropriate medical treatment but can recur if the individual returns to cannabis.

Marrow, *see* **Bone marrow and transplants**

Massage

Massage is as old as history itself. Ancient Greek, Chinese and Indian writings all refer to its benefits. Physicians such as Hippocrates and Galen described a variety of massage techniques for preventing and treating minor ailments.

A special form of massage has developed over the centuries in the Far East. Chinese physicians and therapists use massage to redistribute the flow of life energy (called *chi*) in the treatment of illness; the Chinese form is called *acupressure* and the Japanese *shiatsu* (*see* ACUPUNCTURE). Massage is accepted as part of everyday life in most Eastern cultures, especially in China, Japan, Indonesia and India.

In Western countries, there is no long-standing tradition of massage, but its use was popularized in the 19th century by the Swede Per Henrik Ling. His method was developed at institutes of 'Swedish massage' in various centres around Europe. Most massage therapists in Europe have been trained in Swedish massage, although many now use *shiatsu* techniques as well.

People in Western societies are more inhibited about touch. Yet physiological experiments demonstrate the calming, reassuring and relaxing effects of touch (*see* RELAXATION). Massage can not only have profound effects on the person being massaged, but also help the person giving the massage, who will become more relaxed.

The most immediate and obvious benefits of massage are derived from the relief of muscular tension and a consequent calming effect. Aching, tired or tense muscles can feel much better after a massage. But specific medical problems may also be helped – especially those which are STRESS-related. For example, a headache can be relieved by neck and back massage; even a person with high BLOOD PRESSURE may be helped by a massage.

How massage works

Massage has two main actions, one relaxing, the other stimulating, and it can be adapted to produce the desired over-all effect. A person suffering from cold hands and feet and pain in the legs while walking obviously has poor CIRCULATION. This could be aggravated by tension, with a general over-contraction of muscles reducing the flow of blood, or to prolonged immobility, lack of exercise, obesity or nervousness. In the former case, the massage would be designed to relax the tissues, producing an over-all relaxation with a sedative effect, and as tension is removed, the circulation would respond. In the latter example, the object of the massage would be to stimulate the tissues and the circulation simultaneously, and speed up a sluggish METABOLISM.

The healing effect of massage is to make the superficial tissues of the body relax or return to normal, so that they stop bombarding the spinal cord with abnormal nerve signals. This relieves pain and tension and prevents them from establishing a 'vicious circle' of reflexes, in which, for example, persistent tension and hunching of the shoulders can create headache and nausea, which in turn give rise to more tension.

Western (Swedish) massage

The Western approach, sometimes called Swedish massage because it has always been popular there, is the best known and most often used. It is characterized by the various types of strokes and the use of oil and talcum powder to reduce friction against the skin. The technique, used mainly by PHYSIOTHERAPISTS, masseurs and beauticians, can be summarized in four main actions:

Effleurage: Stroking lengthways up the back, chest and limbs, with a light-to-moderate pressure exerted by the whole hand. The effect is to warm the tissues, reassure the person who is being massaged and tone the circulation. It is especially valuable for redistributing accumulations of fluid in the limbs and abdomen and for encouraging the pores in the skin to open to allow proper elimination.

Petrissage: A firmer stroke with moderate-to-deep pressure, and most of the contact made through the heel of the palm, one hand reinforcing the other. Sometimes the thumbs are used to give denser local pressure in certain areas.

Kneading: Deep manipulation, directed especially at stiff, contracted areas. It can be done with the thumbs only, or between thumb and fingers, with a gesture like kneading dough. When the skin and subcutaneous tissues – those just under the skin – are picked up, pulled away from the body and rolled between the thumb and fingers, the action is known as 'skin rolling'. It is especially useful for joints such as the wrists, ankles and elbows and helps to remove possible accumulations of waste products.

Friction: A series of deep, often circular motions, using thumbs, knuckles or fingertips. Pressure is concentrated on a small area through repeated strokes and is as deep as necessary without causing pain. Relaxation of tense muscles marks the time to move on to another area: prolonging massage at the same point would restimulate the muscle, and could cause pain.

Aromatherapy

When giving a massage, it is essential to use talcum powder or oil to reduce friction between the fingers and the skin, and most masseurs prefer oil. The oil can be scented with aromatic extracts of herbs or flowers, which can give an extra dimension to massage. These extracts are called 'essential oils' and can be purchased from some cosmetics shops or health shops.

Herbalists have for years pointed out that the scent of certain essential oils has beneficial physiological effects. For example, apple extract has been shown to reduce blood pressure. Small amounts of an essential oil can be added to a light vegetable oil for use in a massage. Pour a little vegetable oil into a dish and add a few drops of an essential oil. Camomile, orange blossom (neroli) and sandalwood are calming; bergamot, geranium and rose have antidepressant effects; sage, eucalyptus and rosemary are stimulating and refreshing.

Mastectomy

Cancer is a frightening disease wherever it strikes. Women, though, find the idea of BREAST CANCER particularly distressing. This is partly because it is the most common kind of cancer to be suffered by women, and partly because they fear the treatment, which usually involves some form of mastectomy (breast removal).

Mastectomy is not the only option open to doctors who discover a woman has breast cancer, but it is the most common solution currently used because most doctors feel that it provides the best chance of cure. The purpose is to stop the cancer spreading through the body by taking all the adjacent tissue from around the growth. Some doctors just remove the lump and then administer a course of RADIOTHERAPY or drug treatment as a follow-up. However, this is of little value if the tumour has spread; doctors usually want to remove some tissue from around the breast to try to estimate the degree of spread.

Types of mastectomy

There are various kinds of mastectomy, depending on how far the disease has spread, and sometimes the particular policy of the doctor or the hospital.

Simple mastectomy involves removal of the breast and nothing else. It is sometimes the choice of operation when the cancer seems to be confined to a single lump and has not spread beyond the affected breast.

Modified radical mastectomy is used when the cancer has spread through the LYMPHATIC system. In breast cancer, the first glands or lymph nodes to be affected are those under the arm, and these are removed at the same time as the breast so that the spread may be checked.

Radical mastectomy is a much less common operation nowadays. It includes removal of the pectoral muscles under the breast, which go to form the 'flap' above the armpit.

Diagnosis

Every woman should examine her breasts regularly, and should see her doctor immediately if she notices a lump or anything else different about one or both of them (*see* p. 118).

If the woman has a lump on her breast, a needle BIOPSY may be performed. This often reveals the lump to be a fluid-filled CYST, which is then drawn off through the needle. If the lump is solid, it still might be possible, with a local anaesthetic, to take out a core of the solid material and to test it to see whether there are any cancer cells. When this is not possible, it is usually decided to perform a surgical biopsy. For this, the patient is admitted to hospital and, under general anaesthetic, a small cut is made in the breast, some tissue is removed and analysed immediately. More than 85 per cent of lumps turn out to be benign. In the remainder of cases, it is usually decided to perform a mastectomy.

A common fear among women is that they will go in for a surgical biopsy and wake up minus a breast. Fortunately, however, this does not have to happen. Although many women do sign a consent form giving the doctor the right to proceed with the mastectomy in the event of cancerous cells being found, they are quite within their rights to ask the surgeon to wait and tell them the results of the test so that they can prepare for the operation, and adjust to the idea of having a breast removed.

The operation

Once consent has been given, the biopsy cut will be lengthened, and the surgeon will remove the breast and any associated tissue that is affected or may be affected. The cut is then stitched, and when it is healed, a single scar remains which gradually fades to a thin line. To promote healing, a tube to drain liquid from the site of the operation is inserted and will be there when the patient wakes up.

The patient is usually encouraged to be up and about the day after the operation, although she will be expected to stay in hospital for another ten days. In the majority of cases, the wound is healed within six weeks, although it could take a good three months before the woman feels fully recovered.

Often there will be post-operative follow-up tests, and radiotherapy (radiation treatment) or chemotherapy (drug treatment) may also be suggested.

Many women are prescribed a hormone drug called *tamoxifen*, to be taken (as tablets) after the operation. This drug is known to reduce the risk of recurrence of breast cancer, but must be taken on a regular basis. But it is not necessarily effective or suitable for every women who has had a mastectomy.

Psychological effects

The immediate response to the loss of a breast is one of grief. Coming to terms with a mastectomy has to include a period of mourning for the breast, and this cannot be hurried up by well-meaning people telling the patient to 'cheer up and look on the bright side'.

The grief often comes after the woman has been released from hospital. The shock of the brush with cancer has subsided, the ward routine is no longer there, and neither are the medical staff and the other patients who have been helping to cushion the final blow. And it is in her own home that the woman often feels most desolate. At this time, most women need to talk about their feelings. They need to be reassured by partners, family and friends that they are loved and wanted more than ever before. Meeting and talking to other women who have had mastectomies performed and now lead full and happy lives is also a great help.

The problem worrying most women initially is how the operation will affect their sex lives. Partners may also share that worry. The fact is that most couples find it draws them closer together.

Learning to cope

A woman with a strong supportive family is well on her way to learning to cope with her mastectomy. But there are also practical considerations which are very important.

After the operation, the woman is usually given a lightweight false breast of the same size and shape as her own. This is comfortable and easy to wear while the scar is healing, as it protects the incision. It is often a good idea to wear it at night as well, inserted into a sleep-bra, to protect against accidental knocks in the first weeks after the operation, and to help the body adjust to the sudden loss of the breast.

When the scar is fully healed, the woman should think about getting a more permanent false breast. There are now many good types available. The most popular kind is made of silicone gel, similar to that used for breast implants, and looks and feels very much like a real breast. All of the false breasts come in all shapes and sizes so that a good match can be made with the woman's own breast. When dressed, it is impossible to tell that the woman has had a mastectomy.

Breast reconstruction

Sometimes a surgeon is prepared to consider a breast reconstruction as a more permanent and more natural alternative to a false breast. The reconstruction may be carried out during the mastectomy operation itself or, more usually, some months later.

In some cases, surgeons remove the breast leaving the skin and nipple intact, and insert a bag of silicone gel, as in breast augmentation. Another technique involves the use of part of the muscle from the back of the chest which is transferred to the front to fill in the space left by removal of breast tissue. A very natural appearance can be achieved, and often no false breast is required – or only minimal padding.

Mastitis

At some point in their lives, many women suffer from mastitis, or inflammation of the BREAST. This condition has several forms and it is probably so common because of the structure of the breast and the purpose it serves. The breast is a sponge-like structure made up of thousands of sac-like glands or alveoli which can manufacture milk. Each gland forms a small, totally enclosed pocket, an ideal breeding ground for bacteria which can feed off the milk the breast secretes.

There are two main types of mastitis, acute and chronic. Though both cause inflammation, pain and tenderness in the breast, they are totally different in cause, features and treatment.

Acute or infective mastitis

This occurs when bacteria get into the breast and multiply. The breast is protected from infection by the skin enclosing it but infection can enter through a break in the skin, usually a small wound or a crack or fissure in the area of the nipples. This is particularly likely to occur during breastfeeding. The baby can suck too hard, causing the skin of the nipple to become raw and open, or accidentally scratch the nipple when grasping the breast during feeding.

Sometimes infection develops during breastfeeding without there being any wound or sore. This is because the openings of the milk ducts in the nipple are much wider and more exposed than normal, so it is relatively easy for any bacteria on the nipple to get into them. The bacteria spread down the ducts and, as each collects milk from all the glands in a particular section of the breast, the whole segment may become infected.

When mastitis occurs during breastfeeding, it is often called *puerperal mastitis*. Infection is first indicated by tenderness in the nipple and area behind it. Often is it too painful to have the baby sucking on it. Then the breast begins to ache and a hard, very tender red area develops. Pus may come out of the nipple, either on its own or mixed with the milk. Sometimes infection develops in a segment of the body of the breast rather than the nipple area. If treatment is delayed an ABSCESS may develop in the breast tissue. It may be necessary to drain this by making an incision under anaesthetic. Any illness following childbirth should be avoided at all costs as the mother needs all her resources at this time. Antibiotics, usually a type of penicillin, are used to kill off the infected bacteria, but these will not be effective if an abscess has formed, when surgical drainage is required. Hot flannels around the breast will help ease discomfort, but PAINKILLING drugs may be needed too. It is usually possible to resume breast feeding once the mastitis has subsided.

Chronic mastitis

This is rather inappropriately named as the condition is not serious, although it is certainly a nuisance and can be extremely worrying as women may associate the symptoms with cancer. This condition may be known by other names, such as 'benign breast disease', 'benign mammary dysplasia' and 'fibrocystic disease'.

It usually occurs in women in their 30s and 40s and seems to be related to changes in the amount of hormones from the OVARIES circulating in the blood. It is a mystery why some women develop it and others do not and no connections have been established between chronic mastitis and breastfeeding, contraceptive pills or breast stimulation during love-making.

The symptoms are either a dull aching pain, most marked before and during menstruation, or a lump. It is essential to see the doctor immediately to ensure these symptoms do not indicate something serious. A doctor may be able to make a positive diagnosis by examination alone but a patient cannot.

Any doubts can be resolved by mammography involving either X-RAYS or a special type of ULTRASOUND examination. As a final resort, a small BIOPSY operation is performed to remove a sample of tissue for examination under a microscope. If the lump is caused by an underlying CYST, which occasionally results from MUMPS, this is usually removed as a precautionary measure by a minor surgical procedure which leaves only a very small scar.

Treatment for chronic mastitis may be difficult. The condition tends to come and go of its own accord and may disappear altogether. Pain may be relieved by cyst drainage. Cyclical breast pain is sometimes helped by drugs that affect hormones, but these may have unwanted side-effects. Evening primrose oil may also be helpful.

ME, *see* **Myalgic encephalomyelitis**

Measles

Children most often catch measles between the ages of one and six. A baby has what is known as natural immunity, or inborn resistance, inherited from the mother, which gives protection for several months.

From the age of about one year, all children are at risk. In those areas where few children have been immunized, epidemics, or mass outbreaks tend to occur, for reasons not fully understood, during the spring every two or three years. In older children and adults, measles is rare.

Having the disease once provides immunity for life and in most Western countries, it is now routine to offer IMMUNIZATION against measles to all children in their second year of life.

Progress of the disease

The virus is passed from person to person, like many others, on the tiny droplets of moisture we constantly breathe out and in. Following contact with an infected person, there are generally no symptoms for between seven and 12 days, during which the virus is incubating or multiplying in the cells of the throat and passages leading down to the lungs.

Then follow the two stages of measles proper. The first is known as the 'catarrhal stage', because the symptoms are produced by infection of the mucous membranes lining the eyes, nose and mouth. The patient develops what appears to be a heavy cold with a husky cough. The nose is runny with catarrh, and the eyes are red and watery. There may even be a fine, red RASH which lasts a few hours, then disappears. Parents usually notice the child is upset and 'off colour'. Most children have a temperature rising to 100.4°F (38°C). There is loss of appetite and possible sickness and diarrhoea. If the inside of the mouth is examined at this stage, tiny, white spots are seen lining the cheeks. Known as *Koplik's spots* (after the man who first identified them), these identifying spots are unique to measles. In this initial period, some have no fever at all, and the other symptoms may be extremely mild.

On the third or fourth day (occasionally five to seven days), the temperature falls and the rash appears. This is typically a dusky, red colour, with slightly raised spots which group together in patches to give the blotchy appearance typical of measles.

It starts to form on the face, then spreads to the neck and forehead, eventually covering the face and trunk, and, in severe cases, the limbs. This usually happens over a period of about 24 hours. There is only slight itching, sometimes none at all. Over the next three days, the rash disappears in the order in which it appeared. A brownish staining of the skin remains, which usually disappears with peeling of the skin.

After the rash starts to appear – and on the same day – the temperature rises once more. It is the time when the patient feels most ill and, in severe cases, absolutely wretched. The cough and inflammation of the eyes are at their worst, light is likely to be irritating to the eyes, and complications, if they are to occur, will begin to develop now.

The dangers

In a tiny minority of cases, the patient just happens to have a low resistance to measles. In these, the temperature rises uncontrollably, and there is the danger of bleeding, either in the skin affected by the rash, or in certain organs. Known as *haemorrhagic measles*, it needs hospital treatment if the patient's life is to be saved. Tiny haemorrhages sometimes occur in the rash of mild measles, and these should cause no alarm. But if bleeding is widespread, a doctor should be called without delay.

Ear and lung infection: The measles virus temporarily destroys the lining of the passage leading to the lungs, and paves the way for bacterial infection of adjoining or connected areas such as the EARS and LUNGS. Some cases develop infection of the middle ear, with earache and a discharge of pus. Report this to a doctor without delay – antibiotics will prevent any spread of the infection and clear it up.

A chesty or wheezy cough developing in a measles patient is a sign of BRONCHITIS, or chest infection. Some coughing is normal enough, but if it produces phlegm and is a wheezing one, rather than dry, hacking and unproductive, antibiotics are essential to prevent lung damage. Once again, do not delay in calling the doctor so that proper treatment is given.

In young children, measles sometimes leads to bacterial infection of the LARYNX, the 'voice box'. The passage of air is obstructed, and a 'croupy', or hoarse, croaking cough is produced. This is a serious complication: call the doctor without delay.

Mild CONJUNCTIVITIS – irritation (producing pinkness) of the 'whites' of the eyes – is normal in measles. If there is bacterial infection as well, the discharge produced is thick and sticky – containing pus and other matter. Untreated, this can cause scarring of the conjunctiva and blindness. Again, call the doctor if this condition develops.

Encephalitis: This is the most dreaded complication of measles. It means inflammation of the brain and central nervous system as a response to the virus's presence; the symptoms are drowsiness, hallucination and delirium occurring about ten days into the illness. In these times of immunization, it is rare – developing in only one in 1,000 cases – but it needs urgent hospital treatment if it does develop because the consequences are so severe.

Treatment

Mild measles needs no treatment, other than appropriate home nursing. The patient will retire to bed when feeling too ill to stay up. This is quite normal and should not be cause for alarm. Some doctors give antibiotics to all cases; others reserve them for the most severe, and for complications. Severe cases need intensive home nursing and plenty of reassurance that they will come to no harm; but even these need only retire to bed if feeling too poorly for anything else.

Meckel's diverticulum, *see* **Ileum**

Meditation

For centuries, Eastern religions such as Hinduism, Buddhism, Taoism and Islamic Sufism have used meditation as a path to enlightenment. Today, the great interest that meditation arouses in the West is only partly based on its spiritual value: more and more people are becoming interested in the technique as a way to improve mental and physical health and, in particular, to reduce STRESS.

Meditation in medical practice

Increasingly, doctors and other health workers have come to recognize that meditation can have important calming effects on both the mind and the body. Simple, straightforward techniques of meditation – without any deep religious significance – can be learned by anyone. It is clear that people who practise meditation regularly are able to cope with everyday life in a calm, unhurried manner, and there is some evidence that meditation can protect people against most stress-related medical disorders.

In hospitals and clinics, meditation has been used with good effect to help wean patients off drugs such as TRANQUILLIZERS, or to help in cases of ALCOHOLISM. Patients with high BLOOD PRESSURE or CORONARY HEART DISEASE may also be helped by meditation. One of the more interesting lines of investigation concerns the effect of meditation on CANCERS.

Techniques of meditation

Meditation is a simple and natural practice. A quiet place should be chosen, and you should sit comfortably in an upright chair that supports your back (an armchair sometimes encourages sleep). Breathing should be slow, deep and regular. Some methods stress breathing, and suggest that you concentrate your mind by counting your exhaled breaths from one to ten, and then repeat the process. Your body should be poised and free from tension, but not rigid. Finally, a subject for meditation can be chosen. This could be a plant, a word or phrase (called a *mantra*) or a sound, such as the ticking of a clock.

If you have not tried meditation before, the easiest way to begin is simply to concentrate on making your breathing absolutely regular. You could concentrate on the sensation of air passing in and out of your nostrils, or concentrate on the rise and fall of the centre of the abdomen, just below the umbilicus (which should move absolutely regularly and rhythmically as you breathe).

Ideally, meditation should take place with your eyes closed. If a visual subject is used, then you can close your eyes for a few minutes and concentrate on its 'after-image'. At all times, your mind must focus on the chosen subject. It is inevitable that distracting thoughts will enter your mind, but these should be gently eased aside and your attention returned to the subject. You should remain as still as possible and meditate for 20 minutes at a time, preferably twice a day.

The aim of meditation is to free the mind of all distracting thought and to remain in a state of restfulness while fully alert; with practice it is easily achieved. Many people, at least to begin with, prefer to learn from a teacher and to meditate in a group.

Physical changes

Clinical research has recorded a number of changes in the body and brain during meditation. EEG (ELECTROENCEPHALOGRAPH) tests show electrical waves which are neither those produced in sleep nor wakefulness. They indicate a slow rhythm, with orderly waves recorded from different parts of the brain. This orderliness can continue after meditation if the practice is maintained.

The depth of RELAXATION is indicated by a fall in the basal metabolic rate (energy changes necessary for processes such as the heartbeat) which is twice as much as in deep sleep. There is a reduction in the activity of the AUTONOMIC NERVOUS SYSTEM – a factor which is important in combating stress. The respiratory rate shows a marked decrease, but the amount of oxygen in the blood remains the same, which suggests that the body cells are using less. It is claimed that many of these beneficial effects can become permanent if meditation is practised regularly.

Meiosis, *see* Cells and chromosomes

Melanin and melanoma

Melanin is a dark-coloured pigment found in the SKIN, the HAIR and in the iris of the EYE. It is formed in melanin-making cells, called *melanocytes*, situated in the basal layer of the skin. A *melanoma* is a type of skin cancer formed from melanocytes which have become malignant.

Irrespective of racial type, the same number of melanocytes are found in the skin of every human being. The amount of melanin produced by these cells, however, varies greatly. In dark-skinned races, the melanocytes are larger and produce more pigment.

Function and formation

Melanin's function is to protect the skin from the harmful rays of the sun; the darker the skin, the less likely it is to suffer from SUNBURN.

The complex chemical process of the body which converts the amino acid, *tyrosine*, into melanin, takes place on the outer part of each melanocyte. Once formed, the pigment moves to the centre of the cell to cloud over, and thereby protect, the highly sensitive nucleus. Exposure to ultraviolet light, either from artificial sources or sunlight, stimulates melanin production by the normal process of tanning. Melanin is formed, the cells expand and the skin darkens in colour. Response varies from individual to individual, but all persons except albinos can eventually become pigmented when exposed to enough sunlight.

Melanin disorders

Disorders of melanin are rare and are mostly concerned with absent pigmentation or increased pigmentation.

Skin conditions such as ECZEMA and PSORIASIS which cause severe itching, and therefore scratching and skin abrasions, can lead to increased melanin production in the affected areas. Even constant friction from tight clothing can stimulate melanin formation. The affected skin becomes generally darker – especially in dark-skinned people. The change may last for many months, but can occasionally be permanent.

A rare medical condition known as *Addison's disease* occurs when the ADRENAL GLANDS do not function properly. This causes over-secretion of the hormone ACTH (adrenocorticotrophic hormone), which is produced in the PITUITARY gland and has some activity similar to MSH (melanocyte-stimulating hormone). The patient gradually becomes darker skinned as the melanin forms in response to the hormone and the pigmentation of the skin can be patchy.

In the inherited condition of *albinism*, there is an absence of the ENZYME which converts tyrosine to melanin. And, although the correct number of melanocyte cells is present in the skin, no melanin can be produced. Albinos have snow white hair and pink eyes. Moreover in hot climates, because the protective function of melanin is lost, albinos are at much greater risk from sunburn and sun-induced CANCERS.

In the condition of *vitiligo*, the cause of which is unknown, there is a spontaneous and patchy loss of skin pigment even though the melanocytes are still present in the affected skin. Areas of skin remain unpigmented for months or even years in some cases, and then may suddenly return to normal.

Treatment usually depends on identifying the cause of the increased or decreased pigmentation. There is no treatment for patients with albinism, but treatment for vitiligo is sometimes possible. The melanin can be encouraged to reform in the affected skin by the use of drugs called *psoralens*. After the patient is given one of these drugs, ultraviolet light is shone on to the area. Following a number of such treatments, the melanocytes can begin to produce melanin again, although results are not always satisfactory and are rather unpredictable. Topical steroids may also produce pigmentation, so a trial for 6–8 weeks is justified.

Moles and freckles

Moles are small areas of skin in which there is an abnormal growth of one or more types of skin tissue. Sometimes moles contain abnormally dilated blood vessels, but usually they contain large numbers of melanocytes and a high concentration of melanin which gives them a dark brown or black colour. Everyone has at least a few moles – including both white- and dark-skinned people, although they are more obvious in white-skinned ones. Some people are born with moles, but most develop during childhood and early adult life. The average number of moles on the skin of an adult is 20 or so, but some people have as many as a hundred or more.

There are several different types of moles. Most are flat and only a few millimetres across. Others may be slightly raised, and some form quite prominent lumps on the skin which may grow coarse hairs.

Moles are formed by an abnormally high concentration of melanocytes, but *freckles* are areas of skin with a normal concentration of melanocytes but a higher than usual content of melanin.

In Western countries, freckles are most common in red-headed people of Irish, Welsh or Scottish ancestry. The freckles become more prominent and more numerous after exposure of the skin to sunlight.

Melanoma

Very occasionally, melanocytes in moles become cancerous and start growing in an uncontrolled way to produce a melanoma, which is a type of skin cancer. Usually the cells continue to produce melanin, and irregular, dark patches appear in and around the original mole. The cells may eventually spread to other parts of the body causing cancerous growths elsewhere. Occasionally, however, melanocytes that have become cancerous lose their ability to produce melanin and the growth is not coloured. Although many melanomas begin in a pre-existing mole, this is not always so; they can appear where there were no moles before.

There is no doubt that melanomas can be triggered off by excessive exposure of the skin to sunshine. It appears that the ultraviolet rays of the sun can damage genetic material inside melanocytes and trigger off a cancerous change in the cell. The cell then multiplies in an uncontrolled manner until a melanoma appears. Occasionally, however, melanomas appear in skin that has never been exposed to sunshine, and some other factor must be responsible for them.

People with very fair skin are most at risk of developing melanomas, especially if they spend a lot of time in the sunshine. Melanomas are most likely to occur in those areas of skin which have received most sunlight – for example, the head, the forearms or, in women, the lower legs or feet. However they also occur on those areas of skin which are only infrequently exposed to the sun. But such areas are more likely to have become sunburned as a result of occasional exposure. It is likely that repeated sunburn can also trigger off melanoma even if the skin is never exposed to the sun for very long. A two-week beach holiday in the sun every year with a bad dose of sunburn could be as risky as regular exposure to the sunshine all the year round without any sunburn. Dark-skinned people are much less likely to develop melanomas, but they may occur on the palms of the hands and soles of the feet where the skin is not naturally pigmented.

In Britain, less than 1 per cent of all cancers are melanomas, but the incidence is increasing as more and more people take beach holidays in hotter countries every year. However, white-skinned people who live near the equator, in countries where the sun is stronger, are much more likely to develop melanoma. In Australia, more than 7 per cent of all cancers are melanomas. The northern state of Queensland has the highest incidence, with a rate of new cases per year of 40 per 100,000 people.

Appearance of melanomas

There are at least three types of melanomas. *Superficial* ones spread through the outermost layers of the skin and usually show some variation in density of colour. They are the most common type and tend to occur in the exposed parts of the skin, or on the back. Another type is the *nodular* melanoma which forms a firm lump in the skin, and may penetrate deeply into the underlying tissues. A rarer type develops on the palms of the hands and soles of the feet or around the nails of the fingers or toes. This is the most common form among dark-skinned people.

It is quite unusual to have a mole on the soles of the feet or the palms of the hands. Because such moles can easily be damaged by pressure, there is some risk that they could turn malignant in later life.

It is very important that anyone who thinks he or she might have a melanoma seeks medical advice. The important signs to look for are:

- Increase in the size of a mole, particularly if it grows to more than ¼ in (7 mm) across.
- Irregular edges appearing around a mole, especially if there are other small irregular areas in the pigmentation of the skin nearby.
- Alteration in the depth of colour of a mole or the appearance of irregular colouring of a mole.
- Bleeding or itching of any coloured mark on the skin.
- Ulceration of any skin lumps that fail to heal normally.

Treatment of melanomas

Any suspicious skin lesion which could be a melanoma is surgically removed for microscopic examination to establish exactly what it is. Sometimes the diagnosis remains in doubt until this examination has been carried out.

If the diagnosis is confirmed, further surgery may be necessary to remove an area of skin around the original site of the lesion, to prevent the spread of malignant cells. Sometimes drug treatment is used, and occasionally radiotherapy.

Ménière's disease

This is an affliction of the EAR producing severe attacks of VERTIGO and nausea. It is characterized, too, by deafness during the attacks. With time, the vertigo ceases and, ultimately, DEAFNESS develops.

Ménière's disease is thought to be associated with the fluid endolymph, which fills the chambers and canals of the ear known as the labyrinth (*see* BALANCE). The sound chamber, too, is filled with endolymph.

The cause of the disease is not clear, but there seems to be an increase in the production of endolymph and therefore an increase in the pressure of the fluid.

Symptoms and treatment

There are two ways in which the disease may show itself. There may be a gradual loss of hearing over a period of time which may not be diagnosed as a symptom of Ménière's disease until the first attack of vertigo. Alternatively, the first attack of vertigo may be the first symptom.

The attacks of vertigo seem to follow a pattern. The attack starts with a full or bursting feeling in the ears. This is usually followed by a roaring or hissing noise in the ears (*see* TINNITUS) which develops into increasing deafness. The victim feels extremely dizzy and may not be able to stand since he or she may feel a sensation of somersaulting over and over. The victim may even lose consciousness.

These attacks come on with varying frequency and may last only minutes or for many hours, and there may be unsteadiness for some days afterwards. In between attacks, there is deafness which tends to get worse where there is loud background noise and which makes individual spoken words very hard to distinguish. At first only one ear is affected, but eventually both are involved.

Drugs which sedate the labyrinth are not very effective in preventing symptoms. In about 10 per cent of cases, operations to drain the endolymph from the inner ear are performed and can be helpful in dealing with this problem. For the deafness certain degree of help can be got from a correct type of hearing aid, but this may not solve the problem entirely. Other surgical options include ULTRASOUND destruction of the labyrinth, and severing the nerves from the labyrinth.

Meningitis

The BRAIN is covered by three thin layers of tissue known as the *meninges*. Between the two inner layers is an important fluid which protects and nourishes the brain: *cerobrospinal fluid* (CSF). The meninges extend out of the skull down the spine to cover the SPINAL CORD. The CSF bathes the entire spinal cord as well as the brain.

Meningitis occurs when microbes – either bacteria or viruses – enter the CSF. This irritates the meninges which become red and swollen. Microbes normally enter the CSF via the blood which can carry germs from all surfaces in contact with the outside world (e.g. the nose and throat) or from internal infection (e.g. an ABSCESS). If they are exposed to the air, the meninges can be directly infected.

Certain groups of people are particularly susceptible. First, there are those in whom the meninges can be directly infected. This can occur by accident if the skull or base of the nose is fractured (*see* HEAD AND HEAD INJURIES); it also occurs in SPINA BIFIDA babies who are born with exposed spinal cords. If this condition is not corrected, infection travels up the spine into the brain and the baby will die of meningitis. Another high-risk group is people with poor defence mechanisms, caused either by an immunity-reducing condition such as LEUKAEMIA, or by certain immunosuppressive drugs, particularly the very strong drugs used for treating CANCER. Last, the very young are more susceptible: for example, there are 16 cases of meningitis in every 100,000 children under the age of one, but only 0.3 cases in every 100,000 adults over the age of 25. Incidence of the disease increases again in old age.

Symptoms and signs

The onset of meningitis often occurs in a matter of hours. The most important symptom is severe headache, usually associated with pain in the eyes on looking at light. The patient will feel feverish and unwell, and will probably want to lie quietly, without moving, in a dark room. He or she may complain of a stiff neck, nausea and vomiting, and may become confused and drowsy, or have a fit. In a baby, the main indications are fever, vomiting, poor feeding, general irritability or convulsions.

When a doctor examines the patient for meningitis, he or she is looking for general signs of inflammation and for specific signs that indicate that the inflammation stems from the meninges. The most common important specific sign is neck stiffness caused by inflammation around the brain and along the spinal cord. There will be similar pain if the spinal cord is stretched by bending and straightening the legs. The doctor may also examine the back of the eyes to see if the nerve to the eye has been affected. Meningitis is more difficult to detect in a baby, and the doctor relies heavily on the mother to say if the child is not his or her usual self. In a baby, signs can be bulging in the soft part of the skull (the fontanelle), a stiff neck and a floppy body.

Diagnosis

All patients with suspected meningitis should be sent to hospital for investigation. There doctors will do a simple blood test and perhaps skull and chest X-rays. The most important test for meningitis is the LUMBAR PUNCTURE, when some of the CSF surrounding the spinal cord is drawn off. CSF is normally crystal clear – if it is cloudy, meningitis is likely. The CSF is tested and the infecting bacteria identified.

Types of meningitis

It is important to differentiate between viral and bacterial forms of the illness. *Viral meningitis* is the most common and least dangerous form. Its symptoms can vary from a short flu-like illness with bad headache to more severe symptoms. There is no need for antibiotics and only simple nursing is needed.

The commonest bacterial form is *meningoccal meningitis* which occurs all over Britain, sometimes in local epidemics. It has two forms. The first is very dangerous: onset is sudden, with headache, shock and a rash that looks like bruises all over; death can occur in a very short time – sometimes within 12 hours – so rapid treatment is vital. The second, more common form gives cold-like symptoms for one or two days, followed by severe headache, vomiting and a rash.

Diagnosis is by lumbar puncture, and the meningoccus bacterium can be seen in the CSF. Penicillin is normally used, and recovery chances are good. Meningoccal meningitis is infectious, and patients' close contacts should be protected by antibiotics.

Pneumococcal meningitis is more common in the over-45 age group. It too, is dangerous, and 25 per cent are left with a permanent handicap. Treatment is similar to that described above. It is not very infectious and does not occur in epidemics, so contacts do not need protection.

Haemophilus influenzae meningitis occurs in children under the age of four. It is very similar to other types of bacterial meningitis, but correct diagnosis is important because it does not respond to penicillin; other antibiotics must be used. Babies and young children are now routinely offered IMMUNIZATION against type B of this strain of meningitis with the Hib vaccine (which also affords protection against some other infections).

A rare but important form is *tuberculous (TB) meningitis*, which often occurs in immigrants from countries where TB is common. Babies and adults with malnutrition are particularly at risk. The onset of this form of meningitis is slow. The symptoms are often vague, and it may be several weeks before the patient becomes very ill. It may then, if not treated, progress rapidly to cause death or disability. Again diagnosis is by lumbar puncture, and treatment involves the administration of antibiotics for an extended period – up to one year. Checks are made to see if any of the patient's contacts have TUBERCULOSIS – to prevent spread of the disease.

Treatment and outlook

Treatment for most forms of the disease involves high doses of ANTIBIOTICS given as soon as possible after diagnosis, usually by drip into a vein. If the CSF is cloudy, treatment is often begun before the laboratory tests are ready. Chloramphenicol and penicillin are the two antibiotics most commonly used, depending on the bacterium involved.

The patient requires careful nursing in isolation, and other drugs may be used to make him or her comfortable; PAINKILLERS for headache, anti-convulsants for fits and SEDATIVES and anti-emetics if he or she is restless or vomiting. Antibiotics are continued by drip for several days until the temperature is normal; they may then be taken by mouth to ensure the bacteria are eradicated from the body. The patient should then be ready to return to normal life after a short convalescence.

Recovery from meningitis is usually good, with complete return to normal health after a few weeks. However, it is a dangerous disease: 6 per cent of those who contract it die, and some survive only with serious disability. Later handicap is most common in the very young. There may be DEAFNESS, mental deficiency, CEREBRAL PALSY or EPILEPSY. Occasionally the circulation of fluid around the brain is disturbed giving the child a huge expanding head, known as HYDROCEPHALUS. Children who have had meningitis are checked after recovery for any of these problems. Any patient who has had more than one attack of the disease is investigated closely to find if he or she belongs to one of the high-risk groups, and to prevent it recurring.

With all types of meningitis, early diagnosis saves life. Anyone with the symptoms should immediately consult his or her doctor, who will be aware of the possibility of meningitis, and will send any case to hospital for urgent investigation and treatment.

Menopause

The menopause, or 'change of life' as it is very often called, is the moment in a woman's life when she stops ovulating (*see* OVARIES) and her menstrual PERIODS stop. It generally comes between the ages of 45 and 55, but it may happen a good deal earlier, or be delayed until the late 50s. The bodily changes which it brings about are a process, not a sudden event, and the times during which they happen – a matter of some years – is called the *climacteric*. Its main effect is that a woman can no longer become pregnant because it marks the end of her fertility.

In many women, the menopause happens suddenly. Others may find their periods becoming irregular, scanty or brief, or a combination of all three. (If periods become more frequent or heavier during the middle years, it is important to seek medical advice.)

Problems of the menopause

The commonest physical problems are hot flushes and a decrease in the moisture and elasticity of the VAGINA (called vaginal atrophy).

A hot flush is a sudden feeling of feverish heat in the body, sometimes accompanied by patches of redness on the skin. When it is over, the body often feels chilled. Flushes may happen infrequently, or many times in the course of 24 hours – often at night, when they may disturb sleep.

Dryness and inelasticity of the vagina, which generally occur in the latter part of the climacteric, are caused by a reduction in the secretions of the vaginal walls. This can produce irritation and increase the likelihood of vaginal infection, and can also at times make sexual intercourse uncomfortable.

Research has shown that it is only these two physical symptoms which are quite plainly caused by menopausal changes in the body. Other troublesome physical discomforts, such as swollen ankles, headaches, palpitations and dizziness, may be connected to the body's adjustment to a change in the level of oestrogen, but so far, the link is not clear. A woman whose hormone level is normal or only a little altered during the menopause may have hot flushes, dizziness and so on, while another with a low hormone level may have hardly any symptoms.

The connection between oestrogen level and mental well-being is also still unclear. There is some evidence that a reduction in oestrogen can cause DEPRESSION, but it is possible that the embarrassment and discomfort of hot flushes create tension and anxiety.

One positive step towards an untroubled menopause is to look upon it as a natural stage in life and emphatically not as a form of illness. Women who are by temperament optimistic and relaxed will find it easier to do this than women who tend always to expect problems, and it is the 'natural worriers' who are likely to feel fearful of ageing, becoming unattractive or ill. These anxieties create STRESS, and stress creates physical symptoms – headaches, and insomnia, problems with sexual intercourse, backache, tingling sensations –

until an ordinary physiological event turns into a frightening spiral of stress, discomfort and more stress.

Women who feel anxiety about the menopause need the support and understanding of family and friends, and the knowledge that their fears will be accepted as real, and not dismissed as 'nerves'.

Dealing with difficulties

Despite good intentions to maintain a positive attitude through the menopause, difficulties may arise which need to be resolved. Although some of the possible problems can be helped by HORMONE REPLACEMENT THERAPY (HRT), there are other simpler approaches which can be useful.

One of the more obvious and common problems is that of 'hot flushes'. They tend to be worse in hot, stuffy rooms or if the woman is wearing heavy winter clothes indoors. So it is a good idea to wear light clothes, particularly indoors, or at social gatherings where the atmosphere is likely to be hot and humid. However, hot flushes may occur at any time of day or night and can be potentially embarrassing. It is then worth asking a doctor for advice. A drug called clonidine may then be prescribed to help.

Vaginal dryness may make intercourse difficult or even painful. A water-soluble lubricating jelly which can be obtained from any chemist will help. However, if pain persists despite the use of a lubricating jelly, it is worth asking for medical advice. The vagina is still prone to infections around the time of the menopause, and the pain may be caused by a vaginal infection such as THRUSH, which needs specific treatment. Thrush may result in an irritating discharge; other infections may produce a smelly discharge. The doctor may prescribe antibiotic pessaries or tablets to deal with any infection, but he or she may find that inflammation is caused by atrophy of the vaginal skin. This can be remedied by the use of pessaries or creams containing oestrogen.

Urinary infections are more common around the time of the menopause and may cause discomfort or burning when passing urine. A course of antibiotics is usually necessary to cure the infection.

Psychological difficulties at the time of the menopause are not uncommon, but anxiety or depression should never be dismissed as being simply a result of 'the change' without full assessment by a doctor or other professional. The middle years are often a time of great activity in many women's lives, and consequently there is always the risk of excess stress from family upheavals, difficulties at work or financial worries. All forms of stress can add to the psychological burden and may cause anxiety, PHOBIA, depression or even breakdown. Careful assessment of any psychological symptoms is therefore vital so that specific treatment can be given. Often, the symptoms may decrease following a thorough discussion of problems with a counsellor, but in some cases, treatment with anti-depressant drugs is necessary if depression is severe.

Contraception at the menopause

Although the menopause marks the end of a woman's reproductive life, fertility does not suddenly disappear, but declines gradually over a period of time. Most women ovulate irregularly and may have irregular periods at the beginning of the menopause, but ovulation may still occur some months after the periods have virtually stopped. It is thus possible for a woman to become pregnant during the menopause. For this reason CONTRACEPTION should be continued until at least a year has passed since the last period. Medical advice should be obtained about the most appropriate method.

Hysterectomy and the menopause

If a woman has had a HYSTERECTOMY at a time in her life when she was having periods, the effect on her hormone levels will depend on whether or not both the ovaries were removed at the same time as the hysterectomy was carried out. Usually, if a hysterectomy is carried out for a benign condition such as FIBROIDS, the surgeon leaves the ovaries in place. They continue to produce hormones regularly up to the time that the woman would normally have her menopause, and so symptoms of the menopause may appear at any time between the ages of 45 and 55. However, because periods will have stopped with the hysterectomy, there will be no obvious sign that the menopause is occurring. Nevertheless the symptoms may be just as severe as those experienced by a woman who has not had a hysterectomy.

If the surgeon removes both ovaries at the time of the operation, the woman is likely to experience menopause symptoms immediately after the operation. It may be possible for the doctor to prescribe hormone replacement therapy after the operation to replace the hormones which would otherwise be supplied by the ovaries. However, in some circumstances, particularly if the hysterectomy was carried out for a cancerous condition, this is not possible.

Menstruation, *see* **Periods and period pain, Premenstrual syndrome.**

Mental illness

A mental illness is a disorder of the mind. But this definition really begs the question of how one can recognize such a disorder. Many people have emotional upsets of one sort or another during the course of everyday life, and yet one would not call them mentally ill if they can otherwise cope perfectly well with their lives. Somebody with a mental illness has a disability that interferes with his or her life and which is caused by a disorder of thought, emotion or behaviour. Most mental illnesses are only temporary, and improve with simple treatments. But at the other extreme, there are serious disorders which may last for years and prove to be difficult to treat.

Causes of mental illness

Despite much research, no one single cause has been discovered for any of the most common mental illnesses. It seems that, in any individual case, there are a variety of causes which add up to produce illness. For example, several illnesses undoubtedly have a genetic or hereditary basis because they tend to run in families. Yet some members of the family may escape the illness entirely.

It is likely that, in most mental illnesses, there are certain predisposing factors that determine whether or not a particular person will suffer from a mental illness. For example, the way somebody has been brought up, the circumstances in which he or she lives, difficulties in relationships with other people, problems at work or with money may all be predisposing factors. Finally, there may be some 'trigger factor' which actually starts off the illness. Again, this may be an event in the person's life such as losing a job, a bereavement, or even a physical illness such as a bad dose of flu.

Some mental illnesses are caused by specific disorders of biochemistry in the brain from drugs, injury or degeneration of the brain tissue itself.

Neuroses

The *neuroses* are among the most common mental illnesses. They include anxiety neurosis (*see* STRESS), PHOBIAS, compulsive neurosis, HYPOCHONDRIA and eating disorders (*see* ANOREXIA AND BULIMIA). The patients are usually quite aware of their problems and are often keen to get better. Occasionally, however, they may be so 'locked in' to a pattern of abnormal behaviour that they cannot see for themselves any way of improvement, and they may be resistant to other people's attempts to provide help.

The symptoms of neuroses are excessive reactions to stresses that the person has experienced in the past. Genetic factors with neuroses have a background of insecurity, often starting in childhood, which indicates that upbringing is a significant factor.

Anxiety neurosis: The main symptoms of anxiety neurosis are an almost constant sense of fearfulness or dread and irritability, with poor concentration. Many patients experience physical symptoms as well, such as palpitations, dizziness, sweating, a dry mouth, difficulty in swallowing and tension headaches. The sufferer's work and social life may be seriously affected as well as relationships with other people. Symptoms may temporarily worsen in certain situations with overbreathing and panic – so-called 'panic attacks'.

Anxiety neurosis affects about three women in every 100, but is a little less common among men.

Phobias: A phobia is an intense dread of a certain situation or an object. When confronted with the feared situation, the patient experiences intense anxiety symptoms such that they just cannot cope with the situation and feel they have to escape. They may feel dizzy, have palpitations or even faint.

Hysteria: Although the word 'hysteria' is commonly used to mean uncontrolled excitement, it is used medically to describe a particular type of neurosis in which the patient may appear totally calm. Somebody with hysteria has a 'real' physical symptom that occurs as a result of some stressful event in his or her life. The symptom may be quite serious, such as paralysis of an arm, blindness in an eye, numbness in the body, difficulty in swallowing, vomiting, pain or even fits. The symptom is quite genuine, and the sufferer cannot control it in any way by a conscious effort. (Non-hysterical patients who are malingering, on the other hand, really are consciously imitating a symptom for effect, and can stop pretending if they want to.)

Hysterical symptoms often help the person, subconsciously, to avoid some activity of which he or she is afraid. But the patient may also seem blissfully unconcerned about the problem, or fail to recognize its existence.

Obsessive–compulsive neurosis: Many people can be described as obsessional in that they always want to do things properly or in a set routine. A sufferer from obsessive–compulsive neurosis has an overwhelming need to follow certain set patterns or routines which may be extremely complicated and even tiring. This problem also seems often to be triggered by some stressful event in the patient's life.

One particular type of obsessive neurosis is intense jealousy of another person. A man, for example, may become intensely jealous of his wife or girlfriend so that he cannot let her out of his sight and cannot get out of his mind the thought that she might be unfaithful. This condition has been called the 'Othello syndrome'.

Some sufferers develop ritual behaviour, which may start as normal but become exaggerated out of all proportion to any real need. Obsessive hand-washing after going to the toilet is not uncommon, and may be repeated an exact number of times – often as many as 20 or 30. Other common ritual behaviours include checking on safety, such as a ritual checking to see that windows are shut or gas taps turned off. Again the checking may need to be repeated many times over so that, for example, a sufferer may have to spend up to an hour checking the house before leaving to go out.

Hypochondria: A hypochondriac has a persistent and unjustified fear about his or her physical health. In its mildest form, it is quite a commonplace disorder, but when severe, it can be a very serious problem both for the patient and for his or her doctor. Often the main symptoms are pain, which may be in the chest, abdomen or elsewhere. The pains defeat any attempted cure, such as drug treatment. Some sufferers even convince doctors so well that they have numerous operations in order to investigate or cure the pains. The symptoms only abate when the stress in the patient's life has been properly recognized and treated appropriately.

Eating disorders: Disorders of eating are most common among young adult or teenage women. Anorexia nervosa is a fear of food. Often, however, this condition is associated with excessive over-eating (bulimia) which becomes quite bizarre and compulsive. The two conditions often alternate. The causes of eating disorders are not very well understood, but they can be very serious and may, in a small percentage of cases, even be fatal.

Affective disorders

These are disorders of mood, which in medical terms is called 'affect'. The commonest disorder is DEPRESSION, but mood may also become abnormally high or elated – a condition called 'mania' or, in a mild form, 'hypomania'. Some patients alternate between periods of depression and periods of hypomania.

Mania: This is much rarer than depression but can cause a fairly alarming set of symptoms. The patient feels 'on top of the world', and rushes around doing things at an enormous pace. He or she may spend extravagantly, or start up all kinds of unsound business schemes without realizing the implications. Uninhibited sexual behaviour may occur. Usually the patient sleeps little, talks non-stop and is totally unaware that anything is wrong.

Personality disorder

This is one of the less precise terms used in PSYCHIATRY because it is difficult to define the various different problems that can arise in a disordered personality. The word 'personality' refers to the way in which a person behaves in a variety of different settings – at work, at home or in a social setting. Various disorders are recognized in which the person can be said to react abnormally to the circumstances in which they find themselves, causing difficulties for themselves and for others. So somebody with an obsessional personality is unreasonably rigid in his or her views, is often full of guilt and finds it difficult to relax. A person with a paranoid personality is over-sensitive and reacts adversely to the slightest criticism.

Perhaps the most worrying personality disorder is the psychopathic (or anti-social) personality disorder. Somebody suffering from this problem cannot enter into any loving or caring relationship, acts impulsively, fails to learn from experience and shows no sense of guilt or shame for any anti-social acts. Often such people have a series of criminal convictions and cannot keep a job.

Schizophrenia: This is one of the most difficult mental illnesses to treat. It tends to be long-lasting and, when severe, can destroy the individual's life and work.

SCHIZOPHRENIA may first appear as a sudden 'breakdown', in which the patient starts to behave in a very bizarre and unusual fashion, and he or she may not be able to think logically. Often there are hallucinations (noises, voices or visions in the mind) or delusions – a false belief held against all reason. The patient may be unaware that anything is wrong at all.

Alternatively, the patient may gradually become withdrawn, slow and apathetic. He or she may also be suspicious of other people – paranoid – or feel that their lives are controlled by some external force or being, such as radio waves or a god of some kind.

The illness may improve on its own after a few weeks, but often the symptoms recur. In about a quarter of cases it lasts for many years in a chronic state.

Organic brain disease

The BRAIN may be damaged by injury, the effects of physical illness or by toxic drugs. Symptoms depend on the nature of the damage and whether or not it is permanent. A serious HEAD INJURY can ultimately lead to a permanent change in personality, difficulty in concentrating and possibly some loss of intellect. Serious symptoms can cause temporarily irrational behaviour, which can be misinterpreted as a mental illness such as *hypomania* (*see* MANIC DEPRESSION).

Dementia: About one person in ten over the age of 65 develops dementia, known as *senile dementia.* Occasionally, younger people develop the condition, then known as *presenile dementia.* Early symptoms usually involve forgetfulness, and difficulty in reasoning. Longer term memories may be preserved for some time, but as the disease progresses these too gradually fade. Ultimately there are personality changes, the patient is confused, DEPRESSED and withdrawn. Physical deterioration can also be severe, so that the patient becomes unable to wash, dress or otherwise look after themselves. They may become INCONTINENT. Treatment consists mainly of caring for the patient, and keeping them as contented and active as possible, and may involve TRANQUILLIZING drugs. Certain infections and vitamin deficiencies may be treated by drugs.

The commonest type of dementia (about 75 per cent) is the condition known as *Alzheimer's disease,* which usually begins late in life. Patients with Alzheimer's develop abnormalities in the nerve cells in certain areas of the BRAIN. The cells degenerate and cease to function, tangled masses of abnormal fibres also occur in the damaged tissue. Although much research has been done, so far the cause of this disease has not been definitely established.

A second common cause of dementia is circulatory disorder, caused by hardening of the ARTERIES (arteriosclerosis) or small blood clots (thromboses) in the arteries serving the brain. Other, less common, causes include brain TUMOURS, poisoning (including ALCOHOLISM), recurrent HEAD INJURY, vitamin deficiency, infections such as SYPHILIS and AIDS, and Huntingdon's chorea, a degenerative NEUROLOGICAL complaint.

Treatments for mental illness

A doctor must first assess the patient carefully so that the type of illness can be defined. Treatment may be given by a general practitioner, perhaps with the assistance of a psychiatric nurse or psychologist. Drugs may be used, especially for affective disorders or schizophrenia, but for many disorders psychotherapy (*see* MENTAL THERAPIES) is used. A psychiatrist may be involved for more complicated or serious illnesses. Admission to hospital is considered for any patient whose behaviour is seriously disordered.

Outlook

Most patients with mental illness have a relatively mild disorder which improves with rest and appropriate treatment. Only a minority of patients have persisting problems which may cause long-term disability. The treatments for mental illness are developing and the stigma of mental disorder is decreasing so that more people can live useful and happier lives in the community even though they may still have some residual symptoms of mental illness.

Mental therapies

The choice of treatment for a MENTAL ILLNESS depends on the nature of the problem and the individual concerned. Therapies may prove to be helpful in assisting recovery or in enabling people to come to terms with their difficulties. They include physical treatments, such as drugs, and the talking or behaviour-based therapies in which the patient plays a far more active role. Each person reacts differently, so the doctor may try various treatments in turn to find the one that is most suitable. Or he or she may suggest a combination of treatments in order to tackle different aspects of a problem.

It is easy to pin unrealistic hopes on a particular treatment and expect rapid improvements. Although some treatments may work quickly for a few people, recovery, when it occurs, is more likely to be a slow process.

Seeking help

Most people with mental health problems are treated by their family doctor. It is important to consult the doctor as soon as it is suspected that something is wrong, because the earlier such problems are identified, the easier they are to treat. The doctor will be experienced in dealing with these difficulties because between a quarter and a third of all patients visiting a doctor's surgery have problems related to mental health. If the doctor wants a second opinion, or considers that more specialist help is required, he or she may refer the patient to a PSYCHIATRIST.

In most cases, a psychiatrist will recommend treatment either as an out-patient or through the patient's own doctor. The aim nowadays is to enable people to lead as normal a life as possible within the community while receiving treatment. Patients may be admitted to hospital, however, if it is thought necessary to keep them under constant observation before deciding on treatment, for example, or if they are so distressed that they are quite unable to cope. Patients able to live at home but nevertheless requiring considerable support and treatment may be recommended to attend a day hospital.

Drug treatment

The discovery of a number of useful drugs since the 1950s means that the symptoms of the more serious mental health problems can frequently be alleviated. As a result, most people suffering from SCHIZOPHRENIA, MANIC DEPRESSION and severe DEPRESSION need no longer spend long periods in hospital, but can live within the community, providing that sufficient support is available. Although such drugs have proved to be very beneficial, and even life-saving in many cases, they are not the complete answer. They are, unfortunately, not effective for everybody, they cannot solve the problems that contribute to the illness, and they do have side-effects which are sometimes distressing.

It is important that anybody who is prescribed drugs for mental illness discusses them carefully with the doctor, as soon as they feel able to, in order to understand their aims, advantages and possible drawbacks. The doctor will want to see the patient fairly frequently at first to check the effects of the drug and any side-effects, and to adjust the dose or change the drug if necessary. Because of side-effects, such drugs should be used with caution and the doctor will prescribe the minimum dose for each individual patient.

Drugs often take some time to build up in the body, so it may be several weeks before any improvement is felt. People taking drugs for mental illness should not alter the dose or cease taking the drug suddenly without consulting their doctor. They may need to remain on the drug for some time after they feel better to avoid the risk of a relapse, and then to come off it slowly under the guidance of the doctor; otherwise distressing withdrawal symptoms may occur.

Until the early 1980s, many doctors prescribed TRANQUILLIZERS and SEDATIVES for mental health problems arising from anxiety (*see* STRESS). It is now known, however, that these drugs lose their effectiveness after quite a short time and that, even more worryingly, people taking them run the risk of becoming addicted. Doctors may still prescribe such drugs to help people through a few days of acute stress or to enable them to get a couple of nights' sleep, but people should not expect a prescription for more than a week's supply.

Electroconvulsive therapy

When somebody is severely depressed and fails to respond to drug treatment, a psychiatrist may recommend *electroconvulsive therapy* (ECT). It might also be recommended for depressed patients for whom drugs might be too risky, as when they are suffering from heart disease, for example, or for those who are in such a state of deep depression by the time they seek help that their lives are in danger. In general, ECT acts more quickly than antidepressants to relieve depression.

Although it is not yet clear how ECT works, it does seem to be effective in alleviating severe depression in most cases. Moreover, most of its side-effects are very short term. A few people do complain of some long-term memory loss, but whether this is caused by the ECT or occurs for other reasons is not certain.

Most people have between six and twelve sessions of ECT. They are given a short-acting general ANAESTHETIC and a muscle relaxant, and then a very mild electric current is passed through the brain, causing a minor CONVULSION. The patient then rests for several hours after coming round. Contrary to popular belief, most people who have undergone ECT have not found it distressing.

Behaviour therapy

Many people misunderstand what behaviour therapy is and associate it with techniques such as brain-washing. Nothing could be further from the truth. Behaviour therapy is a commonsense and practical approach in which the cooperation and motivation of the person concerned is crucial. It focuses very much on the present and on the symptoms and reactions that are causing distress, and it aims to enable people to find alternative ways of behaving that will help them to cope. It has proved extremely useful for a range of problems, including PHOBIAS, compulsive rituals and sexual difficulties.

It is not a long-drawn-out form of therapy, and it is usually clear at an early stage whether or not it is likely to be helpful. Sessions with the therapist are usually once a week for an hour at first, and then less often as the person gains in confidence. In early sessions, patients will probably be asked to give a detailed account of their behaviour leading up to, during and following the period of distress. They may be asked to keep a diary and to monitor their anxiety throughout the day on a scale of one to ten. In this way, it is often possible to identify the 'triggers' for the anxiety and the strategies that the person uses to deal with it.

Treatment may consist of talking to the therapist, carrying out a number of everyday tasks that cause anxiety, often with the support of the therapist and friends, or learning an appropriate behaviour therapy technique.

It is often suggested that because behaviour therapy tackles only the symptoms and not the causes of anxiety, problems will simply recur in a different form. In fact, this does not appear to happen. People who overcome difficulties in this way seem to gain in confidence generally.

Talking therapies

Talking to an understanding friend can be a great relief for people who are mentally distressed. But often this is not enough. They need a skilled outsider who is experienced in listening to problems and who will not be shocked by the strength of their feelings. Sometimes a few sessions of talking to a doctor or psychiatrist, or to somebody on a telephone helpline, for example, may be sufficient to get things in perspective. In other instances, a talking therapy such as *counselling, psychotherapy* or *group therapy* may be suggested. These therapies offer people the opportunity to look at their problems in greater depth in order to understand some of the reasons for their feelings or behaviour.

Group therapy can be useful for a wide range of problems, but it is particularly helpful for people who find it hard to mix or make relationships. Groups, which normally meet once a week, usually consist of six to ten members and one or two therapists. The therapists' aim is to encourage members to share their difficulties and help each other work through their problems. Looking at problems with others who are trying to do the same provides support and overcomes feelings of isolation. Many people find it easier to accept the need to change their attitudes or behaviour when suggestions come from others who are struggling to do the same.

Cognitive therapy involves learning to think and therefore to behave in a more positive way and has proved very helpful for people with moderate depression or anxiety. During therapy, the patient works with the therapist to identify the negative thoughts and beliefs that reinforce the depression or anxiety. These might include the idea that friends do not really like you or that you are unable to cope. The patient will learn to challenge these assumptions and replace them with more positive approaches which he or she will then test in practice. It is not a lengthy therapy.

When children or young adolescents have difficulties, other members of the family are usually closely involved. Each sees the situation in a slightly different way, and *family therapy* gives everybody the opportunity to express his or her feelings. It often turns out that stresses within the family are contributing to the problem. Therapy helps the family to sort out for itself the best way of tackling the problem.

There are many different types to training for counselling and psychotherapy, and frequently the two overlap. However, generally in counselling the emphasis is more on what is happening in people's lives at present, whereas psychotherapy concentrates more on the past and the early underlying cause of distress.

Counsellors and psychotherapists will not advise people what to do. Their role is to listen carefully to what people have to say without making judgements, and to help them to work through their problems at their own pace.

Anybody can set up as a counsellor or psychotherapist, so people who consult one privately should ask their doctor or somebody they trust for a recommendation. It is important, too, to check on fees first because these vary widely.

Mesenteric adenitis, *see* Appendicitis

Mesenteric occlusion, *see* Intestines and intestinal disorders

Mesothelioma, *see* Sarcoma

Metabolism

The complex processes that help keep our bodies functioning normally are efficiently controlled by body chemicals called ENZYMES and HORMONES. Enzyme activity influences chemical conversions so that necessary substances are made available to body cells, while hormones control activities such as growth and the utilization of energy reserves.

Efficient metabolism, which is essential to normal body functioning, requires a suitable supply of raw materials. Therefore a bad diet, overeating or undereating (*see* NUTRITION), heavy consumption of ALCOHOL, and even certain drugs can cause troublesome or potentially dangerous metabolic disturbances.

The two processes

Metabolism is the product of two quite distinct and complementary processes, called *catabolism* and *anabolism*. Catabolism consists of the breakdown of CARBOHYDRATES, FATS and PROTEINS and a number of waste products, such as cells and tissues, to provide energy. The energy released by catabolism is converted into useful work through muscle activity, and a certain amount is lost as heat. Anabolism involves constructive processes by which food materials are adapted and stored as energy or used by the body in growth, reproduction and defence against infections.

Many hormones work to regulate the metabolism of food. Often, hormonal activity acts to maintain a 'steady state' of important body chemicals, increasing the production of a chemical if its level falls too low, but directing the chemicals into a catabolic or anabolic pathway if its level rises too high.

Body inputs and outputs

In a growing child or adolescent, the energy input derived from the breakdown of food outweighs the energy output, to provide for the energy requirements of growth. In adults, any excess of energy intake will be converted into fat; conversely, too much energy expenditure will result in weight loss.

All energy content and output is measured in kilojoules (1 kilojoule is equivalent to approximately 4.2 kilocalories or big 'C' calories).

Metabolic rate

The amount of energy a person burns up – his or her *metabolic rate* – has two components. The energy a person expends when he or she is completely at rest is called the *basal* (or resting) *metabolic rate* and consists entirely of energy needed to keep the body 'ticking over'. An average-sized man has a resting metabolic rate of about 7110 kJ/day (1700 kcal/day) and an average-sized woman has a rate of about 5850 kJ/day (1400 kcal/day), but the rate can vary by up to 1470 kJ/day (350 kcal/day) between different adults.

The second component of metabolic rate consists of the amount of energy expended in muscular activity, and varies from close to zero for someone lying perfectly motionless to 2920 kJ/hour (700 kcal/hour) for someone engaged in heavy work or a strenuous sport.

Because of these different components of metabolic rate, people vary widely in how much energy they burn up in a day. For example, a girl engaged in light secretarial work may expend about 8360–10,460 kJ/day (2,000–2,500 kcal/day), while a man engaged in heavy manual labour may expend 16,730–20,900 kJ/day (4,000–5,000 kcal/day). Therefore some people have to eat twice as much as others to provide for their energy requirements.

Carbohydrate breakdown

Much of our energy requirement is provided by the breakdown of carbohydrates – found in foods such as bread and potatoes – into sugars. The most common sugars obtained from food are glucose, fructose and galactose. These are first transported to the LIVER, where fructose and galactose are converted into *glucose*.

Glucose in the liver can be used in a variety of ways – some is used for energy, some becomes *glycogen*. Once the glycogen storage areas are filled up, the glucose is converted into fat. When needed, the glycogen or fat can be converted back to glucose to meet extra energy requirements.

Cells obtain energy from glucose by breaking it down into a substance called *pyruvic acid*. The energy released by this process is temporarily stored as a high energy compound called *adenosine triphosphate* (ATP).

Fat and protein breakdown
Fats and proteins are an important part of the food we eat, and if carbohydrate intake is low, fats and, less commonly, proteins may be used as energy sources.

When carbohydrate sources of energy run out, the fat molecules are split up again into *glycerol* and *fatty acids* which are catabolized separately. Glycerol is converted in the liver into glucose and thus enters the pathway of glucose metabolism.

Proteins contained in the diet are broken down into *amino acids* which are required for growth, and also the enzymes needed to accelerate each cell's metabolic processes.

Migraine

Migraines – violent HEADACHES accompanied by nausea, vomiting and disturbances of sight, hearing, feeling and speech – can affect anyone.

Although the causes of migraine are not fully understood, it is thought to be the result of the blood vessels in the head narrowing down and then expanding. This affects the flow of blood to the brain and so triggers off the disturbances in perception (affecting particularly vision) and the painful headache.

Research has suggested that a migraine attack is triggered by changes in the body in 'vaso-active amines', which are amines affecting blood vessels. These amines are normally present in the body tissue but their level may be raised by a person consuming certain types of foods, or released when sufferers are under STRESS and when their blood sugar level is low as a result of going too long between meals. Foods such as yoghurt, chocolate, cheese, meat and yeast extracts, and some kinds of red wine, contain *tyramine*; some migraine sufferers lack a vital enzyme which breaks this down, so that when they eat these foods, tyramine builds up in their blood and sets off a chain of chemical events that can result in a migraine. In addition, a substance called *serotonin* is raised by the 'positive ions' which are found in the air of stuffy, smoky rooms and in hot, dry winds and this can trigger off a migraine in some susceptible people.

Additionally, it has been found that migraine sufferers are deficient in the 'mono-amine' enzymes which are responsible for breaking down the amines. This may explain why sufferers may be so badly affected by the hormone changes of the menstrual cycle (*see* PREMENSTRUAL SYNDROME) and by the hormones in the contraceptive pill, resulting in worse migraines at the time of their menstruation or while taking the pill.

There are several other factors which contribute to causing migraine. People who already have a tendency to migraine – which can be inherited – may experience more frequent and severe attacks if they develop high BLOOD PRESSURE, or if they are involved in an accident which results in an injury to their head or neck (*see* HEAD AND HEAD INJURIES). When the salt and water content of body tissues is raised (*see* OEDEMA), attacks may be precipitated; this can occur in both sexes, but especially in women before and during their periods. Child sufferers generally have abdominal migraine with only a mild headache, and half grow out of them before adulthood.

Symptoms vary considerably between individuals and from one attack to another. However, there are certain characteristic features that separate migraine from ordinary headaches. These include a headache above or behind one eye or mostly on one side of the head, nausea and vomiting, and blurred vision, flashing lights or an extreme sensitivity to light and sound.

Sufferers may also shake and feel giddy, have difficulty in speaking and seeing normally and experience intense 'other worldly' sensations.

The classical migraine is usually preceded by a warning 'aura', with feelings of exaggerated well-being or visual disturbances. This symptom usually fades with the onset of a headache and is most common in adolescence or in early adulthood.

Treatment

The best treatment for migraine is prevention. First, isolate the factors which trigger migraine. This can be done by keeping a 'migraine diary': note everything you ate and any stressful factors in the 24 hours preceding the migraine. You may be able to identify foods which have an adverse effect, either by eating them or omitting them from your diet for a month. If eye-strain seems to be causing problems, have your spectacle prescription checked: dark glasses or polaroid lenses may reduce general glare or dazzle. Overtiredness, crowds, stuffy places should be avoided if these contribute.

Generally, migraine sufferers need to accept that they may be more sensitive than other people: they need to rest adequately, eat regularly and well, and take life at a gentle pace. Stress at home, in personal relationships and at work can contribute to the severity of migraine, and sufferers should learn not to 'drive' themselves and to avoid situations where they are under pressure. Many migraine sufferers tend to 'bottle up' their feelings, and talking about them may ease some of the tension. Regular gentle physical exercise such a swimming and yoga can help by relaxing the body and making it less likely to become tense. Regular MEDITATION has also been found helpful.

As a preventive measure, some doctors prescribe SEDATIVES to keep stress at bay and anti-depressants to relieve DEPRESSION. Others prescribe drugs to control the nervous impulses controlling blood vessel diameter or to counter the potentially harmful effects of serotonin.

Simple PAINKILLERS such as soluble aspirin, codeine or paracetamol are also suggested for pain relief when an attack occurs. However, as the stomach becomes inactive early in an attack, drugs may not be well absorbed and may be vomited back. For this reason, anti-vomiting and anti-nausea drugs may have to be taken first.

For most people, however, the headache is the most painful part of the attack and is often quite unaffected by simple painkillers; for this reason, drugs derived from the fungus, *ergot,* which constrict the swollen blood vessels in the head, are often prescribed and taken early in an attack. These drugs need to be used with extreme care. They should never be taken during pregnancy and the recommended dosage should never be exceeded.

Because many of the prescribed drugs are unsatisfactory in treating attacks, have unpleasant side-effects and may cause long-term dependence, other methods of treatment should be tried. These are often most effective in the early stages of an attack.

Sufferers should lie flat on a bed, without a pillow, in a quiet, darkened room. At this stage, gentle MASSAGE may help to loosen tension at the neck and base of the skull, on the back and shoulders and on the stomach. Finger pressure on the bridge of the nose, or on the pulse points at the temple and behind the ear may relieve the pain temporarily. Going to sleep early in the attack often helps to shorten it. Trying to 'fight it off' may make it worse.

You could also try HOMOEOPATHIC medicine or ACUPUNCTURE, where fine needles are inserted at different points in the body. Research is also currently under way into the effectiveness of a herb called *feverfew* which has been claimed to relieve migraine if three leaves a day are eaten over a period of months. You can obtain it from most health food shops.

Anybody who suffers from regular migraines should consult his or her doctor about possible long-term preventive treatment. Several different drugs have been found to relieve the frequency of attacks, including propranolol and pizotifen, but they must be taken regularly. There may be minor side-effects with these drugs, such as possible gastro-intestinal disturbances and mild depression with propranolol or drowsiness and weight gain with pizotifen.

Minerals

These are an essential part of the DIET, and they perform a great many functions in various tissues of the body, from building strong BONES and TEETH to forming a key part of BLOOD and some HORMONES.

There are two different sorts of minerals in the body – those which are found throughout the tissues and cells, and those which are only found in specific places in the body and cells where they are an essential part of the single key process. In the first category, there are three main substances: sodium, POTASSIUM and CALCIUM. They are all metals in their purified forms, but in the body they are in the form of SALTS.

This group of metal salts – perhaps with the addition of magnesium – is essential in different types of processes. There is considerable energy expended by the body in controlling all of its functions. For example, the amount of sodium that is found in the fluid surrounding the cell is much greater than that within the cell membrane; with potassium, the reverse is the case. This basic imbalance establishes a tension that is responsible for living cells being able to respond to stimulus. Many essential activities are electrical – muscle contraction (including the heartbeat) and nerve conduction are

The body's minerals

Mineral	Role	Mineral	Role
Sodium and chloride	Found in all tissues, involved in control of fluid balance in kidney. Found in all foods and added in cooking as salt.	Magnesium	Important for metabolism and muscle strength. Sources as for phosphorus.
Potassium	Acts with sodium to control electrical activity of nerves. Found in fresh fruit and vegetables.	Iodine	Needed for thyroid. Found in all seafoods.
Calcium	Essential component of bones and teeth, needed by nerves and muscles. Found in meat, eggs and dairy products.	Iron	Essential for haemoglobin in blood. Found in liver and other meat.
Phosphorus (phosphate)	Basic energy store in all cells, combined with calcium in bones and muscles. Found in meat, dairy products, pulses and cereals.	Copper	Needed for oxygen metabolism in cells. Found in seafood and meat.
		Manganese	As for copper, and for fat metabolism. Sources as for phosphorus.

examples. About 70 per cent of the oxygen that we use to provide energy is needed to keep sodium and potassium on the right side of the cell membranes.

Calcium is the most abundant mineral in the body and it is an essential ingredient in building a healthy bone structure. Exercise is essential to achieve the right balance of calcium in the body, and people who are bedridden, for example, are exercised as much as possible to reduce the risk of fractures.

In contrast, the other minerals may only be required for a few specific purposes in the body. IRON, for example, is an essential component of haemoglobin which carries the oxygen from the lungs to the tissues, while IODINE's only role is in the THYROID hormone – this exerts control over the body's metabolism.

What can go wrong?

The essential minerals are found in the soil and are therefore present in vegetables and animal foods. The two minerals which are most likely to be deficient in natural circumstances are iron and iodine. Iron deficiency, which causes ANAEMIA, is extremely common in underdeveloped countries where diet is inadequate. Even in developed countries, there are some women who become anaemic because of the iron they lose each month during their PERIODS. Foods rich in iron include liver and other types of red meat. Iodine deficiency is avoided by adding its compounds to table salt.

There are complex systems to control the levels of sodium, potassium and calcium in the body. Although we think of the KIDNEY as the organ for the disposal of waste material, it uses most energy in making sure that not too much sodium and potassium is lost in the urine.

Deficiencies of the other minerals are very uncommon. Zinc deficiency does occur though, and may be responsible for the slow healing of skin wounds or ulcers.

It is actually more common to encounter poisoning with minerals such as manganese and copper. Copper poisoning – *Wilson's disease* – results from an inherited defect in the way that the body absorbs and stores copper. Practically all the minerals in the diet can be poisonous in excess. Fortunately, it is rare for people to suffer from toxicity unless they have taken a deliberate or accidental overdose. An overdose or iron (which is a medicine often found in the home) is one of the more common and serious types of poisoning in children. Any iron tablets which are kept at home should be well locked up and out of the reach of young, active children. Potassium, given as a medicine, can be dangerous in excess, and the amount given to patients has to be closely monitored.

Miscarriage

No one knows exactly how common miscarriages are since if one happens in the early weeks of PREGNANCY, the woman herself may be unaware that she was ever pregnant. It is estimated that between 10 and 25 per cent of all pregnancies miscarry in the first three months (first trimester), and that an average of 30 per cent of women will miscarry during a pregnancy at some stage during their reproductive lives. An early miscarriage may be experienced like an unusually heavy period that is a few days late. It is often nature's way of rejecting an embryo that is genetically abnormal or malformed.

Doctors usually refer to a miscarriage as a 'spontaneous abortion', which is strictly the correct medical term. A termination of pregnancy is called an 'induced abortion', although many people only use the word ABORTION when referring to a termination. So do not be upset if your doctor uses the word abortion when referring to a miscarriage.

Causes

A miscarriage in the first 28 days of pregnancy is often caused by a HORMONE imbalance. Instead of producing enough of the hormone that will maintain a pregnancy, the body goes through similar hormonal changes as it does during the menstrual cycle, resulting in what is called a 'partially suppressed period'. The threatened miscarriage often starts at the time of the month at which the woman would normally have had her PERIOD. There may be some bleeding, either heavy or light, accompanied by backache or a heavy ache around the uterus (womb). Hormone deficiencies can also result in problems with the placenta, causing it not to develop adequately to sustain the pregnancy.

About half of all early miscarriages have been shown to be the result of a genetic abnormality in the embryo. Chromosome abnormalities (*see* CELLS AND CHROMOSOMES and GENETICS) can be detected in the cells of many aborted embryos, which are unable to survive because of the abnormality. The abnormality may have occurred because of some genetic problem with the ovum (egg; *see* OVARIES) or SPERM, or because of an abnormality which has arisen during division of the cells in the embryo.

A miscarriage can also be caused by a CERVIX (neck of the womb) that is 'weak'. If the muscles of the cervix have been damaged in any way (either by previous surgery or a difficult previous childbirth), they may not be able to support the pregnant uterus; the cervix is then described as 'incompetent'.

Lastly, miscarriage may occasionally occur if the mother is suffering from a serious illness or from severe MALNUTRITION.

Signs of miscarriage

A miscarriage is likely to start with bleeding and/or pain, which will vary in its severity depending on the length of the pregnancy. The blood may become brighter red in colour, and contractions of the uterus may begin to expel the pregnancy. This could take anything from under an hour to a number of hours and the amount of pain experienced will vary from woman to woman.

Any bleeding from the vagina during the first six months of pregnancy can indicate a 'threatened' miscarriage, although occasionally slight bleeding is caused by other problems, such as infections in the vagina. At first, the bleeding is usually light, although it may be bright red. Sometimes bleeding stops after a few hours, and pain is minimal. If the cervix remains closed, it is quite possible for the pregnancy to continue.

Once the cervix starts to open up, the pregnancy is bound to miscarry, and this situation is then termed an 'inevitable' miscarriage. Bleeding may become more severe, and there is usually quite marked pain, especially low backache which may come in waves. Heavy blood clots can be lost from the vagina.

Once the whole of the foetus, placenta and amniotic sac has been passed from the womb, the miscarriage is said to be 'complete'. Bleeding diminishes quite rapidly and any pain soon lessens.

Sometimes, however, only part of the embryo or foetus is expelled, and some of the amniotic sac or pieces of placental material may remain in the womb. This is an 'incomplete' miscarriage. The woman is then likely to continue bleeding and may continue to have pain. An incomplete miscarriage is more likely after the eighth week of pregnancy – earlier miscarriages are more often complete.

Missed miscarriage

This is an uncommon type of miscarriage. The foetus dies but is not expelled from the uterus. There may be slight bleeding from the woman's vagina but often there is none. The symptoms of pregnancy – breast fullness, nausea, weight gain – rapidly disappear and the woman usually then realizes that something is wrong because she no longer feels pregnant. Eventually the foetus may be expelled, some weeks after it has died, but this may not occur. There is then a danger of complications, such as infection or disturbance of the blood-clotting system of the mother caused by toxins from the dead foetus, which then has to be removed by an operation.

Treatment

Once a threatened miscarriage is suspected, the woman is advised to rest, avoid doing housework and stay in bed until any bleeding subsides. If the bleeding is not too heavy and there are no obvious signs of an incomplete miscarriage, the doctor may allow the woman to stay at home. Many patients with a threatened miscarriage stop bleeding after a day or two.

If there is pain or heavy bleeding, hospital treatment is usual. An internal examination may be performed to see if the miscarriage is inevitable or incomplete, and if so a curettage (scraping of the inside of the womb) may be carried out under anaesthetic to remove the remaining pieces of dead tissue. If there is doubt about whether or not the pregnancy will survive, an ULTRASOUND scan may be carried out which will show up exactly what is present in the uterus: if a live foetus is present, it can be seen, and the heartbeat will be detected.

A woman with an inevitable or incomplete abortion may lose considerable quantities of blood and go into SHOCK. A blood transfusion may then be required.

If the doctor suspects a missed abortion, it is not essential that a curettage is carried out immediately because the embryo or foetus may eventually be expelled naturally, but an operation may be necessary if complications are suspected.

Repeated miscarriages

If a woman miscarries during three or more pregnancies, this is described as 'recurrent' miscarriage. Each miscarriage may have a different cause, so thorough tests are very important – for both the woman and the man concerned. This is because the health of the father's sperm may be poor. Some women miscarry at the same point in each pregnancy. If this happens three or more times it is described as 'habitual' miscarriage. This could be for a number of reasons depending on the time of miscarriage. Internal problems, such as FIBROIDS in the uterus, may be the cause, and these can be treated.

Many miscarriages may be caused by particular circumstances such as a single malformed ovum, which are unlikely to happen again. Doctors usually advise women to wait for three months or so before beginning another pregnancy, although sexual intercourse can start once internal recovery is complete, which may be a matter of weeks.

If recurrent miscarriage is caused by weakness of the cervix (cervical incompetence), a stitch can be inserted around the cervix to make it more secure. The stitch is removed a couple of weeks before the baby is due.

Mitosis, *see* **Cells and chromosomes**

Moles, *see* **Melanin and melanoma**

Mongolism, *see* **Amniocentesis, Down's syndrome**

Mononucleosis, infections, *see* **Glandular fever**

Morning sickness, *see* **Pregnancy**

Motion sickness, *see* **Travel sickness**

Motor neurone disease

Nerves from the brain responsible for moving muscles are called *motor neurones* (*see* NERVOUS SYSTEM). They have only two components to transmit the electrical message rapidly: the upper portion, known as the *upper motor neurone*, runs from a cell station in the brain called a *Betz cell*, down the SPINAL CORD to a level where it leaves as a spinal nerve supply to particular MUSCLES. At this point, there is a second cell station from which a *lower motor neurone* takes over and runs out to the muscles which move our limbs. Motor neurone disease is an incurable condition in which these cell stations and neurones waste away.

Causes

Motor neurone disease affects about five people out of every 100,000 and is found throughout the world. Men and women are affected equally, and the onset of symptoms usually occurs between the ages of 30 and 60, although, rarely, younger adults may be affected by this wasting disease.

As yet no cause has been discovered for this unpleasant and distressing illness. Since older people are usually affected, it appears that it could be the result of a long-term degeneration process in the motor neurones, but how this is triggered off remains a mystery. Studies of sufferers have shown that there may have been some accident in the past which has caused injury to a limb, but the relevance of this is unclear. A number of sufferers have also been found to have used vibrating power tools during their working lives. Other theories concern the possibility of the disease being caused by a toxic substance, perhaps exposure to high quantities of lead, mercury or selenium. Some studies suggest that it is more common among people who have worked in the leather industry.

Research has also indicated that naturally occurring substances called glutamates may harm the neurones when the brain fails to regulate their concentration correctly. Current drug investigations may lead to a way of slowing the progress of the disease with 'anti-glutamates'. It has also been suggested that motor neurone disease may be the result of a slowly progressive virus infection (the Coxsackie B virus has been implicated), but there is still no proof that a virus is part of the cause rather than an effect. Finally, in 1993 an international team identified a gene on chromosome 21 (*see* GENETICS) that may be responsible for an inherited form of the disease, which accounts for 5–10 per cent of cases.

Symptoms

The earliest symptoms are usually quite slight. The patient may notice difficulty in using one hand – for example, in turning a key in a lock. Or he or she may have some weakness of a foot. Wasting of the muscles in one hand or one arm, or cramps in the hand or arm, may occur. Another characteristic symptom is intermittent twitching of muscles in the upper arm or shoulders. Any weakness in the hand or leg becomes greater with exertion.

As the disease progresses, both the arms and legs are likely to become affected by weakness, stiffness and muscular twitching – called *fasciculation*. Walking may become increasingly difficult, and the power in the hands diminishes. The grip weakens, and it may become difficult for the patient to hold anything at all between the fingers and thumb.

Perhaps the most distressing symptom for the patient is difficulty with control of speech and with swallowing. At first, the speech may be slurred but eventually it becomes virtually unintelligible. The patient will tend to choke on food, and may even have difficulty swallowing saliva, with dribbling from the corner of the mouth occurring almost continually. The chest muscles can become weak, and breathing may be difficult, especially at night.

Despite the severe disabling physical symptoms of motor neurone disease, the sufferer remains mentally alert and there is no impairment in thinking or reasoning whatsoever. Virtually all patients realize within months of the first symptoms that the course of the illness is of inevitable physical deterioration. They often feel trapped inside a useless body, and become increasingly frustrated by their inability to do the things they want to do.

Diagnosis and treatment

Once the disorder is suspected, investigations are usually carried out in hospital. Special electrical tests on the muscles or nerves can confirm the diagnosis.

Because there is no treatment that will influence the course of motor neurone disease in any way, treatment consists of trying to reduce any disability, relieving troublesome symptoms and, ultimately, providing skilled nursing care.

In the early stages of the disease, PHYSIOTHERAPY may be helpful. Gentle swimming may help to keep the muscles active. If there is weakness in the hands, splints may be made to help with grip. While the patient can still walk, he or she will be encouraged to do so, but relatives will be shown how to help the patient if he or she falls over. Drugs may be prescribed to help relieve muscular jerking. There are numerous aids available to help the patient get the most out of whatever movement he or she has.

Many patients soon need help with feeding. Semi-solid food is usually easiest to swallow – better than thin liquids or hard solids. Most food will need to be mashed or liquidized. Liquids may, however, be taken in sips.

Most patients deteriorate progressively, and most of them die within three to four years of the first symptoms. One patient in five, however, lives for more than five years, and a few – including the brilliant theoretical physicist Dr Stephen Hawking – live for over ten years.

Mouth ulcers, *see* **Ulcers, skin**

MRI (magnetic resonance imaging) scans, *see* **Neurology and neuro-surgery, X-rays**

Multiple birth

By far the most common multiple birth is that of twins, but women have produced as many as ten babies from one PREGNANCY. However, the largest multiple birth where all the babies survived was of sextuplets (six) in South Africa in 1974.

Statistically, the birth of twins can be expected once in every 50 to 150 pregnancies, depending on the race of the parents – black women have the highest number of twins and oriental women have the lowest. Triplets are born about once in every 6,400 pregnancies and quadruplets (four) only once in every 500,000 pregnancies.

Causes of multiple births

Multiple births can occur in two different ways. One is when the fertilized egg (*see* CONCEPTION) splits in half to form what is known as *monozygotic* (identical) twins; each part can then subdivide to form triplets and so on.

The other way a multiple birth can occur is when more than one egg is released during ovulation and each one is fertilized by a separate sperm. Twins born from separate eggs are called *dizygotic* (fraternal); they are more common and their occurrence is influenced by heredity, race, the age of the mother and by the number of children she has already had. For instance, in the absence of any other influencing factors, a woman in her late 30s with four children is more likely to bear twins than a woman in her 20s, pregnant for the first time. Where twins run in families, the genes are generally handed down on the mother's side. They tend to miss every other generation, so that children of dizygotic twins are more likely to bear twins, than be born twins themselves.

The fertilization of more than one egg can also arise if a woman has been given a fertility drug (*see* INFERTILITY) which causes several eggs to be released at once. Between 8 and 10 per cent of these women go on to have multiple births.

Babies born from a divided egg will be of the same sex, have the same blood group and physical characteristics. Babies born from different eggs, however, have no more in common than brothers and sisters born in different years.

The multiple pregnancy

Where pregnancy has followed the use of a fertility drug, the possibility of a multiple birth will be considered as a matter of course. In other cases, there may be indications which lead a doctor to suspect that a woman is carrying more than one baby. Her uterus may be over-large for the number of weeks of conception or there may be excessive sickness or exceptional weight gain. Confirmation of the initial diagnosis is usually made by ULTRASOUND examination at the hospital clinic. With the increasing use of this technique, some previously unsuspected twin pregnancies are discovered.

One of the main problems of multiple birth is that the babies are often born early and have low birth weights. Therefore, an early confirmation of more than one foetus is important and will help to ensure that the babies receive the best possible care during pregnancy.

All pregnant women must watch the IRON content of their blood, and when there are several babies taking all their nourishment from one mother, this is additionally important. Extra iron, VITAMINS (including folic acid) and PROTEIN should all be taken as advised by the doctor or midwife. A multiple pregnancy is not, however, a licence to overeat. The additional weight gain should not be more than 50 per cent of the weight of a single pregnancy. The pregnant woman may find that smaller, more frequent meals will help to ease the increased pressure on her stomach.

A woman carrying more than one child must ensure that she gets sufficient rest every day to help prevent high BLOOD PRESSURE developing (*see* ECLAMPSIA AND PRE-ECLAMPSIA). Resting in bed relieves some of the pressure on the neck of the womb and also maximizes the blood flow to the foetuses.

During pregnancy, the placenta is normally situated in the upper part of the womb, but when there are several foetuses to be accommodated, one may be what is known as *'placenta praevia'* – lying near the opening of the birth canal. Any sign of bleeding must be watched for closely. If it occurs the doctor will recommend total bedrest. If this is not possible at home, the woman may be admitted to hospital.

The more foetuses there are, the smaller they will be and regular visits to an antenatal clinic are vital. After 14 weeks, a multiply-pregnant woman should be seen by a doctor at least once a fortnight, and weekly after the 29th week of pregnancy.

Delivery

Although CHILDBIRTH is a natural process, complications can and do arise, and these can be magnified when there is more than one baby. It is essential, therefore, that multiple births are conducted in hospital where there will be sufficient staff to care for the mother and babies.

Several babies can be delivered quite normally through the vagina or birth canal, one following the other fairly quickly because they are smaller.

When there are several babies in the womb, it may be necessary to deliver them by CAESAREAN section. The babies may be lying in awkward positions for delivery or the womb may be so overstretched that it does not contract efficiently.

After a multiple birth, the babies may be kept in incubators in a special nursery where the mother can visit and feed them when she is feeling strong enough. This close contact is encouraged by hospital staff as it promotes the vital bonding between mother and infants.

Multiple sclerosis

This illness affects the central NERVOUS SYSTEM. It is unpredictable and can result in only minor physical impairment as well as in severe disability. As yet no one fully understands its cause and how its progression can be arrested. It tends to strike between the teens and middle 30s. Women seem more likely to get multiple sclerosis than men – two out of every three sufferers are female. The illness is more frequent in temperate climates, but no one can explain this environmental factor. It is interesting that Northern Europeans born and brought up in the tropics are unlikely to get the disease.

The first parts of the nervous system to be affected are those that control physical sensation, coordination and movement. This tissue in the nervous system is called the 'white matter' and it carries sensory messages to the BRAIN, as well as impulses from the brain to the muscles. The fibres are surrounded by the *myelin sheath*, which insulates and protects them. In multiple sclerosis, the myelin sheath becomes inflamed, sometimes causing damage to the nerves themselves. The nerves may make faulty connections with each other or be so damaged that they will not work at all. As the disease progresses, patches of 'demyelination' can occur in any part of the nervous system but particularly in the SPINAL CORD at the level of the neck and in nerves from the eye.

The 'grey matter' of the nervous system which makes up a section of the brain – the part that is conscious and can think and remember – is not normally affected.

Causes

Although the cause of multiple sclerosis remains a mystery, considerable research has been carried out to try to find why it occurs, with the hope of providing some effective treatment for sufferers.

Perhaps the most important observation is that people of a certain genetic make-up are more susceptible to multiple sclerosis than others. This genetic susceptibility has been discovered as a result of 'tissue typing' people with the illness. Two or three particular tissue types are clearly associated with multiple sclerosis. Relatives in a family who share a particular tissue type are all more prone to it, but this does not mean that multiple sclerosis is inherited or passed on to children in the same way that hereditary diseases are usually transmitted.

However, HEREDITY cannot fully explain why some people of a particular tissue type develop the disease and others do not. Some researchers believe that sufferers may have an abnormality in the way their bodies treat FATS. Myelin consists largely of fat, and it is thought that myelin in multiple sclerosis sufferers may have been formed abnormally. This could be a result of an inborn biochemical error, or possibly associated with a diet high in animal fat. Another theory is that multiple sclerosis may be an auto-immune disease, with the formation in the circulation of antibodies to myelin. A disease similar to multiple sclerosis can be produced experimentally in animals when they are artificially stimulated to produce antibodies to myelin.

Lastly, some researchers believe that multiple sclerosis may be the result of a 'slow' VIRUS infection. Virus-like particles have been discovered in patients with multiple sclerosis. Similar diseases are known in cattle and sheep which have been proved to have a viral cause and which produce symptoms like those of multiple sclerosis. However, there is no evidence that multiple sclerosis can be passed on from one person to another.

Symptoms

The illness takes the form of repeated exacerbations. For no known reason, the exacerbation usually stops of its own accord and a period of remission follows when the disease is not active.

During a remission, the nervous system tries to heal itself and scar tissue forms around the affected areas. But the scar tissue cannot perform the functions of the destroyed myelin sheath and may cause more harm to the affected nerve, sometimes leaving permanent damage. Scar tissues are called *scleroses* and can occur in various parts of the nervous system: hence the name of the illness.

The severity of the illness varies enormously from person to person. In most patients, there is an interval of months or years following the first attack before there is a relapse, but sometimes there is progressive deterioration from the initial attack, and disability occurs early. The pattern of exacerbation followed by remission can mean that one person can lead a completely able-bodied life while another may be unable to co-ordinate movement and be confined to a wheelchair. Many find that they are weak and easily tired for most of the time – indeed, this can be a major problem. Blurred or double vision may occur, particularly when the sufferer is fatigued. Sometimes the first symptom is a severe disturbance of vision in one eye. This may disappear after a time, but it may recur later along with other symptoms.

A common physical symptom is tingling in the hands, arms, feet, legs or trunk. The feeling is like 'PINS AND NEEDLES' and may produce a sensation of numbness. These feelings are not painful but can become uncomfortable.

There is unlikely to be anything wrong with the nerves of the affected areas: the site of the damage may well be in the upper part of the spinal cord. This means that incorrect nerve messages are getting through to the brain – hot bath water may feel cold to the feet, for example.

Some sufferers from multiple sclerosis find that they cannot move or coordinate a limb. One foot may drag, making walking difficult. Some lose control over their hands so that it becomes difficult to write or hold cups or cutlery. If any of these symptoms become severe, it may be difficult to walk or stand unaided and a wheelchair may be necessary. Nerves in other parts of the body, too, can become affected and cause problems with BLADDER control, giddiness and tremors.

It is possible for any number of these symptoms to occur during an exacerbation. During the subsequent remission, individuals may find themselves as physically able as ever they were before the attack.

Treatment

There is, at present, no cure for multiple sclerosis, which is often so distressing for relatively young adults, but there are a number of ways in which symptoms can be relieved. The understanding and support of family and friends is, of course, crucial.

STEROID treatment (*see* ADRENAL GLANDS) – given as tablets of *prednisolone* – may speed up recovery from sudden relapses, but the amount of function that the person recovers after the relapse is not influenced by the drugs. Unfortunately long-term treatment with steroids does not appear to be effective in halting the general progression of the illness, and there is always a risk of side-effects such as thinning of the bones or the skin, and weight gain.

Doctors have been hopeful that therapy to damp down the reactions of the IMMUNE SYSTEM could benefit patients with multiple sclerosis. This type of treatment is known as 'immunotherapy', and several trials have been conducted in various parts of the world, but none has shown any really conclusive benefit. Drugs such as cyclophosphamide, azathioprine and interferon have all been tested, but there is no evidence of any lasting benefit to patients with multiple sclerosis.

Since metabolism of fat is thought to be abnormal in multiple sclerosis, some trials have involved modification of patients' diets. The blood level of a fatty acid called linoleic acid is abnormally low in patients, so the aim of dietary treatment is to increase it. Recommended diets are usually high in vegetable oils, with very little saturated fat (mostly found in animal products). Patients may take supplements of sunflower oil, which contains linoleic acid, or of evening primrose oil.

Some sufferers have claimed that their symptoms improve if they avoid gluten, which is found mainly in wheat flour. However, again the evidence for any benefit is unsubstantial.

Perhaps the most interesting and controversial treatment used in the last few years has been high-pressure (hyperbaric) oxygen treatment. The patient is treated in an oxygen chamber at increased pressure – up to twice the normal atmospheric pressure – for an hour or two every day. Although early results of this treatment seemed promising, long-term results again unfortunately do not appear to show lasting benefit.

Perhaps the most important part of treatment, however, is regular PHYSIOTHERAPY and maintaining a generally positive approach to life. Many sufferers inevitably become depressed as a result of exacerbations in their condition and they may need treatment with drugs for their DEPRESSION.

Disturbances in the control of the bladder or BOWEL may need sympathetic help from skilled nurses and doctors so that the patient can remain socially active. Aids such as devices to assist with gripping objects or wheelchairs may be needed.

Outlook

About one sixth of all patients with multiple sclerosis have relatively mild symptoms and live for up to 30 or 50 years after the diagnosis has been made, with virtually no disability. Another one sixth of patients have few symptoms for a period of 10 or 15 years, but then may deteriorate.

The remaining patients – about two thirds – have fairly pronounced symptoms, but life expectancy is unpredictable. Patients who have their first symptoms at a relatively early age and who have relapses and remissions tend to live longest. On the other hand, the outlook is poor when more elderly patients develop the disease, especially if the symptoms are progressive without any remissions.

Mumps

This is a very common acute viral infection which produces fever and swelling of the salivary glands. The illness is most common in children aged 5 to 14. Only a small percentage of adults contract it, but the symptoms can be severe and complications more common.

Mumps is also known as *infectious parotitis*, because it is the parotid glands which most commonly become enlarged and tender. The mumps patient is infectious from about two days before the swelling appears, and for three days afterwards.

Causes

Mumps is caused by a specific VIRUS that is similar to the INFLUENZA virus. The virus spreads from person to person by contact with the moisture expelled in the coughs, sneezes and breath of the infected person, or by direct contact. It enters the body through the mouth or respiratory tract and then begins to affect the gland tissues.

Symptoms

The first symptoms noticed are slight fever, a sore throat, headache and shivering, and these can often be mistaken for influenza. The gland which is first affected is generally the parotid, the large salivary gland located between the ear and the angle of the jaw. It becomes tender and swollen, making opening the mouth wide and eating extremely painful. Fever increases and the temperature can rise to 103°F (39.4°C).

Often only one gland will be swollen, but the swelling can spread to the other salivary glands developing under the jaw or even under the tongue. Commonly both sides of the face become swollen at the same time, but sometimes one side is not affected until the other is almost better. The swelling increases for two or three days and then gradually subsides. The temperature also begins to fall. The patient makes a complete recovery and returns to normal eating.

The outlook for cases of uncomplicated mumps is excellent. The patient feels better once the fever subsides and the swelling starts to go down. Even severe swelling rarely lasts more than three or four days, and within a week there is complete recovery.

Dangers and complications

It is very rare for mumps to be dangerous, but the virus can cause inflammation in other glands and the nervous system.

Orchitis: Inflammation of one or both TESTES occurs in about 20 per cent of male cases of mumps. A week after the virus has caused swelling of the salivary glands, there is a painful enlargement of the affected testis. In rare cases, this can even occur without fever or swelling of the salivary glands.

Most testes return to normal size within a week, and even in the most rare cases, where both testes are involved and they shrink in size following the infection, sterility is uncommon, and IMPOTENCE virtually never occurs even with shrinkage of the testes.

Oophritis: This inflammation of the OVARY is uncommon but can produce severe lower abdominal pain and bouts of vomiting. The complication subsides within two or three days and has no long-term effects.

Mastitis: The mammary glands (*see* BREASTS) rarely become inflamed because of mumps. However, if affected, the patient complains of pain and swelling of one or both breasts.

Pancreatitis: The mumps virus can cause inflammation of this gland (*see* PANCREAS). It produces symptoms of pain in the upper part of the abdomen, fever and vomiting. Severe cases can need hospitalization. The inflammation settles within three or four days, and the outlook is excellent.

Meningitis: Mild viral MENINGITIS – inflammation of the membranes of the brain – is found in about 5 per cent of cases. It is the most common site to be infected outside the salivary glands, and occurs about ten days after the initial symptoms of mumps. The patient complains of mild neck stiffness, headache and possibly vomiting. The symptoms subside within three or four days on recovery.

Encephalitis: This is an extremely rare inflammation of the BRAIN and is the only really serious danger from mumps. The patient develops severe headaches, high fever and vomiting. In most cases, the trouble is short-lived and full recovery usually occurs. In a small proportion of cases, there is permanent disability or even death.

Treatment

There is no curative or specific treatment for mumps. In mild and moderate cases, simple PAINKILLERS (paracetamol, not aspirin, for a child) are the best treatment and confinement to bed unnecessary.

In more severe cases, the patient should stay in bed, keep warm and drink plenty of fluid during the feverish period. When gland swelling is severe and eating is painful, bland food and adequate fluid are recommended. Pain-killing tablets are needed to reduce the discomfort and frequent mouth-washes with weak salt water are needed to keep the mouth clean and prevent bacterial infection of the gums or salivary glands.

Prevention

Mumps can be reliably prevented with a vaccine, which can be given to children or adults. In many countries, including Britain, children in their second year or life can be given a 'mixed' vaccine that contains individual vaccines against measles, mumps and rubella – the MMR vaccine (*see* IMMUNIZATION).

Muscles

There are three different kinds of muscle in the body. The first, *voluntary muscle*, is under the control of the brain. Together with the BONES and TENDONS, it is responsible for all forms of movement, from a smile to running up a flight of stairs. The second is *smooth muscle* (so called because of the way it looks under the microscope), concerned with the involuntary movement of internal organs such as the guts and bladder. The third is the *cardiac muscle*, which makes up the main bulk of the HEART.

The location of muscles

Voluntary muscle is distributed throughout the body, making up a very large proportion of its weight – up to 25 per cent, even in a newborn baby. It controls the movement of the different part of the skeleton, from the tiny *stapedius* muscle which works on the stapes, a minute bone in the inner ear, to the huge *gluteus maximus* which forms the bulk of the buttock and controls the hip joint.

The muscles are attached to the skeleton by means of tendons. The end of the tendon nearest to the centre of the body is called the 'origin' of the muscle, and is, in general, shorter than the 'tendon of insertion' at the other end. It is usual for the origin to be on one side of a joint and the insertion to be on the far side, so that, by shortening, the muscle brings about a movement of the joint.

The structure of muscles

Voluntary striped muscle can be visualized as a series of fibre bundles, gathered up to make a complete unit.

The smallest of these fibres – and the basic working unit of the muscle – are the *actin and myosin filaments,* so tiny that they can only be seen with the aid of an electron microscope. They are made of protein and are sometimes known as the 'contractile proteins'. The muscle shortens in length when all the myosin filaments slide past the actin filaments.

The filaments are gathered into bundles called *myofibrils.* Between these are the deposits of muscle fuel in the form of *glycogen,* and the normal energy factories of the cell, the *mitochondria,* where oxygen and food-fuel are burned to make energy.

The myofibrils are gathered into further bundles called muscle fibres. These are really the muscle cells, with cell nuclei along their outside edge, and each one has a nerve fibre (*see* NERVOUS SYSTEM) coming to it to trigger it into action when necessary.

The muscle fibres themselves are grouped together in bundles, in an envelope of connective tissue, rather like the insulation surrounding the copper strands of an electric cable. A small muscle may consist of only a few bundles of fibres, while a huge muscle like the *gluteus maximus* is made up of hundreds of bundles of fibres.

The whole muscle is contained in a fibrous tissue covering, again like the insulation round a multi-core cable.

The structure of smooth muscle does not show the same orderly arrangement of filaments and fibres, built into a complicated geometrical pattern, although its contraction still depends on sliding filaments.

The structure of cardiac muscle, however, when it is seen under the microscope, is the same as that of voluntary muscle, except that the fibres which make it up form cross bridges with each other.

How a muscle works

Nerves run down the SPINAL CORD from the motor (movement controlling) parts of the cerebral cortex of the BRAIN, and pass out of the cord into the individual nerves to the muscles. If a muscle is deprived of its nerve supply, it not only loses its ability to contract but also starts to waste away.

There is an area on the surface of the muscle fibres where the nerves are plugged into the muscles. The electrical force of the nerve impulse when it arrives at the junction with a muscle is absolutely tiny, whereas the electrical changes that take place in muscles when they contract, are, by comparison, quite large, so some form of amplification is necessary. The transmission of the impulse to contract takes place at a special 'motor end-plate' at the point where the nerve fibre meets the muscle fibre. The electrical impulse travelling down the nerve does not stimulate the muscle directly, but releases a transmitter chemical called *acetylcholine,* which causes contraction.

Some of the body's main voluntary muscles

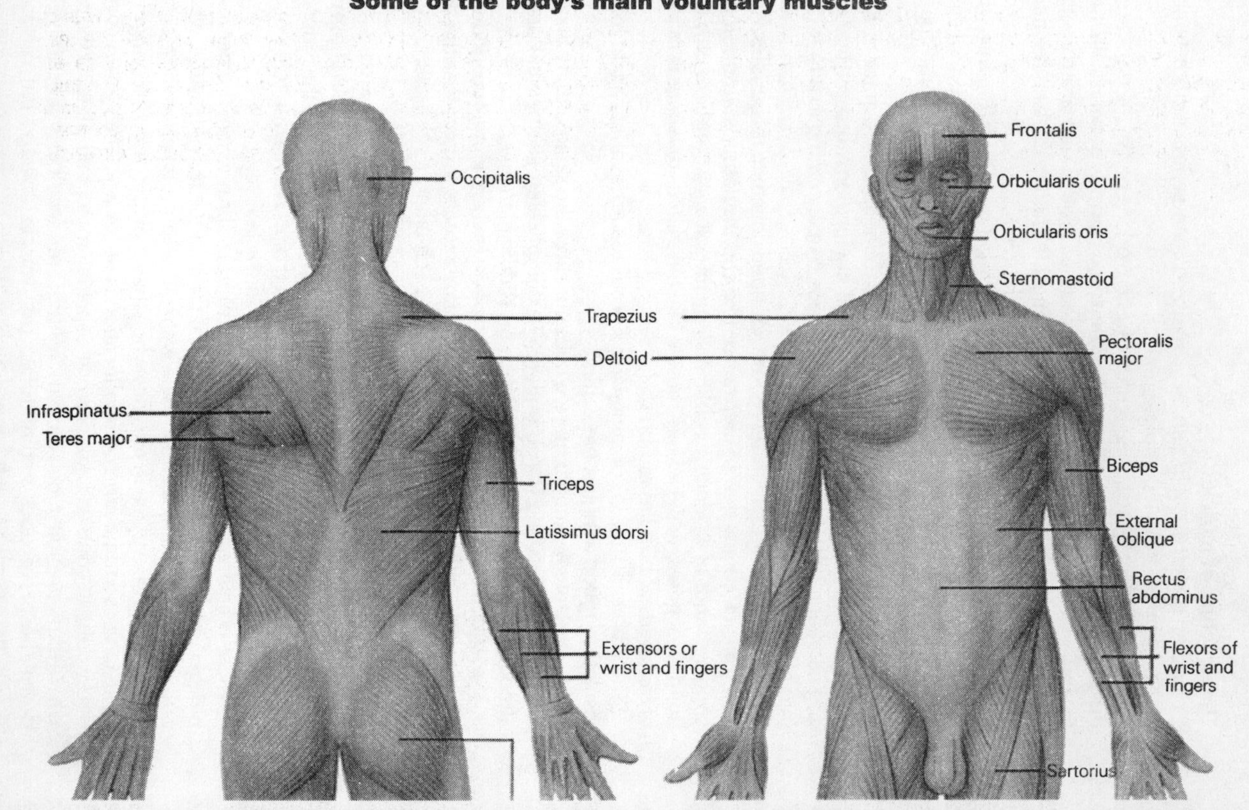

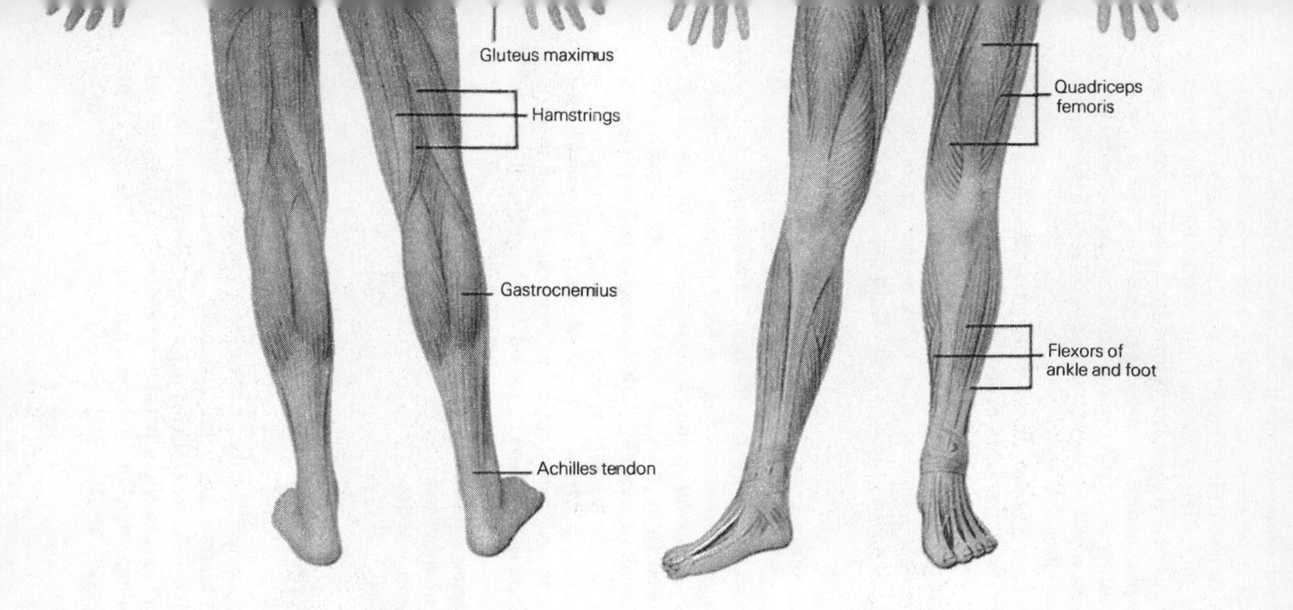

Voluntary muscles are also called striated (striped) muscles because the arrangement of fibres which form them gives them a striped appearance under the microscope. They produce their effect by shortening, a process called contraction. They have to be able to produce sudden, explosive contractions of the kind that leg muscles make when somebody jumps into the air, and to stay contracted to hold a particular posture.

Involuntary muscle – or smooth muscle, as it is usually called – is made up of long spindly cells instead of fibres. It is not under the conscious control of the brain, but is responsible for the muscular contractions required in processes such as digestion, when the peristaltic waves in the intestines, moving food, are caused by smooth muscle contraction. Cardiac muscle, found only in the heart, has a similar structure.

The sliding of the myosin filaments over the actin filaments is a complicated process, in which a series of chemical bonds between them is continually formed and broken. This requires energy, provided by the burning of oxygen and food-fuel in the mitochondria, and stored and transferred as a compound called ATP (adenosine triphosphate), which is very rich in high-energy phosphate. The process of muscular contraction is started by a flow of calcium (one of the common minerals of the body) into the muscle cells through a whole series of little tubes running between the myofibrils, called the *microtubules*.

The muscles also contain a set of fibres which registers the force of contraction and another inside the tendons leading from muscle to bone, which gauges and limits the amount of stretch.

The information is relayed through the nerves back to the brain and is obviously vital in preventing injury: a cat without this measuring equipment could leap about 100 ft (30 m) into the air – and would then explode!

What can go wrong?

Pulled, strained and torn muscles are all, in fact, the same thing: an injury which gives rise to pain and difficulty in using a muscle, arising from muscle fibres being torn, and from bleeding inside the body of the muscle.

Diseases that cause muscle problems are rare. Most people with muscle weakness actually have a disorder of the nervous system which controls muscle movement, caused by a STROKE, for example. Occasionally, the muscles themselves are weak – a condition called a *myopathy*. The commonest cause of this is disease of the HORMONE system, but it can also be brought about by VITAMIN D deficiency and by some forms of CANCER. Inflammation of the muscles – *myositis* – can have a viral cause, but more often seems to result from an abnormal reaction of the IMMUNE SYSTEM. Like myopathy, it may be linked with a tumour.

The rest of the major muscle disorders, of which MUSCULAR DYSTROPHY is the best-known example, are inherited.

See also MULTIPLE SCLEROSIS, PARALYSIS.

Muscular dystrophy

The term 'muscular dystrophy' describes a group of disorders that produce weakness in the MUSCLES themselves, rather than a weakness resulting from disorders of the nerves that make the muscles work. The dystrophies make up only a small number of all the disorders that affect the muscles alone, and are characterized by two things: they do not appear to be a consequence of disease elsewhere in the body, and they are always inherited (*see* GENETICS and HEREDITY).

Causes

Although the cause of the disorder is unknown, it is fairly certain that the problem arises in the muscle cell. When the muscles of people affected with the disease are examined under a microscope, the cells are seen to be in varying stages of destruction.

Just like any other cell in the body, a muscle cell has to convert food and oxygen into energy. In addition, it has to convert energy into physical power by contracting. An abnormality in any one of the many processes involved in this activity could result in muscular dystrophy. Also, it seems likely that the various types of the disease each result from a different abnormality.

Symptoms

These depend on the type of dystrophy which is present. Generally, symptoms appear earlier in the more severe types than the less severe ones.

There are approximately 20 different types of the disease, but only four of them occur at all commonly.

Duchenne's dystrophy is the most severe form of the disease, and may occur in quite young children. About one in every 5,000 male babies is affected. It is a sex-linked disease inherited on the X chromosome, so that when only one X chromosome is present – as it is in boys – the disease becomes evident. Where two X chromosomes are present, as they are in girls, the disease is prevented by the other 'normal' chromosome. However, girls can carry the disease and pass it on.

The disease starts with weakness of the thighs and pelvic muscles, which causes difficulty in standing, walking and climbing. Weakness may be obvious at a very early stage, even before the boy can walk. However, it is more usual for it to come to light between the ages of two and seven. Continuing progression affects the neck, shoulders and back so that loss of power may eventually lead to deformities of the spine and to difficulties in breathing. The heart, which is also a muscle, may become involved, and this combination of difficulties in BREATHING and HEART function can lead to a very early death, often before 20 years of age.

Becker's pseudohypertrophic dystrophia is a similar type but comes on later, usually after the age of ten. People are much less severely affected and can live on into their 30s and 40s.

The face, shoulders and upper arms are the areas that are worst affected in *fasciosapulohumeral dystrophy*. It can occur in both males and females, and affected individuals will have at least one parent with the disease. Anyone with this type of dystrophy has a 50 per cent chance of passing it on.

The face is affected first, with difficulty in puffing up the cheeks or blowing up a balloon being an early sign. Normally the symptoms appear in the teens, but it is possible to find signs of the disease in people in their 50s who did not know that they were ill. The heart is usually unaffected, although people with this condition can occasionally have all the problems that are associated with Duchenne-type dystrophy. As a rule, however, it does not diminish life expectancy and people can be quite old before they suffer a significant disability.

Myotonic dystrophy (or *dystrophica myotonica*) differs significantly from the dystrophies described above, and is the type people are most familiar with. Myotonia means an inability to relax a muscle after it has contracted. This is the earliest symptom that patients will experience and it may occur in the teens. The disease often affects the hands and an inability to relax a hand shake is one of the first signs. In later life, the muscles of the face, neck and hands may become wasted and weak, and this may eventually spread to the legs. Unlike all other types of the disease, myotonic dystrophy may produce symptoms in other parts of the body. For example, BALDNESS (in both male and female patients) and CATARACTS are common. It is also the most variable of the dystrophies, with symptoms ranging from a minor degree of failure in muscle relaxation in a person who lives out a normal life span, to severe weakness that comes on in early life.

Treatment and outlook

Unfortunately there is no treatment that will stop the progression of weakness in the dystrophies, although drugs such as quinine are used to aid relaxation in myotonia. However, patients are encouraged to take as much EXERCISE as possible (*see* PHYSIOTHERAPY). This will keep those muscles in good condition functioning normally.

If you think that you are a carrier (because you have a brother with the disease), you can have a blood test to find out for sure.

Myalgic encephalomyelitis

This is also known as 'chronic fatigue syndrome' or 'post viral fatigue'. The term myalgic encephalomyelitis or ME is misleading, as there is no evidence of encephalitis, and myalgia is not always present.

Symptoms

ME is characterized by prolonged periods of lethargy, usually after an episode resembling a viral illness. Sufferers also complain of HEADACHES, muscular aches and swollen lymph nodes. Symptoms are usually made worse by exercise.

Diagnosis

No specific cause of this condition has been found, and so it can be difficult to diagnose, as there are no specific tests to perform. The doctor usually makes the diagnosis after listening to the symptoms and in the absence of any other proven illness.

The relationship of ME with DEPRESSION is complex. In some patients the symptoms of the depression develop and benefit from antidepressant treatment. More commonly, the patient becomes depressed as a result of the illness.

Treatment

Reassurance that no other diseases have been found and non-specific support are the mainstay of treatment. Contact with other sufferers via support groups may help. Most patients recover within weeks rather than months, but a few may continue to suffer for over a year.

Mycoplasma, *see* **Non-specific urethritis, Pneumonia, Reiter's disease**

Mycoses, *see* **Fungal infections**

Myelitis, *see* **Spinal cord**

Myelogram, *see* **Laminectomy, Neurology and neurosurgery, Slipped disc**

Myocardial infarction, *see* **Arteries and artery disease, Heart attack, Infarction**

Myocarditis, viral, *see* **Heart disease**

Myopathy, *see* **Muscles**

Myositis, *see* **Muscles, Paralysis**

Myotonic dystrophy, *see* **Muscular dystrophy**

Myxoedema, *see* **Thyroid**

N

Naevus, *see* **Birthmarks**

Nails, finger and toe, *see* **Skin and skin diseases, Whitlow**

Nappy rash

The most common form of nappy rash is called *ammoniacal* DERMATITIS and is a direct result of the chemical breakdown of urine by bacteria in the faeces. The ammonia produced by this process has a burning effect on soft baby skin.

Babies fed on cow's milk may be more prone to ammoniacal dermatitis as their stools are more alkaline than those of breastfed babies – and the bacteria in the faeces thrive in an alkaline medium. However, the main contributory factors of this particular type of nappy rash will apply to all babies.

Ammoniacal dermatitis most commonly occurs if soiled nappies are not removed immediately or urine-soaked nappies are left on too long. It may also arise if towelling nappies are not washed and sterilized thoroughly so that bacteria are still present.

Rough, hard nappies that rub against the skin, making it sore and less resilient to the harsh effects of ammonia, can often trigger off a bout of nappy rash. And the condition can be aggravated by plastic pants, which prevent moisture evaporating, keeping the wetness next to the baby's skin.

Another common cause of nappy rash is from the fungus infection THRUSH (*Candida albicans*). A baby contracts thrush in the mouth either at birth from a mother who has vaginal thrush or when feeding from an unsterilized teat. The bacteria of the thrush fungus travel down from the mouth and out of the anus in the baby's faeces.

Occasionally, cradle cap (*seborrhoeic dermatitis*) can cause nappy rash. The condition may spread from the scalp to other parts of the body, including the nappy area.

Symptoms

Ammoniacal dermatitis starts in the form of moist red patches around the genitals. It can also be identified by the smell of ammonia that is given off. Unchecked, it can spread over the whole nappy area, and beyond. Within a matter of hours the rash can develop an extremely red and angry-looking appearance. During the stages that follow, the skin becomes thicker-looking and more wrinkled. It develops a papery texture and may peel. Eventually, the skin becomes raw and ULCERS may form.

Nappy rash caused by thrush starts around the anus and, as it progresses, may spread across the baby's buttocks. The thrush fungus can also be seen inside the mouth as white patches, similar in appearance to milk curd, on the tongue, palate and inside the cheeks.

The rash caused by seborrhoeic dermatitis is a brownish-red colour and is likely to be found on other parts of the body as well as around the nappy area.

Home treatment

Always cleanse your baby's bottom thoroughly, using soap and water, or baby lotion or oil if the baby's bottom is very sore. Zinc and castor oil cream or a silicone-based barrier cream should also be applied before putting on a nappy.

Leave off nappies and plastic pants whenever possible, as this will help the evaporation of moisture and aid healing. If nappies have to be worn during the day, make sure they are changed as often as possible. Disposable nappies are sometimes less absorbent than washable ones, so try to buy a good brand if you use them regularly.

Wash, rinse and sterilize terry nappies thoroughly. Avoid harsh detergents and make sure that all traces of the washing powder have been removed; never use biological washing powders. A final rinse in an acidic solution will discourage the breakdown of urea. This solution can be bought or made at home by simply adding about 1 fl oz (30 ml) of vinegar to 10 pint (4.5 litre) of water.

Medical treatment

If a rash persists and does not seem to be getting any better, consult your doctor as more specific treatment may be required. Left untreated, the rash could become infected, and this in turn could lead to other infections in the genital area.

If your baby's rash is caused by the effect of ammonia on the skin, your doctor will prescribe an ointment to soothe the burning. Some creams may clear up the rash more effectively than others. So once a cream has been found that works for your baby, make a note of its name in case the rash returns.

If the rash is caused by thrush, the treatment usually involves applying an antibiotic cream to the nappy area. In addition, your doctor may prescribe drops or gel to cure the thrush in the mouth.

Nappy rash caused by seborrhoeic dermatitis can be cleared by a prescribed ointment. A medicated shampoo should help to get rid of the cradle cap.

Narcolepsy, *see* **Hypothalamus, Sleep and sleep problems**

Narcotics, *see* **Heroin, Morphine, Painkillers**

Nausea

This feeling of sickness is produced by the stimulation of a collection of nerve cells in the BRAIN, called the 'vomiting centre'. If the stimulation is severe enough, the nausea is followed by actual VOMITING. In most cases, nausea requires little or no treatment. If it persists, or is accompanied by other signs such as pain or weight loss, it is vital to consult a doctor.

Causes

The vomiting centre can be stimulated not only by nerve impulses coming from the STOMACH or bowel but also by nervous impulses from the BALANCE organs in the EAR and by certain chemicals circulating in the bloodstream. Hence there are many varied causes of nausea.

Stomach problems: Any condition that blocks the normal flow of food out of the stomach will cause nausea. Inflammation of the stomach lining is also a cause. One of the commonest causes is simply eating too much food. Overeating distends the stomach and slows down the normal passage of food into the next part of the bowel – the DUODENUM. Indigestion accompanied by a feeling of nausea is the result. Usually the discomfort settles within a few hours.

If there is a physical blockage inside the stomach, nausea may persist. Such a blockage may be caused by a cancerous growth in the stomach, or by constriction of the pylorus, which is the valve leading from the stomach to the duodenum. This condition is known as *pyloric stenosis* and, in adults, is usually the result of scarring from a duodenal ULCER. (Babies may occasionally be born with pyloric stenosis, which can produce persistent vomiting in the early weeks of life).

Inflammation of the stomach lining is known as gastritis (*see* GASTROENTERITIS). This condition may be temporary but sometimes lasts for weeks or months. Drinking too much alcohol may cause gastritis, and nausea is one of the inevitable features of a hangover. Virus infections or FOOD POISONING can also cause a gastritis and this will produce nausea – possibly vomiting as well. People who are tense and worried (*see* STRESS) tend to produce excessive stomach acid which in the long run may cause a gastritis and recurring nausea. Ultimately a stomach or duodenal ulcer may develop, which tends to produce not only nausea but quite severe indigestion pain as well.

Inner ear problems: The inner ear is not only concerned with hearing but also controls the sense of balance. Nerves from the inner ear pass to balance centres in the brain, and they also go to the vomiting centre. Disturbances in the inner ear produce VERTIGO – a sense of spinning or falling in space – accompanied by severe nausea, and occasionally even vomiting.

The inner ear can be quite easily disturbed temporarily by unaccustomed motion. Many people develop vertigo and nausea temporarily after going on a fairground ride. TRAVEL SICKNESS is another form of disturbance of the inner ear.

Regular up-and-down or sideways motion seems to be the most likely to cause travel sickness, especially if there is no fixed point that the sufferer's eye can fix upon to maintain the sense of balance.

Many virus infections can affect the inner ear – including INFLUENZA – but some cause a condition called labyrinthitis, which is an acute infection in the inner ear. This can result in sudden severe vertigo and nausea, which may last for several days.

MÉNIÈRE'S DISEASE is a condition which causes recurrent attacks of vertigo and nausea, and particularly affects middle-aged and elderly people.

Raised intra-cranial pressure: If the pressure inside the skull rises for any reason, one of the first symptoms is nausea – probably because the vomiting centre is very sensitive to the effects of increased pressure. Infection around the BRAIN (MENINGITIS) or within the brain (encephalitis) can both result in severe nausea. Growths in the brain can also cause an increase in pressure with nausea, and often other symptoms as well such as disturbance of nerve function in the limbs or severe headaches.

Migraine: People who suffer from MIGRAINE usually develop nausea early on in the attack. This is probably the result of changes in the circulation of blood to the vomiting centre as the attack develops. Later a severe one-sided headache can develop with worsening nausea or vomiting.

Pregnancy: Between the eighth and sixteenth week of PREGNANCY, many expectant mothers suffer nausea and possibly vomiting. The nausea appears to be a result of the hormonal changes which occur in early pregnancy. These changes seem to directly affect the vomiting centre in the brain. Nausea is often worse first thing in the morning. Some researchers have pinpointed a link between a high intake of fat in the diet and nausea in pregnancy, so keeping off fatty foods may well help to reduce the problem.

Anxiety: People who become anxious for any reason often feel nauseated. This is because the nervous system reacts to stress by halting the activity of the stomach and the bowel. The stomach may then become distended. With severe anxiety, some people may even vomit.

Pain: Any very severe PAIN may be accompanied by nausea. The pain of a serious injury or of a HEART ATTACK can produce nausea, although the mechanism is not entirely clear.

Drugs: Certain drugs may cause nausea as a side-effect, usually as a result of a direct effect on the vomiting centre. Some drugs produce nausea if the dose is too high for the patient: the heart drug digoxin is one example. Other drugs cause nausea whenever they are given – for example, drugs to treat CANCERS.

Treatment

Certain types of nausea need little treatment other than rest, until the condition passes. The nausea of indigestion, or of an illness such as influenza, is best treated with an antacid and plenty to drink. With children, it is advisable to do no more than to provide comfort, keeping a bowl to hand. If vomiting occurs they usually feel very much better.

The nausea of pregnancy is best managed with small frequent meals, avoiding fatty foods. A dry biscuit first thing in the morning often helps to relieve the worst pangs of nausea. Drugs are best avoided unless there is persistent vomiting – when medical advice is essential.

Nausea from other causes may be treated by drugs. Several different types of anti-nauseant drugs are available which work best for certain categories of nausea. Motion sickness may be prevented or treated with drugs such as *hyoscine* or *cyclizine*, which are usually available over the counter in a chemist's shop; most other drugs need a doctor's prescription. For Ménière's disease, *prochlorperazine* is usually prescribed. Nausea or vomiting associated with gastritis may be treated with a drug such as *metoclopramide*.

Nephritis

This is the general term used for inflammation of the KIDNEYS. Inflammation of any organ often results from infection by bacteria, and the kidney is no exception. Nephritis which arises from bacterial infection is called *pyelonephritis*. However, nephritis may result from changes in the structure of the kidney tubules (tiny tubes), particularly the glomerulus – a part of the tubule that filters the blood and extracts the waste products that are then expelled as urine. This second type of kidney inflammation is called by the medical name *glomerulonephritis*.

Pyelonephritis

There are two forms of pyelonephritis: *acute pyelonephritis*, a feverish illness that usually results from an infection (normally CYSTITIS) lower down in the urinary system; and *chronic pyelonephritis*, which results from repeated infection of the kidney. Chronic pyelonephritis causes the affected kidney to become scarred with fibrous tissue. It has recently become clear that, in the majority of cases, the damage is done early in childhood. The kidneys do not necessarily deteriorate at this stage, but once the process of fibrosis and shrinking begins, it leads to a slow deterioration in the function of the kidneys which may not cause problems until adulthood.

Chronic pyelonephritis occurs in a very small proportion of children who have a deficiency at the end of the ureter where it empties into the BLADDER. This allows the URINE to flow back up into the ureter and therefore to carry infection towards the bladder. This 'reflux' shows up on a special X-ray taken during the passing of urine. Any child who has had urinary infection needs special tests to establish whether there is any risk of reflux. Chronic pyelonephritis and repeated attacks of acute pyelonephritis can also occur in people who have some abnormalities in the structure of their kidneys and ureter.

The symptoms of acute pyelonephritis are a feverish illness, pain over the kidney and in the loin, and both pain and burning on passing water. Chronic pyelonephritis does not cause pain. The first indication that it is present may be when the patient's kidneys stop excreting all the body's waste products. This leads to tiredness and general ill health, and is known as *chronic renal failure*. Alternatively, the disease may cause high BLOOD PRESSURE. A characteristic feature of this disease is the presence of BLOOD and PROTEIN in the urine.

Glomerulonephritis

This is a group of disorders, all of which result from inflammation of the kidney material in general and the glomerulus in particular. It is only by examining kidney tissue under a microscope that the various forms of the disease can be differentiated.

Glomerulonephritis can result from a wide range of different diseases, for example a sore throat caused by a streptoccal infection, or it may be associated with the rheumatic disorder, LUPUS ERYTHEMATOSUS. More frequently, however, the disease has no obvious cause, in which case it is described as 'idiopathic'.

The disorder comes to light as one of two syndromes (a group of symptoms that occur together and produce a characteristic picture). In the first, *acute nephritis*, there is some reduction in the amount of urine that is passed, together with some retention of fluid. This leads to swelling (OEDEMA), often around the face and ankles, and even to *pulmonary oedema*, fluid in the lungs which results in breathlessness. Blood is always present in the urine and the blood pressure is often raised a little. When waste products cleared by the kidneys are measured in the blood, some degree of deficiency in kidney function may be found through the tests.

The second disorder that glomerulonephritis may cause is called the *nephrotic syndrome*. It is quite common in children: about 30 children in a million have the condition compared with 8 adults in every million. Nephrotic syndrome differs from acute nephritis in the higher amount of protein that is lost in the urine. As in acute nephritis, swelling is the first symptom, and indicates a large accumulation of fluid in the tissues. It can appear on any part of the body, but is more common in loosely knit tissue such as the skin around the eyes and the male genitals. The legs and ankles may also swell. The syndrome usually occurs when about ⅙th oz (5 g) of protein is lost in the urine every day, although in severe cases, five times this amount can pass out daily. The loss of protein permits fluid to leak out of the blood vessels into the body tissue.

Most young children with the nephrotic syndrome have what is called 'minimal change disease'. This means that, when the kidney tissue is examined under a microscope, very little difference can be seen from normal tissue. Minimal change disease is so common in young children that doctors do not always perform a BIOPSY for this age group, whereas they do for all older patients. It is also most unusual for this type of glomerulonephritis to fail to get better on its own, although STEROID treatment may be needed if protein loss is high – this will correct the protein 'leak' in 95 per cent of all cases.

Dangers

The main danger of any type of kidney disease is that it will develop into kidney failure. In such cases, patients are unable to survive unless the kidneys are helped to clear waste products with the aid of a kidney machine (*see* DIALYSIS), or he or she is given a kidney transplant.

Acute pyelonephritis is not likely to develop into kidney failure, but chronic pyelonephritis and most types of glomerulonephritis may. Generally, the chances of kidney failure are increased with high blood pressure. Since high blood pressure alone can damage the kidneys, its effect on a diseased kidney is much greater. However, careful control of blood pressure with drugs can help to lessen the risk.

Treatment and outlook

Acute pyelonephritis can normally be treated with antibiotics and an increased intake of fluids. However, recurrent attacks of acute pyelonephritis, particularly in children, can indicate a reflux of urine back to the kidneys from the bladder. In this case, it is possible to perform an operation to reimplant the ureters into the bladder and stop this happening. Children who have repeated urinary infections may be treated with prolonged courses of antibiotics to reduce the chance of kidney scarring.

In order for the correct treatment to be given for glomerulonephritis, the exact form of the disease must be known. Some get better without medical treatment; others are divided into those that respond to steroids and those that do not. Diuretic treatment in the form of water tablets helps reduce swelling, and diet is altered to limit the intake of SALT, which contributes to the swelling. Protein intake sometimes needs to be restricted to lessen the work load of the malfunctioning kidneys. However, where cases lead to kidney failure, no form of treatment seems able to halt this progress, and the patient is put on a kidney machine or, alternatively, is given a kidney transplant.

The outlook in pyelonephritis is generally quite good and people often do not run into any trouble until later in life. They may then develop both a raised blood pressure and some degree of failure of the kidneys.

Nervous system

The nervous system is essential to sight (*see* EYES AND EYESIGHT) and HEARING, our perception of PAIN and pleasure, control of movements, regulation of body functions such as DIGESTION and BREATHING and the development of thought, language, memory and decision-making.

The 'working parts' of the nervous system are millions of interconnected cells called neurones, whose function is similar to the wires in a complex electrical machine: they pick up signals in one part of the nervous system and carry them to another, where they may be relayed on to other neurones or bring about some action, such as the contraction of muscle fibres.

Neurones are delicate cells, easily damaged or destroyed by injury, infection, pressure, chemical disturbance or lack of oxygen. Furthermore, since neurones cannot be replaced when destroyed, such disorders tend to have serious consequences.

The nervous system falls into two interdependent parts. One, the *central nervous system*, consists of the BRAIN and SPINAL CORD. The other, the *peripheral nervous system*, consists of all the nerve tissue outside the central nervous system. Both the central and peripheral nervous systems are further divided into a number of components.

The central nervous system

The brain and spinal cord form the central processing unit of the nervous system. They receive messages via the sensory fibres from the body's sense organs and receptors, filter and analyse it, then send out signals along the motor fibres which produce an appropriate response in the muscles and glands.

The analytical, or processing, aspect may be relatively simple for certain functions carried out in the spinal cord, but analysis in the brain is usually highly complex, involving the participation of thousands of different neurones.

Peripheral nervous system

The peripheral nervous system has two main divisions: an outer system called the *somatic nervous system* and an inner one, the AUTONOMIC NERVOUS SYSTEM, which is concerned with the regulation of our internal organs and glands, such as the heart, stomach, kidneys and pancreas.

The somatic system has a dual role. First, it collects information from the body's sense organs and conveys this to the central nervous system. Second, it transmits signals from the central nervous system to the skeletal muscles, thus initiating movement.

It has two main components, the *sensory* and *motor* systems. Information about the outside world is picked up in the sensory organs such as the eyes, which contain special receptor cells. There are similar cells for pain, touch and SKIN temperature.

Signals from these receptors are carried towards the central nervous system in the sensory nerve fibres. The pattern of signalling in these fibres, which may mount to millions of impulses every second, gives us essential data about the outside world.

Just as the sensory fibres carry information towards the central nervous system, so the motor fibres transmit signals away from it towards muscles.

Both sensory and motor fibres are themselves just part of the sensory and motor neurones. All neurones have a cell body, as well as a number of projecting fibres. The motor and sensory fibres of the peripheral nervous system are merely the longest fibres of their respective neurones. The sensory fibres have their cell bodies just outside, and the motor neurones within, the brain or spinal cord.

The motor and sensory fibres carrying messages to and from a particular body organ or area are gathered together in a bundle called a *nerve*. Different

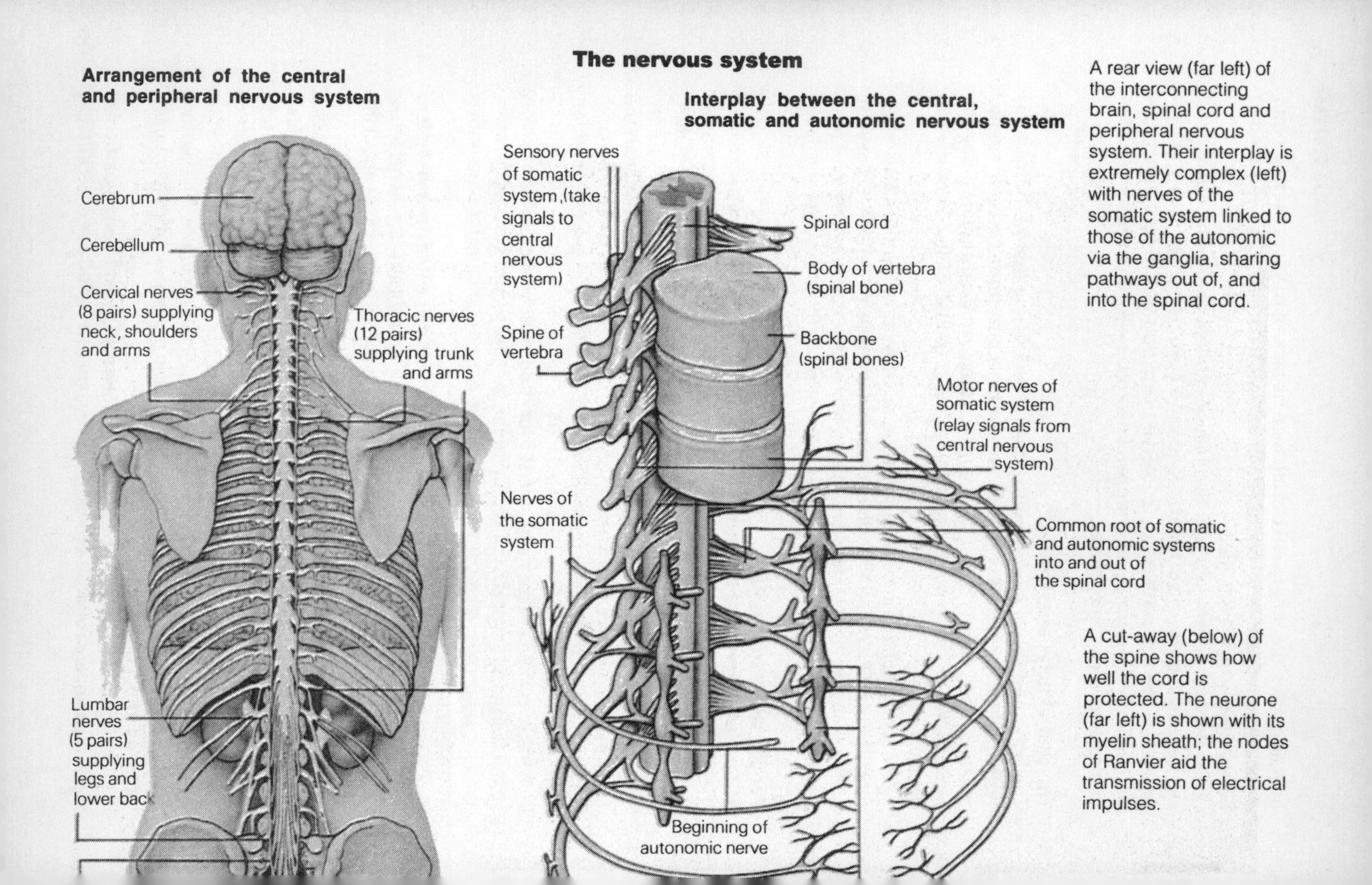

A rear view (far left) of the interconnecting brain, spinal cord and peripheral nervous system. Their interplay is extremely complex (left) with nerves of the somatic system linked to those of the autonomic via the ganglia, sharing pathways out of, and into the spinal cord.

A cut-away (below) of the spine shows how well the cord is protected. The neurone (far left) is shown with its myelin sheath; the nodes of Ranvier aid the transmission of electrical impulses.

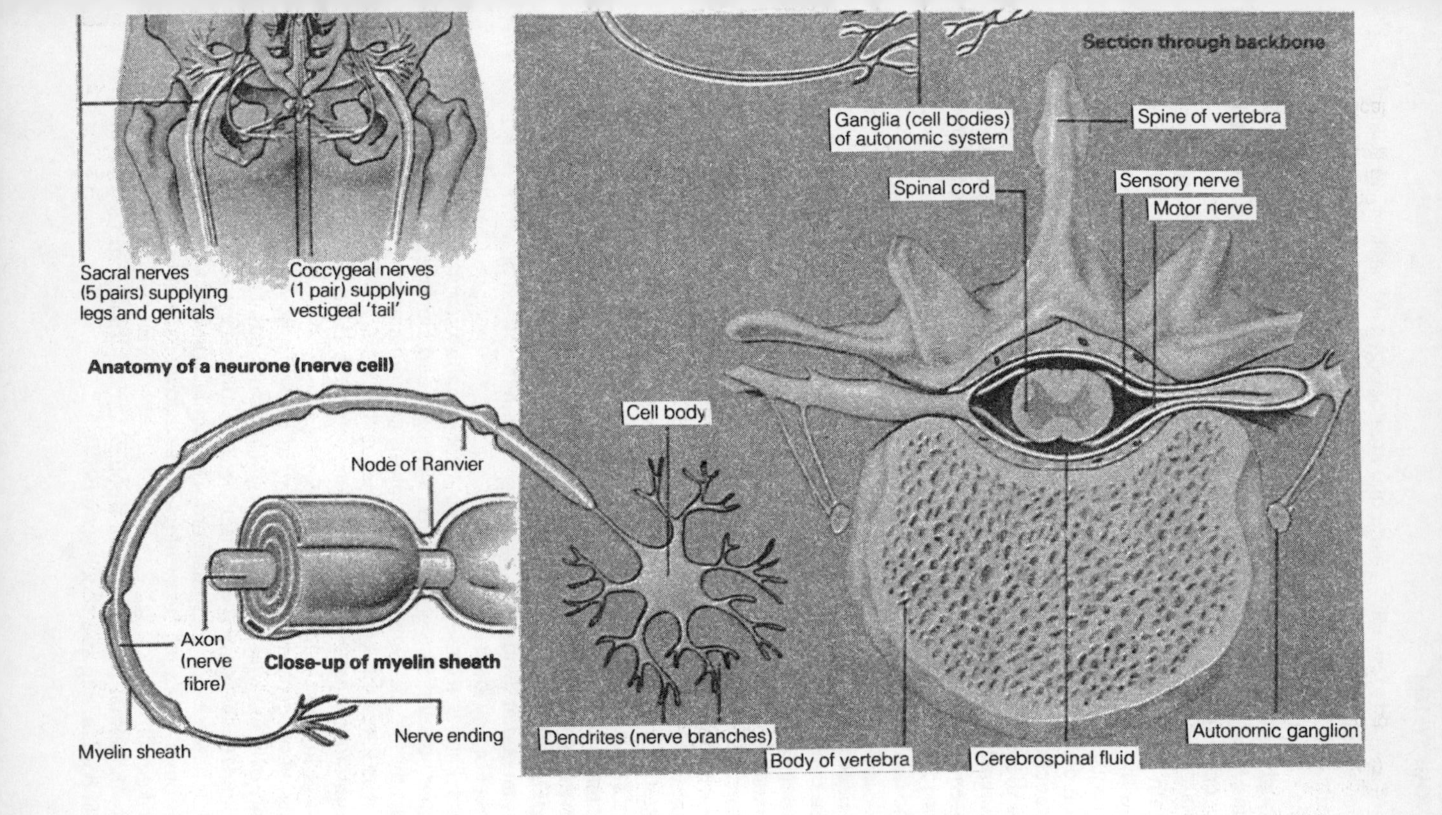
Sacral nerves (5 pairs) supplying legs and genitals
Coccygeal nerves (1 pair) supplying vestigeal 'tail'
Anatomy of a neurone (nerve cell)
Node of Ranvier
Axon (nerve fibre)
Close-up of myelin sheath
Myelin sheath
Nerve ending
Cell body
Dendrites (nerve branches)
Section through backbone
Ganglia (cell bodies) of autonomic system
Spine of vertebra
Spinal cord
Sensory nerve
Motor nerve
Body of vertebra
Cerebrospinal fluid
Autonomic ganglion

nerves are said to 'supply' a particular area or organ. Altogether, 43 pairs of nerves emerge from the central nervous system: 12 pairs of cranial nerves from the brain and the remaining 31 pairs from either side of the spinal cord.

The cranial nerves mainly supply sense organs and muscles in the head, although a very important cranial nerve, the *vagus*, supplies the digestive organs, heart and air passages in the lungs. Some cranial nerves, such as the optic nerve to the eye, contain only sensory fibres.

The spinal nerves emerge at intervals from the spinal cord and always contain both motor and sensory fibres. They supply all areas of the body below the neck. Each spinal nerve is attached to the spinal cord by means of two roots, one of which carries motor fibres, and the other sensory fibres. At a short distance from the spinal cord, each spinal nerve splits into a number of branches.

So the peripheral nervous system acts only to relay sensory and motor messages between the central nervous system and the body's muscles, glands and sense organs. It plays virtually no part in the analysis of sensory signals, or the initiation of motor signals. Both these activities, and much else, occur in the central nervous system.

The neurones

These cells, so central to the working of the whole nervous system, deserve a closer look.

Actually, they are not the only type of cell to be found in the nervous system; another type, called *neuroglia* (simply meaning 'nerve glue') are present in large numbers. Their job is to bind, protect, nourish and provide support for the neurones.

Neurones come in various shapes and sizes, but they all have the same basic structure. Like all cells, they have a nucleus, or 'centre', which is contained in a roughly spherical part of the neurone called the *cell body*. From the cell body, a number of fine, root-like fibres project. These are called *dendrites*. Also projecting from the cell is a single, long fibre called the *axon*. At its far end, it divides into a number of branches, each of which ends in a number of tiny knobs.

Each knob is in close proximity, but not actually touching, a dendrite from another neurone. This gap is called a *synapse* and messages are transmitted across these gaps by means of chemicals called *neurotransmitters*. When a signal reaches the knobs at the end of the axon, it may, under certain circumstances, jump across the synapse to the dendrite of an adjacent neurone and so continue its journey.

The whole central nervous system has to be maintained with a plentiful supply of blood which provides oxygen and nutrients. It is also protected by two kinds of covering. The first is bone: the skull enclosing the brain, and the backbone enclosing the spinal cord. The second consists of three membranes of fibrous tissue called the *meninges*. These cover the whole of the brain and spinal cord.

Cerebrospinal fluid circulates through various spaces in the brain and spinal cord, acting as a shock absorber.

See also BRAIN AND BRAIN DISEASE, DEMENTIA, EPILEPSY, MÉNIÈRE'S DISEASE, MULTIPLE SCLEROSIS, NEURALGIA, NEUROLOGY AND NEUROSURGERY, PARALYSIS, PARKINSON'S DISEASE, PINS AND NEEDLES, POLIOMYELITIS, SCIATICA, SHINGLES, STROKE.

Nettlerash, *see* Allergy

Neuralgia

This means 'PAIN along a nerve'. It is not itself a disease but rather a condition that occurs in several diseases which all give rise to sensations of pain along the course of particular nerves (*see* NERVOUS SYSTEM).

Neuralgia is felt in a specific area of the body; it is not a general 'overall' pain. It is also usually quite severe – a nagging pain that can interfere with sleep or concentration. Sometimes the sensation can be sharp and intense with waves of pain shooting down the affected nerve and causing the sufferer to wince or, in some cases, to writhe in agony.

Causes

Neuralgia is caused by irritation of a nerve and interference with its normal working. It can be brought about by inflammation of a nerve (NEURITIS); a common example of this is the form that often accompanies SHINGLES. Another cause is an area of infection or an ABSCESS close to a nerve and irritating it, as when an abscess in the root of a tooth brings on severe toothache (*see* TEETH).

If something presses on a nerve, this will also give rise to pain. Examples include a broken or displaced bone, an area of bleeding or swelling in a confined space, or the growth of a TUMOUR. SCIATICA occurs when one of the cartilage discs between the vertebrae in the lower back 'slips' and presses on the roots of the sciatic nerve in the spine.

Most people will experience minor types of neuralgia sooner or later. The pain may be brought on by abruptly twisting some part of the body and thus stretching or temporarily trapping a nerve tract, or it may be caused by inflammation resulting from a cold draught. These conditions require no special treatment apart from pain relief and usually last only a day or two. But if the pain persists for more than a few days, you should report it to your doctor.

Symptoms

Facial neuralgia (*trigeminal neuralgia*) is one of the most common and most painful types. The severe pain causes a quick, spasmodic contraction of the muscles of the face. It occurs most often in elderly people. The pain occurs in spasms that usually last less than a minute, but does not usually occur at night. The forehead, cheek, lips and jaw can be affected almost always on one side of the face only. Each attack is brought on by stimulation of a specific area on the face – the 'trigger zone' – by actions such as washing, shaving or eating, or even being touched by a cold wind.

Severe neuralgia is a feature of advanced SYPHILIS. The pain is sudden and sharp and is known as 'lightning pain'. It is usually felt in the legs, chest or abdomen, and may resemble a heart attack or abdominal emergency.

The form of neuralgia linked with shingles is probably the most often encountered. It usually occurs a few days before the appearance of the redness and blisters that are typical of shingles. These symptoms usually develop in a band along the course of the affected nerve. Any of the major face, neck, chest or lumbar nerves may be affected.

After the shingles has cleared, severe neuralgia may still be felt in that area, especially the face.

Treatment

The drugs *phenytoin* and *carbamazepine* are widely prescribed to give relief. Otherwise it may be necessary to put the nerve out of action. This can be done temporarily by the injection of a long-acting local anaesthetic or alcohol. A more permanent relief may be obtained from a phenol injection or from surgery, but at the risk of possible permanent numbness.

If these is something pressing on the nerve, such as a SLIPPED DISC, the pressure has to be relieved by PHYSIOTHERAPY, MANIPULATION or perhaps surgery. Aspirin, paracetamol or a stronger analgesic (*see* PAINKILLERS) prescribed by your doctor will also help to alleviate pain.

Neuritis

This means inflammation of nerves, which may be *motor* nerves going to and from muscles or *sensory* nerves carrying information from sense organs.

There are numerous causes of neuritis, ranging from viral infections to poisons (including alcohol), and the resulting symptoms depend upon how many nerves are involved, whether these are motor or sensory, and the severity of the inflammation.

The severity of the condition can range from something as trivial as NUMBNESS at the tips of the fingers to a much more serious, rapidly progressive PARALYSIS involving the respiratory muscles and sometimes associated with the development of sudden BLINDNESS.

Causes

Perhaps the most common cause of neuritis is injury. At one time or another, most of us have experienced a feeling of numbness of the arm or fingers when waking in the morning. The cause is stretching or crushing of one of the nerves of the arm – commonly the ulnar nerve – by lying on it. As the nerve recovers, we experience an unpleasant tingling sensation, which is commonly known as 'PINS AND NEEDLES'.

When more severe crushing injuries are sustained, these symptoms persist, and some permanent loss of sensation or motor function may result. On occasion, the nerve is crushed by tissue which surrounds it. One nerve which runs through the palm of the hand is especially prone to this and gives rise to pain and tingling in the palms, especially at night. The condition is more common in women and is more liable to affect people with an underactive THYROID, during PREGNANCY, with DIABETES, following fractures of the wrist, or with RHEUMATOID ARTHRITIS. It is known as *carpal tunnel syndrome*.

Infection with a number of VIRUSES can cause a type of neuritis which is striking in the suddenness with which it develops. It progresses rapidly from the nerves supplying the most distant parts of the body to involve the trunk and the muscles used in respiration. The condition has become known as the *Guillain-Barré syndrome* after the doctors who first described it. It has been known to follow shortly after an infection with MEASLES, MUMPS, RUBELLA (German measles), INFLUENZA, CHICKENPOX, GLANDULAR FEVER, HEPATITIS B and even IMMUNIZATION (especially with influenza virus).

In the past, household and industrial poisons were also responsible for neuritis. Nowadays heavy metals such as arsenic and lead are very rarely the cause. Lead used to be the major constituent of weather-resistant white and red paint. This paint was also used to coat household items, such as children's playpens and cots. Poisoning resulted when the child gnawed at the paint while teething.

One of the main causes of neuritis is the consumption of too much ALCOHOL, and persistent heavy drinkers may develop neuritis in the arms and legs. Drinking quite small quantities of wood alcohol (methanol) can cause neuritis of the optic nerve, ultimately resulting in blindness.

Neuritis may also be an unfortunate side-effect of some forms of drug treatment. Large doses of anti-cancer drugs can have this effect, as can some anti-tubercular drugs that somehow interfere with the way the body utilizes certain B vitamins.

The B VITAMINS are essential for nourishment of the nerves, particularly thiamin, riboflavin and vitamins B_6 and B_{12}. Normally there is such an abundance of B vitamins in the food we eat that this type of deficiency is never seen, even among those on a poor diet (*see* NUTRITION). However, failure to absorb specific vitamins may cause neuritis during the course of certain diseases. COELIAC DISEASE is an example where the intestine fails to absorb vitamins due to an ALLERGY to gluten, a principal constituent of all foods containing cereals. Failure to absorb vitamin B_{12} due to loss of an essential factor produced by the stomach, called intrinsic factor, causes a disease known as PERNICIOUS ANAEMIA in which neuritis is also a complication.

Sudden disturbance of vision or even blindness can result from neuritis of the optic nerve which supplies the retina. Optic neuritis may develop during the course of MULTIPLE SCLEROSIS or in certain inflammatory diseases related to rheumatoid arthritis. Neuritis also occurs during the course of diseases such as CANCER, rheumatoid arthritis itself, or in cases of KIDNEY failure and in DIABETES.

Dangers

One obvious danger is blindness caused by optic neuritis. The Guillain-Barré syndrome, too, is dangerous when there is risk of BREATHING becoming paralysed. This happens rapidly and is the only reason why a patient with the symptoms of neuritis which is spreading upwards (known as ascending polyneuritis) should be admitted to hospital for observation. Care must be taken since loss of sensation renders distant parts of the body susceptible to damage, burning or injury.

Treatment

Clearly the most important part of treatment is to remove the cause, if this is known. Trapped nerves, for example, are best treated surgically by cutting the tissue through which the nerve runs. Good control of diabetes can improve diabetic neuritis.

Difficulty arises when the exact cause of the neuritis is not known. Recent evidence suggests that STEROID medicines may not be as effective as once was thought. However, if neuritis involves the optic nerve, large doses of steroids may save the sight of the patient. In most cases, there is no treatment apart from ensuring that the patient takes a sufficient quantity of B vitamins.

In the majority of cases, the neuritis gets completely better. Exceptionally, if patients suffer from neuritis following viral infections, this either improves very slowly or fails to improve at all. Sudden blindness due to poisoning of the optic nerve with wood alcohol is permanent. Peripheral neuritis due to alcoholic poisoning may improve when the patient stops drinking.

Neurology and neurosurgery

In many European countries and some parts of the US, there is no clear distinction between neurology and PSYCHIATRY. In Britain, however, neurologists are mainly concerned with disorders that are clearly a result of some physical malfunction of the NERVOUS SYSTEM. The same disorders become the province of neurosurgery when they need surgical treatment. Neurologists and neurosurgeons often share the same hospital unit because their work overlaps so much.

Symptoms of neurological disorders

The symptoms that may occur as a result of disorders of the nervous system are many and varied. A particular difficulty for neurologists is that some of the symptoms may be quite minor or even vague and yet, at times, indicate possible severe disease. On the other hand, some minor symptoms, such as NUMBNESS, may be caused by relatively trivial conditions or even, at times, result from anxiety (*see* STRESS). Disease in the BRAIN may become obvious because of fits (*see* CONVULSIONS), or difficulty in controlling movements. Other symptoms may include patches of numbness in the arms or legs or weakness in certain groups of muscles. Visual disturbances may occur, and changes in the senses of smell or hearing. In some patients, there may even be personality changes.

Diseases of the SPINAL CORD or peripheral nerves may become obvious because of areas of pain, numbness, weakness or difficulty in coordination of the arms or legs. Neurologists are also concerned with certain muscular disorders which may first show themselves through weakness in the muscles.

The neurological examination

A neurologist begins a consultation by taking a detailed history. Often, the exact nature of the symptoms gives an important clue to the type of disorder from which the patient is suffering. Questions about general health and lifestyle follow. SMOKING and drinking habits may be questioned in some detail, because certain disorders of peripheral nerves occur more often in people who smoke or drink heavily (*see* ALCOHOLISM).

Next, the neurologist examines the patient. Sometimes a meticulous examination of the function of virtually every nerve in the body is undertaken, especially if the symptoms have not given the specialist much information about the possible nature of the disease.

The nerves supplying the sense organs are usually examined first. EYESIGHT, HEARING and sense of SMELL may be tested. The muscles controlling the eyes are tested by asking the patient to look from side to side and up and down. The specialist examines the retina at the back of the eye using an ophthalmoscope. The nerves supplying sensation on the face and the movement of the facial muscles are tested.

Next, the muscles controlling swallowing and the movement of the TONGUE may be examined before the doctor turns his or her attention to the trunk and limbs. MUSCLE function is tested by asking the patient to tense various muscle groups in turn, and then sensation is tested. A small ball of cotton wool is brushed against the SKIN to test for light touch, a pin is used for PAIN sensation. In certain conditions, test-tubes containing hot and cold water may be used to test for temperature sensation. The sense of vibration is examined by using a large tuning fork held against a bony point – for example, at the ankle or elbow. Coordination of movement may be tested by asking the patient to carry out a variety of simple movements or by asking the patient to walk.

One of the more well-known neurological tests is for the REFLEXES. A small hammer is used to tap a tendon in the arm or leg. If the peripheral nerves are all intact, the muscle nearby contracts, producing a 'reflex jerk'.

Sometimes special types of examination are needed. If the neurologist suspects a problem with the optic nerve, the main nerve carrying vision from the eye, a special test of 'visual fields' may be carried out. The information from this detailed examination can help to pinpoint exactly the site of any damage to the optic nerve. Should the patient be suffering from defects of memory or personality change, psychological tests may be needed. A PSYCHOLOGIST may be asked to make a full assessment of the patient using a variety of standard tests, often in the form of a long questionnaire.

Diagnostic tests

Neurologists use a range of tests, some of which assess the structure of various parts of the nervous system while others assess function. In the first group are the various X-ray and scanning techniques; in the second are tests of the electrical activity of the nervous system.

X-rays: Ordinary X-RAYS of the skull and spine are frequently performed in the initial assessment of many complaints, since the bones of the head and back may show signs of what is causing the trouble. If is often necessary to use X-ray dye to show up arteries, veins or the space round the spinal cord, in order to make a diagnosis: this is called *angiography*.

When dye is introduced into the space round the spinal cord, via a LUMBAR PUNCTURE, the procedure is called myelography. It is used to assess disorders of the spinal cord, especially when it is thought that there may be pressure on the nerves coming out of the spinal cord – as there is in the leg pain called SCIATICA, for example (*see also* SLIPPED DISC).

Brain scans: 'Isotope' scans pick up the minute amount of radiation given off by a radioactive chemical injection, and 'translate' it into pictures indicating the amount of blood circulating in the various compartments of the brain. As some diseases affect the circulation of the radiochemical, the scan will show evidence of growths or other diseased areas.

Computerized tomography (CT) scans (also known as CAT – computerized axial tomography – scans) use a computer to assemble the information obtained by passing a series of X-rays through thin 'slices' of the head, building it up into a map or picture of the inside of the head.

Magnetic resonance imaging (MRI) scans produce pictures of the brain by picking up minute disturbances in the way its component molecules behave when they are subjected to a strong magnetic field. No radiation is used and no harm can come to the patient. CT or MRI scans are now the main forms of investigation for assessing neurological disorders in the brain and spinal cord.

A *positron emission tomography (PET) scan* examines the chemical and physical process going on minute by minute in slices of the brain of a living person, giving information on function as well as structure.

Tests of nervous system function

These tests are designed to detect faults in the electrical working of different parts of the nervous system. The ELECTROENCEPHALOGRAM, for example, is used to test people who may be having fits: it is now possible to record EEGs over periods of 24 hours, so picking up signs of fits which may have escaped notice on the ordinary EEG.

In *nerve conduction studies,* the electrical functioning of the peripheral nerves is tested by stimulating them with a small electric current and measuring the speed with which this is conducted down the nerves. Both the EEG and nerve conduction studies are entirely harmless and painless.

Electromyography (EMG) tests the condition of the muscles by passing very fine needles into them and recording their activity. This causes only slight discomfort and gives useful information about inflammation or any other disorder in the muscles or their nerves.

Treatments for neurological disorders

Many patients with neurological disorders are investigated in out-patient clinics, where EEGs, CT scans and other straightforward tests can be carried out.

Many neurological disorders are treated entirely at home. Conditions such as EPILEPSY require drug treatment, often with careful monitoring of the progress of the disorder, and regular blood tests to assess the adequacy of the drug treatment. If the condition involves weakness, PARALYSIS or other disability, services such as PHYSIOTHERAPY, SPEECH THERAPY and OCCUPATIONAL THERAPY can all be provided in the home, backed up where necessary by the district nurse. A patient's own doctor generally supervises all these arrangements for therapy and care, with the help and advice of specialist colleagues. For example, many patients who have had a STROKE may be looked after entirely at home.

Sometimes, however, investigation in hospital may be necessary for more serious conditions or if complicated tests are necessary.

Neurosurgery

Neurosurgery deals with disorders, including injuries to the nervous system, which require some kind of operation for their treatment. The range is wide, taking in various congenital abnormalities such as SPINA BIFIDA (in children), HEAD INJURIES caused by war or traffic accidents, and the removal of TUMOURS.

Neurosurgeons, having first been trained in the techniques of general surgery, then undergo a long specialized training. The most important advance in surgery in general and neurosurgery in particular over the last few years has been the development of microsurgery.

Operations on the nervous system use some very special techniques, such as entering the brain by means of a bone flap in the skull, which can then be replaced after the operation. When part of the skull itself has to be removed or has been severely damaged, a replacement can be made out of plastic or light alloys such as titanium. Tumours inside the brain can often be removed completely, or abnormal blood vessels removed. Some strokes are caused by leaking blood vessels in the brain, or *aneurysms* – swellings on ARTERIES – which can be treated by neurosurgery. Neurosurgeons are also involved in treating patients with severe head injuries. Some skull fractures can be left to heal naturally, but if any fragments of bone have become dislodged and are pressing on the brain, surgery is essential to remove or replace the fragments.

Neurosurgeons also operate on disorders of the spinal cord, for example they may remove tumours from the spinal cord or help to deal with injuries to the spine, often in conjunction with ORTHOPAEDIC surgeons. They also operate to remove SLIPPED DISCS from the spine in the neck.

Neuroses, *see* **Mental illness**

Non-specific urethritis (NSU)

This is the most common yet one of the more puzzling of all SEXUALLY TRANSMITTED DISEASES. As its name implies, NSU is a *urethritis* – an inflammation of the URETHRA, or urinary passage – that is not caused by any particular germ. This distinguishes it from GONORRHOEA, the other main cause of urethritis. Indeed, NSU may also be referred to as NGU, or non-gonococcal urethritis.

A final explanation of its cause has yet to be made. However, two different types of micro-organism are thought to be responsible for most cases – CHLAMYDIA and ureaplasmas, but other organisms may be involved.

Symptoms

The main symptom of NSU is a discharge from the end of the urethra, at the tip of the PENIS. The discharge is usually clear white to grey in colour – as opposed to the creamy yellow matter that is characteristic of gonorrhoea – and is often quite similar to semen in appearance. Again, in contrast to the generally very profuse discharge in gonorrhoea, the discharge in NSU varies: it is usually fairly light and may amount to no more than a moistness at the tip of the penis.

The second common symptom is pain on passing urine. Again, the severity of this may vary: it may not occur at all or be no more than a mild irritation.

Women who are infected by NSU may have no symptoms whatsoever, but may develop a slightly excessive vaginal discharge or pain on urination. Occasionally there may be a copious discharge and pain in the lower abdomen.

Possible causes

NSU is contracted during sexual intercourse. However, no one single bacterium or virus seems to be responsible for NSU, and it differs from other sexually transmitted diseases in several ways.

Although NSU is sexually transmitted, occasional cases seem to arise without any new sexual contact by either partner. Another unusual feature of the disease is that some women do not apparently develop the infection even though their partner is infected.

About 40 to 50 per cent of all cases of NSU are caused by a type of micro-organism known as *Chlamydiae*. These organisms are more like viruses than a bacteria, and do seem to pass easily from one person to another.

About 30 per cent of cases are thought to be a result of infection with an unusual type of bacterium called *Ureaplasma urealyticum*. Men usually show symptoms if the infection is caused by this organism, but women rarely seem to suffer from any symptoms. Indeed it has been found that up to one in five normal women may have a type of *Ureaplasma* present in the vagina, without any symptoms. The latest research suggests that only certain sub-types of the organism are responsible for NSU. Some men and women may be partly resistant to the effects of the organism, and never develop symptoms even when exposed to it.

A few people with NSU may have an infection involving either a yeast or a virus such as the *Herpes simplex* virus, but such cases are uncommon.

In about 30 per cent of cases, however, no micro-organism can be isolated and the cause remains a mystery. It is possible that other micro-organisms may in time be found to cause the symptoms.

Treatment and prevention

If a man suspects he has NSU because he has developed a discharge or pain on urination, he should consult his doctor. It is quite likely that the doctor will refer him to a specialist clinic for genito-urinary medicine (GUM), or he may prefer to make his own appointment at the GUM clinic (sometimes called merely a specialist clinic). All people seen at a GUM clinic are treated in the strictest confidence.

At the clinic, the patient is asked for details of recent sexual contacts, to establish a possible source of infection. Next, samples of the discharge and blood specimens are taken for analysis. An immediate examination of a smear of the discharge will probably be made under a microscope to exclude the possibility of gonorrhoea.

Once the tests have been made, a course of an ANTIBIOTIC is prescribed – either tetracycline or erythromycin. In addition, the patient is told to avoid sexual activity until the treatment has been completed. This is to give the lining of the urethra time to heal, but also to avoid spreading infection to a sexual partner. The patient is also told to avoid alcohol because this seems to interfere with recovery. It is very important that the patient returns to the clinic after treatment for follow-up tests.

A woman who has an unexplained vaginal discharge, particularly associated with low abdominal pain, should see her doctor for a full examination and investigation. Although there are other possible causes, examination of specimens may reveal that she has an infection caused by *Chlamydiae* or ureaplasma, in which case she will receive the same treatment as a man.

There are two things that can be done to prevent a man from contracting NSU (and from spreading it himself) – but, unfortunately, there are no guarantees. The first is to use a condom when having intercourse. The second thing is to get into the habit of passing urine fairly soon after intercourse – by this means he stands a good chance of flushing out of his urethra any material from his partner, such as vaginal secretion, to which he may be sensitive.

Outlook and dangers

Most men, treated with antibiotics, are free from the symptoms of NSU within a few days and the condition is then completely cleared. Occasionally, however, symptoms do not clear up and a different antibiotic may then be required. It is, however, essential that the patient completes the course of antibiotics; otherwise symptoms may return – and with possible complications. These may include internal ABSCESSES in the TESTES, or chronic infection in the PROSTATE GLAND, giving rise to a painful chronic condition called prostatitis. Chronic infection may also cause a narrowing (stricture) of the urethra. A less common complication is the development of REITER'S DISEASE, in which joint pains (ARTHRITIS) and sore eyes (CONJUNCTIVITIS) develop as well as the urethral discharge. All of these complications will settle after prolonged treatment with antibiotics.

More worrying, however, are the possible complications for women who may become infected with *Chlamydiae* as a result of sexual contact with a man who has NSU. Unless the woman is treated with antibiotics, she may develop a hidden infection, with few symptoms, which can grumble on for months but can eventually cause inflammation of the Fallopian tubes and subsequent INFERTILITY. Occasionally surgery may then be required in addition to antibiotic treatment.

It is vital that any woman whose partner has NSU should take the antibiotics advised by the doctor to avoid such long-term, serious complications.

Nose

The nose is one of our most important sensory organs, although we probably rather take it for granted. It has three main functions. It is the natural pathway by which air enters the body in the normal course of BREATHING. The air is warmed, moistened and filtered there before entering the lungs. The nose also acts as a protective device. If irritants such as dust enter, they are expelled by sneezing and do not have a chance to damage the lungs. Finally, of course, the nose is the organ of SMELL.

Structure

The external nose consists partly of BONE and partly of cartilage. The two nasal bones, one on each side, project downward and also form the bridge between the eyes. Below them, the nasal cartilages and the cartilages of the nostrils give the nose firmness, shape and pliability.

Inside, the nose is divided into two narrow cavities by a partition running from front to back. This partition, the *septum,* is made of bone and cartilage. It is covered with a soft, delicate membrane called a mucous membrane, which is continuous with the lining of the nostril. The nostrils themselves are lined with stiff hairs that grow downwards and protect the entrance. They are quite noticeable in some people, especially men.

The two cavities created by the septum are called *nasal fossae.* They are very narrow, less than ¼ in (6 mm) wide.

At the top of the fossae are thin plates of bone (called *turbinate bones,* or *nasal conchae*), with numerous small receptors from the olfactory nerve. When we have a cold, these receptors get covered in thick mucus, which reduces our sense of smell and taste.

Warming and moistening the air

The cavity at the back of the nose is divided into sections by three ridges of bone called the nasal conchae. They are long and thin and run lengthwise, sloping downwards at the back. The passage between each concha is called a *meatus.* It is lined with mucous membrane having a very rich blood supply, and it is this which moistens and warms the air that is inhaled.

This membrane secretes just under a pint (0.5 litres) of mucus every day and is covered with thousands of tiny hairs called *cilia.* The mucus and cilia trap dust particles, which are moved on by the cilia to the back of the THROAT where they are usually swallowed.

Sinuses and tear ducts
The sinuses – spaces at the front of the skull – are connected with the inside of the nose. They are located behind the eyebrows and behind the cheeks, in the triangle between the eyes and the nose. Sinuses help cushion the impact of any blows to the face.

Two other passages lead off the meatuses. Tear ducts carry away tears from the eyes (which is why we have to blow our nose when we cry). The other,

Sections of the nose

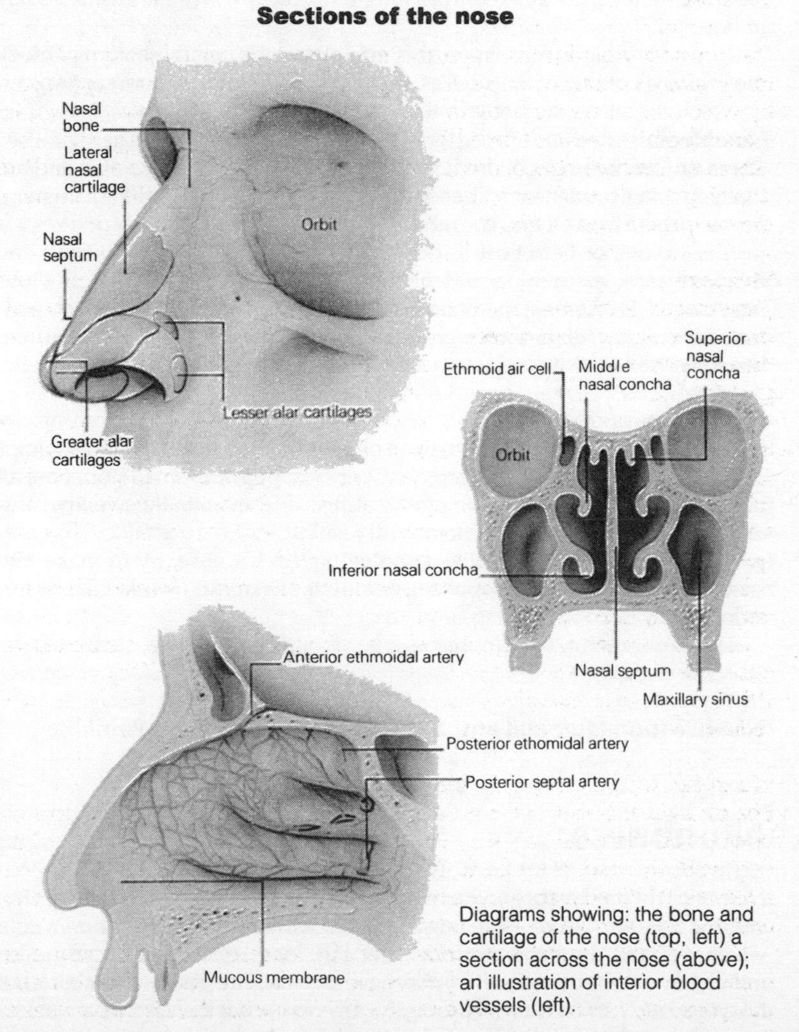

Diagrams showing: the bone and cartilage of the nose (top, left) a section across the nose (above); an illustration of interior blood vessels (left).

the Eustachian tube, is at the back of the nose near the junction with the throat. It leads to the middle EAR, which explains why we sometimes get earache when we have a sore throat.

Injuries and malformation

A broken nose is one of the most common sports injuries. For the first few days, it may be difficult to assess how misshapen a broken nose is due to the swelling, so it is usual to wait until the swelling has gone down before deciding on treatment. When a nose is reset early, this can be done under local anaesthetic, but treatment of a long-term injury will require a night's stay in hospital.

If the nose is badly misshapen, this may distort the central septum or block the openings of one of the sinuses and so cause chronic CATARRH or SINUSITIS.

Nosebleeds

These are common in children, perhaps because they are so active and are likely to suffer sudden knocks and blows. However, some children are more prone to them than others. The most frequent cause is when the blood vessels just inside one or both nostrils burst, after having become weakened and enlarged through rubbing and picking, or perhaps because of previous nosebleeds. Pressure on the brain is not the cause, but in adults, nosebleeds may be due to high BLOOD PRESSURE, so anyone over 40 who has recurrent nosebleeds should see a doctor to have a blood pressure check.

Foreign bodies

Small children are often likely to push objects up their noses. Peanuts, lumps of foam from stuffed toys, buttons, wax crayons, peas and small stones are all used. They may cause no symptoms at first, but eventually swelling, discharge, headache and facial pains will result.

If you think a child has stuffed something up his nose, try to make him sneeze while blocking the opposite nostril. If this doesn't work, take him to a doctor.

See also ADENOIDS, COLD (COMMON), HAY FEVER, POLYPS, RHINITIS, SLEEP AND SLEEP PROBLEMS, SNORING.

NSAIDs (non-steroidal anti-inflammatory drugs), *see* Painkillers

Numbness

Numbness of one sort or another is something all of us have experienced. The cause is usually obvious – banging a finger or working with bare hands in cold weather – and the condition does not last long. However, it can be an indication of some disease which may have unpleasant consequences if it is not taken seriously and dealt with promptly. Any numbness that lasts for a week or more should therefore be reported to the doctor for further investigation.

In the medical sense, numbness means a loss of sensation and it usually refers particularly to interference with the sense of touch. If the loss of feeling is complete the condition is called *anaesthesia*; if it is only partial, as in the familiar sensation of 'PINS AND NEEDLES', it is called *paraethesia*.

Causes

Basically, numbness is due to some problem in the working of the sensory nerves (*see* NERVOUS SYSTEM). These pass messages to the BRAIN about what is happening in and around a particular part of the body. If the sensory nerve is damaged or interfered with in some way, the message cannot reach the brain and numbness will result.

Damage to the sensory nerves may be accompanied by a loss of function in the motor nerves that serve the same part of the body. When the brain receives the message from the sensory nerves, it activates the motor nerves to carry messages to the muscles so a specific movement can be made. Loss or interruption of function in the motor nerves will result in the inability to move the part concerned – PARALYSIS – or weakness and loss of power if the effect is not total. Numbness and paralysis can occur together since, in many parts of the body, the sensory and motor nerves run close to each other and are likely to be affected by similar types of damage.

Common disorders

Numbness can result from several disorders of the sensory nerves. One of the most obvious is when the nerve is cut. A deep cut or gash in the skin, for example, will sever the nerves that are present in the area, causing a feeling of deadness.

Sustained pressure on a sensory nerve can also cause numbness, and is usually preceded by 'pins and needles'. A common example of this is often found with a SLIPPED DISC. One of the cushioning discs between the vertebrae of the spine becomes displaced in such a way that it presses on a major nerve trunk as it leaves the SPINAL CORD. The patient feels the pain along the course of the nerve, and may have numbness in the area of skin supplied by the nerve.

The normal working of a nerve can be interrupted by NEURITIS (inflammation of a nerve). Disorders in which neuritis may occur include DIABETES, MALNUTRITION, ALCOHOLISM and other chemical poisonings, and certain VIRUS infections. The nerve can also cease to function because the supply of blood is cut off. If a piece of string or an elastic band is wound tightly around the base of the finger, it will, in the course of a few minutes, become quite numb. This is due to the pressure around the finger being great enough to squeeze the walls of the blood vessels together, thus cutting off the blood supply.

Nutrition

This is the study of different kinds of foods and how the human body makes use of them.

A look at the list of the body's components will give some idea of the complex chemical structures of which we are made. For the 'average' man, they are: protein (17 per cent); fat (13.8 per cent); carbohydrate (1.5 per cent); water (61.6 per cent); minerals (6.1 per cent). The cells of the body are, in effect, factories which use chemical reactions to change the components supplied to them in our diet into the products necessary for life and growth.

There are about 48 substances which must be supplied ready-made in the diet, including OXYGEN and WATER. All the rest can be manufactured, given these basic essentials. In addition, the body must be supplied with enough fuel-foods for the body's furnaces to be fired. For nutrition to be adequate, it is not only important that these nutrients are supplied in the diet but also that the digestive system absorbs them properly (*see* DIGESTION).

Fuels for the tissues

The basic fuels of the body are fats and carbohydrates. The energy they produce is measured in calories or kilojoules. We take in these fuels from animal and plant products and in the body they are converted into readily-usable forms that can be taken into our cells.

FATS are converted into fatty acids and triglycerides which are carried in the blood as complex lipoproteins. These basic fat-fuels are then either taken to the adipose (fatty) tissues for storage or, if needed, they can be 'burned' chemically as fuel.

CARBOHYDRATES are mainly converted by the digestive processes into various sugars, especially glucose. This is the type of fuel that the body prefers since it is easy to transport and cells can use it conveniently. Glucose can also be made in the LIVER and other tissues by breaking down protein. Some cells, especially in the BRAIN, need glucose as an energy source. This is stored in the form of glycogen (mostly in muscle and the liver), and can be readily converted to glucose when needed. This is important since a minimum level of glucose must be kept up for the brain cells to function.

PROTEINS are broken up in the gut into their basic components, amino acids. From these, the cells make their own proteins. These are not usually used as fuel, but when other sources of energy are lacking, they can be metabolized for this purpose. In cases of prolonged starvation, the muscles waste away as the body burns up these protein components in an effort to maintain the glucose level of the blood.

Essential nutrients

The body also requires some chemicals which it cannot make for itself. However, these can usually be stored, and so we may be able to survive for months or even years without them before the effect of any deficiency in the diet is felt. The nutrients we need are: vitamins, essential elements and minerals (including those which are only required in minute amounts), fatty acids and amino acids.

VITAMINS are needed to help the ENZYME systems which drive the cell factories. Some, such as vitamin D, work in different ways. Once in the body, vitamin D acts like a HORMONE, coordinating the distribution of CALCIUM and the growth of BONE. Others, such as vitamin K, help control such activities as the clotting of BLOOD. Vitamins are soluble (can dissolve) in either water or fat. This difference is important because if the absorption of fat is abnormal (*see* MALABSORPTION), due to some disease in the intestines, the fat-soluble vitamins won't be absorbed.

Other constituents of the diet may interfere with the absorption or use of vitamins. It has been suggested that the nicotinic acid which is present in cereals may be chemically bound to some of the constituents, making it unavailable for use. Food preparation may also affect some water-soluble vitamins. Folic acid is often destroyed in this way through prolonged cooking or in canning. (Nicotinic acid and folic acid are included in the B-vitamin group.)

MINERAL elements needed for adequate nutrition include some, such as carbon and hydrogen, that are so abundant that deficiency is practically impossible.

Sodium and chloride, the constituents of common salt, are essential to our biochemistry. SALT is widely distributed in foods and deficiencies are only found when the body's requirements are greatly increased through abnormal losses. When people living in hot climates sweat excessively, salt loss may be sufficient to require extra dietary supplements.

CALCIUM is an important constituent of bones and other tissues. The body's calcium turnover is carefully regulated by a complex hormone system which includes vitamin D.

IRON is essential for the manufacture of haemoglobin, the vital oxygen-carrying substance in red BLOOD cells. Some iron is also essential in the makeup of some of the important enzyme systems in cells which provide energy to be used by the cells' factories.

Minute quantities of other elements (trace elements) are also needed. IODINE, for example, is essential to the manufacture of THYROID hormone.

It is claimed that fluorine, contained in fluoride, is necessary to prevent tooth decay (*see* DENTAL CARE) and this is often added to water supplies. Other TRACE ELEMENTS such as copper, cobalt and manganese are needed for various enzyme systems.

Amino acids are the nitrogen-containing compounds which are the basic building blocks of the much larger, protein molecules. Our cells can manufacture many of these, but nine must be supplied ready-made in the diet. Different foods have different proportions of these essential substances – so a mixture of food proteins is needed in order to have an adequate diet.

Fatty acids, which are composed of carbon, hydrogen and oxygen, are the main fuel needed for muscular activity. Most of those required as fuel stores and in the makeup of cells can be made in the body. One generally thought to be essential is linoleic acid; deficiency of this is rare.

What is healthy nutrition?

For good health, the diet must include all essential nutrients in sufficient quantities. All the vitamins and minerals must be present, with a sufficient supply of calories to maintain energy output and enough protein to maintain the structure of the body. However, a healthy diet must contain an appropriate *balance* of nutrients.

Energy can be obtained from carbohydrates, fats or proteins. Normally carbohydrates and fats are the main sources of energy, but if there is insufficient carbohydrate or fat in the diet to fulfil energy needs, proteins will be broken down instead. So the metabolism of the body can adjust to different levels of fats, carbohydrates and protein in the diet to maintain a sufficient supply of energy.

Although it has been known for many years that shortage of vitamins and minerals can cause various diseases, it is only within the last 20 years or so that medical attention has focused on the importance of an appropriate balance in the diet between the different types of carbohydrates, fats and protein. The present-day diet has progressively contained more and more fat, particularly fat of animal origin, and it is now clear that this has been responsible, at least in part, for an increased rate of CORONARY HEART DISEASE in many Western countries. High-fat diets are also thought to play a part in causing some other disorders, such as gallstones (*see* GALL BLADDER) and BREAST cancer.

Over the years, the type of carbohydrate in the diet has also changed. 'Natural' sources are starchy foods, such as potatoes or flour-based products, which are all rich in fibre and usually contain other nutrients such as vitamins and minerals. However, refined sugar has often replaced starches in the modern diet. If pure sugar (sucrose) is a major component of the food eaten, it is probably part of a diet that is low in fibre, and possibly deficient in other nutrients as well. A low-fibre diet may cause diseases such as DIVERTICULITIS (an inflammatory condition of the large bowel), and may be a factor in the development of bowel CANCER. Too many sugary foods, taken too frequently during the day, can also be one cause of tooth decay.

Another problem of modern nutrition for some people is simply taking too many calories altogether. Anybody who eats too much food for his or her energy expenditure inevitably becomes overweight. High BLOOD PRESSURE, ARTHRITIS and many other disorders are associated with OBESITY.

Many international and national committees have proposed guidelines for a 'balanced' or a 'healthy diet'. Each set of guidelines varies slightly, but they all have many features in common. Typical recommendations were made by the British National Advisory Committee for Nutritional Education in 1983. Briefly, their recommendations were as follows:

- Energy intake (calorie content of food) should not be excessive for any individual and obesity should be avoided.
- Fats should provide no more than 30 per cent of total energy requirements.
- No more than 10 per cent of energy requirements should come from 'saturated' fats (fats of animal origin such as dairy fats or fat on meat).
- Sugar (sucrose) should be kept below 44 lb (20 kg) per year, including all sugar in snacks, soft drinks, confectionery, cakes and biscuits.
- Dietary fibre intake should be around 1 oz (30 g) per day.
- Vitamin and mineral intake should match the required minimums for each essential nutrient.

By keeping to these guidelines, everybody can ensure that he or she is eating healthily, and can reduce the risk of many of the disorders that are known to be associated either with deficiencies in nutrition – or with dietary excesses.

In practice, following these guidelines probably involves some changes in diet for most people. A reduction in fat content can be achieved by avoiding fatty foods, by grilling instead of frying, and by using low-fat milk and low-fat dairy products. Sugar in the diet can be reduced by avoiding shop-bought sweets, puddings, confectionery and soft drinks. Fresh fruit, vegetables and wholemeal grain products will provide fibre, carbohydrates, plenty of vitamins and minerals, and should comprise a major part of a healthy diet.

See also MALNUTRITION.

Nystagmus, *see* Blindness, Eyes and eyesight

O

Obesity

This can be defined as: a weight that is 20 per cent over 'ideal' body weight. Using this definition, approximately 1 in every 6 men and 1 in every 4 women in the UK are obese. Obesity can happen to anyone – no class or sex is exempt. It can be prevented by proper calorie management, although once the condition occurs, it is difficult for obese people to get down to their ideal weight. But it is not impossible.

Causes

Fatness is caused by eating too much. 'Too much' means more than your body uses, in the course of everyday life and to maintain itself. What is often difficult to grasp is how little 'too much' can be when overeating is spread out over many years and the surplus fat is not burned up. For example, if you eat one slice of bread more than you need every day, after ten years the stored food will weigh roughly 40 lb (about 18 kg), and you will be that much over what should be your ideal weight.

To a certain extent, obesity can run in families. This may be due to genetic INHERITANCE – some people are more liable to become obese than others, given the same food intake and energy expended – but often obesity occurs from acquiring bad eating habits from the family.

Very rarely a medical problem is found to be the cause of obesity. An underactive THYROID gland or overactive ADRENAL GLANDS may result in weight gain, as will even more rare medical causes such as congenital syndromes involving hormonal abnormalities and birth defects which affect appetite regulation.

Finally, emotional factors play an important part in causing obesity. When people are depressed, they often turn to food for comfort and, over time, obesity will result. Their size may then be a cause of DEPRESSION and they will eat more and get fatter.

Development of obesity

When an excess of food is eaten over the needs of the body for fuel or essential building blocks, the surplus is converted into fatty acids by the liver, taken into the bloodstream to the fatty or adipose tissues located around the body and then converted into storage fats.

When fat is laid down in excess, it appears where the tissue is most abundant – usually in the buttocks and stomach initially, followed by the thighs and arms. Different people may develop fat deposits in slightly different places and at different rates of speed, but most follow this general pattern.

Dangers

Being slightly above your ideal weight – by 5 per cent or so – is probably not a great risk, but if your weight is much over this, you will start being liable to a variety of other complications.

The extra weight the obese person carries and its distribution mainly in the central parts of the body puts extra strain on the JOINTS, particularly in the knees, hips and some of the joints in the back. This leads to the early development of osteoarthrosis (wear and tear of the joints), which will become a painful problem (OSTEOARTHRITIS) in early middle age. The extra weight will also cause the arches to drop – therefore flat FEET.

More serious problems arise when the efficiency of the stomach muscles is impaired by the fatty infiltration. Movement of the DIAPHRAGM is inhibited and this makes BREATHING inefficient and may lead to LUNG disorders and shortness of breath. A similar reason underlies the high incidence of lung complications in obese people if they have an anaesthetic before an operation.

Obesity can cause mild DIABETES, which in turn may cause serious complications in the small blood vessels of the EYES and KIDNEYS. Because there is an increase in the available fats, especially cholesterol, in the circulation, the obese person tends to develop gallstones (*see* GALL BLADDER) and, to a lesser extent, GOUT.

Because of the tendency to have high blood fat, there is an increased risk of developing atherosclerosis of the ARTERIES – a thickening and hardening of the arteries which impairs blood circulation in the body. The result is likely to be an increased chance of THROMBOSIS of arteries supplying such vital organs as the brain and heart – resulting in STROKES and HEART ATTACKS. Obesity can lead to high BLOOD PRESSURE, which also contributes to an increased chance of heart attacks, strokes and even kidney failure.

Because of these many complications, obese people have a considerably reduced chance of living to a ripe old age. Indeed insurance companies have calculated that if a man is about 25 lb (11 kg) overweight, his life expectancy will be reduced by one quarter.

Treatment

The mainstay of treatment for obesity is sensible dieting and activity. This is never easy, particularly as it requires the strenuous exercise of willpower and the changing of eating habits acquired over a lifetime. Many obese people try a variety of shortcuts, none of which is effective in the long term.

In general, the success rate for very obese people in losing significant amounts of weight and keeping to their ideal weight is low. However, with perseverance, it can be done – bringing benefits to health.

Obsessive–compulsive neurosis, *see* Mental illness

Occupational hazards

Quite apart from the personal toll that occupational disease and injury can bring, there is a heavy economic price to pay. In Britain, millions of working days are lost each year through work-related injuries and illness.

Many of the most serious occupational hazards have been brought under control by the Factories Acts and the Health and Safety at Work Acts. Accidents with machinery can never be totally avoided because of human error. However they can be minimized if employers ensure that the standards of safety are maintained, and if workers familiarize themselves with and adhere to safety regulations.

Types of hazards

Hazards may be in the form of gas, liquid or solid. They can enter the body through the lungs, by contact with the skin and by ingestion through the mouth.

Dangerous metals: Lead, the most notorious toxic substance, is used in the manufacture of batteries, rubber, paint, roofing and soldering material. It can enter the body through inhalation of small dust particles and fumes, or by ingestion. The first symptoms may include tiredness, headache, loss of appetite, constipation and mild abdominal pain. Extreme poisoning – rare nowadays – can result in severe abdominal pain, muscle weakness, convulsions, coma and death.

Mercury, a silver-coloured liquid used in thermometers, is another hazardous metal. It is utilized in the electrical industry in the manufacture of fluorescent lamps and of precision instruments, and in dentistry. It is also found in the small 'button' batteries used to power watches and cameras. Poisoning causes jerky movements starting in the fingers, irritability, drowsiness and, in the final stage, madness. Other symptoms are sore throat and gums, vomiting and diarrhoea. Compounds from mercury can also be dangerous when they occur in the form of industrial effluents which are absorbed – for instance, by the fish we eat. These can cause blindness, mental deterioration, lack of coordination, birth defects and death.

Cadmium, a soft metal used for increasing the hardness of copper and as a protective plating for other metals, is particularly dangerous because, once someone has inhaled or ingested a certain amount, there is no known cure. Poisoning can be gradual because the amount of metal in the body slowly builds up. At a critical point, the lungs and the kidneys cease to function properly and death can result.

Chromium, a silver-white, hard, brittle metal, is used to make various steels, including stainless steel, and high-speed tools. Its compounds are used in chrome plating, in the production of pigments in paints and inks, in leather tanning agents, in timber preservation and in photography and dyestuffs. The danger of chromium is that even slight contact with dilute solutions can cause skin ulcers and the inhalation of fine droplets or mist containing chromium salts can cause ulcers inside the nose. Although lung cancer has not been associated with chrome plating, it has been linked with the manufacture of chromates. Asthmatic symptoms can also occur, as can chrome sensitivity: a strong reaction to chrome following symptoms of exposure.

Solvents: There are many liquids classed as solvents, and workers in nearly all occupations are exposed to them, from the office typist to the engineer. Solvents evaporate very quickly, and the vapours can enter the body by being inhaled through the lungs, through the skin and, more rarely, through the digestive system. Once they enter the body, they can attack the liver, the heart, the lungs and the nervous system.

Solvents are found in inks, varnishes, glues, cleaners, dry cleaning fluids and many other substances. Some of the most dangerous ones may be very pleasant to smell, whereas others that are foul-smelling may be quite harmless.

Trichloroethylene smells very nice but it can lead to loss of consciousness and death. *Benzene* is another pleasant smelling solvent used in the manufacture of artificial leather, lino detergents, pesticides and paint removers. It can cause dizziness and coma or, when poisoning is chronic, aplastic ANAEMIA.

Because of the dissolving properties of solvents, they can attack the skin and cause dermatitis. Contact with solvents should be strictly limited.

Unlike solvents, all *isocynanates* are dangerous. They are used in the manufacture of polyurethanes which make foams, adhesives, lacquers and paints. Over-exposure to isocynanates in the air can lead to skin inflammations, eye irritations and breathing difficulties, including severe asthma. People can also develop isocynanate-sensitivity.

Dusts: Dust is the biggest killer in industry. However, some dusts are relatively harmless.

There are four basic categories of dust. The first is *nuisance or inert dust* such as plaster of Paris, starch and Portland cement. These can accumulate in the body without producing a serious reaction. *Toxic dusts* include lead and chromium compounds. They can have serious effects on specific organs in the body like the kidneys and the nervous system. *Dusts that produce allergic-type reactions,* such as some wood dusts and fungus spores from grain, can cause asthma and eczema. Finally *dusts that change lung tissue,* such as ASBESTOS and coal dust, make the lungs inefficient, and each year cause death and serious disability in hundreds of people.

Chronic lung diseases caused by dust in industry is known as *pneumoconiosis.* The most common type is coal miner's pneumoconiosis. The lungs become damaged by inflammation and ultimately by *fibrosis.* The normal lung substance is replaced by dense patches of thick fibrous tissue. At first these patches can be quite small and will show up on an X-ray as small spots no more than a few millimetres across, but in the most severe cases, large areas of lung tissue may be replaced by progressive massive fibrosis. This is the name given to the most severe form of pneumoconiosis. The sufferer will, by this time, be breathless and have a chronic cough.

Asbestos workers can develop a form of lung disease called *asbestosis*, although there is also a risk of lung cancer developing after exposure to asbestos, particularly 'blue' asbestos. For this reason, all asbestos work is now controlled by very strict legislation. People who work with silica – for example, in mines – may develop *silicosis*, yet another form of pneumoconiosis.

Noise: In many industries, working with a deafening din was accepted as part of the job. Nowadays noise, though inescapable in many industries, is viewed as an occupational hazard for which there are controls and preventive measures.

The basic preventive measure is to cut the noise of machinery at source by deadening its sound, and by instructing workers to wear appropriate ear muffs or plugs. Though many workers resist wearing them, they drastically reduce the sound reaching the ear. (*See also* DEAFNESS.)

Occupational skin disorders

The most common type of occupational disease is skin disease. Since many types of work often involve handling heavy or rough tools and a wide variety of different chemicals, ranging from soaps and detergents to acids, it is hardly surprising that skin disorders are so common.

Occupational DERMATITIS is a rash which is exactly like eczema. The skin becomes roughened, cracked and sore. There may be small blisters in the skin as well, especially if the hands are affected. Most commonly, hand dermatitis is caused by contact with strong detergents, lubricants, oils, acids or alkalis, paints or varnishes. All of these substances can directly damage the skin surface. Repeated contact causes greater damage unless some protection is provided. Those industries where dermatitis is a particular problem include mining and quarrying, engineering, chemicals and commercial cleaning.

Another form of dermatitis is caused by an ALLERGY to some agent to which the individual is sensitive. Often only one particular substance triggers off the reaction. Hairdressers, for example, may become allergic to the chemicals in permanent waving solutions and come out in a rash when they are exposed to a particular solution. Some people become allergic to nickel and cannot handle any articles made of that metal.

People who work in dusty, unhygienic or very damp conditions are prone to occupational skin infection such as infections under the fingernails (*see* WHITLOW). Oil-soaked overalls may also trigger off a type of ACNE on the areas of skin which are in contact with the oily clothing. This is particularly a problem for garage workers and diesel fitters.

Very rarely skin cancers can arise from prolonged contact with certain chemicals or oils – particularly some types of mineral or vegetable tar.

Radiation

Ultraviolet and infra-red light are both types of light radiation which may be hazardous to those exposed to them. Arc welding, for example, is a source of ultraviolet light which may cause burns to the eyes of a welder ('arc eye') if there is sudden unprotected exposure to an arc, and in the long term, repeated exposure to ultraviolet light may cause CATARACTS.

However, the most dangerous form of radiation is 'ionizing' radiation – X-rays and gamma-rays which are given off by some radioactive isotopes. High doses of ionizing radiation can cause RADIATION SICKNESS which, in severe cases, such as nuclear power station accidents, can be rapidly fatal. Low doses of ionizing radiation can also have damaging effects, especially if somebody is exposed repeatedly. The effects are cumulative. The main risk is from the development of cancers later in life – particularly LEUKAEMIA.

Working with animals

Although agriculture is often regarded as a safer industry than many others, farm workers may be at risk from infections transmitted by farm animals. For example, brucellosis can be transmitted from cattle and causes an acute illness. Certain types of CHLAMYDIA may be transmitted from sheep and can cause abortion in pregnant women farm workers. Farmers may also develop lung problems as a result of allergy to fungi which grow in damp straw and hay – a condition known as 'farmer's lung'.

Veterinary surgeons and those who work with laboratory animals are at risk of certain other infections. Rats, cats, dogs and monkeys all carry various diseases which may be transmitted to people who work with them.

Occupational injuries

A proportion of occupational accidents occur through the use of unguarded machinery. Although all machinery must by law be guarded, some employers, in an attempt to cut corners, do not ensure that this is done. Moreover some workers, such as those on piecework, who believe that the guard is slowing their output and losing them pay, deliberately prevent guards from working – preferring to risk losing a limb.

Machinery maintenance is especially hazardous because guards often have to be removed for access. Mistakes such as failing to switch off the power supply cause serious injuries.

Over 12,000 injuries in British factories each year are caused through the use of handtools. Particularly common are eye injuries from fragments of metal flying off drills or chips of stone or metal split off while hammering. Wearing eye protection – however much disliked – will prevent this type of injury.

Certain types of handtools such as chainsaws can be responsible for a disease known as 'vibration white finger'. The symptoms are pallor spreading down from the fingertips and a tingling sensation. This can progress to a blue tingeing of the fingers and sometimes pain or loss of sensation. There is unfortunately no known cure for white finger. Workers using vibration tools should wear padded gloves and keep their hands warm.

Finally, falls in factories account for a high proportion of occupational injuries. Most of these falls occurred on a level floor, and were mainly due to gangways being cluttered with boxes, spilt liquids not mopped up and sheer untidiness.

Falls also account for half of the 5,000 serious injuries suffered by office staff in Great Britain every year. Trailing wires, filing cabinet drawers left open, and poorly lit stairs are all traps. Many injuries can be prevented by following safety regulations, better office and factory housekeeping and simple care.

Occupational therapy

This is the use of selected activities to help people of all ages with a disability or handicap reach their maximum level of function and independence in all aspects of daily life. Some occupational therapists work mainly with physically disabled patients. They are concerned with mobilizing stiff joints, strengthening muscles, improving coordination and building up stamina. Therapists may use activities such as planing wood to exercise a weak back, treadling a foot-powered lathe to exercise the legs or working a hand printing press to strengthen an arm.

Therapists also help patients who have difficulty with day-to-day activities such as getting in and out of the bath and cutting up food. In most occupational therapy departments, there will be a kitchen, bathroom and bedroom section where patients can try out aids and practise new techniques.

Occupational therapists also treat MENTALLY ILL and mentally handicapped people. Therapists use such activities as painting and music which provide opportunities for self-expression, and discussion groups and social activities to help shy and withdrawn patients express themselves better and relate to others. They use shopping and cooking and work activities to help patients cope with living in the community.

Occupational therapists work with social services departments to help the handicapped live at home. This may mean arranging for the provision of aids such as extended legs to make an armchair higher, or adaptations such as a second banister rail. Or their duties may include working with architects to plan major alterations such as a downstairs bathroom suitable for someone who is in a wheelchair.

Equally, occupational therapists may work in day centres where patients with a physical disability, mental illness or mental handicap can go to meet other patients and enjoy a change in environment.

Oedema

All blood vessels leak just a little fluid which collects outside them. Normally this fluid is removed by an efficient drainage system, the LYMPHATIC vessels, but when the system fails, the fluid builds up and causes puffiness or swelling of the tissues. When this occurs, the condition is known as oedema.

Causes

Fluid passes out of blood vessels because the walls of the vessels are thin and the BLOOD that circulates around the body is being pumped by the heart under considerable pressure. Fluid returns to the blood vessels by a process known as *osmosis.*

Osmosis takes place when a weak solution passes into a strong solution across a semi-permeable membrane. The walls of blood vessels form semi-permeable membranes, and within these vessels flows a strong solution of proteins, dissolved in the plasma, the natural constituents of blood. It is the presence of these proteins that is responsible for the sucking back in of a lot of the fluid that has seeped out.

Lack of protein in the blood resulting from MALNUTRITION or LIVER disease is a common cause of oedema. Obstruction of the drainage system – either the lymphatic vessels or the veins – also leads to the accumulation of fluid because of a build-up in pressure. As a consequence, THROMBOSIS and VARICOSE VEINS are sometimes causes of ankle swelling. HEART failure can lead to a backlog of blood in the veins. When the KIDNEYS fail to remove excessive SALT from the blood, or if we take in too much salt with fluids, the volume of fluid in the blood vessels increases greatly, and so does the rate at which fluid leaks out.

The rate at which salt is passed into the URINE – assuming the kidneys are functioning properly – is regulated by the ADRENAL hormones. The balance of these is altered during PREGNANCY and menstruation (*see* PERIODS): at these times, slight oedema may result from salt retention.

Special types of oedema

Gravity determines where oedema occurs. The most common place is around the ankles, but after a patient has spent a long period in bed, oedema fluid may collect around the buttocks or sacrum.

Severe heart failure, liver failure or obstruction of any of the large veins in the abdomen cause fluid to collect inside the abdominal cavity. This is known as *ascites.*

Similarly, fluid accumulates in the lungs if the left side of the heart fails (pulmonary oedema). This causes severe breathlessness with a cough and frothy sputum and requires emergency attention.

Symptoms and dangers

Ankle oedema is easy to see if the ankles are grossly swollen, but slight swelling can be more difficult to detect. Fluid tends to collect first on the inner side of the ankle, just behind the ankle bone. Breathlessness at rest is a symptom of pulmonary oedema.

Ankle oedema is not dangerous in itself but it may be a symptom of a more serious condition such as heart disease which requires treatment. However, pulmonary oedema, if severe, is a medical emergency, for if not treated quickly the patient will become extremely short of breath, as if drowning in his or her own oedema fluid. Prompt drug treatment will lead to almost certain recovery.

Treatment

Oedema caused by leakage from ageing and thin blood vessels can be controlled by wearing an elastic stocking which squeezes the fluid out of the ankles. If the fundamental cause is heart failure, however, the main approach is to reduce the volume of blood circulating around the body to reduce the strain on the heart. This is done by taking tablets, known as *diuretics*, which make the patient pass water and reduce the level of salt. The process is aided if the patient refrains from adding salt when cooking. It is sometimes necessary to take extra POTASSIUM with diuretic treatment.

Pulmonary oedema is treated with a fast-acting diuretic which is given intravenously. Oxygen given through a mask may also be necessary. Thrombosis of the veins is treated by thinning of the blood with anti-coagulants. Varicose veins can be removed surgically.

Oesophagus

The oesophagus, or gullet, is the tube that connects the back of the mouth to the STOMACH. Its only function is to carry food from the mouth to the parts of the ALIMENTARY CANAL in the abdomen where it will be broken down by the various digestive processes and then absorbed into the bloodstream.

Structure

The top of the oesophagus lies immediately behind the trachea (windpipe). Just below the level of the notch at the top of the chest, the tube bends slightly to the left and passes behind the left bronchus (airway in the lungs). It then goes through the DIAPHRAGM and connects with the upper end of the stomach.

The entrance to the stomach is controlled by a muscular ring (sphincter) that closes to prevent food being forced back up the oesophagus by the forceful contractions of the stomach.

The oesophagus is an elastic tube about 10 in (25 cm) long and about 1 in (2.5 cm) in diameter. Like the rest of the alimentary tract, the oesophagus is made up of four layers – a lining of mucous membrane to enable food to pass down easily, a submucous layer to hold it in place, a relatively thick layer of muscle consisting of both circular and longitudinal fibres, and finally an outer protective covering.

Problems and treatment

Perhaps the most common problem in this area is inflammation of the oesophagus (*oesophagitis*). This is usually caused by acid coming up from the stomach and results in a burning feeling behind the breastbone after eating. This condition, known as 'heartburn', occurs frequently in pregnancy, and is a common symptom of a hiatus hernia (*see* DIAPHRAGM). Treatment of oesophagitis normally depends on antacids and drugs to reduce stomach acid.

Those with cancer of the oesophagus often have a poor prognosis because it is usually only diagnosed when the patient has difficulty swallowing and this usually occurs late in the disease. If the cancer is diagnosed early, an operation may be possible to remove it. However, often this is not the case, and treatment is aimed at keeping the patient swallowing as best as possible.

If the cancer is in the lower part of the oesophagus, the operation will consist of removing the cancerous section and bringing up the stomach to be joined with the cut end. Growths in the upper part of the oesophagus used to be much more difficult to deal with because there is not so much room for manoeuvre. But nowadays it is sometimes possible to overcome this difficulty by transplanting part of the colon to act as a replacement for the diseased section of the oesophagus.

Oestrogen, *see* **Breast and breast cancer, Contraception, Exocrine system, Hormone replacement therapy, Menopause, Ovaries, Periods and period pains, Premenstrual syndrome**

Omentum, *see* **Peritoneum and peritonitis**

Ondine's curse, *see* **Reflexes**

Ophthalmia neonatorum, *see* **Conjunctivitis**

Opium, *see* **Heroin, Morphine, Sedatives**

Oral contraceptives, *see* **Contraception**

Orchitis, *see* **Mumps, Testes**

Orgasm, *see* **Penis, Sex and sexual intercourse**

Orthopaedics

This is the surgical speciality which treats diseases and injuries to BONES and soft tissues. A broken bone left to its own devices will usually heal or, in medical terminology, unite. The orthopaedic surgeon tries to make sure that the FRACTURE unites in a good position so that the limb will function well afterwards. He or she also makes certain that no complications develop while the fracture is healing.

Treatment of fractures

A limb fracture (breakage) is usually diagnosed in the casualty department of a hospital by the casualty officer. An uncomplicated fracture will be set there and then, often under an anaesthetic, and a plaster may be applied to hold the set in place. The patient will not generally see the orthopaedic consultant until he or she visits the fracture clinic to have the plaster inspected and X-rays taken – to ensure that the bone ends are fitting firmly together and that the splint is holding up to everyday wear and tear.

The consultant will decide if a new plaster needs to be applied and when the old plaster is ready to come off. Most simple fractures of the arm need to stay in plaster for between four to six weeks. A leg fracture, however, takes twice as long because the bones are larger and the limb is weight-bearing.

Plaster is the most commonly used method of treating fractures. It has its limitations, though: some areas of the body, such as the shoulder and hip, are difficult to hold in plaster; in addition, plaster covers the skin, which may itself have suffered severe injury and need careful watching. It also stops JOINTS moving and they may become stiff.

Plaster of Paris is the traditional material for a cast, but it is rather heavy and occasionally it cracks. An alternative material is fibreglass, which is not only lighter but also stronger, although it is more expensive.

Reduction and internal fixation

The orthopaedic surgeon may decide that a fracture needs to be operated on. This may be necessary when it is clear that the bones cannot be brought into a satisfactory position by other means, or when the fracture would confine the patient to bed for a long time.

In this sort of operation, an incision is made in the skin along the length of the bone which is then exposed by pulling back the muscles surrounding it. The periosteum – a layer of tissue which coats the bone – is peeled back from the fracture, and the ends of the bones are carefully cleaned and fitted together, or 'reduced'. The ends are joined together with a piece of metal; this is called internal fixation. Usually a strip of metal is screwed along the length of the bone, crossing the fracture site – a procedure known as 'plating'. On some occasions, a long nail is used and this is driven up through the hollow shaft of the bone.

Pin-and-plate operation

When fixing the head of the thigh bone, a pin is driven in from the side of the femur and up the centre of the broken neck, ensuring that the pin stops just short of the joint. This is then held in place with a metal plate screwed to the side of the femur. This procedure is known as a 'pin-and-plate' operation. The great advantage of fixation by pinning or screwing is that the patient can be up and about within days of the operation and a plaster cast is usually unnecessary. The pin-and-plate operation is particularly suitable for elderly people who fall and fracture their hips. The metal used is inert and can stay in the body for life without causing any trouble or discomfort to elderly patients.

Traction for fractures

This is used almost exclusively for fractures of the leg. After such an injury the muscles tighten up and pull the bone ends past each other, so that the lower fragment rides up to lie alongside the upper fragment. Unless the bone ends are pulled apart against the tension of the muscles and correctly aligned this will result in union of the fracture with some shortening of the limb.

Traction is applied to the lower bone fragment by means of a weight hung from a steel pin which is driven through the shin bone or heel with the patient under anaesthetic. The weights are usually suspended from an arrangement of pulleys placed at the end of the bed. Obviously a 14-stone man needs heavier weights than a six-year-old child, and to prevent the weights pulling the patient out of bed, the foot end is sometimes placed on blocks. The advantage of traction is that the joints are free to move, and wounds can be watched.

Bone grafting

Some fractures, particularly those of the tibia, fail to unite. In such cases pieces of bone may be taken from another part of the patient's own SKELETON and 'grafted'. A favourite site for the donor bone is the pelvis, high up on the hip. Here a strip of bone up to 4 in (10 cm) long can be cut away without any damage or interference to the skeleton. The un-united fracture is cleaned thoroughly and small pieces of bone graft are placed in the fracture. This causes the body to form strong new bone around the bone graft, and sound union of the fracture takes place over a few weeks.

Compound fractures

A compound fracture – where broken bone ends have penetrated the overlying skin – carries a high risk of infection and must be treated carefully. This involves cleaning the wound thoroughly by means of an operation. All the dead muscle and skin is cut away, removing the possibility of infection with bacteria that can cause gangrene. After the wound is cleaned, the bone ends can be brought together and the skin sewn back into place.

Back injuries

Serious BACK injuries may involve fractures of one or more vertebrae in the spine. If the ligaments holding the vertebrae together remain intact, the spine is unlikely to become distorted, and recovery from the injury is then usually fairly straightforward and uncomplicated. However, sometimes the spine fractures right across and the vertebrae can move out of alignment. There is then a risk of damage to the SPINAL CORD, the main trunk of nerves from the brain which lies just behind the vertebrae. PARALYSIS of the limbs can result from such an injury, the extent of paralysis depending on the exact site of the fracture.

If a fracture is diagnosed, it may be necessary to stabilize the spine. This can be done by traction, which is applied to the legs or the pelvis if the fracture is low down the spine, or to the skull if the fracture is in the upper part of the spine or neck. For the most serious spinal injuries, an emergency operation may be carried out to stabilize the fractured bones using metal supports, placed alongside the spine, which are screwed or wired to the bones.

Joint dislocation

Reduction of dislocation is usually a simple matter when the patient is fully relaxed under anaesthetic. However, problems arise when repeated dislocation occurs – for example, after a shoulder injury where the original dislocation has weakened the surrounding tissue. Here surgical reconstruction of the joint capsule is required. Joint injuries often cause stiffening, and PHYSIOTHERAPY may be necessary to improve movement and the strength of muscles after these injuries.

Joint replacement surgery

In recent years, advances in engineering and the development of new material have made it possible to replace entire joints. The commonest such operation is hip joint replacement, where a metal ball and plastic socket are cemented into the thigh bone and hip socket with acrylic cement. This operation is very successful in relieving the pain and stiffness of wear-and-tear arthritis. Since it is not yet certain how long the artificial hip joint will go on working before it wears out or loosens, surgeons are cautious of doing this operation on people under 40.

Bone diseases in children

Some orthopaedic surgeons specialize in children's bone disorders. A few babies are born with congenital deformities or birth defects which require careful surgery. SPINA BIFIDA is a rare condition affecting the spine which may be associated with paralysis in the legs. Early surgery may be required, or further operations later in life to correct deformities. More common is the condition of congenital dislocation of the HIPS, which occurs in about one child in 700.

Older children may develop deformities as they grow. They may develop curvature of the spine, or deformities of the legs, such as bow legs or knock knees. Most of these get better on their own in time, although in the most severe cases, operations may be necessary.

Another condition that affects some growing children and teenagers is *osteochondritis.* A growing bone, for some unknown reason, starts to disintegrate internally and becomes painful, and eventually may become deformed. This condition may affect the hips (PERTHES' DISEASE), the knees (*Osgood–Schlatter's disease*) and sometimes the wrist or ankle bones. Rest is usually required to prevent the development of deformity, sometimes with prolonged splintage in plaster.

See also ARTHRITIS, TENDONS.

Osgood–Schlatter's disease, *see* **Orthopaedics**

Osteitis, *see* **Paget's disease**

Osteoarthritis

This is one of the commonest forms of ARTHRITIS. In fact, half the population over the age of 50 have some signs of the disease, which can also affect some people in their 30s and 40s. Although it is possible to get osteoarthritis, or OA, in almost any JOINT in the body, there are some joints where it is particularly likely to occur. These include the HIPS, the KNEES, the hands, the BACK and the neck.

Osteoarthritis is painful and, in some cases, can be crippling since it reduces the amount of movement in severely affected joints. Treatment is with aspirin or other PAINKILLERS, but in severe cases, surgery can be performed to modify the joint surfaces or to replace some of the affected joints.

Causes

Although a great deal if known about how osteoarthritis develops once it actually occurs, the causes of the disease are obscure. Some research indicates the IMMUNE SYSTEM may be involved.

Joints between bones are lined with a membrane called the *synovial membrane*. This forms a kind of bag surrounding the joint which is filled with synovial fluid. The actual parts of the joint where the bones are in contact with each other are lined with cartilage, and it is the two cartilage surfaces coming into contact with each other that bear the load of the joint. Cartilage itself is made up of a hard network of fibres that contain cartilage-producing cells and fluid, so that it provides an excellent lubricated surface for the moving parts of the joint. Osteoarthritis is a disease which results from the alteration in the structure of this cartilage.

In the first stage of osteoarthritis there is flaking and erosion of the surface of the cartilage, followed by the appearance of a number of small clefts, and there is also an increase in the number of cartilage-producing cells. At this stage, the patient may not notice any symptoms or only experience some very slight degree of pain and stiffness.

In the next stage, the cartilage caps on the bone ends begin to wear thin until finally there is no cartilage left and the bone ends bear directly on to one another. There may be considerable destruction of the bone as it is worn away by movements of the joint, and also a thickening of the capsule of the synovial membrane that surrounds the joints.

Unlike cartilage, though, bone is able to repair itself as it gets eaten away. However, the way in which bone does this around an osteoarthritic joint is disorganized. This can sometimes lead to rough deposits, which do more harm than good to the joint.

It would appear that the cause of osteoarthritis is the continual stress on the joint – hence the common name 'wear and tear' arthritis. But this theory does not explain the fact that joints which bear the same amount of weight are not equally affected: that is, the hip and knee are likely to be involved, whereas the ankle is not.

Some factors, however, may predispose a patient to osteoarthritis. For instance a background of repeated small injuries may be a causative factor:

people who play a great deal of sport – footballers, for example – eventually develop more osteoarthritis than normal, particularly in the feet.

Deformity of the limb or a joint may be another contributing factor, and this may lead to stresses on the joint that are so severe that they amount to repeated injury.

However, the fact remains that there is no obvious cause in the majority of patients with the disease.

Symptoms

The main symptom of osteoarthritis is pain. This can vary in severity from a dull ache in an affected joint to an excruciating pain which may make patients practically immobile. Usually the pain from an osteoarthritic joint is worse during movement. There may also be pain of a duller aching character when the joint is at rest. This pain is thought to result from the disorganization of the way that the veins drain blood from the joint: rest pain may well be due to the joint being congested with blood.

The pain tends to become steadily worse, although the severity of the joint's involvement is not always a good indication of the degree of pain. Further, the pain may not actually be felt in the joint involved: it is common for osteoarthritis of the hip to come to light as a result of pain in the knee on the same side, or in the back.

Osteoarthritis also causes stiffness. This is usually worse in the morning, but tends to get better within a few minutes. The affected joints may also swell in some cases.

As the disease progresses, there may be considerable deformity of the joints. Badly affected hips and knees creak; doctors call this *crepitus*. The range of movement decreases as the arthritis progresses, and in some cases the joint may become almost fixed.

Osteoarthritis may affect one joint in the body or it may affect several. If only one joint is involved, it is likely to be a big one such as the knee or hip. Occasionally the only joint involved is where the palm and wrist meet on the thumb side. Other common sites for multiple affected joints are the hand and the spine.

Dangers

Serious problems can arise when the disease affects the spine in the neck, causing pain and stiffness. This condition is known as *cervical spondylosis*. Three problems can arise from this.

The first is pain and stiffness of the neck. The second and third, which are serious but rare, arise from attempts of the bone to repair itself, leading to bone overgrowth. Pressure on the blood vessels to the lower part of the brain will cut off the blood supply, leading possibly to blackouts and dizziness. Pressure on the spinal cord or its nerves will lead to weakness in both the arms and legs.

Treatment

For drug treatment, joint replacement surgery and aids, *see* ARTHRITIS.

Apart from joint replacement, an operation called an *osteotomy*, where the bones on either side of a joint are remodelled, can be of great value as it improves the way the joint carries weight. This operation tends to be used in younger patients, since no one is certain how long artificial joints last, and there is always the option of replacing the joint at some later stage.

Finally the joint can be completely fused so that it cannot move and cannot cause pain. Although this sounds drastic, it can be extremely successful in some patients. It can bring tremendous pain relief, often without much loss of function in the affected limb, which probably was fairly stiff in the first place.

Osteochondritis, *see* **Orthopaedics**

Osteomalacia, *see* **Bones and bone diseases, Rickets**

Osteopathy

This is a system of medicine which concentrates its diagnosis and treatment essentially on the BONES, MUSCLES, ligaments and JOINTS in the body (*see* MANIPULATIVE THERAPIES). At the same time, however, it is a therapy which recognizes all parts of the body and takes into account people's health, life-style, environment, NUTRITION and STRESS factors in regard to treatment.

Osteopaths are highly trained practitioners who use their hands to treat the body when illness arises; to restore body control mechanisms: relieve PAIN and discomfort; and improve the flexibility and the range of movement of every joint in the body.

Although MASSAGE and manipulation have existed since ancient times, the art and science of osteopathy originated in the United States in the late 19th century. The founder, Andrew Taylor Still, had qualified as a doctor, but like many of his contemporaries, he was deeply sceptical of many of the methods then in use. He had begun to develop a consuming interest in the structure of the body during his childhood, and he chose 'osteopathy' (bone disease) as the name for his system of healing to underline the principle that 'structure governs function.' Although this was doubted by the medical profession of his day, modern research has lent some truth to the principle. The self-regulating activities which keep numerous body functions within proper limits (HOMOEOSTASIS) are closely related to the structural components by different reflexes of the NERVOUS SYSTEM. By working to bring back to normal the relationships of joints (especially of the intervertebral joints of the spine; *see* BACK AND BACKACHE), muscles, ligaments and connective tissue, the osteopath is able to produce far-reaching, and sometimes dramatic, effects for the whole body.

Scope of osteopathy

Most people who consult an osteopath do so because they have pain and restricted movement somewhere – often in the lower back, or the neck, or perhaps the shoulder. These injuries arise for many different reasons ranging from accidents to RHEUMATISM.

Medicine divides diseases into the principal categories of 'organic' and 'functional'. Organic illnesses are those in which destruction or permanent alteration of some body tissue or system occurs – for instance, tuberculosis, cancer, diseases of bone, cirrhosis of the liver or coronary artery disease. Functional illnesses occur when the body is not working properly, either because of infection, changes in blood pressure, or by recurring symptoms of migraine or asthma, for example. Many illnesses called 'PSYCHOSOMATIC' are given this label because no obvious medical reason can be found for the disorder. The presence of anxiety, stress, and emotional or personality problems often accompanies these disorders with the resulting symptoms of muscular tension, disturbed circulation, and altered nerve and hormonal supply. Osteopathy, by treating these associated symptoms manually, has a constructive and powerful role to play in the healing process.

Osteopathic treatment is suitable for people of all ages, male or female. It is especially applicable to growing children since, if potential disorders are detected and treated at this stage, future disability can be prevented. Strains, sprains, falls and other minor injuries generally are only painful for a time, but long-term effects caused by muscular and ligamentous shortening, fibrosis and minor derangements in joints are common. Eventually, lack of exercise, OBESITY, increasing age, or a subsequent injury can reveal these weaknesses. Increased susceptibility to injury or the onset of ARTHRITIS are common developments of these earlier problems if they are left untreated.

Training

Osteopaths undergo a four-year training in specialized colleges after first studying the biological sciences. They study medical disciplines including anatomy, physiology, pathology, biochemistry and NEUROLOGY, as well as the specialized subjects of osteopathic diagnosis and treatment. The distinctive feature of the training is the development of great sensitivity of the hands.

Practitioners who have completed a formal training will be Members of the Register of Osteopaths (MRO), although they may also have other professional qualifications such as DO (Diploma in Osteopathy).

Treatment

It is not necessary for you to be referred by your doctor. You can actually just make an appointment to see an osteopath yourself. Osteopaths practise under common law in Britain and their services are therefore not generally available through the health service (although some fund-holding GPs may 'buy them in'. The names of qualified osteopaths may be obtained by consulting one of the professional osteopathic associations.

A typical session lasts about 20 to 30 minutes. Once the cause of pain or illness has been determined, the osteopath will decide if manipulation is safe and desirable, and if so, what type of treatment to apply. Frequently, any specific spinal manipulation is preceded by soft tissue work, massage, stretching and putting the joints through their range of movement. Some osteopaths practise a specialized form of manipulation applied to the head and upper neck (*cranial osteopathy*). This is a gentle treatment and is particularly useful for young children and for treating functional disorders such as MIGRAINE, SINUSITIS and visual disturbances.

The number of sessions needed varies widely among individuals, but most osteopaths prefer to give a course of treatment sufficient to resolve the main problem, improve general mobility and health and to prevent further problems in the future.

Diagnosis of a problem can involve initial X-rays, blood and urine tests and referral to specific specialists.

Dangers

There are a number of diseases and conditions for which manipulation is undesirable, or even dangerous. The skill and experience of the practitioner should determine whether treatment of spinal disc herniation or prolapses (SLIPPED DISC), OSTEOARTHRITIS or severe SCIATICA is attempted. However, TUBERCULOSIS, CANCER, FRACTURES, acute ARTHRITIS, various diseases of bone and severe cases of prolapsed discs which cause neurological symptoms should not be manipulated under any circumstances. A qualified osteopath is able to detect these conditions and make appropriate referrals, but others may not. Repeated manipulation of the same joints is also inadvisable, since this can lead to stretching of the ligaments and instability of the joint.

Osteoporosis

The BONES in our bodies are not, as some people imagine, dead, but living material which is constantly changing. When such change involves a significant loss of bone, it is described as osteoporosis.

Causes

The most common cause is, in fact, age. From middle age onwards, everyone's bones become lighter. This change is more marked in women after the MENOPAUSE or 'change of life', but in both men and women, lighter bones are normal in old age. It is only when an excessive amount of bone is lost that symptoms of osteoporosis arise.

Osteoporosis is much more common in women than in men, and affects white people more often than black people.

There are other, more complicated causes of osteoporosis, most of which are rare. In these cases, the loss of bone is usually a result of drastic changes in the body brought about by another illness. In this case, the osteoporosis is described as secondary, since it is an effect of the initial, or primary, illness which will disappear if that illness is cured. Many of these rare causes are diseases of the hormonal system.

There is, however, one relatively common secondary cause, generally described as immobilization, which simply means that the patient is 'laid up' for some reason. Thus osteoporosis is often seen in the bones of a single limb which cannot be moved because of pain, paralysis or a broken (fractured) bone.

Symptoms

The condition may cause no symptoms at all or alternatively, it may give rise to bone PAIN OR BACKACHE.

Advanced cases suffer from deformities such as loss of height or a bent spine. The bones will tend to break rather easily, even as a result of some minor accident or trivial strain.

The commonest fracture associated with the condition is collapse of one of the vertebrae (small bones) of the spine. This may not hurt, or it may give rise to severe pain over that bone, which tends to improve without treatment over the next two or three months. In the long term, several of these fractures may occur, and as a result, the spine becomes shortened and bent, giving the person a characteristic stoop – known in elderly women as a 'dowager's hump' and medically as KYPHOSIS.

The other common fracture sites are the HIP and WRIST. The hip is more than usually vulnerable in old people whose poor balance and general stiffness make them liable to fall. If an elderly patient has osteoporosis, a relatively minor blow – or, as the doctors say, trauma – will often be enough to break the hip-bone.

Diagnosis

The diagnosis of osteoporosis is confirmed with X-rays and blood tests. Often an X-ray taken for some other reason will reveal it. On the processed X-ray film, the affected bones look blacker, and hidden fractures may be found.

The blood tests are done mainly to check whether the patient has other diseases that have similar symptoms, or whether there is a disease which can cause secondary osteoporosis, such as thyrotoxicosis – an overactive THYROID.

Dangers

Although osteoporosis itself is not a fatal condition, it is a major cause of pain and disability among the elderly, particularly women. Repeated fractures may confine an osteoporosis sufferer to a wheelchair.

A hip fracture is a serious injury requiring hospital treatment and often an operation, which invariably carries certain risks for an elderly person.

The back troubles associated with the condition may affect the nerves leading from the spine to the limbs, giving pain and weakness. In the most advanced cases, the back can become bent almost double, and there may be considerable breathing difficulty.

Treatment

Maintaining mobility in later life keeps the bones strong: regular exercise can prevent osteoporosis in both men and women. If it does occur, the aim of treatment is to keep the patient mobile. Exercise promotes strong bones, and prevents their deterioration, so following a fracture the patient is encouraged to get moving as soon as possible.

To give the bones the best conditions for growth, an ample protein diet is advised, and the raw materials for bone – CALCIUM and VITAMIN D – are given. Several drugs have been tried, as yet without proven benefits.

HORMONE REPLACEMENT THERAPY is given to women who suffer symptoms from the 'change of life' and involves giving the hormone oestrogen, which the body stops producing naturally at the menopause. There is no doubt that osteoporosis in women is largely the result of lack of natural oestrogen. Hormone replacement therapy does help to prevent it, but it must be commenced at around the time of the menopause and needs to be continued for several years. There is a possibility of side-effects of the treatment, but most doctors agree that benefits outweigh the risks.

Osteosarcoma, *see* **Sarcoma**

Osteotomy, *see* **Osteoarthritis**

Otitis externa, Otitis media, *see* **Deafness, Ears**

Otosclerosis, *see* **Deafness, Ears**

Ovaries

These are the parts of the female reproductive system which are designed to make and release mature *ova*, or egg cells. When an ovum is fertilized by a SPERM from a man, it marks the start of a new human life. From the first PERIOD to the MENOPAUSE, normal ovaries release one egg about once a month. They are also essential parts of the body's hormonal, or ENDOCRINE SYSTEM.

Location and structure

The ovaries are two grey-pink, almond-shaped structures each about 1.2 in (3 cm) long and about 0.4 in (1 cm) thick. They are found in the pelvis, the body cavity bounded by the hip bones, and lie one on each side of the UTERUS (womb). Each ovary is held in place by strong, elastic ligaments. Just above each ovary is the feathery opening of the Fallopian tube which leads to the uterus. Although they are very close to each other, there is no direct connection between the ovary and the tube opening.

In a mature woman, the ovaries have a rather lumpy appearance. The reason for this can be seen by looking at the internal structure under a microscope. Covering the ovary is a layer of cells called the *germinal epithelium*. It is from the cells in this border layer that the eggs, or ova, form: thousands of immature eggs, each in a round casing or *follicle* (the egg sac) can be seen clustered near the ovary edge.

Much more noticeable, however, are the follicles containing eggs in various stages of maturation. As these follicles enlarge, and after their eggs have been released, they produce the characteristic bumps on the ovary surface. The centre of the ovary is filled with elastic fibrous tissue which acts as a support for the follicle-containing outer layer.

Ovulation

Under a microscope, maturing follicles of the ovary can be seen as tiny balls enclosing a small mound of cells. In the centre of the mound is the egg cell in its final stages of maturation. When the follicle is ripe and the ovum mature, the cells at the follicle edge allow the ovum to leave. Exactly how this happens

Site, structure and function of ovaries

The ovaries are covered by a layer of cells. The cells which are destined to become eggs pass into the substance of the ovaries, where they are surrounded by a follicle membrane. Each month a single follicle matures, bursts on one ovary's surface and is released. If fertilized, the corpus luteum – which develops at the site of the egg's follicle – grows and secretes hormones that maintain pregnancy.

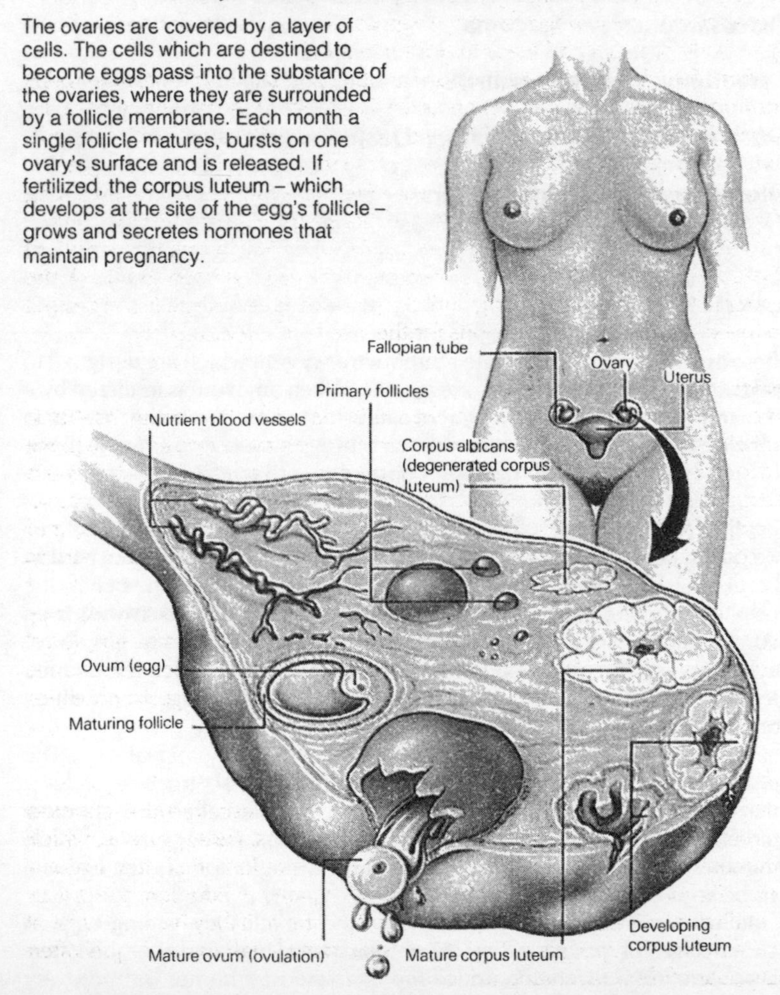

is still a mystery. The ovum is then wafted by the feathery ends, of *fimbria*, of the Fallopian tubes into the tube openings.

Some women feel a dull pain in their abdomen at the time of ovulation. This is what is known as *Mittelschmerz* (German for 'middle-pain'). The pain occurs when the egg is released. Not every woman experiences this, so it is not a reliable indicator of whether or not she is ovulating.

In their role as egg producers, the ovaries also act as hormonal or endocrine glands. The ovaries function under the control of the PITUITARY gland at the base of the brain. The pituitary first makes *follicle-stimulating hormone* (FSH) which travels in the bloodstream to the ovaries. FSH stimulates follicles and ovum development but it also brings about the secretion of the hormone *oestrogen*. Under oestrogen influence, the lining of the uterus thickens in preparation for receiving a fertilized egg. Oestrogen also stimulates the build up of body proteins and leads to fluid retention.

After a follicle has ripened and burst another pituitary hormone, *luteinizing hormone*, or LH, goes into action and brings about the development of the *corpus luteum* ('yellow body') in the empty follicle. It makes and releases its own hormone, *progesterone*. If the egg is not fertilized within a fortnight, the *corpus luteum* shrinks, progesterone production is turned off, and the lining of the uterus is shed as the monthly menstrual PERIOD. FSH production – which is lower during the second half of the cycle – rises just before the period, to begin ripening another follicle. If, however, the egg has been fertilized, the *corpus luteum* goes on working until the placenta is established, and there is no bleeding and no more periods for the whole of the PREGNANCY.

Ovary development

Ovary development is largely complete by the time the female foetus is in the third month of life in the womb, and few major changes will take place until puberty. By the time a baby girl is born, her ovaries contain, between them, from 40,000 to 300,000 primary follicles, each containing an immature egg. At most only 500 or so of these eggs will ever be released, and probably no more than half a dozen – if that – will develop into new human beings.

At the MENOPAUSE, the ovaries stop making hormones and, as a result, they also stop releasing eggs. The many mature eggs remaining in them simply fail to develop any further. As the years after the menopause pass, the ovaries gradually shrink and become full of fibrous tissue which largely obliterates the remaining eggs.

What can go wrong

Apart from the normal failure of the ovaries at menopause, the most common problem of the ovaries is the formation of ovarian CYSTS. These growths, which are usually benign, may grow to such vast proportions that they make a woman's abdomen swell up as if she were pregnant; in addition, some may be malignant. Cysts may cause pain if they rupture, or if they become twisted and their blood supply is cut off. However, many small ovarian cysts often disappear of their own accord.

Ovarian cysts are most common between the ages of 30 and 60, but can occur beyond that. There is evidence that some cysts may arise as a result of the changing hormonal balance as the menopause approaches.

See also ECTOPIC PREGANANCY.

Examining the ovaries

From the outside of the body, the only way a doctor can examine the ovaries is by feeling, or palpating, the woman's abdomen with his or her hands. Lumps in the ovaries may be felt more easily and be better assessed by performing a vaginal, or internal, examination.

A more thorough assessment of the ovaries can be carried out using an ULTRASOUND scan – a completely painless examination performed in an out-patient clinic. The scan machine builds up a television-type picture showing the size, shape and density of the ovaries. Cysts can be easily detected. Alternatively, a laparoscopy can be performed. A small instrument rather like a slim telescope is passed into the abdomen through a small incision while the patient is under an anaesthetic (*see* ENDOSCOPY). The doctor can then look directly at the ovaries and if necessary take tissue samples.

Ovulation, *see* Ovaries

Oxygen

This makes up about a fifth of the air that we breathe, and the work of the LUNGS, the HEART and the blood vessels is primarily concerned with carrying oxygen from the air to the body's tissues, where it is needed to produce the energy that they require in order to stay alive.

Oxygen is an odourless, tasteless and colourless gas. Its main source on Earth is from living green plants.

What oxygen does

Oxygen is essential for the production of energy. Just as a car burns petrol with oxygen, and a coal fire uses both coal and the oxygen in a room to produce heat, so the body's CELLS use oxygen in exactly the same way: they burn up their fuel – which usually comes in the form of sugar – with oxygen to produce energy. The waste products of this chemical reaction are the same in both the body's cells and the car – namely, carbon dioxide and water. Although some of the body's cells are able to function for a while without oxygen, the BRAIN cannot.

Oxygen from the air is inhaled, then absorbed by the lungs and carried in the BLOOD to the body tissues. When the amount of oxygen needed for a particular physical task is greater than can be supplied at the time, an 'oxygen debt' results. A person makes up the supply by panting and breathing deeply so as to take in as much oxygen as possible immediately after the period of exertion.

Oxygen deficiency

There are two main groups of people likely to suffer from a shortage of oxygen in the blood: those with lung disease, and those with the sort of heart complaint that keeps the lungs short of blood.

A lack of oxygen shows up as a blueness around the lips and tongue, which is known medically as *cyanosis. Haemoglobin,* the red pigment in blood which takes up oxygen in the lungs, carries it to the tissues where it is released. Saturated haemoglobin is haemoglobin that has its full amount of oxygen; it then is red in colour. But haemoglobin with insufficient oxygen tends to be more purple. Hence a preponderance of low-oxygen haemoglobin leads to the blue look of cyanosis.

Almost any sort of lung condition can lead to a low level of oxygen in the blood. Chronic BRONCHITIS is perhaps the most common. It is often combined with EMPHYSEMA, a disease in which the lung tissue is destroyed to such an extent that fewer air-sacs than normal are available for the exchange of oxygen between blood and tissues.

A lack of oxygen is also associated with acute attacks of ASTHMA. Severe PNEUMONIA, too, may also lead to cyanosis. And it may be necessary to give oxygen to people who have suffered a HEART ATTACK, as the flow of blood – and hence the delivery of oxygen to the body's tissues – will have been drastically reduced.

Oxytocin, *see* Induction, Pituitary

P

Pacemaker

We rely on the regular beating of the HEART to stay alive. This regular heartbeat depends upon the heart's own natural pacemaker – the part of the heart called the *sino-atrial node.* This initiates impulses that then spread through the heart via a system of specialized electrical conducting tissues. The entire electrical timing system is the conducting system of the heart.

Who needs a pacemaker?
Unfortunately, the heart's own pacing system can sometimes go wrong. This can occur as a result of CORONARY HEART DISEASE, a hardening or blocking of the coronary ARTERIES. Alternatively, a HEART ATTACK may give rise to conducting system difficulties, requiring a pacemaker to be put in as a matter of urgency. Often these pacemakers are only temporary as the heart may recover its ability to control its own timing. If and when this occurs, the pacemaker will be removed in a simple operation.

The majority of patients who require a permanent pacemaker are those in whom the conducting system has broken down entirely. There is no obvious cause for this – it is almost as though the conducting system has worn out. The condition is more common in the elderly. In fact, most patients who need pacemakers are over the age of 65 (*see* HEART DISEASE).

When the heart stops conducting electrical impulses properly, the heart rate slows down; this is known as *heart block* or *arrythmia.* The condition may be variable, leading to sudden attacks of fainting and UNCONSCIOUSNESS. The heart may even stop completely, and if emergency treatment isn't given, death will result. On the other hand, patients may suffer from a continuously slow pulse rate. Although this is enough to keep patients well while they're resting, it leads to lethargy and breathlessness on exertion, which is disabling.

How a pacemaker works
The basic principle in all the various sorts of pacemaker is exactly the same. Two parts make up the pacing system. First, there is some electronic means of producing regular electrical impulses that are of the correct strength and duration to cause the ventricles, the main pumping chambers of the heart, to beat. This impulse is conducted to the heart by a wire, called a *pacing lead,* whose tip is implanted somewhere in the substance of the ventricles. Provided the impulses are strong enough, and there is good electrical connection between the wire and the muscle of the ventricle, a heartbeat will result from each impulse.

To coordinate the timing of the heartbeat, an *impulse generator* or *pacing box*, sends electrical impulses to the heart via the pacing lead. This enables it to 'know' when there has been a heartbeat so that it doesn't send another impulse until the heart is ready. This is called 'demand pacing', and is almost always the system used as it allows the heart specialist to programme the pacemaker.

What happens then is that the pacing box is set at a given rate – say, 60 beats per minute. This means that the box will produce an impulse every second, unless it senses that the heart has produced a beat on its own. If the heart does do this, the pacing box will then wait for another second before producing its next impulse, and so on.

Putting in a pacemaker

Two sorts of pacing systems are used, and both are inserted with the patient having local anaesthesia. The first is a temporary system. A pacing lead is passed through the skin via a special needle and into a large vein, usually around the shoulder. It is then passed into the right atrium, through the tricuspid valve and into the tip of the right ventricle, where it makes contact with the heart muscle. The position of the wire is followed on an X-ray so that it can be guided into the right place. If it is fixed to the skin, it is fairly unlikely to be dislodged. The other end of the wire is attached to a pacing box which remains outside the patient's body.

For a permanent system, the same principle is used. Once the wire is connected to the pacing box, and the electrical connection between the wire and heart is shown to be adequate, the pacing box is sewn into a special pocket under the skin of the chest. Although the pacing box is only the size of a matchbox, it contains enough battery power to keep producing impulses for years – more than ten years in some cases. However, pacemakers are 'serviced' regularly by hospitals.

Paget's disease

Osteitis (inflammation of BONES) exists in several forms, but by far the most common is Paget's disease, or *osteitis deformans*, where the bones are often deformed and weakened. The disease was first described by Sir James Paget in 1870. Much has been learned since about the symptoms and treatment, but the causes of the disease still remain a mystery.

In Britain, Germany, Australia and most other Western countries, Paget's disease affects about 3 per cent of the population over 40 years of age, and it is equally common among men and women. It is rare, however, in Asia, Africa and the Middle East. As yet no genetic factor has been proved, but the disease does sometimes appear to run in families.

Symptoms

Many of the people suffering from Paget's disease have no symptoms at all.

But sometimes these can be unbearably severe and complications can develop.

The disease is diagnosed on X-ray by the alternate light and dark areas of bone. The bones most commonly affected are the skull, the vertebrae of the backbone, the pelvis and the femur and tibia of the leg. Deformity in the long bones is most obvious – the bones bow outwards under the weight of the rest of the body as the bone loses its strength and softens. Strange irregularities in the bone structure show up on X-rays. A 'shepherd's crook'-shaped lump is typical on the top end of the femur. Also, the skull becomes lumpy and also much thicker.

These changes occur because bone cells become super-active and bone resorption (the normal destructive process balanced by growth) proceeds at 10 to 20 times the normal rate. The new bone that is laid down is usually more fragile and less elastic. This means that a small knock can cause a fracture. In very bad cases, bones can break on their own.

Pain is one of the worst symptoms of osteitis: nerves squashed by the enlarging bone may be one cause, but changes in the actual bone structure cause stresses and strain that trigger the pain pathways of the body.

Bone pressure on the auditory nerves coming from the ears can cause DEAFNESS. Sometimes the same result occurs through deformation of the auditory ossicles, the three tiny sound transmitting bone structures in the ears. Beethoven's deafness is said to have been caused by Paget's disease.

BLINDNESS can also be caused by bones pinching the optic nerves. But most of all, the bone at the base of the skull occasionally softens and sticks into the brain-stem. The person may then lose control over vital functions such as breathing.

Treatment

In the past, treatment was not very satisfactory. Drugs are now available that can control the symptoms of disease without the dangerous side-effects that accompanied early therapy.

A hormone called calcitonin (*see* CALCIUM) is the most successful treatment to be given to people with Paget's disease. This is because the main problem in the disease is an imbalance in the function of bone growth and resorption (in normal bones this is a process which is going on all the time). Calcitonin helps by adjusting the balance between these two important processes to a normal level.

With this drug, the rate of bone turnover drops and the temperature of the skin over the diseased bone falls back to normal. Often this drug will be effective against pain, too. Injections have to be given daily and sometimes nausea is a side-effect.

Another drug called Etidronate, which can be given by mouth, may also be prescribed. It is particularly effective in relieving bone pain. It may be given as an alternative to calcitonin, and in some cases the two drugs are used together.

Pain

A large section of the NERVOUS SYSTEM participates in the sensation which we call pain – from the peripheral nerves to the most sophisticated thinking areas of the cerebral cortex in the BRAIN. There are many different types of pain: these depend on the variety of stimuli by which they are caused, and the way in which these stimuli are analysed by the nervous networks in the SPINAL CORD and brain. In addition, cultural and social factors play an enormous role in determining our mind's response to the perception of pain.

How pain comes about

Painful stimuli inside and outside our bodies excite otherwise unspecialized nerve endings in the SKIN and elsewhere. These nerve endings are attached to nerves of two different types. One is fast-conducting and conveys its information rapidly to the spinal cord; the other also takes its information to the spinal cord but in a more leisurely fashion. This helps to distinguish between two types of pain: the immediately felt – and therefore reacted to – tapping or pricking pain, and the deep, dull, aching pain.

These nerve endings make many contacts with the network of fibres in the spinal cord which are responsible for the initial analysis of our sensations and pain in particular. A second nerve fibre then takes this more organized information upwards to the brain. Again this happens by two different pathways: one makes fairly directly for the thalamus (the main sensory relay station deep in the brain), while the other leads a more meandering course, making many connections with centres in the brainstem before also arriving at the thalamus. This enables the cortex (the part of the brain with which we actually perceive the pain) to obtain both direct, fast reports of the painful situation plus more slowly arriving but more heavily analysed information by the slow pathway.

The thalamus, which analyses this information for presentation to the cerebral cortex, has rich connections with the areas of the brain concerned with the maintenance of emotional tone and those concerned with arousal. So before our perceiving brain receives any information – but especially painful stimuli – it is heavily tinged by our emotional state and affected by our level of arousal.

The final arbiter as to whether we perceive pain is the cerebral cortex. It seems that large areas of this part of the brain participate in this complex perception. The frontal lobes, especially those parts of them concerned with the analysis of emotions (that is, the parts of the frontal lobes which connect with the 'limbic system'), seem to be important for our perception of painful stimuli as unpleasant. People who have lost this part of their brains report that they can feel pain but are not upset by it. The parietal lobes of the brain seem to be important in the localization of the painful stimulus, but they also participate in perception of the sensations associated with pain.

Psychological aspects of pain

As large areas of the nervous system participate in our feelings and responses to painful stimuli, it is not surprising that the state of a person's mind is an important factor in his or her perception of pain. This state of mind is strongly influenced by the situation in which the pain occurs and the cultural and social background against which our attitudes to pain have grown up.

In the heat of a battle, a soldier may feel no pain even though he has suffered substantial injuries because his mind may be so occupied with the battle. Later, when the wound is being dressed, the pain may be severe, although the injury is unchanged. With practitioners of yoga in India, the mind may be so diverted away from the painful stimuli by contemplation of other things that what appear to be great feats of endurance – such as lying on beds of nails – can be achieved. It is likely that such people are not actually feeling the pain in the same way as we would, rather than enduring it: they have managed to divert their minds from the unpleasant significance of the stimuli undoubtedly reaching their brains.

The other side of this coin is the psychological effect that pain can have on us. Prolonged severe pain can start a vicious cycle whereby the mental ability to cope with pain is progressively eroded and often appears to change a person's personality. It makes them pay attention to the pain to a greater degree, perceiving it as more and more severe.

It is therefore wrong to consider pain as only being 'in the mind' because all pain is a mental process to a greater or lesser extent, depending on the circumstances.

Painkillers

The medical term for a pain-relieving drug is an *analgesic*. Doctors usually divide pain-killing drugs into two categories – narcotic and non-narcotic. Narcotics, such as morphine and heroin, which are derived from opium, and their synthetic relations such as pethidine and methadone, act principally on the brain and often produce drug dependence. Non-narcotic drugs, such as aspirin, are rarely addictive as such and act on the site of the pain. Narcotic drugs are usually used in highly controlled conditions such as in hospital, to give relief for pain in internal organs. The non-narcotic drugs are used to control pain felt in the joints, muscles, bones or skin.

Aspirin

Aspirin is probably the best known and most widely used drug. Not only does it relieve pain, it also reduces fever and has an anti-inflammatory effect on joints (*see* INFLAMMATION). This is why doctors often prescribe aspirin for INFLUENZA – not necessarily to kill any pain the patient may be feeling – which is often more discomfort than pain – but to reduce the temperature and to help ease the aches in joints often experienced in such an illness. Aspirin is used for ARTHRITIS, often over extended periods, because of this anti-inflammatory property. Aspirin and another, more recent painkiller, ibuprofen, belong to a group of drugs called 'non-steroidal inflammatory drugs' (NSAIDs).

However, aspirin can also be extremely dangerous to some people in certain circumstances. It is an irritant and can cause stomach pain, with nausea and vomiting. But far more important, if swallowed whole, an aspirin tablet will not just irritate the stomach lining but may even cause bleeding. For this reason, aspirin should never be taken on an empty stomach without a drink of water. Never take more than 12 tablets (3.6 g) in 24 hours. Aspirin can be extremely dangerous to old people on poor diets, especially if they are low in iron, and to patients who are weak from an illness.

Some people may react badly to aspirin, and others may have a definite allergy. Since aspirin is present in many commercial drugs, either as aspirin or under chemical compound terms such as *acetylsalicylate* it is important to read the list of ingredients on preparations you buy for mild illnesses, to check that you are not giving it by mistake to someone who is allergic to it, or to someone who suffers from indigestion.

Children under 12 should not be given aspirin because it may cause severe side-effects, particularly when given during certain viral illnesses such as influenza or chickenpox.

Other common analgesics

If, for any reason, a patient should not take aspirin, paracetamol is often a good alternative. Paracetamol is also a mild pain reliever and can reduce the temperature, although it has no effect on inflammation. It does not irritate the stomach lining and so can be used for abdominal pain. However, paracetamol can affect the function of the kidneys and the liver and so should not be taken in very high doses over long periods. In fact, paracetamol can cause enough liver damage to kill several days after an overdose.

Codeine is an opium-derived drug, often used as part of anti-diarrhoea and cough suppressant medicines. As well as being a mild pain reliever, it slows down the action of the bowel and suppresses the cough centre in the brain. Codeine is rarely used on its own but is often combined with other drugs, commonly aspirin and paracetamol. It increases their effects, and adds a mild pain-relieving action on the brain while aspirin or paracetamol affects the site of the pain itself.

MORPHINE is made from opium. If taken repeatedly it becomes addictive, and the painkilling effect lessens as the patient builds up a tolerance to the drug. Despite this problem, morphine is the most effective painkiller available.

Because many drugs cross the placenta to the baby, pregnant women should be cautious about taking painkillers (or any other drug). As a general rule avoid all drugs during the first three months of pregnancy. After that, the *occasional* dose of aspirin or paracetamol during pregnancy is generally regarded as being quite safe. But ask your doctor's advice if you have persisting headache or backache before taking any such drugs for more than a day or so.

Pain should be looked on rather like a burglar alarm. It would be foolish and harmful to switch off the alarm and then leave the burglars rampaging through your house: so in most cases, the cause rather than the symptom should be sought and cured. But, just as many burglar alarms go off because of passing interference, we sometimes feel pain for temporary and passing reasons which do not need the care of a doctor. In these cases, the right painkiller is necessary and beneficial. However, it is not advisable to continue taking over-the-counter painkillers for longer than two to three days. If the pain persists, medical advice should be sought.

Alternatives

It is worth noting that analgesics are not the only way to relieve pain. Non-chemical methods such as applying cold water (for burns and bruises), or heat and MASSAGE (for aches) can bring relief, while techniques on the fringes of orthodox medicine such as ACUPUNCTURE, electrical stimulation, MEDITATION and biofeedback are well worth trying in really chronic cases.

Palpitations, *see* **Heart disease, Psychosomatic disorders, Tachycardia, Thyroid**

Palsy, *see* **Parkinson's disease**

Pancreas

The pancreas, one of the largest GLANDS in the body, is really two glands in one. Almost all its cells are concerned with secretion. It is an ENDROCRINE gland secreting HORMONES, of which insulin is the most important. It is also an *exocrine* gland – which secretes into the gut, rather than the blood.

Position and structure

The pancreas lies across the upper part of the ABDOMEN, in front of the spine and on top of the aorta and the vena cava (the body's main artery and vein). The DUODENUM is wrapped round the 'head' of the pancreas. The rest of it consists of the 'body' and 'tail', stretching out over the spine to the left.

The basic structures in the pancreas are the *acini,* collections of secreting cells round the blind end of a small duct. Each duct joins up with ducts from other acini until all of them eventually connect with the main duct running down the centre of the pancreas. Among the acini are small groups of cells called the 'islets of Langerhans': these constitute the whole 'other life' of the pancreas as an endocrine organ secreting the insulin which is needed by the body for the constant control of its sugar level.

The exocrine pancreas The pancreas produces essential alkali in the form of sodium bicarbonate to neutralize the heavily acid contents of the stomach as they enter the duodenum. It also produces a number of important ENZYMES which help to break food down into its basic chemical constituents; these are then absorbed through the wall of the intestine.

The fact that most of the main enzymes for the DIGESTION of PROTEIN are produced by the pancreas creates something of a problem, because the pancreas itself, like the rest of the body, is basically a protein-based structure. There is, therefore, quite a risk that it might digest itself, but this is avoided by the main protein-digesting enzyme – *trypsin* – being secreted in an inactive form called *trypsinogen*, which changes to the active form once the pancreatic juices reach the duodenum. The pancreas also produces *amylase* and *lipase*, important enzymes which break down CARBOHYDRATES and FATS respectively.

These digestive juices are powerful, and cannot be released into the intestine safely unless there is food there for them to act upon. There is, therefore, a very sophisticated control system acting on pancreatic secretion. The *vagus nerve* – the main nerve of the parasympathetic system (*see* AUTONOMIC NERVOUS SYSTEM) – stimulates the first small secretion as a result of the thought, taste or smell of food. Further secretion is stimulated by distension of the stomach, but most of the secretion takes place when the food finally reaches the duodenum. As this happens, cells in the wall of the duodenum release two separate hormones into the bloodstream, *secretin* and *pancreozymin*, which travel in the blood to the pancreas and speed up secretion. (Secretin was, in fact, the first hormone to be discovered, in 1902.)

The endocrine pancreas The most important pancreatic hormone is, of course, insulin, produced by the beta cells of the islets of Langerhans, to lower the level of blood SUGAR and to prevent DIABETES.

The islets also produce a hormone called *glucagon* which has the effect of *raising* rather than lowering the level of sugar in the blood.

What can go wrong?

The main problem that occurs with the pancreas is when it ceases to produce insulin, resulting in diabetes.

There are really only three diseases that cause trouble on the digestive side of the organ's activity, all of them rather rare.

The first is *acute pancreatitis*, inflammation of the organ that can cause an emergency, with sudden pain in the abdomen and collapse. The second is a related disease called *chronic pancreatitis*, where there are recurrent attacks of pain, and failure of the pancreas to produce adequate amounts of digestive juice. The third is the inherited disease CYSTIC FIBROSIS, in which many of the glands, including the pancreas, are unable to produce proper secretions.

When there is inadequate secretion of digestive juice, MALABSORPTION results. One of its commoner causes is chronic pancreatitis, which is accompanied by pain in the abdomen, sometimes so severe that the pancreas has to be removed. Eventually the endocrine part of the pancreas will become involved; and this will lead to diabetes. Since chronic pancreatitis is often associated with excessive ALCOHOL consumption, avoidance of alcohol can improve the symptoms, and problems of malabsorption can be lessened by taking an extract of pancreas with food.

Acute pancreatitis also may be associated with alcohol, but the disease can often occur without an apparent cause. Sometimes acute pancreatitis is caused by a virus – very occasionally MUMPS can trigger off an attack. Gallstones (*see* GALL BLADDER) may be a factor in both acute and chronic pancreatitis, presumably because they cause inflammation or blockage at the point where the pancreatic duct and the BILE duct empty. Acute pancreatitis seems to result from a sudden tendency on the part of the pancreas to release active digestive juices inside itself, leading to a breakdown of its own substance, and resulting in severe pain in the stomach and collapse. The treatment is to support the patient's circulation with fluids while the problem settles down of its own accord.

Finally, the pancreas can produce a CANCER, which usually grows in the head of the organ near the duodenum, and is, unfortunately, very difficult to treat because it is usually rather advanced before it becomes apparent. Its symptoms are rather vague, although it can produce considerable pain and discomfort. If the point at which the bile duct drains becomes involved, JAUNDICE may be the feature that brings the cancer to light. Surgery may be necessary to re-establish the drainage of bile, but it is only undertaken to try to cure the disease in those cases where the cancer has not spread.

If the pancreas has to be removed, the body can still function satisfactorily. Insulin, which is essential to life, can be taken in the form of injections; digestive enzymes can be sprinkled on food; or, alternatively, the stomach can be prevented from producing acids with the drug cimetidine.

Papules, *see* **Moles, Rash**

Paracetamol, *see* **Liver and liver diseases, Painkillers**

Paraesthesia, *see* **Numbness, Pins and needles**

Paralysis

This involves the temporary or permanent loss of some muscular activities, and can be a serious threat to a person's independence – or life. In paralysis, the complex 'motor system' (*see* NERVOUS SYSTEM) which governs our movements can be attacked on a number of levels by many different diseases as well as by injuries. It is also important *where* the motor system is attacked, as well as by *what*.

What is paralysis?

Simply put, paralysis is the loss of normal functioning of the MUSCLES to a part of the body. When this happens, you will feel a weakness when you try to use that part of your body. This is obvious when paralysis affects your arm or leg muscles: walking will be difficult, or your grip will lose its strength. If, however, the muscles affected are the ones which make SPEECH possible, then paralysis may show itself in slurred or incoherent speech. Or, if the eye muscles are affected, double vision may be experienced. The common factor in all these symptoms is that some or all of the muscles are not working to their desired strength.

How does paralysis come about?
Our muscles are made up of tiny fibres grouped together in bundles. These bundles are each connected to the fibre of a single motor nerve cell, or 'motor neurone' in the SPINAL CORD. These motor neurones are closely connected with many other nerve networks in the spinal cord, and also with the fibres of the nerves descending from the BRAIN.

Paralysis can come about as a result of damage or malfunction of *any* part of this chain of command. Which component is damaged will have a great bearing on the character and distribution of the weakness that is experienced.

The muscles
When paralysis is caused by a disease of the muscles, the effect is usually felt on both sides of the body, generally affecting the shoulder and hip muscles most strongly. Diseases that affect the muscles and cause paralysis may be present from birth, such as MUSCULAR DYSTROPHY; or the cells of the muscles may become inflamed: this disease is called *myositis*. When these diseases strike, in addition to weakness the muscles often waste away, making the affected part of the body look thin. Walking may be difficult because the hip muscles are involved, and if the disease is severe enough, the leg muscles may become totally paralysed. Paralysis of the shoulder muscles will make shaving and brushing hair more difficult, even if the hands retain their ability to grip things. Of course, the diseases of the muscles that cause a degree of paralysis vary enormously in their severity, and very often the paralysis is only partial. In myositis, weakness may be accompanied by pain, since the inflammation causes the muscles to swell.

The muscle–nerve junction
The connection between the surface of the muscle fibres and the nerve fibres that come to them is not direct: instead there is a very short gap across which tiny quantities of a chemical transmitter 'jump' when the nerve is activated. In a disease called *myasthenia gravis*, the 'receptor' on the muscle fibres on to which the transmitter jumps is damaged, and a weakness ensues. This paralysis is progressive: the muscle gets weaker the more it is used, but will recover with rest.

The muscles that may be hit by this progressive paralysis vary, but often in addition to the shoulder and hip muscles, those governing the voice, swallowing and BREATHING may be involved. Breathing, for example, may become very difficult, so that artificial help is needed. When the throat muscles are affected, a drink may be regurgitated or 'go down the wrong way' into the lungs, causing the patient to choke.

Damage to the motor nerves
Weakness and paralysis of some groups of muscles can come about as a result of damage to the nerves serving those muscles. For example, in some people the ulnar nerve which passes down the arm is rather exposed close to the elbow and may be damaged if the elbow is jarred continually. This will lead to paralysis in the muscles of the hand. The grip will become weaker because

the thumb cannot be brought across the hand to meet the fingers when something is grasped.

Individual motor nerves may be damaged by SLIPPED DISCS in the spine: as the nerves emerge from the spinal cord the slipped discs may put pressure on them. Here the paralysis affects only part of the leg or arm, and unless the damage is severe or prolonged, relieving the pressure on the motor nerve will remove the paralysis.

The spinal cord

Damage to the spinal cord usually involves damage to the nerve fibres carrying the brain's instructions down both sides of the body. Where the spinal cord has been damaged will determine what parts of the body are paralysed. Both legs may be paralysed (paraplegia) or all four limbs if the damage is in the neck (*tetraplegia*). The spinal cord may be damaged in an accident where the BACK bones or neck are broken or displaced; or there may be blood vessel damage due to clots or haemorrhage; or alternatively there may be inflammation as in MULTIPLE SCLEROSIS. Occasionally if the cause of the paralysis – such as a depressed fragment of bone pressing on the spinal cord – can be removed quickly, there may be immediate relief.

Diseases of the spinal cord can also cause paralysis. For example, POLIO, which used to be very common, is an infection of the spinal cord by a virus. It starts with paralysis of an arm or a leg and may go on to involve the entire body.

The brain

The nerve fibres from the brain to the spinal cord that carry instructions to the muscles cross over from one side to the other at the bottom of the brain-stem as it meets the spinal cord. Damage to the nerves above this crossing-over will therefore cause weakness in the *opposite* side of the body. One of the most common causes of this type of paralysis is a STROKE, which is caused by failure of the blood supply to parts of the brain. If the part of the brain supplied by a particular blood vessel which has become blocked or has burst includes the motor nerves, then paralysis on the opposite side of the body will result. Strokes usually cause this paralysis very suddenly, and the brain's powers of recovery are considerable. Paralysis caused by brain TUMOURS develop more slowly and can be distinguished from strokes because of this. *See also* CEREBRAL PALSY, OCCUPATIONAL THERAPY, PHYSIOTHERAPY.

Paraphimosis, *see* Penis

Parasites

These live in or on their 'hosts', depending totally upon them for survival. People and animals are troubled by numerous types of parasites – they can be as small in size as a single cell, such as the MALARIAL parasite, or up to 65 ft (20 m) long, like the fish tapeworm. Parasites can damage their hosts in different ways. Some feed directly upon their tissues, such as the LIVER fluke, which feeds on liver cells; or the hookworm, which lives on its host's blood (*see* WORMS).

In Britain, parasites are not as common as in many other parts of the world (*see* TROPICAL DISEASES). Threadworms (*see* WORMS) are perhaps the most common – they live in the large INTESTINE, and lay eggs around the anal skin during the night, which causes intense itching. Children are most commonly affected.

Fleas, head and body LICE, and mites are also relatively common. They differ from other parasites because they live outside the body and feed exclusively on their hosts' blood.

The parasitic life-style

Parasites have adapted and modified their way of life in accordance with the life-styles of their hosts. They can overcome IMMUNE defences, so the body can do very little to fight the parasite.

They have voracious appetites. Each tiny hookworm, for example, consumes 8,000 times its own weight of human blood each day. The main reason for this is that parasites need to produce eggs or larvae at a colossal rate to ensure that reproduction takes place, and that new hosts are to be infected.

Ascaris is one of the most common parasitic worms – it infests a billion people around the world, and lives in the small intestine. The infestation is transmitted when the host eats food which has been contaminated with infected faeces.

Parasites which live in the tissues or in the bloodstream usually depend on mosquitoes or other biting insects – known as *vectors* – for transmission. Their larvae or reproductive cells are microscopic, and so have to be produced in huge numbers to make sure that an insect becomes infected each time it bites.

How parasites are spread

The eggs, cysts, or larvae of many parasites are to be found in the faeces of their hosts – whether animal or human.

In some countries, human faeces are still an important source of fertilizer and are spread over the land: in others, facilities for disposal of sewage are simply inadequate. Flies and cockroaches spread eggs directly from the faeces of one host to the food of another – so do dirty hands. Water from wells and rivers is easily contaminated by unhygienic disposal of faeces, and may also be contaminated by sewage.

Soil which has been contaminated with faeces often harbours larvae which are able to penetrate the bare feet of the next host – this is how hookworm is transmitted. Faeces may also contain eggs or cysts which infect secondary hosts – such as cows or pigs, in the case of the tapeworm, and fresh-water snails, in the case of schistosomiasis (bilharzia). In this way, the parasites multiply and are spread further afield.

Is it obvious that better sanitation, treatment and more careful disposal of faeces would interrupt the life cycles of all these parasites, and help bring the diseases that they cause under control. Better hygiene and more care when handling food are essential to prevention.

Meat infestation can be massive – pork may contain one million larvae of the parasite *trichinella* in a single gram (a fraction of an ounce) – and even a small quantity of such meat may be very dangerous. Thorough cooking is necessary to make meat safe.

The other important route of spread for parasites is by insect vectors. A vector becomes infected when it bites the host; the parasite multiples within it, and the infected vector is soon able to pass the disease on to new hosts with each bite. In this way, amoebic dysentery can be spread by flies, and malaria is spread by *Anopheles* mosquitoes. One way of controlling such diseases is by attacking the insect vector. This can be done by destroying breeding grounds, by draining mosquito-ridden swamps, and by the use of insecticides.

Effects of parasites

Some of the ways that parasites cause harm have already been mentioned. Often, however, the damage done to the host is really not obvious at all, or only appears after a long time.

Infestation with ascaris or tapeworms, which live in the intestines and feed on partly digested food, is often not noticed by a healthy host. But in poor countries, where food is scarce, such parasites are an important contributing factor in MALNUTRITION.

Treatment

Drugs are available to treat nearly all parasitic diseases, and treatment is often a simple matter. In some diseases, however, where the host suffers damage over a period of many years, treatment to kill the parasite may come too late – drugs cannot undo the liver damage which occurs in schistosomiasis, or the deformity of elephantiasis (*see* LYMPHATIC SYSTEM).

Drug treatment is not always as practical a solution for the treatment of large communities. Some drugs are too toxic for use on a large scale, and have to be carefully supervised. And sometimes it is simply pointless to give treatment to kill parasites when immediate re-infection is quite inevitable. Prevention is often where the emphasis should lie – e.g., improving sanitation and hygiene.

See also HOLIDAY HEALTH.

Parasympathetic nervous system, *see* Autonomic nervous system

Parathyroid

These are four tiny glands situated behind the THYROID glands, which in turn is found just below the LARYNX. They play a major part in controlling the levels of CALCIUM in the body. Calcium is a vital mineral: not only because it is the major structural element in the formation of bones and teeth, but also because it plays a central role in the workings of the muscles and nerve cells. The body's calcium levels have to be kept within pretty constant boundaries; otherwise the muscles stop working and fits may occur. This is where the parathyroid glands come in: they keep the calcium levels in balance.

The absorption of calcium into the bloodstream is controlled by VITAMIN D, which we get from sunlight and some foods, and an important hormone produced by the parathyroids called *parathyroid hormone* or PTH. If the level of calcium is too low, the parathyroids secrete an increased quantity of the hormone, which actually releases calcium from the bones to raise the level in the bloodstream. Conversely, if there is too much calcium, the parathyroids reduce or halt the production of PTH, thus bringing the level down.

The parathyroids are so small that they can be difficult to find. The upper two are situated behind the thyroid gland; the lower two, however, may actually be *inside* the thyroid or occasionally right down inside the chest.

Like most ENDOCRINE (hormone) glands, the parathyroids can cause two main problems. They can be overactive, and this leads to a high level of calcium in the bloodstream, or they can be underactive, allowing the level to get dangerously low.

Overactive parathyroids

Overactive parathyroids – *hyperparathyroidism* – are quite a common problem. It has now become usual practice to measure the level of calcium in the blood as a routine part of the biochemical screening test that is carried out on practically all hospital patients, and also on many patients by their own doctors. As a result, rather more instances of unexpectedly high blood calcium levels have been found – in the past, the level of calcium in the blood was measured only when an abnormality was suspected. It is now thought that as many as one person per 1,000 may have some degree of parathyroid overactivity.

Symptoms

A raised blood calcium level *may* be caused by hyperparathyroidism. It is important to realize that there could be other causes. For example, the other common cause of high levels of blood calcium is a CANCER that gives rise to secondary deposits of cancer tissue in the bones. This causes the bones to be eaten away and a lot of calcium is released into the bloodstream. An excessive intake of vitamin D, too, can also cause a raised calcium level.

Generally speaking, the two main symptoms of a raised calcium level are thirst and passing a lot of water. There may also be feelings of tiredness and poor concentration. Loss of appetite and vomiting may also result. Where overactive parathyroids are the cause of the high blood calcium, many patients develop KIDNEY stones. In this disease, the urine contains a lot of calcium and it tends to settle out in the kidneys to produce stones. People with overactive parathyroids also seem to suffer from indigestion. In about 10 per cent of cases, the amount of calcium that is released from the bones as a result of the high levels of PTH is so great that the bones themselves begin to show signs of strain – there may be bone pain, some loss of height and even spontaneous fractures (*see* OSTEOPOROSIS). X-rays will show a characteristic picture of cysts in the bones, particularly the hands. The combination of the bone problems, kidney stones and indigestion has led to the old saying among doctors that the disease causes problems with 'bones, stones and abdominal groans'.

Treatment

The only really effective treatment for the disease is surgical removal of the overactive gland or glands. In most cases, all the glands are found to be bigger than normal (hypertrophied), and standard surgical procedure is to identify all four glands and then to remove three-and-a-half. The remaining half gland provides enough PTH to keep the calcium level under control.

The parathyroid glands are very small organs, and not surprisingly they are extremely difficult for a surgeon to find during an operation. But oddly enough they take up a dye, called methylene blue, and one technique is to inject the patient with this dye before the operation. The parathyroids absorb the dye and can be seen more easily and distinguished from surrounding thyroid and other tissues.

In the remainder of cases, there is a tumour. Usually this affects only one gland, and only a tiny minority of patients will be found to have a tumour that is malignant (cancerous).

Underactive parathyroids

In contrast, underactivity (*hypoparathyroidism*) is very rare – unless, of course, the parathyroids are removed during surgery on the thyroid. People suffering from this disease are often rather tired; they may start having fits and there may be signs of *tetany* – a muscular spasm which affects the hands.

There also may be marked mental problems. Many patients will have DEPRESSION, but a surprising number show irrational overactivity – known as *mania*. As well as all the symptoms of low blood calcium, people with hypoparathyroidism are susceptible to candida infection of the nails (THRUSH).

Fortunately this disease can be combated effectively by taking vitamin D by mouth, although a careful eye has to be kept on the calcium level.

Paratyphoid, *see* Typhoid and paratyphoid

Parkinson's disease

This is a disease of the middle-aged and elderly and is fairly common, but treatment can, to a great extent, postpone the onset of disability for years.

In most cases, Parkinson's disease is caused by premature ageing of deep-seated BRAIN cells in what is known as the *basal ganglia*. These cells normally form a complex control system that coordinates the MUSCLE activity which allows us to perform specific types of movement freely and unconsciously. This sort of muscle activity is involved in various common actions such as the swinging of our arms when we walk, in facial expression and in the positioning of limbs before we stand up or walk.

Difficulties occur when the brain cells that allow the body to perform these tasks die off prematurely.

Symptoms

The old names for Parkinson's disease – *paralysis agitans*, or shaking palsy – help to describe one of its most common symptoms. They usually develop very slowly and are often assumed to be part of the normal process of ageing. At the beginning, they seem to occur on only one side of the body. Ultimately, however, both sides are usually affected.

Most noticeable is the trembling of the hands, which shake in a 'pin-rolling' tremor as if the person is rolling something between his or her fingers and thumb. It is most evident when the arm is inactive, for the shaking usually stops as soon as movement begins – when reaching for a cup, for example.

The muscles of people afflicted with the disease become unusually stiff. In the early stages, it causes aching shoulders and discomfort first thing in the morning, after hours of rest. The face is also less mobile than usual, which gives the person a 'dead-pan' expression.

Walking is also very difficult. After a hesitant start, a person with Parkinson's disease moves forward quickly in a shuffling manner. He or she takes small steps and leans forward in a stoop. This difficulty in walking can sometimes lead to severe falls if the usual automatic reaction of using the hands to break the fall is also impaired – as is often the case.

Initially the intellect is not affected, but after some years, the patient may gradually lose the ability to perform higher mental tasks. In this advanced stage of the disease, every physical movement becomes increasingly difficult. Yet, curiously, many instances have been recorded of a person with Parkinson's disease being impelled to act very quickly – running away from a fire, for example.

The disease is accompanied by a drop in BLOOD PRESSURE when the patient stands up, which results in fainting – this is called 'postural hypotension' – and by slurred and distorted speech, caused by damage to the relevant muscles.

Treatment and outlook

The usual treatment is the drug L-Dopa, which is given in tablet form. It replenishes the brain's supply of dopamine, the chemical 'transmitter' produced by cells in the basal ganglia, and alleviates many symptoms of the disease.

Another drug called *selegeline* may, if given early in the disease, prevent or delay progression of Parkinson's symptoms. A new drug called *apomorphine* can be given by injection to patients whose symptoms stop and start suddenly – something known as 'on/off phenomenon'.

Although degeneration of the brain cells cannot be reversed, drug therapy, regular exercise and proper nourishment will allow the patient to lead a full life for at least ten years from the onset of the disease. After this period, it becomes more difficult to control the symptoms.

New treatments

Surgery to the basal ganglia may be attempted: part of this region is destroyed using stereotactic surgery which does not cause any damage to other parts of the brain (*see* NEUROLOGY AND NEUROSURGERY). Although such an operation may relieve the shaking of Parkinson's disease, it does little to relieve other symptoms.

Recently an extremely controversial operation has been developed in which a small piece of brain tissue taken from an aborted human foetus has been transplanted into the basal ganglia. It appears that the transplant is able to restore normal function to this area of the brain, and in the few cases where the operation has been attempted, the results appear to have been dramatically successful. Yet there are opponents to this operation who do not believe that it is ethically justified to use brain tissue from an aborted foetus for a transplant.

Paronychia, *see* Thrush, Whitlow

Pelvic inflammatory disease (PID), *see* Hysterectomy, Infertility, Salpingitis, Sexually transmitted diseases

Pemphigus/pemphigoid, *see* Rash

Pendred's syndrome, *see* Thyroid

Penis

The penis consists of a central tube – the URETHRA – down which urine passes when a man relieves himself (urination, or micturition), or down which semen passes during SEXUAL INTERCOURSE. The urethra connects the bladder, where urine is stored, to a hole at the tip of the penis (the *meatus*). Semen enters the urethra during intercourse through a pair of tubes called the *seminal ducts* or *vasa deferens* which join it shortly after it leaves the bladder. A tight ring of muscle at the opening from the bladder into the urethra keeps the passage closed so that urine only emerges when this is intended.

The penis usually hangs down in front of the scrotum, the wrinkled bag that contains the TESTICLES, in a slack or flaccid state. Its length varies from 2½–5 in (6–12 cm). When sexually stimulated, it becomes stiff and erect, usually pointing slightly upwards. It is then 4–8 in (10–20 cm) long. The tip of the penis – the *glans* or 'helmet' – is the most sensitive area. The valley behind the glans is the *coronal sulcus*, the main length of the penis is the *body* or *shaft*, and the area of the penis where it joins the lower abdomen is called the *root*.

Erection and ejaculation

During the sexual process a man's penis goes from its normal, unaroused state

The anatomy of the penis

Immediately below is a detailed view of the penis, showing all its parts. The illustration below right shows the male genitalia, both internal and external. The section through the shaft of the penis (centre) shows the three groups of tissue responsible for erection. The bottom illustration shows a longitudinal section of the penis. The path of the urethra is clearly seen.

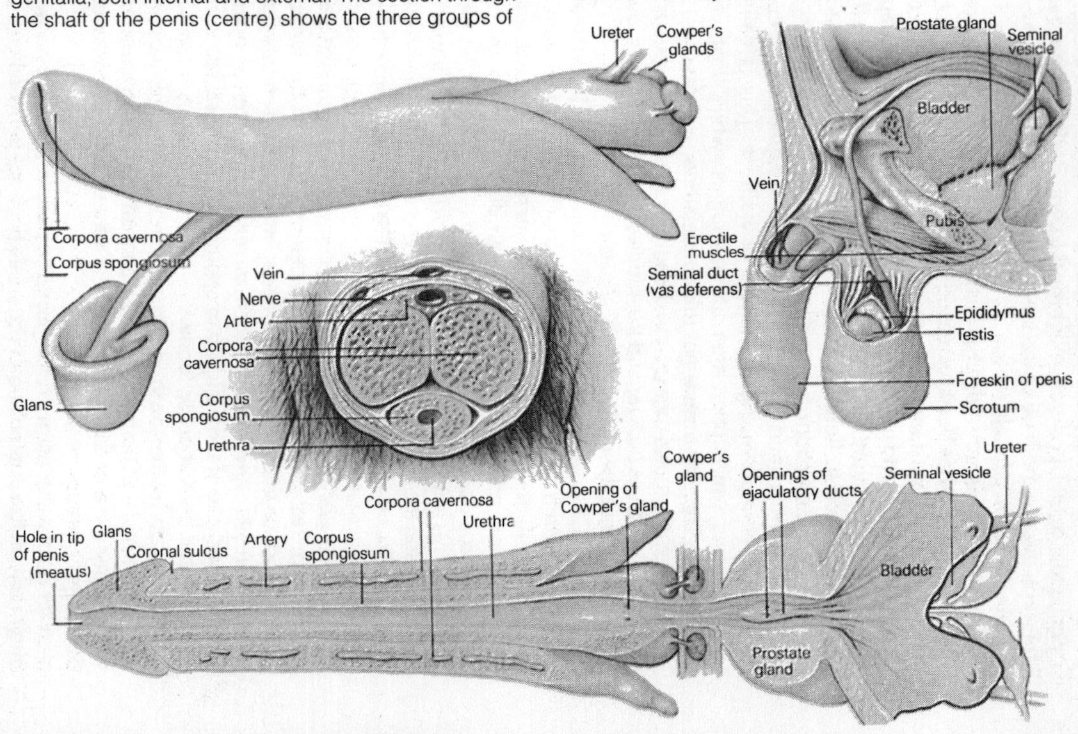

to orgasm, where sperm is discharged. There are four stages in this orgasmic cycle: arousal, plateau, orgasm and resolution.

Sexual *arousal* is usually associated with an arousing thought, though physical stimulation is required actually to reach orgasm. The stimulation may either be indirect, kissing, stroking, fondling parts of the body that are not specifically sexual, or direct, touching the penis itself. A nerve message from the BRAIN goes to the base of the SPINAL CORD, which in turn sends a message of arousal to the genitals.

Once the man is aroused, the penis becomes larger and more erect because the blood supply has been increased by the action of nerves. A new system of blood flow comes into operation. Blood vessels which have lain close together now expand to allow a generous blood flow to be pumped into the penis. The blood flow continues, and special veins expand to allow a small amount of blood to flow back into the body's general circulation without decreasing the erection.

Sometimes men (and babies and young boys) experience erection without any sexual stimulation, either direct or indirect. This is called a reflex erection, and can happen after lifting weights, while dreaming or upon awakening. This response is not fully understood.

During the arousal phase, the heartbeat and BLOOD PRESSURE increase, breathing becomes heavier and the nipples may harden and grow erect; this lasts throughout the cycle.

During the *plateau* phase, the penis is fully erect, having increased in both length and width. The glans darkens in colour because of the increased blood flow. The testicles increase in size by as much as 50 per cent, and rise up to enable a more powerful thrust of the penis during intercourse.

A few drops of semen may appear at the opening of the penis and be released. This is one reason why *coitus interruptus* or the withdrawal method (withdrawing the penis from the vagina before orgasm) can be an unreliable method of CONTRACEPTION, as sperm are often present in this small amount of seminal fluid that is released initially.

The ejaculatory climax – *orgasm* – occurs in two stages. First, sperm travels up from the testicles through the vas deferens to meet the seminal vesicles which produce the seminal fluid. The sperm and the seminal fluid are then mixed together, and the fluid then travels to the internal opening of the urethra. Because of the build-up of sperm in the urethral entrance, the man will feel that he is about to 'come'.

In the second stage, the fluid is forced through the urethra by the rhythmic contractions of the urethra's muscles, and out of the external opening. There are usually three or four main bursts of semen, followed by weaker, more irregular contractions.

After ejaculation comes *resolution*. The penis and testicles slowly return to their normal size and position. The penis once again becomes flaccid as the blood drains away back into the body, and the blood vessels return to their non-aroused state. Some men may find that the head of their penis is particularly sensitive at this time. If the plateau phase has been long, or the penis remains inside the vagina, the penis may stay erect for a considerable time.

Problems with erection and ejaculation

One of the most common difficulties is *premature ejaculation,* in which the plateau phase is very short and ejaculation takes place almost immediately. This is usually due to worry, either about sexual performance, or problems within the relationship. Often this STRESS has to be worked through before the problem can be solved. One self-help technique is simple distraction: when you are at the point of orgasm, think of something totally unconnected with sex; this may delay your orgasm. Alternatively, there is the 'squeeze' technique, developed by the sex therapists Masters and Johnson in the US. When you are at the point of ejaculating, your partner should squeeze the *fraenulum,* which is a thin, triangular mark located on the underside of the point where the glans of the penis meets the shaft. If you are uncircumcised, draw back the foreskin to see it. The pressure should be fairly firm and should be maintained for three or four seconds, and then released. This should stop ejaculation, but if your erection diminishes, your penis should be stimulated again.

Some men find it difficult to maintain an erection or reach orgasm when they are with a partner, but they are perfectly able to do so through masturbation. This is known as *impotence.* Frequently the reason is psychological: they are worried about letting their partner down and 'failing' sexually.

Both premature ejaculation and impotence are usually based on emotional factors rather than physical ones. Your doctor may, if necessary, refer you to a psychosexual specialist.

Infections

The chief hazard to which the penis is exposed is infection, particularly SEXUALLY TRANSMITTED DISEASES, often called venereal diseases. Inflammation of the urethra – when it discharges pus, usually accompanied by discomfort or pain in passing urine – is called *urethritis.* It can be caused by GONORRHOEA, when the discharge is copious and yellow, or NON-SPECIFIC URETHRITIS (NSU), where the discharge is likely to be less and more mucous in appearance. These conditions are potentially dangerous – both to the patient and his sexual partner – and they should be treated as soon as possible.

Another, even more serious – but fortunately less common – disease that makes its initial attack on the penis is SYPHILIS. This normally shows itself as a single ulcer near the head of the penis. It may be no more than a painless 'cut' or fissure in the skin, and will probably go away by itself in a few days, but unfortunately this is only the first stage. Left untreated, syphilis will develop over a period of years, sometimes with disastrous consequences.

Other conditions which may affect the penis are: *phimosis,* where the foreskin is too tight to peel back during erection or sticks to the glans; *paraphimosis,* where a tight foreskin has retracted and forms a band around the coronal sulcus, causing the tip of the penis to swell up; and HERPES *genitalis* – small ulcers, similar to COLD SORES, appearing on the penis. All these conditions except *herpes genitalis,* which is persistent, respond well to treatment. *See also* WARTS.

Pericarditis

When people suddenly suffer from a bad pain in the middle of the chest, they often imagine that they are having a HEART ATTACK. This may, in fact, be the case, but in a small proportion of people, it is pericarditis that is causing the trouble. Pericarditis is inflammation of the fibrous membrane (*pericardium*) in which the HEART sits. It may arise from a number of different causes but virus infection is the most common.

The pericardium can also become full of fluid as a result of inflammation; this may give no symptoms, although it can be picked up on a chest X-ray. In a small number of cases when there is fluid in the pericardial sac – *pericardial effusion* – there is a build up of pressure on the heart that stops it working properly. The only other way that a pericardium can give rise to trouble is when it becomes very much thickened following an infection such as TUBERCULOSIS; this, too, restricts the action of the heart and can lead to heart failure.

Other causes

Pericarditis can suddenly attack perfectly fit people. The symptoms are very like those of a heart attack – severe central chest pain that is worse on sitting forward – and it can sometimes be rather difficult initially to tell them apart, even with an ECG (ELECTROCARDIOGRAM). This situation is made more complicated by the fact that there are two different sorts of pericarditis that can come on *as a result* of a heart attack. The first is death of heart muscle which can give rise to inflammation around the heart as the body attempts to clear away the damaged tissue. The second, which is more rare, is known as *Dressler's syndrome*: this follows about a week after the heart attack when an abnormal response in the body's IMMUNE SYSTEM leads to antibodies being formed against the heart.

Occasionally CANCER can involve the pericardium; this does not usually arise from the pericardium itself, but spreads from elsewhere – particularly the lung. It may often give rise to a big pericardial effusion, and this, in turn, may lead to restriction of the heart's movements and so to heart failure (*cardiac tamponade*). This can also occur when the pericardium is thickened as a result of tuberculosis.

Pericarditis also happens in severe KIDNEY failure and in diseases such as systemic LUPUS ERYTHEMATOSUS where there is a generalized inflammation in various parts of the body because of a disturbance of the immune system.

Dangers

The heart failure that results from a collection of fluid in the pericardial sac – *tamponade* – is a serious condition, and the pressure on the heart has to be relieved. This can normally be done by passing a needle through the wall of the chest and into the pericardium. When the constriction of the heart is a result of a very thick pericardium – as it is in TB – an operation is necessary to remove the thick lining.

Treatment

Aspirin-like drugs, particularly one called indomethacin, are the best form of treatment and help relieve the pain. In Dressler's syndrome, indomethacin may not be quite enough and STEROID drugs can often be needed to reduce the inflammation. In diseases such as systemic lupus erythematosus and kidney failure, there can be inflammation but no pain, so no additional medication is required apart, of course, from treatment for the underlying condition.

The outlook in viral pericarditis is really very good. The types of pericarditis that follow a heart attack do not really make the outlook any worse for the patient than the attack itself. In TB, the operation to strip all the thickened pericardium from the heart is a big undertaking, but it has very good results.

Periodontal disease, *see* Dental care

Periods and period pains

The time from the first day of one period to the first day of the next is known as the *menstrual cycle*. During this cycle, the reproductive organs undergo a series of changes which make it possible for an egg to be released from the OVARY and travel to the UTERUS (womb). If this egg is fertilized by a SPERM, it will be nourished by secretions from the cells lining the womb until it burrows its way into the lining of the womb and is nourished from the mother's blood supply (*see* PREGNANCY).

If the egg is not fertilized, the lining of the womb is shed in the menstrual flow, or *menses*. This allows a new lining to grow, ready to nourish the next egg.

The menstrual cycle

This intricate cycle or activity is controlled by a centre in the brain called the HYPOTHALAMUS, which acts as a menstrual clock. The clock operates through a small gland called the anterior PITUITARY gland, situated at the base of the brain. This gland releases several HORMONES, two of which are particularly important for reproduction. One stimulates the growth and maturation of several small eggs in the ovary, while the other stimulates the release of these ripened eggs.

The eggs which mature during the menstrual cycle are surrounded by hormone-producing cells. The egg, together with these cells, is called the *Graafian follicle*. The main hormone produced by this follicle is *oestrogen*. During the cycle, the surge in oestrogen production is responsible for stimulating the growth and formation of glands in the lining of the womb. It also changes the secretions at the neck of the womb (CERVIX) making it easier for sperm to swim into the womb and so meet the egg. Approximately 15 days before the next period is due, the pituitary gland releases a large amount of *luteinizing hormone* (LH) which stimulates the release of an egg from the ovary about 36 hours later. The egg then travels down a Fallopian tube into the womb. Fertilization usually takes place in the Fallopian tube.

The cells in the ovary which have formed the Graafian follicle now undergo changes, which include taking up fat. They are now referred to as the *corpus luteum* ('yellow body'). They still produce oestrogen, but now also produce a hormone called progesterone. Progesterone has two main functions in the menstrual cycle. The first is to alter the mucus at the neck of the womb, making it too thick for sperm to swim into the womb; the second is to make the glands lining the womb secrete a fluid which will nourish the newly fertilized egg.

If the egg is not fertilized, the *corpus luteum* degenerates. Small blood vessels in the area go into spasm so that cells lining the womb no longer receive oxygen and die. They are then shed together, with some blood, as *menstruation*, and the cycle is complete. All the hormones released during the cycle can influence the menstrual clock.

Duration

The length of the menstrual cycle is controlled ultimately by the pituitary gland, and can vary from 21 days to three months in normal women. Most women have a cycle of around 25 to 30 days. When periods first start at puberty, it is common for the cycle to be quite irregular; many teenagers find that it is impossible to predict when their periods are going to start. After a few years, however, the cycle usually settles down into a set pattern.

Ovulation occurs only once in the menstrual cycle, so a woman who has a long cycle – say, of 10 or 12 weeks – is inevitably less fertile than a woman who has a short regular cycle. Ovulation usually occurs about 14 days before a period is due, and is usually marked by a rise in body temperature. The fertile time of the cycle for a woman with a 28-day cycle starts around the 10th or 11th day of the cycle and lasts until the 16th or 17th day. A woman who has a 10-week cycle will probably not become fertile until the seventh week of her cycle. However, ovulation timing may vary from month to month. Careful timing of sexual intercourse can help to achieve a pregnancy (*see* INFERTILITY); abstinence during the time of fertility can be used as a method of CONTRACEPTION, but advice from a family planning specialist is required if this 'rhythm' method is to be used successfully.

Menstrual flow

Average blood loss during menstruation is between 0.7 fl oz (20 ml) and 2.8 fl oz (80 ml) over a few days. Women taking the contraceptive pill tend to lose less blood. We do not really understand why some periods are heavier than others. Heavy periods can be caused by inflammation of the womb, the use of intra-uterine contraceptive devices (the IUD), and certain endocrine diseases, such as an under-active THYROID gland. Occasionally, the surface area of the lining of the womb is increased by FIBROIDS, also causing heavy periods.

Menstrual flow often has an unpleasant odour, largely due to the action of bacteria on the blood and cells which have been expelled from the womb.

During menstruation, it is important to pay particular care to personal hygiene. If a tampon is left in the vagina for too long or forgotten completely, it can give rise to a foul-smelling vaginal discharge (*see also* TOXIC SHOCK SYNDROME).

Not all blood loss from the vagina is necessarily due to menstruation. Blood loss can occur from the neck of the womb if the tissue is very weak (a condition called cervical erosion); it can also occur from a POLYP in the womb, or from a CANCER. Should you experience bleeding after intercourse or between periods, it is always wise to consult your doctor about the problem.

Period pains

We are not sure of the exact cause of menstrual pains (*dysmenorrhoea*). Possibly the muscle of the womb goes into spasm; a substance released from the cells lining the womb called *prostaglandin* is another possible cause. Often a mild PAINKILLER such as aspirin or paracetamol, or gentle heat from a warm hot-water bottle will help; more painful periods can sometimes be cured by taking the contraceptive pill, although some women continue to have period pains even when taking it.

Another simpler approach is to take an anti-inflammatory drug during the period. These drugs block the effects of prostaglandins and help to relieve menstrual pain, as well as reducing blood flow. *Mefenamic acid* (Ponstan) is often prescribed by doctors; *ibuprofen* (Brufen, Nurofen) is an anti-inflammatory drug that can be obtained over the counter in a chemist's shop.

In the past, many women had a D & C – dilation and curetage, or 'scrape' – in an attempt to cure the problem on the theory that the stretching of the neck of the womb will make expulsion of the menstrual blood easier. Unfortunately there is no real evidence to support this theory, and painful periods could return a few months after the procedure.

If painful periods are caused by the conditions called *adenomyosis* and ENDOMETRIOSIS, in which small areas of womb-lining tissue occur elsewhere in the abdomen, surgery may be necessary, but this is very rare.

Dangers

Probably the most worrying problem occurs when a period is unusually heavy (*menorrhagia*) or painful (*dysmenorrhoea*). This can mean that the woman is having a MISCARRIAGE, especially if the period is a few days late. She should always seek her doctor's advice if this happens, as a D & C may be necessary to clean out the womb.

If a woman usually has very heavy periods, she may gradually lose so much blood that she becomes ANAEMIC. This can be diagnosed very simply by the doctor, and can usually be cured by taking iron tablets. However, it is more sensible to try to cure heavy periods by diagnosing the cause and giving appropriate treatment.

Menstrual problems

Many menstrual problems will simply resolve themselves, but if they persist, it is worthwhile for a woman to seek reassurance from her doctor.

A frequent worry is when periods do not occur (*amenorrhoea*). This takes two forms: primary amenorrhoea, when menstruation does not start at puberty, and secondary amenorrhoea, when for some reason periods stop. If periods have never occurred there may well be delayed puberty and associated hormonal problems. If there is secondary amenorrhoea, the primary cause could be pregnancy, but if this is ruled out, emotional factors may be responsible for upsetting the normal cycle. Eating disorders, particularly ANOREXIA nervosa, can cause amenorrhoea. This is often affected by stress – for example, after leaving home, changing jobs or a broken love affair. A visit to the doctor for a simple test will establish whether or not a woman is pregnant; otherwise, infrequent periods are generally of no concern. In an established menstrual cycle, periods may be uneven in quantity, prolonged or occur at differing time intervals. This pattern of menstruation is described as *metrorrhagia*. Excessive periods are called *menorrhagia*.

In younger women, serious disease of the reproductive system is uncommon and most problems such as heavy or painful periods can be treated with tablets once examination, which may include a pelvic (vaginal) check, has conclusively established the cause.

Effects of contraceptives

It is thought that, during the reproductive years, some menstrual problems may be associated with a woman's choice of contraceptive.

The contraceptive pill works by interfering with the control of ovulation by the pituitary; if it is taken properly, according to the instructions, ovulation does not occur at all. A period occurs at the end of each packet, when the pill is stopped for seven days. But the bleeding at this time is not a natural period; it is an artificial one brought about by the reduction of progesterone and oestrogen intake. Bleeding is usually lighter than would occur with a normal period, and menstrual pains are often less. Occasionally, bleeding may occur between periods when a woman is on the pill; this usually indicates that the dose of hormones in the pill could be too low for her. If such bleeding does not settle after a month or two, the doctor usually prescribes a pill with a higher dose of progesterone. However, such bleeding may occasionally have other causes and should be reported to a doctor.

The mini-pill, or progesterone-only pill, works in quite a different way from the ordinary pill. Ovulation may still continue; the pill works by blocking the thinning of cervical mucus which normally occurs in the middle of the menstrual cycle so that sperm cannot travel up into the uterus. Irregular bleeding is a very common side-effect with this pill, but it does not indicate any reduction in effectiveness. There may be small amounts of bleeding between periods: sometimes the periods come much more frequently. Any woman on the mini-pill should keep a chart of her periods and any other bleeding that may occur, to show to her doctor. If bleeding is troublesome, a higher dose of pill may be prescribed.

Progesterones may also be given by long-acting injections once every three months for contraception. Again, menstrual irregularity is very common. Often periods stop altogether after the second or third injection, although in the early weeks after the first infection, there may be very frequent and irregular bleeding.

Women who use the coil (IUD or intra-uterine device) may find their periods become a little heavier. This may be most noticeable in the first few months after the coil is fitted, but then the periods may settle down. However, if the IUD causes severe discomfort or heavy bleeding, it may have to be removed and a different contraceptive used. Your doctor or family planning clinic can advise you.

When to see your doctor

Four problems are of particular importance and would justify an early visit to the doctor. These are: very heavy prolonged periods which occur at the usual time (menorrhagia); bleeding after intercourse; bleeding from the vagina between periods; bleeding from the vagina after the MENOPAUSE. All of these symptoms, although usually caused by a minor problem, can occasionally be early symptoms of cancer of the womb, which can be cured if diagnosed and treated at an early stage.

As women become older, menstrual disorders are more often associated with disease of the reproductive organs. Diagnostic tests, such as a D & C, are performed to exclude this possibility; otherwise the condition may be treated with synthetic sex hormones such as progesterone. At the time of the menopause, periods usually become more and more infrequent, before finally stopping. This is normal and needs no further treatment.

A frequent disorder at this time is menorrhagia (heavy periods). Doctors often try prescribing hormonal tablets to control their severity. Unfortunately, this treatment does not always work, and a hysterectomy (removal of the womb) may be suggested as an alternative. This is a difficult decision for the patient to make. She has to decide whether her symptoms are severe enough to warrant a major operation or if she is prepared to tolerate her heavy periods.

See also PREMENSTRUAL SYNDROME.

Peristalsis, *see* Alimentary canal, Colon and colitis, Constipation, Digestion, Ileum, Intestines, Jejunum, Malabsorption, Oesophagus, Stomach

Peritoneum and peritonitis

This is a thin MEMBRANE which lines the abdominal cavity, and also covers all the organs contained within the ABDOMEN. Thus, the LIVER, the STOMACH and the INTESTINES are covered with peritoneum, as are the SPLEEN, GALL BLADDER, PANCREAS, UTERUS (in women) and APPENDIX.

In spite of its being such a thin layer – when separated away from, say, the stomach, it would be transparent – the peritoneum is very strong, and the way it is attached inside the abdominal cavity creates various spaces where fluid could collect in the event of a leak from one of the abdominal organs, such as the pancreas, bladder or intestines.

The function of the peritoneum

In the normal, healthy person, the main function of the peritoneum is to allow the various structures inside the abdomen to move about freely. When you eat a meal, for instance, the stomach and the intestines become mobile, and the muscle in their wall contracts so that the food is both mixed and propelled along. During this process, the stomach and intestines will slide over one another, helped by the fact that they are both covered with peritoneum, separated by a thin layer of fluid which lubricates them.

While the peritoneum covers organs such as the stomach, it also lines the abdominal cavity. The former is known as the *visceral peritoneum*, and the latter as the *parietal peritoneum*. The parietal peritoneum has an extremely sensitive nerve supply, so that any injury or inflammation occurring in this layer is felt as an acute localized pain.

The visceral peritoneum is not so sensitive and pain is only experienced if, say, the intestine is stretched or distended. For instance, a stab wound that penetrates the intestine causes little or no pain. Even then, the pain is not well localized and is felt as a dull ache, usually in the centre of the abdomen. These differences have an important bearing on the symptoms of various disorders of the abdominal contents.

The omentum

One structure which should be mentioned when describing the peritoneum is the *omentum*. Shaped rather like an apron, it consists of fat with a rich blood supply, covered with peritoneum. It hangs down from the stomach, and its lower part is free to move about in the space between the abdominal organs and the abdominal wall. It is thus between the visceral and parietal peritoneum, outside the intestines.

Ascites and adhesions

Two of the ways in which the peritoneum can be affected by disease are *ascites* and *adhesions*. In ascites, there is an excess amount of the lubricating fluid normally present between the parietal and visceral layers. It is caused either by an imbalance in the mechanism controlling the amount of fluid produced (such as occurs with LIVER disease) or it comes about when the peritoneum is irritated to a minor degree over a long period of time (such as can happen with a slow-growing TUMOUR). A person with ascites usually has a very distended abdomen, although often the distension is not accompanied by any sort of pain.

Normally, the various abdominal organs such as the stomach and the intestines are attached by *mesenteries*, membranes containing a series of branching arteries, veins, lymph vessels and nerves. The mesentery is the lifeline of the organ to which it is attached. Otherwise, the organs are free to move about to a certain extent. Adhesions occur where a part of one of these organs becomes stuck to the abdominal wall or another organ and can happen after any operation on the abdomen, or after peritonitis. The effect of adhesions is twofold. First, the mobility of the organ involved is impaired, which may lead to obstruction of the bowel; and second, the bowel may twist around an adhesion, cutting off its blood supply and, if left untreated, leading eventually to gangrene of the bowel.

The symptoms of someone with adhesions vary considerably, but they can range from recurrent attacks of abdominal pain to complete obstruction of the bowel with pain, abdominal distension and constipation. Bowel obstruction caused by adhesions sometimes rights itself without surgery, but if it continues for more than a few hours, an operation is needed to divide the adhesion and to check that the bowel has not become gangrenous. Unfortunately, adhesions after an abdominal operation cannot be prevented, so some people tend to experience recurrent problems.

Peritonitis

A third disease which can affect the peritoneum is peritonitis. The peritoneum becomes inflamed due to infection, irritation with harmful substances, or injury. The main symptom is pain, which differs from other pains in that it is constant and may be well localized. The patient with peritonitis usually lies still and any movement of the abdomen is extremely painful – even coughing and breathing may cause severe pain.

With abdominal pain due to other causes, such as obstruction with adhesions, the patient experiences waves of pain; when the pain reaches its peak, he or she tends to roll around in agony, changing position frequently. It is very unusual for a patient with peritonitis to do this.

When the peritonitis has been present for some hours, the peritoneum on the outside of the intestine becomes inflamed and the normal movements of the intestines (peristalsis) cease altogether. This is known as *paralytic ileus* (*see* ILEUM). Eventually, because nothing is passing through the alimentary tract, the stomach fills up with digestive juices and undigested food which will eventually cause the patient to vomit.

The spread of peritonitis can be prevented by the omentum which has the property of being able to stick on to areas of inflammation, 'wall off' infection and prevent it spreading to the rest of the abdominal cavity.

When a doctor examines a patient with possible peritonitis, he or she looks for lack of movement of the abdominal wall, a feeling of rigidity when the abdomen is pressed, and an absence of bowel sounds. The patient may show signs of SHOCK: low pulse, low blood pressure, pale and clammy skin.

Causes of peritonitis

Peritonitis can be caused by various diseases, including acute APPENDICITIS. Another cause of peritonitis is a perforated duodenal ULCER. A hole is made by the ulcer through the wall of the duodenum, so that bile, pancreatic juice and gastric juice flood out into the space between the visceral and parietal peritoneums. These digestive juices have a corrosive effect, and if the resulting peritonitis is not treated at an early stage, it becomes infected and the patient becomes very ill with bacterial peritonitis.

Among the other causes is a condition known as perforated DIVERTICULITIS in which a little diverticulum, a blind-ending sac on the side of the bowel, becomes inflamed and bursts, with similar consequences to a ruptured appendix.

Peritonitis can also be caused by injury, such as stabbing, or from a kick or a car accident. There are also cases which result from infected Fallopian tubes in women, and peritonitis can be a complication of pancreatitis (*see* PANCREAS).

Treatment and outlook

The treatment of peritonitis will obviously depend on the underlying cause. Most causes require an operation but there is one, pancreatitis (diagnosed by a special blood test), where operation is thought unnecessary and even dangerous. Because the patient has often been vomiting, he or she will be given fluid through an intravenous needle. If infection is playing a part, antibiotics will be given. A tube is usually passed into the stomach to draw off excess fluid.

Most people make a complete recovery from peritonitis and, within a few months, are completely back to normal. Occasionally the patient is troubled by adhesions, which may require a further operation. In cases of peritonitis involving the peritoneum in the pelvis, women can have problems with fertility, as the Fallopian tubes may become blocked (*see* INFERTILITY).

Pernicious anaemia

It would be difficult to invent a disease that causes both severe ANAEMIA and disorders in the NERVOUS SYSTEM simply by attacking the lining of the STOMACH. Nevertheless, pernicious anaemia is just such a disease.

It results from the formation of antibodies, by the body's own IMMUNE (defence) SYSTEM, to the cells that make up the stomach's lining. As a result, no *intrinsic factor* (the substance VITAMIN B_{12} depends upon for its absorption) is produced, and because of this, a vitamin B_{12} deficiency occurs. Vitamin B_{12} and folic acid (another B vitamin) are necessary for the BONE MARROW to make an adequate number of red cells; when the deficiency occurs, the number of red cells is reduced, and those that remain are larger and more irregular than normal (*megaloblastic anaemia*). Additionally a lack of vitamin B_{12} results in a reduction in the amount of white (infection fighting) cells.

Although the term 'pernicious anaemia' only refers to the disease when antibodies to the stomach wall are produced, there are other reasons why the body may run short of B_{12} and folic acid. The human body contains about 3 mg of vitamin B_{12} – an infinitesimal amount – and the average daily requirement is only one thousandth of this. B_{12} is only found in food of animal origin, so people who never eat anything of animal origin – strict vegetarians (vegans) – may run short of the vitamin, but otherwise dietary deficiency is rare.

People can also become deficient in vitamin B_{12} if they have an operation to remove their stomachs: this may result in a shortage of intrinsic factor. Intestinal disease may also produce pernicious anaemia, particularly if the ILEUM (the last part of the small intestine where vitamin B_{12} is actually absorbed) is involved. An inflammation of the intestine known as Crohn's disease (*see* COLON AND COLITIS) is the most common reason for this.

Folic acid deficiency can be due to a lack of fresh vegetables in the diet. Intestinal disease can cause folic acid deficiency much more commonly than vitamin B_{12} deficiency. Folic acid may also be lacking in pregnant women, so an additional amount is given.

Symptoms and dangers

Symptoms include paleness, lethargy, tiredness and breathlessness. Nosebleeds may also occur and, in extremely severe cases, heart failure. As well as the anaemia symptoms, patients exhibit a number of other characteristic features: prematurely grey hair and yellow skin.

Pernicious anaemia develops over a very long period: this means that the level of haemoglobin (the red oxygen-carrying pigment in the red blood cells) falls very slowly so the body is able to adjust to its effects. Often the haemoglobin level has to get to a seriously low level before the condition comes to light.

Without treatment, anaemia due to any cause may be fatal. However, death is very unusual since the condition is easy to recognize and can be treated promptly by giving a blood transfusion.

Since pernicious anaemia is associated with stomach antibodies, there is also a loss of the normal hydrochloric acid production by the stomach. Though this produces few symptoms, there may be a slightly increased risk of stomach CANCER.

Perhaps the most serious complication of pernicious anaemia is its effect on the nervous system. A lack of vitamin B_{12} causes problems in the SPINAL CORD, resulting in failure of those parts of the cord which carry sensation from the legs. There is a tingling in the legs, followed by a numbness, weakness and difficulty with balance. In later stages, the arms are affected. This complication, called *subacute combined degeneration of the cord,* responds well to treatment with vitamin B_{12} injections.

Treatment and outlook

With pernicious anaemia, the missing vitamin B_{12} has to be given on a regular basis (either monthly or every three months) by injection. And since the cause of the missing vitamin is the stomach's failure to secrete intrinsic factor – a disorder that will never improve – the treatment lasts for life.

Perspiration

Normal temperature (*see* FEVER) is, by tradition, 98.4°F (37°C), though there are variations and daily fluctuations from person to person. It is essential, however, that the body's core temperature is kept more or less constant. If the outside temperature rises too much, the core temperature is maintained largely by losing heat through perspiration.

A small amount of body heat is lost each day directly through the LUNGS and through the SKIN without involving the sweat glands at all. But, as can be imagined, this is a fairly inefficient way of losing heat. It is not a very flexible method, because you cannot increase your breathing – like a panting dog – if it gets very hot.

In fact, most of the heat loss that occurs every day results from perspiration – sweat production from the sweat glands. However, the liquid sweat usually evaporates from the skin before it can be noticed, and for this reason, it is known as 'insensible perspiration'. It is this evaporation that allows heat to be lost. It works on the principle that liquid needs energy to evaporate – like turning boiling water into steam. In human beings, that energy comes from the surface of the skin, and the effect of evaporating sweat is to use up some of the heat and energy in the skin, thereby leaving you cooler. Once you have become so hot that the sweat is beginning to pour off your skin, the system has actually reached the stage where it can only just cope.

The sweat glands

The body is covered in sweat glands that produce liquid. Before puberty, only one set is functioning – the *eccrine* GLANDS which are all over the body except the lips and some parts of the sexual organs. There are many of these glands in thick-skinned areas such as the palms of hands and the soles of the feet, and their activity is controlled both by the NERVOUS SYSTEM and some HORMONES. This means that as well as responding to changes in temperature, they also react under other conditions, hence the sweaty hands of excitement (*see* STRESS) and the unexpected hot flush of the MENOPAUSE.

The other glands, the *apocrine* glands, are much more complicated than the eccrine glands. Under a microscope, they look like worm casts – highly complicated coils. They develop and start to function during adolescence and are found in the armpits, the groin and the areola of the breast. They are not associated with the nervous system, and they produce a thick milky substance which contains more protein and fat than the secretions of the eccrine glands.

See also SUNSTROKE.

Body odour

Everyone produces some natural aroma from the skin. It is known that some people can recognize members of their family, friends or lovers by their smell. Research has shown that we all excrete tiny quantities of chemicals called *pheromones* in sweat, which can have a direct effect on the metabolism of other people. For many animal specialists, it is clear that such chemicals play an important part in allowing members of a herd to recognize each other and stay together, but they can also act as a powerful sexual attraction. In human beings, too, natural body aromas are often described by others as pleasant or even sexually stimulating – especially the natural aroma from a person of the opposite sex (*see* SEX AND SEXUAL INTERCOURSE).

However, sometimes body odours become unpleasant or even offensive to others. There are a number of possible reasons. Strongly flavoured foods such as chilli, curries or garlic can all add their own aroma to both the breath and the sweat of people who have eaten them. But the most common reason for body odour is simply poor hygiene. The secretions of the apocrine glands in the groin and armpits contain substances which the natural bacteria on the skin convert into foul-smelling by-products

Deodorants either mask the smell or inhibit the action of the bacteria, while antiperspirants stop the sweat glands working by contracting the skin so that the sweat cannot flow. Both types of protection are never 100 per cent effective and may cause irritation for people with sensitive skins. There is no substitute for regular washing with soap and water and wearing natural rather than synthetic fibres.

Hyperhidrosis

This is a relatively uncommon but unpleasant condition in which the sweat glands are continually overactive, even when the person is in a cool environment and does not need to perspire to keep the body cool. Often the condition affects just one area – frequently the armpits, but sometimes the groin or the feet.

Typically a sufferer of hyperhidrosis in the armpits needs to change his or her shirt or blouse several times a day simply because sweat constantly pours down from the armpits and soaks the person's clothes down to the waist on each side. A strong antiperspirant, such as aluminium chloride in alcohol, may be prescribed by a doctor for this condition. Used over a period of weeks, it reduces the activity of the sweat glands and is generally effective. In the most severe cases, surgery may be needed to remove the affected sweat glands.

Hidradenitis suppurativa

Apocrine sweat glands in the armpits or groin may become blocked and deformed, giving rise to recurrent infections in these areas. Repeated blind BOILS occur (which often smell revolting) and the skin becomes permanently reddened and inflamed – a condition known as *hidradenitis suppurativa*. This is a most distressing problem which cannot easily be cured by simple treatments. Prolonged courses of antibiotics may be prescribed to damp down infections, but ultimately many sufferers need surgery. The whole area of skin affected has to be removed and allowed to heal naturally. Despite the large areas of skin removed, there is very little scarring.

Pertussis, *see* Whooping cough

PET (positron emission tomography), *see* Neurology and neurosurgery

Pharynx

This is the part of our body we commonly called our 'THROAT' – the area at the back of the mouth, extending a little way down inside the neck, that gets sore when we have a COLD or TONSILLITIS. Deep-lined with muscles, it is shaped, very roughly, like an inverted cone, extending for about 5 in (12 cm) behind the arch at the back of the mouth to where it joins up with the gullet, or OESOPHAGUS, which leads to the stomach.

The upper and wider part of the pharynx is given rigidity by the bones of the skull, while at the lower and narrow end, its muscles are joined to the elastic cartilages of the voice-box or LARYNX. The outermost tissue layer of the pharynx, continuous with the lining of the mouth, contains many mucus-producing glands which help to keep the mouth and throat well lubricated during eating and speaking.

The parts of the pharynx

Anatomically, the pharynx is divided into three sections according to their positions and the jobs each is designed to perform. The uppermost part, the *nasopharynx*, gets its name from the fact that it lies above the level of the soft palate and forms the back of the nose. Below, the nasopharynx is bordered by the soft palate itself: upward movement of this palate closes off the nasopharynx when you swallow to prevent food being forced up and out of the nose.

In the roof of the nasopharynx are two clumps of tissue, particularly prominent in children, known as the ADENOIDS. The nasopharynx also contains, either side of the head, an entrance to the Eustachian tube, the passage between the middle EAR and the throat. The problem, however, is that disease-causing micro-organisms of the mouth, nose and throat have easy access to the ears and commonly cause middle-ear infections.

The part of the pharynx at the back of the mouth, the *oropharynx*, is part of the airway between mouth and lungs. Much more mobile than the nasopharynx, the squeezing actions of the muscles of the oropharynx help shape the sounds of SPEECH as they come from the larynx. With the aid of the tongue, these muscles also help to push food down towards the entrance to the oesophagus. The most important organs of the oropharynx are the notorious tonsils, two mounds of tissue which are often implicated in the sore throats common in childhood. Like the adenoids, the tonsils are composed of lymphoid tissue characteristic of the body's IMMUNE SYSTEM and which produces specialized white blood cells which engulf invading bacteria and viruses.

The lowermost or *laryngeal* section of the pharynx is involved entirely with swallowing. This section lies directly behind the larynx and its lining is joined to the thyroid and cricoid cartilages whose movements also help to produce the sounds of speech. Again, squeezing actions of muscles help to propel mouthfuls of food through this part of the pharynx on their digestive journey. Just above the laryngeal part of the pharynx is the *epiglottis*, a flap of tissue which closes down over the entrance to the airway as you swallow and so prevents food from getting into the lungs and choking you.

What can go wrong?

By far the most common problem of the pharynx is inflammation, known medically as *pharyngitis* and experienced as a 'sore throat'. Pharyngitis can either come on suddenly (acute), or it can persist over several months or years (chronic).

The most usual cause of acute pharyngitis is the common cold – the sore throat is the tell-tale sign of an impending infection even before the first cough or sneeze. While the common cold is caused by a virus, there is also a bacterium called streptococcus, which can cause a form of pharyngitis known as 'strep throat'.

The chief culprits in chronic pharyngitis are SMOKING and excessive drinking. Too much of either can certainly result in pharyngitis, and cutting down or, especially in the case of smoking, stopping altogether, is needed to effect a permanent cure. Another common cause of chronic pharyngitis is post-nasal drip – a constant drip of fluid from the back of the nose. This results from persistent mouth-breathing owing to a blocked nose. The causes of this are many and so need diagnosis by a doctor.

Treatment

Treatment of pharyngitis depends, of course, on its cause, but in general falls into two categories: first, there is the treatment of those cases caused by viruses, such as the common cold virus, which do not respond to antibiotics; and second, the treatment of cases such as 'strep throat' which are caused by bacteria and so can be cleared up quickly with antibiotics.

As well as being a direct infection, the acute form of pharyngitis may result from the spread of infection elsewhere in the throat. Thus inflammation of the larynx (laryngitis), sinuses (SINUSITIS) and tonsils (tonsillitis) may all involve pharyngitis as well. SCARLET FEVER, also confined to the nose and throat, is associated with severe pharyngitis. Other more general infections such as GLANDULAR FEVER, MEASLES and RUBELLA may have a sore throat with pharyngitis as one of their symptoms.

Phenylketonuria (PKU)

This is a rare inherited disease, which affects about one in every 10,000 babies. It is one of a group of diseases that are known as the 'inborn errors of METABOLISM'. This means that the disease, which is present from birth, is one where the body is unable to handle some particular chemical constituent. In phenylketonuria, this chemical is *phenylalanine*. Normally, the enzyme phenylalanine hydroxylase acts on this amino acid to turn it into another amino acid called tyrosine. Because of the deficiency of phenylalanine hydroxylase, high levels of phenylalanine accumulate in the blood as none of it can pass into the next stage of processing by the cells.

The high level of phenylalanine causes brain damage in the developing brain, which is particularly susceptible to the effects of a raised phenylalanine level. Additionally, because the phenylalanine is not being converted to tyrosine, which is responsible for making the body's dark pigment, MELANIN, there is a lack of this amino acid in the tissues. As a result, affected children have blue eyes, blond hair and fair skin.

PKU is one of 50 known inborn errors in the handling of amino acids, and is inherited in a recessive way (*see* GENETICS and HEREDITY). That is, the abnormal gene has to be inherited from both parents. If a couple have one child affected with PKU, there is a 25 per cent risk that any further child will be affected.

Babies affected by PKU are normal at birth. Brain damage only begins when they start to take in phenylalanine with their feeds (including human breastmilk). It they remain untreated, 97 per cent will be severely brain-damaged individuals, with an IQ of less than 30. PKU babies often have bad ECZEMA. They might also suffer from fits and they tend to take no interest in other people.

Dangers

Phenylketonuria is dangerous in that it can affect children unnecessarily. Women who were born with the disease and treated with a special diet must go back on that diet before becoming pregnant, and the level of phenylalanine in their blood must be kept within strict bounds during their pregnancy so that the developing foetus is not affected.

People with PKU are unlikely to pass the disease on to their children unless they marry a carrier of the abnormal gene. The same applies to the brothers and sisters of affected people. Nevertheless genetic counselling should be sought if there is PKU in the family.

Treatment and outlook

All babies are screened at or around the fifth day of life with a simple heel prick test (*Guthrie test*). If positive results are obtained, the treatment is then started immediately.

Children are given a special feed that is usually made of a mixture of amino acids and is low in phenylalanine. Protein is avoided, including human and cow's milk, since phenylalanine is a common constituent of the amino acid protein in both animal and vegetable foods.

At three months, the situation is reassessed. Some babies, who have a minor form of the disease and can tolerate normal levels of phenylalanine in their feeds, can begin to eat more normally; others, who have a high level of phenylalanine, have to remain on a special diet.

When weaned, children are allowed more normal foods, though they can have no high-protein ones other than the special feed. Breakfast cereals, milk and potatoes are strictly rationed because they contain a lot of phenylalanine, but butter, jam, sweets and drinks can be taken in unlimited amounts as they are low in phenylalanine. Children are also permitted special brands of breads, flours, biscuits and pastas.

Between the age of six and 12, the diet is allowed to return to normal, although any deterioration in schoolwork or general behaviour requires urgent reassessment and restarting of the diet if tests show that the blood levels of phenylalanine are very high.

Pheromones, *see* **Perspiration, Sex and sexual intercourse**

Phimosis, *see* **Penis**

Phlebitis

The word 'phlebitis' is derived from the Greek word *phlebos*, 'VEIN', and ending *-itis*, 'INFLAMMATION'. So phlebitis means any condition where there is inflammation of a vein. The word is commonly used to mean inflammation either of the superficial veins in the LEGS or of the veins deep in the muscles of the leg or the pelvis. Because inflammation of a vein often leads to clotting of blood in the vein, or THROMBOSIS, the word *thrombophlebitis* is sometimes used to describe the condition where there is inflammation of a vein, followed by thrombosis.

Superficial thrombophlebitis

In this condition, the veins that are usually visible under the skin become inflamed – red, swollen and extremely tender to the touch. It often starts in one part of the vein and then spreads upwards along the limb as a tender red line. Often the inflamed vein can be felt, hard and cord-like, just beneath the skin. There is often considerable local pain which may keep the patient awake at night, and if it is not treated, the pain gets worse as the area of inflammation becomes larger. Eventually, there is a long line of inflammation which is extremely tender. The patient may also have a raised temperature and the limb may be swollen.

The commonest place to find a vein affected by superficial thrombophlebitis is in the lower leg. Usually the veins involved are widened and twisted. Veins in the arm can also be affected, but this is much more unusual.

The most common cause of superficial thrombophlebitis is VARICOSE VEINS. This condition, which runs in families and is much more common in women, usually occurs in young adulthood and becomes worse over the years. The superficial veins of the leg are enlarged so that they become thin-walled, wide and twisted. The blood-flow through them is very sluggish. It is then much more likely to lead to clotting of the blood in the vein itself, probably the first stage in phlebitis. After the blood has clotted, the wall of the vein becomes inflamed to try to dissolve the clot. At this stage, the patient notices pain, tenderness and redness.

Phlebitis sometimes follows an injury. The thin-walled vein, only just beneath the skin's surface, is bumped, for instance on the edge of a coffee table. Normally, the vein is lined by a thin layer of cells which help to prevent the blood from clotting. If this lining is damaged, then as soon as the blood comes into contact with the raw surface, it tends to clot.

Varicose veins are often made worse during PREGNANCY. There are two reasons for this. First, the pressure of the uterus on the pelvic veins tends to make the veins in the leg swell up. Second, hormones released during pregnancy tend to loosen all the supporting tissues in the body. In the case of varicose veins, the supporting tissue around the veins is lost, and they become stretched.

The presence of an intravenous needle can also cause superficial thrombophlebitis. Someone in hospital suffering from some other condition may have to have fluids put into a vein for a prolonged period of time. The little plastic tube, which is inserted into the vein and is connected up to the drip bottle, probably irritates the lining of the vein, leading to thrombosis and then inflammation.

Other causes include abnormalities of the blood itself, where for some reason the blood is more prone to clotting, and immobilization, particularly during and just after a major operation and in any condition where the patient is immobile for a prolonged period. With certain types of CANCER, notably cancer of the PANCREAS, a person who has never had any trouble with varicose veins or phlebitis may suddenly develop areas of superficial phlebitis on the legs.

Deep-vein phlebothrombosis

In this condition, the large veins which travel up the leg inside the muscles become blocked with a blood clot and then become inflamed. The clot (thrombosis) occurs first, and then the phlebitis follows. Pain is felt deep in the calf and is sometimes made worse by moving the ankle; the tissues around the ankle may swell. There may be no external evidence of the phlebitis at all, unlike superficial thrombophlebitis, in which there is often a tender red area. Except that varicose veins are not usually involved, the various causes of deep-vein phlebothrombosis are similar to those for the superficial type – poor flow through the veins, a change in the composition of the blood or some damage to the wall of the vein itself.

It has been suggested that SMOKING may increase the incidence of deep-vein thrombosis. There also tends to be a higher incidence of deep vein trouble in women who take a high-dosage oral CONTRACEPTIVE, particularly if they are over 35, overweight and smoke. The lower-dosage contraceptive pill, now more commonly prescribed, does not have the same effect.

Dangers

There is very little serious danger with superficial thrombophlebitis. The vein involved may end up as a fibrous cord with no blood inside it, but this does not cause any symptoms as the blood finds its way back via a different route. Recurrent attacks may occur, but are not a serious health hazard.

In contrast, deep-vein phlebothrombosis can have very serious effects. First, the blood clot in the vein may grow until it is of considerable length. A piece can then break off and finds its way up into the main CIRCULATION. It would then pass along the *vena cava* (the large vein at the back of the abdomen draining all the blood from the lower half of the body) and enter the HEART, from where it would be pumped into the main artery which supplies blood to the LUNGS. Depending on its size, it would then block off one or more of the branches of this artery. This condition is known as a *pulmonary embolus*. If large enough, it could cause a complete blockage, leading to immediate death. A smaller one would find its way into the periphery of the lung and cause less severe damage.

The second effect of a deep-vein thrombosis is to cause damage to the little valves that are found into the veins of the leg. This would lead eventually to permanent swelling of the leg, and possibly even skin problems, leading to ulceration (*see* ULCERS, SKIN).

Treatment

As there is no serious risk to health, the treatment of superficial thrombophlebitis is aimed at alleviating the symptoms only. The first thing to do is to elevate the leg whenever you sit down. This helps to reduce swelling and the effects of inflammation. A bandage or a support stocking may help, as this encourages more rapid blood flow in the veins by compressing them, and helps to support the inflamed area. Some doctors use drugs such as aspirin and ibuprofen, which have a direct effect on inflamed tissue and reduce the pain and the swelling. Rubbing the affected area with a special cream may also help.

Treatment for deep-vein phlebothrombosis is usually instituted early on to prevent the clot getting bigger and causing a severe blockage to the vein. Anticoagulant drugs are frequently prescribed to 'thin' the patient's blood and prevent further clot formation. There are two types of anticoagulants in use at the present time: *heparin*, which is given by injection and works immediately, and *warfarin*, which is given by tablet and takes two or three days to take effect. Heparin is given first and then warfarin is started after a few days and continued for at least three months. Occasionally special drugs are given to try to dissolve away the clot, or the clot may have to be removed surgically.

If treatment for a deep-vein thrombosis is started promptly, there should be no effects. However, there are some patients who can develop the so-called 'post-phlebitic' leg in spite of treatment. The leg remains permanently swollen at the ankle, and ulcers may form later on. Treatment consists of the wearing of support tights or stockings, the administration of tablets to reduce body water (diuretics), and possibly surgery to help heal ulcers. In some cases, the valves in the veins of the lower leg are destroyed by the phlebitis, and this leads to the formation of large veins connecting the superficial to the deep system. A surgical operation to tie off these veins may heal the ulcer.

Even when the post-phlebitic leg does not develop, the pain and swelling following a full-blown deep-vein thrombosis may persist for several weeks. Eventually the swelling subsides, but it may be found that the affected limb swells slightly towards the end of the day. The wearing of support hose and elevation of the leg are again helpful, as is exercise, although in the early stages it may be difficult to walk very far.

Phlegm

Phlegm – or *sputum,* as it is called medically – is a term used to refer to any material which is produced as a result of COUGHING. It may contain mucus, saliva, pus, BLOOD, particles of inhaled dust or fibre, shreds of tissue from diseased parts of the respiratory tract – or any combination of these things. It is usually clear or white in colour. When it is green, this is usually a sign of lung infection, requiring antibiotic treatment.

See also CATARRH.

Phobias

A phobia is an intense, irrational fear of an object or situation, which the sufferer *knows* is perfectly natural. The word comes from the Greek *phobos,* which means extreme fear or terror. The fear can be of things that are truly harmless, such as mice, open spaces, running water or sex. On the other hand, it may concern things or situations which may be harmful under certain circumstances but are generally unlikely to constitute a danger. Examples of this kind of phobia are an exaggerated and irrational fear of cats and dogs, thunder, spiders and snakes, choking or drowning, heights, enclosed spaces or darkness.

Fears cannot be classified as phobias when there is good reason to be afraid: a soldier who is terrified in battle cannot be said to have battle phobia. However, if long after he has been demobilized he is unable to walk past a soldier in uniform without becoming anxious, then a phobia can be said to be present.

Similarly, an obsession is not the same thing as a phobia. People who are obsessive do not fear an actual object or situation – they fear its *consequences.* The person who is obsessive about cleaning the kitchen doesn't have a phobia: he or she fears the possibility of contamination.

Who gets phobias?

In contrast to many other PSYCHOLOGICAL upsets, phobias are surprisingly common among the general public. It has been estimated that nearly 8 per cent of all adults have a phobia of one sort or another. Admittedly, not all phobias are regarded even by their possessors as a problem, and surveys have shown that only about 1 per cent of the population regard their phobias as interfering seriously with their life-styles.

Many sufferers nevertheless feel that their phobia is something to be ashamed of, or impossible to explain, and the situation isn't helped by the general lack of understanding about phobias. Take, for example, a young man with a phobia about spiders. He is otherwise carefree and reasonably popular with his friends. He knows that, in his locality, harmful spiders just do not exist, but all the same, he shows panic signs if a small, harmless spider crosses the floor in front of him, or he comes across a picture of a spider in a newspaper. In general, the reaction of his friends may well range from amusement or frank disbelief to irritation – and this attitude can only fuel the shame which he already feels about his phobia.

Phobias are usually associated with the emotional or introverted personality. The age at which the phobia begins varies according to its nature: animal phobias and a fear of going to school start in childhood, while agoraphobia (fear of open spaces), social phobias involving a fear of meeting other people, and general phobias such as a fear of illness, traffic, heights, sex and the like generally develop after puberty.

Signs and symptoms

It is difficult to someone who is untroubled by a phobia to realize quite how intense the person's anxiety is and to sympathize with his or her plight. In the presence of the object or situation which causes the phobia, especially if the sufferer cannot escape easily, there is not merely a well-bred distaste, but the possibility of abject pain.

Increased and uneven heartbeat, pallor, sweating, muscle tension, a tightness in the chest and difficulty in breathing to the point of fainting are not uncommon (*see* STRESS). Of course, the person does not have to go through such distress at each encounter with the feared stimulus, for he or she will often have developed ways of avoiding it – long before other people have noticed he or she has a phobia at all. Nevertheless, its unexpected appearance in, for example, a TV advertisement may be enough to set the train of reactions into motion, and the sufferer's discomfort will be all the more intense because he or she has not even had the opportunity to prepare for and thus resist the fear.

Treatment

There are differing opinions about how to treat a phobia. Basically there are two schools of thought – one maintaining that phobias can be treated by *psychoanalysis* (*see* PSYCHIATRY), the other suggesting that behavioural therapy (*see* MENTAL THERAPIES) is more effective.

Psychoanalysts take the view that phobias are symbols for deeply rooted conflict. The fears associated with objects or situations are based on childhood experiences and relate to conflict about one's sexual feelings or aggression. Analysts always try to find the *real* source of the problem so that the patient can understand and change his or her thinking and behaviour.

Behavioural therapists, on the other hand, believe almost exactly the opposite: that a phobia is actually an acquired habit of responding with fear to an object or a situation, and that the habit can be broken by training the sufferer to respond without fear.

Psychoanalysis takes a considerable time to achieve a result because the analyst usually needs to consider not only the whole of the person's present emotional problems but will also delve into the past. Behavioural therapy concentrates on treating the phobia itself and usually achieves a result – if the treatment is to be successful – within a few sessions.

Phosphorus, *see* **Minerals**

Physiotherapy

Physiotherapy is a necessary adjunct to many treatments of disease, disability and injury. In addition to its traditional role of treating rheumatic aches and stiff joints, physiotherapy is concerned with restoring limbs to function after an injury; helping pregnant women prepare for CHILDBIRTH; and teaching children with disabilities to control their limbs.

Equally importantly, physiotherapy also helps many post-operative and bedridden patients to breathe; trains those who have suffered brain or spinal damage to relearn mobility skills; and teaches paralysed patients to use other muscles so that they can become more independent.

Physiotherapists are highly trained medical personnel. They study anatomy (the structure of bones, muscles, blood vessels and nerves); physiology (how the body works, including breathing, digestion and circulation); pathology (how disease affects the body); psychology; and therapeutic exercises and techniques of healing.

In addition to their wide variety of manipulative skills, they have at their disposal a whole battery of machines and aids. The treatments they use range from the simple to the highly complex, and they employ various techniques to strengthen MUSCLES, mobilize JOINTS, relieve aches, pains and stiffness, and teach coordination and walking.

Methods

Physiotherapists essentially work around three 'Ms' – MANIPULATION, mobilization and MASSAGE – to get the patient and his or her limbs moving.

Manipulation is a method used to make joints and tissues more flexible. Finger and hand movements are used to apply pressure – for example, in cases where joints, while not dislocated, have moved slightly out of alignment and have become stiff or fixed. Many back complaints benefit from this treatment. Forceful, finely isolated pressure can relieve pain where a nerve has become inflamed or 'nipped'. A great deal of skill is needed to know precisely where and how to apply pressure to obtain a satisfactory result. Unskilled manipulation can be positively dangerous.

In mobilization, similar skills are used to get joints moving and relieve pain. Often less force and gentler pressure are needed and the benefit comes not from one or two particular manipulations by the physiotherapist, but from repeated movements where the patient has to work with the therapist. Exercises are used to restore strength to weakened muscles.

In massage, the masseur's hands are used to manipulate soft tissues around the joints to improve the blood flow, thus assisting limb movement. A great deal of modern massage is now based on Swedish methods.

Techniques

In addition to manipulative skills, physiotherapists can use a wide range of equipment in their treatment. The most modern is electrotherapy: electricity of a low or high frequency, which has a healing effect on the skin, muscles and other tissues.

Electrotherapy comes in a variety of forms. *Short-wave diathermy* is a high frequency current which penetrates deep into the tissues and is used to relieve deep-seated pain in, for instance, the hip joint. *Pulse magnetic field therapy*, where pulses of magnetic energy are passed through the limb, is used in FRACTURE healing. A combination of high- and low-frequency currents which penetrate deep into the tissues is used in *inferential therapy* to increase circulation and reduce pain. Low-frequency currents initiate muscle contractions in limbs that have been affected by disease or injury. PAIN reduction is also achieved by *transcutaneous nerve stimulation*: passing a low electric current through the tissues, thereby stimulating nerves near the skin's surface.

Other techniques include ULTRASOUND, where sound waves are passed into the body at very high speed. It decreases inflammation, improves circulation and gets movement in the fluid components of the tissues. For pain relief and improved circulation, *infra-red irradiation* from a lamp can be used.

There is, in addition, a wide range of traditional treatments. *Cold therapy* is usually applied in the form of ice in towels or crushed ice in water, and is used to suppress pain and relieve swelling. Like heat therapy, cold therapy can stimulate circulation, but it can be a more convenient method of treating hand, feet and knee injuries.

Hydrotherapy consists of exercising in warm water in special swimming pools, where the heat helps muscles relax and relieves pain. The special exercises aim to restore muscle power and make movement easier. Hydrotherapy is widely used for PARALYSIS and rheumatic disorders.

The time-honoured treatment of *paraffin wax* can be used to treat painful joints in the hands. The wax is moulded around the fingers, and as it prevents heat loss, the heat is retained for a long time.

Finally, there are *facilitatory techniques* that can be used for improving movement, either for the body as a whole or for an individual part. Facilitatory techniques are used when there is abnormal or no movement of limbs; the aim is to make the limb more efficient by working through nerve reflexes and nerve stimulation.

Physiotherapists work very closely with their colleagues in the health care team, including the OCCUPATIONAL THERAPIST and, where there has been a stroke, possibly the SPEECH THERAPIST. All of these could be involved in assessing patients' needs in preparation for their return home from hospital.

PID (pelvic inflammatory disease), *see* **Salpingitis**

Piles

In a medical context, the word 'piles' refers to several different conditions of the anal canal, each of which has different symptoms. Most commonly, the word refers to *haemorrhoids*, or internal piles, but it is often used also to denote anal fissure, thrombosed external haemorrhoids and simple anal skin tags.

There is some confusion about the treatment of these conditions, probably because of the patient's difficulty in visualizing what the problem is. The result is that any condition of the anal canal that consists of bleeding, pain or the presence of a lump is referred to as 'piles'.

Problems of the anal canal

The anal canal (or anus) is a short tube, about 1½ in (3.8 cm) long, which connects the RECTUM (the last part of the large bowel) to the outside. Its upper (or innermost) half is lined with mucous membrane – the type of lining found throughout the gut. The lower half is lined with skin. This lower half is extremely sensitive to painful stimuli, whereas the upper or inner half is insensitive to pain.

The whole of the anal canal is surrounded by a ring of muscle, the *anal sphincter*, which can relax during the passage of a bowel motion, but which normally remains tightly contracted so that continence of faeces is maintained.

Different conditions of the anal canal occur in different parts of it and, as such, produce different symptoms.

Internal haemorrhoids are swellings that arise from the upper part of the anal canal (the insensitive part) and gradually become larger over a period of years. They are probably caused by prolonged straining to pass small, hard faeces, but they are made worse by PREGNANCY.

Essentially, piles are the result of an interference in the return flow of blood from veins in the anal region. During late pregnancy in particular, the presence of the baby in the womb tends to obstruct the return flow of blood. This causes a swelling of the veins in the anal area.

Internal haemorrhoids used to be thought of as VARICOSE VEINS, but are now thought to be made of spongy tissue rich in small blood vessels. They generally occur in threes, and the first symptom is usually bleeding. The blood is bright red; the amount of bleeding is small, occurs at the end of defaecation and does not usually cause any pain.

Patients with small internal haemorrhoids have bouts of bleeding on and off over several years, and because of the length of time they have had the symptoms, they are perfectly used to the fact that they have haemorrhoids. Also, they may never have more than minimal symptoms. If the haemorrhoids become larger, as well as bleeding during defaecation, they may come out of the anal canal and be visible as a lump. The lump may only be evident during defaecation, or, if the haemorrhoids are very large, may be present all the time. The essential thing about the lump is that it appears to emerge from inside the anal canal.

Anatomy of the anal canal

The diagram (right) illustrates how networks of veins – called plexuses – are concentrated in certain areas of the rectum. It is in these areas that piles may occur, either as internal haemorrhoids (below) or as external haemorrhoids (bottom). Skin tags are not true haemorrhoids, although they may be treated as such; they seldom cause any problems.

Internal haemorrhoids

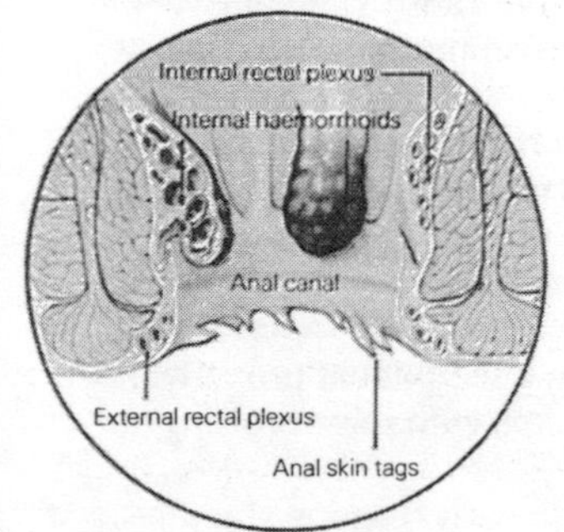

External haemorrhoids

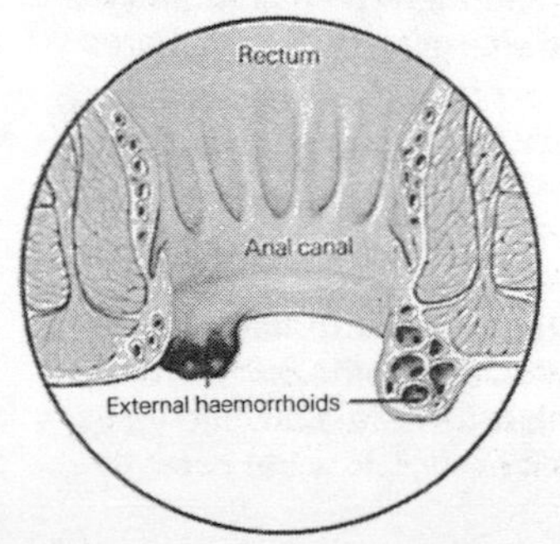

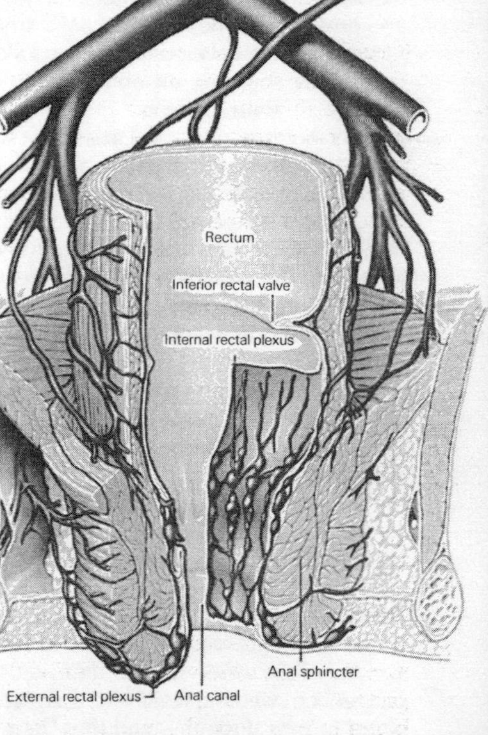

Occasionally, these kinds of haemorrhoids can become painful. When this happens, the patient usually notices a large tender lump that becomes excruciatingly painful and, without specific treatment, lasts for several days. This is what is known as an 'attack of piles'. It must be stressed, however, that haemorrhoids are not usually painful, and when they are, it is because they have become strangulated, or squeezed by a tight anal canal.

Anal fissure bears no relation to internal haemorrhoids. It is due to a split in the skin of the anal canal in a longitudinal direction. This condition is probably caused by straining in a person who has CONSTIPATION. Because the split is in the highly sensitive skin of the anal canal, it is extremely painful. The usual story given by the patient with an anal fissure is that of extreme pain during defaecation, together with the passage of a small amount of blood, often only on the toilet-paper. The pain may be so severe that the patient is afraid to have a bowel action. A vicious circle of pain and constipation arises.

This condition, which is common after pregnancy, is often diagnosed as 'piles' and therefore treated inappropriately. If a careful case history is taken from the patient, there should be no doubt about the diagnosis. Anal fissures can sometimes heal up spontaneously and at other times can become severe and prolonged enough to warrant a small operation.

Some people develop tags of extra skin around the anal canal. These are not strictly speaking an abnormality, but they do cause problems with hygiene in some patients. They are, however, commonly diagnosed as haemorrhoids or piles, and treated as such.

Thrombosed external piles is a condition in which a blood clot forms when a small vein under the skin bursts, setting up local inflammation. The patient experiences severe pain during defaecation and the pain persists after it is finished. Some time later a painful lump is noticed. This becomes red and inflamed. The condition is easy to treat but, like anal fissure, relies on the doctor taking a careful case history and examining the patient properly. A thrombosed external pile can be seen as a lump, often with some bruising on it.

The condition known as *anal fistula* is also occasionally diagnosed as piles, but really should never be confused with the above condition. The main symptom is a discharge of fluid, often like pus, and there is seldom much bleeding, a lump or pain. Anal fistula is usually the after-effect of a tiny ABSCESS in the lining of the anal canal. There is an abnormal connection between the skin next to the anal canal and the inside of the canal. Secretions therefore leak out through this channel.

Treatment

If haemorrhoids PROLAPSE (appear as lumps), sitting in a warm bath with a handful of salt dissolved in it often helps a lot. Salt baths soothe the area and can reduce swelling; while taking an ordinary bath softens the skin, allowing water to pass through – and thus increasing swelling – salt water actually draws water out of the area.

When to seek medical help

- If the bleeding is persistent or profuse.
- If there is pain in the abdomen.
- If there is a change in the normal bowel habit – for example, an increase or decrease in frequency persisting for more than two weeks.
- If there is persistent pain in the anal region.
- If symptoms attributable to 'piles' start in a person over the age of 50.
- If the blood from the area is dark in colour.

Occasionally, when haemorrhoids beome thrombosed, a polythene bag full of crushed ice applied to the enlarged haemorrhoids may help as well.

Treatment of true internal haemorrhoids takes several different forms. Initially, the doctor will want to make sure that there is no other serious cause for the bleeding by examining the lower part of the rectum.

The haemorrhoids can be injected with a special substance that makes them shrivel up. This may sound painful but if done properly should not hurt at all as the injection is put into the upper insensitive part of the anal canal. Other methods of treatment are to use a special freezing instrument called a cryoprobe which shrinks the haemorrhoids, or to put tiny rubber bands around them that cut off their blood supply.

None of these treatments is in any way painful and can be done in the out-patient department of a hospital. As well as these treatments, a high-fibre diet is recommended. It is thought that lack of fibre, or roughage, in the diet is one of the main factors in the formation of haemorrhoids.

Because anal fissure is so frequently confused with haemorrhoids, many patients soldier on with severe pain when they could easily have simple treatment.

The treatment of an anal fissure depends on whether or not it is a small, recent one, or a larger one of some months' duration. In the mild form, the use of some local anaesthetic cream, together with the intake of increased amounts of dietary fibre, may allow the fissure to heal up. In the more severe cases, the pain on defaecation causes intense spasm of the ring of muscle around the anal canal, making it more difficult to pass a motion. This in turn aggravates the condition even further.

In these cases, there is so much pain that it is usually impossible to examine the patient properly. The surgeon will give the patient a general anaesthetic before attempting an examination. If a fissure is found, a 'canal stretch' is performed: the ring of muscle around the anal canal is stretched so that it is unable to contract strongly. This allows the patient to have an easy bowel action, and the fissure to heal up quickly. Most patients notice an immediate relief in the amount of pain after the anal stretch has been performed.

Thrombosed external piles can easily be treated under a local anaesthetic. After cutting through the skin, the blood clot is removed, with instant pain relief.

The condition of anal fistula can also be easily treated, but again, it has to be correctly diagnosed first. Most cases can be treated by opening up the abnormal track on to the surface of the skin. Sometimes a longer operation is necessary but this is very rare nowadays.

Pimples, *see* **Acne**

Pink eye, *see* **Conjunctivitis**

Pins and needles

Most of us have experienced pins and needles at some time or another – that prickly feeling we get when our limbs have 'gone to sleep' after a long time in a cramped position, and normal sensation is just beginning to return.

Though most often felt in everyday situations, the same or similar feelings can accompany various diseases, especially of the peripheral nerves (*see* NERVOUS SYSTEM). Abnormalities of the BRAIN and SPINAL CORD can also cause pins and needles when the areas of these which analyse the messages coming from the nerves are damaged. In these more serious cases, however, the prickly feelings of pins and needles may not pass and may be accompanied by other symptoms, depending on the particular cause.

The most common cause of pins and needles – known medically as *paraesthesia* – is pressure on the peripheral nerves. When our legs and arms feel normal, they do so because the brain is constantly getting messages from many different nerves in the limbs, and making out of all this a picture of what is going on there. The nerves that are involved in sending in the information on which this picture is based are varied in type and size and so differ in how they respond to any damage, however slight. When our legs are crossed for a long time, for example, the nerve to the foot, which is close to the surface at the inside of the knee, sustains pressure from the leg underneath it, and some of the nerve fibres work less well. Since there are different types of nerves, they respond quite differently to this pressure. The spinal cord cells and those of the thalamus in the brain (which carry out sophisticated analysis of the incoming messages) start getting an incorrect combination of messages and, therefore, the sensations they relay to our conscious brain are jumbled. The nerves which convey messages of pricking and pinpoint pain get their messages through more effectively than the others, so the sensations they convey tend to be felt alone.

Diseases of the nerves

Many diseases of the nerves (*see* NEUROLOGY AND NEUROSURGERY) can cause pins and needles at some time in their course. This may be as a result of inflammation of the nerves (*see* NEURITIS), damage from poisons (including ALCOHOL), DIABETES or, more rarely, as a remote effect of a CANCER elsewhere in the body. The pins and needles occur because the disorder causing the damage tends to disturb the function of different types of nerve fibres to a different degree, causing the brain to receive confused messages. Usually these diseases cause damage to many nerves, and the pins and needles are therefore felt in both feet or all four limbs and do not recover when the person moves around or changes position.

Other damage can result from pressure on a nerve from nearby bones or other structures. This commonly occurs in the wrist where the median nerve is compressed as it passes through the tunnel made by bones and ligaments. The result is pins and needles in the hands which classically occur in the middle of the night or when the hands are being used in sewing or other intricate handiwork. This common condition, called *carpal tunnel syndrome,* is easily treated either by splinting the wrist or by surgery to reduce pressure.

Poor blood supply can slightly damage some fibres of a nerve and cause pins and needles in the same way as pressure.

Overbreathing, which some people do when they are exceptionally upset or excited, causes too much carbon dioxide to be exhaled. This results in chemical changes in the blood, which make some nerve fibres work less well, especially in the fingertips and around the mouth, and produces the prickly sensation of pins and needles.

See also NUMBNESS.

Pituitary

The pituitary gland is found in the base of the BRAIN. It is connected to the HYPOTHALAMUS by a stalk of nervous tissue and works closely with this area of the brain. Together the pituitary and the hypothalamus control many aspects of the body's METABOLISM – the various chemical processes that keep every part of the body functioning.

Structure and function

The pituitary sits inside a protective bony 'saddle' called the *sella turcica* (a Latin word meaning 'Turkish saddle'). The *sella turcica* – or *sella,* as doctors refer to it – can be seen clearly on an X-ray of the skull; enlargement of the *sella* is a good indication that something is wrong with the pituitary gland.

The gland is divided into two halves, each of which is quite separate from the other in the way that it acts. The back half, or *posterior pituitary,* is connected to the hypothalamus through the pituitary stalk. It is concerned with the production of only two main HORMONES, which are actually produced in the hypothalamus. From there, they travel along specialized nerve cells to the posterior pituitary and are released when the hypothalamus receives appropriate messages about the state of the body. The posterior pituitary and the hypothalamus are therefore very much a self-contained unit.

The anterior pituitary produces the hormones that activate other important glands in the body as well as producing one or two important hormones that act directly on the tissues. Although it is not linked directly with the hypothalamus, it is still very closely bound up with it in the way that it works.

Since the anterior pituitary has no direct nerve paths to link it with the hypothalamus, it has to depend on a series of special releasing and inhibiting factors to control hormone release. Some of these factors are themselves specialized hormones that are released by the hypothalamus and act on the pituitary gland a few millimetres away. They are carried in a special set of blood vessels called the *pituitary portal system*, which runs between the hypothalamus and the pituitary.

Although many of the instructions to release hormones come from the hypothalamus, the anterior pituitary itself also has a good deal of independent control over their release. The release of some of the secretions is inhibited by substances that are circulating in the bloodstream. An example of this is the hormone TSH (*thyroid-stimulating hormone* or *thyrotrophin*) which stimulates the THYROID gland in the neck to produce its hormones. The release of TSH by the pituitary is inhibited when high levels of thyroid hormone are in the blood. This is an important principle in the control of many of the pituitary hormones and is called 'negative feedback'. It means that the levels of the final hormone produced in glands remote from the pituitary (but dependent on it) can never rise too high, since negative feedback on the pituitary will turn off the production of stimulating hormones. Low levels of hormones in the blood have the opposite effect of switching the pituitary back on.

Hormones of the pituitary

The posterior pituitary produces two hormones called *antidiuretic hormone*, or ADH, and *oxytocin*.

ADH is concerned with the control of water in the body. It acts on the tubules of the KIDNEY, affecting their ability to retain or release water. That is, the kidney tissue is able to suck more or less water, as necessary, out of the urine as it leaves the tubule. When ADH is secreted into the blood, the kidneys tend to conserve water. When the hormone is not secreted, more water is lost from the body in the urine.

The role of oxytocin is less clear. It is concerned with starting off labour and causing the uterus to contract (*see* CHILDBIRTH). It also plays an important part in starting the secretion of milk from the breasts during lactation. In males, it is thought that oxytocin may be concerned with generating an orgasm (*see* PENIS).

The anterior pituitary produces six main hormones. Four of these are concerned with the control of other important glands in the body: the thyroid, the ADRENAL GLANDS and the gonads (the TESTES in the male, the OVARIES in the female).

The activity of the thyroid gland is triggered off by TSH, while the cortex (outer part) of the adrenal gland is affected by the hormone ACTH (*adreno-corticotrophic hormone*). The overall levels of thyroid hormone and cortisone from the adrenal glands is maintained by a combination of negative feedback acting on the pituitary and extra signals that come from the hypothalamus – for example, in times of STRESS.

The anterior pituitary also releases the hormones FSH (*follicle-stimulating hormone*) and LH (*luteinizing hormone*). These are known as gonadotrophins – hormones that affect the sex glands. They stimulate the production of two major sex hormones, oestrogen and progesterone, which, in the female, control the menstrual cycle (*see* PERIODS AND PERIOD PAINS). In the male, FSH and LH stimulate the production of male hormones and SPERM.

The hormone *prolactin* is one of two hormones of the anterior pituitary that seem to act directly on the tissues without stimulating some other gland. Like the gonadotrophins, prolactin is very much concerned with controlling the means of reproduction. Similarly, prolactin has a much more complicated role in the female than in the male. In fact, its role in the male is not clear, although when present in excess it can have ill effects.

In the female, prolactin stimulates the breast to produce milk. When it is present in large amounts, it also inhibits ovulation and the menstrual cycle. This explains the fact that women who are breastfeeding are unlikely to conceive (although breastfeeding is not a foolproof means of CONTRACEPTION).

The other hormone that the anterior pituitary produces is called the *growth hormone*; its role, as its name suggests, is to promote normal growth. While this is of most importance during childhood and adolescence, the hormone continues to have some importance in later life, as it determines the way that body tissues handle CARBOHYDRATES.

A number of other hormones are also produced by the anterior pituitary, although as yet their role in the body is not clear. These include lipotrophins, endorphins and enkephalins, some of which are present in the brain during times of stress or when somebody is in PAIN.

What can go wrong

As the pituitary plays such an important role in the working of the body, any malfunctions of this gland can be quite serious. However, problems associated with the pituitary are rather unusual.

The pituitary may give rise to problems in three ways. Like any other gland, it may be either overactive or underactive; it may also be the site of a TUMOUR. Since it lies in the base of the brain, tumours cause problems by growing outwards from the *sella* and pressing on important structures. For example, immediately above the *sella* is a structure called the *optic chiasma*. This is where the optic nerves, carrying all the information from the EYES, cross over. Pressure on the optic chiasma from a pituitary tumour can lead to progressive loss of sight.

Tumours arising in the pituitary gland itself fall into two categories: those that produce excessive amounts of the various hormones, and those that do not. The commonest type are called *prolactinomas* – these may be very tiny but produce the high levels of prolactin that cause problems. In women, high levels of prolactin will lead to amenorrhoea (absence of periods), INFERTILITY and sometimes galactorrhoea (milk production from the breast). In men, it can lead to IMPOTENCE and sterility.

A second type of hormone-producing tumour leads to very high levels of growth hormone in the blood. If this starts before puberty, it leads to gigantism, although this condition is very rare. It is much commoner for the condition to start in adulthood when the long bones of the arms and legs are no longer capable of growing, but the hands and feet may grow thicker and the features may become gradually coarser as a result of the new growth of the facial bones. The non-bony parts of the body may also grow large, and this leads to weight gain and thickening of the skin. When an excess of growth hormone causes all these problems, the condition is called *acromegaly*.

Another hormone-producing tumour makes ACTH, the hormone that stimulates the adrenal gland. This gives rise to *Cushing's disease*, in which the adrenal glands produce too much cortisone. The condition results in obesity which characteristically is confined to the abdomen and chest. At the same time, there tends to be wasting of the muscles, leading to thin arms and legs. The skin is thin and bruises easily, and stretch marks, similar to those that occur in pregnancy, may develop.

Tumours in the pituitary itself may press on the rest of the gland so that it can no longer produce its normal hormones. This can also occur when other types of tumour in the region of the pituitary start to interfere with the function of the gland. All these problems can lead to *hypopituitarism*, in which the gland no longer secretes enough hormones.

In an adult, hypopituitarism may produce a reduction in the amount of gonadotrophins that are secreted; this leads to a falling-off of sexual function in men and amenorrhoea in women. Although this may severely interfere with people's lives, it is unlikely to be fatal.

If the adrenal glands or thyroid gland stop working properly, serious illness or even death can result. This is why doctors are anxious to investigate anyone who may have a pituitary tumour. The main role of cortisone in the body is to enable it to respond to stress, and it cannot do this if there is no ACTH to simulate the adrenal glands when stress occurs. Doctors test this system by giving an injection of insulin to lower the blood sugar; if the adrenal glands are working normally, the level of blood cortisone will be raised.

The posterior pituitary may also fail to produce hormones, although it is only the lack of ADH that causes difficulties. When this is absent, the body cannot retain water, and this results in excessive thirst, while at the same time large amounts of urine are passed.

In children, an underactive pituitary means that normal growth may be very slow, or may stop altogether. A lack of gonadotrophins will also delay the onset of puberty. Tumours affecting the pituitary can occur in childhood, leading to these problems, but are extremely rare.

Treatment

In the few cases where the pituitary produces diseases, successful investigation depends on careful investigation of the underlying hormonal problems. This can be exacting for both doctor and patient.

Prolactinomas are sometimes treated by surgery on the pituitary, but more often the prolactin levels can be kept under control with a drug called *bromocriptine*. This inhibits the release of prolactin. When there is an excess of the growth hormone, surgery is required more often than when prolactinomas are present: the tumours tend to be larger.

If the patient has Cushing's disease, a complicated series of tests has to be performed to see whether the problem arises as a result of too much ACTH being produced by the pituitary, or whether the adrenal glands themselves are the source of trouble. When the pituitary is at fault, an operation may be necessary to remove the tiny pituitary tumour.

For cortisone deficiency, cortisone tablets can be given by mouth. Thyroid hormones, as well as sex hormones in women, can also be administered in this way by using preparations that are similar to the contraceptive pill. In men, sex hormone replacement is best given by long-lasting injections, or implants, of testosterone – the male hormone.

A deficiency of ADH is remedied by giving the hormone in the form of snuff or a nasal spray.

Pityriasis rosea, *see* **Rash**

Pityriasis versicolor, *see* **Fungal infections, Rash**

Plantar wart, *see* **Verruca**

Plasma, *see* **Blood**

Plastic surgery

The term 'plastic surgery' simply means any surgery that changes the shape of the body, but it is also used now to mean surgery where tissues are moved from one part of the body to another. Because SKIN is one of the very few body tissues that can be moved relatively easily, plastic surgery and skin grafting have tended to become synonymous, but many other techniques are used by the plastic surgeon.

Reconstructive surgery forms the major part of plastic surgery. While *cosmetic surgery* may be more widely publicized, it is only a small part of this important and skilful branch of medicine.

Conditions requiring treatment

Plastic surgery deals with a wide range of conditions, including congenital abnormalities (those people are born with), injuries such as crushed hands and burns, and disfigurements and scars resulting from diseases such as CANCER of the skin or lining of the mouth.

Congenital abnormalities that are brought to the attention of the plastic surgeon include CLEFT PALATE AND HARE LIP, conditions that can occur together. Correction of these defects not only makes a truly remarkable improvement in appearance, but is necessary for the normal development of speech and the proper growth of teeth. A hare lip is usually corrected when the baby is about three months old, although some surgeons prefer to make the repair when the infant is much younger. The palate is repaired at about nine months to one year, before the time when speech development begins.

Children with BIRTHMARKS are often referred to plastic surgeons. Many of these marks, such as the 'strawberry' naevus, do not normally require surgery because they often disappear as the child grows older. However, an operation may be required if complications arise, such as bleeding from the birthmark or obstruction of the baby's eyesight.

There are a number of other deformities that children are born with that may require plastic surgery, although none of them are common. A baby may have extra fingers or toes (*polydactyly*), fingers that are joined together (*syndactyly*) or extra tags around the earlobes (*accessory auricle*). Occasionally the PENIS is slightly abnormal, with the opening on the underside instead of at the tip (*hypospadias*). As none of these conditions is dangerous, there is no urgency to correct them, and surgery is usually left until the child is older – when he or she is ready to go to school. At this age, the operation and the administration of anaesthetic are a little easier.

Severe burns may require the attention of the plastic surgeon both in the immediate stage and at a later date to improve the scars that may develop. If the burns are of partial thickness – that is, the deeper layers of skin are not damaged – the burns will heal by themselves. Areas where the burns are full thickness, when even the deepest layers in the skin have been damaged, will require skin grafts. It is remarkable that, once the burned area is covered with skin, it becomes much less painful.

Severe burns often require a series of plastic surgery operations, first to cover the area with grafts but later to free tissues that may have contracted after the burns. Special techniques may be used to move skin from one part of the body to another to rebuild the face, or to free the fingers from tight scar tissue. Careful prompt treatment can save the lives of severely burned patients, but the operations which are subsequently needed to restore the function of the body may take place over a period of several years.

Head and neck

Severe injuries to the face and jaws are usually treated jointly by plastic surgeons and maxillo-facial surgeons who are trained both in dentistry and in surgery. Simple lacerations may need very careful treatment to avoid scarring; plastic surgeons always pay particular attention to the technique of suturing wounds to minimize subsequent disfigurement. If the face or jaw has been fractured, special techniques may be needed to wire the pieces of bone together. In the most severe cases, the jaw FRACTURE may be stabilized externally by a system of metal struts fixed to a metal plate encircling the skull. This plate, sometimes referred to as a 'halo', is in turn fixed to the skull using screws and is left in place until the jaw fracture has united – a period of several weeks.

Some of the most remarkable operations carried out by plastic surgeons involve the correction of severe deformities of the skull or the face. Such operations usually involve a team of surgeons including a maxillo-facial surgeon, a neurosurgeon and sometimes an ear, nose and throat surgeon as well. Usually these operations are carried out on older children or young teenagers. They may involve moving the whole of the face to realign it with the skull or remodelling the shape of the skull. The operation is planned meticulously beforehand using numerous X-rays of the patient's head. Computer techniques have recently been developed which allow the surgeon to test the effect of moving particular areas of bone on a computer model of the head before undertaking the operation.

One of the most complicated types of operation is the surgical treatment of a condition known as *hypertelorism,* in which the forehead tends to be low and the eyes very far apart, resulting in an extremely bizarre facial appearance. The face is separated into several pieces during the course of the operation, and the eyes in their sockets moved closer together.

Surgical removal of cancers of the jaw, the tongue or the neck often involves removal of a large part of the bones of the face. The plastic surgeon can often reconstruct the face in stages after such a procedure, using bone grafts from other parts of the body and skin transferred from the chest wall.

Hand surgery

Although some surgery to the hand is also carried out by orthopaedic surgeons, many plastic surgeons have developed special skills in dealing with hand injuries and hand deformities. If tendons or nerves are damaged as a result of severe lacerations to the hand or forearm, they must be repaired carefully to restore full function to the damaged limb. Often they are repaired using a special operating microscope and tiny surgical instruments (microsurgery). Arteries and veins may need to be repaired in the same way. Similar techniques are used for 'replantation' – sewing back a finger, a hand or even an arm which has been accidentally amputated – for example, by a chainsaw. During the operation, bones, arteries, veins, tendons, nerves and skin all have to be repaired accurately. It is unusual, however, for a patient to regain completely normal function or feeling in the limb or digit after such a severe injury.

Plastic surgeons may also operate on patient's hands which are severely affected by ARTHRITIS. Tendons may need to be released and sometimes artificial joints are inserted into the knuckles or in the fingers.

Skin lesions

A number of skin problems are also treated by plastic surgeons. Large unsightly MOLES may be removed and any defects left in the skin may need covering with skin grafts. Various types of skin cancer are treated by removal and grafting, although RADIOTHERAPY (X-ray treatment) or drug therapy may be required as well. Large sores such as bedsores (*see* ULCERS, SKIN) can sometimes require skin-grafting to promote healing.

Vascular abnormalities in the skin – for example, *haemangiomas,* which show up as large red lesions – may also require removal by a plastic surgeon.

Cosmetic surgery

Cosmetic operations can improve the features of the face, such as straightening or reducing the size of a nose or tightening sagging tissues under the chin, cheeks or eyelids. These operations are usually done under a general anaesthetic and the patient usually spends a day or two in hospital.

Breasts may be increased in size by inserting artificial implants or 'prostheses' deep into the breast tissue. These prostheses are plastic bags filled with silicone gel or saline and are designed to mimic the texture and shape of a real breast. Sensation in the nipple may be temporarily changed, but breastfeeding is not altered by the operation as breast tissue is not damaged.

In contrast, an operation to make the breasts smaller involves cutting through the breast tissue and breastfeeding is therefore no longer possible.

Operations have also been devised for reducing the amount of fat and loose skin on the stomach, thighs and buttocks. These are major operations usually requiring a week or more in hospital. The plastic surgeon tries to make the long scars that result from these operations as unobtrusive as possible – for example, by putting them in the 'bikini' area.

Strictly speaking, cosmetic surgery is a branch of plastic surgery and should therefore be performed by a qualified plastic surgeon. However, in Britain, some cosmetic surgery is performed by people who are not trained plastic surgeons. This situation has arisen because of the large demand for cosmetic operations in recent years, which provides tremendous financial incentives for some cosmetic clinics. In such cases, it is in the interest of every potential patient to find out who will perform the operation, what his or her qualifications are and whether he or she is a member of the British Association of Aesthetic Plastic Surgeons.

Platelets, *see* Blood

Pleural effusion, *see* Lungs and lung diseases

Pleurisy

In the past, the very mention of pleurisy frightened people. This was because it was invariably associated with yesterday's great killer of young children – lobar PNEUMONIA. Nowadays, however, this is a rare disease and one which in any case can be controlled with ANTIBIOTICS. In modern parlance, pleurisy is a name given to problems involving inflammation of the pleura – the delicate lining membrane of the LUNGS. It can be associated with all sorts of diseases.

The pleura

Each lung is surrounded by a lining membrane, which is called the *visceral pleura*. It covers the whole of the surface of the lung and even lines both sides of the fissures (cracks) that divide the lung into its various lobes. The inner surface of the chest wall is lined with another layer called the *parietal pleura*.

In healthy people, the visceral and parietal layers of pleura are always in contact with each other, and they slide over each other as the lung moves in the act of BREATHING. Of course, there is some space between the two layers. In healthy people, this 'potential' space is minimal: just enough to accommodate tiny amounts of fluid that help to lubricate the two layers as they glide over each other. In one type of pleurisy, however, the space can fill up with large amounts of fluid: this is called a *pleural effusion*.

Unlike the lung, the pleura is equipped with the nerves that allow it to feel pain, and it is this pain that is characteristic of pleurisy. Any sort of inflammation will make the surface of the pleura raw, and the pain will arise as the visceral and parietal pleura slide past each other in the process of breathing.

Pleurisy can cause permanent damage to the lungs or the pleura. This happens particularly in tuberculosis. In this disease, pleural infection tends to leave thick scars on the surface of the pleura. Sometimes the scarring becomes even thicker as a result of infiltration by calcium, and in very rare cases, this process can lead to the lung becoming encased in a hard, bony cage.

Causes of pleurisy

Viruses may cause the pleural membranes to become inflamed and sore in the same way as they affect the membranes of the nose when you have a cold. Like any other sort of viral infection, pleurisy can occur in small epidemics. Painful chest muscles, together with pain on breathing are the hallmarks of the disease. Viral pleurisy settles without treatment or complications.

Bacteria can also produce pleurisy, although they usually do this as a result of underlying pneumonia. As infection spreads through lung tissue, it eventually leads to inflammation on the outer surface of the lung. This then leads to the symptoms of pleurisy.

Bacteria can also cause pleurisy in TUBERCULOSIS. This disease is really still quite common, particularly in Third World countries. There may be a big pleural effusion, although the painful breathing so typical of many sorts of pleurisy is not nearly as common in cases related to tuberculosis.

Occasionally a pleural effusion turns out to be due to neither infection nor a tumour, but to some other disease. For example, diseases which set up a general level of inflammation in the body as a result of disturbances in the body's immune system can cause a pleural effusion. One such disease is called *systemic* LUPUS ERYTHEMATOSUS.

A pulmonary embolus (*see* LUNG AND LUNG DISEASES) is another possible cause of pleurisy. In this condition, a blood clot which has formed in the leg breaks free and travels in the blood around the circulation to the lung. Inflammation set up by the blood clot can affect the pleura.

Symptoms and treatment

The typical symptom of pleurisy is pain in the chest. This is made worse by breathing – particularly deep breathing – as the two inflamed pleural surfaces rub against each other. Variation in position may also make a difference.

When fluid begins to collect in the pleural space, inflamed layers of pleura are separated, and the pain may disappear. Thus with a large pleural effusion, the main problem is likely to be breathlessness rather than pain.

Your doctor can diagnose pleurisy simply by listening to your description of the pain. He or she will also be helped in the diagnosis if he or she can hear what is called a 'pleural rub' through a stethoscope. A pleural rub is exactly that: the sound of the two inflamed layers rubbing against each other. It sounds a bit like a foot crunching through packed snow with each breath. Chest X-RAYS are also helpful, particularly in cases of patients suffering from pleural effusions.

The sort of treatment depends on the underlying condition. Pleuritic symptoms can be very painful, and will certainly require a PAINKILLER.

When a large amount of fluid is present, this has to be drained. This is a simple procedure: the doctor freezes a small section of the chest with local anaesthetic, and then passes a needle into the pleural space to draw off the fluid. In addition, by using a special needle, your doctor can remove a piece of the pleura for examination under a microscope.

Pneumoconiosis, *see* **Emphysema, Lungs and lung diseases, Occupational hazards**

Pneumonia

Pneumonia means inflammation of the substance of the LUNGS. Although it most commonly occurs as a result of a bacterial infection, it may also arise from a viral or fungal infection, or from inhaling foreign matter. Treatment with ANTIBIOTICS has meant a decline in fatalities, although the elderly, those with chronic lung disorders and those already weakened by other serious illness remain at risk.

Causes

To understand how pneumonia affects the lungs, it is necessary to look at their structure (*see* BREATHING).

The main breathing tube that supplies air to the lungs is the windpipe (trachea). This splits into two branches (the bronchi), which in turn divide into three branches on the right and two main branches on the left. Each of these branches supplies one lobe of one of the lungs: there are three lobes on the right and two on the left, divided from each other by thin membranes of fibrous tissue.

Each of these main bronchi to one of the lobes then splits down into a series of finger branches which supply all the tiny air sacs or alveoli where oxygen finally crosses from the air inside the lungs into the blood.

 When infection strikes the chest, the inflammation it causes may be confined to the bronchi. This inflammation, called BRONCHITIS, results in a thickening of the bronchi's lining membrane and the production of large amounts of secretions from the bronchi's glands.

In pneumonia, the infection occurs in the smaller bronchi and the alveoli. These become solid with secretions, rather than filled with air. This is called 'consolidation' and on a chest X-ray, the affected area shows up as a white patch, rather than a black area as in a normal lung. The congestion may severely affect breathing.

There are two main types of pneumonia: lobar pneumonia and bronchopneumonia.

Lobar pneumonia was, in the past, the commoner of the two. Although it has now become rather rare today in countries such as Britain, it is still common in less developed ones. Lobar pneumonia is nearly always due to the *Pneumococcus* bacterium. Only one lobe of the lung tends to be involved, and this lobe becomes consolidated while the rest of the lung remains relatively normal. (When two lobes are involved, this is commonly known as 'double pneumonia'.)

Bronchopneumonia can be caused by many different types of organism, although normally some sort of bacterium is responsible. Of these, the most common is the *Haemophilus influenzae* bacterium. Other kinds of bacteria that can cause bronchopneumonia include the *Pneumococcus*, and the *staphylococci*, which is the more serious. This kind of bronchopneumonia tends to appear after a dose of the flu, and fatalities may occur in people who previously were well; but it is not very common nowadays.

Bronchopneumonia is characterized by little white patches of consolidation which appear all over the lungs, and though these patches may be concentrated in one lung, or even in one part of one lung, a whole lobe is not involved. Bronchopneumonia can occur at the same time as bronchitis, and often results from bronchitis spreading. This frequently happens to people who have had long-term (chronic) chest problems, but it is also common for people to get acute bronchopneumonia on top of chronic bronchitis.

Viruses can also cause pneumonia, although more often it is a virus infection in the upper part of the respiratory system (the throat and nose) that paves the way for a bacterium becoming established lower down in the chest.

Tiny organisms such as the CHLAMYDIA (which causes psittacosis, a disease caught from caged birds), Rickettsia (which causes TYPHUS and *Q fever*) and the *Mycoplasma* organism can also cause pneumonia.

Pneumonia may also arise as a result of a blockage of one of the main bronchial tubes – for instance, from CANCER of the bronchus. Similarly, chronic disorders of the bronchus, such as *bronchiectasis* (where the bronchi continually produce pus as a result of a chronic infection that also destroys the normal bronchial wall) can produce pneumonia by blocking the tubes and allowing pus to be sucked back into normal lung tissue.

Finally, pneumonia can result from inhaling things such as loose teeth or peanuts into the lungs. However the main kind of 'aspiration pneumonia' occurs as a result of UNCONSCIOUSNESS, as at this time, there is a failure in the COUGHING mechanism that prevents food and other foreign substances from going down the wrong way. For this reason, a careful watch is kept so that no such inhalations occur when an anaesthetic is given, or when emergency resuscitation is needed.

Symptoms

The main symptom of pneumonia is a cough, which varies according to the type of pneumonia. In bronchopneumonia with added acute bronchitis, there may be a lot of infected (yellow or green) sputum produced, while in a viral pneumonia there could be a dry cough with no sputum at all. In bronchopneumonia, there is usually a cough, though it is not the main symptom.

Lobar pneumonia is a feverish illness and unless it is treated with antibiotics, very high temperatures will result. Since the whole lobe is involved, the inflammation may spread to the lining of the pleura, causing PLEURISY, with the ensuing result that pain on coughing or taking a deep breath is often a common additional symptom.

In bronchopneumonia due to bacteria, symptoms tend to vary according to how much extra bronchitis there is. However, there is nearly always more sputum produced in bronchopneumonia, while pleurisy is a less common occurrence. There is usually a temperature but it is not so high as in lobar pneumonia.

Bronchopneumonia is a disease that is more likely to affect the old and the ill or infirm. Often there are fewer symptoms in the elderly than in the young and fit; despite this, when the disease occurs in older people, it may cause death after a long illness.

In the rarer forms of pneumonia due to organisms that are not bacteria, the symptoms vary, but by and large, feverish illnesses are common. Changes in the lungs are obvious in the X-rays, while the cough and sputum production is less than in bacterial pneumonia.

Dangers and complications

One of the commoner complications of all kinds of pneumonia is pleurisy. This may lead to a *pleural effusion* – a collection of fluid within the pleural cavity. This can become infected, leading to a large collection of pus forming in the pleural cavity (*empyema*).

Pockets of pus can also form within the infected lung, causing a lung ABSCESS. This is especially likely to happen in staphylococcal pneumonia and in a rare form of lobar pneumonia called *Klebsiella*. Lung abscesses are a serious problem, and only occur as a result of severe lung infection; they can cause permanent scarring on the lungs.

In general, though, it is pneumonia which is a complication of other diseases, rather than pneumonia which gives rise to other complications. It is for this reason that pneumonia, usually severe bronchopneumonia, may be fatal, because it is so often the final event in the life of someone who is already very weak, ill or elderly.

Treatment and outlook

In fit people, treatment with antibiotics is generally all that is necessary. In older people, or people who already have a chronic chest disease or another illness, it is very important to make sure that the secretions in the lung produced by pneumonia are coughed up and not allowed to remain in the chest where they can cause further problems. The PHYSIOTHERAPIST has a vital role to play in helping people with pneumonia to clear these secretions. Drugs that are inhaled through a vapour in an oxygen mask may help to widen the bronchi, which tend to narrow down in pneumonia.

The outlook in pneumonia depends upon the age and the state of health of the patient.

Pneumothorax, *see* **Lungs and lung diseases**

Poliomyelitis

This disease, commonly called polio, is caused by the VIRUS invading the motor cells of the SPINAL CORD and parts of the BRAIN. The nerve cells involved are principally those that work the muscles of the limbs and those controlling breathing and swallowing. The invasion of these cells stimulates a reaction in the body's IMMUNE SYSTEM; the NERVOUS SYSTEM becomes the field on which the battle is fought and the resulting damage causes the disabling symptoms.

The disease starts with the polio virus multiplying in the lining of the throat and stomach. Often the infection stops here, having caused what only appears to be a mild bout of gastric influenza; or, indeed, there may be no symptoms at all. Then, in a small number of people, symptoms of nervous system involvement may appear after a few weeks. Initially these symptoms are mild and consist of muscle pain and aches. Again, in many people, the illness may have then run its course. If not, more serious signs, such as a MENINGITIS with neck stiffness and over-sensitivity to light, may develop. After this, or sometimes instead of this stage, one leg or arm may become progressively weaker. In some cases, this weakness may be extremely severe, affecting all the limbs and the muscles that control swallowing and breathing: this is probably the most dangerous stage of polio as the patient may be unable to breathe without the aid of a breathing machine. If the brainstem – the part of the brain that controls the automatic functions of the body – is affected, the circulation may collapse, causing a drop in BLOOD PRESSURE and problems with the HEART's rhythm.

After a rather variable time, the acute inflammation which has been causing the symptoms settles down as the body's immune system gets the better of the virus. The weakness and other symptoms may then recover to some extent as the undamaged nerve cells take over the function of those destroyed by the infection. However, any muscle wasting that has already occurred as a result of the loss of the muscle's nerve supply cannot be reversed.

Treatment and outlook

Viruses, unlike bacteria, are very difficult to get rid of once they have entered the body and started an infection, and antibiotics are not effective in destroying these germs. This means that, once someone has contracted polio, treatment has to be restricted to trying to prevent the serious effects on the nervous system causing irreparable damage.

Although there is no specific treatment as such, there is much that can be done. Careful nursing will help to reduce complications such as bedsores (*see* ULCERS, SKIN), and PHYSIOTHERAPY will be given to prevent paralysed limbs from wasting. If breathing is affected, it may be necessary for the patient to breathe using a ventilator.

Fortunately, the vast majority of people who become infected with the polio virus do not get severe symptoms. However, they can and do pass on the virus to others in whom it may cause a far more serious illness.

The chances of recovery are quite good, although children and old people seem to do less well than young adults. Many polio victims may be left with some wasting of muscles, but only a small number become disabled.

Since polio is so difficult to treat once infection has occurred, it is vital that it is prevented. For one thing, increasing attention to sanitation in developed countries has meant that the virus which is shed in the excreta is less readily spread. (However, this also means that very young children – who once developed extremely mild forms of the disease and were then immune – are no longer exposed to polio and may then develop more serious cases when they are older.) And, more importantly, the IMMUNIZATION campaigns of the late 1950s and 1960s – which still continue – have succeeded in nearly wiping out this disease in many developed countries.

Immunization is very simple. Nowadays, the vaccine does not even need to be administered by injection, but can be given orally. Most babies and young children in Britain are routinely vaccinated against polio with their other inoculations. In fact, it is essential for everyone to be vaccinated, particularly in these days of widespread travel, as this is the only way to combat this disease effectively. The immunity given is life-long and the vaccine is very safe.

Polio is now extremely rare in developed countries, and with international immunization programmes being carried out elsewhere, it is hoped that this disease, like SMALLPOX, will soon be eradicated from the earth.

Polymorphs, *see* **Blood**

Polymyalgia rheumatica, *see* **Muscles**

Polyps

Any small lump attached to a stalk and arising from a lining membrane is known as a *polyp*. Most are due to an overgrowth of the membrane at a particular site so that a definite small lump is formed. They may occur singly or in large numbers and be present from birth or develop later in life.

Common sites of polyps are the NOSE, LARYNX, STOMACH, COLON or UTERUS. Most are quite benign, some are potentially malignant (cancerous) and a few are malignant from the beginning.

Nasal polyps

These polyps are attached to the membrane lining the nose and consist of swellings which can grow as big as a grape if left untreated. They occur in people who have frequent COLDS and HAY FEVER but are also a cause of nasal infections in the SINUSES – the cavities in the bones of the face – by blocking the tiny communicating channels between the nasal cavity and the sinuses.

Nasal polyps come to light when one side of the nose becomes blocked or when there is excessive discharge from the nose for a long time. The polyps can be seen by a doctor with the help of a special viewing instrument. They are easily removed under a general anaesthetic by passing a wire loop around each one in turn and 'snaring' it. This is a relatively minor procedure, although further treatment may be needed if more polyps develop.

Polyps in the intestines

Polyps in the INTESTINES occur most often in the large bowel and RECTUM but are sometimes found in the small intestine, especially in certain rare congenital syndromes. In the large bowel, polyps may be single or multiple, very small in size or they may grow as large as 1⅕ in (3 cm) in diameter.

In the condition known as *familial polyposis coli*, hundreds of small polyps develop in the colon (large intestine). Several members of a family may be affected in this way. There is a high risk that one or more of these polyps may turn malignant so the colon is always removed and the small bowel joined to the rectum.

Most cases of polyps in the large bowel are not hereditary, however, and usually appear in the lower part of the colon. A person affected may notice blood or excessive mucus in the motions and lower abdominal pain due to the bowel attempting to pass the polyp along as if it were faeces. This pulls on the polyp, and hence the bowel wall, causing pain.

Polyps in the bowel can be seen with the aid of a sigmoidoscope – a hollow tube passed into the rectum – or a colonoscope (*see* ENDOSCOPY), a long flexible viewing instrument that can be manoeuvred along the bends of the colon. A BARIUM enema, whereby the bowel shows up on X-ray, may also be used to clarify diagnosis.

Polyps must always be removed because of the symptoms they cause or because they are liable to turn malignant if they grow larger than about ⅖ in (1 cm) in diameter. The polyp can be removed with a colonoscope, but if it is large, an operation has to be performed.

When a polyp is removed with a colonoscope, the patient is sedated with an injection and the instrument passed into the rectum. The polyp is identified and a long wire with a loop at the end is threaded through the colonoscope.

The loop is put over the polyp, pulled tight and an electric current passed through the wire. This cauterizes the base of the polyp so that it can be removed without bleeding. The patient can usually go home the same day.

Polyps in the uterus

Polyps may arise in the uterus (womb) either from the membrane lining the inside of the uterus or from the CERVIX (neck of the womb). They may become apparent because of heavy PERIODS or because of bleeding between periods or a vaginal discharge.

These polyps are normally removed by the procedure of dilatation and curettage (D & C). The lining of the uterus is scraped out together with any polyps that are present. Sometimes polyps in the uterus are an indication of FIBROIDS, which are fibrous swellings in the muscular wall of the uterus. In such a case, it may be necessary to remove the uterus to cure the symptoms.

A small polyp would not cause any harm during pregnancy, but a large one, or a group of polyps, might do so, as they can become squashed and suddenly degenerate, causing pain.

Post-natal depression

DEPRESSION after CHILDBIRTH is a very common condition. It ranges from the temporary 'baby blues' to black despair. It can occur after the birth of any child, not just the first, and may last for a long time. The most worrying aspect of this condition is that mothers who are depressed often feel ashamed of their unhappiness and thus neither seek nor receive help.

'Baby blues' are experienced by 80 per cent of all new mothers. It usually occurs between three and four days after delivery, and it takes the form of a general feeling of vulnerability and a persistent weepiness. This feeling normally passes after one or two weeks. If it continues for longer, it is a sign of more serious depression. Twenty per cent of mothers suffer from low-grade post-natal depression, serious enough to make life seem rather grey, but not so severe that they are unable to cope. Probably about one mother in 20 has severe enough depression to require active medical treatment, often with drugs. Very serious psychotic depression occurs in one in every 500 mothers, and usually requires hospital treatment.

The more serious forms of post-natal depression may not start for a long time after the birth. It is not always easy to say at what point a feeling of being low or tired or fed-up turns into a fully fledged depression, but in general if the mood lasts longer than a few weeks or if the symptoms affect the sufferer's life, she should seek help. Relatives may be the first to notice depression because one of the early signs may be difficulty in coping with the baby.

Causes

Post-natal depression is a response to an event that causes great change and STRESS in a woman's life. There is no single cause: just a combination of factors which may be difficult to cope with. There are six main areas of stress:

Childbirth: Giving birth is one of the most important experiences in a woman's life, and a bad birth experience can be damaging emotionally. Problems during the delivery, such as a difficult forceps delivery, may well trigger off a depression. The mother may feel she has in some way 'failed' her baby.

Motherhood: Mothers are both idealized and undervalued. They are told that they are important and yet may be treated as if they didn't exist. Coping realistically with such a situation can be very difficult.

Loss: All depression has an element of grieving about it. The birth of a baby may be an obvious gain, but it also involves a loss of identity for the mother. The inevitable loss of independence may also trigger off a depression.

Isolation: Social isolation is one of the worst problems any new mother has to cope with. Getting out of the house and talking over worries with other adults are very important.

Exhaustion: Broken nights and the lack of regular sleeping patterns can easily produce feelings of disorientation.

Hormonal changes: A woman's body goes through considerable change as a result of pregnancy and birth. This often makes women more vulnerable to stress.

Symptoms

The main symptom of depression is a lack of self-esteem. When you feel really low, you blame yourself for virtually everything. Other emotional symptoms include tearfulness, feeling inadequate and unable to cope, especially with the baby, and feelings of guilt – for not loving the baby enough.

Physical symptoms include loss of appetite and reduced sexual interest. The mother may also have problems sleeping at night – even when the baby *isn't* crying. Nightmares are quite common.

Sometimes anxiety is more marked than depression, and this can take different forms. Anxiety over health – the baby's, your partner's or your own – is common, as is the fear of leaving the house (*agoraphobia*).

Treatment

Most women try to fight depression by hiding it behind a smile and feeling guilty or ashamed about their problems. However, once a mother accepts that she needs help, there are a number of things that can be done to give her the support and care that she needs.

The best course for a mother suffering from depression is never to fight it, but to accept it. Once she has accepted the fact that she can't cope very well without help, it becomes much easier for her to ask for it, and to talk to other people about her feelings. She should try to get out of the house at least once a day and make time to do things that she enjoys, and which have nothing to do with the baby.

Medical treatment with antidepressant drugs can be useful in helping to remove the symptoms of depression. However, both practical support and help with emotional problems are always needed as well.

Post-viral fatigue syndrome, *see* Myalgic encephalomyelitis

Potassium

This is a metallic element (*see* MINERALS) which in the body exists in the form of positively charged ions (atoms which have acquired an electric charge). Together with another simple substance, *sodium* (*see* SALT), potassium plays a vital role in the functioning of individual body cells.

Potassium is essential to healthy NERVE and MUSCLE function. It is found chiefly within cells, dissolved in cellular fluid, while sodium is principally outside cells.

However, the body contains more potassium than sodium. An average 10 stone (65 kg) man has a total of 6 oz (168 g) of potassium in his body, of which 5 oz (136 g) is contained within the cells. On the other hand, there is a total of just 3 oz (89 g) of sodium in the body of which no less than 80 g is in bone or outside the cells. Only about ⅓ oz (9 g) is present in the cells of the body.

Sodium and potassium cannot be considered independently since they have complementary roles in biochemical terms. The cell walls actively keep potassium inside cells, and conversely keep sodium out of them. The result is that there is a very small electrical charge on each side of all cell membranes. Nerve and muscle cells make use of this charge in triggering off both nerve impulses and muscle contractions. The specialized cell walls of these tissues contain a type of electrical relay system which depends on the presence of both potassium and sodium, in the form of electrically charged ions, on each side of the cell wall. Other minerals are also involved in this process – for example, magnesium and CALCIUM.

Control of potassium balance

Appreciable amounts of potassium are eliminated from the body each day in the urine, faeces, sweat and dead cells. The normal intake of food can, however, usually compensate for this, and any excess is excreted. The main controlling mechanism for sodium and potassium levels involves the KIDNEYS and ADRENAL GLANDS. These glands produce a hormone called *aldosterone,* which stimulates the kidneys to excrete more potassium. The amount of aldosterone produced is very carefully and automatically adjusted by the adrenal glands so that the potassium concentration in the body remains precisely the same – unless there are severe problems causing shortages or excesses of potassium.

Potassium depletion and excess

This is the commonest disorder affecting potassium balance. Potassium can become depleted if a person becomes dehydrated from lack of WATER – for example, in a very hot environment with excessive sweating, or if there is no water to drink. The person continues to produce urine containing potassium, and as water is lost, so is potassium. A person who has a bad attack of GASTRO-ENTERITIS can also become potassium deficient because the body can lose considerable quantities of potassium if there is profuse DIARRHOEA; this is particularly dangerous in infants and small children. Some types of kidney and LIVER diseases and severe DIABETES may also cause an excessive loss of potassium. Lastly, certain diuretic drugs may also cause potassium depletion if they are taken over prolonged periods of time.

The chief symptoms of potassium depletion are muscular weakness and mental confusion. The functioning of the muscles is first to become affected, and then the nerves; in severe cases, the patient may even become paralysed. The muscle in the bowel may stop working, giving rise to a condition called ileus (*see* ILEUM). Ultimately the HEART action becomes irregular. Unless treatment is given, death may occur. This is only likely in those rare circumstances such as serious dehydration where medical treatment is not readily available.

It is unusual for an excess of potassium to build up in the body, but it can occur if the patient is suffering from acute kidney failure or severe burns, or after taking certain drugs. It can have dangerous effects on the heart and must be treated urgently.

Treatment

Although dietary shortage of potassium is unusual, there are a number of situations in which extra potassium may be needed. This can often be given in the diet (bananas are an excellent source), or potassium can be prescribed as a medicine or tablets.

Most people feel weak after an attack of gastro-enteritis, and extra potassium will help recovery. Some people even claim that potassium supplements help a hangover.

Potassium supplements may be prescribed for patients who are on diuretics, or a 'potassium sparing' diuretic may be prescribed. In hospital, potassium supplements may be given by an intravenous drip if patients have become seriously short of potassium – for example, as a result of dehydration associated with diabetes or kidney disease.

The treatment of excess potassium involves the intravenous injection of calcium, and the patient may require urgent dialysis in the case of kidney failure.

Pott's disease, *see* Kyphosis

Potts' fracture, *see* Fracture, Leg

Pre-eclampsia, *see* Eclampsia and pre-eclampsia

Pregnancy

This is the remarkable and highly complex process between CONCEPTION and CHILDBIRTH and lasts on average 38 weeks. Because the date of conception is often not known exactly, it is easier to date the pregnancy from the first day of the last menstrual PERIOD, which is usually about a fortnight before conception, making a total of 40 weeks.

The first signs

The first sign of pregnancy is usually a missed period, although this can be caused by other conditions. However, if intercourse without contraception has taken place, pregnancy is the most likely cause. Other early symptoms include a sense of fullness and tingling in the breasts and a need to pass urine more frequently. NAUSEA, and even vomiting, is suffered by many women in early pregnancy. Popularly known as 'morning sickness', it can, in fact, come at any time of day.

If you think you are pregnant

It is important that you should go to see your doctor as soon as you suspect you might be pregnant – say, two weeks after your missed period. Take with you to your appointment a sample of the first urine you passed that morning. A pregnancy test can then be done to detect the presence or absence of a hormone called *human chorionic gonadotrophin* which is produced by the developing egg and excreted in the mother's urine. Simple home pregnancy tests are available from chemists, and these work on exactly the same principle. If you carry out the test yourself, you should still consult your doctor if the result is positive. Most tests are reliable only six weeks after the last period, but there are a few that can be used earlier.

Once your pregnancy is confirmed, your family doctor will arrange for your care during pregnancy and labour. If the baby is to be born in hospital, he or she will arrange a booking examination at the hospital which usually takes place when you are 12 to 13 weeks pregnant. Visits to the antenatal clinic are then arranged on a monthly basis during the first 28 weeks of pregnancy, then fortnightly until 36 weeks and thereafter weekly until the baby is born. Obviously, these arrangements have to be flexible to allow for any unusual circumstances.

Antenatal check-ups may take place entirely at the hospital throughout the pregnancy; or the hospital may send you back to your own doctor after the initial 'booking' examination. You will then be examined regularly at his or her surgery until you are about 32 weeks pregnant, when you will return to the hospital for later appointments. Alternatively, you may choose to attend a local clinic where you will be looked after by midwives during your pregnancy.

Antenatal clinics not only check that the mother and baby are healthy, they also arrange classes on baby care and preparation for labour and childbirth. Most courses include at least one session for the prospective fathers to advise them on how best to help their partners during pregnancy and labour and after the birth.

Morning sickness

Morning sickness is usually confined to the first three months of pregnancy. Most women find that it has stopped entirely by the 14th week, although a very few unlucky mothers-to-be continue to suffer from the sickness until they give birth.

No one knows quite why women should suffer from morning sickness. There are HORMONE changes, particularly the rapid increase in oestrogen, which are thought to be a contributing factor, especially as they are occurring at the same time as metabolic and chemical changes. It is also thought that the fall in BLOOD PRESSURE, typical in early pregnancy, is likely to cause feelings of nausea. Some research suggests that morning sickness may occur more frequently if the woman eats meals high in fat. Psychological factors are sometimes believed to play their part, particularly when the pregnancy is unplanned, although, as many women experience morning sickness, this would obviously comprise only a small proportion.

The effects: Almost all women find that their feelings of nausea are accompanied by a loss of appetite. Some women find that eating a little makes them feel better, others have to make themselves sick before they can carry on. Women can be very frightened when the vomiting is severe. The abdominal muscles usually feel sore afterwards, and there appears to be such internal pressure that it is often thought that the stability of the pregnancy is being affected. In fact, the baby is quite unharmed by the action of vomiting, and even women who have to be hospitalized because they are vomiting to the extreme are there so that their liquid and glucose intake can be monitored – not because a MISCARRIAGE is expected.

The sickness is quite normal, and not dangerous. The most obvious danger lies in taking drugs to control the sickness, for in the early stages this could affect the development of the baby. Nothing should be taken that has not been prescribed by a doctor, and the dose should never be exceeded.

Coping with morning sickness: Most women find that they can control the nausea to some extent by following a few simple rules. They avoid any food or drink that they instinctively feel would make them sick, even if there is pressure on them to take it. Many women are helped by eating and drinking a little half an hour or so before getting up – dry biscuits or toast and weak tea work for some women. This often prevents the uncomfortable dry retching sometimes felt on rising.

Greasy or spiced foods are to be avoided. Occasionally even the smell of them can affect a woman badly, so it would be wise if she kept her own cooking to a minimum while she is suffering from the nausea. Tight clothing can also contribute to a feeling of fullness around the abdomen, so it is better to switch to looser clothes, even if the pregnancy has not yet started to 'show'.

Many women have found that supplements of VITAMIN B_6 are effective in controlling nausea, though as with any vitamin supplement, they should be taken in conjunction with a good balanced diet.

Morning sickness usually disappears entirely by the 14th week of pregnancy, and many women find the rest of their term free of this problem.

Other minor discomforts

Vaginal discharge: Women have an increased vaginal discharge in pregnancy. This is quite normal and, unless offensive or irritating, does not require medical attention.

Backache and cramp may present a problem as the pregnancy advances. A pregnant woman tends to throw her shoulders back in an attempt to counteract the weight of the growing uterus, and this can put undue strain on the back (*see* LORDOSIS). Improved posture and comfortable, low-heeled shoes may relieve it. Leg cramps are common in late pregnancy and may be troublesome at night. They can sometimes be relieved by gently stretching the affected muscle. *See also* BACK AND BACKACHE.

Constipation and heartburn are commonly experienced during pregnancy. They are both the result of the effect of the hormone progesterone, which relaxes the smooth muscle fibres. Unfortunately, its action is not confined to the growing uterus, but affects the bowel, making it sluggish (*see* CONSTIPATION), and the sphincter muscle at the opening from the oesophagus into the stomach (*see* DIAPHRAGM). The latter can allow the stomach contents to be regurgitated and cause heartburn; a mild antacid can help.

Haemorrhoids or PILES are fairly common in pregnancy as the blood flow from the woman's legs and pelvis is partially obstructed by pressure from the baby and womb. Straining through constipation can aggravate it.

Varicose veins may become worse during pregnancy, owing to the effect of progesterone on the blood vessels, or they may appear for the first time. Maternity support tights can prevent them from forming, and they should be put on before getting out of bed in the morning. Women with VARICOSE VEINS should avoid standing still; it is better to walk around to keep the circulation going. When sitting, prop up the feet on a stool or low chair.

Oedema is caused by excess water in the body which causes swelling in certain areas, particularly ankles and feet. Mild OEDEMA is fairly common in late pregnancy; a low salt diet and plenty of rest with the feet up should help. If oedema is associated with raised blood pressure and protein in the urine, however, special treatment will be necessary as this could indicate toxaemia, a serious condition (*see* ECLAMPSIA AND PRE-ECLAMPSIA).

 Skin changes: As pregnancy proceeds, STRETCH MARKS may appear on the abdomen, thighs and breasts. Little can be done to prevent these, but they fade once the baby is born.

Changes in the uterus and breasts

Pregnancy is divided into three 'trimesters', each lasting about 13 weeks. In the first trimester, the uterus is still contained within the pelvic cavity although it is growing rapidly. It is during the second trimester that a woman becomes obviously pregnant. By about 22 weeks the upper edge of the womb, or *fundus*, reaches the navel, and at 36 weeks, most of the abdominal cavity is taken up. The intestines are pushed upwards and sideways so that they press on the stomach and diaphragm. The pressure on the diaphragm means that the lungs cannot expand fully and many women find themselves short of breath.

Around 22 weeks in a first pregnancy and 18 weeks in a later one, the mother will feel her baby's movements. The foetal heartbeat is usually audible through a stethoscope by 24 weeks.

The main change a woman will notice in her breasts during pregnancy is that they grow larger in preparation for feeding. The *areola* – the ring of darker skin around the nipple – gets larger and darker in colour and a secondary areola appears which helps to improve the strength of the skin. From about 12 weeks of pregnancy, the breasts produce a protein-rich substance called *colostrum* and in the last few weeks this fluid may leak. Colostrum provides all the nutritional needs of the newborn baby until the milk appears on the third day after the birth.

Antenatal care

Antenatal clinics are usually attached to a hospital, or your own doctor may provide antenatal care. The first visit should be made between the first 8 to 12 weeks of pregnancy. The doctor will check your medical history. He or she will then give you a general examination and measure your weight, height and blood pressure. You may have an internal examination. Samples of urine and blood will be taken for tests, and a card detailing your medical history, tests carried out and the progress of the pregnancy may be issued. From the blood sample, your BLOOD GROUP will be established, and you will be tested for ANAEMIA, SEXUALLY TRANSMITTED DISEASES and your susceptibility to RUBELLA.

Your next visit will be four weeks later, and then at four-weekly intervals up to the 28th week of your pregnancy. After that, you will need a check-up every two weeks up to the 36th week, then every week until the baby is born.

Each time, after you have been asked how you feel, you will have a urine test, your blood pressure and weight will be checked and your abdomen examined. The doctor will listen to the foetal heartbeat and you may have an internal examination.

Special procedures

When you are about 16 weeks pregnant, a blood sample will be taken specifically to see if there is an excess of *alpha fetoprotein*. This is known as the AFP test, and if you give a high reading, it might – but only might – indicate

The Stages of Pregnancy

6 weeks

At six weeks, the embryo is still not recognizably human, and is only about ½ in (1.3 cm) long. A pregnancy test at this time proves positive and the mother may feel some symptoms such as breast tenderness and morning sickness.

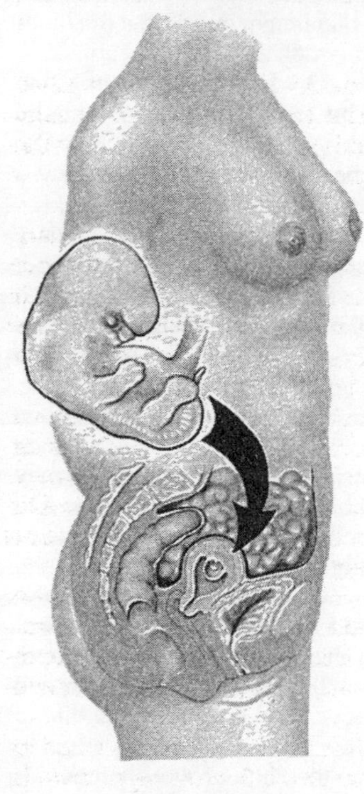

12 weeks

By 12 weeks, the uterus can just be felt above the pelvis. By now all the major foetal organs are formed, and nails are appearing on the fingers and toes. The foetus is about 3 in (7½ cm) long and weighs about ½ oz (14 g).

20 weeks

At 20 weeks into pregnancy, the uterus has reached the level of the mother's navel, and she becomes aware of the baby's movements. The foetus now measures about 8 in (21 cm) and is covered in fine, downy hair.

28 weeks

At 28 weeks, the uterus reaches about halfway between the navel and the breastbone. Foetal movements are vigorous, and the mother may feel painless rhythmic contractions. If the foetus were born at this stage, it could survive. Its skin is covered by a coating of protective vernix, and it can open its eyes. It measures about 15 in (37 cm).

40 weeks

At 40 weeks, pregnancy is full term. The upper edge of the uterus descends from its position high up under the rib cage as the baby's head moves down into the mother's pelvis. This is called 'engagement'. The mother's breathing becomes easier, although pressure on the bladder continues.

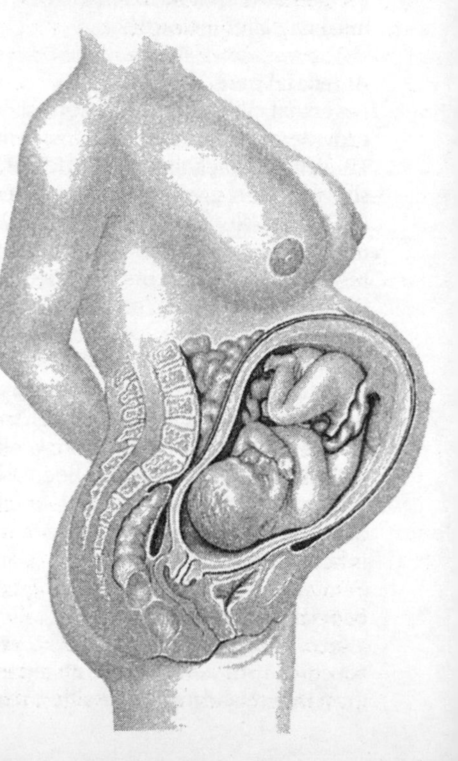

that the foetus has a neural deficiency such as SPINA BIFIDA or an encephaly (when the brain is not properly formed).

AFP increases naturally as pregnancy progresses so it is important this test is done between 16 and 18 weeks. A high reading might only indicate a presence of twins (*see* MULTIPLE BIRTH) or just that you are further on in your pregnancy than you imagined. In this case, a further AFP test will be given and you will probably be offered amniocentesis (*see below*) as well, which will give a more exact diagnosis.

Another blood test called the 'triple' test can be performed at 12 weeks' pregnancy, to assess the risk of having a baby affected by DOWN'S SYNDROME or neural tube defects.

Ultrasound scan: Most women have at least one ULTRASOUND scan during their pregnancy – again, usually at about 16 weeks. The scan can detect neural deficiency, a small-for-dates baby, twins, and *placenta praevia* (where the placenta is positioned very low, possibly right over the cervix).

Amniocentesis: A diagnostic technique, this is used to check for abnormalities in unborn babies who may be at special risk. It involves taking a sample of the amniotic fluid which surrounds the baby, by inserting a hollow needle carefully through the expectant mother's abdomen. This may sound, and indeed look, unpleasant, but if skilfully done, it does not even require an anaesthetic injection, though a local anaesthetic may be used.

The amount of fluid withdrawn is only about 20 cc, the equivalent of two dessert spoonfuls, although this can vary according to the number of tests necessary. This fluid contains cells from the foetus (the developing baby). Chemical and microscopic examinations of these can provide invaluable information, revealing the presence or absence of GENETIC disorders, which at one time could only be guessed at, with often distressing results.

The moment a human egg is fertilized, it has all the inherited information needed to create a new being. Both male and female cells contain chromosomes (*see* CELLS AND CHROMOSOMES), which determine sex and carry the genes that transmit inherited characteristics (*see* HEREDITY), but occasionally these chromosomes are found to be faulty.

From about the 16th week, the doubts and fears which previously had to be endured throughout pregnancy can be resolved. By this stage, there is enough amniotic fluid to allow the test to be carried out – and there is still time for the pregnancy to be terminated (*see* ABORTION) if this is thought to be necessary.

The main disorders which amniocentesis can reveal are spina bifida, an abnormality of the nervous system where the baby either does not survive or is born with severe spinal defects, and Down's syndrome, which used to be known as mongolism. Examining the chromosomes can also reveal the sex of the baby, but the test is not merely to satisfy curiosity without good medical reason. The sex of the baby only becomes medically important where there is known to be a history of a disorder such as HAEMOPHILIA (excessive bleeding from the smallest wound) within a family. Although carried by females, the disease only affects males, and if the test reveals a male child, a further test can confirm whether or not the baby is affected.

Amniocentesis is offered to women over 35 or so because the risk of chromosome defects increases with age. It is also recommended, regardless of age, to women who have already had a baby with spina bifida, Down's syndrome or any rare defect which is detectable by this technique.

It is carried out quite simply in the out-patients' department of a hospital, with no risk to the mother-to-be but a slight possibility of risk to the baby. About one in every 100 babies aborts after amniocentesis, and although many would have died or aborted anyway due to abnormalities, it still means that a few normal babies are lost. Fortunately, the technique of ultrasound scanning is now used together with amniocentesis to give a picture of the position of the foetus in the uterus as the needle is inserted, so making the whole procedure very much safer.

If a serious abnormality is found in the foetus, the parents are told and an abortion is offered to them.

Chorionic villus sampling (CVS): This is also known as chorionic biopsy. A small sample of tissue, taken from the cells surrounding the embryo, is analysed for the presence of genetic abnormalities.

X-rays: These are rarely carried out because radiation carries a small but definite risk to an unborn baby. Sometimes, however, a single X-ray is needed to check on the size of the pelvis to see if it is wide enough for the baby's head to pass through. This is never done before the last four weeks of pregnancy, after the baby has developed fully.

While you are pregnant

It is important that a pregnant woman should eat a sensible, well-balanced diet with plenty of protein (meat, fish, cheese), milk, fresh fruit and vegetables. Too many cakes and biscuits should be avoided as they can lead to excessive weight gain which will be difficult to shed after the birth. The amount of weight gained should not be more than 22 lb (10 kg), but crash slimming diets should never be undertaken in pregnancy, as you will undernourish the baby. If your doctor has prescribed IRON tablets, be sure to take them.

Certain foods should be avoided in pregnancy: soft cheeses and pâtés, because of the risk of the bacteria *Listeria*; liver, because of the risks of excess vitamin A; and very under-done and uncooked meat, because of the risk of food poisoning.

Moderate exercise is a good idea, although pregnancy is not the time to take up a new, strenuous sport. You will be taught exercises at antenatal classes to strengthen your back and muscles.

SMOKING should be avoided if at all possible. Every time a pregnant mother smokes, the blood vessels in the placenta are constricted and the blood flow decreases. As a result, the baby gets less nourishment and oxygen. Smoking even 10 cigarettes a day significantly reduces a baby's birthweight and increases the risk of mental and physical damage to the foetus. In fact, no drugs (and nicotine is a drug) or tablets should be taken without your doctor's advice.

While the occasional alcoholic drink will do no harm, it is not wise to indulge in heavy drinking as this could damage the baby's brain and slow his or her growth.

Premenstrual syndrome (PMS)

Not every woman going through the menstrual cycle (*see* PERIODS AND PERIOD PAIN) has problems in the premenstrual phase. While some women experience changes in their body or moods they do not find these distressing enough to seek treatment; others even report that they feel particularly productive and fit. It has been estimated, however, that over 50 per cent of women suffer from some type of noticeable premenstrual symptoms.

Premenstrual syndrome (PMS) consists of a wide variety of different symptoms. The exact nature of these varies from one person to another. However, many women feel tense and 'uptight' – hence the older term 'premenstrual tension'. But some women predominantly suffer from other symptoms such as bloating or weight gain, so the term premenstrual syndrome is now used.

The menstrual cycle

If you suffer from PMS, or suspect that you might, it is important to understand what happens during the menstrual cycle. The one described below is a 28-day cycle, but this is only an average; the length varies from woman to woman and may be longer or shorter than this.

During menstruation, the lining of the UTERUS is shed and the body gets ready to begin a new cycle. The period lasts for about five days, and as soon as menstruation stops, the PITUITARY gland in the brain sends a hormonal message to one of the two OVARIES, telling it to ripen an egg.

The hormone oestrogen is then produced from the *Graafian follicle* (made up of the egg and the cells surrounding it). One of the functions of oestrogen is to begin preparation of the lining of the uterus for any possible pregnancy. The amount of oestrogen that is produced continues to rise until it is time for ovulation.

On or near the 14th day of the cycle, the egg is fully ripened. The pituitary gland then releases another hormone to stimulate the release of the egg which travels into the Fallopian tube adjacent to the ovary. The follicle left behind after ovulation now starts to produce oestrogen and progesterone. These hormones make the uterine lining thicker and more spongy, ready to nourish a fertilized egg. It is at this stage of the cycle that a pregnancy can occur, but this will be possible for only a day or so.

If the egg is not fertilized, it quickly begins to degenerate. The levels of oestrogen and progesterone begin to fall, and as a result, the uterine lining cannot be maintained. The lining is shed – *menstruation* – and the cycle begins again. It is during the second phase of the menstrual cycle – i.e. after ovulation – that women who suffer from PMS may experience symptoms.

Symptoms and related problems

The physical symptoms of the *premenstruum* (the days immediately preceding menstruation) vary a great deal in type and severity from woman to woman. For example, one woman may experience slight tenderness and swelling of the breasts while another may experience swelling in most parts of her body, making her feel clumsy and awkward. Swelling and bloatedness are related to water retention (*see* OEDEMA): not all of the water that is taken into the body is passed in urine, but some of it accumulates in body cells and tissues. This results in weight gains and some women put on as much as 3–11 lb (1.5–3 kg) just before menstruation begins. Women who suffer from premenstrual weight gain may also experience oedema of the ankles and a considerable increase in their waist measurement. They feel bloated and uncomfortable, but usually all the excess weight disappears once the period starts.

Other physical symptoms associated with PMS are skin problems such as spots or blotchiness, an increase in the likelihood of CYSTITIS and a general feeling of being 'under the weather'. In addition, women who suffer from conditions such as EPILEPSY, ASTHMA, MIGRAINE and CONJUNCTIVITIS may find that the condition worsens at this time. Women who wear contact lenses may find that their lenses become uncomfortable.

The reasons for some of these physical symptoms are not yet fully understood. What is known is that the symptoms are likely to improve dramatically once menstruation begins and will return at the next premenstrual phase.

The psychological symptoms that are related to PMS are also likely to improve as soon as the period starts. A woman with PMS may feel depressed and anxious in the days before her period, suffer from lack of energy and a marked increase in irritability, be less interested in sex or find it difficult to concentrate. Because any one of these problems can exist independently of the premenstruum, this can make it difficult for a doctor to diagnose PMS.

In certain court cases, PMS has been used as a defence for women charged with violent and criminal behaviour, and some women have been acquitted on the grounds of diminished responsibility due to premenstrual syndrome. But the question of whether the premenstrual phase can produce such behaviour is still at issue.

Causes

Although research is not conclusive, many researchers believe that ovulation occurs earlier than usual when women suffer from PMS. Progesterone levels appear to rise early in the cycle but later, towards the end of the cycle, the levels fall more than usual. Some research also suggests that the levels of certain hormones from the pituitary gland – *gonadotrophins* – may be higher than usual in the second half of the cycle. Another line of research suggests that levels of *pyridoxal phosphate* in the brain may be inadequate. This is an important chemical derived from *pyridoxine,* VITAMIN B_6.

However, there may be other factors involved that are not strictly medical. It may be that many women are ashamed of their body's reproductive processes or associate the menstrual cycle with something negative – for example, some women still refer to their period as 'the curse'. But because it is difficult to measure the effect of such ideas on individual women, it is also difficult to arrive at any proof for such theories. There seems little doubt that women are less able to cope with STRESS in their lives when they have symptoms of PMS, but it is difficult to know whether the stress-related difficulties are a cause or an effect of PMS.

Other scientists say that PMS may be caused by a mixture of medical and social factors. While there is no doubt that the body and its chemistry do change throughout the menstrual cycle, this fact alone may not be an adequate explanation of the causes.

Diagnosing the problem

Any problems that particularly occur during the premenstruum may be a sign that you suffer from PMS. You may find that your mood swings and physical symptoms follow a pattern that coincides with the days before menstruation. One way to discover if this is the case is to record these changes in a diary, on a calendar or on a special chart. From this, you may discover that you are especially clumsy, short-tempered or tired in the days before your period. Your record will be useful not only for yourself but for your doctor if you decide to seek medical help. Your doctor or a nurse at your doctor's practice will be able to give you a chart on which to record your symptoms.

Keep your record for at least three months. If you do discover that there is a clear pattern of negative symptoms, you may find that you are able to help yourself.

Self-help

Try to adjust your routine in the days before a period so that you do not put yourself under physical stress. This applies particularly to dieting, which may increase the likelihood of faintness or dizziness. Do not go on a very strict diet during the premenstrual phase and make certain that you eat regularly – little, but often – when PMS problems arise.

A leading expert who has worked for many years on premenstrual problems recommends that your liquid intake should be restricted to about four cups a day if you suffer from water retention. She also suggests a reduction in the amount of SALT in the diet as salt increases water retention.

EXERCISE can also help a great deal and it will make you feel generally fitter. RELAXATION exercises can help with tension, both physical and emotional.

If you find that your premenstrual problems affect your emotions – you feel irritable or depressed, for example – it is important to explain to those who are close to you just what is happening. You may wish to tell them that your reactions to difficulties are likely to be more intense during this time and to ask for their understanding and support. It is impossible to avoid all sources of difficulty during this phase, but forward planning may enable you to avoid particularly stressful occasions and obligations.

Help from your doctor

Many women with severe PMS cannot cope with their symptoms without some medical treatment. If you feel that your symptoms are causing severe difficulties either for you or your partner or family, it is worth making an appointment with your doctor and taking with you a chart of all the symptoms you have been experiencing over a few months. It may also be helpful to take your partner with you so that he can explain the impact which the symptoms are having both on you and the family.

There is no diagnostic test for PMS, and so the doctor will rely heavily on what you tell him or her when deciding whether or not you should be treated. The doctor is likely to ask a number of questions about your life and about your work, hobbies, sleeping pattern and emotional matters. He or she will need to know if you put on weight just before your periods. If you are complaining of mental or emotional problems, the doctor will pay particular attention to whether or not these symptoms are closely linked to your monthly cycle. If they are not, therapy for premenstrual syndrome would be ineffective in solving them. It is unlikely that the doctor will want to carry out any complicated examinations or tests.

Pyridoxine (vitamin B_6)

Pyridoxine is one of the B vitamins which is present naturally in many foods, including yeast, liver, meat, fish, some grain products and certain fruits such as bananas. There is no doubt that we all need a satisfactory supply of such foods to ensure that we do not become deficient in vitamin B_6, but it is unlikely that women who suffer from PMS are actually deficient in these foodstuffs. It does seem, however, that they may have too little vitamin B_6, in the form of pyridoxal phosphate, reaching the deeper parts of the brain.

Numerous trials of vitamin B_6 treatment have demonstrated that it is an effective treatment for many of the symptoms of PMS. In one trial, it completely removed symptoms in 48 per cent of patients and significantly improved them in a further 22 per cent. Only 22 per cent of patients were left with moderate or severe symptoms. Mood change, headache and breast discomfort are particularly helped by pyridoxine; it does not help much with fluid retention.

A minimum dose of 50 mg once every day is required, but some women do not improve at this dose, so if symptoms persist, it is often suggested that the dose be increased each month, stepwise, to 100 mg, 150 mg or 200 mg each day.

Evening primrose oil

This oil contains an essential type of fat called gamma-linoleic acid (GLA), which is used by the body to make chemicals called *prostaglandins*. It is thought that disordered metabolism of prostaglandins could lead to PMS.

A number of researchers have demonstrated that evening primrose oil, taken in a dose of three to six capsules a day, can be effective in relieving some of the symptoms of PMS. The treatment should begin three days before the symptoms usually start, and continue daily until the period begins. The proportion of women helped by this treatment is similar to the result of pyridoxine – about three quarters of all women who suffer from PMS benefit.

Evening primrose oil is particularly successful in relieving breast discomfort, tenderness and swelling. Many women complain of lumpiness or hardness in their breasts just before a period, and evening primrose oil helps to relieve such symptoms.

Diuretics

Women who put on a great deal of weight in the premenstrual phase often benefit from taking a diuretic during this time. These drugs reduce excessive fluid in the circulation and not only minimize weight gain but also help breast discomfort and ankle swelling. Doctors will only prescribe diuretics for severe cases, but when they do, they often prescribe one containing a drug called *spironolactone*, because it has been shown to help the condition of 'cyclical oedema' better than many other drugs. However, diuretics do not help other symptoms of PMS.

Hormone therapy

Of the various treatments used for PMS, hormone therapy is the most reliable and predictable in relieving symptoms. But many doctors and patients prefer to commence with a simpler treatment, such as pyridoxine, and consider changing to a hormonal treatment only if there is no improvement.

The commonest type of hormone treatment prescribed is a progesterone. A natural type of progesterone may be given by injection, but commonly a synthetic form of progesterone such as *dydrogesterone* or *norethisterone* is given in tablet form to be taken daily, usually from the 12th day of the cycle until the 28th day.

The majority of symptoms of PMS are relieved by progesterone treatment, although weight gain and bloatedness may not be affected very much. Nearly 70 per cent of patients benefit considerably, with another 20 per cent experiencing significant improvements.

The contraceptive pill contains both progesterone and oestrogen and it may certainly help some women who suffer from PMS, but by no means all (*see* CONTRACEPTION). Many doctors recommend the use of pyridoxine as well if PMS remains a problem for women who are on the pill.

Recently another treatment for PMS has become available. Called *danazol*, it is a drug that interferes with the production of the gonadotrophin hormones from the pituitary gland, which in turn control the menstrual cycle. The drug must be taken every day, and sometimes has side-effects such as nausea. It is an extremely expensive drug but does work very well in cases of disabling PMS.

See also HORMONE REPLACEMENT THERAPY.

Pressure sacs, *see* Ulcers, skin

Prickly heat, *see* Perspiration

Proctalgia and proctitis

Proctalgia means any pain in the RECTUM, and usually it is no more than a nuisance. *Proctitis*, an inflamed rectum, may indicate a more serious condition.

The rectum is the lowest part of the large bowel, and when pain occurs here, it may be for a variety of reasons. It may be present almost continuously or for only a short time, and is a symptom that should not be ignored. In proctitis, the normal smooth pink lining of the rectum becomes swollen, angry-red and ulcerated. It bleeds easily and weeps fluid. Again, there are a number of causes for this, few of which are serious and all of which can be treated.

Causes and treatment of proctalgia

Where pain occurs during defaecation and perhaps lasts for several hours afterwards, the proctalgia is usually caused by an anal fissure – that is, a split in the skin of the anal canal (*see* PILES). This may also give rise to the passage of a small amount of bright red blood.

CONSTIPATION can sometimes cause considerable pain. This will only happen if the constipation is very severe, since the rectum is capable of being greatly distended before pain is felt.

Occasionally a patient with a TUMOUR will complain of pain in this region, although most cases of tumour manifest themselves by a change in bowel habit or the passage of blood or mucus in the stool. There are some extremely rare tumours which can occur in the tissues around the rectum and these might occasionally cause proctalgia.

Proctalgia fugax, which means a fleeting pain in the rectum, describes such pain for which there is no known cause. It may be severe enough to make the patient double up and can come on at any time. It usually lasts for only a few minutes and may be relieved by the passage of wind or faeces.

A doctor should investigate all cases of proctalgia so that the cause can be identified and treated. Proctalgia fugax is very difficult to treat since the cause is largely unknown, but once any serious underlying condition has been ruled out, the patient can be safely reassured and this sometimes helps the pain to disappear.

Causes and symptoms of proctitis

Proctitis may be part of the inflammation associated with ulcerative colitis (*see* COLON AND COLITIS), a disease affecting the large bowel. It may also occur in conjunction with Crohn's disease, another inflammatory disease which may affect any part of the intestine. Finally, it may be an isolated incident involving inflammation confined only to the rectum.

Proctitis may cause a severe disturbance of the normal bowel habit or there may be minimal change. The patient tends to pass loose motions with mucus and, in severe cases, large amounts of blood. Another symptom is *tenesmus*, whereby the patient has the constant desire to defaecate but is unable to do so.

Treatment of proctitis

Some cases of proctitis clear up spontaneously after a short time. Others persist for days or weeks and can lead to quite severe illness. However, the illness is never as severe as when the whole colon is affected.

A doctor should be consulted if the symptoms continue for more than a day or two. He or she will examine the rectum with a special viewing instrument called a *sigmoidoscope*, or refer the patient to a specialist who will do so. This procedure will reveal the severity and extent of the inflammation.

If the rest of the large bowel seems to be involved, the doctor may suggest that a BARIUM enema X-ray is carried out. This means that a special dye is passed into the rectum so that X-ray pictures can be taken.

He or she will probably also take a tiny piece from the lining of the rectum for examination under a microscope. This may pinpoint the cause of the proctitis, and help in treatment.

Some cases of proctitis would probably settle down of their own accord but various drugs can help. Salazopyrin, which is a drug similar to aspirin, can be taken by mouth three times a day, although sometimes people are found to be allergic to it.

The most effective way of overcoming an acute attack is by the use of cortisone (*see* STEROIDS) and its related compounds taken in the form of an enema.

Most cases of proctitis settle rapidly with treatment. It may recur or it may form part of the more serious disease, ulcerative colitis. After one attack, however, many patients never have any further trouble or recurrence of inflammation.

Prolactin, *see* **Breasts and breast cancer, Endocrine system, Hormones, Pituitary**

Prolapse

This means literally to 'fall forward' and can be applied to any organ which has been displaced from its normal position through weakness in supporting tissues. However, the term is most often used to describe this condition in one or more of a woman's reproductive organs.

The fibrous and muscular sling which lies across the bones forming the pelvic girdle is called the pelvic floor. This has to support the weight of all the contents of the abdominal cavity such as the gut and the BLADDER and, in women, the UTERUS (womb) as well. Occasionally, if the support system becomes weakened, the womb may slide down into the VAGINA. This is called a *uterine prolapse*. Other organs which are positioned on each side of the vagina may also be involved in a prolapse, including the bladder.

Causes

Anything which exerts too much weight or pressure on the pelvic floor, or weakens it, will make a woman more likely to develop a prolapse – for example, coughing, heavy lifting or regular straining to open the bowels. Frequent PREGNANCIES, especially if the babies are large or the labour prolonged, will weaken the mother's pelvic floor. It may also become weaker if the woman is overweight.

The supporting tissues seem to need a supply of the female sex hormone called *oestrogen* to retain their strength. This is mainly released from a woman's OVARIES. After the MENOPAUSE, the ovaries no longer secrete large amounts of oestrogen, the pelvic floor becomes weaker and, as a result, the woman is in greater danger of developing a prolapse.

Types of prolapse

One of the commonest types of prolapse is uterine prolapse. The CERVIX (neck of the womb) tends to lengthen slightly, and as the supporting tissues on each side of the uterus weaken, the uterus descends lower in the vagina. Although this type of prolapse does occur after CHILDBIRTH has weakened the pelvic floor, it may also occur in middle-aged or elderly women who have never borne children.

Three degrees of severity of prolapse are described. A *first-degree* prolapse occurs where the cervix is situated very low in the vagina, but always remains in the vagina. *Second-degree* prolapse indicates that the cervix actually protrudes beyond the vagina when the woman coughs or strains. *Third-degree* prolapse is a rare but severe form of prolapse in which the whole of the uterus protrudes from the vagina and the vagina itself becomes turned inside out.

The next most common form of prolapse involves the front wall of the vagina. Immediately in front of the vagina is the bladder and the URETHRA, the short tube that allows urine to pass out of the bladder. The front wall of the vagina, containing part of the bladder, and often the urethra as well, prolapses downwards into the entrance of the vagina. This form of prolapse is called a *cystocoele* if it contains part of the bladder, or a *urethrocoele* if it contains the urethra. It is a common problem after prolonged or difficult labours, although it may not show up for several years. Often there is some degree of uterine prolapse as well.

If the back wall of the vagina is involved in prolapse, part of the RECTUM may fall forward; the prolapse is then called a *rectocoele*. Rarely a prolapse comes from the higher part of the posterior wall of the vagina and contains some small bowel. This type of prolapse is called an *enterocoele*. It may be combined with a rectocoele.

Symptoms of uterine prolapse

The symptoms which a prolapse produces depend on its severity and whether or not the bladder or bowel are involved. Many women have no symptoms; some simply experience a downward pressure in the vagina. Others feel a lump (the womb) in the vagina or something 'coming down'. In those cases where there is a third-degree uterine prolapse, the entire womb will be protruding from the vagina. Obviously this makes walking and sitting very uncomfortable but, fortunately, it is very uncommon. If the bowel is involved in the prolapse, the woman may find it difficult to pass a motion without first pushing the womb back into the vagina.

If the bladder is part of the prolapse, the woman may find she is unable to pass urine without replacing the womb in the vagina. However, a much more common problem is that the woman leaks urine if she runs, laughs or coughs. This is called *stress* INCONTINENCE and may occur if there is a cystocoele or urethrocoele.

A prolapse does not cause vaginal bleeding nor does it cause pain, but occasionally women may notice a dull backache at the end of the day which is relieved by lying down.

Fortunately, prolapses in women are becoming less common, partly because women have better nutrition, and tend to have smaller families, but largely due to better antenatal preparation.

Prevention and treatment of uterine prolapse

It is important to try to prevent prolapses occurring. Careful obstetric care during delivery can prevent excessive strain on the pelvic floor by avoiding a prolonged or difficult labour. The muscles of the pelvic floor can also be strengthened by exercises, and women both at antenatal classes and in the post-natal ward are taught these exercises. HORMONE REPLACEMENT THERAPY after the menopause may also help some women to avoid a prolapse.

If a woman's prolapse is very small, it can sometimes be corrected if she loses weight and is prescribed a course of exercise by a PHYSIOTHERAPIST. Elderly or unfit women who wish to avoid an operation for more severe forms of prolapse can be treated by placing a plastic or rubber ring – a ring pessary – in the vagina to hold the uterus in place.

Most women are usually advised to have an operation. However, this is normally delayed until the woman has completed her family. If a woman has another baby by vaginal delivery after an operation for a prolapse, the prolapse is likely to recur.

If the patient has either a cystocoele or a rectocoele, the operation can be straightforward. Excess skin from the vaginal wall is removed and deep stitches placed behind the wall to repair the damaged supporting tissues. When a cystocoele is repaired in this way, the operation is called an *anterior colporrhaphy*; repair of the rectocoele or enterocoele is called *posterior colporrhaphy*. If the cervix is low in the vagina, it may be removed at the same time as a colporrhaphy, without the removal of the body of the uterus. This operation is known as a 'Manchester repair' after the hospital where the technique was first developed.

A second-degree or third-degree uterine prolapse is usually treated by a HYSTERECTOMY – the complete removal of the uterus. The operation is carried out in these circumstances entirely through the vagina without the need for an abdominal incision.

Other forms of prolapse

Although it is customary to think of a prolapse as something that only affects the womb, there are, in fact, other structures which can prolapse. One of the most dramatic but fortunately rare forms of prolapse is a *prolapsed cord.* This means that, in the process of birth a baby's umbilical cord comes out of the birth canal before him or her and may be compressed against the bones of the mother's pelvis, thus interfering with the supply of blood to the baby. Special measures are necessary to deal with this situation and ensure that the baby survives childbirth without damage.

Doctors also talk about a *prolapsed intervertebral disc.* This is normally called a 'SLIPPED DISC' and means that one of the spongy middle sections of the tough discs that lie between the vertebrae has broken through the fibrous ring that surrounds it, and is now pressing on a nerve leaving the spinal cord, causing pain in the back of the legs.

After uterine prolapse, however, perhaps the most common sort of prolapse is that of the rectum. This condition means that the rectum is pushed down through the anal orifice. Since the rectum is a tube which is tethered to the anus, it can be pushed down through it rather like a sock being turned inside out. This tends to happen more frequently in women than in men, but it may also happen in children. When a child is involved, the condition is not usually serious, and the prolapse can nearly always be reduced (pushed back) without much discomfort – it is very rare for an operation to be required in a child. In contrast, in adults there is often a need to operate and the prolapse cannot be reduced so easily. For a severe prolapse, it is usually necessary to open the abdomen and repair the damage from inside.

It is not clear why rectal prolapse should occur. In children, CONSTIPATION and excessive straining to open the bowels may be a cause. When adults are concerned, the condition is usually found in elderly women, although where a male is affected, it can occur at any age. A certain laxity of the muscles of the floor of the pelvis may well be a part of the cause, just as in the case of uterine prolapse, although the rectum does not seem more likely to prolapse if women have had a lot of children. Fortunately, it is not a common condition, and when it does occur, it is usually successfully treated by a surgical repair.

Prostate gland

This is a walnut-shaped structure found only in males. It is situated at the base of the BLADDER and surrounds the URETHRA – the tube through which urine and seminal fluid pass out of the body (*see* PENIS).

This GLAND produces the fluid that mixes with semen to make up part of the seminal fluid. Although the exact function of the prostatic fluid is unknown, it is thought that one of its roles is to help keep the SPERM active so that fertilization can occur more easily.

Owing to its position in the body, problems associated with this gland can often affect the normal functioning of the bladder – although this is more common among elderly men. TUMOURS of the gland – both benign and malignant – can occur, as can infection, which can be sudden ('acute prostatitis') or prolonged and chronic.

Acute prostatitis

This condition is fairly common and can affect adult men of any age. The cause of the infection is usually a bacterium which appears to find its way to the gland through the bloodstream. Occasionally, however, acute prostatitis may arises as a complication of a SEXUALLY TRANSMITTED infection such as GONORRHOEA or NSU (NON-SPECIFIC URETHRITIS).

The first symptoms of acute prostatitis are usually a high fever, muscular aches and pains (caused by the body's general reaction to the infection) and a deep-seated pain in the lower part of the abdomen. Typically there is pain just behind the scrotum in the perineum (between the legs). There is pain on passing urine and possibly on opening the bowels as well. Unless the infection is treated quickly, the patient may become very ill within a day or two. Rarely, an ABSCESS may form on the prostate gland.

Chronic prostatitis

Acute prostatitis may sometimes lead to a persistent low-grade infection in the prostate gland. Sexually transmitted diseases can also cause this problem.

One of the typical features of chronic prostatitis infection is a dull pain in the perineum. There may be discomfort when sitting down. A discharge from the urethra may occur, and there may be pain on passing urine and an

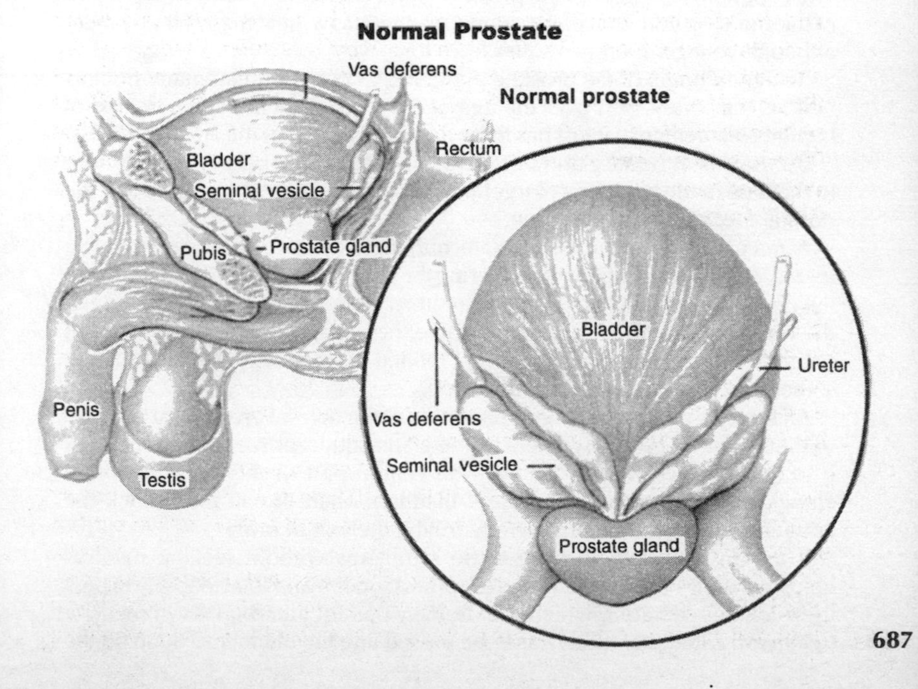

increase in the frequency of urination. It may be difficult to start passing urine. Low backache is not uncommon and there may also be some interference with sexual function – possibly IMPOTENCE.

Infection may spread to other genital organs – the seminal vesicles (located just above the prostate gland) or the epididymis (part of the testicles). The gland may become calcified, and gravel-like stones may be formed within it.

Treatment of prostatitis

To make a diagnosis of prostatitis, the doctor carries out a rectal examination. With one hand on the patient's abdomen and a plastic glove on the other, he passes a finger into the rectum to feel the prostate through the rectal wall. If prostatitis is present, the gland is very tender. By massaging the gland, a small amount of infected secretions may be expressed through the urethra and appear at the tip of the penis. The doctor will take a sample of this secretion for analysis in the laboratory so that the infection can be identified.

Once the diagnosis has been made, the patient will be given a course of antibiotics. Acute prostatitis usually responds to treatment within a few days. Chronic prostatitis may need many weeks or even months of treatment. Surgery is rarely needed, but an abscess in the gland may need surgical drainage.

Benign enlargement

The commonest tumour of the prostate gland is a benign increase in the size of the gland – a non-cancerous condition affecting a great many elderly men, although younger men can suffer from it.

Benign tumours of the prostate gland are so common that many doctors believe that every man over the age of 50 years or so has some degree of benign enlargement – it just has to be accepted as part of the ageing process.

Because the prostate gland surrounds the urethra, and because it is so close to the base of the bladder, enlargement of the gland can seriously impair the normal mechanism of urination.

A man with an enlarged prostate may notice the following symptoms: increased frequency of urination during the day; getting up at night to urinate; the development of a poor urinary stream; a tendency to stop and start, with the sensation that there is more to come; having to stand and wait several seconds before urine starts to flow; dribbling of urine after the stream; and, sometimes, a sudden urge to pass urine.

All these symptoms are due to distortion of the normal anatomy at the base of the bladder. The enlargement of the gland squeezes the urethra, causing it to become narrow. Sometimes, the central part of the gland becomes elongated and extends up into the bladder, where it can then block the entrance to the urethra and thereby inhibit the exit of urine.

If a man continues to have these symptoms without seeking medical help, two things can happen. There can be a sudden and total inability to pass urine (acute retention), which is extremely painful and requires immediate treatment. A catheter (tube) has to be passed into the bladder to drain off the excess urine. Alternatively, the bladder can become stretched so that every time the man passes urine he does not quite empty it and urine remains undischarged.

Because the bladder expands so gradually, there is no pain and the symptoms may go unnoticed for a while. Eventually, he passes urine in a dribble, and may even find that he is permanently wetting his underclothes and his bed. In the end, there is so much back-pressure on the KIDNEYS that they start failing, and waste-products build up in the bloodstream, with extremely serious consequences – a situation known as 'chronic retention of urine with renal failure'.

Treatment

When a patient goes to his doctor complaining of difficulty in passing urine, or, perhaps, passing small quantities frequently, he will be sent for a series of special tests, often including an ULTRASOUND scan of the kidneys and bladder, and blood tests. Special equipment may also be used to measure his urine flow.

If the tests show that the prostate gland is enlarged, surgery would be recommended, as leaving the gland to enlarge further would complicate treatment later on. An operation would also be recommended for a patient who develops acute retention of urine as he would be unable to urinate if the catheter were removed. A permanent bladder catheter can be not only a social problem but a medical one, too, because of the increased risk of infection in the urine.

The operation

The prostate gland is situated in an extremely inaccessible part of the body, and because of this, an operation to remove it can be difficult. Also, because it is near the opening of the bladder, the delicate muscles which prevent urine from leaking in between the acts of urination can be damaged by the surgery if great care is not taken.

Nowadays there are two types of operation. The *retropubic prostatectomy*, also known as the 'open' method, and the *transurethral prostatectomy* or TUR.

The 'open' method is reserved for very large glands and also where an operation on the bladder has to be performed at the same time. It consists of making a cut across the lower abdomen and approaching the gland via the space between the back of the pubic bone and the bladder. The capsule of the prostate gland is opened and the gland is 'shelled out' from inside the capsule. Fluid is then passed via a tube into the bladder to prevent the formation of blood clots. This tube is usually left in the bladder for about five days after the operation, and is then removed if there is no residual bleeding. A patient having this operation is usually in hospital for seven to ten days.

The 'closed' method or TUR, is performed using a fine telescope-like instrument which is passed up the penis into the bladder. This instrument has a viewing-piece and a special cautery (searing) device which has a wire loop on the end. Using this method, the prostate gland is chipped away from inside the urethra, little pieces of tissue being cut away each time the wire loop, which is attached to an electric current, moves through the tissue.

The great advantage of the TUR method is that the patient is spared a surgical incision and there is less discomfort or pain after the operation. As with the 'open' method, a tube is left in the bladder but, here, the tube is often taken out after two or three days. Patients make a much quicker recovery from this operation, because it is less traumatic to the body.

After a prostatectomy, the urinary stream is noticeably better, but there will be side-effects. Because of the anatomy of the prostate gland, patients who have had either type of prostatectomy are unable to ejaculate semen normally. In this condition, known as *retrograde ejaculation*, the semen goes back into the bladder instead of travelling down and out of the penis, in effect making the man INFERTILE. This is because, in removing the gland, the muscle at the base of the bladder has to be cut. This muscle usually contracts during orgasm, preventing semen from going up into the bladder. Sexual performance is most unlikely to be affected by a TUR operation; erection and orgasm are usually unimpaired, although there will be no ejaculation at the time of orgasm. A retropubic operation occasionally does affect potency, but not always.

As this operation is usually performed on elderly men, infertility may not be a problem (sexual performance need not be affected). But a younger man suffering from an enlarged prostate may be worried by the prospect of retrograde ejaculation if he wants to have children. Sometimes the surgeon will be able to postpone treatment until the man has fathered a child, but this is not always possible if the symptoms are very severe. Alternatively, it may be possible for samples of semen to be stored frozen so that they may be used to inseminate the man's partner artificially after the operation has been carried out (*see* ARTIFICIAL INSEMINATION).

Cancer of the prostate

CANCER of the prostate is one of the most common cancers to occur in males. In fact, it has been found in routine post-mortem examination of the prostate gland that nearly all elderly men have a tiny focus of cancer in the prostate gland. Most of these people would not have shown any symptoms nor have known that they had anything wrong.

However, when a malignant tumour does manifest itself during a man's life, it does so in a number of ways. First, it may be found on a routine examination by a doctor who notices a lump in the gland (the gland can be felt through the anterior wall of the rectum). Second, the patient may have difficulty passing urine because the tumour is so close to the urethra and develop symptoms identical to those of a benign tumour of the prostate; the cancer may be diagnosed only at the time of the operation. Third, the patient may have no urinary symptoms, but develop symptoms from the spread of the tumour outside the gland. One of the commonest sites for the secondary spread of the tumour is in the bones. The spread probably occurs as a result of tiny clumps of cells breaking off and circulating in the bloodstream.

Treatment and outlook

The treatment of cancer of the prostate depends on many factors, but one of the most important is the extent of spread of the tumour. Therefore, a patient who is suspected of having a malignant tumour of the prostate will have several tests, including X-rays and radioactive scans of the bones, to determine the exact extent of the spread.

If the tumour has been found quite by accident, and consists of a small nodule confined to the gland itself, many surgeons would treat this simply by observation, with no specific drug or radiation treatment. The majority of these patients will live for years with no problems. If there are symptoms from the tumour, such as a reduced flow of urine or excessive frequency, a TUR operation may be carried out.

If the tests show that the tumour has spread outside the prostate gland, then treatment in the form of HORMONE drugs will be given. Most cancers of the prostate have been found to be dependent on male hormones for their growth; so by counteracting their effect with female hormones, the cancer can be kept at bay. The drug is given in very small doses and often has quite dramatic effects on the primary and secondary tumours. Bones which have been riddled with secondary tumours become normal again, and the swelling in the gland becomes smaller.

The female hormone drug does have side-effects, however. It can promote the loss of hair, increase the growth of breast tissue and decrease libido. It can also cause the body tissues to retain more fluid than usual (*see* OEDEMA), leading to swelling of the ankles, and sometimes heart failure.

These side-effects are troublesome in only a few patients, however, and the benefits of the drug in controlling the tumour far outweigh the disadvantages. Some surgeons, to produce the same effect, remove the TESTES (the glands that produce the male hormone testosterone), as they find that there is the same response from the tumour without the possible side-effects of the drug.

Surgery in cancer of the prostate gland is usually reserved for those patients in whom the growth of the tumour has caused a narrowing of the urethra, so that urine cannot be passed easily. In these cases, the blockage is removed but no attempt is made to remove the whole tumour. Treatment with X-rays is sometimes given, but usually only when the secondary tumours in the bones are causing a lot of pain.

Recently, large operations have been developed that remove the whole prostate gland with the tumour in it; nerves to the bladder sphincter are kept intact to preserve continence. There is a debate as to whether surgery of this sort is justified, when the long-term effects of the disease may be so minimal.

There are a small number of patients whose tumours do not respond to drug treatment. Luckily, though, they are only a very small proportion of the many patients with cancer of the prostate. The outlook for a lot of patients with prostatic cancer is very good indeed. Some men live for many years, taking a small dose of the hormone drug every day.

Protein

The three main classes of food are proteins, FATS and CARBOHYDRATES. The fats and carbohydrates simply supply the energy that the body needs to carry out its daily work, but the proteins are the basic building blocks from which the body is made up. Although they, too, can be burned in the cells simply as a fuel, the minimum basic requirement of protein is necessary to maintain the body's continuing process of reconstruction and repair so that bones, muscles and all the tissues remain healthy.

What is protein?

One essential characteristic of protein is that it contains the chemical element nitrogen in addition to the carbon, oxygen and hydrogen that are the basis of the carbohydrates and the fats. In fact, proteins are made up of chains of smaller compounds called amino acids. There are only 20 amino acids which make up all the protein found in food: eight of them are essential parts of the diet since the body must have them and is not capable of making them from basic chemicals. The other 12 can be made by the body, although its capacity to do this is not always adequate.

When an amino acid chain grows long enough to form a protein, a number of things happen to it. First, the amino acids have to be in the right order: this is called the *primary structure*. The *secondary structure* concerns the way in which the protein is twisted around itself just as the fibres of a piece of wool are twisted to make up a strand. Finally there is the *tertiary structure*: this means that the twisted strand of protein is curled around itself so that it ends up rather like a long plait, or sort of knot. The different structures are very important in the way that a protein works – many of them will not fulfil their function unless the tertiary structure is right.

Where does protein come from?

The protein that is used in the body comes from the basic amino acids that are absorbed from the INTESTINE. These are the products of the DIGESTION of protein in the food we eat. As a food which is rich in protein – such as meat, for instance – passes into the STOMACH, the action of the acid in the stomach starts to break the meat down into individual molecules of protein. When these pass into the DUODENUM, the digestive ENZYMES released from the PANCREAS start to split the protein molecules up into the individual amino acids that make them up. These can then be absorbed by the wall of the intestine so that they can pass to the LIVER and then out into the bloodstream.

Although some of the tissues, particularly the liver, are able to store some of the amino acids that are taken into the body after a protein meal, there is really no major store of protein or of the amino acids that make it up. Fat and carbohydrate, in contrast, can both be stored in the body in considerable quantities.

What does protein do?

Protein has many functions within the body. First and most important is its role as a basic building block. Our tissues are basically made of protein, and the central substance in general connective tissue that holds the various organs and tissues together is a protein molecule which is called *collagen.*

The next important role of proteins is in making the enzymes, protein molecules which act as catalysts for the huge range of chemical reactions that the body depends upon.

As well as the protein that makes up the tissues, there is a fair amount of protein circulating in a dissolved form in the blood. This circulating protein is divided into two main classes – *albumin,* which is made up of rather small protein molecules, and the *globulins,* a group of larger proteins. The blood proteins have a very important role in keeping fluid in the bloodstream and preventing it from leaking out into the tissues. The globulin portion of the blood proteins also contains the *immunoglobulins,* or antibodies (*see* IMMUNE SYSTEM) which form the spearhead of the body's defence against infection. Each one is made up of two or more protein molecules that are linked together.

Some of the body's HORMONES are also proteins, and they too have a vital role in the body's overall function. Insulin is the best example of a protein hormone – it is made of two linked protein chains.

Pruritis

Itching or irritation of the skin, known medically as pruritus, may be brought on by a variety of causes. It can vary from being merely a mild annoyance, easily forgotten, to being so severe and persistent that the patient is unable to sleep because of it. It may involve the entire SKIN surface of the body or be restricted to a small area. Any part of the body can be affected, including the EYES, EARS, NOSE, anus and VAGINA. Pruritus is essentially a manifestation of skin INFLAMMATION in the same way that RASHES, soreness and swelling are.

Causes

Generalized pruritus – itching felt all over the body – is usually an indication of some disease affecting the person as a whole, and should be regarded as an early warning sign. It may be symptomatic of a general condition such as HODGKIN'S DISEASE, for example. It is also common in PREGNANCY, old age, severe JAUNDICE (when it is due to bile salts being deposited in the skin) and CHICKENPOX (when it is associated with the skin eruption).

Generalized pruritus also occurs as a result of an ALLERGIC response. This usually affects only the part of the body in contact with the substance concerned, but if a person is acutely allergic to something there may be a general as well as a local reaction. It may be provoked by food or medicine to which the patient is allergic, and the irritation is often accompanied by a generalized rash and sometimes the kind of weals known as *urticaria* or *hives.*

Most cases of pruritus however are related to small areas of the body. Some skin diseases, such as ECZEMA and DERMATITIS, usually have marked pruritus in the area of affected skin. Some types of eczema and dermatitis accompany VARICOSE VEINS and others result from contact with such substances as detergents, industrial solvents and oils, and metals, particularly nickel.

A wide range of common skin disturbances can also give rise to pruritus. It may occur with FUNGAL INFECTIONS such as ATHLETE'S FOOT and RINGWORM, or with severe DANDRUFF and seborrhoeic dermatitis where excessive grease is secreted on to the skin or scalp. Chilblains or even the accumulation of dirt on unwashed skin commonly cause localized itching and irritation in different areas of the body.

Stings from insects and plants frequently give rise to pruritus, and it exists in a more persistent and intense form with insect infestations as in fleas, LICE or SCABIES. It is often in such cases the main feature indicating the presence of the condition and thus is an aid to diagnosis.

In some conditions, pruritus affects only a specific part of the body. Irritation around the anus (*pruritus anai*) may be caused by PILES or an anal fissure, while vaginal infections such as THRUSH cause pruritus in that area (*pruritus vulvae*). *Pruritus vulvae* is also common in DIABETES. Similarly, irritation occurs around the nose and eyes with HAY FEVER and allergic RHINITIS.

Treatment

Treatment of generalized pruritis consists in treating the underlying condition, so that as this improves the pruritus disappears. Unless there is a rash, any attempt to alleviate the irritation by applying cream or lotion to the skin is usually ineffective. With chickenpox, a soothing lotion such as calamine will help to reduce the itching. If the irritation is very severe, antihistamine tablets or syrup taken by mouth often help.

Where generalized pruritus occurs as part of an allergic reaction, antihistamines are normally used to treat the causative condition. These are again taken in the form of tablets or syrup, but can also be injected for a more rapid effect in severe cases. Antihistamine ointments or creams should never be used on the skin to relieve itching because this can give rise to a skin sensitivity to the antihistamine itself, rendering that substance dangerous and unsuitable for use on a future occasion.

The cause of localized pruritus must also be diagnosed so that an appropriate treatment can be given. For example, various ointments are available to suit different types of eczema. In cases of contact dermatitis, a patient can help by trying to identify the cause so that it can be avoided in future. Meanwhile calamine lotion is useful in soothing the area affected. Alternatively, 1 per cent hydrocortisone ointment purchased from a chemist will calm inflamed skin.

Psittacosis, *see* Chlamydia, Pneumonia

Psoriasis

In psoriasis, the SKIN forms pink-to-dull red patches covered with a characteristic silver scaling. It is usually a chronic condition with acute phases of eruption followed by remissions. About 2 per cent of white-skinned Western populations develop psoriasis, but it is less common among black- and brown-skinned people and in hot countries. Although medical treatments can do a good deal to control the condition, there is as yet no cure for psoriasis.

Causes

There is considerable evidence to indicate a GENETIC inheritance of the disease, and it often happens that a newly diagnosed psoriasis sufferer (psoriatic) finds that a relative also has the condition. Recent research has shown that people with certain tissue types are more prone to psoriasis. Tissue types are inherited in a predictable way, but this does not mean that everyone in the family is likely to develop psoriasis; it simply means that it is likely to occur more frequently than usual within the family.

Many things can trigger the eruption of psoriasis in someone who has this inherited tendency. Physical and chemical trauma can precipitate it, and when it occurs in already damaged skin, it is known as the *Koebner phenomenon*. A general infection such as influenza may also cause a relapse of the disease.

Hormonal changes seem to influence the incidence of psoriasis in that it tends especially to coincide with puberty and the MENOPAUSE. On the other hand there is often a remission during PREGNANCY, with a relapse once the pregnancy is over. Drugs are rarely a precipitating factor, although an association has been noted with certain drugs used to treat MALARIA and with lithium, a drug used to treat DEPRESSION.

Psychological causes are of variable importance in psoriasis. It may perhaps be triggered off by emotional STRESS, such as examinations or bereavement, while some studies done by psychiatrists suggest that psoriasis may be an outward expression of subconscious problems. Equally, understanding and resolution of conflicts may help psoriasis to get better.

Considerable research has been carried out to find out exactly what is wrong with the skin in a person with psoriasis. Normally the skin replaces itself by growing outwards from deeper layers; as skin cells eventually reach the outermost layer they are rubbed off as microscopic flakes and replaced by new skin cells from underneath. The outer layer of skin cells are protective and tougher than those deeper down.

In areas affected by psoriasis, the turnover of cells is speeded up at least tenfold. The cells in the deeper layers multiply abnormally fast and accumulate in the psoriatic lesion. As they reach the surface, the cells fail to develop the normal tough protective coating so those areas affected by psoriasis are not well protected from friction or further damage. Since there is so much skin tissue produced, the excess comes away in large visible flakes.

The exact cause of the abnormal proliferation of skin in psoriasis is still not clear. It is possible that HORMONES or ENZYMES in the body may be responsible for triggering the excessive growth of skin tissue. Recent research has, however, found that even normal-looking skin in a person with psoriasis is not in fact perfectly normal. The biochemical structure of the skin is significantly different from the skin of someone who does not have the disorder. Any slight trigger factor can thus apparently set off a psoriatic action.

Symptoms and types

There are many different types of psoriasis. At its mildest, there may be just one or two very small patches of abnormal skin, but in its severest form, it can cover large areas of the body and make the sufferer quite ill.

All age groups may be affected, but it often starts in early adult life. Typically, there are times when the sufferer has widespread and fairly severe lesions, but then it is quite common for the rash to clear up on its own for many months or even years. One type of psoriasis may occur together with others, or sometimes a sufferer may have one type on one occasion and another later on in his or her life.

The commonest type is *discoid psoriasis.* An area of skin ranging in size from 1 in (2.5 cm) or so up to 3 in (7.5 cm) across becomes raised, reddened and takes on a cracked or fissured appearance. This lesion is called a *plaque* and it throws off copious quantities of silvery scales. The sites most commonly affected by plaques are the elbows and knees, followed by the limbs and the trunk. Psoriasis rarely affects the face. In severe cases, the plaques merge into each other to give quite large areas of abnormal skin. The plaques rarely cause pain, but they can itch and irritate. If they are scratched, tiny bleeding points can be seen where the blood vessels run into the thickened skin.

The scalp is also frequently involved and is usually affected to some degree in most people who have discoid psoriasis. Sometimes, however, it is the only area of skin involved. Apart from some soreness, the main symptom is of copious quantities of large scales pouring from the scalp and matting the hair.

Psoriasis on the palms of the hands and soles of the feet may look somewhat different from psoriasis elsewhere. The scales tend to be thicker and more adherent to the skin and there may also be pustules present. The pustules are small deep-seated micro-abscesses which form in the skin. They are not infected but the result of a deep sterile inflammation associated with the psoriasis rash. Rarely, this type of *pustular psoriasis* may spread to other parts of the body as well.

Flexural psoriasis again has a different appearance. If psoriasis occurs in the groin, the armpit or the genitalia, it tends to be less scaly, but becomes very red and sore.

The nails may also become involved. Many people with discoid psoriasis have at least some changes in their nails. The commonest sign is the appearance of many tiny pits or dimples in the surface of some or all of the fingernails. In more severe cases, the nails can become distorted, or they separate from the nail bed, a condition called *onycholysis.*

Children and teenagers can develop *guttate psoriasis* (*guttate* means 'a drop'). The trigger to this type of psoriasis is often an attack of tonsillitis or a bad sore throat. A few weeks later numerous small spots of psoriasis appear all over the trunk and upper limbs – as if the body were covered in splashes or drops of psoriasis. Each spot is usually only a few millimetres across (¼ in). The rash tends to last a few weeks and then often clears up completely. Sometimes, however, the child or teenager may go on to develop discoid psoriasis, especially if there is a family history of the disorder.

Treatment

No treatment has yet been found that will cure psoriasis, but there are a number of therapies which can keep the condition under control. Unfortunately, some of the treatments are difficult to apply or messy, and so many people with very mild psoriasis and perhaps just one or two plaques choose to put up with the problem.

People with the more severe forms of psoriasis have to come to terms with its implications for their lives. Some people may need to change their job if substances they deal with aggravate the skin. In any case, time must be taken off work to rest during flare-ups. Where stress has a bearing on the occurrence of psoriasis, steps must be taken to resolve the emotional and psychological problems involved.

Many people with psoriasis feel tainted by the unpleasant appearance of the rash and are unwilling to expose even small areas of skin to public gaze, so long sleeves and trousers are often the only clothes which sufferers – both men and women – will contemplate. People with psoriasis may also feel that their rash may interfere with personal relationships – especially those with the opposite sex. They may be afraid to stay in other people's houses or in hotels because, after a night in bed, they leave large amounts of skin scales in the bedding. Some patients find it beneficial to join an association or a group for sufferers where they can benefit from mutual support and advice.

The basis of medical treatment of psoriasis is direct application of creams, oils or ointments to the skin. In an acute attack, bland preparations such as zinc pastes or moisturizing oils and creams are used. STEROID creams have also been prescribed for many years to treat psoriasis. Weak steroid creams, such as hydrocortisone, may be used for short periods (up to eight weeks) for scalp, facial and flexural psoriasis. Stronger creams and ointments have to be used sparingly because of the risk of side-effects. There is also the risk that, although the stronger steroids may suppress the disease in the short term, when stopped they may lead to severe relapse of psoriasis. For this reason, they are seldom used. However, they are sometimes prescribed for flexural psoriasis or for the scalp, hands and feet. These areas are less susceptible to side-effects.

One of the mainstays of treatment for psoriasis is tar. Both coal tar and various wood tars are incorporated into a variety of oils and creams. Tar-based shampoos are often prescribed for the scalp or tar-medicated bath additives to treat the skin of the trunk.

Strong tar ointments can be applied to discoid psoriasis. Such treatment may help to clear quite severe plaques but it is very messy and the smell can be overpowering, so these treatments have largely fallen into disuse.

Discoid psoriasis is usually treated with *dithranol*. This is a drug which effectively reduces the excessive turnover of cells in the skin and can completely eradicate psoriatic plaques. It is used as a cream or paste, or it can be incorporated into a stick rather like a large lipstick. The preparation is carefully applied by the patient to each plaque, and after a specified time, it is washed off again. The original treatments were left on overnight, but dithranol stains clothing so this method proved to be very difficult because it involved bandaging all the treated areas. However, it has now been found that if dithranol preparations are left on the skin for only half an hour, the results are almost as good as those obtained with longer treatments. Dithranol is used daily until the plaques are gone. Although it does stain the surrounding normal skin a brown colour, this fades in time.

For severely resistant cases, a drug called *acitretin* is now available. This will usually only be prescribed by a hospital dermatologist.

It has long been known that sunlight is beneficial for psoriasis. Indeed, it is possible that this is the reason for psoriasis being less common in tropical and subtropical countries. At least three out of four sufferers benefit from natural sunlight. Sufferers can even visit special treatment centres set up in warm sunny climates. There is one such treatment centre at the Dead Sea, which takes advantage of the fact that the sunlight there is filtered through an extra layer of the atmosphere, since the Dead Sea is below sea level. Treatments involving sunlight and special applications of muds or minerals are combined into a therapy known as *climatotherapy*.

In temperate climates, sunlight is often unreliable, so alternative artificial sources may be used. A treatment known as PUVA was introduced in the mid-1970s and has been carefully evaluated. The sufferer is given a drug called *psoralens* and then exposed to ultraviolet A light in a high-intensity type of solarium. UVA tubes are fixed vertically all around the patient who stands in the middle of a solarium 'cabinet'. The treatment is given for 15 to 30 minutes two or three times a week. It is highly effective for the most severe types of psoriasis but it does carry a small extra risk of eventually triggering off small skin cancers, accelerated ageing and CATARACT formation (*see* MELANIN AND MELANOMA). Therefore, any patients treated with regular PUVA must be followed up by a dermatologist for many years.

Complications of psoriasis

A rare severe type of psoriasis can occur in which the whole of the skin becomes red and scaly. This form is known as *erythrodermic psoriasis*. The patient can become quite ill and usually needs treatment in hospital. The loss of skin is so profound that the patient can become PROTEIN deficient and may lose considerable quantities of fluid so that intravenous therapy is required. Treatment is usually with steroids given by mouth, or a drug called *methotrexate* may be prescribed. This drug slows down the excessive division of skin cells but its use must be carefully monitored because it can have toxic side-effects.

Another complication of psoriasis is the occurrence of an ARTHRITIS associated with the condition. About one person in 20 who has psoriasis develops joint problems very similar to RHEUMATOID ARTHRITIS. It can affect many joints in the fingers and toes, and the smaller joints in the hands and feet. Occasionally, people with only very mild psoriasis can develop this complication, although usually the patient's fingernails show some psoriatic pits. Another form of arthritis called ankylosing SPONDYLITIS also occurs more frequently among people with psoriasis. This affects the bones of the back and the pelvis.

Psychiatry

Society's attitude to people suffering from MENTAL ILLNESS has come a long way since the days when anyone who was emotionally disturbed was considered to be possessed by the devil. Psychiatry – a term derived from two Greek words meaning 'mind' and 'healing' – is the branch of medicine which specializes in the study, diagnosis, treatment and prevention of mental disorders.

Diagnosing psychiatric disorders

It has been claimed that 80 per cent of women and 70 per cent of men consult a doctor because of some emotional difficulty: many use minor physical ailments as an excuse for a chat which may allude to underlying psychological problems. This may include a wide range from the very mild, such as shyness in certain social situations, to severe, such as a feeling of near-suicidal helplessness. Less commonly, some people have strange experiences which other people don't share – for example, the novelist Virginia Woolf claimed that she could hear birds singing in Greek.

While all psychiatric problems are a nuisance and interfere with normal life, some can scarcely be classed as illnesses, and respond to simple help and guidance. Others fall into the disease category and may need urgent treatment, often with drugs and sometimes in hospital.

The main diagnostic tool of psychiatrists is simply listening to you and talking with you. They will want to know in depth details about your family background, family health, personalities and relationships. They will also ask about your job, your own health, your feelings towards those you live and work with, and your sex life if it is relevant. It should be stressed here that what you tell psychiatrists is always kept in the strictest confidence.

A lot of information a psychiatrist needs may seem irrelevant: it is not. A psychiatrist has to get as complete a picture of your whole life, and the people in it, as possible; this would include information about your past experiences and reactions.

In addition, it should be reiterated that listening and talking are mainly *diagnostic* tools: treatment itself may involve listening and talking, but once the problem has been isolated, many psychiatrists also use physical methods such as medication, or they may use dynamic techniques such as psychodrama or behaviour therapy.

As patients tell their psychiatrists about, for example, their early life of their families, psychiatrists will be accumulating data concerning the patients' state of mind, their personality and the people they turn to when in difficulty. Most patients will be quite frank in a general sense, but it is a characteristic of psychiatric disorders that the victims themselves cannot understand what is happening to them or why they feel the way they do, particularly in severe cases.

One of the psychiatrist's tools is patients' body language. If patients are depressed, they may droop, speak slowly and blink only rarely. Anxious people may sit on the hard edge of their chairs fidgeting with their fingers, sweating lightly, their voices quiet and high. Those who are angry or resentful tend to lean forward, jut out their chins and speak loudly. Patients suffering from hallucinations may pause to listen or look around – for someone who is not there.

Even what patients do not say may help psychiatrists to understand: a trifling hesitation when patients mention a particular name, or when they attempt to skirt around the subject, can provide vital clues.

Sometimes psychiatrists may want to give their patients a thorough physical check-up. For instance, they may arrange tests for ANAEMIA, or to search out GLANDULAR or other problems. Physical and psychiatric problems are often interconnected, and emotional tensions may lead to bodily symptoms. Equally, physical illnesses can induce psychological disturbances: many people experience DEPRESSION after a bout of INFLUENZA or HEPATITIS.

Specific psychiatric problems

There are three general categories of mental disorders which the psychiatrist may deal with. These are: organic brain disorders, which would include delirium and senile DEMENTIA; psychogenic disorders, which include neuroses, DEPRESSION and other 'affective' disorders, psychoses, PSYCHOSOMATIC and personality problems; and mental handicap.

Organic brain disorders: These disorders are classified as either acute or chronic. Acute brain disorders are temporary disturbances of brain function, involving a disruption of the metabolism of the brain, from which a patient usually recovers. The main symptom of this disorder is delirium – a disordered state of mind with incoherent speech, hallucinations and bewilderment; in its deepest stages, it can lead to coma. The ALCOHOLIC's *delirium tremens* is the best-known manifestation of this disorder.

Chronic brain disorders result from physical changes or damage to the brain tissues. Some are curable, but the commonest form is called Alzheimer's disease, in which a person's memory and sense of time fail progressively. These patients need looking after, and medication usually cannot cure them.

Sigmund Freud introduced the technique of free association of ideas, where patients were encouraged to say anything that came into their minds, and thus provide the analyst with valuable clues. Freud also gave shape to the study of the meaning of dreams, slips of the tongue, forgetfulness and other mistakes and errors in everyday life. His researches suggested to him a new conception of the structure of personality. He divided it into the *id*, the inherited, instinctive impulses of the individual; the *ego*, the part of the mind that reacts to reality; and the *super-ego*, the part of the mind that exerts conscience and responds to social rule. He also stated that conflicts between these three facets led to the arousal of anxiety. The concept of transference was another of his contributions: transference, in the form of deep emotional attachments to parents, is one of the keystones of psychoanalysis. Finally, Freud evolved the *libido* theory: that the development of personality is a psycho-sexual evolution that begins at birth and continues through childhood.

Carl Jung moved away from Freud's theories in a direction that was essentially mystical. Whereas Freud used the term 'libido' to describe sexual energy, Jung preferred to expand its definition, and linked it with what he called the 'collective unconscious': a reservoir of common knowledge.

Melanie Klein expanded the framework of psychoanalysis to include the activities of very young children. She claimed that their spontaneous play activities, utterances and relationships with the people around them could all be material for analysis.

Psychogenic disorders: Psychogenic disorders are defined as mental conditions whose causes are not attributable to a clear physical cause or to structural damage to the NERVOUS SYSTEM. They can produce a range of mental disturbances ranging from the minor to the catastrophic. Some psychiatrists believe that they are due to disturbances of chemical balance in the nervous system.
Psychoses: These are psychogenic disorders in which rational thought in the sufferer is suspended or distorted. Patients may be unable to deal with reality and will create their own special environments in which their perceptions become delusions or hallucinations. Psychotic people may seem totally emotionless.

Psychoses include SCHIZOPHRENIA and MANIC DEPRESSION, both of which may respond well to medication and to other treatment.
Neuroses: Neurotic disorders also come into the psychogenics category: in the general sense, they are understandable but excessive reactions to the difficulties of living and to inner conflicts (*see* NEUROSES). We all feel sad, cross or anxious at times, and these normal feelings are regarded as part of neurosis when they are much more intense and numerous, or last very much longer than apparent STRESS would explain. In this sort of plight, the sufferer needs professional help and will generally respond to it.

There are four main categories of neurotic disorders. These are anxiety states, PHOBIAS, hysterical neuroses and obsessive or compulsive disorders. All need specific treatment.

Anxiety states can take two forms: free-floating and phobic. The first comprises a general, inexplicable feeling of dread: it stops sufferers getting to sleep or concentrating, while their hearts thump and they keep wanting to urinate. Phobic anxiety, on the other hand, consists of panicky feelings only in certain situations, such as might occur on being in a crowd. Medicines and special practical techniques can be very beneficial.

Hysterical illnesses can include physical symptoms and memory disturbances which are brought on through anxiety. Two case studies illustrate this. The first involved a man who was angry with his unfaithful wife, but was afraid that he might hit her dangerously hard. He suddenly developed a weakness in his right arm, so that he couldn't hit her if he tried. The second describes a schoolgirl, who went out with a boyfriend of whom her mother disapproved. She genuinely – but temporarily – lost her memory, so that she did not have to explain her actions.

Obsessive or compulsive neuroses manifest themselves by patients not being able to resist repeating certain actions, even though they know that these are completely unnecessary.

Affective disorders: An affective disorder is one in which the patient's mood or 'affect' is disturbed. The commonest affective disorder is DEPRESSION. A depressive illness is much more serious than simple unhappiness, which is a normal emotion which everybody experiences at times. Depressive illness implies a serious disorder in which sufferers can hardly cope with ordinary life, and are so miserable that they cannot even stir to do anything to help themselves.

Personality problems: Personality – a person's characteristic way of looking at things and of reacting to other people and situations – is unique in every human being. There are numerous distinct personality traits, and all of us have a mixture of these, with the emphasis on one factor or another. Thus one person may have a tendency to shyness, and another to mood changes.

Personality makes people different and interesting; however, when certain traits become exaggerated, they may cause trouble or unhappiness. Personality characteristics seem to be emphasized when people are under stress – for instance, from physical illness or psychological strain. They can also be heightened as a result of psychiatric illness.

Psychosomatic disorders: This category has both physical and mental elements. Certain disorders, such as ulcerative colitis (*see* COLON AND COLITIS), high BLOOD PRESSURE or heart palpitations are thought to have, wholly or in part, an emotional cause that results in physical or psychological changes. The term 'psychosomatic' tends to be used rather loosely, and since disorders of this kind are usually marked by real physical symptoms, only a psychiatrist is qualified to judge – and even he or she may not be sure.

Treatment will involve both body and emotions. For example, if a man is suffering from a peptic ULCER which the doctor suspects is due at least in part to emotional problems, both drugs and psychological treatment may be needed.

Mental deficiency: Mental deficiency, mental subnormality, mental retardation, mental handicap or subnormal intelligence are the result of defective brain development. As a result, the child has learning difficulties and will have trouble leading a normal life. Once the brain has been damaged, the condition is irreversible, but early detection enables special methods of teaching to be used to minimize its effects.

Treatment in psychiatry

There is a wide variety of treatment available for psychiatric problems, from therapy for an individual or group (*see* MENTAL THERAPIES) to different types of medication.

Medication: While other forms of treatment play an important part in psychiatry, it is modern medication that has significantly altered the outlook for mental patients, and brought psychiatric illnesses into line with treatable physical illnesses. No one today need remain miserable for months through depression, nor, as happened in the past with schizophrenia, as a hopelessly deluded hospital inmate for years. Antidepressants and TRANQUILLIZERS may cut short and control the symptoms of many mental diseases.

There are four major types of medicine used in treatment. *Anxiolytics* reduce tension and help the patient to relax; *hypnotics* help the patient to sleep; *tranquillizers* calm and clear the thinking of disturbed patients and, in tiny doses, help combat anxiety; *antidepressants* help to restore a sense of hope and the ability to cope in depression. However, many psycho-active drugs do have side-effects, and the doctor must choose the drug with care for a particular patient. Drug treatments are often combined with other treatments such as supportive psychotherapy.

ECT: Electroconvulsive therapy has a lot of scare stories attached to it, but in cases of severe suicidal depression, it may still occasionally be used. Administered under the most rigidly controlled conditions, it is safe and, in some circumstances, acts more quickly than medication. ECT cannot be given without signed consent. All that patients are likely to remember is the anaesthetic injection. While patients are anaesthetized, a small electrical current is passed across part of their heads for a few seconds: it works rather like electrical treatment for a weak muscle. Some patients experience a little difficulty in remembering small events from before the treatment, but this AMNESIA is usually only temporary.

Psychosurgery: Treating mental disturbances by means of brain surgery, or *prefrontal lobotomy*, is a radical procedure which is performed only after every other form of treatment has proved ineffective. Since the introduction of tranquillizing drugs, very few cases of mental illness warrant such drastic measures.

Psychology

'Psychology' means 'knowledge of the mind' – how it works and why people and other animals think, feel and behave the way that they do. Psychologists are therefore concerned with every aspect of mental life.

Because psychologists deal with all aspects of the mind, only a small proportion of their study is concerned with people's problems. In spite of this, however, discoveries made by psychologists may help to improve the quality of people's lives. Those who specialize in how memory works, for example, may contribute to ways of helping those people whose memory is poor, while those who study how we learn may be able to assist in helping us learn more easily.

Clinical psychology

Unlike PSYCHIATRISTS who are doctors who specialize in mental health, clinical psychologists need not have a medical qualification. However, they will have a degree in psychology and additional qualifications that equip them to work with mental health problems.

Many clinical psychologists are based in psychiatric hospitals and work closely with psychiatrists in the management of patients with psychiatric illnesses (*see* MENTAL ILLNESS), but increasingly, they are also based in health centres or community clinics. Much of their work involves helping people with problems of behaviour which may or may not be associated with psychiatric illness. If somebody has a behavioural problem, such as a serious relationship difficulty, it is quite usual for that person to be seen directly by a psychologist without any involvement from a psychiatrist – unless a mental illness is also present. Clinical psychologists based in the community spend much of their time helping people with personality difficulties or relationship problems. Often the two go together. A person who has an anti-social or psychopathic personality finds it difficult to make friends, and often appears heartless, cold and cruel. The impact of such a personality on relationships can be disastrous, especially if the behaviour of the individual is affecting his or her partner or children.

Other personality disorders include the hysterical (or histrionic) personality, and the paranoid personality. People with hysterical personalities are always looking for attention and are very self-centred, whereas people with paranoid personalities tend to feel that everyone is getting at them, and are argumentative and touchy.

Relationship difficulties may occur, however, even when there are no personality disorders present. Clinical psychologists may see couples with marital problems and also help with specific sexual difficulties (*see* SEX AND SEXUAL INTERCOURSE).

The common *neuroses* are often treated by clinical psychologists. These include anxiety, reactions to STRESS, obsession and PHOBIAS, particularly agoraphobia. Frequently neuroses and stress reactions go hand in hand with some physical symptom or illness such as constant headaches, abdominal pain or, more seriously, stomach and duodenal ulcers, high blood pressure and heart disease. So clinical psychologists may work with general practitioners or specialist physicians in treating patients with such PSYCHOSOMATIC DISORDERS.

Sometimes a clinical psychologist may be able to help a patient who has severe emotional reaction to a HEART ATTACK, the amputation of a limb, the loss of a BREAST or other serious disabling illness. It is often difficult for patients to come to terms with the implications of such illnesses, and they may need psychological help to adapt to a new way of life.

Occasionally, a psychologist may help a patient deal with chronic PAIN. Psychological treatments may diminish the perception of pain and make the patient's life more bearable.

Bereavement can at times set up a chain of severe behavioural difficulties, and here again the clinical psychologist can be most helpful in assisting patients to come to terms with their loss.

In hospitals, clinical psychologists assist psychiatrists with specific treatments for patients with psychiatric illness. Not only neuroses, but also severe DEPRESSION and chronic SCHIZOPHRENIA may be improved by behavioural treatments. Such treatments are often used in addition to drug therapy, but sometimes they are the sole or main treatment for a disorder.

Psychological treatments

Clinical psychologists use a variety of techniques (*see* MENTAL THERAPIES) to decide how best to treat their patients, although most frequently they simply talk to them at length. They need to find out their problems and how these problems are affecting their lives. Sometimes, however, they do use special questionnaires to assess the patient's personality, attitudes or other aspects of his or her life. Needless to say, all the information divulged by the patient is held in total confidence. Like a psychiatrist, a clinical psychologist may need to know about intensely personal details of his or her patient's life.

A technique that is frequently used in behaviour therapy is progressive RELAXATION training, to help the patient to become calmer and to reduce the impact of stress. Used on its own, relaxation therapy may be of great value in stress-related disorders and anxiety.

Clinical child psychology

Some clinical psychologists specialize in behavioural disorders of children and in the assessment of children's development. These psychologists may work from a child guidance centre or with a paediatrician in a hospital. Even very young children may develop behavioural problems such as temper tantrums, sleeping difficulty or problems with feeding or toilet training. Older children can develop various attention-seeking behaviours, including aggressiveness and destructiveness. Adolescents can engage in a variety of anti-social behaviour, which may include stealing and violence, or in drug taking or promiscuous sexual behaviour.

Child psychologists tend to work not just with the child but with the family as well, since often the disordered behaviour has its roots in a deeper family problem or in the way in which the child's parents have been dealing with the child.

Educational psychology

Educational psychologists deal with the school process in general, helping gifted, normal and educationally 'challenged' children, and their parents and teachers, with learning difficulties or problems. This work involves administering psychological tests, as it is sometimes possible to improve the quality of a child's education by carefully sorting out precise areas of strengths and weaknesses and obtaining specialized help if this is necessary. For example, a child who is falling behind at school may be referred to an educational psychologist because he or she is wrongly believed to be lazy, uncaring, generally backward or lacking in concentration. Specialized tests may reveal, however, that the child is actually suffering from DYSLEXIA or some other condition that involves a learning problem but does not affect the child's intelligence in any way.

An educational psychologist is, therefore, more a specialist who tests and diagnoses conditions than one who treats these conditions directly. After diagnosis, the child may be referred to a therapist or other helper. School phobia, emotional or behavioural problems may be dealt with in special classes. Sometimes, however, no referral will be necessary, for a word with the teacher or head teacher may be all that is necessary to steer the child towards making the best use of his or her educational abilities.

Psychosomatic disorders

The word 'psychosomatic' is made up from two Greek words meaning 'mind' (*psyche*) and 'body' (*soma*). It was first used by a German psychiatrist in 1818 in a discussion about the causes of insomnia. Later, certain diseases were called psychosomatic because they were thought to be caused by severe disturbances in the mind. These included asthma and coronary thrombosis.

Recently it has become customary to use the word psychosomatic to describe any illness that is associated with both emotional and physical factors. This does not mean that all pain is 'in the mind' or that it is 'imaginary', but that the pain and the actual physical illness can often accompany the emotional changes taking place in a person. Many people tend to dismiss psychosomatic illness as simply mild symptoms that will recover when a person 'sorts himself out'. But many serious physical illnesses are now known to have – at least in part – some psychological cause or trigger.

The mind's influence on the body

The mind influences the body in innumerable ways, and people have been aware of this for a long time, even before the mechanisms of how this happens were explained. Our language is rich in expressions that show the wide recognition of this. We speak of going 'pale with fear' which can also 'strike us dumb' or even 'paralyse' us. We can be made to feel 'sick with disgust' and may actually vomit; we find it 'difficult to swallow' distasteful facts and cannot 'stomach' something that is totally unacceptable to us.

These are only a small number of ways the mind can affect the body, and usually these changes are short-lived. Often simply confiding in a friend, or talking things over with some suitable companion 'gets it off the chest' – with the result that the unpleasant symptoms will soon disappear.

At other times, the trouble persists, the symptoms get worse and some illness leads the sufferer to the doctor. There may be no awareness that there is any emotional disturbance but only a feeling that an illness needs medical attention. Even direct questioning by the doctor at such times may bring a denial from the patient that there have been any worries or problems.

Illness and emotional stress

There is an increasing amount of evidence that between half and two-thirds of all illnesses reported to general practitioners in Britain are largely dependent to some degree on emotional STRESS. More recently it has been shown that areas with high unemployment are producing increased rates of sickness that need a psychosomatic approach.

Personality is an important cause of psychosomatic disorders. People who 'live in the fast lane' and are sometimes known as 'Type A' personalities tend to suffer more physical disorders – such as HEART ATTACKS – than 'Type B' personalities, who are relaxed, laid-back individuals less vulnerable to stress.

Anxiety plays a very important part in the production of many physical symptoms. These, in turn, produce even more anxiety so that a vicious circle is set up. It is thought that anxiety is essential for the continuation of life. As a result of anxiety or fear, certain HORMONES are produced in the body. These hormones affect part of the AUTONOMIC NERVOUS SYSTEM so that the person in question is prepared for 'fight or flight'.

Normally these changes last only as long as the state of emergency lasts. When, however, such changes are brought about repeatedly by the continuation of emotional tension, these physiological changes persist. This can lead to physical changes in the body that can as a result become pathologically abnormal.

Probably the simplest example of this is seen in the production of high BLOOD PRESSURE. When an animal, including a human, prepares to deal with an external emergency, among the many physical changes which are required is increased circulatory effort. To bring this about, the heart is stimulated to beat more powerfully as well as faster, and the blood pressure is increased. When the emergency is over, the blood pressure returns to normal level. If, however, the blood pressure is raised repeatedly, perhaps continuously, as a response to some emotional stress, secondary changes take place in the blood vessels and in the kidneys and brain so that permanent damage to these structures may result.

It is not only anxiety that can be accompanied by body changes and symptoms. Other strong feelings such as anger, frustration and feelings of guilt as well as stress can also be accompanied by distressing symptoms.

The range of psychosomatic disorders

It is now clear from research that different personality types have variations in the biochemical functioning of the body as well as the differences in the level of 'nervous activity' in the brain. Changes in biochemistry can affect the hormonal system which controls many bodily functions. Stress can not only affect the hormonal system but even the IMMUNE SYSTEM which protects the body against infection, and also seems to have a part to play in protecting against CANCER. So the range of possible psychosomatic disorders is considerable.

MIGRAINE is a very good example of the way the mind and the body interact. The blood vessels around the brain have a tendency to go into spasm, and this is the basis of migrainous headaches. The fact that many people get headaches as they relax after a busy week is typical, and it is almost impossible for a conscientious person with a tendency to migraine to avoid this problem from time to time.

Obvious symptoms such as tension HEADACHES are relatively easily explained, but it is now clear that even some cancers may be triggered by psychological disorders. Stress or depression also seems to be an important factor in the disabling condition of MYALGIC ENCEPHALOMYELITIS (ME). In addition, it has been said that our SKIN frequently mirrors our emotions. Studies have shown that a large number of skin disorders (*see* ECZEMA) are clearly linked with emotional stress.

Diagnosis

When you consult your doctor about any symptoms or illness, it is important that you tell him or her about any recent changes in your life, or recent emotional upsets or problems. If you suspect an emotional cause for your symptoms, do not be shy about revealing it. This will help the doctor considerably in assessing your symptoms. The doctor can then carry out a physical examination to confirm a diagnosis – or sometimes exclude physical conditions.

It is not enough to exclude the presence of physical disease, and then to diagnose an illness caused mainly by an emotional problem. This diagnosis must be made on positive evidence of some actual emotional difficulty that can then be fully explored. If, in spite of a thorough discussion between doctor and patient, there is no apparent emotional cause, the diagnosis must be reconsidered. However, it must be remembered that, on occasion, the emotional content may be repressed – that is, it may not be in the conscious memory. In such cases, only further discussion, perhaps in psychotherapy (*see* PSYCHIATRY), will identify the problem.

Treatment

Once a diagnosis has been made, most psychosomatic illnesses are treated by the family doctor. However, it is never enough simply to treat the physical symptoms with drugs or, perhaps, surgery. The doctor will want to help the patient to reassess his or her life-style and try to eliminate any stress factors.

If the psychosomatic disease is serious – for example, a duodenal ULCER or heart attack occurring at the time of great stress – the patient may be advised to consider a major change in life-style, or a change of job if work has been the major cause of stress. For less serious problems, the patient may be taught RELAXATION therapy, or stress management techniques. Some patients may need detailed psychological or psychiatric help.

One of the most important factors in treatment of psychosomatic disorders is for the patient to accept that there is a psychological basis for his or her illness. Only then can a realistic plan of action be made to remove the underlying cause.

Public health, *see* **Occupational hazards**

Pulmonary embolus, *see* **Infarction, Phlebitis, Thrombosis**

Pulse

When a doctor feels the pulse, he or she is feeling the action of the HEART pumping BLOOD with each beat around the body by means of the ARTERIES. The force of each heartbeat is transmitted along the arterial walls just as a wave travels across the surface of a lake. The walls of the arteries are elastic and expand to take the initial force of a heartbeat. Later in the course of the beat, they contract and, in this way, push blood smoothly along the system.

The body's pulses

The pulse can be felt in a number of the arteries that lie near the surface of the body. The most common is the radial artery in the WRIST which can be felt on the inner surface of the wrist just below the thumb. It is customary to feel this pulse with one or two fingers rather than the thumb, which has its own pulse and can therefore cause some confusion.

The brachial artery in the arm has a pulse which can likewise be easily felt on the inside of the elbow joint almost in line with the little finger.

A doctor may also examine the pulse in the neck created by the carotid artery. This pulse is located about 1 in (2.5 cm) below the angle of the jaw. He may listen to a major artery like the carotid with a stethoscope which can reveal a 'bruit' – a regular whooshing noise with each heartbeat. This may indicate a partial blockage of the artery even though the pulse feels quite normal.

There are also pulses in the groin, behind the knees, on the inside of the ankle and on top of the foot.

What is learned from the pulse?

The first thing a doctor discovers is simply the condition of the arteries themselves. This can be decided on the basis of whether all the pulses are present and normal. It is particularly important to see if the pulses in the legs are present, since the arteries in the legs are most liable to artherosclerosis (furring up of the arteries). If these pulses are diminished or difficult to feel, artherosclerosis may have already developed.

A doctor also uses to pulses to gauge the working of the heart. A regular rhythm suggests that the heart is beating regularly, since the pulse rate gives an exact indication of the heartbeat. Sometimes there can be a discrepancy between the heart rate and the pulse because some of the beats that the heart is making are too weak to be transmitted along the arterial system. This suggests heart trouble.

A fast heartbeat (TACHYCARDIA), of more than 120 beats per minute, occurs as a normal response on exertion, or as the result of a fever. It may also be caused by an abnormality in the heart's electrical conducting system.

A slow heartbeat may be normal, particularly in athletes, but rates of less than 50 beats per minute are abnormal, especially in the elderly. This can mean that there is a heart block due to an interruption of the conduction of electrical impulses in the heart. It can also be caused by overactivity of the parasympathetic part of the AUTONOMIC NERVOUS SYSTEM. This creates the drop in heart rate that leads to a faint.

Even unusual diseases may be pinpointed by an examination of the pulses. When the pulses in the legs are diminished in force and delayed in time compared with those in the arms, a rare congenital problem may be indicated. In this, the body's main artery, the aorta, is blocked as it passes down the chest.

The pulses in the legs, and even in one or both of the arms, may disappear in a commoner disease known as *dissection of the aorta,* where the inner lining of the aorta is torn. This forces blood into the arterial wall, again creating a blockage.

The shape of a pulse wave may also help a doctor in diagnosis. For example, a slowly rising pulse indicates obstruction of the aortic valve, while a pulse which rises fast and falls away again – a 'collapsing' pulse – indicates a leaking aortic valve. Both cases may require surgery.

Purpura

This is the name used to describe the condition of bleeding into the skin. Normally, any tendency to bleed is controlled by the BLOOD clotting and the clot blocking the 'leak' from the damaged blood vessels. Clotting is the result of certain PROTEINS in the blood interlocking to form a mesh. Special cells called *platelets* get caught in the mesh to plug the holes and so make the clot solid. If something goes wrong with this system, purpura may result, as bleeding can thus occur inside the skin.

Purpura may also result from damage to the small blood vessels. In this case, even though the blood clots normally, uncontrolled bleeding may occur because the vessels leak.

Causes

Purpura may be a sign of several diseases. First, there are conditions in which the blood-clotting mechanism may not be working properly. Anti-coagulant drugs, especially designed to reduce the ability of the blood to clot, may cause purpura if taken in too high a dose. LIVER failure, as an end stage of CIRRHOSIS, results in lack of blood-clotting proteins and therefore in purpura.

Second, there are diseases in which the number of platelets in the circulation is reduced. This means that, although the blood clots normally, the mesh is weak and falls apart as the gaps are not 'plugged' with platelets. These platelets are made in the BONE MARROW along with most of the other blood cells. Any disease that affects the bone marrow – such as septicaemia, or blood-poisoning (*see* SEPTIC CONDITIONS), and certain types of CANCER – will therefore result in a reduced platelet count. Moreover, the platelets are often the first structures to be affected by such disorders and so purpura may be the first symptom of a bone marrow disease.

Third, purpura may be due to problems with the blood vessels. In these cases, the clotting mechanism functions normally, the platelet count is satisfactory but the purpura results from blood leaking from the damaged vessels. This is most commonly seen in normal bruising.

This type of purpura may be precipitated by increased pressure in the small vessels due to coughing, vomiting or prolonged standing. It may be a result of decreased support for the blood vessels by the surrounding tissues. This happens particularly in the elderly (*senile purpura*). VITAMIN C deficiency (SCURVY) and the prolonged use of STEROID-containing ointments can also weaken the skin and lead to purpura. Blood vessels may also leak because of various inflammatory reactions within their walls.

Finally, *Henoch-Schönlein purpura* is a childhood illness in which a purpuric rash is the most obvious feature. It is associated with pains in the joints and in the abdomen. The rash is seen mainly on the front of the legs, the buttocks and the outside of the arms and face. It may also be more itchy than is usual for purpura. The disease sometimes involves the kidneys. It is quite common, though not as widespread as measles or chickenpox, and often follows a throat or ear infection.

Symptoms

Everyone knows what a bruise looks like: a large dark patch under the skin which may or may not be associated with some pain and swelling. Usually, purpura is just the same kind of coloured patch but there is no swelling or pain unless it is a result of physical damage. Many old people do not notice the purpuric spots on their skin unless they are pointed out.

Purpura can be distinguished from other red RASHES because rashes usually disappear temporarily when pressure is applied to them, but this does not happen with purpura. This is because the blood is outside the blood-vessels and so cannot easily be carried away. With rashes, the colour is from dilated blood-vessels but the blood is still inside and is therefore easy to squeeze away.

Generally, purpura due to clotting defects will give rise to large red patches. There may be other signs of bleeding such as NOSEBLEEDS. Low platelet counts do not cause such extensive purpura but more usually small spots, as the blood can still clot but the clot leaks. Problems with blood vessels produce typical bruises.

Treatment

The treatment of purpura depends on the underlying cause. In the case of senile purpura, bruising and purpura induced by the effects of pressure, there is little that can be done. Vitamin supplements may help strengthen the tissues.

Purpura caused by some form of disease must first be investigated to decide what the disease is. A simple blood test will show if the platelet count is adequate. The bleeding time can be measured: this is the time taken for a pinprick to stop bleeding. It is usually three to six minutes and depends both on the blood clotting and the platelets plugging the mesh adequately. Finally, the clotting time (the time it takes for blood to clot in a tube) is measured. This is independent of the platelets and shows whether the clotting mechanism is functioning properly.

If purpura is found to be secondary to some other problem, this must be treated first. When the bleeding tendency is serious, it will most likely be treated with a blood transfusion that contains platelets and the blood-clotting proteins. In cases of purpura where no other factor appears to be involved, the condition may respond to treatment with steroid tablets. If that fails it has been found that operating and removing the SPLEEN often helps. However, this type of purpura may also improve without treatment.

Pustule, *see* Rash

Pyelitis, *see* Cystitis, Kidneys and kidney diseases

Pyelogram, *see* Kidney and kidney diseases

Pyloric stenosis, *see* Nausea, Stomach, Ulcers, peptic

Pyoderma gangrenosum, *see* Colon and colitis

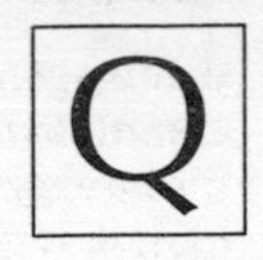

Q fever, *see* Pneumonia

Quadriplegia, *see* Cerebral palsy

Quinine

This drug was first discovered by the South American Indians and then brought over to Europe by the Spanish in the 17th century. Although it took some time for the value of this powerful – but potentially dangerous – drug to be understood, it eventually became the major treatment for MALARIA and remained so until the late 1920s. This remarkable drug can also treat some MUSCLE and HEART disorders.

Quinine is, in fact, derived from the bark of cinchona trees which are found in Peru and elsewhere in South America. And it was through the South American Indians that the Spanish learnt that quinine had a valuable effect on fevers. However, they would not have known that quinine's real power lay in its action against the dreaded disease of malaria.

Quinine was therefore one of the first drugs to be used successfully against an infectious disease. It was of immense value since malaria was extremely common in hot climates in those days – in fact, in world terms, it still remains one of the most virulent infectious diseases.

Uses

The cinchona bark actually contains many related active compounds. Today we use only two of them with any frequency – they are *quinine* and the closely related compound *quinidine*.

Quinine still has a place in the treatment of malaria, but as what doctors call 'a second line drug'. The reason why it has been superseded by synthetic drugs in some ways is that there is only a small margin between the amount of quinine needed to treat an attack of malaria and the toxic dose. However, in many parts of the world, it is an important treatment for falciparum malaria (malignant malaria), and it is also safe for pregnant women to take. In one other respect, though, it remains an extremely important drug – this is in the treatment of the type of malaria that is resistant to other drugs. Despite intensive work on anti-malarial drugs, the drug least likely to encounter a resistant organism remains quinine.

Quinine also has very valuable effects on the heart as it can help to suppress abnormalities of the heart rhythm. In practice, however, it is usually the related drug quinidine that is used for this purpose, since it seems to have a slightly greater effect on the heart than quinine itself, although the two are almost identical in chemical structure.

The way that the drug interferes with the electrical activity of the heart muscle is probably closely related to the way in which quinine helps with various problems in ordinary muscle. It can help to produce a greater degree of relaxation in congenital muscle disease such as myotonia and in relieving the annoying night cramps that many people suffer from as they grow older.

Quinsy, *see* Tonsils

Rabies

This is one of the most terrifying diseases in the world. It is transmitted via the bite of an animal driven to a frenzy by the disease – perhaps the most chilling way that any disease is transferred from victim to victim. The horror of the disease is intensified by the knowledge that, once symptoms of the disease begin, the outcome is usually fatal.

Although there are only a handful of cases every year in developed countries, rabies remains a very important disease in worldwide terms. In India alone, there are around 15,000 deaths every year from the disease. Almost all human cases are caused by the bite of an infected dog, the reason being that the dog is the creature most likely to come into contact with humans. Nevertheless, there are many species of animals that can have rabies, and in northern Europe, for example, the fox is the most common carrier.

Causes

Rabies is caused by a VIRUS and is found almost everywhere in the world, although in most places it is confined to the wild animal population, and only very rarely does it actually spread to human beings.

Transmission of the disease occurs when an infected animal bites another animal. The animal that attacks and bites will die of the disease, so the rabies virus ensures its survival by altering the behaviour of the animal that is infected so that it makes this uncharacteristic attack. The madness of the 'mad dog' with rabies is therefore an important part in the survival of the virus, and is no doubt brought about in part by *hydrophobia*, the thirst for water that is accompanied by terror and spasms at the very sight of it. Indeed, hydrophobia is the most characteristic sign of the disease in humans, and it used to be the name by which rabies was commonly known.

Once the infecting virus has made its way through the skin, it may lie dormant for some time, with the incubation period extending in some cases to years. Generally, though it ranges from 20 to 90 days. After the skin stage, the virus enters the nerves of its victim and works its way up them through the nerve cells until it reaches the brain. Once it has become established in the brain, the symptoms of the disease break out. The fact that the virus has to make this journey through the nerves explains why the incubation period seems to be longer in those people who are bitten on the foot compared with those who are bitten on the hand or the face: the further the virus has to go from its site of entry to reach the brain, the longer it is going to take.

A bite is not the only way that the disease is spread. It is possible for the virus to get in through a cut or scratch in the skin, so even a lick from an infected animal can produce the disease. It has also been known for people to get an infection by inhaling droplets of virus-carrying liquid.

Symptoms

Rabies is basically a form of encephalitis, that is, the symptoms are due to infection of the tissues of the BRAIN.

The best known and most horrifying symptom is hydrophobia. This symptom is unique and quite characteristic when it occurs – which it does in 50 per cent of patients. They may be thirsty, and may be longing for a drink, but as the water is brought to them, they will recoil and have spasms of the throat. This may progress to terror at the sight or mention of water, generalized convulsions and the sort of back-arching spasms that are found in patients suffering from TETANUS.

Hydrophobia doesn't come on until the disease is quite well developed. The disease usually starts with a few days of ill health, fever, sore throat and muscular aches. Although this may sound like the start of any other virus infection, a kind of restlessness and insomnia that is typical of rabies accompanies it. Another clue in the early stages is that there has been pain and tingling at the site where the person has been bitten.

After the hydrophobia has come on, the disease progresses to a generalized involvement of the NERVOUS SYSTEM. Spasms get more frequent and any one of them can end in death. The patient may have episodes of wild, confused excitement alternating with lucid periods. There is often an exaggeration of such automatic functions as salivation and sweating – the equivalent of the frothing at the mouth of a typical rabid dog. Eventually the victim lapses into a coma and dies 10–14 days after the onset of symptoms. This form of the disease is known as 'furious rabies' and it is the pattern that most patients follow. However, the progress of the disease is different in about a fifth of patients with PARALYSIS being the major feature. The paralysis begins by ascending the body from the legs upwards in a symmetrical pattern. Hydrophobia may occur, but it tends to happen later in the disease.

Recently, new, useful tests have been developed that use fluorescent antibodies to identify rabies antigen in saliva.

Treatment

There is no cure for established rabies, and it appears almost inevitable that people with the disease are going to die. However, most cases of the disease occur in developing countries where there are few facilities for the intensive care that the more technologically advanced countries are able to give patients.

Treatment of rabies consists of putting patients on a ventilator (breathing machine) and maintaining support of their vital functions such as their heartbeat and the urine output of their kidneys in the hope that they may recover. There have been only three such recoveries recorded, all in patients who have been vaccinated shortly after their exposure to the disease. There is also some hope that the anti-viral substance interferon may be of some value in treating the disease. Despite all this, however, the hopes for someone with the established disease must be considered very, very faint.

One of the problems that a doctor will face in a country such as Britain is in proving the diagnosis with a laboratory test. Samples of blood and other body fluids are not as much use as one might expect since the level of antibodies to the disease (which give the diagnosis) does not begin to rise until fairly late, after the symptoms have started to develop.

Another test which can be done is to take a small sample of skin, preferably from the hairline, which, when treated in a special way, will reveal the rabies virus in the tiny nerves. Finally there is the old-fashioned way of making the diagnosis: this involves the rather drastic measure of making a hole in the patient's skull and taking some brain tissue for examination under the microscope. This shows conclusive signs of the disease.

It is very important that the diagnosis should be confirmed. In a country such as Britain, where rabies is so rare that there is, on average, less than one case per year, it is very unlikely that a case of the disease will actually turn up under the care of a doctor who has seen it before. Considerable public health programmes may have to be undertaken as the result of a single case, so it is very useful to have confirmation. Fortunately doctors in Britain can get help with the diagnosis from the Public Health Service reference laboratory.

Prevention

The basis of rabies control must be prevention since cure of the disease seems very unlikely. People at risk are given IMMUNIZATION, and those who may have suffered a bite from an infected animal (or one that might have been, if it has been impossible to capture the animal) are not only given a course of this, but may also be given protection in the form of immunoglobulins (antibodies) prepared from the blood of someone who is well immunized against the disease. In countries which cannot afford human immunoglobulin, it is standard procedure to use antibodies raised in horses, although this carries the risk of a reaction to the horse serum itself.

In the past, the common vaccine that was used contained viral matter raised on nervous tissue. This required large amounts of vaccine to be given, and it carried the risk of a reaction to the nervous tissue itself which could, in a very few cases, prove fatal. This vaccine is still the most widely used in worldwide terms, but there is another sort of vaccine which is raised on tissue in a cell culture which has the advantages of being safer, and of needing fewer injections.

In spite of the fact that there are now good vaccines available, the best thing that can be done is to try and keep a country totally free of the disease.

Radiculogram, *see* **Slipped disc**

Radiation sickness

Today, radiation sickness is most commonly seen in the treatment of CANCER when it is an unpleasant, yet controllable side-effect of RADIOTHERAPY: controllable because the extent of damage to cells and tissues depends on the dose of radiation received. And, even where large amounts of radiotherapy are necessary – for instance, in the treatment of a large tumour deep in the abdomen – doses are split to minimize the unpleasant effects of radiation sickness.

In the case of a nuclear disaster, on the other hand, such as nuclear war or a major accident at a nuclear power plant, exposure to radiation would be massive and the ultimate effects both far-reaching and devastating.

The effect of radiation on the body depends on the exact dosage received. A relatively high dose of radiation causes nausea and perhaps vomiting within an hour or two of exposure. Higher doses produce a more rapid onset of symptoms. The vomiting may settle after four to six hours, but other symptoms may occur.

Effects of radiotherapy

When radiation sickness develops during the course of radiotherapy, the first symptoms are tiredness and weakness, headache, nausea and vomiting. It is thought that these symptoms may be partly due to the release of toxic products into the bloodstream from tissues damaged by radiation.

Other unpleasant effects of radiotherapy depend on the sensitivity of various parts of the body. The most sensitive areas are those in a constant state of self-renewal, such as the SKIN, the cells in the BONE MARROW which produce new blood cells and the cells which line the STOMACH and the INTESTINES. This growth process is easily damaged by radiation, and radiotherapists make use of this effect to destroy the malignant cells of cancerous tumours.

Following a sufficient dose of radiation, the skin becomes red and sore. Hair roots are damaged and the hair eventually falls out, although it usually regrows within two to three months. Sweat glands are damaged as well, so the skin also becomes very dry. Higher doses cause more redness and blistering, followed by scab formation. Healing from this stage takes about three weeks. In the bone marrow, the cells which produce white blood cells and platelets are most easily damaged, so frequent blood tests are necessary during treatment to make sure that the white blood cell and platelet counts do not fall too low. Ulceration, diarrhoea and bleeding follow exposure of the stomach and intestines to radiation. Patients receiving radiotherapy may also suffer from dryness of the mouth and soreness of the throat which may make swallowing difficult.

There is no doubt that these side-effects are unpleasant and unwanted, but it is usually possible to take steps to treat or at least minimize most of them. In any case, they are temporary and generally considered worth putting up with when weighed against the effectiveness of the treatment.

Whole-body irradiation

Irradiation to the whole body may result from accidents in the nuclear industry or from nuclear explosions. The initial effects of a severe exposure depend on the dose received, but nausea and sickness are again the first and most obvious symptoms. After a day or so, once the initial sickness has improved, further intestinal symptoms develop. The lining of the bowel normally grows at a rapid rate, so it is among the first tissues to suffer from ill-effects of radiation. Absorption of food from the bowel decreases, so the victim loses weight rapidly, and develops nausea and diarrhoea.

Bone marrow cells are also affected immediately by whole body irradiation. If the dose is low, there is just a temporary drop in the numbers of white blood cells. But with higher doses, the bone marrow virtually ceases functioning altogether. As the white cells drop in numbers, the person loses resistance to infections.

Eventually, if the person survives for more than a week or two, they also become anaemic. The ANAEMIA may be worsened by internal bleeding or easy bruising because the platelets, responsible for triggering off blood clotting, are also damaged by irradiation.

Severe exposure to whole-body radiation produces not only rapid nausea and sickness but also confusion and disorientation. These effects are largely a result of disordered action of the brain. Coma and early death occur as a direct result of brain damage by radiation.

If people survive whole-body irradiation, long-term effects may be evident years later. Several types of cancer are much commoner as a result of such radiation, particularly LEUKAEMIA, skin cancer, THYROID cancer and BREAST cancer. Even relatively small amounts of excess radiation may increase the risk of cancer later in life. It is now believed that background radiation, which comes from cosmic rays and natural radioactive materials and gases such as radon and thoron, is actually responsible for some cases of cancer in the population.

Treatment of radiation sickness

A person receiving radiotherapy treatment receives very careful doses of radiation under medical supervision. The doses can be planned to minimize radiation sickness, but if it does occur, drugs can be used to relieve the symptoms. If the sickness becomes intolerable, the radiotherapist may delay the next treatment or replan the treatment to minimize side-effects.

In the event of a major nuclear accident similar to that at Chernobyl in 1986 or an accident with a nuclear-powered ship or submarine, it would be possible to provide treatment for those severely affected by radiation. The first priority for doctors would be to relieve sickness with drugs and to estimate the degree of damage caused by irradiation. Blood tests would be taken to assess the effect of irradiation on the white blood cells. More sophisticated tests on the chromosomes in the blood cells can also be used to gauge the level of exposure. The patients would have to be kept in a germ-free environment because they would be more susceptible to infections. They would be given sterile food and regular doses of antibiotics to prevent germs in the bowel from reaching other organs. If the victim became anaemic, a bone marrow transplant could be carried out.

For those less severely affected, a programme to administer IODINE would be commenced. This prevents radioactive iodine from the nuclear accident from becoming concentrated in the thyroid gland, which could precipitate thyroid cancer in later life. The bone marrow could also be restimulated by the use of vaccines such as TETANUS vaccine.

After an accident involving radioactive dusts or solid materials, it is very important to try to remove as much of the material as possible. The victim's skin must be washed thoroughly. If radioactive dusts have entered the lungs it is even possible for doctors to wash out the trachea and bronchial tubes in the lungs using a special instrument called a bronchoscope (*see* ENDOSCOPY). This procedure would be carried out under anaesthetic.

Radiotherapy

The use of radiation in the treatment of disease is an effective weapon against many forms of CANCER. The two main sources of radiation are X-RAYS and gamma-rays; both belong to the same 'family' as radio waves and light waves. Radio waves carry energy from radio stations to radio sets in our home, and we can feel the effects of the heat energy that is carried in rays of sunlight. X-rays and gamma-rays are also invisible rays or waves that carry very large amounts of energy.

X-rays are produced artificially by bombarding a small tungsten 'target' with electricity in a device called an X-ray tube. Gamma-rays are not produced artificially but are naturally emitted by radioactive substances such as radium, cobalt and caesium.

When X-rays were first discovered in the early years of the twentieth century only weak sources were available and only skin tumours could be successfully treated with radiotherapy; the low-energy X-rays from these sources were just not capable of penetrating further than a very short distance into the tissue. Over the years, new technology has revolutionized this branch of medicine and increased its scope. Today we know much more about the different forms of radiation and how they work.

How radiotherapy works

Radiotherapy is used to control the growth and spread of abnormal body cells. All living cells are damaged when they absorb energy from X-rays and gamma-rays but growing or dividing cells are damaged more easily than others. It is because cancer cells grow more rapidly than normal cells that they are slow to recover from the effects of radiation. Radiation from X-rays and gamma-rays also destroys small blood-vessels on which TUMOUR cells depend for nourishment, so that following radiotherapy, these cells are more susceptible to the body's own natural defences.

While surrounding normal tissue is more resistant to this type of radiation, it is still easily damaged. More than any other factor, damage to healthy tissue limits the doses of radiation that may be used in treatment.

Types of radiotherapy

The many types of X-ray machines in everyday use differ in the amount of energy or power of the X-rays that they produce. If a tumour lies in or close to the skin, it would be unwise to use high-energy X-rays that would penetrate deep into the body and damage normal tissues. Conversely, there is no point in using low-energy X-rays to treat a lung tumour, for example; the X-rays will not penetrate to a sufficient depth. So there are superficial-voltage X-ray machines that are used to treat skin cancers, deep X-ray therapy units that are used to treat tumours up to a depth of 4 in (10 cm), and megavoltage or supervoltage machines that are used to treat deep-lying tumours.

Because it is difficult to produce very high-energy radiation from X-rays, gamma-ray sources are more often employed for this purpose. Cobalt or caesium are the substances in most common use. A gamma-ray unit consists simply of a quantity of a radioactive isotope of caesium or cobalt encased in thick lead shielding. A small aperture in the shielding is opened during treatment, allowing a gamma-ray beam to emerge.

When powerful X-ray and gamma-ray beams are used, it is essential to take great care to protect normal tissue from exposure. The narrowest possible X-ray beam which will encompass the whole of the tumour is used. Healthy areas are covered with lead shielding and when this is technically difficult – on an irregular surface such as the face, for example – a lead mould or mask is specially made to fit over the entire region, with a 'window' cut out over the area to be treated. With a deep-lying tumour, the X-ray dose to the surface tissues can be reduced by selecting different points of entry for the beam, treating the tumour from several different angles in turn. This technique is known as *overlapping field therapy*.

It is also possible to give radiotherapy by placing radioactive sources within the body. Needles, tubes, wires, or tiny seeds of radioactive material may be placed in close contact with, or implanted in the tumours. Because only low-energy sources are used, the radiation emitted has only a limited penetrating power and normal tissues are unlikely to be damaged. In treatment of cancer of the CERVIX (neck of the womb) and of the UTERUS (womb), tiny radium sources are placed inside the upper part of the vagina and the uterus, giving a much higher dose of radiation than would be possible using other techniques directly to the tumour. Radioactive implants are also used to treat some forms of BREAST cancer.

Although overactivity of the THYROID gland is usually not a cancerous condition, it does nevertheless respond to a special form of radiotherapy. Unlike other parts of the body, the thyroid gland selectively stores iodine. The patient is given a small amount of radioactive iodine to swallow and the amount of radioactivity which passes into the thyroid gland is sufficient to destroy the overactive tissue without harming other parts of the body.

Choosing the right treatment

Just as there are many different types of infectious diseases, each with its own most effective form of treatment, so there are many different types of cancer. The most appropriate treatment depends not only on the precise nature of the cancer, but also on how far advanced it has become. Treatment may involve surgery, radiotherapy, drugs (chemotherapy) or any combination of these three.

Surgery is usually undertaken when a tumour is considered to be accessible and readily removable, provided that there is no evidence that it has spread to other parts of the body through the bloodstream. Chemotherapy may be preferable if spread is suspected because, unlike either radiotherapy or surgery, the effects of anti-cancer drugs reach the whole body and are not solely confined to the site of an operation or the site of radiation treatment.

In some radio-sensitive tumours, radiotherapy alone is often sufficient to achieve a cure. More often, however, it is used in combination with other treatments. It is also an especially good way of relieving any unpleasant symptoms in patients for whom a complete cure is not considered possible; this is known as *palliation*.

Treatment is planned by the radiotherapist in conjunction with a radiation physicist. Together they will map out the location of the tumour on an X-ray film or a scan of the diseased area, and using a special computer will calculate precisely the energy, dosage and position of the treatment beams that will be required. The beam positions, or 'fields', are marked on the patient's skin using indelible ink or sometimes tattoos. This permanent method of marking the skin is done so that the patient can be accurately repositioned under the beam each time treatment is given.

The course of treatment is usually spread over three to six weeks and is given in divided doses three to five times per week. It is actually the total dosage that determines how many tumour cells are destroyed, but dividing the doses allows much better recovery of normal tissue and increases the total dose that can be tolerated.

Most patients do not need hospital admission during the course of radiotherapy but can be treated as out-patients. The treatment itself is quite painless and involves lying or sitting quite still on an X-ray table beneath the radiation beam for a few minutes at a time, in a special room shielded with lead and concrete. The staff who work in radiotherapy departments are at special risk from long-term effects of exposure to radiation and are therefore not allowed to remain in the room while treatment is being given.

Side-effects

The most common side-effect of radiotherapy is redness and soreness of the skin overlying the treatment field. When this occurs, patients are instructed not to wash or shave affected skin for a few days until it improves, since soap and drying with a towel make the soreness much worse.

If the field includes an area of scalp, the patient may lose some of his or her hair, but it will usually grow back after treatment has been completed.

Any exposure of the mouth, gullet, stomach, or intestines may cause loss of appetite, dryness of the mouth, vomiting or diarrhoea. A high-calorie, easily assimilated diet is often necessary until these effects wear off.

Radiotherapy can cause sterility, though this can often be avoided if the reproductive organs are protected with lead shielding. But ability to enjoy sexual intercourse and achieve orgasms is not affected.

In addition, any exposure to radiation carries a very small but very definite risk of causing cancer, perhaps years later, which depends on the dose received. The risks of getting LEUKAEMIA and cancer of the lung, breast, thyroid, and skin may all increase following exposure to radiation.

Blood counts taken during treatment are used to monitor harmful effects of radiation on the bone marrow. RADIATION SICKNESS is treated with anti-nausea drugs and sedation.

Ramsay Hunt syndrome, *see* Shingles

Rash

A rash may be an outward sign of a condition affecting the body as a whole. Thus infectious fevers, emotional disorders and ALLERGIES all may have accompanying rashes.

They may equally, however, be an indication of a localized disorder in the skin – the kind of inflammation that is commonly called DERMATITIS. Included in this kind of local inflammation are NAPPY RASH, prickly heat, ECZEMA and FUNGAL INFECTIONS of the skin.

Rashes can take many different forms. The rash which is present at the beginning of an illness is called the *primary rash.* It may subsequently change in character and appearance during the natural course of the causative disease, or as a result of complications or in response to treatment. New rashes or changes in the appearance of the original rash are called *secondary eruptions,* and each has its own set of characteristics that may require different treatment.

Primary rashes

The commonest of the primary rashes are areas or spots of redness which doctors call *macules.* Any abnormal change in the colour of the skin over a limited area qualifies as a macular rash, the redness itself being given the name *erythema.* Sometimes, as in the early stages of MEASLES, the rash consists of hundreds of tiny red spots, each separate or 'discrete' from each other.

In other cases the spots enlarge until they run into each other, joining up to form blotchy patches. This is called a *confluent rash.* Usually if you press your thumb on a part of the rash it will not fade, but sometimes it will temporarily leave a white area. This is an important diagnostic feature and is characteristic of several conditions including SCARLET FEVER and TYPHOID FEVER in particular.

Rashes caused by skin infection or allergy

Cellulitis	A bright red raised area of skin which aches and may throb. Usually localized to one small area of the body. Caused by bacterial infection. Sometimes called *erysipelas*.
Dermatitis herpetiformis	Intensely irritating groups of blisters over the trunk, elbows or knees. Associated with allergy to wheat flour (gluten). *See* DERMATITIS.
Eczema	Scaly reddened areas of skin with cracking. Almost anywhere on the body but often hands or feet, fronts of elbows and backs of knees. *See* ECZEMA.
Herpes simplex	Usually known as 'cold sores'. Itchy blistering rash around the mouth or on the nose (Type I herpes). Sometimes affects the genital area in men and women ('genital herpes' – caused by Type II *herpes simplex* virus). *See* HERPES.
Impetigo	Small areas of blistering rash with yellow discharge that crusts. Very contagious – spreads easily. Caused by bacterial infection. *See* IMPETIGO.
Lichen planus	Small purple-coloured areas of raised, fissured skin. Usually on wrists, legs. Unknown cause.
Pemphigus	Large blistering lesions occurring almost anywhere on the skin surface. A similar condition is called *pemphigoid*; both are 'auto-immune' diseases.
Pityriasis rosea	Flat spots on the trunk and upper limbs which rarely hurt but may itch. Fades after 2 or 3 weeks. Caused by a virus.
Pityriasis versicolor	Pale brown scaly patches on trunk or limbs. Do not become brown with sunbathing, so then stand out as white patches. Caused by a fungus infection.
Psoriasis	Thick 'plaques' of reddened, scaly skin. Often on backs of elbows, fronts of knees, and scalp, but may affect virtually any area of the body except the central part of the face. *See* PSORIASIS.
Ringworm	Areas of red raised patches; scaly with a prominent margin and paler centre. Tends to grow outwards, enlarging over days. Caused by a fungus infection. *See* RINGWORM.

Rashes associated with infectious diseases

Chickenpox	Small flat spots turning into pimples then small blisters. These become pustules which burst to form scabs. The rash starts on the trunk, itches and lasts about a week. *See* CHICKENPOX.
Rubella	Tiny red spots, often very faint, appearing first on the face and spreading down to the trunk. Also called German measles. *See* RUBELLA.
Measles	Tiny red spots first on the forehead and behind the ears, spreading down to the chest and abdomen. The rash is preceded by small white spots inside the mouth, takes two days to develop fully, and starts to fade after about a week. *See* MEASLES.
Scarlet fever	Flat red spots or small blotches, most marked at the armpits, and elbow and groin creases, leaving a clear area around the mouth. Pressing on skin leaves a light mark. *See* SCARLET FEVER.
Syphilis	A faint copper-coloured rash appears in the secondary stage of the disease, most often on the trunk, palms of the hands, soles of the feet and the forehead. A blood test can confirm the diagnosis. *See* SYPHILIS.
Typhoid and *paratyphoid*	Successive crops of a dozen or so 'rose-spots', about ¼ in (0.5 cm) across, on the chest and abdomen, lasting two to three days. *See* TYPHOID AND PARATYPHOID.

The second common type of rash consists of spots which are not necessarily red but project above the surface of the skin. They can be felt as small raised pimples if a fingertip is run over the skin (rather like goose pimples), in contrast to a macular rash which is not raised. These little pimples are known as *papules,* and the rash as a *papular rash.* A maculo-papular rash is halfway between a macular and a papular one.

When the rash is made up of pimples containing a clear or milky fluid doctors refer to it as *vesicular,* with each pimple being a vesicle. CHICKENPOX and SMALLPOX are typical examples.

A rash may also consist of raised areas of skin much larger than papules. These are known as *weals,* and they are usually white at the centre and pink or red at the outer edge. This type of skin eruption – called *urticaria* or, more commonly, nettlerash or hives – is usually highly irritant and indicates an allergic reaction which releases histamine into the skin to cause the inflammation.

You can usually tell the difference between a rash due to an infectious disease and one due to an allergy. The rashes of the common infectious diseases differ from each other in appearance, and rarely form weals or irritate as acutely as those due to an allergy. Also, a person with an infectious disease will probably have a fever and feel ill, while those with an allergy usually feels quite well in themselves.

Secondary rashes

In some cases, the primary rash, whatever its type, simply fades away or 'resolves' as the condition improves, without going through any secondary stage and without leaving scars or any other after-effects. Secondary eruptions are common with some infections, however, and may take a variety of forms.

Often the area of skin covered by the rash peels away. This normally occurs if the original rash was a dry macular or papular one, or a mixture of the two.

The type of rash usually seen in the later stages of chickenpox is, by contrast, pustular, which means that the spots have become infected pustules, containing pus. This type of moist lesion will dry out to form a crust or small scab. New skin will grow under the scabs which will eventually separate and drop off. If the deeper layers of skin have been affected – as when chickenpox spots are scratched – there may be permanent scarring in the form of pock-marks, which form tiny pits in the skin.

Other types of secondary rash include thickening of the area of skin concerned, giving it a leathery look and feel which is characteristic of long-term or chronic inflammation. Similarly, permanent discoloration or pigmentation of the skin may develop.

Finally, entire areas of skin may break down, exposing the underlying or subcutaneous tissue. Without the protective covering of skin, the ULCERS so formed frequently become infected by bacteria from the atmosphere, especially in moist, heavily contaminated situations. This sometimes happens with nappy rash, COLD SORES or SHINGLES.

Chronic rashes

Apart from temporary rashes associated with infectious diseases or an intermittent allergy, certain types of rash can occur on the skin as part of an ongoing skin disorder. These disorders tend to be long-lasting, or 'chronic'.

One of the commonest skin disorders is eczema and its associated condition, dermatitis. These disorders produce a reddened, scaly rash which may affect the hands or feet, fronts of the elbows, backs of the knees or, when severe, almost any part of the body. Dermatitis is the name given to a type of eczema triggered off by sensitivity or allergy to chemicals, soaps, dusts or even metal jewellery containing nickel. Housewives or anyone whose hands are in water for long periods may develop dermatitis.

PSORIASIS is a condition which produces areas of red, thickened, scaly skin. Other chronic rashes may be caused by a variety of disorders, the origin of which often remains obscure.

Treatment

The rashes of infectious diseases rarely need any specific treatment but, where necessary, the underlying condition will be treated. If itching is a problem, a simple cooling lotion such as calamine lotion may be helpful.

Mild allergic disorders or small patches of dermatitis can be treated safely with 1 per cent hydrocortisone cream, which can be bought in a chemist's shop.

Chronic rashes, however, usually require medical assessment and treatment. If your family doctor cannot identify the rash, he or she may refer you to a dermatologist for further assessment. In some cases a small piece of skin may be removed under local anaesthetic for examination in the laboratory so that the rash may be identified. Treatment is usually with creams or ointments. For dermatitis and eczema, steroid creams are often prescribed; for psoriasis, dithranol or tar preparations.

Raynaud's disease

Raynaud's disease – sometimes called 'white finger' – most frequently affects women, starting in the teens or early 20s. It has very similar symptoms to and is a progressive form of Raynaud's *phenomenon*, which occurs in association with other conditions or illnesses such as RHEUMATOID ARTHRITIS and *scleroderma*. It can also happen in people whose work exposes their hands to continually prolonged periods of vibration.

Causes

Raynaud's *disease* results from an abnormality in the small blood vessels of the fingers. Occasionally the toes are affected as well, but this is less common. The blood vessels become extra-sensitive to the cold. Normally exposure to it causes a slight reduction in blood flow to the skin, but if a person has Raynaud's disease, the blood flow virtually stops as a result of the tiny blood vessels constricting very tightly. The underlying reason for this is, however, completely unknown. Apart from the abnormality in the small blood vessels in the hands, nothing else seems to be affected by this condition and the rest of the circulation remains perfectly normal.

Raynaud's *phenomenon* is a similar problem but is always associated with some other condition. One of the commonest causes is repeated vibration that affects the hands. It can occur in professional pianists or chain-saw operators whose hands are regularly subjected to vibration. The vibration probably damages the nerves running to the small blood vessels in the fingers, so affecting the response of the blood vessels to cold.

Some forms of ARTHRITIS, such as rheumatoid arthritis, and various other connective tissue disorders may also trigger off Raynaud's phenomenon, but again the underlying reason is unclear.

If the larger blood vessels running to the hands or feet become blocked by fatty deposits – the condition called *atherosclerosis* (*see* ARTERIES) – the circulation to the feet or hands suffers. An early sign of such trouble can be the occurrence of Raynaud's phenomenon in the limb.

Certain rare blood disorders may also be a cause of Raynaud's phenomenon. Abnormal PROTEINS can occasionally be produced by the BONE MARROW and LYMPH SYSTEMS, and they then circulate in the bloodstream. These proteins – called *cryoglobulins* – coagulate at a temperature which is only slightly lower than the body temperature. So if a patient suffering from this condition (*cryoglobulinaemia*) is exposed to the cold, he or she shows the signs of Raynaud's phenomenon. The symptoms may be very widespread, affecting both the hands and the feet.

Finally, a rare cause of Raynaud's phenomenon is an overdose or the accidental ingestion of a drug called *ergotamine*. This drug is used occasionally to treat MIGRAINE and its dose must be very carefully controlled.

Symptoms

In a patient with Raynaud's disease, usually the fingers of both hands are affected, although sometimes only two or three are involved. The usual pattern of events is that the sufferer experiences attacks when going out of doors on a cold day, or attacks may occur after putting the hands in cold water. First, the affected fingers become almost completely white and cold, and they also become quite painful. Usually there is a sharp line at the bottom of the fingers between the area of skin affected and the normal skin on the palms and the back of the hand. After a variable time – perhaps half an hour or more – the fingers start to go a dark blue colour, before turning purple and dark red and then eventually returning to normal.

If the person has Raynaud's phenomenon associated with a problem of the nerves running to the fingers, the affected area only is involved. Similarly if there is disease caused by atheroma in the larger blood vessels, only the limbs affected develop the symptoms of Raynaud's phenomenon. The symptoms or ergot poisoning tend to be widespread.

Investigation

If a young woman with typical symptoms of the symmetrical attacks of Raynaud's disease attends her doctor, it is very unlikely that the doctor will carry out any special tests beyond perhaps a simple routine blood test. But if there are unusual factors, then the doctor may want to carry out extensive investigation. The reason for this is that the patient may be suffering from Raynaud's phenomenon. The symptoms could then be the first sign of some more serious underlying disease. For example, if a middle-aged man suddenly starts developing the signs of Raynaud's phenomenon in one hand, it is quite likely that there may be an underlying nerve disorder or a disorder of the circulation to the hand. Investigations may therefore include special blood tests to detect underlying protein disorders in the blood, X-rays of bones or joints and sometimes a special X-ray called an *angiogram*.

Treatment

The most obvious and important thing for a sufferer of Raynaud's disease to do is to avoid the cold. If it is unavoidable to go out in cold weather, then one or even two pairs of really warm gloves are essential. You can also now obtain special gloves that are heated.

If the attacks are repeated, severe and painful, a doctor may prescribe vasodilator drugs such as *nifedipine*. The drugs may have to be taken regularly to be effective. If drug treatment fails, a last resort is an operation called *sympathectomy*. This blocks the nerve impulses to the fingers that cause the blood vessels to constrict.

If the problem is Raynaud's phenomenon, the most important aspect of treatment is that of the underlying condition. Vibration 'white finger' will be helped by avoiding the use of vibrating tools. Most of the other causes of Raynaud's phenomenon respond to specific therapy for the underlying problem, but vasodilator treatment may be needed as well.

Rectum

There is much confusion among lay people about the difference between the rectum and the anus. The anus is only the short narrow tube surrounded by a ring of muscle which joins the rectum, the lowermost part of the large intestines, to the outside. The main function of the anus is to maintain continence of FAECES (stools) while the rectum acts as a reservoir for them. With the normally functioning anus and rectum, a person can evacuate his or her bowels when it is socially convenient and not just when faeces happen to have passed through the whole of the large bowel.

The rectum itself, like the rest of the bowel, consists of a muscular tube lined with a special membrane which is known as *epithelium*. In the rectum, this epithelium contains glands which produce mucus to lubricate the faeces and make their passage easier. The muscular part of the rectum contracts during defecation to expel the faeces, but at other times, is capable of stretching. It is this potential for increasing in size which enables the rectum to act as a reservoir.

What can go wrong?

There are several conditions which affect the rectum, including PROCTALGIA (pain) and PROCTITIS (inflammation), PROLAPSE and POLYPS. By far the most serious disease which can occur in this part of the body is that of cancer (*carcinoma*) of the rectum.

This is a malignant tumour which arises from the epithelium. A patient with a carcinoma of the rectum is usually middle-aged or elderly, although on rare occasions, the disease can occur in early adulthood. It shows itself in several different ways. First, there may be bleeding, the blood normally being bright red and mixed in with the bowel motion. Second, there can be an excess of mucus during defecation, probably caused by an irritation of the lining of the rectum. Third, the patient experiences a sensation of wanting to defecate, because there is a tumour in the rectum; however, there is no resulting bowel action. This means that the patient finds he or she is constantly going to the toilet, with no result. These symptoms are described by the medical term *tenesmus*. Finally, the tumour may have spread to other parts of the body, without very much in the way of symptoms in the rectum itself.

There seems to be a link between cancer of the rectum and hereditary factors. In addition, if there is a history of polyps in the rectum, this can sometimes be a strong factor in the subsequent development of a cancer.

The doctor will first examine the rectum to make the diagnosis. Some growths can be felt easily with a gloved finger, but others can only be diagnosed by passing a metal tube into the rectum and inflating it with air. This examination, called a *sigmoidoscopy*, is painless, and means that the doctor can see the growth, and perhaps take a tiny piece with forceps so that it can be examined closely (BIOPSY).

The only successful treatment for a carcinoma of the rectum is surgery. The type of surgery involved depends on the situation of the growth in the rectum. Basically, if the growth is in the upper part, then it can be removed and the bowel ends joined together. However, if it is at the lower end, near the anal canal, then the lower rectum and anal canal have to be removed. This means that the patient has to have a permanent COLOSTOMY, or opening of the bowel on the front of the abdomen (*see* STOMA CARE).

One of the newer developments in the field of surgery for carcinoma of the rectum is the use of a special stapling device, known as a stapling 'gun', to join the two ends of bowel together. Using this, much lower joins can be made and thus some patients who would have had to have a colostomy are spared one.

Some patients have a temporary colostomy further up the large bowel, for a few weeks after the operation to remove the tumour. This acts as a safety valve until the join between the colon and the rectum has healed up properly.

Reflexes

A reflex is an automatic response to a specific stimulus which is not under conscious control. For a reflex to occur there must be: a sense receptor; nerves to convey the report of the stimulus (*see* NERVOUS SYSTEM); an apparatus to convert this information into a response; and, finally, MUSCLES or GLANDS to provide the response – usually some type of movement. Any response which follows this pattern of automatic reaction to a stimulus is called a reflex

Conscious behaviour is not reflex because, between the stimulus and the response, an analysis takes place – we relate the stimulus to our previous experience, mood, present desires and so on. This means that the same stimulus may produce different responses each time it is encountered; a reflex response, on the other hand, is the same whenever the stimulus is presented. A conscious reaction can overcome some reflexes – for example, if we are foolish enough we *can* keep our hand on the hot stove, but we would have to apply conscious effort to do so. Reflexes thus provide the body with protective, quick responses, especially to harmful stimuli. Some reflex movements, such as BREATHING, are so important that while they can be stopped by conscious effort for some time, they eventually break through that control.

Different types of reflexes

There are numerous different types of reflex: some control our muscle movements, our basic bodily functions, and our correct orientation while standing or sitting. Other, more complex, reflexes are programmed responses to dangerous or frightening situations.

Muscle reflexes: These are more accurately called 'tendon reflexes' since it is vibration in the tendons which sparks them off. When the doctor 'tests your reflexes' by striking your knee with his or her tendon hammer, the vibration is noticed by tiny receivers in the muscles which send messages to the SPINAL CORD and fire the nerve cells there controlling the muscles which make your leg jerk. These reflexes are part of a very complex set of machinery in the spinal cord which controls the tone of our muscles – that is, their readiness for action.

The spinal cord machinery is in turn controlled by the more 'senior' parts of the movement control hierarchy in the BRAIN. So the spinal reflexes can be brisker or more sluggish according to the 'setting' imposed on them from above. The same spinal cord machinery is tied into PAIN receptors in the skin and elsewhere so that swift reflex responses can be made when harmful stimuli are received.

Orientation reflexes: If a cat falls from a few feet above the ground, the animal will always land perfectly on its feet (and come to no harm!). This is an example of the speed with which the reflexes controlling our posture and orientation can work. Similarly, if you slip on an icy pavement, your body twists to right itself and your hand often shoots out to stop your fall.

These more complex responses are programmed by more advanced parts of our motor system. Sensitive receivers in a special part of the EARS monitor our position in space (*see* BALANCE). When we start to fall, messages from these receivers are quickly relayed to the cerebellum at the base of the brain which selects the correct series of commands to the muscles of our arms and legs. All this occurs in a far shorter time than if we had consciously to sort out the right set of movements. Primitive examples of this type of orientation reflex are seen in small babies. For example, if the baby's head is suddenly released, he or she will outstretch the arms in a sort of grasping movement. This is called the *Moro reflex* (after the doctor who first described it): it disappears after some weeks if development is normal.

Bodily function reflex: Children still in nappies have no conscious control over the passage of urine from their BLADDERS. When the bladder is full the pressure inside signals the spinal cord to put into effect a reflex to empty it. As a child develops, he becomes able to suppress this reflex until the appropriate opportunity to pass urine arises. However, even fully mature adults cannot suppress the reflex indefinitely: a point will be reached when the bladder empties by reflex 'on its own' (actually with the spinal cord's help).

Similar reflexes control many basic bodily functions, including breathing. Some – like bladder control and, to a lesser extent, breathing – can be consciously controlled; others like the control of our heartbeat (*see* PULSE), are purely automatic.

Behavioural reflexes: These are the most sophisticated reflexes in the body and are used to prepare its behaviour responses in a standardized way when faced with extreme situations. The best example is the so-called 'fight-or-flight' reaction (*see* ADRENAL GLANDS) – a pattern of reflex responses which are produced in answer to a threatening situation. When we are suddenly confronted with a mugger, for example, we will either fight or run away; similarly, an animal faced with an aggressor has these two choices. The needs of the body are similar whether our brain decides to run or to stand and fight. Accordingly, this complex of reflexes produces automatically the optimum conditions of heartbeat, breathing and so on which will then be available for whichever course of action is chosen.

The same set of responses includes sweating (allowing heat loss during the fight or the flight) and paleness of the skin (pale because blood is pumped away from the skin to the more important muscles). This same reflex can be induced by the mere *thought* of any frightening or threatening situation, when it becomes part of a so-called *conditioned response* (*see also* STRESS).

Conditioned reflexes: A reflex is called conditioned when it is brought on by a stimulus different from that which first (or naturally) produced it, and becomes 'attached' to that different stimulus. This happens when the second stimulus occurs repeatedly with the normal stimulus.

The famous Russian psychologist Pavlov first described this type of reflex when he noticed that, if he rang a bell each time he gave a dog some food, after a time he could produce the response of salivation in the dog by ringing the bell alone – initially, only the food would prompt this reflex response.

If reflexes are lost

The reflexes vary in their relative importance in everyday life. Losing a 'knee jerk' by itself does not make much difference, although the underlying reason for the loss may be causing some other symptoms. However, other reflexes are more vital, such as the orientation reflex. These may be lost in some diseases of the cerebellum, and the person concerned will have considerable trouble maintaining balance unless he or she concentrates. Similarly, if the blink reflex is lost, the eye can become seriously damaged by particles which land on it and are not swept away by the blink.

People who lose the automatic reflex to breathe get into serious trouble at night when the voluntary breathing system will no longer be working. Rarely, children may be born without the proper breathing reflex – a condition dramatically called 'Ondine's curse' – which means that they can breathe only when conscious, and need a ventilator at night when asleep. People who have lost such important reflexes must be protected by special treatment until the cause of the lost reflex can be put right.

See also HEAD AND HEAD INJURIES.

Reiter's disease

The symptoms of Reiter's disease always appear after a previous infection. Usually the infection is a SEXUALLY TRANSMITTED DISEASE such as NSU (NON-SPECIFIC URETHRITIS) or GONORRHOEA. Three different micro-organisms can be responsible for NSU – CHLAMYDIA, mycoplasmas and ureaplasmas. However, sometimes Reiter's disease can follow an attack of dysentery caused by germs such as SALMONELLA or *Shigella*, both of which are frequent causes of severe diarrhoeal illnesses. These germs can be transmitted by contaminated food or in water supplies.

But only a small proportion of people who suffer from NSU, gonorrhoea or dysentery ever develop Reiter's disease. Men are much more likely to have it – the ratio in Britain is 13 male cases to 1 female case. Young adult men between 16 and 35 years of age also appear to be the most susceptible. However, Reiter's disease can occur at virtually any time of life – even young babies can develop Reiter's disease after an attack of dysentery.

It has been found over the years that there is an inherited tendency to develop this disorder. Recently this tendency has been linked to certain 'tissue types'. So it seems that people who possess a particular GENETIC makeup (described as HLA-B27 tissue type) are in some way more likely genetically to react to certain types of infection by subsequently contracting Reiter's disease.

Symptoms

The frequency with which Reiter's disease occurs is very low. After an attack of dysentery, the risk of developing it is only about one in 500. There is a higher risk after an attack of NSU – about one in 50. In Britain, the United States, Australia and New Zealand, most cases of Reiter's disease occur after sexually transmitted infections, but in Africa and many parts of Asia, dysentery is the more common cause.

The first symptom to occur in a man is usually a slight discharge from the URETHRA at the tip of the PENIS. Women may have some internal inflammation affecting the CERVIX at the top of the VAGINA. But often this goes unnoticed. These symptoms are called *urethritis* or *cervicitis*, and while they are almost always present after sexually acquired infection, they do also occur when Reiter's disease follows an attack of dysentery, although not in every case.

After a few days the urethritis may worsen and then the second major symptom occurs – ARTHRITIS. Often the onset of arthritis is quite sudden and disabling. One or more joints can become hot, swollen and intensely painful. The knee and ankle joints can be involved – but usually one at a time – and, less frequently, the wrists or elbows.

The third major symptom is inflammation of the front of the EYE – CONJUNCTIVITIS. The whites of the eye becomes inflamed, reddened and painful. Sometimes a more serious inflammation called *anterior uveitis* can occur, in which deeper tissues in the front of the eye become inflamed. This can lead later to scarring of the iris or cornea if it is left untreated.

Apart from the three major symptoms – urethritis, arthritis and conjunctivitis – a number of other distressing symptoms may also appear. About one patient in five with the condition develops a skin RASH called *keratoderma blenorrhagica*. This rash is rather like PSORIASIS, a thickened fissured area of skin which can occur on the soles of the feet, or on the limbs and trunk. A painless rash may also occur on the genitalia – in men, particularly noticeable on the penis.

The TENDONS and ligaments in the feet may become affected. The Achilles tendon at the back of the foot or the connective tissue in the sole of the foot can become inflamed and tender. About one patient in five is affected.

The initial attack of Reiter's disease can last several weeks or even months, but the symptoms tend to clear up. But then further attacks can occur at intervals over many years. Each attack may start with urethritis, just like the first, but in some cases recurrent arthritis or conjunctivitis may be the only sign of the return of the disease. Some patients with recurring Reiter's disease (about one in ten) develop inflammation of the sacro-iliac joints, which are located at the bottom of the spine where the spine joins the pelvis (*see* SPONDYLITIS). Fifty per cent of sufferers will go on to develop arthritis or ankylosing spondylitis in later life.

Treatment

Initially doctors may have some difficulty diagnosing a case of Reiter's disease. The symptoms are variable, and occasionally the disorder displays only two out of three classic symptoms. An added problem is that there is no specific test for the disease. Diagnosis depends entirely on recognition of the typical pattern of symptoms after an attack of NSU, gonorrhoea or dysentery. Blood tests show certain non-specific changes – for example, a rise in the number of white blood cells in the blood. If the doctor checks the patient's tissue type and finds HLA-B27 is present, the diagnosis is more likely.

Once a diagnosis has been made, a course of tetracycline or similar ANTIBIOTIC will probably be prescribed. Because it is known that the disease is an abnormal reaction to an infection, it makes sense to get rid of any lingering infection which may be present. Indeed some doctors believe that many cases of Reiter's disease are caused by persistent infection in the tissues as a result of poor immune response to the original infection.

Next, treatment will depend on the extent and nature of the symptoms. If arthritis is present, anti-inflammatory drugs may be prescribed. For conjunctivitis or anterior uveitis, soothing eyedrops or steroid medication can be given.

Rejection of tissue

TRANSPLANT surgery is one of the great success stories of modern medicine. What seemed unthinkable a few years ago is now being regularly achieved. KIDNEY transplants are a basic part of the treatment of a long-term kidney failure, while transplantation of HEARTS, LUNGS, LIVER and BONE MARROW has developed rapidly. But the problem of tissue rejection – the IMMUNE SYSTEM rejecting 'foreign' tissue – still remains the major hurdle in any transplant procedure.

What is rejection?

If you graft a piece of skin from one mouse on to the skin of another mouse, it will appear to settle into its new home for a day or two with few problems. As time goes on, though, the situation will deteriorate. The blood vessels that have grown at the base of the graft will stop growing, and between the third and ninth day, microscopic examination of the new skin will show that the cells of inflammation – the body's storm troops in the fight against foreign invaders – have moved in. Once this has happened, the graft begins to die, and it is sloughed off by about the tenth day. Moreover, if you tried to repeat the experiment on the same mouse, the result would be the same – but reaction would be even quicker than before. This is what rejection is, and it is exactly what would happen in a kidney transplant, for example, if precautions were not taken to reduce the extent of the possible rejection, and if treatment to damp down the rejection were not available.

How does rejection occur?

Rejection results from activity of the body's immune system. The immune system helps to fight infection by 'recognizing' something that is not a normal body constituent and then turning its activity against the invader. This means that the system has to be able to recognize what is a normal constituent, and this ability to differentiate between 'self' and 'non-self' is actually its most basic characteristic.

The immune system consists of an interconnected collection of cells and small organs. It includes the LYMPHATIC SYSTEM, the BLOOD-borne lymphocytes and related cells in the tissues, the SPLEEN, the BONE MARROW and the THYMUS gland in the neck.

The lymphocytes – particularly the T-lymphocytes, which are dependent on the thymus gland – are the immune cells that actually carry out the work of rejection. This has been proved by experiments which show that an animal which has had its thymus removed at birth is not able to reject a graft in the usual way. These experiments have been extended: a mouse with its thymus removed at birth can actually be made to reject a graft in the usual way if it is given a transfusion of lymphocytes from another mouse that has normal thymus function. In most cases, it is this *T-lymphocyte response* – called *cellular immunity* – that is responsible for rejection.

Some organs, such as the cornea in the eye, can be transplanted without any problems with rejection. This is because the corneas (the clear cover at the front of the eye) do not have any blood vessels running through them. This, in turn, means that the cells which control the body's immune system cannot come into contact with the newly transplanted part – and so there is no chance of rejection taking place.

Pig heart valves are about the only sort of non-human tissue that can commonly be transplanted. The valve is made up of fibrous tissue, and it is prepared very carefully before it is inserted into a human heart. (The preparation is rather akin to tanning leather.) Since they contain no living cells, and have no direct blood supply, these valves are not accessible to the body's immune system in the same way as a transplanted human organ would be. Thus, they do not carry a risk of infection. Pig valves are actually one of the most successful types of replacement valve.

Symptoms of rejection

The most commonly transplanted organ is the kidney. Many recipients of kidneys have one or more minor episodes of rejection, although sometimes the process is more severe. Basically there are three things that can happen. First, there may be a very brisk response to the transplant, occurring within minutes of the graft taking place. This is called *hyperacute rejection* and is unlike other sorts of rejection in that it seems to depend on antibodies rather than on any cellular immunity. It is normally possible to detect these antibodies in the blood and to avoid this kind of problem..

Second, and most common, is an *acute rejection episode*. Transplant patients are given drugs designed to suppress these episodes, and usually an increase in the dosage of these drugs will control them. The clues that an episode is happening vary: patients often feel feverish and experience pain, and this may be accompanied by a deterioration in the function of the transplanted kidney, so that blood and protein appear in the urine and the level of waste products in the blood rises.

Finally, there may be a slow and steady deterioration in the function of the transplanted kidney, giving rise to what is known as *chronic rejection*. This tends to be more difficult to treat than episodes of acute rejection.

One of the most extraordinary aspects of rejection occurs not in the transplantation of kidneys, but in bone marrow transplants. This astonishing operation has been developed to treat people whose bone marrow is not working or is diseased. In these cases, the body no longer produces normal blood cells, which are, of course, essential for life. Bone marrow is taken from a donor – nearly always a close relative – and simply injected into a vein. This marrow settles in the bone and liver of the recipient and will start to work normally if all goes well. In fact, what sometimes happens in this situation is that the patient has his immune system destroyed (since, without bone marrow, lymphocytes, the basic immune cell, cannot be produced) and then has someone else's immune system put in! Since all the lymphocytes that are produced from the new marrow are foreign and will not recognize their new body as 'self', they may start to attack the body in which they find themselves.

This is called the *graft versus host reaction*, and may feature rashes, intestinal upsets and kidney trouble.

Preventing rejection

Recently great strides have been made in 'grouping' tissues in much the same way as BLOOD GROUPS are classified, and this has made dealing with rejection much easier. When you talk about a blood group, in fact what you are saying is that the blood cells carry a kind of marker, called an antigen, on their surfaces. This antigen will react with antibodies from the blood of another person who has a different blood group. Thus if, for example, you are blood group A, you will have the 'A' antigen on the surfaces of your blood cells.

In tissue grouping, or typing, there is a similar but much more complicated system of cell-surface antigens called the HLA system. In the normal blood group classification, there are only four possible groups: A, B, AB and O. In the HLS system, however, there are four main classes of antigen – A, B, C and D – and literally thousands of subsidiary combinations, governed principally by heredity. Thus typing a tissue group is extremely complex.

Most kidney transplant surgeons will try to get a reasonable match between donor and recipient, although it is not essential that the match be exact. In difficult situations – transplanting bone marrow, for example – it is much better to get a reasonable match with tissue from a member of the immediate family rather than an exact match with tissue from someone unrelated.

The treatment of rejection

The basis of the treatment of rejection is to use drugs which damp down the whole immune system. There are basically three drugs that are widely used today. The first is prednisolone, a STEROID drug closely related to cortisone; the second is azathioprine, which is a drug that reduces cell division and therefore reduces the production of lymphocytes. The third and newest is cyclosporin, which is a very powerful immunosuppressant. It is derived from a fungus and its most exciting quality is that it seems to act on one specific part of the immune system – unlike the other drugs, which damp down the whole system. By giving this drug at the right time, it is possible to suppress hostile recognition of the transplant by the lymphocytes of the immune system – meaning, in effect, that reaction is suppressed without depressing immunity to any invading infection.

ATG and OKT3 are newer immunosuppressant drugs, which are now being used successfully.

Obviously, when the activity of the immune system is inhibited, resistance to infection is reduced, and this can be one of the main problems for patients who have transplants. A patient who has received a bone marrow transplant will have no immune system at all until the grafted marrow is functioning normally, and this means that the patient must have the strictest possible protection against infection, living isolated from the outside world.

Relaxation

If you are physically and mentally overwrought, your body may react by becoming a mass of aches and pains. Knowing how to relax your muscles gives you an improved sense of well-being.

Benefits of relaxation

General problems arising from tension include those which affect personal relationships. Irritability, nagging and outbursts of temper increase when a person is under pressure. Also, STRESS is self-perpetuating – that is, if you are taking your feelings of tension out on your husband, wife or children, they will take it out on each other. If you can decrease your tension by being more relaxed, your marriage and family will benefit.

Because a tense person tends to be a clumsy person, cutting down muscle tension improves performance in activities which require coordination. Relaxation also maximizes the effect of EXERCISE; if you relax totally after a jogging or swimming session, for example, you will become fitter much more quickly.

Another bonus from being properly relaxed is an increase in the tolerance of PAIN which is linked with an ability to recover more quickly from illness.

How to relax

As well as developing a sensible approach to your life, and trying to cut back on your commitments if you are already doing too much, it is also sensible to learn some simple techniques of relaxation for those times when you feel uptight. One of the most important lessons to learn is that periods of intense activity must always be balanced by relaxation. But there are also techniques for ensuring that you do not become too tense in the first place – in other words, by adapting a more relaxed approach to whatever you are doing.

Posture

A correct, well-balanced posture is of vital importance in everyday life. Tension in the muscles of the body shows itself in an unbalanced, tense posture. Some people hold themselves very rigidly – like a soldier on parade – and then wonder why they get backache. The position of the head is particularly important. Your head is heavy – it weighs around 14 lb (6 kg). If you constantly hold your head to one side or drop your head forwards, the muscles become tense and you start to have tension headaches. You should always try to 'balance' your head so that it is neither falling to one side or the other, nor flopping forward or jutting out.

Many people gain considerable benefit from learning the *Alexander technique*. This is a method of training which helps to improve bodily posture and which is claimed to have an overall calming affect on the body. The method not only helps to provide a relaxed approach to life but can also help to relieve many of the symptoms of stress-related disorders.

In everyday life, it is important to remember that the way you sit or stand

and the postures you adopt at work can all contribute to tension. You should try to ensure that your chair is comfortable and well-supporting. A very low easy chair that provides insufficient support can actually contribute to muscular tension simply because it forces the body into unnatural postures and sets up abnormal muscular activity in an attempt by the body to keep the bones and joints in alignment. Good, 'ergonomic' design reduces tension by ensuring that the worker adopts good postures.

Breathing and meditation

Many different methods of relaxation rely on careful control of BREATHING to restore calmness to the body and mind. Certain types of yoga teach breathing techniques, and MEDITATION can begin with a focus on calm, regular breathing.

You can try a simple breathing exercise yourself. Settle in a comfortable, but fairly upright, chair and place your feet squarely on the floor, with your arms relaxed by your sides. Gently close your eyes. Then concentrate on the sensation of the air flowing in and out of your nose. Feel the air passing over a spot in the middle of your nose, just inside the nostrils. Then imagine a clock face with a single big hand. The hand sweeps around the clock from the top to the bottom as you breathe in and then goes back to the top again as you breathe out. The clock hand moves all the time, regularly in time with your breathing, round and round. Keep this up for ten minutes or so. Practising a couple of times a day will help to calm you down. Try this technique in your lunch break at work or in your tea-break if you are having a heavy day.

If you want to learn a more sophisticated approach to breathing exercises, you could enrol in a yoga class. In most areas, transcendental meditation is taught by qualified teachers. Once the technique has been learned, it can be incorporated into your daily routine.

Muscular relaxation

If your muscles are tense, you will feel tense. But there is a vicious circle at work here because if you feel stressed, your muscles tense up too. To break the circle, you have to learn to relax your muscles. Some people find that active participation in a sport or physical exercise such as a game of squash, jogging or swimming leads to complete relaxation afterwards. This works for many people – provided the participation is not too competitive. A driving ambition to win or out-perform an opponent can of itself cause excess tension.

There are, however, a number of straightforward techniques to aid muscular relaxation. You can practise simple muscular relaxation for yourself at home sitting in a chair or lying on the floor. Concentrate on each muscle group in turn working from the head downwards to the arms, the trunk and the legs. A technique called *progressive relaxation* relies on the fact that when one muscle group contracts the opposite muscle group (which moves the limb in the opposite direction) relaxes. Contraction of each muscle group in turn is followed by deep relaxation. This technique is not difficult to learn. At health shops, you can buy audio cassette tapes that give simple directions for this type of relaxation. The tape can be played while you relax lying on the floor, or sitting in a chair.

Autogenic training is another method in which you train yourself to give directions to your muscles, in turn, to gently relax.

Massage

One of the best and most effective techniques for relaxation is MASSAGE. Gentle massage has a considerable power to ease mental and emotional tension, whereas deep massage works at the muscles themselves. Local massage can relieve specific aches and pains. For example, a tension headache can be eased by massage of the muscles at the back of the neck. Usually massage is given by one person to another; learning massage provides you with a wonderful gift you can give to your partner, family and friends. But you can also learn to massage yourself to ease away tension, aches and pains. *See also* AROMATHERAPY.

Relaxation in everyday life

Once you understand the importance of relaxation to keep tension under control, you can help yourself by incorporating a few relaxation exercises into your everyday life. If you feel yourself stiffening up, do a few simple exercises, bending and stretching. Travelling in a bus, car, train, or plane often forces you into cramped, unnatural postures. A few exercises at half-hourly intervals will help. Stretch your legs and arms, move your feet up and down and roll your head from side to side. If you are driving, stop for a few minutes every hour or so for a stretch and a brief walk.

Renal disease, *see* Kidneys and kidney diseases

Renin, *see* Blood pressure

Repetitive strain injury

This is a syndrome that came to light in the 1980s and first affected office workers who spent long periods of time using a keyboard. It produces symptoms of pain in the affected joints which is difficult to relieve and is aggravated by movement of the joint. It can also affect a variety of workers in other jobs. The treatment is with rest and painkillers. Some doctors have doubted the existence of repetitive strain injury because there is no test than can be performed to diagnose it and there are no specific X-ray changes.

There has been considerable recent controversy in legal cases where sufferers have failed to convince the judge and jury of RSI's existence and so have failed to gain compensation.

Respiration, respiratory system, *see* Breathing, Lungs and lung diseases

Retinitis pigmentosa, *see* Blindness

 Retinopathy, hypertensive, *see* Blood pressure

Rhesus factor

There are two main BLOOD GROUP systems: one is the ABO system; the other is the Rhesus factor (Rh in medical shorthand). In certain circumstances, incompatibility of two Rhesus factors between a mother and her baby can cause a disease which breaks down the red cells in the bloodstream of the foetus or newborn baby. Left untreated, it can be fatal.

The Rh factor

The Rhesus system of blood groupings is based on the presence or absence in the BLOOD of several different biochemical molecules, or factors. Of these factors, the most important to the Rh system is one always designated as 'D' when it is present and 'd' when it is absent. We all inherit a pair of Rhesus genes: one from our mother, the other from our father. As a result, a person can be DD (both parents Rh positive); Dd (one parent Rh positive, the other Rh negative); or dd (both parents with an Rh-negative gene). Because D is dominant over d, which is carried on a recessive gene, a person who is Dd will have the D factor in his blood, and so be Rh positive. Only dd individuals make no D factor at all, and they are known as Rh negative in this grouping.

The basis of incompatibility

The Rhesus factor causes problems when, for some reason, Rh-positive blood gets into the bloodstream of an Rh-negative person. The body then reacts as if it has been invaded by a disease-causing organism and begins to make antibodies ready to attack and eliminate that organism. On the first occasion that the blood types mix, only the antibody-manufacturing equipment is made. In this situation, the Rh-negative blood is said to have become 'sensitized' to the presence of Rh-positive blood.

If this sensitized blood subsequently becomes mixed with Rh-positive blood again, even 20 to 30 years later, then the antibody-making machinery goes into action immediately to make anti-D antibodies. The antibodies multiply and begin to attack the red cells of the Rh-positive blood, breaking them down into chemical fragments, making the blood unable to do its job of carrying oxygen round the circulation.

Pregnancy and problems

The likelihood of Rhesus incompatibility in PREGNANCY only arises if the ovum of an Rh-negative woman is fertilized by a sperm from an Rh-positive man. If the developing foetus has Rh-negative blood (which it may do if the father is Dd, and the baby inherits his d rather than his D gene), then there is no problem. But if the foetus is Rh positive, which is more likely because of the greater frequency of the D gene in the population, then trouble is likely, although it does not happen immediately.

When an Rh-negative mother is carrying an Rh-positive foetus, occasionally blood cells manage to escape from the foetal circulation, cross the placenta and enter the mother's blood. This transfer can occur if a woman has a threatened MISCARRIAGE, a miscarriage or an abortion, but is most likely to take place during delivery.

The resulting sensitization in the mother's blood does not affect the first baby, but subsequent Rh-positive babies are definitely in danger. In response to the presence of Rh-positive blood cells from the foetus, the sensitized mother's body begins making vast quantities of antibodies which are small enough to cross the placental barrier. Once inside the baby's bloodstream, they begin the process of breaking down the red cells in its Rh-positive blood.

If left untreated, this situation will damage the foetus. In the most severe cases, the foetus dies in the womb, usually because of extremely severe ANAEMIA and heart failure. This condition is known as *hydrops foetalis*. Alternatively, the baby may be born alive but with a weak heart or with severe JAUNDICE. The yellow colour of the baby's complexion is caused by the release of yellow BILE pigments (bilirubin) from the destroyed red blood cells. This jaundice places the baby at risk because of the toxicity of the bile pigments.

Prevention of Rhesus disease

Luckily Rhesus disease is now extremely uncommon because a reliable technique has been developed for stopping the production of antibodies by the mother. It depends on an injection of anti-D antibodies, which can destroy any Rh-positive blood cells from the baby before the mother becomes sensitized. So any Rh-negative woman who gives birth to an Rh-positive baby is given the injection soon after the delivery, destroying any cells from the baby that have remained in the mother's bloodstream and so safeguarding future pregnancies. The same injection must also be given to an Rh-negative woman who suffers a threatened miscarriage, an actual miscarriage or has a termination of pregnancy.

In the rare instances where a baby affected by Rhesus disease is born, the baby can be treated by 'exchange transfusion', which replaces the red cells destroyed by the mother's anti-Rhesus antibodies and removes the offending antibodies from the baby's blood. It entails taking a small volume of the baby's blood and replacing it with an equal volume of fresh donor blood. The procedure is repeated until the total volume of the newborn child's blood has been exchanged.

Rheumatic fever

This used to be a common disease in Great Britain, but nowadays it has become quite rare. It is caused by an infection and usually follows a sore throat. Rheumatic fever affects different systems of the body, with the result that it has different effects on those who have suffered from the disease.

Although it almost invariably occurs in children and adolescents, the damage it causes to the heart may persist, leading to long-term heart trouble. Indeed cardiac surgeons are still performing operations to repair heart valves that were damaged years ago by the disease.

Causes

Rheumatic fever is caused by a *streptococcus* bacterium belonging to a strain known as Lancefield Group A. Only a small proportion of the population are at risk of getting the disease even if they develop a sore throat due to this type of bacterium. Unfortunately there is no way of knowing who is susceptible.

Why the disease should follow on from a streptococcal sore throat is unknown. The bacterium itself does not play any part in the direct causation of the various problems associated with rheumatic fever. The body's IMMUNE SYSTEM is almost certainly involved, as there is a reaction between normal tissue and the immune system at the basis of the rheumatic problems. This immune activity is probably triggered off by the streptococcal infection in susceptible people, who can be shown to develop higher levels of antibodies to the organism than would normally be expected.

Symptoms

Rheumatic fever produces a variety of different symptoms. It is characterized by a generalized feeling of illness, with fever and tiredness, paleness, loss of appetite and loss of weight.

Rheumatic fever causes an inflammation of the joints (similar to that of RHEUMATOID ARTHRITIS, hence the name). The disease mainly affects the larger joints of the hips and knees and has the curious tendency to spread from one joint to another – so-called 'flitting arthritis'.

The disease also affects the skin, producing a typical RASH consisting of a red line enclosing palish areas (*erythema marginatum*). Additionally, nodules can be felt under the skin over bony protrusions such as the wrists, knees, elbows and ankles.

Most importantly – and more worrying – rheumatic fever affects the HEART. There is inflammation of the fibrous lining of the heart and the heart muscle, which may lead to heart failure. The inner lining of the heart, or *endocardium*, may be affected: this is potentially serious for it can lead to abnormalities of the heart VALVES.

Finally, the disease affects the nervous system, causing *chorea* or *St Vitus's dance*. This is characterized by odd writhing movements of the trunk and the limbs, and facial grimacing. The movements are made worse by excitement and disappear when the child is asleep. It is commoner in girls.

Dangers

The main danger is that the child will have repeated attacks of the disease, and this can lead to the development of problems with the heart valves. In the past, it was this that led to people becoming 'cardiac cripples', often at a very young age. Although disease due to the furring up of the heart's arteries is now the commonest heart problem, this was not always the case; rheumatic heart disease once held this distinction. There are many people still alive with long-term heart troubles from rheumatic fever, but new cases in the Western world are rare. However, it is still a significant problem in developing countries.

Treatment and outlook

Once the diagnosis has been made, the mainstay of treatment consists of bedrest together with regular large doses of aspirin. Where heart failure has occurred, children are often given STEROID drugs instead of aspirin to cut down the inflammation of the heart. Generally, it takes about six weeks to recover.

Once the child is well, it is important to prevent further attacks, since every bout can cause additional injury to the heart. For this reason an ANTIBIOTIC, usually penicillin, is given until the age of 18.

Rheumatism

This is a vague term used to describe aches and pains in JOINTS and their surrounding structures such as MUSCLES, TENDONS and ligaments. It is not a specific condition in itself; it is more a collection of symptoms.

Rheumatoid arthritis

To most people, rheumatoid arthritis conjures up horrific pictures of patients in wheelchairs, crippled by their disease and, worst of all, living out the remainder of their lives racked by pain. This concept is now out of date, and while it is still true that people may be severely disabled by the disease, this is certainly not so in the vast majority of cases.

Early diagnosis, improved methods of treatment and rehabilitation where appropriate make the life of a patient with rheumatoid arthritis easier in every respect. By controlling the progression of the disease, relieving pain and preventing the development of deformities the patient is able to lead a normal or as near normal a life as possible.

What is rheumatoid arthritis?

Rheumatoid arthritis is a disease which mainly affects the JOINTS but may, in severe case, affect many other organs such as the HEART, LUNGS, NERVOUS SYSTEM and the EYES. It occurs in both men and women but is more common in women, generally occurring in a ratio of about three to one. The usual age of onset is from the middle to late 20s until late middle age. However, it may also occur outside this age range in both younger and more elderly people.

Rheumatoid arthritis is a chronic condition which is frequently punctuated by periods when, for no apparent reason, the symptoms become worse, lessen or disappear. The disease itself may even disappear completely, in which case it is sometimes referred to as 'burnt out' rheumatoid arthritis.

Rheumatoid arthritis in children

Rheumatoid arthritis can occur in children – a condition called *Still's disease* – but it is fortunately rare. Two main age groups are affected – between the ages of 2 and 3, and between 10 and 15. The inflammation starts gradually and, in about one third of cases, occurs in one joint only, commonly the knee. It can also affect the hands, wrists, feet and ankles.

This disease is slowly progressive, but burns itself out in late adolescence. The chances of a cure depend on the severity of the case, how early it is diagnosed and how quickly treatment is begun. It should be started early to prevent permanent stiffening and joint deformity.

Cause

Although the basic cause of rheumatoid arthritis has not been discovered, it is known that the disease occurs when the body's defence mechanisms (the IMMUNE SYSTEM) react to the presence of the initiating agent and try to eliminate it.

This immune response causes an accumulation of inflamed cells within the synovial membrane that lines the synovial joints. Enzymes that are released from the inflamed cells lead to the breakdown of bone and cartilage within the joint, causing characteristic symptoms. Unless treatment is given fairly promptly, the joint will eventually become deformed.

Two particularly interesting results of this inflammatory response are the production of the *rheumatoid factor* and the development of *rheumatoid nodules*. Rheumatoid factor is an antibody produced in large amounts in people with the disease; this doesn't occur in other forms of arthritis. By doing a blood test, the amount of rheumatoid factor in the blood can be measured, and this forms the basis for a simple test which can be performed to see if a patient has the disease.

Rheumatoid nodules are lumps which may occur over the elbows or on the backs of the hands and feet. They are composed of collections of inflamed cells similar to those seen within the joints and, if present, are a further aid to diagnosis.

Symptoms

Pain, swelling and stiffness of the affected joints are the main symptoms of rheumatoid arthritis. Characteristically the small joints of the hands and feet – for example, the knuckle joints and the balls of the feet – are affected first, but other joints may become involved, particularly the wrists, knees, ankles, elbows, shoulders and, eventually, the hip joints. The number of joints affected depends on the severity of the disease which may vary enormously from one individual to another.

A characteristic feature that distinguishes this form of arthritis from others is the symmetry of the disease: that is, if a joint on one side of the body is affected, the same joint on the other side is usually involved. This is called a *symmetrical polyarthritis* and is typical of rheumatoid arthritis, particularly when the disease occurs in a young to middle-aged woman.

Usually the stiffness that occurs in the joints is most pronounced first thing in the morning on rising, and it may last for varying lengths of time – from a few minutes to a few hours. This is often accompanied by a general feeling of malaise and tiredness which reflects the fact that the disease affects the whole body and is not confined to a particular area. Patients will experience difficulty in gripping things such as cups or eating utensils because of the stiffness in their hands. Dressing, particularly doing up buttons, may also become a problem, and in addition, patients begin to experience pain in the affected joints.

As well as joint symptoms, patients may complain of symptoms which relate to other organ systems, although this is unusual. One of the commonest of these involves the eyes. The most common complaints are of soreness and redness resulting from inflammation in the various parts of the eye.

Symptoms will characteristically fluctuate so that they are much worse at certain times without there being any obvious reason for this.

Dangers and complications

The complications and dangers of the disorder relate largely to the joints; through incorrect use and positioning during acute stages, deformity may develop leading to loss of use of the affected part. A patient may thus develop contractions of a joint resulting in limited movement and function. Alternatively the joint may become unstable owing to the destruction of the ligaments and this may result in its dislocation.

In addition to these specific joint complications, the involvement of other organs in the body may complicate the picture further. In particular, patients with rheumatoid arthritis are more liable to infections generally, especially chest infections and bacterial infections of the joints. Other complications relating to the loss of function may also arise, so that the patient has difficulty carrying out normal physical movements.

Treatment

The treatment of rheumatoid arthritis requires making a close assessment of the problems of each individual patient and planning an appropriate programme of treatment to meet his or her needs. The usual approach involves prescribing a PAINKILLING drug such as ASPIRIN, ibuprofen or a closely related compound that has the same or a similar effect. *See* ARTHRITIS for further details.

If the disease begins to take a relentlessly progressive course (usually shown on X-rays as increasing destruction of bone), it may well be necessary to begin 'second line' therapy. This usually involves using slightly more toxic drugs which have been shown to slow or halt the progress of the disease. STEROIDS may have to be used initially to damp down the inflammation. Then the second-line agents may be introduced. These include gold salts and penicillamine. The former is usually given as weekly, fortnightly or monthly injections; it can produce, as a mild side-effect, what is known as a 'gold rash'. Penicillamine is taken in tablet form. Both of these compounds seem to modify the disease and, in some individuals, may even stop it completely. However, they can have serious side-effects which involve the kidneys and the blood, and it is for this reason that most patients given these compounds have weekly blood and urine tests. In this way, abnormalities induced by the drugs can be detected early before any serious damage is done and the drugs can then be stopped.

Other second-line drugs include the anti-malarial chloroquine and suphasalazine. They may be less effective than gold or penicillamine but have slightly fewer side-effects.

When a joint becomes inflamed, fluid leaks out of the synovial membrane that lines the joint space and this collects in the joint cavity. The fluid is called an *effusion* and it is this that causes the joint to swell. If the joint is large and a larger effusion is present, it is often possible to remove the fluid with a needle and syringe. This can give the patient considerable relief from pain and stiffness in that joint.

Surgery can be useful as an addition to drug therapy. Occasionally, the inflamed joint lining (the synovial membrane) is removed, although the effect of this operation, called *synovectomy*, is not permanent and the problem will recur.

Joint deformities may be improved by operations such as repair of the TENDONS and ligaments around the involved joints. The most important type of surgery now done is replacement of the diseased joints by artificial joints, particularly the hips, knees and knuckle joints.

Both PHYSIOTHERAPY and OCCUPATIONAL THERAPY also play a major part in the treatment of rheumatoid arthritis. Exercise maintains muscle strength and joint movement and also helps to prevent joint deformities. In addition, patients may be trained by the therapists to perform everyday activities such as dressing, cooking and washing. The therapists will also provide aids where necessary. These enable patients to deal with many essential tasks much more easily.

Rheumatology, ***see*** **Arthritis, Joints, Osteoarthritis, Rheumatoid arthritis, Spondylitis**

Rhinitis

This is the medical term for inflammation of the tissues that line the inside of the NOSE. Although not a disease in itself, it is often unpleasant, can be caused by a number of complaints and is the central feature of both the common COLD and HAY FEVER.

Rhythm method, ***see*** **Contraception**

Rickets

This is a condition that occurs when an insufficient amount of CALCIUM is laid down in the BONE as it is growing. It results from a lack of VITAMIN D in children, and is a disease that is more common in northern countries since vitamin D is made by the SKIN in response to sunlight.

Vitamin D is responsible for facilitating the absorption of calcium from the diet, and ensuring that it is passed from the blood into the bone when more bone is laid down. Since children have growing bones, vitamin D deficiency has a greater effect on them than it does on adults, although exactly the same sort of deficiency can happen in adults, when it is known as *osteomalacia*.

At one time, rickets was commonplace in British cities because of the poor nutrition of children, and the fact that what little sunlight there was was cut off from the ground by a layer of fog and haze. Over the years, these situations were greatly improved and rickets became increasingly rare. Today, however, it has returned and has become a major problem among the children of Asian families in British cities. One study in Bradford found an indication of rickets in 45 per cent of the Asian children examined. The reason is that dark skin is less sensitive to light and needs a far higher concentration of sunlight in order to make vitamin D. This, combined with a lack of vitamin D in traditional Asian diets, has contributed to the incidence of rickets among Asian children and osteomalacia among their mothers. Health campaigns are now under way to ensure that Asian communities are aware of the need to supplement their diet with vitamin D.

Causes

The control of the level of calcium in the body is managed by both the PARATHYROID glands in the neck, and by vitamin D. In fact, it is wrong to think of vitamin D as an ordinary vitamin, as it can be made in the body by the skin as a result of the effects of sunlight, and it is also handled in a special way by both the LIVER and the KIDNEYS. These organs are responsible for making a series of changes to the D compound so that it can be switched into active and inactive forms according to the levels of calcium in the bloodstream.

As the level of vitamin D starts to fall, the level of calcium in the blood will fall also since it cannot be absorbed without this vitamin. The level of blood calcium cannot be allowed to fall too low. If it did, *tetany* (muscle spasms) would result. So, to prevent this happening, the parathyroid glands make sure that calcium is released from the bones and comes back into the bloodstream. The result of this, however, is to leave the bones weakened through lack of calcium.

Although both rickets and osteomalacia are usually caused by a straightforward deficiency of vitamin D, they can also result from disease elsewhere in the body – in the liver or kidneys, for example.

Symptoms

In addition to general weakening of muscles, rickets causes softening and deformity of the bones. Since the newly developing bone cannot be made strong with calcium, the latter is replaced by large amounts of the bone's background substance – osteoid. This osteoid is laid down in large amounts at the points where the bones are growing, so that the wrists, knees and ankles tend to grow bigger than normal. There may also be a chain of osteoid bumps, known as a 'rickety rosary'. These osteoid bumps are located at the front end of the ribs.

The bones of the skull tend to become soft. And as the disease progresses, the long bones such as the tibia in the lower part of the leg will start to become bent, leading to bow legs or knock knees. In more severe cases, the backbone and pelvis will be affected and may unfortunately even become deformed.

Treatment and prevention

Where the disease is already present, extra vitamin D must be given in the form of drops or tablets. In more complicated cases arising from disease elsewhere in the body, it may be necessary to give more advanced forms of vitamin D where the chemical change that is normally made on the substance by the kidneys has already been carried out.

Although treatment may well improve matters in rickets, there is a definite chance of permanent deformity – and for this reason, its prevention is essential. This can be done simply and effectively by taking the minute amount of vitamin D that is required. Young babies get all the vitamin D they need from breast milk or from the newer fortified feeds. In the winter months, however, they may benefit from supplementary doses of vitamin D drops. Children under five and women who are either pregnant or breastfeeding are often prescribed vitamin D supplements to make sure that they are not lacking in calcium. For the rest of us, however, a balanced diet containing sufficient milk, cheese and fish should be adequate, but if in doubt check with your doctor.

Large quantities of cod liver and other fish oils used to be given to prevent rickets, but it is now realized that this is not a good idea. Fish liver oils are certainly a good source of vitamin D and they will therefore prevent rickets – but be careful. High levels of vitamin D can be very dangerous as they lead to high levels of calcium in the blood.

Rigid spine disease, *see* **Spondylitis**

Ringing in the ears, *see* **Tinnitus**

Ringworm

This is a common SKIN disease whose name is somewhat misleading. This condition has nothing to do with worms and certainly does not always manifest itself in the shape of a ring. It is, in fact, caused by a contagious infection of the body with one of a variety of fungi (*see* FUNGAL INFECTIONS). The areas of the body most likely to be affected are the feet, nails, scalp, armpits, genital areas and groin. Ringworm is usually caught from other people, but it may be transmitted by contact with animals – dogs, cats or even cattle.

Areas of infection

Ringworm of the scalp is the condition that helped give the disease its name. This is because the fungus usually grows outwards in a ring, and as the inner area begins to heal up, the red, itchy area spreads in a circle of ever-increasing diameter. As this spreading takes place, the hairs in the centre snap off and leave a stubble overlying the scaly skin. As the skin heals in the centre of the ring, new hairs begin to grow, giving the scalp an even more mottled appearance. Ringworm of the scalp is usually due to an infection by the *Microsporum* fungus. It is particularly common in childhood and spreads rapidly through schools.

The fungus that usually infects the feet is called *Trichophyton* and causes the common condition known as ATHLETE'S FOOT.

The *Epidermophyton* fungus causes ringworm of the genital or groin areas, commonly known as 'dhobi itch' and medically as *Tinea cruris*. Like the other ringworm fungi, this one thrives in damp, warm conditions, which explains why infection is most common in people who wear tight-fitting underwear and trousers. Sometimes ringworm appears on the trunk, causing slowly growing red patches with a paler centre.

Treatment and prevention

The exact treatment of ringworm depends on the site of the infection and the infecting fungus. For athlete's foot there are various anti-fungal powders, creams and sprays available. Ringworm of the scalp is treated with the antibiotic *griseofluvin*, although mild cases may respond effectively to anti-fungal creams. With dhobi itch, in addition to using anti-fungal preparations, cleanliness, thorough drying after washing and wearing sensible clothes are essential. Most cases of ringworm respond to anti-fungal antibiotics in cream formulations, but careful attention to hygiene is also important.

Roughage, *see* **Carbohydrates, Constipation**

Rubella

Also called German measles, this is a common, mild VIRUS INFECTION which occurs mostly in children. Infection appears to be most likely in the spring or summer months and to run in four- to six-year cycles of minor epidemics.

The virus itself causes virtually no serious illness in an adult or child. Once the diagnosis is confirmed the illness can usually be forgotten. However, the virus can be extremely damaging to a foetus developing in the mother's womb (uterus), causing serious abnormalities if the mother catches it in the early months of PREGNANCY. For this reason, it is important to make sure that pregnant women do not catch rubella.

Cause

Rubella is caused by a virus found in the nose and throat of the patient. Like most viruses living along the respiratory tract, it is passed from person to person by the tiny droplets in the air breathed out. It is transmitted from a mother to her developing baby through the bloodstream via the placenta.

The virus has an incubation period of about two to three weeks, during which it is getting established and the patient shows no symptoms.

Symptoms

The illness's alternative name refers to measles because, in some cases, the initial symptoms are similar – a runny nose and mild CONJUNCTIVITIS followed by a RASH. But whereas measles can be a serious illness, German measles – more properly called rubella (from the Latin for 'reddish') – is often so mild that an attack passes unnoticed.

In most cases, there are only two symptoms. A rash appears on the face and neck, spreading to the trunk and limbs, and some of lymph nodes ('glands') swell and become tender.

The rash looks like fine pink dots under the skin. It appears on the first or third day of the illness and disappears within four to five days with no staining or peeling of the skin.

The doctor will usually look at the rash and feel for enlarged nodes at the back of the neck to confirm the diagnosis. In older people, nodes may also swell in the armpit or groin. The nodes enlarge because they are producing antibodies to destroy the virus.

Some patients develop a low fever, but this rarely rises above 100°F (37°C) and medical complications are rare although they are more common if the patient is an adult. Joints may become inflamed, particularly the ankle joints, but this goes after a period of rest. Very rarely, nerves may become affected with accompanying weakness or numbness.

Cases are often difficult to diagnose because the symptoms are so mild. Similar symptoms can be produced by other viruses, but the rubella virus is the only one known to damage developing babies.

There is no treatment which will cure the disease and only the body's own defences will end infection. Although most patients hardly know they are ill (apart from the rash), some may get a sore throat. Aspirin gargles will help (but must not be given to children under 12), as will painkilling drugs. For the average case, there is no treatment other than to rest if the patient feels unwell. A large proportion of adults will be able to continue work and most children will be able to attend school – depending on the school rules – and play normally throughout the illness. The rash disappears after a few days.

Risks

The earlier in pregnancy the virus infects the foetus, the greater the risk of damage. If it is caught between CONCEPTION and four weeks, 50 per cent of babies are affected; between five and eight weeks, 35 per cent are affected; and between 9 and 17 weeks, 12 per cent of babies are affected. Older foetuses are well enough developed for the virus not to harm them.

The defects the virus can cause include retarded growth, EYE defects, HEART defects, DEAFNESS, NERVE defects (which can cause mental backwardness), encephalitis (inflammation of the BRAIN), BONE defects and enlarged SPLEEN and LIVER. Often two or more of the defects occur together.

The reason developing babies are so susceptible is that, while they are forming, they have no defence against such viruses (*see* IMMUNE SYSTEM) and the breeding virus disrupts the developing cells. The mother's antibodies cannot help because they (unlike the virus) do not all cross the placenta into the foetus's bloodstream.

Vaccination

A vaccination is available which gives life-long protection against rubella. A single dose is all that is necessary, and has no side-effects.

Because rubella can be so mild that it goes unnoticed, it is important for girls to have the injection even if they think they have had German measles. The only people who should not have it are those on steroid drugs or with a serious illness. If in any doubt, your doctor will be able to advise you whether you run any risk.

In the past, only girls were given the rubella vaccine. Now, however, all children – boys and girls – are given a vaccine during their second year of life which protects against measles, mumps and rubella (MMR) in one single injection. Vaccination of only girls would only protect all women if 100 per cent of all women have the vaccine – and even then, the vaccine is only 95 per cent effective, so some women will always be at risk. If boys and girls are all vaccinated, it is very likely that rubella will die out altogether in the near future, so then all women will be safe, even if a few are not fully protected by vaccination. In those countries where this vaccine has been used for a number of years, rubella is now very rare.

See also IMMUNIZATION.

S

St Vitus's dance, *see* Rheumatic fever

Salmonella

FOOD POISONING is something that many of us experience at some time in our lives, and the BACTERIA responsible for causing it are often members of the salmonellae group. Although food poisoning can be quite a mild disease, it can occasionally be serious, particularly in babies. Typhoid, on the other hand, is nearly always serious, and this too is caused by one of the salmonellae bacteria.

Over the past few years in Britain and in some other European countries, the incidence of salmonella food poisoning has been increasing. Good hygiene in food production and preparation are crucial if outbreaks are to be avoided.

What are salmonellae?

The salmonellae are a group or family of small, rod-shaped bacteria – technically called *bacilli*. These are divided into two main groups. The first group are the typhoid organisms, *Salmonella typhi* and the various types of *Salmonella paratyphi*. These produce typhoid fever or, in the case of *Salmonella paratyphi*, a disease very much like it called paratyphoid fever. The typhoid group of salmonellae only infect humans, and they are not caught from animals, except under very unusual circumstances. (*See* TYPHOID AND PARATYPHOID for further details.)

The second group of salmonellae cause food poisoning. Nearly all infect more than one sort of animal, although they may be found in one species more commonly than in others. There are at least 1,400 different types of these food poisoning salmonellae, but only a small number regularly cause any serious trouble in humans. Food may become infected with these at almost any point along its journey from the farm to the table.

Spread of salmonella infection

Salmonellae always enter the body through the mouth. In the case of food poisoning, they then pass down through the stomach and into the intestines where they cause DIARRHOEA. Symptoms come on within 48 hours of eating contaminated food.

Salmonellae are killed by being heated, so that freshly cooked food should be quite safe provided that it has been heated right through: cooking for four minutes at a temperature above 165.6°F (75°C) should be sufficient to kill nearly all varieties. Conversely, freezing does not kill these organisms; rather, it only inhibits their ability to grow. When food is recooked, the salmonellae then return to normal. This is why it is essential to take precautions with frozen food: make sure that you do not refreeze meat without having cooked it right through, and do not allow any sort of contamination between the time you cook it and put it into the freezer.

Certain foods can be a serious risk. The first of these is chicken, although poultry in general seem to be particularly likely to harbour the disease. Some battery-reared poultry appear to have been infected through chicken feed containing salmonellae. Both fresh and frozen chickens are quite likely to have salmonellae present on the flesh, although recent improvements in both feeding practices and hygiene in preparation of chickens should reduce the problem. The salmonellae will be killed if the meat is thoroughly cooked, but this does not always happen, particularly if the chicken is cooked on a rotisserie. Also, if the chicken is not thawed fully, cooking will be insufficient to kill the salmonellae.

For some years, it has been known that duck eggs can be contaminated with salmonellae, and thorough cooking of duck eggs is always recommended. More recently hen eggs have occasionally been found to be contaminated as well. Laying flocks of hens are now regularly tested to check that they are free from salmonellae, but since there is still a small risk of contamination, it is suggested that raw fresh eggs should not be used for home-made ice-cream or mayonnaise – especially if the dishes are to be served to young children or the elderly, who are especially susceptible to the effects of food poisoning.

Symptoms and treatment

The main symptom of salmonella food poisoning is diarrhoea, which is often accompanied by pain in the abdomen. There may be a little vomiting, but this is not often severe. In a few cases, some of the organisms may spread through into the bloodstream and cause the sort of feverish illness that typhoid causes; however this is rare. Occasionally there may be an infection in odd places like the membranes of the brain (MENINGITIS) or an infection in the bone (osteomyelitis).

There is no really effective treatment for salmonella food poisoning. Medicines to stop the diarrhoea such as kaolin mixture or codeine phosphate tablets are often given. However, it is possible that damping down of the normal movements of the intestines (*peristalsis*) may lead to salmonella becoming established in the intestinal wall and so have the opposite effect of prolonging the infection.

Salpingitis

This is a major gynaecological problem. It means inflammation of the Fallopian tubes (the oviducts), the tubes that the eggs normally pass through on their way from the OVARIES to the UTERUS (womb) and where fertilization of the egg occurs. It is thought that the inflammation is caused by bacteria, but doctors can usually only isolate bacteria from about half of the Fallopian tubes that they examine. Salpingitis is sometimes also called *pelvic inflammatory disease* because it is quite common for infection to spread to other organs in the pelvis. Doctors may simply use the abbreviation PID.

Chronic and acute conditions

Salpingitis is usually described as acute or chronic. During acute salpingitis, the Fallopian tubes become congested with blood and so look deep red and swollen. Later they may return to normal or they may release a sticky secretion. This can either stick the walls of the tubes together and block them, or make the tubes stick to other structures in the abdominal cavity such as the bowel.

The Fallopian tubes can also swell into a bag of pus which occasionally will burst, causing severe inflammation to spread throughout the abdominal cavity (*see* PERITONEUM AND PERITONITIS). Fortunately this is very rare. It is more common for the pus in the tube to be replaced by a clear, watery fluid so that the Fallopian tube becomes a thin-walled, mis-shapen structure distended with fluid, rather than the normal tubular structure down which an egg can pass. This condition is called *hydrosalpinx*.

Chronic salpingitis may follow acute salpingitis. In this case, the inflammation decreases but never completely disappears. The chronic condition may also be a result of continuous mild inflammation which never becomes severe enough to damage the tubes seriously.

Because there is a rich supply of LYMPH channels between the Fallopian tubes, infection in one tube nearly always travels to the tube on the other side of the uterus.

Causes of infection

The Fallopian tubes may become infected by BACTERIA carried in the blood. This was commonly the case in the past when some women contracted TUBERCULOSIS in their tubes. Today it is more usual for the infection to spread directly from the vagina or the uterus. For example, gonococci, the microorganisms responsible for GONORRHOEA, may be introduced into the vagina by a woman's partner during sexual intercourse and then spread up the genital tract to the Fallopian tubes. Another organism which may be spread in this way is *Chlamydia trachomatis* (*see* CHLAMYDIA). This is a germ which is rather more like a virus than a bacterium; it is now thought to be the cause of at least 30 per cent of all cases of salpingitis – particularly the chronic type. Men can carry this organism and it may give them symptoms of NSU – NON-SPECIFIC URETHRITIS – which usually include a burning sensation on passing urine and a discharge from the penis. But some men may have practically no symptoms from *Chlamydia* even though they are carrying it, and can infect a sexual partner.

Infection may also enter the Fallopian tubes after CHILDBIRTH, an ABORTION or a MISCARRIAGE, causing inflammation in both the vagina and the tubes.

Finally, there may also be a spread of infection from a nearby abdominal organ – for example, from an infected APPENDIX.

It is probable that the increase in sexual freedom, together with the large number of abortions performed today, have increased the risk of women contracting salpingitis. It is also known that women who are fitted with an intra-uterine contraceptive (IUD) (*see* CONTRACEPTION) are at slightly greater risk of developing salpingitis. All intra-uterine devices in common use have a plastic thread which is left protruding from the cervix so that the device can be removed easily. However, infection may spread along this thread; the presence of a 'foreign body' in the uterus also seems to encourage infection to develop.

If an IUD is fitted to a woman who has never had a baby, the risk of salpingitis is two or three times greater than the risk to a woman who has had a baby and uses an IUD. The chances of infection are also greater among younger women who use an IUD whether or not they have had children. For these reasons, most doctors are unwilling to fit an IUD to a woman who has never had children, especially if she is under 25 years of age.

Symptoms

Acute salpingitis usually develops quite rapidly – over a day or two. The first symptoms are a deep-seated pain low in the abdomen which may be associated with backache, and a thick, unpleasant vaginal discharge. The woman feels generally unwell and often develops a temperature. Any attempt at sexual intercourse produces a worsening of the pain, and deep penetration is excruciatingly painful. If the condition is not treated quickly the woman may become very ill, with severe lower abdominal pain made worse by moving, and she may start to vomit. The pain may be confused with that caused by an ECTOPIC PREGNANCY, but the latter usually occurs on only one side of the lower abdomen, whereas salpingitis will cause pain on both sides.

Chronic salpingitis (or 'chronic pelvic inflammatory disease') may follow an acute attack or it may appear without any previous symptoms at all. Occasionally chronic salpingitis is diagnosed when a woman is investigated for INFERTILITY; she may never have had any symptoms at all other than the fact that she is infertile. More often, a woman with chronic salpingitis has an intermittent dull ache in the lower abdomen, and probably an excessive discharge. Intercourse may be uncomfortable, especially in certain positions which allow deep penetration. Symptoms are often worse just before the woman's period is due and during the period.

Investigations

After taking a full medical history, the doctor will carry out an internal examination. He or she will be checking for tenderness in one or other of the Fallopian tubes and also for the presence of swellings on either side of the uterus which may indicate either an abscess or a hydrosalpinx. If salpingitis is suspected, it is important for the germ causing the infection to be identified if at all possible. It is assumed that any germs found in the CERVIX of the uterus will be the same as those higher up, in the Fallopian tubes. Therefore the doctor will take several swabs from the cervix, using a vaginal speculum to expose the cervix to view. Swabs will be taken to check for the presence of *Chlamydia* and other organisms such as gonorrhoea.

In more severe cases or where diagnosis is in doubt, hospital investigation may be needed. An instrument called a laparoscope is used. This surgical instrument is like a telescope and can be inserted into the abdomen through a very small incision. The gynaecologist can then see directly if the Fallopian tubes are inflamed. Bacterial swabs can be taken directly from the tubes.

Treatment

A woman with severe acute salpingitis is usually treated in hospital. She requires bedrest and large doses of the correct ANTIBIOTIC. This may be given by intravenous drip if she is too ill to take much by mouth.

Usually, however, a woman with salpingitis is treated by her own general practitioner with antibiotics taken by mouth. While waiting for the results of tests, the woman is often given two different antibiotics to be taken together, so that there is a very good chance of dealing with any possible germ. Chronic salpingitis tends to take some time to improve so it is quite usual for antibiotics to be prescribed for three weeks or more.

Dangers of salpingitis

Many woman who have salpingitis make complete recoveries, but there are many possible consequences of the condition. A woman may become infertile because the tubes are so severely damaged that the eggs are no longer able to meet and be fertilized by sperm. Repeated attacks of salpingitis leads to an increasing likelihood of infertility.

When damage is less severe, the egg may be fertilized in the tube but will not travel on to implant in the womb; instead it implants in the damaged tube. This is an ectopic pregnancy and both the embryo and the tube must be surgically removed.

The sticky secretion released from an infected tube can make the bowel become attached to the tubes. This can give a patient discomfort, especially if she is constipated. The ovaries, which normally float in the pelvis, can also become stuck down behind the womb. These are always tender when touched; usually during sexual intercourse, they move and so avoid pressure, but after salpingitis, this may no longer be the case. As the ovaries may be exceptionally tender, sex becomes uncomfortable. Finally, the woman may be left with small areas of infected tissue that can occasionally spread and cause further pain.

Salt

This is a very simple chemical compound composed of two elements, *sodium* and *chlorine*, which give it its chemical name, sodium chloride. In the body, it is dissolved in water, and in this state, the sodium and chlorine parts separate and move independently as sodium and chlorine ions (electrically charged particles similar to atoms).

The body's salt content occurs in the ratio of three parts of sodium to two of chlorine. In practice, when doctors refer to salt retention and loss, they mean sodium retention and loss, with the assumption that chlorine always coexists with sodium.

Where is salt found?

Salt is found in all the body's fluids, but there is much more in the blood and the extracellular fluid than in the fluid inside cells, and for good reason.

There is a balance maintained between the extracellular fluid containing sodium and the similar solution inside cells which contains the complementary element POTASSIUM. All cells have a mechanism for pumping sodium outwards while keeping potassium inside. This is aptly called the 'sodium pump', and most of the body's energy is taken up in the ceaseless activity of these tiny pumps. The cells therefore act in a similar way to single-celled animals in the sea which keep their salt levels low compared with the water around them.

Function and sources of salt

Salt has the important function of maintaining the body's fluids (*see* WATER) at an optimum level. This comes about because the volume of a fluid depends directly on the amount of salt dissolved in it. Thus, since the amount of salt in the body is itself rigidly controlled, the volume of blood and other fluids is thereby regulated.

We take salt in its pure form, but it is also present in meat and vegetables, and in large quantities in some processed foods such as potato crisps and peanuts.

How the salt level is controlled

The body loses salt in the urine and sweat (*see* PERSPIRATION). The plasma, or liquid part of the blood, passes out into the urine and the important parts are then taken in by the KIDNEY tubules. Salt is reabsorbed from the tubular fluid in the kidneys, and the water also needed by the body tends to follow by osmosis, the process whereby a substance (such as water, in this case) passes across membranes from a weaker solution to a stronger one. Water will therefore leave the kidney tubules when they have lost salt, and pass into the blood which has a higher salt content than the kidneys.

The kidneys are thus very important in controlling salt levels in the body, and the balance will tend to be disturbed particularly by factors acting directly on the kidneys. For example, the steroid hormone aldosterone makes the kidneys retain more salt than usual, while other steroid hormones, such as cortisone, have a similar but less marked effect.

Since the volume of blood is controlled chiefly by the salt level, any fall-off in the amount of blood reaching the kidneys will give the impression that the salt level is too low. Therefore the kidneys will tend to retain salt in an effort to restore the blood to its normal level. The kidneys behave in this way when there are HEART problems. The salt levels then increase, giving rise to greater amounts of fluid in the circulation. Eventually there is too much blood for the heart to cope with and heart failure sets in. This explains why diuretic tablets, or water pills, are used to control heart failure since their function is to make the kidneys lose sodium in the urine.

Salt loss through sweating is less easily controlled, so that – in a hot climate, for example – more salt than usual should be taken or serious illness can result.

Salt loss

When there is salt loss, the body tries to keep enough fluid in the circulation for the heart to work effectively. Eventually it is unable to meet the body's requirements and collapse follows.

Dehydration through sweating, vomiting and diarrhoea can all do this, particularly in the case of babies and small children who have low salt levels in their bodies and so can afford to lose much less. Treatment is to give large doses of salty water (saline) preferably into a vein. Salt loss and water loss nearly always go together and so are treated accordingly.

Salt loss also occurs with a failure in the production of steroid hormones, although this involves less water loss. A low BLOOD PRESSURE and a tendency to collapse are among the symptoms of such failure, which is known medically as *Addison's disease.*

Too much salt

It is commonly said that too much salt causes high blood pressure. The exact cause of this is not known. However, the disease is commoner in countries where there is a high salt intake, and there is anyway little doubt that the body's salt-retaining mechanisms are involved in setting the level of blood pressure higher than normal. Very low salt diets can also be successful in lowering blood pressure, so it would seem that salt plays an important part in the disease, even if it is not the sole cause.

Sarcoma

A sarcoma is a certain type of malignant TUMOUR (*see* CANCER). Its name comes from the Greek word meaning 'flesh', because many of these tumours are fleshy in nature.

The body tissues are divided broadly into *epithelium,* which is the tissue that forms lining membranes, and *connective tissue,* which makes up the main substance of the body, and includes MUSCLES, BONE, fibrous tissue and FAT. Malignant tumours which arise from the epithelium are known as *carcinomas,* and malignant tumours which arise from the connective tissue are known as sarcomas.

Types of sarcoma
As a group of tumours, sarcomas are far less common than carcinomas, and tend to affect a much younger age group. Different sarcomas present different problems depending on their exact anatomical location; they can occur anywhere there is muscle, bone, fibrous tissue, fat or lymph tissue.

Chondrosarcoma is a tumour of cartilage – the gristle which covers the ends of bones and lines the joints. These tumours are very rare; they occur most commonly between the ages of 50 and 70 years. The first symptom is often pain in a joint. A lump is unusual.

Fibrosarcoma is a tumour in fibrous tissue. These rare tumours may occur within muscles and the fibrous connective tissues that join them together. Other sites include the deeper layers of the skin and the external surface of bones, which are covered in a fibrous tissue called *periosteum*. Most typically, fibrosarcomas occur in patients over 30 years old. The first sign of the tumour is often simply an unusual lump which may ache. The lump grows fairly rapidly.

Kaposi's sarcoma was once an extremely rare tumour affecting the lining (endothelium) of SKIN blood vessels. It causes rather unsightly purple lumps in the skin of virtually any part of the body. Many sufferers develop lesions on the face, particularly on the tip of the nose.

In 1981, American doctors noticed that the incidence of Kaposi's sarcoma had begun to increase dramatically, and it soon became clear that patients with AIDS were very likely to develop this tumour. For some reason, the immune damage caused by AIDS appears to predispose to the development of Kaposi's sarcoma, which now affects 18 per cent of all adult patients with AIDS.

Leiomyosarcoma is a tumour of the type of muscle found in the stomach, small intestine and uterus (womb). These are therefore the usual sites for this type of tumour.

Liposarcoma is a tumour that develops in fat cells and is the commonest sarcoma occurring in humans; it may rarely occur in a previously benign tumour called a LIPOMA.

Mesothelioma is a type of sarcoma that arises in the thin membrane (pleura) that lines the chest cavity and the surface of the lungs. Although this tumour is very rare, it was found some years ago to occur more commonly in people who worked in the asbestos industry. It appears that exposure to certain types of asbestos fibre, particularly 'blue' asbestos, can trigger a mesothelioma which may come to light many years after the exposure. The use of asbestos is now carefully controlled in all industries, and workers must be protected from asbestos dust.

Osteosarcoma is one of the better known types of sarcoma, arising from bony tissue. Osteosarcomas can occur in any bone of the body but most commonly they occur at the ends of the long bones, typically just above or below the knee, at the ankle or occasionally in one of the long bones of the arm. Usually they affect young people between 10 and 20 years of age but they may affect elderly people in their 60s or 70s.

The first symptom of an osteosarcoma is pain, and if the tumour is developing in a leg, a limp. Although the tumour has usually grown to a size of several inches across by the time it is diagnosed, it frequently does not cause a particularly obvious swelling of the skin surface because much of the tumour growth is internal, within the bone. However the size of the tumour can often be appreciated by feeling the limb. Sometimes the skin surface is shiny and there may be obvious veins running over the tumour.

Because most people with osteosarcomas are teenagers, it is not surprising that the first symptom may be a fracture at the site of the tumour, caused by a sudden sprain, possibly from some fairly normal sporting activity.

Rhabdomyosarcoma occurs in the muscles of the skeleton, in so-called 'voluntary muscles' and, rarely, in the heart.

Treatment

The main treatment of a sarcoma is surgical removal wherever possible. In the treatment of an osteosarcoma, however, at the lower end of the femur, it may be necessary to amputate the leg. Of course, other sarcomas in more superficial parts of the limb may be removable without such a radical operation.

If a sarcoma spreads, it usually does so via the bloodstream, so that secondary growths may occur in the lungs or the liver. When this happens, it is obviously not possible to perform further surgery. In this case, the patient would be treated with special drugs known as *cytotoxic* (anti-cancer) drugs. These drugs work by killing cells which are rapidly dividing, such as tumour cells. Some of them are given as a course of injections, and some are given as tablets.

The results of the treatment of sarcomas depend very largely on the exact site and how quickly surgery is performed. In the past, an osteosarcoma was considered to be almost invariably fatal, even with amputation. But now cytotoxic drugs are usually employed in addition to amputation, and many teenagers' lives have been saved by early treatment. Complete cure is possible. The results of treatment of other types of sarcoma are not so promising, but combinations of surgery and cytotoxic therapy may occasionally prolong life and even, on occasion, bring about a cure.

Patients with AIDS who have Kaposi's sarcoma are usually treated with cytotoxic drugs, but often their poor general condition makes it impossible for the doctors to use sufficiently high doses of cytotoxics to be really effective.

Scabies

These are tiny insects – also known as *mites* – which live on the skin surface and feed on the dead scales which slough off in the normal shedding process. All the stages in the life-cycle of the mite take place on or just under the skin, especially of the hands.

How scabies is caused

When breeding, the fertilized female mite digs a burrow in the surface layers of the skin and lays her eggs along the tunnel. The female then dies but the eggs subsequently hatch into larvae. These eat their way out of the burrow to the surface again, where they mature into new adult mites after several days.

In the course of this maturation, they often transfer to other humans, or even animals, who come into close enough contact for migration to occur. In practice, they do not live long on animals or clothing, so this means of transmission is relatively uncommon. They are most commonly spread by close personal contact, such as when people share a bed or bedding.

When the mites have matured, they mate, and though the male soon dies, the female goes through the breeding cycle, thus perpetuating the infection. The whole cycle, from the time that eggs are laid to the maturation of fresh mites, takes about two weeks.

Symptoms

There are no symptoms until the females start their reproductive burrows, which are dug most frequently on the hands and wrists. They usually appear as a thin red line between the fingers, and this virtually clinches a diagnosis. The elbows, feet, ankles, penis, scrotum and nipples are also common sites for burrows. They are rarely found on the chest and back, and mites seem to avoid the head altogether. The burrows may itch, or may pass unnoticed even after the larvae have hatched into new mites.

After a few weeks, the body develops an allergic response to the insects' repeated burrowing, and this shows itself in a generalized skin RASH consisting of red itchy spots and blotches. The itching (*see* PRURITUS) is the worst problem and leads to intense scratching, particularly at night and when the skin is warm. The skin may even bleed from being scratched so much, and bacterial infection may then create a further complication. It is therefore sensible to seek treatment before the skin has been damaged too much.

The burrows continue to appear wherever a female is laying eggs. They are usually $^1/_5$–$^3/_5$ in (0.5–1.5 cm) in length and may be curved or S-shaped. The average female moves under the skin very slowly so that a new burrow can take up to a week to form. A clear little blister may appear at the end of the burrow where the female dies.

Diagnosis and treatment

Anyone suffering from scabies soon seeks medical help because of the irritation. By this stage, the rash is a confusing picture of allergic patches of inflammation, scratch marks and burrows. The diagnosis is confirmed by extracting a female mite from her burrow by means of a needle, and examining her appearance under magnification.

Once the diagnosis is certain, treatment is simple and effective. A lotion of *benzyl benzoate* or *gamma benzene hexachloride* is used to kill the mites on the skin surface; provided reinfection is avoided, all the symptoms will subside. The mites are quite resilient so the lotion must be left on the skin for 24 hours. After a course of treatment has been correctly followed, the scabies should be cured, although the allergic response of a red itchy rash may take several days to clear up completely.

Anyone who has been in close personal contact with an infected person should also be treated since the mites spread easily in this way. In the latent period between infection and the development of symptoms, fresh mites may be released before the newly infected contact has sought treatment. Therefore everyone in the family or household should be treated to prevent an outbreak.

Scarlet fever

This is an infectious disease which is caused by a BACTERIUM. It is characterized by a sore throat and a red – if not actually scarlet – RASH. Treatment with penicillin or another suitable ANTIBIOTIC will prevent complications and effect a complete cure.

Scarlet fever used to be a common cause of death among children, but nowadays you rarely hear about it. It seems as though the streptococcus has become a lot less virulent – that is, it causes less serious symptoms. This change in the pattern of behaviour of the streptococcus began at the end of the nineteenth century, well before antibiotics were invented. Nobody knows why this change happened. However, although scarlet fever is now very rare in Western countries, it is still a major cause of illness – and even of death – in the Third World.

Causes

Scarlet fever (or 'scarlatina', as mild cases used to be called) is caused by the *Streptococcus pyogenes* bacterium. To differentiate one type of bacterium from another, they are grown separately on bacteriological plates that contain blood. Some types break down the blood, leaving a clear ring around the little colonies of bacteria. This is called *haemolysis* ('blood breaking'). The type of streptococcus that causes scarlet fever produces a type of haemolysis referred to as *beta-haemolysis.*

In doing so, it indicates that the streptococcus must be producing and excreting a toxic substance, since the bacterium is having an effect beyond the bounds of the colony itself. In fact, it is the organism's ability to produce toxins that leads to scarlet fever, since the organism itself only infects the throat, but the effects of its toxins show up all over the body.

Symptoms

Scarlet fever usually starts within two to four years of incubation, but the limits of the incubation period are between one and seven days.

Traditionally, one of the most characteristic aspects of the disease was that it started in a dramatic manner, with a sudden temperature accompanied by vomiting and a sore throat. At this stage, the tonsils became infected, and had a whitish crust (exudate) on them. Less serious infections don't cause vomiting, and nowadays the disease can be so mild that children don't even have a sore throat.

The day after the disease starts, the rash which gives it its name breaks out. This is a diffuse reddening of the skin caused by all the little blood vessels opening up. If you press down over an area of affected skin, the skin will whiten with the pressure, and it will stay white for longer than normal. The rash starts on the face and then spreads down to affect the rest of the body. The farther away from the face it gets, the likelier it is to form actual spots rather than a uniform redness: these spots tend to be found on the legs and to a lesser extent on the hands. The rash usually lasts for about two or three days.

While the rash is appearing and then fading away, there are a series of changes that affect the TONGUE. First, there is a creamy white exudate all over it with the tongue's little papillae pointing up through it. This is known as 'white strawberry tongue'. As the exudate peels off, the tongue is left rather red and raw with its papillae still showing prominently to make it look like a strawberry. This is called 'red strawberry tongue'.

One of the most typical and striking effects of the disease then occurs as the rash begins to fade. The skin starts to peel off and, in more serious cases, it may peel off in great sheets (desquamation). In the past, it was not uncommon to see an entire cast of a hand in the form of dead skin, although nowadays such occurrences are extremely rare.

Dangers

Infection can spread to the EARS causing *otitis media* and to the LYMPH glands, producing a serious abscess-forming illness. Infection may also lodge in the nose: this is a trivial complication with little or no symptoms, but it can lead to the spread of the disease as a result of 'droplet infection' when one of the carriers sneezes.

Other problems are a result of the body's IMMUNE SYSTEM having an abnormal response to the streptococcus and producing one of the two types of sensitivity reaction. The first is nephritis, where the KIDNEYS become inflamed, and the second is acute RHEUMATIC FEVER where a rash, joint pains and even heart damage may occur.

Treatment

Scarlet fever is treated with penicillin or another antibiotic: these drugs kill the bacteria in the throat and stop them producing toxin that gives rise to the disease. The patient improves rapidly with treatment as long as it is given reasonably early in the course of the illness. Even minor cases are treated this way because, after 24 hours of the antibiotic, the organism is no longer infectious.

Scheuermann's disease, *see* **Kyphosis**

Schistosomiasis, *see* **Tropical diseases, Worms**

Schizophrenia

This is one of the most serious MENTAL ILLNESSES. The term 'schizophrenia' was first used by a Swiss psychiatrist in 1908 to describe 'a rending or splitting of the psychic function' and the disease has been described in layman's terms as 'having a split personality'. It may include withdrawal from reality, disorders of thought processes, abnormal behaviour and a gross inability to communicate with other people. It is the most common type of psychosis (*see* PSYCHIATRY) and affects up to one person in every 100. Modern treatment has meant a revolution in its outlook, although not too long ago, about one third of those in mental hospitals suffered from this condition to some degree.

The symptoms and manifestations of schizophrenia are diverse, so much so that some clinicians prefer to talk about 'the schizophrenias' in the plural rather than as if it were just one condition. A variety of treatments have enjoyed vogues, but as yet, none has been found to be universally effective. The condition can sometimes gradually disappear even without treatment; but even if schizophrenic behaviour improves spontaneously, in some cases it may recur at a later stage and be serious enough to require specialist treatment.

Symptoms

The common denominator in most forms of schizophrenia is irrationality in thought or behaviour, often, rather surprisingly, mixed with other behaviour which is natural and reassuring. Thus, Mr Smith may reply easily and courteously to questions – yet assert that his mind is controlled by X-rays coming from the hospital radiators.

Someone suffering from schizophrenia may have delusions about ordinary happenings, and will say, for example: 'Because that woman put my shoes under the bed, I know I must go home to meet the Queen.' Alternatively, he may have delusions of attack: 'The police are projecting rays that enter the back of my neck and stop me getting an erection.' Or he may feel that thoughts are being implanted in his mind: 'I can't think my own thoughts any more. I have to think thoughts my dead father is having.'

Some sufferers may have difficulty in concentrating: 'I can't watch television because I can't sort out what's happening and understand the words at the same time. I just feel overwhelmed.' Others may have delusions of hearing voices: 'As soon as I think of something, this voice says it out loud a few seconds later. Or sometimes it contradicts what I say and argues with me.'

All the examples given so far are those of disorders of thought. Sometimes, however, there will be irrational behaviour – strange facial expressions, repeated gestures of a pointless yet complex nature, flailing of limbs and twitching. Alternatively, there will be a strange immobility called *catatonia*, where the patient stays unmoving in an unusual position (to curl up in a ball is quite common), often for several hours. In certain cases, the patient will show what is called 'waxy flexibility'. This is when his limbs can be moved into any position by another person, and will retain that position for a long time afterwards.

The patient suffering from schizophrenia may also show unusual emotional patterns, either exhibiting inappropriate emotion (giggling when told that a friend has died, flying into a rage because someone walked by past his shadow) or none at all.

As can be imagined, the diversity of schizophrenic symptoms sometimes make diagnosis of the condition difficult. Diagnosis is also not helped by the fact that, in some cases, the behaviour is normal *but inappropriate*. This presents special difficulties when the person being examined comes from a different culture from that of his doctor. For example, in some societies it is normal for a religious person to talk out loud to God and to believe that God answers; yet the unthinking clinician could easily construe this as 'delusional thought and hallucination', and thus as incipient schizophrenia.

It is clear that, even when the diagnosis has been made carefully and precisely, certain patterns of illness emerge. 'Acute schizophrenia' is the term given to a common form of the illness in which the individual remains quite active but has hallucinations and delusions. The patient may look fairly normal and go about daily life with some vigour. Often the person hears voices, which may be talking about him or her, or telling him or her what to do.

'Chronic schizophrenia', on the other hand, is characterized by slowness and withdrawal. The patient usually behaves quite abnormally, and often has a dishevelled appearance, seeming to be emotionally flat with slow, hesitant speech. Catatonia is quite common in this form of schizophrenia. Some people also become depressed.

Who develops schizophrenia?

Schizophrenia is no respecter of persons; young or old, male or female, rich or poor alike can become its victims. There is nevertheless powerful evidence that it runs in families, and careful research has established that this is not necessarily due solely to patterns of upbringing or to the way a schizophrenic parent behaves towards his or her offspring, but is due in part to genetic transmission.

Overall in Europe, between two and five people in 1,000 have schizophrenia at any one time. The prevalence does, however, vary from place to place. In parts of Scandinavia, particularly in remote areas, the rate is higher but this may be a result of migration: people who are emotionally and physically fit tend to move away from such areas, leaving schizophrenics behind.

The risk of any one individual developing schizophrenia at some time in his or her life is about 7 in 1,000.

Childhood schizophrenia

It is extremely important to realize that disturbed behaviour, imagined events, inappropriate emotion and bizarre thought patterns in childhood can occur without schizophrenia or indeed any mental disorder being present. However, schizophrenia can occur in children, but generally not before the child is three or four years old. (This makes it different from AUTISM, with which it is sometimes confused, because autism generally appears quite soon after birth.) It is marked by poor emotional relationships with others, and a lack of belief in his or her own identity. For example, when schizophrenic children are asked if they want to go out, they may say 'Yes, *he* wants to put on *his* coat to go out,' as if they are talking about someone else.

Children suffering from schizophrenia may show acute, excessive and illogical anxiety, loss of speech, distortions in the way they see or hear things, bizarre movements and a determined resistance to change in their environment. A test often used is the so-called 'whirling response', in which if a child's head is turned fairly quickly to one side by an adult standing behind him, instead of only the head moving, the rest of the child's body tries to turn as well.

Causes

There are many theories about what causes schizophrenia. Factors cited have included genetic, chemical, family upbringing and later social pressures. The psychiatrist R. D. Laing, for example, argued that schizophrenia is not an illness at all, but occurs as a defence against intolerable pressures produced by society.

Laing's theory is ingenious, and he produced examples of patients for whom his ideas may well be true. However, there is little other evidence to support the view that environment is a major cause of schizophrenia; it is probably more accurate to say that it may well precipitate an attack in someone who was already predisposed to schizophrenia.

Heredity is probably the most powerful influence on the development of schizophrenia. Numerous studies indicate that the condition tends to run in families – but it should be stressed that this is not necessarily proof that schizophrenia is hereditary, since a poor heredity and an unfavourable environment usually go together. In addition, most psychiatrists and psychologists agree that what *can* be inherited is a *predisposition* to schizophrenia: under severe pressure, a predisposed individual is more likely to develop the condition than others.

The hypothesis that schizophrenia is hereditary gets strong support from the fact that identical twins, who come from the same egg, show more tendency to schizophrenia than fraternal twins, who come from different eggs produced at the same time.

But environmental factors cannot be discounted entirely. The schizophrenic parent may transmit the disorder to his offspring by means of faulty child-rearing rather than faulty genes. And two parents suffering from the condition would surely provide a more abnormal environment than just one.

A theory proposed over 50 years ago postulated that physical constitution may contribute to the development of schizophrenia. It was suggested that people suffering from the condition were more often slim and wiry than very muscular and plump. Research has shown this theory to have some basis: the narrower the physique, the more marked the thought disorder and the earlier the onset of the condition will be. This, however, may be the genetic influence in another form, since genes control body build.

Body chemicals are also important in schizophrenia. Research with drugs that produce schizophrenic symptoms artificially have suggested that chemicals present in the bodies of some people render the person liable to the development of schizophrenia. Unfortunately, if such chemicals do exist, they have yet to be identified, and there is some doubt whether it is the chemicals that produce the condition – or the condition that produces the chemicals. And where does the 'instruction' to produce the chemicals come from? This, too, may be genetic.

Finally, some researchers believe that schizophrenia may be triggered off by a stressful event in a person's life (*see* STRESS). A physical illness does on occasion seem to precede the diagnosis of schizophrenia, or some psychological trauma such as a divorce or loss of a job.

Treatment

The primary treatment for schizophrenia is drug therapy. Nowadays the phenothiazine derivatives are commonly used, such as chlorpromazine or another class of drugs such as haloperidol. These have the property of blocking certain chemical transmitters in the brain.

In the acute phase of schizophrenia, the phenothiazine drugs can be dramatically effective and may restore the obviously disturbed patient to virtual normality. However, there is some controversy over how long they should be used. Some patients with chronic schizophrenia can clearly be helped by long-term maintenance therapy in that their behaviour becomes more normal and they become more sociable. Often the drugs are given by long-acting injection every few weeks.

Phenothiazines are not without their problems, however. Some patients develop a muscular tremor while they are on these drugs. The tremor – which is rather similar to that which occurs with PARKINSON'S DISEASE – can be controlled by the use of anti-Parkinsonian medication and usually stops once the phenothiazine is discontinued. Of more concern to psychiatrists is a side-effect called *tardive dyskinesia*. This causes abnormal writhing movement of the limbs, which the patient is quite unable to control.

Drugs are generally prescribed for several months. As and when the symptoms abate, social and psychological treatment (*see* MENTAL THERAPIES) can begin, involving 'talk out' sessions, work therapy, social involvement practice and OCCUPATIONAL THERAPY. These activities are important both in promoting recovery and, in severe cases, in preventing deterioration.

Some psychiatrists believe that both acute and chronic schizophrenia can be managed with little or no drug treatment. Apart from psychotherapy, it also appears that providing a supportive, stable environment for the patient is important. It may actually be better to provide a good institutional environment for the patient than to return him or her to an unhappy and emotionally unstable family. If the patient is returned home, regular support by a community psychiatric nurse is vital.

Hospital studies show that about one in five patients recover completely, two-thirds will have relapses and one in ten will become seriously socially disabled. The outlook may even be better than these figures imply, for many who may *in the end* deteriorate seriously have long periods when they can return to the outside world with success, even though they may have to be looked after by the people around them.

Sciatica

This occurs most often as the result of a SLIPPED DISC. Although it may affect nerves in the arms and the legs, it is the particular pressure on certain nerves on their way to the back of the leg which causes the sharp, stabbing leg pain that is characteristic of sciatica. The pain may come on suddenly or more gradually, and may be recurrent if the disc between the vertebrae does not heal up.

Most people who suffer from sciatica do so because the discs in the backbone become weakened, either through age or as a result of excessive strain.

Occasionally sciatica is caused by other disorders of the SPINAL CORD such as a TUMOUR or inflammation. These problems are very rare, however, and would be detected by examination and X-rays.

The effects

Pain low in the middle of the back is often the first thing that is noticed when the discs start to bulge out or 'slip'. This may happen suddenly during a bending or stretching action, or may come on more gradually during days of hard work such as doing housework, washing or lifting heavy objects. As the bulging disc presses on the nerves in the spinal canal, a sharper pain is felt going down the back of the leg into the foot. This is because the nerves most often pressed on are those which form the major component of the sciatic nerve which supplies this part of the leg and foot. Most of the pain is usually felt deep in the buttock and the back of the thigh. If the trouble gets worse, the slightest movement – even coughing or sneezing – will bring on or intensify these pains.

Pressure on the nerve roots, which causes the pain felt in sciatica, can also produce other changes, some of which may be noticed by the sufferer, others may only be picked up by the doctor.

Often one or other of the reflexes in the leg becomes diminished as the nerve conducts its messages less well. This does not cause the patient any problem on its own: it is, in fact, a useful sign as it enables a doctor to know exactly which nerve is being affected. If the pressure is severe, some weakness may occur. More often the sensation over the outer side of the foot may be diminished so that the skin feels slightly numb or some pins and needles may be felt in this area. This is because the nerve root involved in sciatica supplies this part of the leg.

A serious symptom is the development of urinary incontinence or faecal incontinence, which may indicate pressure on the nerves to the bladder or anus. This may require an urgent operation as damage can be permanent if the pressure from the slipped disc persists.

Treatment

The treatment of sciatica is the same as for slipped disc.

Scleroderma, *see* Raynaud's disease

Scoliosis, *see* Kyphosis

Scrofula, *see* Tuberculosis

Scurvy

This results from a deficiency of VITAMIN C, which is found mainly in fresh fruit and vegetables. It was once such a common disease that it found its way into the English language as a term of abuse. Like all diseases of inadequate NUTRITION, it is now rare in Western countries although it certainly still occurs. There are many people with a diet that is deficient, and they may find themselves on the borderline of developing scurvy.

Symptoms

Most of the symptoms of the disease are related to abnormal bleeding. In adults this tends to affect the SKIN and the gums (although the gums are only involved in people who still have all their TEETH). In the early stages of the disease, there is bleeding from around the base of the teeth. After this, the gums retract from the teeth and eventually the teeth are lost.

In the skin, the bleeding usually takes the form of large bruises which tend to occur in the thigh. However, the areas of bleeding may be much smaller – sometimes there are little red haemorrhages visible around the roots of body hairs – and these are generally concentrated around the legs.

As the disease progresses, bleeding may occur in deeper tissues such as the muscles or the intestines and stomach. As well as causing bleeding, scurvy also seems to interfere with the formation of BLOOD cells, resulting in a form of ANAEMIA in the sufferer.

Vitamin C is essential for the skin to heal properly, and another characteristic of scurvy is that wounds may not heal. This is because vitamin C is required to lay down collagen, the basic protein that makes up all fibrous tissue. Collagen is also required to make BONE, and the bones may become softened.

Scurvy is a most unpleasant condition, and if the teeth are still present in the mouth, it can be very painful. The pain of scurvy is most striking in babies, though: the disease causes bleeding into the periosteum – the fibrous covering of the bones – and this is so painful that the baby may adopt a characteristic frog-like posture.

In countries such as the UK, scurvy is now very uncommon and it almost always affects either the elderly or those whose social isolation leads to a deficient diet. Fortunately it is rare in children and infants. In the past, children who were bottle fed were more likely to be affected: this is because cow's milk contains almost no vitamin C.

Although the disease does occur in elderly women on inadequate diets, in the UK at least it seems to affect men in particular. The typical sufferer from scurvy these days is a man living alone who smokes heavily.

The treatment is simple – give vitamin C by mouth. Improvement will be immediate and will continue over the course of a few weeks. It is obviously important to look for signs of other vitamin deficiencies, and in practice, most doctors will prescribe a mixture of vitamins.

Sedatives

In the general sense, sedatives are drugs which relax and calm people, and so relieve anxiety. They are the most commonly prescribed sort of drug in the world – and there is a very real danger that they are overprescribed. Nevertheless they have been found to be effective, and used properly, they can be effective in helping STRESS and SLEEPING problems.

Types of sedative

The first important sedatives to be used were opium and ALCOHOL. *Opium* and its derivatives (*see* HEROIN and morphine) are rarely prescribed today because of the very high risk of addiction. Alcohol, too, is not often prescribed as a sedative, but it is an ingrained tradition in millions of homes that the stresses and strains of work are relieved by a drink at the end of the working day. Although this habit is relatively harmless in people who are not prone to anxiety, it can be the quickest road to ruin in anyone who is inclined to worry.

In the early part of the 20th century, *bromides,* which have a depressant action on the central NERVOUS SYSTEM, were widely used as sedatives. However they had serious side-effects: administered over a long period, they caused drowsiness, loss of sensation and slurred speech. Bromides were replaced as sedatives by barbiturates. In the past they were used for treating epilepsy, but are not commonly used for this nowadays, and are most usually given as part of an anaesthetic. They are not prescribed as sedatives or sleeping pills because they are frighteningly addictive.

The next major group of drugs to appear on the scene were the *phenothiazines,* which were developed in the early 1950s. The main value of these drugs lies in treating the more serious types of mental disorder such as SCHIZOPHRENIA, but they can be used to treat severe anxiety, as can their modern derivatives.

A group of drugs called the *benzodiazepines* – or TRANQUILLIZERS – were now developed. The first one of these, chlordizepoxide (more commonly known as Librium) was made in 1947, but its value in the treatment of anxiety was not recognized and applied until 1964. Since then tranquillizers have become the most widely prescribed – and overprescribed – group of sedative drugs. The best known and most often used is diazepam (Valium).

Another major family of drugs that have sedative action is the *anti-depressants,* which, as their name suggests, are used mainly in the treatment of DEPRESSION. Of course, it is not at all uncommon for patients to suffer from a mixture of both anxiety and depression, and the anti-depressants – particularly those known as the *tricyclic anti-depressants* – are very valuable in treating this sort of problem.

Finally, a group of drugs whose sedative action is almost a side issue is the *beta-blocking drugs.* These are important in treating diseases affecting the HEART and the CIRCULATION. For example, they are used widely in the treatment of both BLOOD PRESSURE and ANGINA. These drugs certainly help to relieve anxiety, particularly when the symptoms of the condition include sweating, palpitations and the like. They work by blocking the effects of the AUTONOMIC NERVOUS SYSTEM, rather than by acting directly on the brain – unlike the other drugs.

How do sedatives work?

Alcohol and the barbiturates work by having a generalized suppressive effect on the action of the nerve cells in the brain. Although we tend to think of alcohol as a drug which exhilarates and liberates, this effect is brought about by suppressing parts of the brain that ordinarily act to inhibit various types of behaviour. It is obvious that, if enough alcohol is drunk, it will so inhibit brain function that unconsciousness results.

The mechanism by which the benzodiazepines or tranquillizers act was largely unknown until quite recently, although their sedative qualities were easy to demonstrate. Benzodiazepines have been shown to reduce the aggressive instincts in animals.

Are sedatives addictive?

In general, the answer to this question is yes. Alcohol, barbiturates, morphine and heroin are all sedative drugs to some extent and they are also highly addictive. With the benzodiazepines, however, addiction in the sense of physical dependence is less common. *But* they can very easily be habit-forming, so that people who have been on these drugs even for only a week or two may not feel right without them and may soon come to depend upon them.

The anti-psychotic drugs such as *chlorpromazine* are used to treat severe anxiety. While they may have more side-effects than benzodiazepines – for example, drowsiness and sometimes abnormal muscular tremors – they are less addictive than benzodiazepines.

Who needs sedatives?
Stress and anxiety of some sort is an unavoidable part of everybody's life. The question that faces doctors is: When does anxiety stop being normal, and become a disease?

There is never a simple answer to this question, although the main criteria that a doctor will consider concern the extent to which anxiety interferes with somebody's life. Even when a doctor decides that a patient *does* suffer from what is called 'pathological' anxiety, it is by no means definite that drugs will help. In any case, resolution of the underlying problem, by counselling or some other form of psychotherapy (*see* MENTAL THERAPIES), is preferable.

Perhaps the main value of sedative drugs is to help someone settle down enough to take stock of the situation, and to give him or her a little time to work through his or her problems, often with the help of some sort of counselling.

Septic conditions

Micro-organisms exist everywhere – on our bodies, in our clothes, in the air and in the soil. They are not a problem unless they get the upper hand in their constant struggle with the body's defences against INFECTION (*see* IMMUNE SYSTEM). The moment these defences are overcome, the micro-organisms can invade, thus establishing an infection and producing *sepsis*, commonly known as a septic condition.

Causes
This invasion by BACTERIA happens typically across the skin. A cut through the skin will push the germs on the surface into the wound. Some of the underlying tissue will also be damaged and bleed, providing a pool of blood high in nutrients in which the germs can multiply. They can then invade directly beneath the skin.

On the other hand, if the skin is quite clean the number of germs introduced will probably be too small to start an infection. The white cells (*see* BLOOD) released by the cut can mop up a reasonable number of germs and so prevent sepsis. It has been found that about 100,000 micro-organisms need to get through the skin for an infection to become established. Because they are so small, this number could be carried on a pinhead.

Germs also breed in injured tissue even where the skin has not been cut through. Injury means that nutrients are released as the cells die, so that bacteria have an ample source of food. For example, in osteomyelitis – a septic condition of bones usually affecting children – there may be a history of injury to the bones prior to the development of sepsis. In most cases, there appears to be no local place where germs have entered, so they have probably spread from INFLAMMATION elsewhere via the bloodstream to become lodged in the damaged area.

Common septic conditions

One of the most common septic conditions is a BOIL. It starts when germs enter a hair follicle on the SKIN surface and set up an infection deep inside the skin. Boils may occur virtually anywhere on the surface of the body, but they are more common in areas where there are large pores in the skin, such as the armpit and the area around the groin. Infected boils in these areas are sometimes caused by a condition in which there is an abnormality in the structure of the skin glands called *hidradenitis suppuritive*. Boils or ABSCESSES may also occur in the BREAST or around the anus.

Any wound in the skin surface provides a ready-made entry point for germs to get into the body. A wound that is contaminated with dirt is particularly likely to become septic. Wounds caused by spikes or long sharp objects are especially prone to sepsis because germs may be driven deep into the tissues.

Sometimes sepsis can arise deep within the body – in an organ or body cavity. The germs may have been carried in the bloodstream, but often there is also some structural abnormality which interferes with the body's normal protective processes. Middle EAR infection is a good example of the process. During a COLD, CATARRH from the back of the throat can track up into the middle ear via the Eustachian tube (which connects the throat to the ear). The middle ear becomes filled with catarrh and infection can then spread up into it. A child with earache caused by middle ear infection has the equivalent of an abscess deep inside his or her ear.

Sepsis may also occur in the LUNGS as a complication of PNEUMONIA, in the KIDNEYS, and in the BONES – a condition called osteomyelitis. The bowel in elderly people may be affected by a condition called DIVERTICULITIS, in which sepsis occurs alongside the bowel in small pockets of tissue called diverticulae. APPENDICITIS is caused by sepsis in the appendix.

Deep-seated sepsis may on occasion follow surgical operations, especially after long and complicated operations on the bowel. In these cases, the infection usually comes from the bowel itself: because the bowel is full of bacteria, it is often difficult for the surgeon to avoid some internal contamination of other tissues during the operation.

Symptoms

The most obvious sign of a septic condition is pus. This is formed by a combination of dead white cells, bacteria and tissue fragments, the white cells being attracted to the site of the inflammation to fight the infection.

PAIN occurs due to distension of the tissues and also to the firing of pain nerves by various chemicals which are released by the white blood cells. Swelling results when the blood vessels leak out antibodies and white cells from the circulation. Redness is also a symptom of the dilation of blood vessels due to inflammation.

Symptoms of sepsis may sometimes be present throughout the body. This happens when the local infection is out of control so that micro-organisms and the toxic substances produced by them travel in the CIRCULATION to other parts of the body. FEVER is common, caused by poisons from the infection, and creates a feeling of being unwell. More seriously, the spread of micro-organisms in the blood, known as blood poisoning or *septicaemia*, can lead to a generalized collapse of the circulation so that the BLOOD PRESSURE falls and the patient becomes pale and shocked. This condition is called 'septic shock' and can be a lethal condition unless treated with intravenous ANTIBIOTICS.

Prevention

Since septic conditions are caused by micro-organisms, prevention concentrates on excluding or destroying them. In general, simple washing with soap and water is sufficient to reduce the number of germs on the skin to the extent that cuts will not go septic unless they are made by a dirty instrument.

Putting antiseptics in an open wound may help, but if the skin was contaminated before the injury, they will be ineffective, since the dirt and germs already on the skin will have been pushed deep into the wound. Therefore all wounds should be thoroughly cleaned and any dirt and damaged tissue removed physically so that germs have nowhere to breed and establish an infection. Using soap and water prevents most septic conditions which can arise in the home.

Essentially antiseptics work in three ways. There is, first, a cleaning action from scrubbing and washing which reduces the number of germs. Then their cell walls may be either dissolved by alcohol preparations or broken down by detergents. Finally, the organisms may be attacked chemically by oxidizing compounds such as chlorine, iodine, hydrogen peroxide and chlorhexidine.

Before any medical procedure, a very high standard of cleanliness is essential to prevent sepsis. Doctors use antiseptics such as iodine or chlorhexidine to clean their own skin as well as the patient's. All surgical instruments are carefully sterilized before use. Likewise, feeding teats should be sterilized in a mild antiseptic because babies have a poor resistance to infection.

During an operation, only the surgeon and his assistants may touch the operating-field – which is sterile – and the surgeon himself must not touch anything that has not been sterilized.

Serum, *see* **Blood**

Sex and sexual intercourse

Sex is a fundamental driving force of human life. Even so, the complex relationships between the biological need to reproduce, cultural influences, love, affection, and the sex drive itself are still not fully understood. Much of what we know about human sexuality has only been researched and written about this century, and there is still great controversy about many of its aspects.

As our society has developed, much of what was once considered taboo is now part of normal sexual behaviour and can be discussed freely. In the past, a common premise was that women were interested in sex only for the sake of fulfilling the maternal instinct or pleasing their partners. Nowadays, however, it has become clear that women have as powerful a need for sexual satisfaction and fulfilment as men. Men used to be seen as less emotional and sensitive, wanting sex only to gratify some basic animal urge, but we now know that emotional expression in sexual activity is equally important to men and women.

Sexual intercourse

This is the entering of the PENIS into the VAGINA. Often, the act of intercourse culminates for one or both partners in orgasm (sexual climax). CONCEPTION may take place if the woman is ovulating. PREGNANCY is not intended by most couples every time intercourse takes place, however, and thus the act becomes part of an expression of their mutual love and sexuality.

Masters and Johnson, the American sex therapists, describe four stages that the body goes through during the orgasmic cycle.

The excitement phase

Arousal usually begins with the emotional wish for sex, triggered off by feelings of being attracted to the partner. The complex hormonal scents known as pheromones may play a part in this attraction. The body quickly responds to the mind.

The sexual organs of both men and women become engorged with blood. In a man, this will result in the erection of the penis, which swells and becomes darker in colour. The internal sexual organs of the woman will also become filled with blood, and so will the vulva (external sexual organs).

The vagina expands in length and width, and its walls begin to produce a lubricant which eases the entrance of the penis. The clitoris, most sensitive part of the female genitals, becomes erect.

The skin of both the man and the woman becomes more sensitive, particularly around the erogenous zones: lips, nipples, buttocks and genitals. This, in turn, heightens arousal if those parts of the body receive stimulation during foreplay. Breathing becomes deeper and faster, and the pupils of the eyes may dilate. Both the man and the woman may develop a fine flush on the chest and neck. Intercourse may begin at this stage.

The plateau phase

Excitement continues to increase for both partners. The vagina becomes about 2 in (5 cm) longer than normal, and the entrance to the vagina narrows to grip the penis. The clitoris draws itself back into its hood.

The penis will have expanded to its maximum size, and the TESTICLES become larger and rise up towards the body. Small drops of seminal fluid may appear on the glans (head of the penis).

The penis and the vagina move together rhythmically to produce the maximum pleasure and sensation for both partners. This movement causes friction on the penis, as well as on the clitoris and inside the vagina, depending on the position. Both the man and the woman will feel highly aroused, and their bodies will tense a little.

Orgasm

The female orgasm starts as a rush of sensation that begins in the clitoris, spreads to the vagina and throughout the body. The muscles around the vagina, vulva and anus go into a series of contractions lasting for a number of seconds. This is an intense physical experience – the climax of pleasure in lovemaking.

The man will experience a build-up of feeling in his genitals. SPERM will have travelled from the testicles and will meet the seminal fluid produced from the seminal vesicles. The sperm and seminal fluid are then forced to the internal entrance of the URETHRA leading to the penis by the action of the PROSTATE GLAND.

The muscles in the penis that surround the urethra produce a series of contractions, and ejaculation begins. The amount of sperm and seminal fluid will be between 0.07–0.20 fl oz (2–6 ml). The internal contractions, as well as the build-up which immediately precedes them, are intensely pleasurable.

The resolution phase

This phase begins immediately after orgasm. The body will relax and breathing becomes more gentle. The clitoris will immediately return to its non-aroused state, and the blood that has been engorging the internal organs will slowly reduce in quantity. In women, this will take about 30 minutes. The man's penis will lose its erection and go back to its non-aroused state. The testicles will also get smaller.

During the resolution phase, both the man and the woman will feel a sensation of release and calm. They may wish to rest or fall asleep for a short time.

Male orgasmic problems

Most men find that reaching orgasm is relatively easy. Problems can stem from the inability to maintain the plateau phase, when the penis is erect. This can result in either *premature ejaculation* (when a climax takes place very quickly after arousal has begun) or the loss of erection (*impotence*). Rarely there is a physical reason for this, though in some cases other factors such as drugs for treating DEPRESSION or high BLOOD PRESSURE, or over-indulgence in ALCOHOL, can make arousal or orgasm difficult. A man who is experiencing any of these problems should consult his doctor to see that all is well physically.

The most common reason for difficulty with orgasm is psychological. A man may find it easy to maintain an erection and have a satisfying climax by masturbation, but fail to do so when he is with a partner. Some men worry about their performance and fear failure; others find that lovemaking makes them feel so nervous and over-excited that they climax before sexual intercourse begins. Both of these problems can begin after one unsatisfactory occasion, leading to anxiety from then on.

Female orgasmic problems

Women often find it more difficult to have orgasms. In some cases, there may be a physical problem such as an unusually over-developed hymen, or an inflammation of the vagina or bladder or a shrinkage of the vaginal lining after menopause, all of which can produce pain on intercourse (*dyspareunia*). In other cases, the *libido* (sex drive) can be affected by drugs the woman is taking, including the contraceptive pill. Women who are experiencing such difficulties should see their doctor.

Women are sometimes worried that sexual intercourse will cause pain, or they associate intercourse with a painful experience in the past. This fear of pain in intercourse can cause *vaginismus,* an involuntary contraction of the muscles around the vagina, which makes it impossible for the penis to enter. Women who have recently given birth, or who have gynaecological problems, may feel protective about their bodies and resistant to intercourse.

Many women are able to have orgasms through masturbation on their own, but find it impossible to climax when they are with their partner. This may simply be a question of technique: the woman may need direct clitoral stimulation, but her partner may only be willing to have intercourse and nothing else.

Other women find it difficult to ask for what they want, so their partners are unaware that different techniques are needed. The unvarying pattern of cursory foreplay followed by intercourse can also cause difficulties, since what a man may consider to be merely the preliminaries to 'real' sex – that is, sexual intercourse – may be what the woman finds most pleasurable and stimulating. She may be just about to reach climax, but because direct clitoral stimulation ceases, she is unable to do so. To overcome this, either the woman or her partner should continue to stimulate her clitoris manually during intercourse.

Some women have never had an orgasm, either alone or with a partner. The reasons for this – called *general sexual dysfunction,* or, more commonly, 'frigidity' – are various and include simple lack of knowledge and a fear of insisting that their partner help to satisfy them. Therapists advise women who have never had an orgasm to explore their bodies and find out about their sexual response through masturbation, either manually or by using a vibrator. Once they begin to have orgasms, they can communicate their desires and appropriate techniques to their partners.

Sexual therapy

Although specific problems such as premature ejaculation and vaginismus can be treated by well-established physical methods, nearly all sexual therapy takes the form of specialist counselling, together with a programme of events designed to restore a full sexual life.

Involvement of both partners: Except when a client has no stable sexual relationship, sex therapists know that what may be wrong almost always concerns the partner of that person as well, and both partners must thus be involved in the therapy.

 Sex education: Clients for sexual therapy are often unaware of basic aspects of sexual physiology and techniques. Education helps reduce the fear of the unknown in sex and thus reduces anxiety.

Attitude change: Therapists try to counter negative attitudes towards sex and help clients to be happy about seeking the sexual pleasure they have previously denied themselves.

Anxiety reduction: The direct methods of reducing anxiety used in behaviour therapy can effectively be used where sexual anxiety is concerned (*see* MENTAL THERAPIES).

Sexual communication: Some couples are afraid to communicate their sexual needs, desires and preferences to each other for fear of being rejected or despised. Therapy can help them overcome this fear and to avoid any rejection which otherwise might have occurred.

Prescribing changes in behaviour: Although the idea of a set programme may seem strange, a graduated series of sexual activities to encourage a couple's enjoyment of body contact and sexual versatility is often prescribed. Such a programme helps to overcome the shyness some couples feel.

Sensate focusing: For men with potency problems or women with general sexual dysfunction, therapist-guided sensate focusing aims to take the worry and fear out of sex over the course of a few weeks. With gentle caresses of each other's bodies, initially avoiding the genitals, the partners learn to concentrate on their own pleasurable sensations. By removing the potential 'stress' of intercourse, relaxation occurs. After several sessions, genital caressing is allowed. Eventually full intercourse can be attempted.

Sexually transmitted diseases (STDs)

This is a collection of many quite different conditions that are grouped together because they are all acquired as a result of sexual intercourse with a person who has already contracted the infection. They were previously known as *venereal diseases* (VD).

There are four common diseases that are particularly troublesome: SYPHILIS, GONORRHOEA, NON-SPECIFIC URETHRITIS and genital HERPES. Less serious venereal diseases include TRICHOMONIASIS, THRUSH or monilia, pubic LICE and genital WARTS. The HIV virus, which causes AIDS, may also be spread by sexual contact. If the infection eventually leads to the development of AIDS, there is at present no certain cure, and the illness will ultimately prove fatal.

Casual sex and STDs

In spite of modern and effective treatment, more people in Europe and North America today have sexually transmitted diseases than at any time in the past

30–40 years. The reason for this increase, especially among young people, is that the development of new CONTRACEPTIVES has led to an alteration in views and habits in sexual behaviour, and, consequently, greater sexual freedom at an earlier age. Within the past few years, HIV infection has spread at an alarming rate, and virtually no part of the world is unaffected now. Although HIV infection may be spread by contamination on hypodermic needles or blood products, sexual transmission is still the commonest method of spread in most parts of the world, including Europe, North America, Australia and the Far East.

Prevention

What, if anything, can you do that will improve your chances of not getting a sexually transmitted disease? Ideally, of course, STDs are best avoided by being faithful to one lover. Certainly you should think about the risk before you have sexual intercourse with somebody you do not know very well, and take certain precautions. The use of a condom will give both of you a considerable degree of protection against all forms of STDs, including AIDS.

There are certain situations that are especially risky in terms of the possibility of exposure to STDs or AIDS. Both male and female prostitutes are very likely to have one or more infections. In some parts of the world, over half of all local prostitutes are HIV-positive. A prostitute who uses drugs (and many do) may have contracted HIV from an infected needle or syringe. Anyone travelling away from home should also remember that a casual fling or brief holiday romance may pose considerable risks. In all these situations, a condom will provide essential protection.

Some people have come to believe that urinating after intercourse may help protect against sexually transmitted disease. It does not. Nor does washing. Women may resort to using douches of antiseptics. Such practices are unwise, possibly dangerous and provide negligible protection against infection. The only realistic form for most people is to enjoy 'safer sex' – avoiding any exchange of sexual fluids. This means avoiding oral sex (especially involving ejaculation by the man) and always using a condom during intercourse – both male-to-male and male-to-female intercourse.

Where to go for help

If you think that there is the *slightest* chance that you might have an STD, go to a 'special' clinic to find out for sure. Such clinics – sometimes called STD clinics or genito-urinary departments – exist in most towns, and you can find out the time they are open either by telephoning your local hospital or from public notices.

In most, you will be seen without an appointment or a letter from your own doctor. Everything that takes place at the clinic is strictly confidential and you will usually be referred to by a number, so that your anonymity is completely preserved. No information will be given about you in response to queries from your spouse or partner, friends, parents, school, employer, or anybody else. The clinic notes are kept quite separately from any medical records that may exist about you in some other part of the hospital, so that there is no possibility of cross-reference between them. The staff are not there to judge you, and the atmosphere in most clinics is friendly and helpful.

Shiatsu, *see* **Acupuncture**

Shick test, *see* **Diphtheria**

Shingles

This is a very painful disease that tends to affect the elderly and the ill. It is not dangerous and complete recovery nearly always occurs. The medical name of the virus responsible for the condition is *Herpes zoster* – which is Greek for a 'creeping girdle' – and the disease shows up as a belt-like rash around the body.

Causes
Shingles and CHICKENPOX are both caused by the same virus, although the two diseases are quite different. Their only similarity is that they both produce a RASH with vesicles (fluid-filled clear spots) on the skin.

Chickenpox and shingles tend to occur in very different age groups. Chickenpox primarily affects children, while shingles is very rare in childhood; most cases crop up after the age of 40. Many doctors think that everyone who gets shingles must have had chickenpox in the past, but it is difficult to prove. Chickenpox may be caught from shingles, but the reverse does not seem to happen.

Symptoms
Shingles starts with PAIN felt on the surface of the skin where the disease is going to strike. This pain may get worse over the next few days, and the skin will redden. At this point, the rash starts to break out, with little vesicles forming on the skin. The pain tends to diminish as the rash advances, but it may still be quite severe. The rash will often creep around one side of the body, causing the clear belt- or band-like condition that characterizes the disease. The areas most commonly affected are the chest and upper part of the abdomen; the lower abdomen, limbs, neck and face are involved less often.

The disease has this band-like appearance because the virus spreads down sensory nerves from the SPINAL CORD. These nerves emerge in pairs from between each of the vertebrae in the backbone, and each one supplies a band of skin – known as a *dermatome* – on one half of the body. There is no truth in the belief that, if a band of rash meets in the middle, the patient will die.

Once the rash has appeared, it will persist for several days, and the vesicles may even run together to form a mat of affected skin with a crust over it.

Eventually, though, the rash will clear, leaving normal skin behind. Sometimes there will be minor scarring or depigmentation. The pain usually disappears with the rash or soon after.

Aside from affecting mainly older people, shingles is also typically found in patients suffering from other diseases which tend to suppress the activity of the IMMUNE SYSTEM. Examples of such diseases are LEUKAEMIA or a LYMPHOMA.

Unusual forms of the disease

There may be variations in the disease. It is thought that shingles can actually occur without the tell-tale rash. This is very difficult to prove, but it is a likely explanation for the occasional patient who has a nasty pain in the area where one would expect shingles to develop.

Sometimes the disease is not confined to the sensory part of the nervous system, and muscle weakness may occur with an attack of shingles. This suggests that the motor nerve as well as the nerves of sensation are involved.

Shingles can also affect areas supplied by the nerves of the head which do not in fact arise from the spinal cord, but from the brain. Although any area of the face can be involved it usually affects the ophthalmic branch of the trigeminal nerve – the main nerve of sensation in the face. Generally the skin around the eye is affected, but occasionally the eye itself is involved. A collection of nerve cell bodies, called a ganglion, may be affected in the ear, and is called Ramsay Hunt syndrome. This produces deafness and paralysis of the muscles on one side of the face (Bell's Palsy).

Dangers

The main danger of the disease is the development of post-herpetic NEURALGIA. This means that the pain associated with the condition does not abate as the rash disappears. This is more likely to happen when the trigeminal nerve of the face is involved. This form of the disease may also be dangerous, since the eye may become involved, leading to inflammation and, in rare cases, even BLINDNESS.

Treatment

Several different anti-viral drugs have been developed which can shorten a bout of shingles. They must be used early in the attack for maximum effectiveness, preferably on the same day that symptoms first appear. Acyclovir is usually given as a course of tablets. Another drug called idoxuridine is applied to the affected area as a paint. Both of these drugs can reduce the likelihood of post-herpetic neuralgia.

See also HERPES.

Shock

There is a big difference between the way that most people use the word 'shock' and the way that doctors use it. In the ordinary way, we talk about the sudden event giving rise to an unpleasant surprise – a shock, in fact. To the doctor, shock is a medical condition in which the collapse of the CIRCULATION, for one reason or another, is a central feature. Sometimes, the different uses of the word cause confusion.

What is shock?

Shock develops because of the way the HEART and circulation work together. If for some reason the heart either fails to pump properly or there is not enough BLOOD for it to pump, then insufficient blood will be circulating to sustain the vital functions of the body. This can be brought on by several things, ranging from loss of large amounts of blood to failure of the heart itself.

For the heart to pump in the correct manner, it has to be primed with blood, and there has to be a certain amount of blood in the system for the heart to get up enough pressure to push the blood round (*see* BLOOD PRESSURE). Normally, blood leaves the heart and travels out through the arteries until it gets to the tissues. In the tissues, there are tiny arteries called arterioles which have thick muscular walls.

If the pressure of the blood goes down, these arterioles can constrict (become narrower) so that there is less space for the blood to flow through – this causes the pressure to rise again because the blood is being squeezed into a smaller space than before. This system of constriction of the arterioles, called *vaso-constriction*, is the body's way of maintaining the correct blood pressure when things go wrong. If the pressure falls too low, blood cannot flow around all the tissues. In fact, when the system fails – after excessive bleeding, for example – shock develops.

Causes

Loss of blood after accidents is one of the commonest causes of shock. But trauma is not the only way in which large amounts of blood can be lost. It is not uncommon for there to be quite serious bleeding from ULCERS in the stomach or the duodenum when large amounts of blood are either vomited or passed through the rectum. Patients with this sort of gastro-intestinal bleeding can arrive in hospital in a very shocked state. Another time of large blood loss can be during CHILDBIRTH.

Some sorts of infection can also cause shock, although in this case, the mechanism underlying the shock is different. Infection in the blood usually by bacteria may lead to the production of toxins (poisons). These toxins seem to have a direct effect on the blood vessels in the tissues causing the venules (the very small veins) to become widened. Blood becomes pooled in the venules and not enough returns to the heart so it does not have enough to pump and so the blood pressure falls. This is known as *endotoxic* or *septicaemic shock*.

The other major cause of shock is when it results from disease of the heart itself. The main cause of this is an extensive HEART ATTACK. The heart muscle is destroyed by the heart attack, and the more that is destroyed, the more severe the effects of the attack will be. When more than 40 per cent has been destroyed, shock is likely to develop because the remaining heart muscle simply lacks the power to pump enough blood. This is called *cardiogenic shock.*

Symptoms of shock

People with shock tend to have a similar appearance. They are pale and often cold and clammy to the touch; when the blood pressure is measured, it is found to be very low – critically so.

The paleness is caused by the lack of blood in the skin – all the blood has been forced from the skin by the vaso-constriction. The coldness is also because the blood – which carries body heat – has been sent back into the core of the body.

It might seem strange that people are sweaty at the same time as being cold, but the AUTONOMIC NERVOUS SYSTEM, which is responsible for controlling the body's unconscious functions, not only causes the vaso-constriction but also increases the activity of sweat glands, as do the substances released by the adrenal glands. The trauma involved in shock stimulates the body's 'flight and fight' response, one part of which is increasing sweating.

Effects of shock

As well as the immediate, dangerous effects – the prostration and grave illness – shock can create other, long-term problems. The two most important of these affect the KIDNEYS and the LUNGS.

When shock develops and there is insufficient blood passing through the kidneys, acute renal failure can develop. The kidneys stop passing urine, and waste products – particularly urea, a breakdown product of protein – start to build up in the blood. If the shock is dealt with relatively quickly, the kidneys are very likely to recover speedily. However, the process can be rather slow and dialysis may be required for days or even weeks.

But if shock has stopped the kidneys working, the situation may deteriorate even further. The blood supply to the brain may become inadequate, and consequently, confusion and then UNCONSCIOUSNESS may set in. The skin can sometimes progress from being cold and clammy, and gangrene results because of the poor blood flow. When it has gone this far, there is unfortunately very little hope for the patient.

The effect of shock on the lungs is a comparatively newly recognized condition. The effect, called *shock lung,* can occur even in apparently fit young people who have had large-volume blood transfusions following an event such as a car accident. Patients who have this complication become breathless and the level of oxygen in the blood starts to fall. There is also extensive shadowing on chest X-rays.

The exact sequence of events that cause shock lung are poorly understood, but the end result is an increase in the leakiness of the capillaries (the smallest blood vessels) in the lung and a build up of fluid in lung spaces. This is a difficult condition to deal with, and the basis of most treatment is to take over the function of the lungs by placing the patient on a respirator, or breathing machine.

Treatment of shock

The aim of treatment of shock in all its forms is to try to return the volume of blood in the circulation to normal so that the heart can pump normally and an adequate amount of blood flow to the tissues. When blood loss has been the cause of shock, the treatment is simply a transfusion of the correct amount of blood to bring the volume back to normal. When the shock is due to septicaemia (*see* SEPTIC CONDITIONS), the body still needs fluid even though the blood is pooled in the blood vessels. So here, clear fluids in the form of salt or sugar solutions, or protein-containing fluids such as plasma are used. The infection is also treated with high doses of antibiotics, often given into the intravenous drip.

But there can be problems in giving large amounts of blood or fluid to older patients since these 'extra' fluids can overload the heart and lead to heart failure. Doctors have to get round this problem, and to do this, they have to keep a balance between having too much and too little fluid in the circulation. They measure this by checking the pressure in the part of the heart that 'primes' it – the right atrium.

This pressure measurement is called the *central venous pressure* (CVP). To take the pressure, a fine tube is passed into a vein in the arm or neck and the pressure is measured outside the body using a simple column of water. If the pressure is too high, there is too much fluid; if it is too low, there is not enough.

Shock caused by a heart attack – cardiogenic shock – cannot, however, be treated by a blood transfusion. Common forms of treatment include drugs which make the heart work harder and drugs which lessen the amount of work it has to do. But drugs that make it work harder can place an even greater strain on a heart weakened by an attack.

One technique which has been tried to get round these problems is the balloon pump. A long sausage-shaped balloon is put at the top of the aorta, the biggest artery from the heart, and connected by a tube to a pump outside the body. The balloon is blown up between heartbeats and helps force blood along the arteries. When the heart has recovered, the balloon is removed again.

Sickle-cell anaemia

OXYGEN is carried in the BLOOD by the *haemoglobin* molecules in our red cells. Each of these molecules is made up of a central *haem* portion – an iron compound responsible for carrying oxygen – attached to which are four chains of *globin* molecules. The structure of the globin molecules determines that the haemoglobin will take up oxygen from the lungs and release it into the tissues where it is needed. Sickle-cell anaemia results from abnormalities in the globin structure.

This particular type of abnormal haemoglobin is called haemoglobin S, as distinct from normal haemoglobin A which is found in the blood in large quantities after birth.

There are many other kinds of abnormal haemoglobin which can all give rise to problems. It is quite possible to inherit the genes for two different types of abnormal haemoglobin from your parents. This leads to diseases where both abnormalities are found. In fact, the combination of haemoglobin S and another abnormal haemoglobin C is quite common, and is called SC disease. There are over 300 kinds of abnormal haemoglobin, but by no means all of them give rise to any problems.

Causes

This abnormality is GENETIC, which means that it is passed from parent to child at conception. Every characteristic in the body is controlled by a pair of genes, one of which is inherited from the mother and one from the father. In the case of haemoglobin, if you inherit one normal gene, the BONE MARROW will make a mixture of normal haemoglobin A and abnormal haemoglobin S. This is known as the *sickle-cell trait*. When both the controlling genes are abnormal, the full-blown disease will result, with the red blood cells containing a very high proportion of abnormal haemoglobin. People affected in this way are called *homozygotes*; those with one abnormal gene are *heterozygotes*.

Sickle-cell disease is found in all parts of the world where MALARIA is, or has been, prevalent. Thus it is common in Africa, and in people of African origin who live in the West Indies and North and South America. It is also a problem in Britain among West Indians who originally came from Africa; and it is found in the Mediterranean, India and western Asia generally.

The inherited abnormality is thought to be so common because it may also give protection against malaria. Thus the process of evolution has not tended to act against people carrying the sickle gene, unless they are seriously affected. In other words, people with the sickle-cell trait, which usually produces no symptoms, will have a greater chance of surviving because of their greater resistance to malaria, at the expense of the relatively few individuals who have the full-blown disease which will cause serious problems in most cases.

Symptoms

With homozygous sickle-cell disease – the disease resulting from two abnormal genes – the effects are very variable. In Africa, probably about 10 per cent of children with the problem reach adult life. At the same time, it is possible for the disease to produce no symptoms, and only be discovered on a routine blood test.

Chronic ANAEMIA can result from the continuous breakdown of red blood cells, but the greatest problem is the incidence of 'crises' which occur when the oxygen-level of the blood falls too low. The haemoglobin molecules in the red cells then 'sickle' or become twisted into an abnormal shape, making the cells themselves twisted. These are known as 'sickle cells' and give the disease its name.

The deformed cells tend to block off small blood vessels, making the blood clot and thus stopping the tissues from receiving oxygen. Painful infarctions (areas of tissues which have died because of blocked circulation) then occur.

The bones are often affected in this way. People with the sickle-cell trait may also be liable to crises under certain circumstances, such as during an ANAESTHETIC.

The SPLEEN can become enlarged as it separates abnormal cells from the blood. As time goes on, however, infarction of the spleen will result so that it can no longer be felt in the abdomen. People with sickle-cell anaemia are also more prone to infection, arising particularly from pneumonoccus bacteria which cause lobar PNEUMONIA. The disease also leads to ULCERS on the legs.

Treatment

Treatment consists chiefly in treating the crises as they arise by rehydrating the patient with plenty of fluids and giving oxygen when necessary. It is also possible to give exchange transfusions so that sickle cells are replaced by normal blood, although sickle cells return as the person makes his or her own blood.

Outlook

Advances have been made in the prevention of the disease through genetic counselling, and by testing the blood of potential parents for the abnormal sickle cell trait. For example, in Britain it is now routine for all women who have African, West Indian or Mediterranean parentage to be offered screening should they become pregnant. However, it is far better if the test is carried out before PREGNANCY, and that both the prospective parents are screened. Indeed there are good reasons for carrying out a sickle-cell test on everyone who may be at risk. Emergency anaesthetics carry some risk for a person with sickle-cell trait.

Another preventive measure is to use the technique of amniocentesis to obtain and examine samples of foetal blood in early pregnancy. In this way, it is possible to locate an abnormality of the haemoglobin. If it is found, a termination of the pregnancy may be advised by the doctor.

SIDS (sudden infant death syndrome), *see* **Cot death**

Sinews, *see* **Tendons**

Sinusitis

This infection of the air cavities in the front of the skull is a common problem. The *sinuses*, or sinus cavities, contain air, thus contributing to the skull's lightness, and because they are linked with the NOSE and upper THROAT, they are vulnerable to the spread of infection from these areas. There are two kinds of sinusitis – acute and chronic – with differing symptoms.

Causes

The nose and sinuses are lined with special cells which produce mucus to

Position of the sinuses

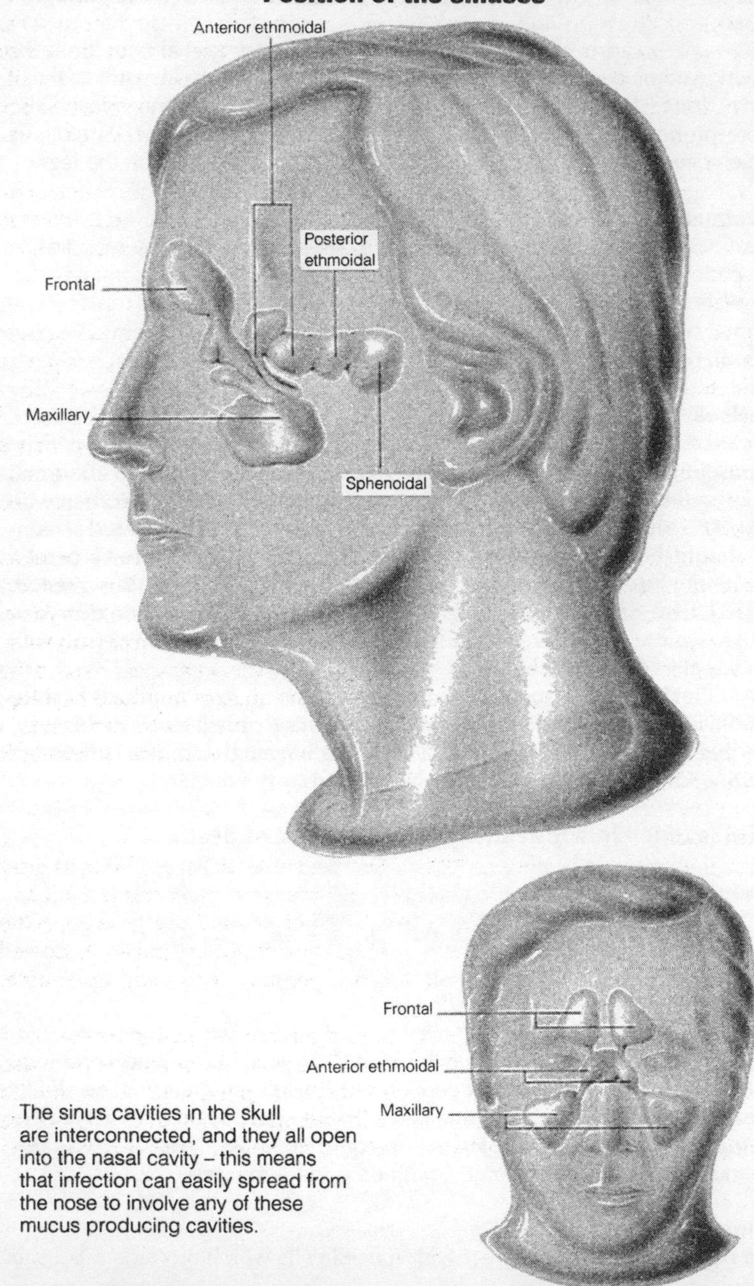

The sinus cavities in the skull are interconnected, and they all open into the nasal cavity – this means that infection can easily spread from the nose to involve any of these mucus producing cavities.

combat an initial infection – for example, from a COLD or INFLUENZA virus. When the virus enters the body, this mucus production increases – which makes the linings of the nose and sinuses swell and block up the communicating channels between them. The mucus can no longer escape, pressure builds up and the infection in the sinuses is trapped. Bacteria which normally live in the nose and sinuses now multiply, and the sinuses become filled with yellow or green pus. It is this pus which, being under pressure, creates the symptoms of sinusitis.

Dental infections, fractures of the facial bones or gunshot wounds may also bring about sinusitis. Poor drainage of the nose, and enlarged, infected ADENOIDS and TONSILS are likewise contributory factors of this condition.

Symptoms and dangers

Acute sinusitis gives rise to pain, and sometimes redness and swelling over the sinus. The patient may have a severe localized headache, depending on which sinus is affected. *Frontal* sinusitis, for example, produces pain above the eyes. With *maxillary* sinusitis – of which 10 per cent of cases are caused by tooth abscess or dental extraction – there is pain in the cheeks, which is often throbbing and made worse by stooping or moving the head. The nose is blocked on the affected side but there may be very little discharge. The senses of smell and taste are usually reduced.

Chronic sinusitis produces nasal discharge, low-grade pain, a blocked nose, cough and, in children, a tendency to EAR infections. The infection continues for weeks or months, and often follows an acute initial infection.

Sometimes infection of one of the frontal sinuses spreads around the eye, causing double vision, swelling of the eyelids or even an abscess behind the eyeball pushing it outwards. MENINGITIS or a brain abscess may also develop. Middle ear infections often occur with maxillary sinusitis and can result in deafness in the case of children. The infection may also spread downwards causing laryngitis or PNEUMONIA.

Treatment

It is important that sinusitis and all related infections are treated very thoroughly to prevent the development of possible serious complications.

An X-ray may be taken to locate trapped fluid. POLYPS – overgrowths of the mucus membrane lining the nose – may be present. Acute sinusitis is treated with antibiotics, decongestant nose-drops perhaps containing ephedrine, menthol inhalations and painkillers.

In some cases, it may be necessary to drain out the pus from the sinus through a small hole made on the inside of the nose. An operation may also be of use in chronic sinusitis or where there are polyps. In children with sinusitis, it is often best to remove the adenoids and tonsils. Washing out the sinuses with a salt water solution can also be helpful after pus has been drained off.

Skeleton

Some 206 BONES go to make up the skeleton of the average adult. The bones have a hard, thick, strong outer layer and a soft middle or marrow. They are as strong and as tough as concrete and can support great weights without bending, breaking or being crushed. Linked together by JOINTS and moved by MUSCLES which are attached at either end, they provide cages to protect the soft and delicate parts of the body. However, the way that all the parts are structured still allows for great flexibility of movement. In addition, the skeleton is the framework or scaffolding on which the other parts of the body are hung and supported.

Structure of the skeleton

Each of the different parts of the skeleton is designed to do a particular job. The skull or cranium (*see* HEAD) protects the brain and also the eyes and ears. The lower jaw and teeth are attached to it, enabling us to eat. There are holes for the eyes, ears, nose and mouth, and also one in the base of the skull where it joins the spinal column; the spinal cord passes through this, connecting the brain to every other part of the body.

The backbone or spine (*see* BACK) is made up of a chain of small bones, rather like cotton reels, called vertebrae, and forms the central axis of the skeleton. It has enormous strength, but because it is a rod made up of small sections, instead of being one solid piece of bone, it is also very flexible. This enables us to bend down and touch our toes and to hold ourselves stiff and upright. The vertebrae also protect the delicate spinal cord which passes through the middle. Between the vertebrae are discs of cartilage which act as cushions and help to protect them from rubbing on each other and becoming damaged as we bend down and straighten up. The bottom end or tip of the spinal column is called the *coccyx*. In some animals, such as the dog and cat, it's very much longer and forms a tail.

The rib-cage is made up of the ribs at the sides, the spinal column at the back and the breast-bone, or sternum, in front. It is designed to protect the heart and lungs which lie inside it, since damage to these organs could prove fatal. The rib-cage also expands to alter the volume of the lung cavities and this plays an important role in respiration.

The arms are joined on to the central axis of the spinal column by the shoulder girdle which is made up of the scapula (shoulder-blade) and the clavicle (collar-bone). The big bone of the upper arm is called the humerus and is joined at the elbow to the two bones of the forearm: the radius and ulna. The hand is made up of a large number of small bones. This makes it possible for us to grip things and to carry out delicate, complicated movements in which each of the many parts of the hand moves in a different, but highly co-ordinated way.

The LEGS are attached to the spine by the pelvic girdle, which shields the reproductive organs and the bladder and gives protection to the develop-

Skeletal growth

The proportions of the human skeleton change dramatically as people grow. In a baby, the mid-point of the skeleton is at the navel, whereas in an adult it is at the pubic symphisis, just above the genitals. Scaling the baby to adult size (below) shows just how large a baby's head is in relation to its body.

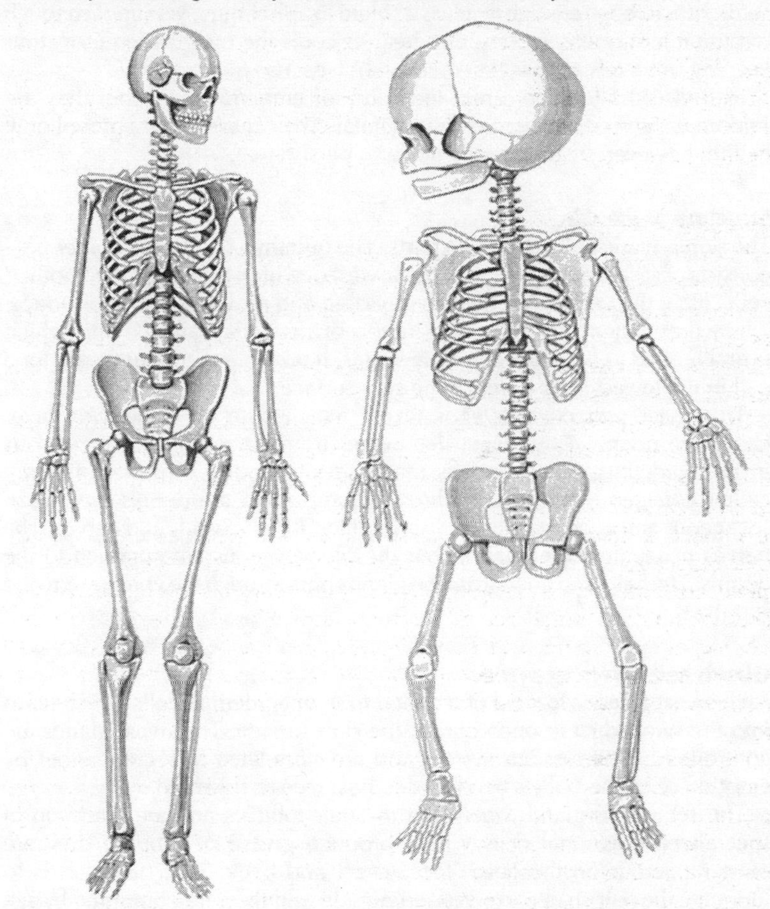

ing baby which lies in this part of its mother's body. The femur – the thick bone of the thigh – is the longest bone in the body. Its round head fits into the socket in the pelvis to form the HIP joint which is designed to maximize freedom of movement of the leg. There are two bones in the lower leg – the shin bone or tibia and the much thinner fibula. The foot (*see* FEET), like the hand, is made up of a complicated arrangement of small bones. This enables us to both stand firmly and comfortably and also to walk and run without falling over.

Skin and skin diseases

The skin is much more than a simple wrapping around our bodies. It is an active and versatile organ which is waterproof so that we do not dry up in the heat or melt in the rain, and it protects us from the damaging radiation of sunlight. It is tough enough to act as a shield against injury, yet supple enough to permit movement. It conserves heat or cools the body as required, thus keeping our internal TEMPERATURE constant (*see also* HOMOEOSTASIS).

Skin diseases may be a nuisance and an embarrassment, but they are seldom dangerous and are very rarely fatal. They cause a vast amount of ill health, however, by their frequency and persistence.

Structure of the skin

The skin is made up of two main parts. The outermost part – the *epidermis* – consists of several layers of cells, the lowest of which are called the 'mother' cells. Here the cells are constantly dividing and moving up to the surface, where they flatten, die and consist largely of a material called *keratin* which is finally shed as tiny, barely visible scales. It takes three to four weeks for a cell in the lowest layer to reach the skin surface.

This outer protective layer is firmly attached to an underlying layer called the *dermis.* Tiny, finger-like bulges from the dermis fit into sockets in the epidermis. The dermis is made up of bundles of protein fibres – called *collagen* – and elastic fibres. Embedded in the dermis are sweat, sebaceous and apocrine glands, HAIR follicles, blood vessels and nerves. The nerves penetrate the epidermis but the blood vessels are confined to the dermis. The hairs and ducts from the glands pass through the epidermis to the surface.

Glands and nerves

Each sweat gland is formed of a coiled tube of epidermal cells which leads into the sweat duct to open out on the skin surface. The sweat glands are controlled by the nervous system and are stimulated to secrete either by emotion or by the body's need to lose heat (*see* PERSPIRATION).

The sebaceous glands open into the hair follicles and are made up of specialized epidermal cells which produce grease or sebum. They are most numerous on the head, face, chest and back. Their function is to lubricate the hair shaft and surrounding skin and they are controlled by sex HORMONES.

The apocrine glands develop at puberty and are found in the armpits, breasts and near the genitals. They are odour-producing and are a sexual characteristic. When they begin to function, they secrete a thick milky substance.

There is a fine network of nerve endings in both layers of skin, and they are particularly numerous at the fingertips. They transmit pleasurable sensations of warmth and touch, as well as cold, pressure, itching (*see* PRURITUS) and PAIN which may evoke protective reflexes.

Hair and nails

Hair and nails are both specialized forms of keratin. Although nails are produced by living skin cells, the nail itself is dead and will not hurt or bleed if it is damaged. The visible part of the nail is called the 'nail body', and its shape is partly determined by genetic factors. The bottom part of the nail – the 'root' – is implanted in a groove in the skin. The 'cuticle' overlaps the root, which is the site of active growth. As the cells divide and move upwards, they become thickened and toughened with keratin, and when they die, they become part of the nail itself.

Hair is formed by cells in the hair follicles. There are two types: fine, downy hair, which is found over most of the body except the palms of the hands and soles of the feet; and thick, pigmented hair, which is present on the scalp, eyebrows, beard and genital areas.

Skin colour

Skin colour is due to the black pigment MELANIN which is produced by pigment cells in the lowest layer of the epidermis. There is the same number of pigment-producing cells in the skin of all races, but the amount of melanin produced varies. In dark-skinned people, more melanin is created than in light-skinned people.

Other factors contributing to skin colour are the blood in the blood vessels of the skin and the natural yellowish tinge of the skin tissue. The state of the blood within the blood vessels can greatly change skin colour. Thus we become 'white' with fear when small vessels close off, 'red' with anger due to an increased blood flow, and 'blue' with cold when most of the oxygen in the blood moves out to the tissues as the blood flow slows down.

Skin conditions in children

BIRTHMARKS are marks which are present on a baby's skin at birth or appear soon afterwards. They include strawberry marks, moles and port wine stains. Many birthmarks do not require treatment and disappear of their own accord. Strawberry marks, for instance, appear a few weeks after birth and grow rapidly for a while, but the majority disappear completely by the time the child goes to school.

MOLES are not usually present at birth but develop in childhood, gradually increasing in size during adult life and possibly disappearing in old age. They are formed from collections of the pigment-producing cells in the skin, and their significance is that they may very occasionally become malignant.

Babies and children have their own particular complaints – these include infant *cradle cap* and NAPPY RASH. Cradle cap is a normal collection of scales and grease which stick together and adhere to the scalp. It can be removed by gentle shampooing after the scales have been softened with olive oil the night before.

Infection of the skin frequently occurs in childhood since the skin's natural defences have not yet been built up against BACTERIA, VIRUSES and FUNGI. IMPETIGO is a bacterial infection of the superficial layers of skin which is particularly likely to happen where skin is already damaged. It starts as a little red spot that enlarges and blisters to form a honey-coloured crust. It is easily treated with antibiotics.

RINGWORM is caused by several kinds of fungi and gets its name from the ringed appearance of the rash. Sites most commonly affected are the scalp, groin and feet. It is rare in adults because of their greater immunity, and it is thought that the sebaceous glands on the scalp may have some protective effect. Treatment is with anti-fungal preparations.

WARTS are the commonest virus infection of the skin. They tend to be found on the hands, knees and soles of the feet (*see* VERRUCA), since the virus enters wherever the skin is broken. It lives in the outer layer of skin and causes very little damage so a wart may pass unnoticed for months or even years. When the body becomes aware of its presence, it mobilizes its defences and the wart may disappear as if by magic – hence the success of many wart charms and cures.

The hormonal changes which occur at puberty affect the skin chiefly by activating the grease-producing glands. Sweating and blushing can be annoying problems for teenagers. Excessive sweating of the armpits and hands which is caused by emotion and heat can be treated with aluminium chloride deodorants applied locally. Blushing is not usually treated but tends to diminish as confidence increases. Most teenagers develop a few ACNE spots which sometimes require medical attention.

Skin conditions in adults

As the skin ages, there is a falling-off in the production of natural emollients and it becomes dry. This drying process results in cracks in the skin, leaving it open to irritants at work or at home. People who work with chemicals, oils or detergents often get skin conditions. Industrial DERMATITIS is a commoner cause of absence from work than any other industrial disease. ('Dermatitis' is the term used for ECZEMA which is thought to be due to an external cause.)

Eczema is also common, giving rise to discomfort and disability at all ages. It presents different appearances at different stages and may last from a few days to a lifetime. Initially there is reddening of the affected skin with itching followed by pinhead swelling. Blisters then form and there is weeping and scaling.

Skin allergies are often manifested in the development of *urticaria*, or 'hives'. The RASH consists of white weals surrounded by reddened skin which itches, but it does not last longer than a few hours. New weals may appear, however, so that the condition persists for days or weeks. The cause is often something that has been eaten – fruit or shellfish, for instance – while some people are allergic to preservatives and synthetic dyes.

The commonest fungus infection of the skin is ATHLETE'S FOOT. The first signs are itching and peeling of the skin between the toes which are often worse on one foot. Relapses are common in the summer, but the condition usually settles in cool weather, and remedies are simple and effective.

As the skin ages, it not only dries out but it also loses its elasticity and does not heal so easily. Wounds leave only slight scars which may be barely visible in a few months. Many people also develop skin tags, sun-induced keratoses

Structure of the skin

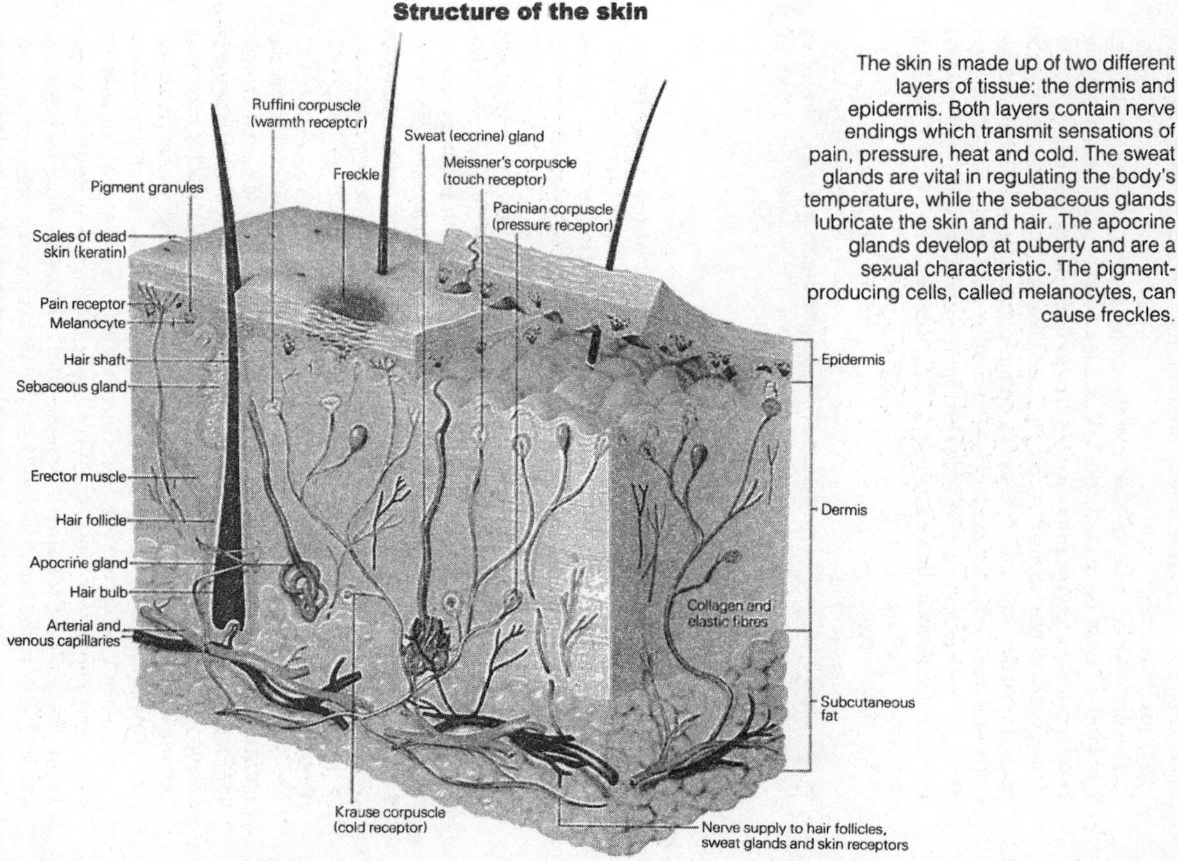

The skin is made up of two different layers of tissue: the dermis and epidermis. Both layers contain nerve endings which transmit sensations of pain, pressure, heat and cold. The sweat glands are vital in regulating the body's temperature, while the sebaceous glands lubricate the skin and hair. The apocrine glands develop at puberty and are a sexual characteristic. The pigment-producing cells, called melanocytes, can cause freckles.

– greyish patches of skin – and *seborrhoeic warts.* These are brownish-black warty lesions which commonly appear on the covered parts of the body after the age of 50. They are easily treated by freezing or scraping off with a specialist instrument.

The commonest type of skin cancer is the *rodent ulcer* or basal cell carcinoma. These do occur in the UK, but are even more commonly found among fair-skinned people who live in sunny climates, such as Australia. They usually occur on the face and neck and are slow-growing. Usually the patient notices that a small crusty lesion has been present for some months and forms a new scab when the crust is removed. As it enlarges, a depression forms in the centre and a rolled edge becomes visible. They are easily treated by local excision if small enough or by RADIOTHERAPY, and are the least dangerous of all cancers.

See also SUNBURN.

Skull, *see* Bones and bone diseases, Head and head injuries, Skeleton

Sleep and sleep problems

During a normal working day, we use up energy and tire ourselves both physically and mentally, and if we try to do without regular periods of rest, we become exhausted. The most complete form of rest is sleep: for our bodies and minds to be fresh and healthy and to work efficiently, each of us needs to spend a part of each 24 hours in sleep.

Of course, our bodies and minds don't stop working altogether while we are asleep – we go on breathing and our hearts continue to beat. Indeed, many parts of our bodies never rest: our eyelids flicker, we usually turn over several times and kick about, and some of us talk and even walk about in our sleep. But even though the vital processes of living, such as respiration and the circulation of blood, still continue, they do so at a much slower rate.

What happens to the brain?

The sleep/wakefulness controls are located in the brain-stem. Unless the cortex of the cerebral hemispheres, the 'thinking' part of the BRAIN, is activated by the brain-stem, it is too torpid for intellectual activity and we say it is asleep. When we are awake, the cerebral hemispheres are at a high pitch of activity, enabling us to understand and respond to the things we see and hear. The SPINAL CORD is also highly tuned: it receives instructions from the brain to fire off carefully adjusted nerve messages which travel from the spinal cord cells along nerves to the muscles that make our limbs move. Responsiveness in the cerebral cortex and in the spinal cord is brought about by electrical influences from the brain-stem. When we are awake, the brain-stem pours these currents along nerve channels. Just as, when the sun shines, insects and plants become active, so the brain-stem 'activates' the cerebral hemispheres and spinal cord and we wake up.

Waking or sleeping?

What causes the brain-stem sleep/wakefulness centre sometimes to bring about wakefulness, sometimes sleep? Among other things, a sort of chemical clock makes us sleepy every 24 hours. The clock setting is quite difficult to change, as one discovers after a long flight to a country in a different time zone – for example North America where clocks are set five to eight hours behind those in Britain. For the first week, one finds oneself nodding off in the late afternoon but waking and feeling bright in the early hours of the local morning. The sleep/wakefulness centre is also much affected by lack of sleep. But overriding everything else is the effect of the things going on around us and their significance. No matter how sleepy you are, if someone pulls your hair or sits you up, you will almost certainly wake up. In other words, the brain-stem centre is stimulated by physical sensations, and especially *change* of sensation. But it is not only nerve messages from the body's sense organs that are stimulating. The sleep/wakefulness centre also receives messages from the cortex of the cerebral hemispheres, so that a worrying thought going round and round in your mind bombards the brain-stem with stimulating messages which keep you awake.

Also important in keeping us awake is variety. If the sights and sounds around us are monotonous and we are immobile, there is nothing new to stimulate the brain-stem and sleep comes easily. Some continuous rhythm, like the drumming of train wheels, adds to the effect. A warm temperature will also help to bring about relaxation. The brain-stem centre is also affected by chemicals and drugs – some, such as amphetamines, will prevent sleep, and others, such as alcohol or sleeping pills, will have the opposite effect and make you drowsy.

There are rare people who regularly devote less than three hours to sleep and others who demand more than nine hours – everyone is different. The majority of adults average just under eight hours' sleep, although children sleep longer and old people less.

You can, over a short period, build up a 'sleep-debt' and, if forced to make do with short hours of sleep for a spell of days or weeks, will take more than the average eight hours at the weekend or holiday break. Although at times you may manage to keep going on a reduced sleep ration, you probably do not feel really well and almost certainly are not quite so efficient nor so attentive to detail in your daily tasks.

Dreaming

Not only do we need sleep, we need two different kinds. There is a definite pattern of events during prolonged sleep, with increased restlessness, change in the electrical brain waves (*see* ELECTROENCEPHALOGRAM), and spells of *rapid eye movement* occurring about every one-and-a-half hours – and lasting about 20 minutes each time. If people are deliberately woken during the rapid eye movement periods, they usually say they have just been dreaming. If woken at other times, they usually say they have not been dreaming and, indeed, have apparently forgotten the dream which presumably accompanied the previous rapid eye movement period.

The rapid eye movement phase of sleep is also known as REM or *paradoxical* sleep. In these phases, the electrical brain waves are faster than in the orthodox, non-rapid eye movement (NREM) phases. The heart rate, breathing and blood pressure undergo rapid fluctuations during REM sleep, especially at the time of a sudden flurry of eye movements. Most bodily muscles are completely relaxed, the usual reflexes are absent, in men the penis is often erect, the blood flows more rapidly through the brain and less flows through the muscles. At these times, there is dreaming.

In the NREM phase of sleep into which we always first pass for an hour or so before switching into the REM phase, the brain waves are large and slow. Electrical activity of most individual brain cells is lessened. During this phase, the body's cells and tissues repair and renew themselves wherever this is necessary. In babies and children, it is known that growth occurs most actively during this phase of sleep.

Sleepwalking

Sleepwalking – *somnambulism* – is a disorder that occurs most commonly in children, but it may also involve adults. It is thought to affect about 2 per cent of the population. It was once believed that sleepwalking was actually 'acting out' a dream, and that it took place during periods of shallow sleep. However, experiments have revealed that sleepers walk during the *deepest* phases of sleep. Episodes last from 30 seconds to a few minutes.

Sleepwalkers observed in laboratories walk with open, but expressionless eyes, giving them a blank or dazed look. Some do no more than sit up in bed and lie down again, while others walk around aimlessly, in a rigid, robot-like fashion. They often rub some object repetitively. Most eventually go back to bed of their own accord, and all may eventually be led back without difficulty. In every case, when they wake up they remember nothing about the incident.

Although many people believe that sleepwalkers have some deep psychological problem, this is rarely so. In most cases, sleepwalking should just be regarded as a normal variant of the sleeping pattern. Children normally grow out of sleepwalking, and sleepwalkers seldom harm themselves, but precautions are advisable. Doors and windows should be locked, and things such as electric fires and sharp objects should be taken out of the sleepwalker's room. If you find someone walking in his sleep, help him back to bed. Don't wake him unless you have to: he may become disorientated and confused.

Insomnia

Difficulties in sleeping are a common and disturbing adult complaint. Insomnia may manifest itself as difficulty in getting to sleep, interrupted sleep, or waking up too early. Worry, STRESS and DEPRESSION are by far the commonest causes: but PAIN, uncomfortable surroundings, fever, breathing difficulties on lying down (*orthopnoea*), a need to pass urine frequently and INDIGESTION may also give rise to it.

There are many ways you can help yourself over sleeplessness. It is important to make sure that no unresolved tensions are left over from the day, because these are virtually certain to interfere with your sleep: if possible, settle all family quarrels before you go to bed. When you are in bed, go over all the events of the day in your mind – from the time you woke up. Things happen to us so fast during the day that often our minds cannot 'digest' them properly. That 'undigested' material is a disturber of sleep.

Surroundings matter, too – quietness, warmth and a firm mattress are good investments. Adequate physical fatigue can be important; it helps if your body is tired as well as your mind. If you don't get much exercise in your job, a late night walk is often a successful way of dealing with insomnia. And if something is going round and round in your mind so that you can't sleep, half an hour downstairs with a good but unexciting book or listening to music is much more effective than tossing and turning.

Any difficulty in sleeping that goes on for more than two weeks should be referred to a doctor – by this time, the cause needs to be identified and treated. Sleeping pills and TRANQUILLIZERS can only be regarded as a temporary aid to sleeping problems – they are never a permanent solution. They easily give rise to addiction, and make you less of a person than you would otherwise be – less alert, less aware, less alive.

See also RELAXATION and SNORING.

Sleeping sickness, *see* Tropical diseases

Slipped disc

BACK problems are an extremely common cause of PAIN and suffering. It is estimated that more days of work are lost in the UK through backache than through strikes. There are many causes of backache, of which slipped disc is only one of the range of possibilities.

What is a slipped disc?

The discs are pads of tissue situated between each of the vertebrae which make up the spine. Each disc consists of a tough, fibrous outer layer and a softer, jelly-like inner layer called the nucleus. The function of the disc is both to act as a strong connection between the vertebrae and as a cushion to absorb loads on the spinal column.

A slipped disc doesn't really slip; the tough outer layer cracks open and the softer inner layer protrudes, or prolapses out through the crack, like toothpaste coming out through the crack in a toothpaste tube. For this reason, doctors prefer to speak of a disc protrusion or prolapse rather than a 'slipped disc'.

The soft inner layer of a disc is softest and most like jelly during childhood. Over the years, this material gradually dries out so that, by middle age, it is like crab meat. As age increases, it becomes even firmer. In the elderly, the disc is really just a section of scar tissue. Disc protrusion therefore becomes more uncommon as age increases and it is really a disorder affecting young and early middle-aged adults.

The disc protrusion occurs where the outer layer of the disc is weakest, that is just in front of the nerve roots which emerge from the SPINAL CORD at each vertebrae level. If a person has a slightly narrow spinal canal, the protruding disc material presses on the nerve root at that level and causes the symptoms of a slipped disc.

By far the commonest level of the spine to be affected is the lowermost part of the back. Here the greatest strains occur so it is not surprising that most discs which fail are at this level. It is possible, however, for discs to protrude at any level along the length of the spinal column – in the back or neck.

The disc begins to protrude when a crack develops in its tough outer layer. This is usually a result of wear and tear in the back as a result of normal ageing. One particularly heavy or awkward lift, a fall or even a sudden cough or sneeze may force some soft disc nucleus to protrude, giving rise to sudden symptoms.

Symptoms

When a protruding disc presses on a nerve root, symptoms occur both in the back and in the area which the nerve root supplies; in the lower back, this means the legs.

Symptoms in the back can include severe backache which the sufferer will not be able to localize very accurately. He or she may also develop painful muscle spasms in the muscles that lie along each side of the spine, particularly in the early stages. The patient will feel more pain when moving about and some relief when lying flat. Coughing or sneezing can cause the protruding disc material to bulge out suddenly, causing a sharp pain in the back or legs. In addition there may be a curvature of the spine – the patient unconsciously 'leans away' from the side of the disc protrusion to try to take the pressure off the nerve root that is involved.

If the pressure on the nerve root is not too severe, the nerve will continue to work but will be painful. The brain cannot tell that the painful pressure is coming from the area of the disc, but instead interprets the information as pain originating in the nerve end. In a lower back disc protrusion, the sciatic nerve can therefore be irritated and the individual may feel pain in the thigh, calf, ankle or foot; this pain is called SCIATICA.

More severe pressure on the nerve root may cause the nerve to stop functioning altogether. Areas of skin which this nerve supplies will become numb, so that a light touch or even a pinprick cannot be felt. Muscles supplied by the nerve will become weak or even completely paralysed. The reflexes such as the knee-jerk reflex may disappear. If only one nerve root is involved, this is not too serious, since each nerve supplies only a small area of skin or a limited number of muscles. If the nerves to the bladder or genitals are affected, however, their function can be permanently lost and such cases need urgent medical attention to relieve the pressure on these nerves.

Treatment

Well over 90 per cent of people with acute disc protrusions get better simply by resting and waiting for nature to cure them. The soft inner disc material tends to dry up and shrink once it has undergone protrusion, thus relieving the pressure on the nerve root.

The main form of treatment therefore is rest. Once the doctor has examined the individual and confirmed that there is a straightforward disc prolapse, he or she will advise the patient to rest by lying flat in bed. In the horizontal position, the pressure within the disc which acts to force out the soft inner material is minimal. In the standing position, this pressure is higher, and when the back is bent – for example, when sitting or bending over – the pressure is much higher. A saggy bed also bends the back so it is best to put boards under the mattress or even to put the mattress on the floor.

PAINKILLING drugs are of help in dulling the pain in acute disc protrusion, although they will probably not take it away altogether. Drugs which relax the muscles, such as chlormezanone, help to settle muscle spasm. Sedatives such as Valium (diazepam) may also help muscle spasm and interrupt the cycle of pain and spasm.

Most patients will get better if strict bedrest is undertaken for a few days to three weeks. Great patience is required – there is no way that nature's healing processes can be speeded up. Getting up too soon will often result in a relapse.

Patients who fail to make a recovery after a proper course of rest may need further treatment. This may entail a period of rest in hospital, perhaps with traction to the legs to help relieve the pain. If this fails, a special X-ray may be necessary. Ordinary X-rays show only the bones of the spine – the disc itself appears only as a space between the bones and this space is not altered in an acute disc prolapse. The special X-ray is called a *radiculogram* or a *myelogram*. A dye which shows on X-rays is injected into the space just outside the spinal canal; if the disc is protruding, it shows as an indentation in the column of dye. Nowadays CT scans or magnetic resonance images (MRI) of the spine are commonly used to detect slipped discs instead of myelograms.

An operation to remove the protruding disc material may be necessary if an adequate course of rest fails to improve symptoms, if there are signs of rapidly worsening function of nerve roots or if the nerves to the bladder or the genitals are involved.

The operation – a LAMINECTOMY – involves making a small opening in the bones surrounding the spinal cord and gently pushing it aside along with the nerve roots in order to remove the disc material. Patients can usually get up within two weeks of this operation.

An alternative to a full laminectomy has been developed which saves a long stay in hospital. With the patient under anaesthetic, the surgeon places a needle through the back muscles right into the disc, using X-rays to locate it properly. An injection of a drug called papain is made into the disc, whose tissues are dissolved away. The success rate of this technique is not quite as high as a laminectomy, but it is a much simpler alternative for the patient and avoids the scar of laminectomy.

Many people suffering from disc prolapse receive other forms of treatment such as PHYSIOTHERAPY and MANIPULATION. Physiotherapy may consist of heat treatment which temporarily lessens the pain, and traction exercises. TRACTION helps to relieve pain, probably by decreasing muscle spasm. Exercises help to strengthen the muscles of the back and stomach so that they can take some of the strain off the bones and joints in the spine. None of these treatments has been shown to speed up the healing process, but they make the individual more comfortable in the short term.

Manipulation is practised by many physiotherapists, some doctors and all osteopaths. The aim is to move the protruding disc material away from its point of contact on the nerve root and to free the nerve from any inflammation in the area. There is no evidence to show that the soft protruding disc material can actually be placed back into the firm outer casing of the disc – this would be like trying to suck toothpaste back into its tube – but enough movement to take some pressure off the nerve root may be achieved. Manipulation is probably more useful in other types of back disorders, although some individuals receive excellent results from manipulation for prolapsed disc. Treatments should, however, be undertaken by well-qualified practitioners.

Back supports, corsets and plaster jackets are used by some doctors to prevent patients from bending their backs during the recovery period after a disc prolapse. They can provide a valuable temporary support to avoid placing too much strain on the spine again.

Prevention

People who have suffered from disc prolapse and those who are at risk because of their occupation need to learn to look after their backs. Proper lifting procedures such as keeping the back straight, bending at the knees rather than bending the back when picking things up from the floor, and avoiding lifting too much weight are all important. It is also vital not to become too overweight – every pound of weight puts additional strain on the back. Regular exercise will increase the efficiency of the back muscles. Swimming is particularly beneficial since the effects of gravity are eliminated and the discs are not placed under undue strain. A firm mattress helps to prevent the back from sagging into a bent position.

Smallpox

This was once the commonest of the dangerous, fatal VIRUS diseases. But in 1979, the World Health Organization declared the world free of the disease. This is certainly one of the most remarkable successes of preventive medicine that the world has yet seen. But before this, the disease was widespread and many people are still marked by the scars left by the smallpox spots.

A famous eighteenth-century English doctor, Edward Jenner, discovered that people who had been exposed to cows with the disease cowpox seemed to be immune to the effects of smallpox. He invented successful IMMUNIZATION, but it took half a century for the true value of his method to be recognized by the medical establishment.

In the middle 1960s, smallpox was to be found in about 50 countries and no country was entirely free from the disease because of the increased amount of international air travel. By the early 1970s, the number of countries was down to about 20, and the last major outbreak from the disease was finally eliminated from Bangladesh in 1975.

The success of the eradication campaign depended upon mass immunization and the rapid diagnosis and isolation of cases. Of course, this was easy enough to organize in a developed country like the UK but in Bangladesh and elsewhere in the developing world, trained medical staff were few and far between. Despite these difficulties, the World Health Organization was able to educate the population sufficiently well so that they could recognize the disease quickly and isolate cases.

Smell

The sense of smell is probably the oldest and the least understood of our five senses. During evolution, the most primitive sense has kept its connections with the part of the BRAIN which grew to be the sorting house for our emotional responses, intimately linking smells to our emotions.

Our sense of smell also plays an important role in sexual attraction, although this has become considerably muted during human evolutionary development. Its most important roles are those of a warning system and information gatherer: warning us of danger and giving us valuable information about the outside world.

How do we smell things?

As with many organs in the body, the smelling apparatus is duplicated, each circuit acting independently.

The sensory receptors for smell are found in the roof of the nasal cavity (*see* NOSE), just beneath the frontal lobes of the brain. This is called the *olfactory area* and is tightly packed with millions of small cells, the *olfactory cells*. Each olfactory cell has about a dozen fine hairs – *cilia* – which project into a layer of mucus. The mucus keeps the cilia moist and acts as a trap for odorous substances, while the cilia effectively enlarge the area of each olfactory cell and so increase our sensitivity to smells.

It is not clearly understood how the minute amounts of chemical substances which give us smells trigger off the olfactory cells, but it is thought that these substances dissolve in the mucus fluids, stick to the cilia and then cause the cells to fire off electrical signals.

Olfactory nerve fibres channel these signals across the bone of the skull to the two olfactory bulbs in the brain, where the information is gathered, processed and then passed through a complicated circuitry of nerve endings to the cerebral cortex. Here the message is identified and the smell becomes a conscious fact.

The exact molecular mechanism of the sense of smell is still largely unknown. Quite how the receptor cells can detect thousands of different odours and distinguish minute differences between them remains a mystery.

Links between smell and taste

The close link between the sense of taste and the sense of smell is something we are not always aware of. Only when we have a cold do we realize that not only can we not smell things, but the taste of food has also vanished.

Much of what we think of as taste is really smell. In fact, our sense of smell is far more sensitive – 10,000 times more sensitive. The taste buds in the tongue monitor relatively crude sensations of salt, sweet and sour, while the more sophisticated 'taste' sensations are made by the smell receivers in the nose. Faint vapours of whatever we are eating drift into the nasal cavity where the smell receptors add more detail to the information given by the taste buds.

When the nose becomes blocked, the gas and vapours cannot move over the receiver cells; consequently, we cannot smell anything and can only taste the cruder tastes.

'Smelling problems'

A decrease in the ability to smell is most commonly due to trouble in the nose, as in the common COLD or SINUSITIS. Heavy SMOKERS also suffer a loss of smelling ability and this is due to the delicate smell tissue drying up.

HEAD INJURIES can cause a loss of smell, and the injury need not be a serious one. It is thought that the delicate olfactory nerves, which pierce the bottom of the skull, are either bruised or even sheared off by the knock on the head. The loss of smell can be permanent and may affect only one nostril or both.

Diseases within the skull can also be associated with a loss of smell, though these are not very common. A TUMOUR or aneurysm (*see* ARTERIES) pressing on the olfactory nerves may impair the sense of smell, or may just temporarily interrupt the ability to smell. MENINGITIS and internal haemorrhaging may also affect smell.

Smoking

People smoke for a wide variety of reasons. Once they have smoked their first few experimental cigarettes, which can cause coughing, nausea and sometimes vomiting, most smokers get pleasure from the taste and aroma of tobacco and tobacco smoke. They may also get pleasure from the whole ritual of lighting up.

Smokers make two claims for their habit. First, that smoking sedates them, or 'settles their nerves' when they need sedating. Second, that it acts as a stimulant when they need to work. Evidence has shown that these effects are due to nicotine and that both these claims are true, depending on the dose, on what the smoker is doing and on his or her particular psychological and physical make-up.

There may be a true physical addiction to nicotine so that, when deprived of the drug, the person concerned suffers from unpleasant physical withdrawal symptoms which are only relieved by a further dose. We know from research results that smokers of a cigarette with a high-nicotine content who change to a brand with a low-nicotine yield automatically increase their puff rate or smoke more cigarettes to get the same amount of nicotine as they did previously.

Dependence on smoking may be psychological as well as physical; smokers miss whatever they get from smoking but they do not really need it. Often, too, smoking has become such an ingrained habit that smokers smoke a cigarette almost without knowing it.

The climate of opinion in which we live is an important factor in determining smoking. Society was once made for smokers. In our homes and in friends' homes, in cinemas and when travelling, we were surrounded by ashtrays, and it was assumed that we needed and would use them. We were offered cigarettes, and the general assumption was that we smoked. However, things have changed drastically over the last decade. Following a lead from the Americans, British offices, public buildings, cinemas and other gathering places now ban or severely restrict smoking. Non-smokers now feel fully justified in refusing to allow smoking in their homes.

Cigarette manufacturers try to persuade us to smoke. However, with the decline in tobacco consumption, smokers are now in the minority, and even the majority of people who do smoke would like to give up, so the number of people who really feel that their smoking is 'usual' or a good thing for them is very small indeed.

Factors in starting smoking

Not wanting to feel left out is a particularly important factor in considering what happens to make children start smoking. Many children are conditioned almost from birth to the expectation that they will smoke. There are strong connections between children smoking and the smoking habits of their parents and older brothers and sisters.

Children in the early years at school usually disapprove of the tobacco habit intensely, just as they usually disapprove of the habit of drinking alcohol. By the early teens, however, they are at the stage of trying such things out, and this is because of the strong identification formed at an earlier stage between drinking and smoking and being and acting 'grown up'.

Once adolescence has been reached, the influence of a teenager's group of friends and acquaintances begins to exert itself. Young people believe – and they are often right – that the more extroverted, more sexually advanced and 'tougher' older teenagers smoke, while the less precocious but often more academically or athletically successful ones do not. Young people are torn between the two and, depending on what they wish for themselves and what they believe or have been led to believe, they will or will not opt for the smoking habit.

What's wrong with smoking?

Shortly after the end of the Second World War, Professor A. Bradford Hill and Dr (now Sir) Richard Doll published the first of a series of papers leading to the inescapable conclusion that cigarette smoking was the major factor in the rising incidence of LUNG CANCER. They began with a retrospective study – that is, they investigated a large number of patients with cancer of the lung and compared them with a carefully matched control group who did not have this form of cancer. After comparing a number of factors that might have a bearing on the cause of this disease, the only great difference to emerge was that the smoking habits of the two groups varied.

Only one in 200 male lung cancer patients were non-smokers, indicating smoking as the cause. The same sort of statistics appeared for women. Furthermore, there appeared to be a relationship between the risk of getting lung cancer and the number of cigarettes smoked.

Bradford Hill and Doll next set up an investigation that would study the prospective health of smokers. They had 25,000 British doctors give details of their smoking habits as well as a variety of other relevant information. As the years passed, some of these doctors died; Doll and Bradford Hill investigated the cause of death in each case. Some of the deaths were from lung cancer, and two facts emerged quite clearly. First, there was a very clear relationship between cigarette smoking and lung cancer. Second, the chances of dying from the disease increased with increasing cigarette consumption.

As the investigation into British doctors proceeded and the results of other investigations became available, it became clear that cigarette smoking was an important factor in causing other diseases, of which the most important are chronic BRONCHITIS and CORONARY HEART DISEASE. The end result was the demonstration of two important facts: first, cigarette smokers live, on average, shorter lives than non-smokers, and second, that giving up smoking removes this excess risk in proportion to the time elapsed since giving up.

In addition to the three main diseases mentioned above, there is evidence that cigarette smoking can cause other lung disorders, delays the healing of gastric ULCERS, plays a part in the cause of some cancers of the mouth, LARYNX, gullet and BLADDER, and leads to a degree of SKIN wrinkling appropriate to non-smokers who are 20 years older. Smoking is also a cause of IMPOTENCE in men and may contribute to reduced fertility in both men and women (*see* INFERTILITY). Smoking is a major factor in the development of athersclerosis, which not only causes coronary heart disease but also impairs the circulation in the legs, causing pain on walking, ulceration and often gangrene.

For non-smokers, only about one in five will not reach retirement age; for smokers of over 25 cigarettes a day, two in five will not reach this age. In other words, the risk is doubled, and it isn't only that smokers are more likely to die of certain diseases – they are more likely to be disabled by them.

The death rate for smokers is much higher among those who inhale than among those who do not; the earlier you start smoking, the greater the risk;

and the more you smoke, the greater the risk. According to American findings, the use of filter-tipped cigarettes does slightly reduce the risk of lung cancer.

Women and smoking

There are some special risks for women. Any woman who takes the CONTRACEPTIVE pill faces a very small but measurable risk of a serious side-effect, such as THROMBOSIS, STROKE or HEART ATTACK. A number of years ago, it was found that women who are on the pill and smoke are approximately eight times more likely to develop serious side-effects than women on the pill who are non-smokers.

Smoking has also been shown to be particularly damaging during PREGNANCY. The effects on an unborn child can be quite serious. Chemicals in cigarette smoke interfere with the circulation of blood through the placenta so that fewer nutrients are supplied to the unborn baby. As a result of this damage, women who smoke 20 or more cigarettes a day are twice as likely as non-smoking women to suffer certain complications of pregnancy such as MISCARRIAGE and bleeding during pregnancy. Smoking even a few cigarettes a day presents some extra risk – the more you smoke, the greater the risk. On average, a baby born to a smoking mother will be 200 g (8 oz) lighter than a baby born to a non-smoking mother, and there is also an increased risk of the baby dying around the time of birth or soon after.

Research studies have shown that the harmful effects of cigarette smoke on the unborn child can even be detected many years later. At 11 years of age, children born to smoking mothers are on average three months behind in school work compared to children born to mothers who did not smoke at all during pregnancy.

Effects of smoke on non-smokers

There is now quite conclusive evidence that exposure to cigarette smoke in the air can harm non-smokers. In 1986 an authoritative report was published by the Surgeon General in the United States which supported this conclusion, and a year later a similar report was issued by the British government.

The evidence presented in these reports is very detailed. One of the most conclusive findings concerned the risk of lung cancer in the non-smoking husband or wife of a smoker. The spouse of a smoker runs a risk of developing lung cancer which is two or three times the usual risk for a non-smoker. It has also been found that the children of parents who smoke are much more likely to develop bronchitis or PNEUMONIA, especially in the first year of life. Other forms of throat, ear and lung disease are more common among the children of smokers.

So far as adults are concerned, it is clear that certain people are more prone to the effects of smoke in the atmosphere than others. ASTHMATICS may develop acute attacks as a result of exposure to smoke, and other people may develop CONJUNCTIVITIS or a dry irritation of the throat. Indeed, chemical analysis of 'side-stream smoke', which is the smoke given off at the tip of the cigarette directly into the atmosphere, shows that it is more toxic than the smoke inhaled by the smoker.

Snoring

Snoring – breathing heavily through the mouth or NOSE with a vibrating or snorting noise when asleep – is chronic in as many as one in eight sleepers (*see* SLEEP AND SLEEP PROBLEMS). It is a medically innocent occurrence. But at the same time, few things can be quite as irritating as lying awake, listening to someone snore lustily. It's been suggested that this can cause marital disharmony – and it's no wonder, since the noise generated by the snoring partner may rival speaking, and can, at its worst, put a pneumatic drill to shame!

What causes snoring?

Snoring is an involuntary act. The characteristic noise is created when, for some reason, the sleeper begins to breathe through his or her mouth, and the muscles of the soft palate and the uvula are allowed to relax. Thus the passages through which air passes are narrowed, and as the sleeper inhales, the air drawn into the lungs causes the soft palate and the uvula to vibrate.

The quality and the intensity of the snoring will be governed by the shape of the mouth, the elasticity of the tissues and the vigour with which the snorer inhales. Occasionally a person snores so vigorously that he wakes himself up but generally he is oblivious to the noise he is making.

Snoring is most likely to occur when a person sleeps with his mouth open, so a blocked nose or anything obstructing the nasal airways which forces him to breathe through his mouth will make it more likely. A stuffy nose because of a cold, enlarged TONSILS OR ADENOIDS – any of these may make him likely to breathe through his mouth.

If the muscles of the lower jaw and palate relax in sleep, snoring may start. A person who is sitting up and falls asleep loses control over these muscles and they relax. This is why so many people snore when they fall asleep sitting up on trains or in armchairs. Similarly, people who lie on their backs when they are asleep may also be prone to snoring, because the lower jaw drops and the muscles of the palate relax.

People who are overweight are more likely to snore than their normal counterparts, because excess fat is laid down in the pharynx, increasing the obstruction to breathing at night. But it has been shown that if a snorer who is overweight loses a few pounds, there is likely to be a reduction of noise – if not a complete cessation of snoring.

Atmosphere, too, may have an effect. A very dry, centrally heated room can lead to snoring in a susceptible individual, as can a moist, over-humid environment.

Stopping snoring

Since snoring involves breathing through the mouth in sleep, most forms of treatment to alleviate the condition aim at trying to re-establish breathing through the nose. So if someone who does not normally snore contracts a cold and is told – presumably with some irritation – that he has started snoring, all he needs to do is relieve the symptoms of the cold, so that he can breathe through his nose again. In the same way, treating obstructions such as enlarged adenoids in the nasal airways will relieve, if not cure, the snoring.

Unfortunately, colds and nasal obstructions account for only a part of the snoring population, and other forms of treatment have to be tried in more indeterminate cases. Some are commonsense – for example, if a person snores when he is sleeping on his back, he can be persuaded to try to sleep on his side or his stomach.

It has been found that some heavy snorers actually stop breathing for some time at regular intervals through the night, only to start again with a heavy snort. This condition is called the *sleep apnoea syndrome*. It tends to make the person tired and irritable during the day, especially in the mornings. Treatment is with a machine called 'nasal continuous positive airways pressure' (CPAP) which supplies a constant pressure of air through a nasal mask. This holds the airway open, and ensures regular breathing and no snoring. The equipment has to be installed in the patient's bedroom and used every night.

Nasal decongestant sprays can be effective. If a sufferer uses too many pillows at night this bends the neck forward, and decreases the space in the pharynx making the snoring louder. The snorer should sleep on one flat pillow only and raise the head of the bed by putting blocks under the bed.

In extreme cases ENT surgeons can perform an operation for snoring in which the soft palate and uvula (which vibrates and causes the noise of snoring) are removed. This is called an 'uvulopalatopharyngoplasty' or UPPP. It is a painful operation and is not successful for everyone.

Sodium, *see* **Minerals, Salt**

Solvent abuse

Although commonly described as 'glue sniffing', the deliberate inhalation of vapours of organic solvents is better described as 'solvent abuse'. Children and adolescents are the main abusers, and there are a number of deaths each year in Britain from the effects of solvent inhalation. For this reason the dangers must be stressed.

Who does it?

Young people in the 8-to-16 age group are the main abusers; the peak age is 14. Boys are more frequently involved than girls. 'Peer influence' – following the example of other members of a group – is a contributing factor. The practice then spreads through a school or neighbourhood, becoming a fad or craze.

What is involved?

There are three methods of inhalation: putting the glue or other substance into a plastic or paper bag and breathing in and out; spraying the solvent on to a cloth and inhaling it through the mouth; and directly inhaling an aerosol spray – a particularly dangerous method.

If the solvent vapour is inhaled in sufficient concentration, a feeling of well-being or euphoria, comparable in some ways with that of alcohol intoxication, will be produced. Visual hallucinations often also occur. The effects of solvent sniffing are experienced within seconds.

Solvent abuse may become apparent in a number of ways. A child may behave as if he or she were drunk. His breath may smell of solvents, and he may have red nostrils or sores around the mouth. He may appear dreamy and moody, and there may be a loss of appetite. The finding of glue smears on skin or clothes, and paper or plastic bags and tubes or cans of glue or other substances, may confirm that the child has been sniffing a solvent.

Dangers

One of the main dangers of solvent abuse is suffocation, because insufficient oxygen reaches the brain during a sniffing session. Solvents sensitize the HEART to the effects of adrenalin, and a fatal disturbance of heart rhythm can occur. A single deep breath of certain solvents can result in cardiac arrest and instant death. Physical dangers to those who are intoxicated include drowning, falling from a height and road traffic accidents.

Long-term solvent abuse may cause permanent BRAIN damage. This condition, which is known as *solvent encephalopathy*, can produce behaviour disturbances, convulsions and coma. Solvent abuse can damage the BONE MARROW, leading to ANAEMIA, and it can also damage the lungs, kidneys and liver. In some cases, solvent abuse can lead to ALCOHOL abuse.

Treatment

Solvents are not physically addictive, and withdrawal symptoms do not occur, but it is clear that there is psychological addiction in the small proportion who become chronic abusers. No 'drying out' is necessary as there is with alcoholism, but the habit does need to be broken, and medical help is usually needed. Some chronic abusers have been known to use as much as 3½ pints (about 2 litres) of glue daily, and this itself may lead to committing crimes to fund their habit.

Sore throat, *see* Larynx and laryngitis, Pharynx

Spastic colon, *see* Irritable bowel syndrome

Spasticity, *see* Brain and brain disease, Cerebral palsy

Speech

This is one of the most complex and delicate operations that the body is asked to undertake. Ultimately, all speech, talking and comprehension are controlled and coordinated by the BRAIN. In the cerebral cortex, there are areas called the *speech centres* where words are deciphered and signals and instructions are sent out to the hundreds of muscles in the LUNGS, THROAT and mouth that are involved in producing speech. All this complex control is something that we are born with the ability to do, but the actual way we speak and the sounds we make are learned from our parents and the people around us as we grow up.

Thinking and speaking

The cerebral cortex of the brain is divided up into left and right sections called hemispheres; speech, and its associated functions are usually concentrated in one hemisphere. In a right-handed person, this is usually in the left hemisphere, and in a left-handed person, it is usually in the right hemisphere. This area of the brain is divided into the *motor speech centre* which controls the muscles of the mouth and throat, and the *sensory speech centre* which interprets the incoming sound signals coming along the nerves from the ears. Also nearby are the parts of the brain which coordinate HEARING (by which we comprehend what others around us are saying), vision (by which we decipher the written word; *see* EYES AND EYESIGHT) and the complex hand movements used in writing, playing an instrument and so on.

Conversation is a very complicated procedure. The first thing that happens when we hear a person speaking is that the hearing centres, in the cerebral cortex, recognize the jumble of incoming auditory signals from the ears. The sensory speech centre decodes the words so that the other parts of the brain involved in the process can then recognize the words and formulate an answer. Once a reply has been thought up, the motor speech centre and another part of the brain, called the *brain stem*, come into operation. The brain stem controls both the intercostal muscles, between the ribs, which inflate the lungs, and the abdominal muscles which determine the pressure of the incoming and outgoing air. As air is expelled from the lungs, the motor speech areas signal the vocal cords (*see* LARYNX) simultaneously to move into the stream of air in the throat, causing the cords to vibrate and produce a simple sound. This is called *phonation*.

The amount of pressure applied to the lungs during exhalation governs the speed with which the air passes over the vocal cords, and the faster the air, the louder the sound produced. During whispering, the vocal cords are set wide apart so that they do not actually vibrate as the air passes between them, they merely act as friction surfaces. But for the most part, the shaping of words is performed by movements of the lips, TONGUE and soft palate – controlled by the cortex.

Producing speech sounds

To turn the simple sounds produced by the vocal cords into intelligible words, the lips, the tongue, the soft palate, and the chambers which give resonance to the voice all play a part. The resonating chambers include the whole mouth chamber, the nose, the sinuses, the PHARYNX (the part of the throat between the mouth and the oesophagus) and to a lesser degree the chest cavity.

The control of these structures is achieved by hundreds of tiny muscles which work very closely together and at incredible speed. Put simply, speech is made up of vowels and consonants – vowels are all phonated sounds.

The resonant qualities of the various chambers of the mouth and respiratory system provide us with the individuality of our voices. For instance, the so-called 'nasal sounds' like *m, n* and *ng* depend for their correct vocalization on free resonance in the nose; try pinching your nose when you say something – the comic effect shows how the air space of the nose gives our speech roundness and clarity. Different people have different shapes of nose, chest and mouth, hence different people have different sounding voices.

The skull also resonates when we speak, and we hear part of what we say transmitted through the bones of the skull, as well as what is picked up by the ears. This not only provides us with vital 'feedback' about what we are saying, but also explains why our voices sound so strange when played back through a tape recorder – the sounds we then hear being only those transmitted through air.

Speech defects

Because of the great complexity of the whole speech process, involving as it does many areas of the brain, the control of breathing and all the many muscles that manipulate the sound-producing and modifying apparatus, speech problems can be very complicated.

The disorders can be divided into a few basic types: problems of the voice (disorders of the larynx and its parts); problems of voice development; problems caused by damage to the various speech areas of the brain; abnormalities of the mouth; and problems brought on by or associated with DEAFNESS.

Basically, anything that gets in the way of the ability either to formulate speech (in the brain), communicate the commands to the bodily parts (along the nerve network) or execute the commands (in the muscles) can cause some kind of speech disorder.

Occasionally, disorders caused by problems with the NERVOUS SYSTEM are called *dysarthria*. Included in this category are such diseases as CEREBRAL PALSY, shaking palsy and chorea. Deafness can cause mutism because a deaf child will not be able to pick up the language being spoken around him. If the patient is deaf at birth, concentrated speech therapy must be undertaken using visual means to stimulate the correct vocalization of words.

These are some of the areas where there are problems with speech, and treatment of all speech defects depends on the actual cause of the disturbance. The determination of the cause can involve consultation with neurologists, psychologists or any of the other specialists that have some involvement with any of the speech-producing mechanisms. Any eventual treatment may also involve doctors and therapists from many specialities.

See also CLEFT PALATE AND HARE LIP.

Speech therapy

Many people confuse speech therapy with elocution or teaching people how to pronounce English clearly. But a speech therapist is not someone who changes accents or dialects – he or she helps children and adults who have speech or language difficulties that make it hard for them either to understand or to be understood. A speech therapist is responsible for assessment, diagnosis and treatment of any speech or language difficulty, and associated problems with swallowing due to laryngeal and pharyngeal weakness, usually after the patient has been referred by a doctor.

Speech difficulty

The main areas in which people need speech therapy are where they have difficulty in understanding speech or language, difficulty in articulation (pronunciation of sounds), difficulty in expressing ideas through spoken, written or sign language (following a STROKE or an accident perhaps).

Causes of speech or language difficulty in children include delayed development or disorder of articulation (pronunciation of sounds), delayed or disordered development of language, AUTISM, CLEFT PALATE, mental retardation, physical handicap, DEAFNESS, voice disorder and stammering. Adults can suffer from speech or language problems, caused by stroke, PARKINSON'S DISEASE, MULTIPLE SCLEROSIS or cancer of the LARYNX.

Difficulties in understanding and expression of speech and language vary enormously. In children, problems usually result from some kind of damage to the brain or the hearing or speaking apparatus from birth; or delayed and sometimes abnormal development in childhood. Adults have usually lost the ability to speak as a result of brain damage, as a result of damage to nerves supplying the speech muscles, or the deterioration of the muscles of speech through disease. In some cases of cancer of the larynx, the whole voice box is removed, and the patient has to learn to speak using the OESOPHAGUS.

Therapy for children

Unless the child's difficulty is purely in speaking, or the speech problems are very severe, the first area of treatment is language comprehension. In young children between the ages of three and six years, this is usually done through play. The parents also take a major role in continuing therapy in between sessions with the therapist. Typically, language is taught by playing with a doll's house, items of furniture and miniature people. Keeping language short and simple, the child is asked to select items – this teaches nouns. The child is then asked to do things with them, which teaches verbs.

Where children have difficulty in articulating, it is usually because they either do not know how to make the sounds or they do not recognize that certain sounds are different from other similar ones.

Sounds develop until the age of six or seven, so a speech therapist would not treat a four-year-old who has difficulty with only *s* or *r* as these are difficult sounds to say. In therapy, a child is first shown *how* to make the sound. He or she then says the sound by itself before going on to practise it as the first sound in short words. Then he or she says the sound at the end of words and finally in the middle of words in continuous speech.

Therapy for adults

Where speech or language is lost through brain damage as a result of stroke, the patient often recovers some or all of his or her speech spontaneously, usually between six months and two years after the stroke. The speech therapist's role is to guide and stimulate recovery with speech and language exercises. These range from pointing to pictures by name to reconstructing complex, abstract sentences in which written words have been jumbled.

The extent of recovery depends largely on the extent of brain damage. Some patients never recover speech and language. In these cases, other forms of communication are taught. These may include simple gesture or sign language, or just pointing at pictures of what the patient needs.

Dysarthria (slurred articulation), which can be caused by stroke or multiple sclerosis occurs because the tongue cannot move rapidly enough from one sound to another. The patient is told to slow down his speech in order to give himself time to make the sounds accurately. Tongue and lip exercises are practised in order to strengthen the muscles of speech.

Sperm

This is the name given to the male reproductive cell. Its only purpose is to achieve fertilization by union with the female cell, the *ovum* (*see* OVARIES).

Each sperm is about 0.05 mm in length and is shaped like a tadpole. It has three main sections which consist of a head, a mid-section and a tail. The front of the head – the *acrosome* – contains special enzymes which enable the sperm to penetrate into the ovum and so achieve fertilization. The mid-section contains structures called *mitochondria,* which hold the vital source of energy needed by the sperm on its journey to the ovum.

The tail's only function is to propel the sperm, which it does by moving in a whip-like fashion, generating a speed of about 3–3.5 mm per minute.

The sperm is made up of a number of chemicals and GENETIC material. These are the chromosomes (*see* CELLS AND CHROMOSOMES) which carry the genetic blueprint of the father, and which will determine the paternally inherited characteristics of the child. It is the sperm which carries the genetic message that determines the sex of the child.

The manufacture of sperm

The successful manufacture of sperm necessitates a temperature of about 5.5°F (3°C) lower than the rest of the body. Consequently, manufacture takes place outside the body, within the scrotum. Surrounding tissue helps to regulate the temperature of the TESTES (testicles) inside the scrotum by pulling them upwards towards the body in cold conditions, and by a rich supply of blood vessels which dissipate the heat when the temperature gets too high.

Sperm production – at the rate of 10 to 30 billion a month – takes place in the *seminiferous tubules* in the testicles. The newly formed sperm then passes through these into the *epididymis* which is located behind the testicles. This serves as a storage and development area, the sperm taking 60–72 hours to achieve full maturity. The epididymis can be emptied by three or four ejaculations (*see* PENIS) in 12 hours; it takes about two days to be refilled. If ejaculation does not take place, the sperm disintegrate and are absorbed back into the testicles.

Ejaculation

Before ejaculation occurs, the sperm moves along the *vas deferens* – two tubes connecting the testicles to the PROSTATE GLAND – and into a further storage area, the *ampulla*. Here, the sperm receive a secretion from the *seminal vesicles*, two coiled tubes adjoining the ampulla. This secretion, called *seminal fluid*, stimulates the motility (the ability to move) of the sperm, and helps them survive in the vaginal secretion. The prostate gland – through which the sperm pass during ejaculation – produces a small amount of a similar fluid, giving the sperm full motility.

At the moment of ejaculation, the sperm and seminal fluid are forced out of the ampullae and epididymes into the URETHRA by muscular contractions.

If the sperm have been ejaculated into the VAGINA of a woman, they move as fast as they can through the CERVIX and into the UTERUS, where they make their way into the Fallopian tubes. It is in these tubes that fertilization may occur if an egg is present.

What can go wrong

Fertilization is unlikely to take place if the concentration of the sperm is too low, if the sperm are abnormal in form or if they are unable to move or stop moving too soon. The condition of the seminal fluid is another vital factor, as it both nourishes and protects the sperm. A previous infection in the testicles (such as MUMPS) may be a cause of INFERTILITY, as can an injury to the testicles. Even stress and ill health, or very tight clothing, can cause temporary loss of fertility.

The number of normal, healthy sperm in one ejaculate varies widely, but there are normally about 100 million sperms per millilitre (ml) of semen. Most men with a sperm count of less than 20 million per ml of semen are infertile.

Where infertility is suspected a specimen of sperm will be tested in a pathology laboratory, and treatment and advice will depend on the cause. A man with a low sperm count may be advised to save up his sperm for a few days so as to produce the optimum number of sperm in his ejaculate. In other cases, ARTIFICIAL INSEMINATION is recommended. In certain cases of male infertility, drugs may be used and these may improve the sperm count.

See also VASECTOMY.

Spermicides, *see* **Contraception**

Spina bifida

Many people are confused about spina bifida because some affected children are normal whereas others are severely disabled. This is because there are different types of spina bifida – the name simply means that some of the bones in the spine have not joined properly. Many people have such an abnormality without realizing it, because it can be a harmless condition which causes no disability.

Possible causes

Spina bifida occurs more commonly in some families than in others. The reasons for this are not fully understood. But once doctors know a spina bifida foetus has been conceived, they may want to screen other members of the family – even cousins – who have become pregnant, as a risk has already been identified.

It has also been discovered recently that some mothers who have given birth to spina bifida babies – and who have a one in 25 chance of giving birth to another – may have been lacking in certain VITAMINS, and there is now some evidence to suggest that taking *folic acid* tablets before CONCEPTION may substantially reduce the chances of an affected baby being conceived.

Early research suggested that folic acid may be one of the vitamins important in the prevention of spina bifida. This is a B vitamin that occurs naturally in leafy green vegetables such as cabbage and broccoli. In a small trial carried out some years ago, women who had previously given birth to a spina bifida baby were given extra folic acid. The result of the trial showed some reduction in the risk of having a further spina bifida baby. Then a larger trial was conducted in Britain using a combination of several different vitamins. Women were given a multivitamin capsule from the very earliest stage of PREGNANCY, and this also resulted in a reduction in the expected number of spina bifida babies.

It is therefore likely that one of the major causes of spina bifida is a vitamin deficiency in the mother's diet. It is still not clear, however, whether the condition results from a deficiency of just one vitamin, such as folic acid, or of several vitamins. It is also possible that the basic underlying cause could be some other undetected factor which is counteracted by vitamins. Further research is being carried out to try to pin down the cause with greater accuracy.

Types of spina bifida

Sometimes a baby is born with a soft CYST on the back, which is called a *meningocoele*. It is usually on the neck or the bottom of the spine, but can occur at any point, and is an outward bulging of the fluid which surrounds the nerves and SPINAL CORD. The danger is that the skin covering it may be very thin, and may become damaged and liable to infection. Early surgery is very successful in this type of spina bifida, and the baby usually grows into a perfectly normal adult.

Unfortunately most cases of spina bifida are more serious. In these types of 'open' spina bifida, the baby is born with part of the backbone, some nerves and the spinal cord lying exposed at the bottom of the cyst – called a *myelomeningocoele* – which often bursts even before birth. Most of these babies will be handicapped, the severity of the disability depending on the part of the back affected and the amount of damage to nerves.

Since the extent of nerve damage varies greatly, the baby may have little or no disability or, at the other extreme, may be severely disabled. If the neck is affected, the nerves used for breathing are usually damaged and nearly all these babies die soon after birth. If the very bottom of the spine is involved, only a few nerves going to the feet may be abnormal and the baby can be born with nothing more serious than club FEET. This can be cured by PHYSIOTHERAPY which the parents can be taught so that they can treat the baby themselves at home, or by ORTHOPAEDIC surgery. Sometimes a few of the nerves which control the BLADDER are slightly damaged so that the child may be INCONTINENT.

If the middle of the back is affected, the results are far more serious. Generally, the higher the opening in the back, the worse is the outlook. All of these children will have at least some deformity or weakness of the legs – indeed some will never be able to walk and will be confined to wheelchairs. Others will be able to walk after many operations on their bones and tendons, provided they wear callipers for support. Some of the children may be born with joint deformities, such as dislocation of the HIPS, which must be treated by orthopaedic appliances to ensure full movement of the joints later in life.

Many of these children are incontinent of bowel and bladder and may need some form of incontinence control such as a catheter to drain the urine. A severely affected child may also develop curvature of the spine at puberty which can, however, be rectified by a major operation. HYDROCEPHALUS – excessive water on the brain – often accompanies this kind of spina bifida. It has to be drained out into the chest or abdomen through special tubes and valves. For various reasons, some of these children are also mentally disabled to differing degrees.

In another form of spina bifida, the baby is born apparently normal except for a fatty lump at the bottom of the back. The danger of this is that it may be ignored because the baby can move his or her legs when newly born. However, many deteriorate as they get older, so it is very important that a specialist sees them for regular check-ups. An operation may be done to free the trapped nerves at the first sign of trouble, although this is not always completely successful.

Early treatment

An expert should examine a baby born with spina bifida straightaway, even though this may mean that the baby has to be separated from the mother and sent to one of the big regional centres where he or she will be in the care of a paediatric surgeon.

A whole team of specialists can then decide whether or not the baby will benefit from surgery, often carried out before the baby is 24 hours old to achieve the best results and to reduce the risk of serious infection.

The decision whether or not to operate on a baby with spina bifida is one of the most difficult facing a surgeon. It has become clear over the years that most of the more severely affected children will not do well even with surgery. These include babies with a severe spinal deformity at birth, severe paralysis of the legs, and hydrocephalus. Such babies have a poor outlook, and many die in the early years of life whatever treatment is given.

So the decision to operate has to be made as a result of an extremely careful and detailed assessment of the baby. X-RAYS are carried out together with a computerized X-ray scan (CT scan) or ULTRASOUND scan of the baby's head. The results of all the tests are discussed with the parents, who are then asked to agree with one or other of the possible procedures. If an operation is performed, it involves replacing any nervous tissue which is exposed on the surface and closing the defect in the baby's back.

If the baby cannot be helped by an urgent operation, doctors differ in their advice to parents. Some doctors recommend that the parents take the baby home as soon as they feel able to cope. Many of these babies die from MENINGITIS within a few weeks. However, others feed well and the spina bifida heals by itself in about six to eight weeks, although it frequently forms a big cyst which has to be removed several months later. Many of these babies develop fluid on the brain which has to be treated by an operation when they are three to six months old. Alternatively, some doctors think that they are best kept in hospital to be given regular painkillers. Sadly, severely affected babies do not feed well and most die within six months.

Continuing care

If an early operation has been carried out, the child will have to return to hospital for regular check-ups, for hydrocephalus for example. Orthopaedic operations may need to be planned to relieve deformity of the limbs or to help to mobilize joints. Most importantly, physiotherapy must be carried out regularly, and the parents given instructions about keeping the child's legs mobile.

As the child gets older, he or she may have to be taught about bladder function and bladder care if there is incontinence. Some children learn special manoeuvres to expel the urine from the bladder but in some instances, a catheter (a tube inserted into the bladder) may be needed, either permanently or, more likely, intermittently.

Prevention

There is now sufficient evidence concerning the role of vitamins in protecting against not only spina bifida but also other problems in pregnancy that women should ensure that they are eating a good varied diet from the time the decision is made to conceive. To ensure sufficient intake of folic acid, green leafy vegetables should be eaten most days, and also a good variety of other vegetables and fruit to supply other vitamins and minerals. It is now recommended that all women take folic acid supplements while trying to conceive and during the first 12 weeks of pregnancy.

Since the early 1980s, there has been a routine blood test that can reliably detect the more severe forms of spina bifida in 90 per cent of cases. This tests for the presence of alpha-fetoprotein (AFP). A high blood level of AFP during the 16th to 18th weeks of pregnancy indicates a high probability that the baby has a spina bifida, although a high level is also found in normal twin pregnancies (a low level is found in Down's syndrome).

If the result is abnormal, an ultrasound scan be carried out, which can detect twins but can sometimes also detect the more severe forms of spina bifida. Then an amniocentesis may be performed (*see* PREGNANCY). A sample of amniotic fluid, taken from the sac surrounding the foetus, is analysed for the presence of alpha-fetoprotein. If this test confirms the previous blood test result, the mother can be offered the choice of a termination of the pregnancy (*see* ABORTION).

In most hospitals an AFP blood test is now routine procedure at the 16th week of pregnancy; an amniocentesis can also be performed as a routine where there is a history of a previous spina bifida baby. As a result of this screening test, the numbers of babies born with spina bifida is decreasing.

Spinal cord

Running most of the length of the bony part of the spine, this is a vital link between the BRAIN and nerves connected to the rest of the body (*see* NERVOUS SYSTEM). Though often thought of as simply a bundle of nerve fibres to and from the brain, the spinal cord is much more than this. It acts as an important initial analyser for incoming sensations and as a programming station for organizing some of the basic movements of the limbs.

Structure of the spinal cord

The spinal cord runs from the medulla oblongata in the brain to the first or second lumbar vertebra.

It is well protected as it passes through the arches of the spinal vertebrae. Sensory and motor nerves of the peripheral nervous system leave the spinal cord separately just below the vertebrae, and then unite to form 31 pairs of spinal nerves: 8 *cervical,* 12 *thoracic,* 5 *lumbar,* 5 *sacral* and 1 *coccygeal,* each nerve corresponding to the vertebra from which it exits. These nerves branch out from the spinal cord, spreading to the surface of the body and to all the skeletal muscles.

The spinal cord is composed of collections of nerve cell bodies of neurones and bundles of nerve fibres. The grey matter – which is what the nerve cell collections are called – is H-shaped in cross-section, with a posterior (rear) and anterior (front) horn (protuberance) in each half. The anterior is composed of motor neurones, while the posterior horn contains cell bodies of connector neurones and sensory neurones. Motor neurones are so called because they send out impulses to move the muscles of the body. Sensory neurones receive messages which convey sensation.

The grey matter is surrounded by the white matter. This is divided into three columns and contains ascending and descending nerve tracts which connect the brain and the spinal cord in both directions. The descending tracts send motor impulses from the brain to the peripheral nervous system, while the ascending tracts channel sensory impulses to the brain.

Surrounding these nerves and fibres is a series of rough membranes (*meninges*) which are extensions of those membranes that surround the brain. Between the outer two of these three membrane layers is a small gap containing *cerebrospinal fluid*, which circulates around the spinal cord and the brain, providing nutrients to the nerves and acting as a protective buffer.

Functions of the spinal cord

The spinal cord has two main functions: to act as a two-way conduction system between the brain and the peripheral nervous system and to control simple REFLEX actions.

The spinal cord and the brain make up the *central nervous system.* Messages – in the form of electrical impulses created by the firing of interconnected neurones – from the surface of the body connect with the spinal cord via the sensory nerve fibres in the peripheral nervous system. The grey matter in the spinal cord rapidly processes the messages, and then relays some of them up the ascending tract of the spinal cord for more detailed analysis in the brain.

If action is required, the brain sends messages of action – motor impulses – down the descending tract that result in coordinated muscular action involving many different muscles in the body. If an itch is felt in the hand, for example, initial analysis takes place at the spinal cord and further analysis at the brain, which may then send messages in response, instructing the appropriate muscles of the body to move accordingly.

In controlling the simple reflex action, the usual pattern of message transmission to the brain is drastically curtailed. If the skin touches something hot, streams of impulses are passed via the sensory neurones to the posterior horn in the grey matter of the spinal cord. Instead of then ascending to the brain, the messages are immediately processed, and then cross to the anterior horn of the grey matter via connector neurones. These allow messages to be transmitted from sensory neurones to motor neurones, giving an immediate physical response – the hand is rapidly and 'automatically' withdrawn. This is known as the *reflex arc.* At the same time, information will be passed on to the brain, which will determine further action, if any (*see* PAIN).

Many of the body's important functions are controlled through reflex action and these occur at all levels of the spinal cord. Some movements involved in respiration, digestion and especially excretion, for example, are reflex actions controlled in part by the spinal cord.

 Spine, *see* **Back and backache, Spinal cord**

Spleen

This is an important organ of the body. Its main function is to act as a filter for the BLOOD and to make antibodies (*see* IMMUNE SYSTEM); in addition, an enlarged spleen, which doctors can feel through the walls of the abdomen, is often an indication of disease somewhere in the body.

The spleen is also an integral part of the LYMPHATIC SYSTEM – the basis of the body's defences against infection.

Location

The spleen lies just below the DIAPHRAGM at the top of the left-hand side of the ABDOMEN. It is normally about 5 in (13 cm) long, and it lies along the line of the 10th rib. The spleen usually weighs about ½ lb (about 200 g)) in adults, but in cases where it is enlarged, it can weigh up to 4½ lb (2 kg)) or more.

If a spleen is examined with the naked eye, it looks like a fibrous capsule surrounding a mass of featureless red pulp. It may just be possible to make out little granulations called *Malpighian corpuscles.*

The organ is supplied with blood via the splenic artery, which, like any other artery, splits first into smaller arteries and then into tiny arterioles. However, the arterioles of the spleen are unusual in that they are surrounded by a mass of lymphocytes (white blood cells) as they pass through the pulp of the spleen. The arterioles are unique in one other way: instead of being connected to a network of capillaries, they empty out into the substance of the spleen itself, into thin-walled spaces called sinusoids, which in turn drain into small venules.

The odd way in which the spleen is supplied with blood is what enables it to perform two of its basic functions. First, the fact that the arterioles are surrounded by lymphatic tissue means that the lymphatic system comes into immediate contact with any abnormal protein in the blood, and forms antibodies to it. Second, the way that the blood empties directly into the pulp of the spleen also allows the *reticular cells* of the organ to come into direct contact with the blood, filtering it of any old or worn-out cells.

Functions of the spleen

The spleen is one of the main filters of the blood. Not only do the reticular cells remove the old and worn-out blood cells, but they will also remove any abnormal ones. This applies in particular to red blood cells, but white cells and platelets are also filtered selectively when necessary by the spleen.

The spleen will also remove abnormal particles floating in the bloodstream. This means that it plays a major part in ridding the body of harmful bacteria, to give just one example. It is also instrumental in making antibodies – proteins circulating in the blood which bind on to and immobilize a foreign protein, so that white blood cells called *phagocytes* can destroy it. The Malpighian corpuscles, which are collections of lymphocytes, make the antibody.

In some circumstances, the spleen has a very important role in the manufacture of new blood cells. This does not happen in the normal adult, but in people who have a BONE MARROW disease, the spleen and the liver are major sites of red blood cell production. In addition, the spleen makes much of the blood of a baby in the womb.

Enlargement of the spleen

The spleen may enlarge for many reasons, and a doctor will be able to feel it easily when the abdomen is examined. Since one of its main functions is to break down old and worn-out blood cells, those conditions where blood is broken down faster than normal are associated with an enlarged spleen. These diseases are called *haemolytic* ANAEMIAS, and many can be inherited (*see* SICKLE-CELL ANAEMIA and THALASSAEMIA).

Other blood diseases also cause the spleen to become enlarged – in some cases of LEUKAEMIA, for example, the spleen grows so much that it stretches from the top left-hand corner of the abdomen to the bottom right-hand corner.

There are two other diseases that are associated with enlarged spleens: MALARIA and the parasitical disease called *kala-azar*, in which the PARASITES actually inhabit the spleen. Many other infections can cause an enlarged spleen, including GLANDULAR FEVER. The spleen may also become enlarged in some types of liver disease.

Removal of the spleen

There are, however, a number of reasons why the spleen may have to be removed. Despite the fact that it is an important filter of the blood, very few ill effects seem to result from its removal, although it is possible to see changes in peripheral blood, such as the presence of Howell–Jolly bodies. In addition red blood cells may show striking changes in size and shape.

If the spleen is injured as the result of an accident, it may bleed profusely, and this means that it will have to be removed. The spleen may also be removed during laparotomies (investigative operations where the abdomen is opened) to investigate the extent of LYMPHOMAS – lymphatic tumours.

Occasionally the spleen becomes overactive in its function of breaking down blood cells, and this leads to excessive destruction of cells. This is likely to happen only when the spleen is already enlarged for some reason – such as a lymphoma or portal hypertension due to liver disease. In these cases, too, the spleen may be removed.

Spondylitis

BACK problems are a very common source of pain and disability, and the terms *spondylitis* and *spondylosis* are often used when talking about them. These conditions are easily confused, but they are, in fact, quite distinct.

Spondylitis denotes any disease which gives rise to inflammation of the JOINTS between spinal vertebrae as well as the associated ligaments. The joints usually involved are those at the bottom of the spine, between the sacral vertebrae and the pelvic bones.

Spondylosis is a completely different disorder of the spine, resulting from degenerative rather than inflammatory changes in the joints. These changes may lead to outgrowths of small spurs of bone which can irritate nerves, causing pain.

Causes

Spondylitis may arise in the course of a number of different diseases, the best known of which is probably *ankylosing spondylitis.* Other conditions in which the illness can occur include PSORIASIS and some intestinal diseases such as Crohn's disease or ULCERATIVE COLITIS. It sometimes follows certain bowel infections and a genito-urinary disease that is sometimes referred to as Reiter's disease. The exact cause of these diseases is unknown, but they all have in common the fact that they may give rise to spondylitis, and sometimes ARTHRITIS of the limb joints.

It seems likely, however, that these conditions result from an abnormal response by the body's defence or IMMUNE SYSTEM so that inflammatory white blood cells accumulate in the lining of the spinal joints. This is particularly true of ankylosing spondylitis, in which the joint inflammation precedes the formation of bony bridges across the spinal joints. This leads to loss of mobility, and in severe cases, the spine may become rigid along its whole length so that patients cannot bend their backs at all.

This process whereby the spinal joints become fused is known as *ankylosis*, which is how the disease derives its name. However, this severe type of spondylitis is seen only in ankylosing spondylitis – spondylitis accompanying other conditions is rarely so extreme.

Patients with ankylosing spondylitis have been found, in very many cases, to belong to a particular tissue type known as HLA-B27. It is currently thought that some people with this tissue type may be particularly liable to develop spondylitis after certain infections.

Symptoms

The commonest and earliest symptoms are aching and stiffness in the lower back, which are most acute in the morning and wear off during the day.

In more advanced cases, patients may notice restriction of spinal movement and chest pain as the joints between the ribs and the thoracic vertebrae are involved. If there is concurrent arthritis, the symptoms of pain, swelling and tenderness occur in the involved joints – most commonly the hip joints. The other large joints such as the knees, wrists and ankles may also be affected. In addition, *iritis* – red, painful eyes – sometimes develops, and may recur. Prompt treatment is needed to prevent the eye damage which may result.

The main complication of ankylosing spondylitis is the onset of postural deformities which vary from patient to patient. Recurrent iritis may lead to visual impairment and, very rarely, valvular HEART disease develops.

Treatment

The treatment of the patient with ankylosing spondylitis involves the close cooperation of the medical team with the PHYSIOTHERAPIST and OCCUPATIONAL

THERAPIST. The main aim is to relieve pain and prevent deformities by a planned programme of back exercises. Of all rheumatic diseases, ankylosing spondylitis is the one which benefits particularly from exercise. This relieves pain, improves mobility and may prevent or delay the onset of bony ankylosis.

Anti-inflammatory agents are useful in relieving symptoms. The use of these drugs together with physiotherapy forms the mainstay of treatment.

Spondylolisthesis, *see* **Skeleton**

Sputum, *see* **Phlegm**

Squamous carcinoma, *see* **Cancer, Lungs and lung diseases**

Squint

This is the inability to move both eyes in the same direction at the same time. The condition can affect adults, but occurs more commonly in children.

During the first six months of life, a baby's eyes may move about randomly in any direction, but after this age, they should move together. If the eyes are not parallel the child is said to have a squint, or *strabismus.* (This is also commonly called a 'turn' or a 'boss-eye'.) It has no connection with screwing up the eyes, an affectation of no consequence to which young children seem particularly prone.

Normally, children are able to use both eyes together and blend the images seen with each eye into one unified perception with full three-dimensional vision. Children with squints are unable to do this because the eyes are looking in different directions. The children compensate for this by suppressing the image seen by the deviating eye so that they are not troubled by double vision. Because the child's visual system is immature, this suppression results in permanent impairment of vision unless the condition is treated, and the squinting eye becomes 'lazy' (*see* BLINDNESS).

Most childhood squints are *convergent,* with the squinting eye moving inwards. *Divergent* squint, when the eye moves outwards, is more common later in life, as is a *vertical* squint.

Causes and dangers of squint

Some squints are congenital, appearing at birth, but most infantile squints appear between the ages of two and four years, often after a childhood illness and initially only when the child is tired. Many factors are involved in its cause, but it is usually associated with an imbalance between the focusing mechanism of the eye and the muscular control of the eye itself.

A 'lazy' eye is one that has not reached its full visual potential. At birth, the eyes are capable of seeing very little, and it is not until the age of five years that normal vision is fully acquired. Any disorder that interrupts this maturing process will, if untreated, result in a 'lazy' eye with defective vision. Squint is the commonest condition that may result in a 'lazy' eye.

Squint can also occur later in life, although this is less common. Because an adult's visual system is fully developed, this type of squint is accompanied by troublesome double vision which the patient is often unable to suppress. Although there is no risk of the squinting eye becoming lazy, the disorientation caused by double vision – so that the world seems to swim around the sufferer – is severely incapacitating.

A squint in adult life is usually caused by damage to an ocular nerve or muscle and, as such, requires a thorough medical examination to identify the cause. DIABETES, high BLOOD PRESSURE and THYROID disorders are the common culprits.

Getting advice and treatment

If you think that your child may be developing a squint, it is important that you seek medical advice immediately. Fortunately a lot of children only appear to be squinting because of the presence of vertical folds of skin on either side of the nasal bridge. By the time the child reaches school age, the nasal bridge is more developed and the 'pseudo-squint' has disappeared. However, only a specialist can differentiate between a 'true' and an 'apparent' squint and the two may exist together. Do not jeopardize your child's vision: seek advice.

Squints are commonly treated by special glasses, which the child should be encouraged to wear at all times. Some squints are cured by glasses alone.

In many cases, the child will be given exercises to do by an orthoptist, a specialist professional who works closely with ophthalmic surgeons in treating squints. Exercises in the hospital clinic and later at home may help with certain types of squint, and the orthoptist will check regularly to assess progress.

Often glasses only partly correct the condition, and a full correction is only achieved with surgery on the muscles that move the eye. Essentially, this involves weakening the muscles that are overactive and strengthening the underactive ones.

If children develop a 'lazy' eye as a result of their squint, the usual treatment is to cover (occlude) the normal eye with a patch. This will force the 'lazy' eye to work.

Squint operations are routine for the ophthalmic surgeon and necessitate only a few days' stay in hospital for the child. After the operation, there is surprisingly little discomfort, and within three to four weeks the scars will have healed and become virtually invisible.

Squints that appear later in life are treated differently. Any underlying medical disorder must be dealt with, and the initial aim of ocular treatment is to alleviate the troublesome double vision. This can be achieved either by covering the deviating eye with a patch or by incorporating a prism into the patient's spectacle lens which artificially bends the light rays to compensate for the deviation. Adult squints which arise because of an impairment in control of eye movements sometimes improve with orthoptic exercises.

These are designed to increase and strengthen the patient's ability to use the two eyes in unison.

If an ocular muscle is paralysed, surgery may be necessary. However, it is essential that this is deferred for at least six months, as spontaneous recovery can occur in these cases.

Staphylococci, *see* **Bacteria, Diarrhoea, Food poisoning, Impetigo, Infection and infectious diseases, Pneumonia, Toxic shock syndrome**

Starch, *see* **Carbohydrates**

STDs, *see* **Sexually transmitted diseases**

Sterilization, female

The term 'sterilization' is usually used to describe the operation which makes a woman sterile and unable to have children. The equivalent operation for a man is called a VASECTOMY.

Any woman choosing this method of CONTRACEPTION must be confident that she will want no more children even if her personal circumstances change, since with current surgical techniques, it is potentially irreversible.

Methods of sterilization

For a woman to be fertile, she must be able to release eggs from her OVARIES; she must have intact Fallopian tubes along which the eggs can pass to the UTERUS (womb); and she must have a normal womb in which the fertilized egg can embed itself and develop into a foetus and eventually a baby. All methods of sterilization work by permanently blocking one or more of these stages.

Most sterilization operations consist in blocking the Fallopian tubes in one of a number of ways. This method is particularly popular as it involves a relatively minor operation, although it is still a slightly more risky procedure than sterilizing a man by vasectomy. Women sterilized in this way do not have sudden MENOPAUSAL symptoms – as happens when the ovaries are involved – and their PERIODS continue, although these may be slightly heavier.

The function of the Fallopian tubes may be permanently interrupted in a variety of ways. First, they may be completely removed, a method of sterilization which is very unlikely to fail. Alternatively, a portion – about ⅓ in (1 cm) – may be cut away from the middle of each, or they may be cut through or burnt by the method of diathermy. The burn is made in only two places but the effect will travel along the tubes, thus damaging them. In some cases, clips are placed on both tubes, or a loop of each is pulled into a tight plastic ring. All these procedures, except total removal of the Fallopian tubes, are potentially reversible, but any woman undergoing one of these operations should assume that it will make her permanently sterile. They are probably the methods most often used, and there are seldom any complications.

Unfortunately, between one and four women in every 1000 who have this type of operation subsequently become pregnant. This is probably because the tubes get unblocked. Another rare problem is that a fertilized egg can be trapped in one of the Fallopian tubes, where it grows until it ruptures the tube and passes into the abdominal cavity. This is called an ECTOPIC PREGNANCY and is treated by surgically removing the affected Fallopian tube. These problems are nevertheless uncommon, and many women are very happy with this type of sterilization.

There are other methods which are not often used as they are less satisfactory. For example, it is possible to sterilize a woman by removing or damaging her ovaries, but she will then rapidly develop menopausal symptoms such as hot flushes. This method is usually contemplated only if the ovaries are already damaged or diseased.

Women and doctors seldom consider HYSTERECTOMY – the removal of the uterus – an ideal form of contraception because it involves a major operation. However, it may be a sensible choice if the woman has gynaecological problems such as large FIBROIDS or very heavy periods, both of which may be effectively cured by hysterectomy.

Why choose sterilization?

There seem to be three important times in a woman's life when she may consider sterilization as a form of contraception. The first may be when she is having an ABORTION. Although her decision is often completely rational, many doctors prefer not to sterilize a woman at the same time as performing a termination. There are two main reasons for this. First, she runs a greater risk of developing blood clots (*see* THROMBOSIS) in her leg and pelvic veins during the operation, since she still has in her blood the altered levels of clotting factors which are associated with PREGNANCY. Second, many women come to regret the decision they made at a time when they were undergoing much emotional turmoil.

Similar arguments apply against sterilizing a woman immediately after having a baby, as well as the further argument that it is sensible to be certain that the new baby will thrive. Often, however, women and doctors feel that the convenience of the mother being sterilized while still in hospital with the baby outweighs the disadvantages.

Women also choose sterilization as they approach middle age rather than continuing to take the contraceptive pill.

The operation

An instrument called a laparoscope is often used in sterilization. This is a fine rod which allows a clear view of the Fallopian tubes, and along which the necessary instruments can be passed to perform the operation (*see* ENDOSCOPY).

Laparoscopic sterilization is occasionally done while the woman is awake, but, of course, the area where the laparoscope is to be inserted is first made completely numb so that the operation is relatively painless. The majority of sterilizations are, however, performed under general ANAESTHETIC and the woman is allowed home the next day. The scar will be tender for several days and most women prefer to rest as much as possible during this time, although this is difficult if a woman has a large family.

Unlike male sterilization, female sterilization is effective immediately so that a couple need not use any other form of contraception. Most women wait a week or so after being sterilized before having SEXUAL INTERCOURSE so that their scars will have time to heal. If the woman has been sterilized by hysterectomy, her scars will take much longer to heal, and she would be well advised to wait at least a month or even six weeks before attempting to have sexual intercourse.

Reversing the operation

It is possible to attempt to reverse sterilization operations where only the Fallopian tubes have been obstructed. The woman must convince her doctor of the importance to her of having another baby, since this is a major operation, and has only a 50 per cent chance of success. For this reason it is important for women to realize that if they are sterilized, it is very likely that they will ever have another pregnancy even if they are prepared to undergo major surgery in an attempt to achieve it.

Sterilization, male, *see* Vasectomy

Steroids

Produced naturally in the body by the ADRENAL GLANDS, these HORMONES are a normal and essential part of the body's ENDOCRINE SYSTEM. The drugs that are referred to as 'steroids' are either exactly the same as the body's naturally occurring steroids – that is, either *cortisone* or *hydrocortisone* – or else they are very closely related both in their chemical structure and in their effects on the body.

Steroid drug treatment is now widely used to fight INFLAMMATION and disease, and to reduce the activity of the body's IMMUNE SYSTEM. But the treatment can have serious side-effects. Consequently, steroid treatment must be a skilful balancing act.

The use of steroid drugs

One of the natural effects of steroid activity is to damp down excessive inflammation. When the body's defence system responds to infection, some of the cells that take part in attacking the infection have their activity suppressed by the steroids so that their response is not so vigorous as to damage the body itself.

This action is of particular interest with regard to ALLERGY, and steroids are now widely used in controlling the symptoms of those conditions that have an allergic element to them. For example, in the case of ASTHMA, part of the allergic reaction may include severe obstruction to breathing, a sign of the body's defence system over-reacting. This response can be considerably reduced by steroid treatment. It is also possible to reduce the strength of any side-effects by giving the steroids in a locally active form – in an inhaler.

Steroid drugs are also widely used against a group of diseases in which the body's immune system turns against itself – that is, *auto-immune diseases*. These include the generalized inflammatory disease known as systemic LUPUS ERYTHEMATOSUS, and a similar disease, RHEUMATOID ARTHRITIS. There is no doubt that, in the short term, steroids can do much to alleviate the symptoms of these diseases. However, in the case of rheumatoid arthritis, if the treatment is used over a long period, the side-effects usually outweigh the benefits. Consequently, in treating rheumatoid arthritis, it is more usually used as a short-term treatment.

There are many other unusual and ill-explained inflammatory diseases that respond almost magically to steroids. A good example is the condition called *temporal arteritis*, where the lining of the arteries becomes inflamed for no obvious reason. This condition affects the elderly and is most common in the arteries in the head, causing bad headaches and possibly even blindness. But once the diagnosis is made, it settles down within 24 hours of being treated with steroids.

Steroids are also the basis of the treatment of organ REJECTION after transplantation. The patient may be given quite high doses for some time to suppress substantially the body's natural response of rejecting foreign tissue.

Various TUMOURS also respond well to steroids, as do JOINT inflammations like housemaid's knee and TENNIS ELBOW.

Side-effects

The unwanted side-effects of oral steroids occur because they are given in much higher amounts than would normally be found in the body. These side-effects are very similar to the symptoms of *Cushing's disease*, a condition where the adrenal glands become over-active and so produce excessive amounts of steroid hormones in the body.

These symptoms include excessive weight gain – with the tendency for the fat to be found on the face and trunk – and the loss of PROTEIN leading to weakness of muscles, bones, skin and gut linings (leading to ULCERS). DIABETES frequently occurs and the BLOOD PRESSURE is raised; there may even be severe mental disturbance.

However, steroid treatment also tends to suppress the body's own adrenal activity. As the dose is reduced, it is possible for the body to become short of steroids. The main danger of this is that there is a reduced capacity to respond to STRESS, so that there might be a sudden collapse with loss of blood pressure during a minor illness, for example. To avoid this possibility, the dose is very carefully reduced, giving the adrenal glands time to recover their own activity.

ADDISON'S DISEASE results from failure of the adrenal glands to produce an adequate amount of steroids. The missing steroids can be replaced by steroid tablets. Since this is simply replacement treatment which does not raise the level of steroids in the body above normal, there is no risk of side-effects.

It is because of these side-effects that different ways of giving steroids have been developed, such as inhalers or creams which minimize absorption of steroid into the bloodstream and so reduce side-effects.

Still births

At present, the term 'still birth' is used when the death of a baby occurs before it is born, but after 28 weeks of PREGNANCY. Most deaths occur while the baby is still in the uterus before labour begins, but about 10 per cent occur during labour (*see* CHILDBIRTH). If a foetus dies before 28 weeks of pregnancy it is known as a spontaneous ABORTION or MISCARRIAGE.

Causes of still birth

The cause of many still births is unknown, but there is evidence to suggest that some occur when there is an inadequate supply of oxygen in the blood to the baby from the mother via the umbilical cord and the PLACENTA.

In the condition known as *placenta praevia*, the placenta lies too low in the uterus. When labour begins, it can separate from the uterine wall, or be damaged by the baby trying to get out, and cause severe bleeding. This may end in a still birth, although an emergency CAESAREAN section can be performed which can save the baby's life.

Blood vessels in the placenta may clot (*infarction*); sometimes the placenta just does not seem to work very well; or it separates partly or wholly from the wall of the uterus before birth (an *abruptio-placenta*) – all these conditions can predispose to a still birth.

Toxaemia of pregnancy, high blood pressure and kidney disease (*see* ECLAMPSIA AND PRE-ECLAMPSIA) can all cause blockage to the circulation of blood through the placenta, and in some cases, this may be associated with still birth.

There does seem to be a higher still birth rate in those women who smoke and drink heavily during pregnancy, although an occasional alcoholic drink will probably do no harm. Smoking should be avoided completely.

About 20 per cent of still births are caused by an abnormality of the baby – it may have a chromosome disorder such as DOWN'S SYNDROME or a congenital abnormality such as SPINA BIFIDA. There may be heart or kidney abnormalities. These can be diagnosed by chorionic villi sampling, amniocentesis or ULTRASOUND scan, but sometimes the still birth cannot be prevented.

Problems during labour

A still birth can also occur as a result of complications during labour. If the baby is very large compared to the size of the mother's pelvis, or is lying abnormally in the womb, it may be a difficult delivery and the blood and hence the oxygen supply to the baby can become obstructed. The umbilical cord can come out before the baby, or be torn, twisted in a knot or around the baby's neck – again all can interfere with the baby's supply of oxygen from the mother.

Premature babies are much more susceptible to trauma and lack of oxygen during delivery than full-term babies, and hence more at risk of being stillborn.

Symptoms

Many women notice that their baby moves much less in the last few days before a still birth happens. Others feel very jerky movements – 'as though the baby is trying to escape from the womb'. Many do not notice anything. Once the baby has died, no movements whatsoever will be detected.

Death is confirmed by the doctor or midwife being unable to hear any foetal heartbeat, and by there having been no movements for more than 12 hours. This can be checked with an ultrasound scan, or, if the baby has been dead for several days, with an X-ray. If death occurs during delivery, there will be no sign of life (heartbeats, attempts to breathe or movement) at birth.

After the death

Once the doctor is sure that the baby is dead, he or she will tell the parents, preferably when they are together. If the foetus is still in the uterus, labour will be induced as soon as possible. If left alone, it might take several weeks for labour to occur spontaneously; this would be extremely difficult for a woman to bear emotionally. The dead foetus can also cause the mother to bleed if not removed.

Sometimes, especially if the doctors are not sure why a baby died, it is important for a post-mortem to be performed so that they can tell the parents why their baby died and to try to prevent it happening again. Often this is the only way of finding out the cause of death.

Once delivered, the mother should be asked where she would like to go. She may decide to go to the gynaecological ward rather than the post-natal ward. She needs the same care as if her baby had lived, but arrangements for her to go home as soon as possible will be made with her midwife, and an appointment booked for her post-natal check and family planning advice.

The birth must also be registered as a still birth with the local Registrar, and arrangements made for a burial service in accordance with the parents' wishes.

Initially after the death of a baby, there is a phase of shock. This can last about two months, and many parents during this time will need to express their grief, to cry and to talk about any guilty feelings they may have. Other children in the family will also need to be comforted.

Stoma care

A *stoma* is a surgically created opening, usually connected with the bowel (when it is called a *colostomy, ileostomy* or *jejunostomy*), but sometimes connected with the windpipe or throat (*tracheostomy, pharyngostomy*), or the stomach (*gastrostomy*) or part of the urinary tract (*ureterostomy*) or one of the kidneys themselves (*nephrostomy*).

Stomas have various functions, including by-passing a blockage in a tube such as the gut or windpipe, or creating a new opening further along a tube when, for instance, a part of the gut or urinary tract has to be removed, together with its normal opening. A stoma can also be used after gut or ureter surgery to divert the contents of the tube temporarily until the join has healed. Or a stoma, connecting the upper part of the gastro-intestinal tract with the outside, can be used for introducing food into the digestive system of a patient who is otherwise unable to swallow normally.

Care of the stoma will vary according to the part of the body to which it is connected, and the reason for its being fashioned for a patient.

Caring for a stoma

There are a number of different types of stoma, and each requires special care and attention by the patient.

Tracheostomy: A tracheostomy, or an opening between the skin and the trachea (windpipe), can either be temporary (when a hole is made in the trachea and a tube is passed through a hole in the skin into the trachea) or permanent (when the trachea is divided across and the lower end, which leads down towards the lungs, is brought up to the skin surface and the edges fixed to the skin).

Many types of tracheostomy will close over naturally, and so they have to be kept open by means of a tracheostomy tube. This is inserted through the skin and passes some way down the trachea. The tube must be cleaned frequently as it can become encrusted with secretions. Initially this cleaning is done by a qualified medical person, but patients are taught how to do it if the tube is to be permanent (for instance, when the larynx has been removed). Further, since the air passes straight into the trachea, the humidifying effect of the mouth and nasal passages is lost; this can lead to serious drying effects on the lining of the trachea. In the beginning, this can be overcome by humidifying the air the patient breathes, but once the tracheostomy has been established for some time, it becomes less of a problem.

Colostomy: There are many different types of colostomy and each presents slightly different problems. A colostomy is a surgical opening that is made through the skin and the abdominal wall muscles. The cut end or a loop of the colon (large INTESTINE) is then brought through and on to this surface. This enables the contents of the intestines to pass out into a special plastic bag, which fits snugly over the stoma and sticks to the skin.

Care of the colostomy involves ensuring that the bag is the correct size for the stoma, that there is a watertight and gastight fit, and that the skin around the stoma does not become sore. The latter could arise either if there was a leakage under the adhesive, or if the hole in the bag is much bigger than the stoma, allowing skin to rot in prolonged contact with faeces. Most new colostomy patients experience difficulties initially overcoming these problems, but after this, management of the colostomy becomes routine and presents few difficulties.

Patients also learn to deal with opening up a colostomy wound, which has a tendency to close. The problem of the offensive odour, which gave older colostomies a bad name, has largely been solved by the use of plastic and adhesives, and by carefully watching the diet.

Ileostomy: An ileostomy differs from a colostomy in that here the terminal part of the small intestine is brought to the surface; the effluent is liquid, not solid; and the fluid does not usually smell offensive. There are two advantages to an ileostomy: the bag does not need to be taken off the skin, and it can be opened at the bottom end and simply emptied; and the odour is not such a problem, so patients feel safer in company. The fluid from an ileostomy, however, is much more likely to cause damage to the surrounding skin, and so the hole in the bag should be carefully chosen to fit the stoma snugly.

Ileal conduit: Some patients have an ileostomy that is connected to their kidneys so that urine drains into the bag. The bag can be left stuck to the skin for many days, and each time it is full, a little tap can be opened for emptying. At night, the tap can be connected via a tube to a larger bag, so that the ileostomy bag does not fill up.

Stomach

This is a muscular bag situated in the upper part of the ABDOMEN. It is connected at its upper end to the OESOPHAGUS (gullet), and at its lower end to the DUODENUM (first part of the small intestine). The wall of the stomach consists of a thick layer of muscle, lined with a special membrane called the *epithelium.*

Function

One of the main functions of the stomach is to act as a reservoir for food. Virtually all the food eaten during a meal is retained in the stomach until it is thoroughly mixed together by the muscular actions of the stomach wall.

The stomach also secretes large quantities of digestive juices. The juices contain an ENZYME called *pepsin,* which breaks down PROTEINS into small molecules that can be absorbed more easily lower down the digestive tract. This enzyme is similar to rennet, which is used to curdle milk in cheese-making. Any milk in the diet is curdled by pepsin as soon as it reaches the stomach. This accounts for the fact that the milk in a baby's vomit is always curdled.

Stomach juices also contain *hydrochloric acid,* which is produced by the glands in the deep folds of the stomach lining. The acid is almost as strong as the acid used in a car battery. Its functions are to aid in digestion but it also acts as an antiseptic, killing off any germs that may be present in the food. The amount of acid in the stomach juice and the amount of juice produced varies

The stomach: site and structure

The stomach is an S-shaped organ in the upper left part of the abdomen. Food enters it through the oesophagus and leaves via the duodenum. The inside surface is convoluted into numerous folds.

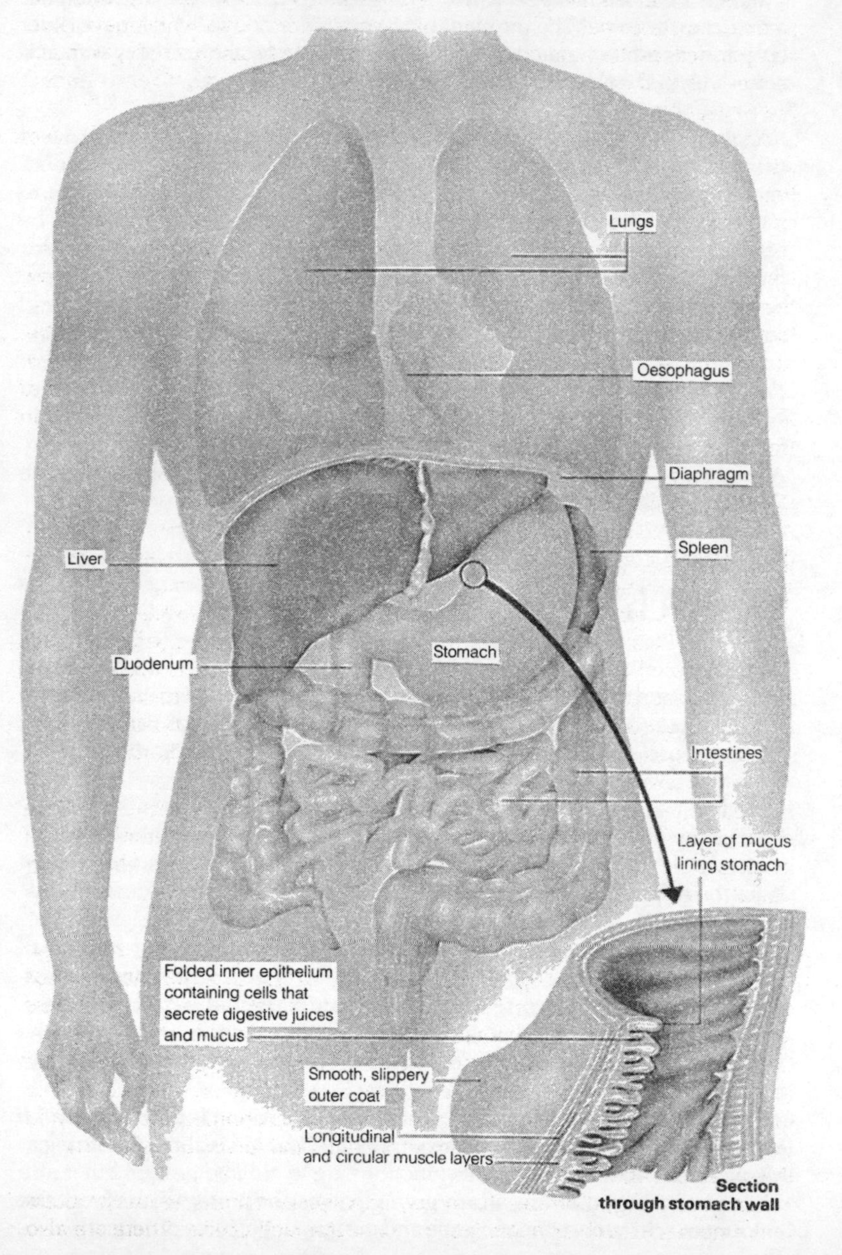

from time to time during the day. There is always about 1 fl oz (30 ml) of fluid in the stomach even when it is empty of food. The sight of food or the thought of a meal increases the flow of stomach juice, ready to act on any food that passes into the stomach. The secretion of juice is partly under nervous control and partly a result of the action of a HORMONE called *gastrin.* During a meal, up to 11 to 14 fl oz (300 or 400 ml) of juice may be secreted. Over 24 hours, 2½ pints (about 1½ litres) of stomach juice are produced.

Apart from food, STRESS is known to increase the secretion of stomach juice and acid. This is particularly so if the stress involves anger or resentment. People who lead stressful lives can have problems, such as ulcers, that are caused by these excess secretions.

Once food has entered the stomach, it is mixed with the stomach juice until it has the consistency of a thick paste. Very little food is actually absorbed into the bloodstream from the stomach, apart from small amounts of sugar. Once it is mixed together, food is forced, in small quantities at a time, into the duodenum. At the junction between the stomach and the duodenum, there is a ring of muscle, the *pyloric sphincter,* which relaxes from time to time to allow the food to pass into the duodenum. The food is then pushed along the intestines to be further digested and absorbed.

Common problems

At some time or other, most of us have experienced that queasy feeling when the stomach contracts forcibly. When this happens, the contents of the stomach may be ejected up into the gullet, an action known as VOMITING.

Frequently, vomiting may be associated with a common condition known as *gastritis.* This is when the lining of the stomach becomes inflamed as a result of a viral infection ('gastric flu'), eating spicy foods, drinking strong alcohol, taking certain drugs, or stress – or for no particular reason at all. A mild attack of gastritis produces symptoms of nausea, vomiting and occasionally some pain in the upper abdomen. More severe attacks can lead to bleeding from the lining of the stomach.

The treatment of gastritis is to remove the cause wherever possible, and to drink plenty of bland liquids. Sometimes drugs which prevent vomiting may be prescribed by a doctor. Fortunately, gastritis is usually a self-limiting condition once the primary cause has been removed. *See also* GASTRO-ENTERITIS.

Often INDIGESTION is simply the result of eating too much food or eating too quickly. Pain is felt in the upper abdomen with slight nausea, but after an hour or two it should pass. A glass of milk or an antacid tablet will reduce the excess acidity in the stomach and help the indigestion to settle. Sometimes indigestion is felt as a pain in the centre of the chest and then it is usually called 'heartburn'. This condition may occur simply as a result of unwise eating or from gastritis. It may be a symptom of hiatus hernia, a condition in which acid from the stomach passes up into the oesophagus and sets up an inflammation there (*see* DIAPHRAGM).

Persistent indigestion can, however, be a sign of a more serious problem in the stomach, such as a stomach ULCER or stomach CANCER. There are also other causes for indigestion, including GALL BLADDER disease, gallstones and duodenal ulcers. Many women have indigestion in PREGNANCY. Sometimes persistent indigestion is simply due to excessive acid production caused by STRESS or nervousness – a condition which may be known as 'nervous gastritis'. This problem is popularly associated with highly stressed businessmen, but, in fact, affects all types of people.

Cancer of the stomach

Gastric cancer is one of the most common malignant tumours, and it affects men more than women. It can start as a small ulcer or as a small polyp and eventually grows big enough to obstruct the passage of food through the stomach.

Because the tumour involves the lining of the stomach, patients may lose blood into the stomach, and it may be ANAEMIA that brings the illness to light. Others feel constantly nauseated and lose their appetites, and consequently lose weight. Other patients may develop pain in the upper part of the abdomen. Because the pain can be very similar to that caused by a benign gastric or duodenal ulcer, these patients can often find that they are treated for a long time with antacids with no relief of symptoms. It is for this reason that any patient over the age of about 50 coming to the doctor's surgery complaining of indigestion is treated with some caution. If he does not respond quickly to conventional treatment for indigestion, further investigation of the case will be essential.

Like a benign ulcer, gastric cancer is usually diagnosed by means of a barium meal X-ray or a gastroscopy (*see* ENDOSCOPY). The sooner this is done, the better, since there is evidence that an early diagnosis improves the overall outlook of the treatment. Wherever possible, the treatment of gastric cancer involves the surgical removal of the tumour – this often means removing the whole stomach. Patients who have had their stomach – or a major portion of it – removed are usually unable to eat large meals, but in other respects should be able to carry on as normal. They do, however, have to be seen at yearly intervals as they are more likely to develop anaemia and nutritional disturbances (especially a deficiency of VITAMIN B_{12}), which can usually be corrected by appropriate diet supplements.

Pyloric stenosis

Sometimes the outlet of the stomach – the pyloric canal – becomes blocked, leading to a build-up of stomach contents and eventual profuse vomiting. In infants, this can occur as a result of overgrowth of the muscle in this region, the cause of which is unknown. In adults, it is caused either by a cancerous growth or by a long-standing duodenal ulcer which has caused fibrous scarring.

Strabismus, *see* **Squint**

Streptococci, *see* **Bacteria, Kidneys and kidney diseases, Nephritis, Pharynx, Rheumatic fever, Tonsils**

Stress

This serves a useful purpose in stimulating effort, inventiveness and high standards. But when there is more than we can cope with, a stress disorder is likely to develop, and this illness may be either mental or physical in its main manifestations. Whether or not we get to a point of breakdown, and how this may affect us, depends on many factors such as the intensity of the stress to which we are subjected versus our capacity to contain and adapt to it. And this in turn will depend on the character features that we inherit at birth, the experience of our formative years and the effects of subsequent successes and failures in coping with life's many ups and downs.

What is necessary for emotional health is a reasonably peaceful and yet fulfilling balance between ourselves and the circumstances in which we find ourselves and with which we have to live. It is important for us to bear in mind that a large number of factors are interacting together and that this creates a constantly changing picture which may hold still hardly long enough for us to grasp it in detail. It is not surprising, therefore, that most of us find ourselves, our state of mind at any particular time and our motives very confusing.

Mental and physical reactions

The ability to cope adequately with stress depends on a combination of constitutional or natural resources, character, training and experience.

Sudden intense stress, which is closely related to fear and represents a direct challenge to our basic instinct for survival, provokes a chemical and, subsequently, a physical response as well as the severe emotional feeling which we call panic. This consists of the production of greatly increased amounts of the hormone adrenalin from the ADRENAL GLANDS, which are situated on top of each kidney. The adrenalin is released directly into the bloodstream and has an immediate effect in preparing the body to take immediate action in the direction of either 'fight or flight'. This surge of adrenalin occurs in response to either physical or emotional stress and prepares a wide variety of body tissues and organs for a vigorous reaction to a crisis which may be severe enough to involve fear or panic.

When necessary, a variety of defence mechanisms may also be called upon, usually subconsciously. This may be done by discounting or refusing to recognize the reality that exists; denying the existence of unpleasant facts such as a major breakdown in a relationship, failure at work or in personal standards; or chronic illness. Aggression, hostility and virtual persecution towards others because of our own failings may occur. We may rationalize failure to achieve an objective by convincing ourselves that we did not really want it anyway. We may compensate for our failure in one direction by exceptional attainment in another. We may displace our distress by displaying friendliness and charm where we actually feel hostility and anxiety or even fear.

Causes of stress

The causes of stress reaction in the body are often referred to as 'stressors', although an individual's response to a given number of stressors is determined by his or her own personal characteristics and mental fitness.

External events are often among the most potent causes of stress in people's lives. It is not just the hectic pace of modern living which takes its toll, but a variety of 'life events'. Some years ago, it was shown that a mental breakdown or suicide attempt was often preceded by a series of life events which built up pressure on the individual.

The events that appear to be most damaging and potentially dangerous are those involving either some form of loss or conflict. The loss may be of a person such as the death of a spouse or close relative or of something important in one's life, such as the loss of a job. Many worries may bring with them the loss of an accustomed lifestyle; a physical illness may mean loss of self-esteem or self-image simply because the person cannot function at work or at home in the normal way.

Conflict may arise at home or at work. Arguments with people you like or respect can be very damaging, especially if the argument is protracted and unresolved. Even family holidays can be sources of conflict because family members spend longer than usual in each other's company – and all may have different aspirations for the holiday itself, leading to rows and arguments.

Conflicts with others often involve a choice between one of two or more alternatives, but more often than not, one alternative is more attractive than the other. If an individual is faced with a choice, the decision itself may actually increase stress levels, but if he or she is denied the preferred choice because of circumstances, a sense of bitterness and frustration can set in. Sometimes people just avoid making any decision in an attempt to diminish stress for themselves, but often this just makes matters worse.

It is increasingly recognized that considerable amounts of stress can be generated at work by bad management practices and ineffective bosses. At work, people expect to be given a clear idea of what they are supposed to do, and helped to achieve the targets they have been set. If something changes in the way work is allocated or in arrangements at the place of work, workers should be consulted first and their ideas taken into account before a final decision is made. Stress can easily arise if workers are unclear about the work they should do, or if they feel that they are simply a 'cog in a machine' and their ideas are never taken into account.

Managers who fail to make decisions are often a source of great annoyance and frustration to the people who work with them, as are managers who fail to compliment workers who achieve the targets that have been set for them.

Apart from external events or the effect of other people on an individual, stress can arise from the way an individual plans his or her own life. Taking on too much at a time when one already has a great deal to cope with can act as the final straw and precipitate a breakdown.

Signs of stress

Once stressors begin to build up in a person's life, there are often early warning signs of 'impending' trouble. These may take the form of minor physical disorders, such as muscular 'tics' or twitches, recurring HEADACHES or

MIGRAINE, some INDIGESTION or occasional bowel irregularity. Excessive use of coffee as a stimulant, SMOKING too much or drinking too much ALCOHOL are also common ways in which people may try to help themselves through a stressful period of their lives, but in fact they are also important warning signals of things going badly.

Acute stress, such as may occur if a person loses a loved one either as a result of separation or bereavement, can be marked by more dramatic symptoms. Loss of appetite, SLEEPLESSNESS, anger, hostility and difficulty in concentrating are all common in such situations.

Once warning signs mount up, then further 'danger signals' may ultimately appear. Persistent difficulty in concentrating, interference with normal relationships with other people (which in a sexual relationship can include IMPOTENCE and frigidity), persistent headaches or other physical symptoms are all worrying signs. Medical help is invariably required once several such signs are present.

Long-term effects of stress

There are a variety of physical illnesses which are undoubtedly related to stress. Digestive disorders such as the IRRITABLE BOWEL SYNDROME and indigestion can be stress related. There is also good evidence that stress can contribute to stomach or duodenal ULCERS. Other long-term effects of stress include high blood pressure, which can ultimately lead to HEART ATTACKS or even STROKES. Skin diseases such as ECZEMA often affect women during periods of stress.

The long-term effects of stress on mental functioning can be quite serious. For example, agoraphobia or other PHOBIAS may arise, as can persistent panic attacks. Ultimately a severe anxiety state or a DEPRESSIVE illness may be the end result of long-term stress.

Recently there has been great medical interest in the effects of stress on the IMMUNE SYSTEM. This normally fights off infections and keeps abnormal cells in the body under control. People under stress are more likely than others to suffer from VIRUS infections and they may take longer to recover from infections.

The illness known as MYALGIC ENCEPHALOMYELITIS (ME) is thought by many doctors to occur as a result of a failure by the body to cope normally with a virus infection. Stress may reduce the immune response to the infection, allowing it to persist and causing long-term muscular and mental fatigue.

Some evidence from research in the United States has also linked stress to the appearance of certain CANCERS. It is possible that the immune system may be damaged enough by stress to allow cancerous cells to proliferate.

Coping with unavoidable stress

The first principle is to avoid throwing up our hands in horror in the belief that nothing can be changed and that all is lost; when we seriously get down to the nitty-gritty of situations, there is always far more in them that can be changed than we had imagined. Job, home circumstances, relationships – we may seem hopelessly trapped and without any room for manoeuvre in any of them; but all can be shifted sufficiently to give survival space if the need is great enough. And action must be taken in this direction, as unselfishly and with as much care of other people's rights and needs as possible, before anything else is considered.

Once we have taken all possible steps to reduce our level of stress to the minimum, we should direct our efforts to ensuring that the impact of that burden is reduced as much as possible. Basically this means adopting – and living out – an attitude of bending as smoothly and gracefully as possible with what we cannot stand up against. Both history and our own contemporaries rightly put a premium on endeavour, but it is far more folly than virtue to lose our life or our health tilting at unnecessary windmills. Wisdom here is to recognize what are essential confrontations in the preservation of mental and moral integrity; and what are really only exercises in personal vanity, based on an unrealistic – and usually disastrously fruitless – determination never to be beaten. Whenever possible, the blows of life should be either side-stepped or bowed to, rather than met in a head-on collision.

Releasing pent-up feelings

There will be some situations in which a considerable degree of stress is absolutely unavoidable. Most of these, since they are likely to seem either unreasonable, unprovoked or unjust, will lead to our feeling angry. This is the most destructive and harmful form of stress, and it is vitally important that steps are taken to deal with it. There are only two satisfactory ways of doing this – by releasing it or by sublimating it. The alternative – repressing stress – merely allows the development of stress-related illness. Releasing anger means giving it open expression by making our feelings known to those concerned – even if this does mean losing our temper. As long as we take the precaution of making sure that we are right, and are not being unjust, this is by far the best course; much more is usually gained in a relationship by clearing the air than is ever lost by the outburst. Our society sets far too much store on preserving peace at all costs, where a forthright expression of feelings, even if accompanied by some heat, would do far more good.

Many people need to learn to be more assertive in their dealings with others. This does *not* mean being aggressive: it means making clear to others how you feel about something. If you are able to express your feelings clearly to others, it is more likely that they will take your views into account. Your own internal conflicts and possibly your frustrations can be relieved if others know how you are affected by their actions.

See also MASSAGE, MEDITATION, RELAXATION.

Stroke

About a quarter of the people registered as physically disabled in the United Kingdom have become so by strokes. Strokes often – though not exclusively – attack the elderly and are one of the most common causes of death in the Western world. Present advances in medical research, however, particularly in connection with the role of high BLOOD PRESSURE in diseases of the ARTERIES, have helped our understanding of this illness.

What is a stroke?

Most people have some idea of what a stroke is, which is a testament to how often the disease occurs. The common factor in all strokes is that, due to disease of the blood vessel which supplies a particular part of the BRAIN, a section of the brain suddenly stops working. This means that the person involved often has little or no warning that something is wrong before he or she is struck down with partial or total weakness or PARALYSIS down one side of the body. This may be accompanied by aphasia – loss of the power of speech – or other problems in higher brain functions. Some strokes can occur away from the parts of the brain that control movement, so that this paralysis – also called hemiplegia – does not happen; but the first type of stroke is much more common.

What causes stroke?

Like the rest of the body, the brain must have a constant supply of BLOOD reaching it through its arteries. If one of these arteries becomes blocked, the part of the brain that it feeds will die because of the lack of oxygen and food which would normally be carried in the blood. Fortunately, in the brain there are many cross-connections between neighbouring blood vessels so that the area of damage is generally restricted. However, even that part of the brain which does not die may swell and damage the rest of the brain.

The other way in which strokes may be caused is when blood vessels in the brain burst. When this happens, the blood rushes into the brain under pressure, severely damaging nerve fibres.

These two basic mechanisms, cerebral infarction (when the artery is blocked) and cerebral haemorrhage (when there is bleeding into the brain) can be brought about by a number of different disorders.

Diseases which cause strokes

Obstruction of an artery in the brain can result from a disease which produces a blockage in the artery itself – a *cerebral* THROMBOSIS – or when a blood clot passes up the blood supply to the brain artery and gets stuck there. This is called a *cerebral embolism*.

Thrombosis – or blood-clotting – most usually occurs when an artery of the brain becomes furred up: fatty material accumulates in the walls of the artery. This is typical of a disease called *atherosclerosis*, which also causes the heart's blood vessels to become furred up and narrowed, resulting in HEART ATTACKS. Occasionally other problems in the arteries can cause thrombosis. These include inflammation of the artery, which can occur on its own or as a result of some serious infections.

Embolisms can be caused by HEART DISEASES or by disorders in the main arteries in the neck from which the blood enters the brain. Thus heart disease and strokes are linked, not only because the same disease of the arteries can cause trouble in both the heart and the brain, but also because in many

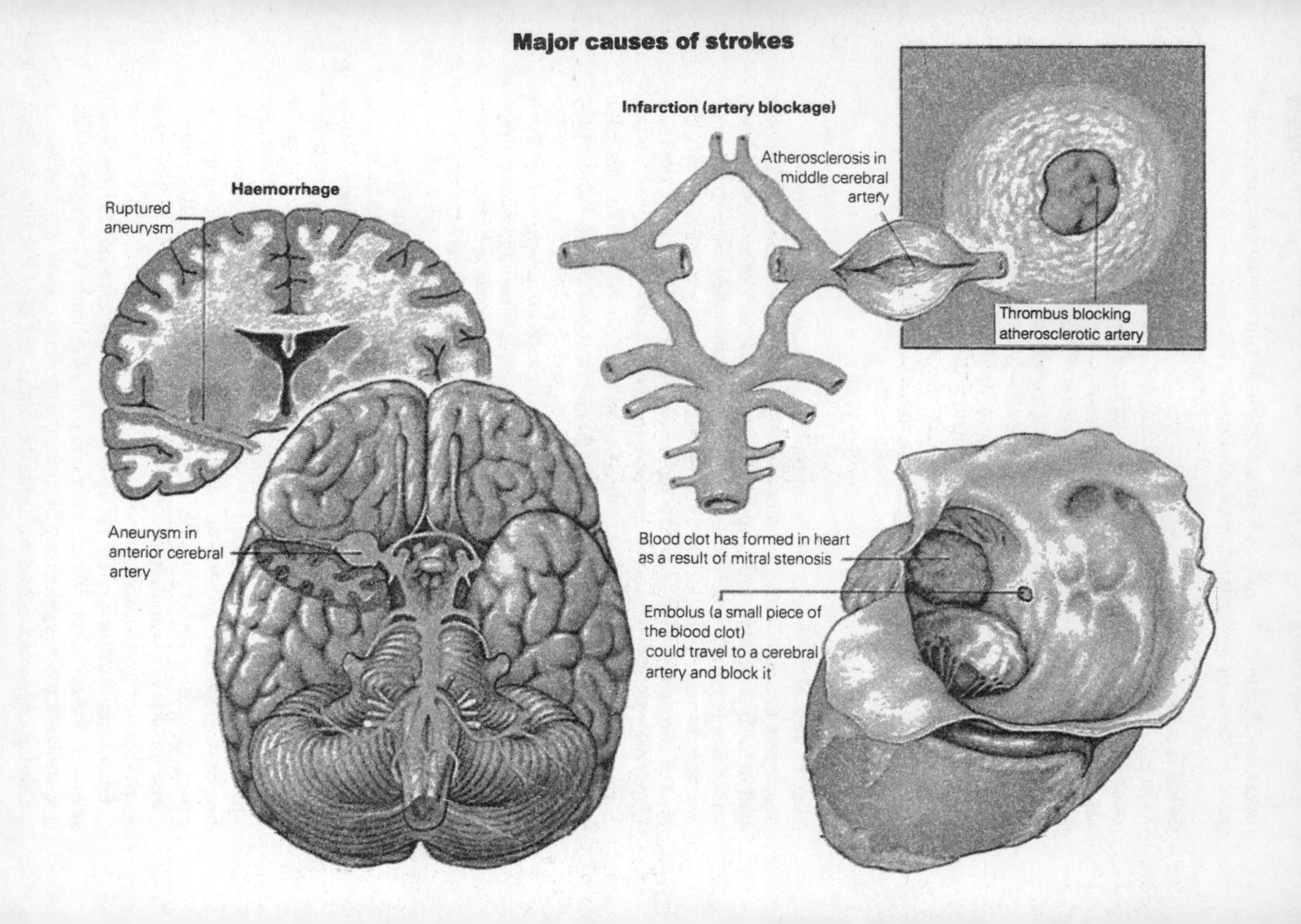
Major causes of strokes
Haemorrhage
Ruptured aneurysm
Aneurysm in anterior cerebral artery
Infarction (artery blockage)
Atherosclerosis in middle cerebral artery
Thrombus blocking atherosclerotic artery
Blood clot has formed in heart as a result of mitral stenosis
Embolus (a small piece of the blood clot) could travel to a cerebral artery and block it

diseases of the heart, blood clots form on the VALVES or on the damaged inside walls of the heart and these then fly off as emboli to cause strokes.

Cerebral haemorrhages – when the blood vessels in the brain burst – also have a number of causes. The most common is when there are weak places – called *aneurysms* – in the walls of the brain's arteries which then burst, often under the influence of a higher than normal blood pressure. In the larger brain arteries at the base of the skull, these aneurysms may be congenital (the patient is born with them), although they may not rupture until late in life if at all.

High blood pressure also has a tendency to produce weak places in the smaller arteries within the substance of the brain from which brain haemorrhage then occurs. Less common causes of cerebral haemorrhage can occur as a result of the presence of small, abnormally formed blood vessels in the brain, rather like the strawberry marks that are a similar abnormality of the blood vessels in the skin. This is called *arterio-venous anomaly* and is again a congenital condition.

Who is at risk?

Certain people have a higher risk of having strokes than others. The main conditions which predispose to stroke are DIABETES, high blood pressure, having a high serum cholesterol and SMOKING cigarettes. In addition, stroke seems to run in some families, though because it is such a common condition, this is difficult to prove. There are also people with heart diseases that can cause stroke by embolism. Thus people with a high risk can often be identified and preventive measures taken to reduce the chances of a stroke occurring.

In a tiny number of women, strokes have occurred while they were on the contraceptive pill. For this reason doctors try to discourage women who smoke, have high blood pressure or who are over 35 from taking the contraceptive pill. There is far less risk in women who are under 35, although doctors will dissuade even these women from continuing with the contraceptive pill if they have a history of MIGRAINE, as in this instance the contraceptive pill does increase slightly the chances of having a stroke at a younger age.

Symptoms

Some stroke patients have a warning attack in the weeks or months before a major stroke. These warning attacks can take the form of short-lived episodes of weakness down one side or transient blacking out of vision in one eye – a sign of blockage in one of the blood vessels to the retina. These are called 'transient iscaemic attacks' or TIAs and resolve completely within 24 hours. Most stroke patients, however, do not get any warning: what really typifies a stroke is the suddenness with which it happens. In most cases, disabilities such as loss of function of one side of the body or loss of speech reach their maximum within minutes, though occasionally it may take hours. In the following days and weeks, there will be an improvement as some of the brain cells recover, and after six months, the disabilities will be considerably less than at the onset of the stroke.

Other symptoms may include loss of vision in the right- or left-hand half of each eye (visual field defect), difficulty in dressing or finding one's way around familiar surroundings, and a host of other subtle difficulties in brain function. If a large area of the brain was damaged at the start of the stroke, the patient may not have a clear awareness of what has happened, or may ignore everything that happens on one side of his body. As the damaged brain swells, he may become drowsy or lose consciousness. This may happen much more quickly in brain haemorrhages, since the surge of blood into the brain causes much early damage to the centres and mechanisms that maintain alertness.

Treatment

Initial treatment consists of limiting the amount of damage that may be caused by the swelling spreading to the unaffected parts of the brain. This is done by paying close attention to the blood pressure and reducing it by administering drugs where necessary. Very seldom can surgeons remove blood clots that are causing pressure because they are often in inaccessible parts of the brain. A CT scan will be performed to confirm whether the stroke is due to a clot or a haemorrhage. If due to a clot, then a source of emboli will be looked for and treatment with aspirin started. In the case of heart valve lesions, anticoagulation with warfarin will be considered.

However, the main care of patients who have had strokes lies in the hands of nursing staff, PHYSIOTHERAPISTS, SPEECH THERAPISTS and OCCUPATIONAL THERAPISTS. Careful nursing is very important to prevent the emergence of bedsores (*see* ULCERS, SKIN) and chest troubles which can seriously impair the recovery from a stroke. During this vulnerable period when the stroke patient is often unable to care for himself, good nursing can literally save his life.

Preventing a stroke

The recent major advances in stroke research have been concerned with prevention. The fact that, in in the US, the number of strokes has declined is indicative of the effectiveness of the research. This is due mainly to the successful identification and treatment of high blood pressure – in fact, it has been shown that careful treatment of high blood pressure can significantly reduce the risk of developing a stroke. Often the difficulty is that most people with high blood pressure feel perfectly well and may need some convincing to take their tablets religiously to keep it down. Generally your doctor will take your blood pressure as a matter of routine when you consult him so that he can detect high blood pressure before it leads to trouble.

After minor strokes from which the patient may have recovered completely, it is an important part of treatment to try to prevent another more serious episode occurring in the future. Sometimes surgery can be performed on the large blood vessels in the neck (i.e. the carotid arteries): this may be done if the blood vessels have roughened parts in their lining from which clots fly off as emboli. Aspirin should be given daily to patients who suffered an embolic stroke since it has been found that relatively small amounts of the drug affect the clotting ability of the blood – not much, but enough to prevent blood from clotting in the brain's vessels.

Other drugs called *anticoagulants* reduce the blood's liability to clot, and these are used to prevent a stroke when one of the predisposing heart conditions is identified. Many other drugs which can prevent stroke in those at risk are now undergoing trials.

Sudden infant death syndrome (SIDS), *see* **Cot death**

Sugars, *see* **Carbohydrates**

Suicide, *see* **Depression, Hypochondria, Manic depression, Tranquillizers**

Sulphonamides, *see* **Antibiotics**

Sunburn

The sun is really a small star and its energy can be compared with a continuous and enormous atomic explosion. Some of its rays are deadly, but these are filtered out by the earth's atmosphere and never reach the earth itself. The rays that do pass through the atmosphere are part of the sun's spectrum. It contains visible rays which we see as light, infra-red rays which we feel as heat, and the group that causes sunburn – the ultraviolet or invisible rays. These are called ultraviolet because they are beyond the violet end of the visible spectrum.

The ultraviolet and infra-red rays are both capable of damaging the human body. However, the infra-red rays do not cause a problem, since they are registered as heat, and an exposed area can be withdrawn before any harm is done. It is the ultraviolet rays that cause sunburn because they can penetrate and damage the SKIN without giving an immediate feeling of warmth.

Effects on the skin

The skin is made up of two layers. In the outer layer – the *epidermis* – cells are continuously being shed from the surface and replaced by new ones which are formed in the lowest level of the epidermis. It is in this outer layer that the effects of sunburn occur.

The epidermis also contains the pigment-producing cells, or *melanocytes.* These are stimulated by ultraviolet light to produce the pigment MELANIN which acts as a very efficient filter of the ultraviolet rays. The new pigmentation – which is seen as a suntan – begins soon after exposure to the sun and builds up during continual exposure. After the period of exposure, the pigmentation will fade at varying rates, and will likely disappear completely within nine months. Sunburn occurs when there is not enough pigment filter present.

There are two types of sun damage – immediate and delayed. The immediate type of damage is sunburn, but like any form of radiation burn, it does not show its effects for some hours. The first signs are redness and a sensation of burning caused by an increase in the blood supply to the skin. This may happen any time up to 24 hours after exposure. Later, small blisters may develop. More severe damage produces large blisters and can actually damage some of the cells in the epidermis – these are called 'sunburn cells'. The degree of sunburn depends on the strength of the ultraviolet rays.

Sunburn itself is not as serious as the long-term damage to the skin. This is caused by repeated sun damage to the cells at the skin's surface and to the supporting tissues below. It takes years to develop, but once it has happened, it is not reversible.

The changes are similar to those of ageing and the obvious effects can be seen in the seaman's or farmer's face, where there is marked wrinkling and a leathery thickening of the skin. Other effects can be very localized, such as patchy increases in the pigmentation and a thickening of the horny covering of the skin. This can give rise to wart-like lumps, called *solar keratoses*, which are common in the middle-aged and elderly.

Widening of the blood vessels of the face and dryness and cracking of the skin are part of the ageing process but are more marked in people who have spent their lives outdoors.

The greatest cause of skin CANCER is repeated exposure to the sun. It was very uncommon in the Victorian era when there was little exposure of the skin, but nowadays it often occurs in sunworshipping nations such as Australia – in fact, Australia has the highest incidence of skin cancer in the world.

Fair-skinned people who can produce enough melanin pigment to give a good tan are still vulnerable to skin cancer. There is a limit to the number of harmful rays that can be absorbed by the pigment filter, and once this has been saturated, these rays can then cause damage. It is therefore not impossible for a tanned person to develop sunburn from excessive exposure. Dark-skinned people suffer the same effects but to a much lesser degree.

Treatment

Once sunburn has occurred, the most important factor in treatment is to prevent further damage by avoiding further exposure. In mild burns, the redness and burning usually resolve in a few days, and are often followed by peeling. Soothing lotions such as calamine are most effective, and if sleep is disturbed, antihistamines may be prescribed – these are mildly sedative but have no effect on the skin. In more severe burns, the symptoms are usually most acute on the second day when blisters may form on the affected areas. STEROID ointments reduce the intensity and duration of the skin reaction.

Prevention

Most people quickly learn how much sun they can take without burning. The body's natural protection is, of course, a tan built up gradually each day by increasing periods of exposure.

The intensity of the sun must also be taken into account. The most accurate way of gauging this is not by the degree of heat or light, but by the angle of

Which suntan cream to use?

Skin type		**Children** Under the age of 12	**Adults** Strong sun or during first few days of exposure	**Adults** After several days of tanning, or in moderate or light sun
		Skin Protection Factor (SPF)		
Type I	Always burns, never tans	15	15	15
Type II	Always burns, sometimes tans	15	12 or 15	12 or 15
Type III	Sometimes burns, sometimes tans	12 or 15	8 to 12	6 to 8
Type IV	Never burns, always tans	8 or 12	6 to 8	3 to 6

This chart can be used for sunbathing in Europe or S. Australia. In North Africa or N. Australia, use stronger SPF numbers and limit exposure carefully.

the sun above the horizon. This determines the amount of ultraviolet light that reaches the skin.

At midday, the sun is directly overhead and the rays pass through less of the earth's atmosphere. When the sun is low, in the morning and evening, the strength of the ultraviolet rays is considerably reduced. You are therefore unlikely to get sunburned in the early morning or after mid-afternoon. Particular care must be taken when swimming, sailing or skiing. Water absorbs the heat rays, but the ultraviolet rays are still being directed on to the skin, and snow gives a feeling of coolness but actually reflects the ultraviolet rays.

There are many sunscreen creams and lotions available, which aid tanning by preventing sunburn. The skin may thus be exposed for longer periods, but these preparations must be applied frequently, and especially just before and after swimming. They protect mainly against the 'sunburn' rays but let through enough of the longer ultraviolet waves to produce a gradual tan. The tan is, however, no deeper than one obtained simply by gradual exposure without a sunscreen. Some sunscreens give almost total protection by stopping all the ultraviolet and visible rays, so that prolonged exposure without damage is possible.

Some parts of the body are more liable to sunburn than others because they are exposed the most. A bald head, the face, top of the ears, forearms and backs of the hands are particularly at risk. A hat should always be worn when the hair is thin and this will also protect the nose and tops of the ears. Otherwise a sunscreen may be used on these small areas. Clothing is an efficient filter of the sun's harmful rays, if it is opaque.

Sunstroke

Although we are all used to thinking of an extremely serious heat disorder as sunstroke – something that only happens to people who stay out too long in the hot sun – it is, in fact, the heat itself that is the problem and not the sun's rays. For instance, people who find themselves in very hot places such as engine rooms and steelworks can suffer the severe effects of 'sunstroke' without ever being near the sun. And, for this reason, doctors tend to talk about 'heatstroke' rather than use the more common term 'sunstroke'.

The body's reaction to heat

The body has two main mechanisms for losing heat. First, the blood vessels to the skin are dilated so that more blood flows to the surface, allowing it to lose heat through the skin into the air. Second, the skin is cooled by the action of the sweat glands (*see* PERSPIRATION). The sweat glands pour out their salty fluid on to the surface of the skin. It evaporates, and heat is lost as vapour.

There are many ways in which the environment can intensify the effects of heat on the body – it is not just a question of the reading on the thermometer. If the air is humid, this reduces the ease with which the sweat evaporates, so that it becomes more difficult to lose heat. Similarly, if the air is very still, then less heat is lost from the surface of the body by convection.

People doing hard physical work in a hot environment are, of course, producing a lot of heat of their own. They may be losing up to one litre of sweat every hour, compared with the one litre per day of the sedentary worker in a temperate climate. This loss of SALT and WATER can contribute to a condition known as *heat exhaustion*, which, unless checked, can lead to the eventual breakdown of the body's temperature-regulating mechanism (heatstroke). Fortunately, however, as the body gets used to working in a hot environment, it adapts and the loss of salts decreases, making the body less vulnerable to heat disorders.

The very young and the very old are most at risk from heat disorders, and consequently from heatstroke. This is because their bodies' temperature-regulating mechanisms are not very efficient. Also elderly people tend to wear too much clothing in hot weather.

However, there are several other predisposing factors. People who are unused to heat, who are very overweight, who drink heavily, or who are suffering from a feverish illness, may – in the right circumstances – all be at a greater risk from heatstroke.

Symptoms and dangers

The three basic signs of heatstroke are: a very high temperature (more than 106°F/41°C); a total absence of sweating; and, most seriously, nervous system problems which lead to coma (*see* UNCONSCIOUSNESS). Disturbances of mood, disorientation and headache, often accompanied by dizziness and difficulty in walking all happen in the early stages of heatstroke until, eventually, consciousness is lost.

Unfortunately, fully developed heatstroke is an extremely dangerous condition, and over 20 per cent of sufferers may die, even with treatment. And those who do recover may have persistent trouble in the nervous system, and their balance and coördination may take months to get back to normal. However, if treatment is prompt – at the first sign of symptoms and *before* consciousness is lost – the chances of recovery are good.

Treatment and prevention
As soon as any symptoms appear, it is essential to call a doctor immediately. Meanwhile, cool the patient down as quickly as possible. The temperature should be brought down to about 102°F (39°C) – no lower as the patient's circulation may go into SHOCK. The best way to cool the patient down is in a bath of cold water. In hospital, special slatted beds on which sufferers can be doused with water and cooled by fans are used.

The most sensible and effective way to fight sunstroke is, of course, prevention. And this can be done quite simply by ensuring that the body is not overheated. This means not staying out too long in the sun; wearing cool, loose clothing and hats in the heat; and taking salt tablets and drinking plenty of liquids when doing physical work in very hot environments.

Sweating, *see* **Perspiration**

Sympathetic nervous system, *see* **Autonomic nervous system**

Syncope, *see* **Unconsciousness**

Synovectomy, *see* **Arthritis**

Syphilis

This is not the commonest SEXUALLY TRANSMITTED DISEASE, but it is potentially very serious if not treated within the first few years. If not diagnosed, it continues – like a life sentence – through three progressively more serious stages. However, in a proportion of untreated patients it appears to clear spontaneously; the reason is unknown.

In the primary and secondary stages, syphilis is an infectious disease of the sex organs and sometimes of the skin and lining of the mouth. It later passes through a dormant or latent period when no signs of the disease can be seen, and the patient has no symptoms of illness. This stage may last from 5 to as many as 50 years, and it is only after all that time that some of those infected enter into the third stage. In these people, syphilis is often a chronic, crippling and killing disease.

Worldwide, syphilis remains one of the most serious public health problems, although in Western countries it is now less common; nevertheless it still occurs.

Progress of the disease
The syphilis germ, which is like a tiny corkscrew, is called *Treponema pallidum* or *spirochaete*. About 1000 of these may be acquired during intercourse with an infected person. Once in the skin they divide rapidly and then soon spread through the bloodstream.

The primary stage: in this stage, the disease usually shows itself by the appearance of an ULCER or sore on or in the sex organs. This ulcer is completely painless and is often neglected for this reason. Occasionally, the primary sore may appear on other parts of the body – for example, in or around the mouth or on the fingers. In homosexual men, the sore may appear in or at the opening of the back passage.

In some women with syphilis, the primary ulcer or sore is internal and may therefore pass unnoticed. Primary sores – there may be more than one – appear about 21 days after the infecting intercourse, but this incubation period may be as short as 9 days or, rarely, as long as 90 days. In some patients, there is nothing to be seen at all, and in a few, the sore may only be a small crack in the skin. Within a week or two of the appearance of the sore, painless lumps which are enlarged glands can be found in the groin.

After days or weeks, the ulcer, even if untreated, heals. This gives those who have not been treated the impression that all is well, but unfortunately this is not so, for if the disease is not treated, the germs may invade almost any organ of the body – something which occurs in about 40 per cent of patients.

The secondary stage: This stage shows itself as a generalized RASH. This is not itchy and may appear anywhere on the body. It can be so slight and faint that it is often ignored. There may also be sores in the mouth or in the throat or around the sex organs. Headache, fever and aches in the bones may occur, and there is often enlargement of the glands in the neck and elsewhere. These symptoms of secondary syphilis come and go if the disease is not treated.

The latent period: If the infection is not diagnosed, or if it is not treated properly, the rash and other symptoms wax and wane and eventually disappear. The disease then enters the dormant or latent period: this can last from 5 to 50 years and will be wholly symptom-free. The disease is no longer infectious and will not be transmitted through sexual intercourse, but women who have undetected syphilis can pass on the condition to their foetus if they become pregnant even several years later. This may result in a baby born dead, deformed or diseased.

The third stage: About a third of those who have undetected syphilis suffer sooner or later from skin ulcers, syphilitic HEART DISEASE, syphilitic PARALYSIS, insanity, BLINDNESS or DEAFNESS. In this stage, so much damage has often been done by the germs over many years that treatment can only halt the progress of the disease; damage to the nervous system or circulatory system will not improve. In the earlier stages, syphilis can be cured completely.

Detection and treatment

In the primary and secondary stages, syphilis can be diagnosed by scraping the primary sore or one of the parts of the rash, taking some of the fluid which then oozes out and finding the tiny corkscrew treponeme in it under the microscope. Six weeks after infection, substances which show that the body's defences are working can be detected by a blood test, but before that time, the blood test will be negative. In the latent period, only a blood test will detect whether a person has or has had syphilis. This test is given to all people attending a hospital's 'special' or GUM (genito-urinary medicine) clinic.

All pregnant women attending ante-natal clinics have a blood test for syphilis as a matter of course, and if the disease is found, they are treated and then have perfectly healthy children. Every donation of blood for transfusion is, by law, tested for syphilis before it can be given to another person.

For all stages, penicillin is the chosen treatment. It is given as a course of daily injections, the patient attending if possible out of working hours. Thereafter, every treated person is asked to attend for two years at monthly, and later three-monthly, intervals for an examination and a blood test. Only in this way can the doctor guarantee that the cure is permanent. Treatment given during the first year of the latent period is curative.

Systemic lupus erythematosis, *see* Lupus erythematosis

T

Tachycardia

Simply put, a tachycardia is an unusually fast heartbeat. An attack of tachycardia may vary in severity from minor palpitations to a possibly fatal illness.

Although tachycardias are usually associated with HEART DISEASE, they often occur in people with no HEART complaints at all. In addition, attacks can begin at an early age: teenagers and, very occasionally, children may suffer.

The human heart beats at an average rate of about 70 beats per minute. This rate is regulated by a sophisticated timing system which delivers electrical pulses that allow the heart to beat either slowly enough, so that the heart muscle can pump effectively without becoming exhausted, or fast, to enable the heartbeat to accelerate during heavy exertion. The heart rate in young people who are exercising hard may go as high as 200 beats per minute, and in children it can go even higher.

The steady electrical pulse that drives the heart is generated from a part of the right atrium called the *sinoatrial (SA) node*. In an adult at rest, one impulse is produced every second or so, and it passes through the atrium and stimulates it to contract. The impulse then reaches the junction between the atrium and the ventricle, where it is 'stored' for a fraction of a second in another specialized conducting structure known as the *atrio-ventricular (AV) node*. The reason the impulse is delayed here is to allow the ventricles to benefit from the atrial contraction.

Once the impulse has reached the ventricles – the main pumping chambers of the heart – it is conducted through to the ventricular muscle via a system of specialized muscle fibres called the *His bundle* and the *Purkinje fibres* or the *His-Purkinje system*. So once the His-Purkinje system has stimulated the muscles of the ventricle to contract, the impulse for that particular heartbeat has completed its journey through the heart from the SA node. When the heart is beating normally, the whole journey takes about one third of a second.

Sometimes, however, another part of the electrically active tissue of the heart may start to produce impulses in competition with the SA node. If only one such impulse is produced, a single abnormal – or 'ectopic' – beat will be the result. But in some cases, this abnormal new source of impulses triggers off at a very high speed, so that the normal circuits never have time to take control. This is one of the mechanisms of a tachycardia. The reason this phenomenon takes place is because the heart's sophisticated conduction apparatus has back-up systems that will fire away on their own if necessary – and this is an important protective feature which will prevent trouble if the impulses from the SA node should stop arriving, which could be extremely dangerous (a situation known as *heart block*). But it requires only the most minute electrical changes in the heart for some area to start to fire away automatically.

Symptoms

One of the major symptoms of a tachycardia is palpitation, which is an uncomfortable, thumping sensation in the chest as the heart beats away at higher than normal speeds. Another major problem associated with a fast heart rate is that, at these speeds, the heart is unable to pump efficiently: as a result, patients may feel very limp and may collapse and lose consciousness as the blood supply to the brain is cut off.

It takes very little to set off a tachycardia, and it may occur as a result of almost any type of heart problem. Many diseases affect the heart, causing it to struggle to pump blood, and this in turn leads to stretching of the two atria as back pressure builds up. Eventually the atria stop working properly, and a background of disorganized electrical activity with no active contraction builds up in them. This then drives the ventricles at a fast and irregular rate.

After heart attacks, parts of the ventricular muscle are poorly supplied with oxygen, and this leads to electrical abnormalities which may cause ectopic beats and tachycardias.

Treatment

Nowadays there are many drugs which alter the electrical activity of the heart cells, and so alter the background which allowed the tachycardia to develop in the first place. The correct drug must be chosen with care after an exact diagnosis of the type of tachycardia has been made by analysing ELECTROCARDIOGRAMS.

Often, however, a fast heartbeat has such a detrimental effect that it becomes vital to re-establish normal heart function. This is done by giving the patient an electric shock across the chest. The shock seems to have the effect of wiping the electrical slate clean and allowing normal activity to take over. Later, drugs may be used to try to prevent the problem from happening again.

See also VENTRICULAR FIBRILLATION.

Tamoxifen, *see* **Breasts and breast cancer, Mastectomy**

Tamponade, *see* **Pericarditis**

Tardive dyskinesia, *see* **Schizophrenia, Tranquillizers**

Taste

Like SMELL, the taste mechanism is triggered off by the chemical content of substances in food and drink. Chemical particles are picked up in the mouth and converted into nerve impulses which are sent to the brain and interpreted.

The taste buds are at the heart of this system. Studding the surface of the

The sense of taste

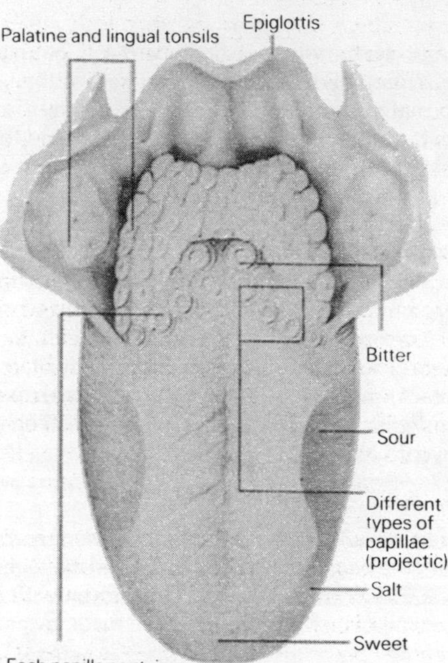

The tongue is covered with hundreds of 'bumps' called papillae, which increase the surface area in contact with food. Except for those in the centre, they include numerous taste buds. These, in turn, contain taste receptors which are distributed so that different parts of the tongue recognize different tastes.

TONGUE are many small projections, called *papillae*. Inside these are the taste buds. An adult has about 9000 taste buds, mainly on the upper surface of the tongue, but there are also some on the palate and even the THROAT.

Each taste bud consists of groups of receptor cells, and each of these has fine hair-like projections – called *microvilli* – sticking out into the surface of the tongue through fine pores in the surface of the papilla. At the opposite end to this, the receptor cells link up with a network of nerve fibres. The design of this network is complex, as there is a great deal of interlinking between nerve fibres and receptor cells. Two different nerve bundles, which make up the *facial nerve* and the *glossopharyngeal nerve*, carry the impulses to the brain.

The taste buds respond to only four basic tastes – sweet, sour, salt and bitter

– and the receptor sites for these tastes are located on different parts of the tongue. The buds that respond to sweet are at the tip of the tongue, while those specializing in salt, sour and bitter are located progressively further back.

Quite how the taste buds respond to the chemicals in the food and initiate the nerve impulses to the brain is not fully understood, but in order to be tasted, the chemicals must be in liquid form. Dry food gives very little immediate sensation of taste, and only acquires its taste after being dissolved in saliva.

At present, it is believed that the chemicals in the food alter the electrical charge on the surface of the receptor cells, which in turn cause a nerve impulse to be generated in the nerve fibres.

The analysis of taste by the brain

The two nerves carrying taste impulses from the tongue (the facial nerve or the glossopharyngeal nerve) first pass to the specialized cells in the brain-stem. This area of the BRAIN-stem also acts as the first stop for other sensations coming from the mouth. After initial processing in this brain-stem centre, the taste impulses are transferred in a second set of fibres across to the other side of the brain-stem and ascend to the thalamus. Here, there is another relay, where further analysis of the taste impulses is carried out before information is passed to the part of the cerebral cortex participating in the actual conscious perception of taste.

The cortex also deals with other sensations – such as texture and temperature – coming from the tongue. These sensations probably are mixed with the basic taste sensations from the tongue, and so produce the subtle sensations with which we are familiar when we eat.

This analysis, carried out in the lower part of the parietal lobe in the cortex, is further influenced by smell information being analysed in the nearby temporal lobe. Much of the refinements of taste sensation are due to smell sensations.

What can go wrong?

Loss of taste itself usually comes about from trouble in the facial nerve. This nerve is connected to the muscles of the face, but a small branch carries the taste fibres from the front two-thirds of the tongue. For the taste part of the nerve to become affected, the nerve must be damaged before the branch. This branch occurs just before the facial nerve passes near the eardrum. In the past, when continued ear infections were common and operations had to be performed for mastoiditis (as antibiotics were not yet known), the nerve was often damaged.

However, even when the nerve on one side of the face is severely affected, the other side will continue to send taste information to the brain. If the nerve that connects to the back third of the tongue is also damaged there may be considerable taste loss.

Taste may also be affected in the much more common *Bell's palsy*, where the facial nerve becomes inactive quite suddenly and for reasons which are not known. It is very rare for all taste nerves to be affected at the same time for any reason; complete taste loss is very rare.

In fact, it is much more common for people who have lost their sense of smell on both sides (for example, in a HEAD INJURY) to complain of loss, or reduction in their sense of taste. This is because, without this sense of smell, much of the subtler refinements of taste are lost.

It is quite common for people who are suffering from DEPRESSION to complain of unpleasant tastes in their mouths. The cause of this is not at all clear, but it may be related to the close relationship of taste and smell. Smell analysing centres of the brain have close connections with the emotional circuitry of the limbic system, and it has been suggested that certain moods can 'conjure up' tastes and smells. Another type of unpleasant taste occurs in some people as the 'aura' or warning sensation before an EPILEPTIC fit. This usually means that the abnormal electrical activity causing the fit is centred either low in the parietal lobe or in the neighbouring temporal lobe.

Teeth and teething

The teeth are hard bone-like structures implanted in the sockets of the jaws. Two successive sets occur in a lifetime.

Each tooth consists of two parts: the *crown*, which is the portion visible within the mouth, and the *root*, which is the part embedded within the jaw bone. The roots of the teeth are usually longer than the crowns. Front teeth have only one root, while those placed further back generally have two or three roots.

The major structural element of a tooth is composed of a calcified tissue known as *dentine*. This is a hard bone-like material which contains living cells. It is a sensitive tissue and gives the sensation of pain when stimulated either thermally (with heat) or by chemical means. The dentine of the crown is covered by a protective layer of *enamel*, an extremely hard cell-free and insensitive tissue. The root is covered with a layer of *cementum*, a substance that is somewhat similar to dentine and which helps anchor the tooth in its socket.

The centre of the tooth is a hollow chamber filled with a sensitive connective tissue known as the *dental pulp*. This extends from within the crown right down to the end of the root, which is open at its deepest part. Through this opening, minute blood vessels and nerves run into the pulp chamber.

Support of teeth

Each tooth is attached by its root to the jawbone; the part of the jaw which supports the teeth is known as the *alveolar process*. Teeth are attached to this by fibres known as the *periodontal ligaments*. This consists of a series of tough collagen fibres which run from the cementum covering the root to the adjacent alveolar bone. These fibres are interspersed with connective tissue which also contains blood vessels and nerve fibres.

The mode of attachment of the teeth results in a very small degree of natural mobility. This serves as a kind of buffer which may protect the teeth and bone from damage when biting.

A zone of crucial importance in this system is at the neck of the tooth where the crown and root merge. In this region, a cuff of gum is tightly joined to the tooth and serves to protect the underlying supporting tissues from infection and other harmful influences.

Types of teeth

There are two series of human teeth. *Deciduous* teeth are those present during childhood and are all usually shed. They can be divided into three categories: *incisors, canines* and *molars.* The *permanent teeth* are those which replace and also extend the initial series. These teeth can be divided into the same types as the deciduous teeth, and in addition there is a further category known as the *premolars,* which are intermediate both in form and position between canines (eye teeth) and molars.

Incisors are characterized by a narrow blade-like 'incised edge', and the incisors in opposite jaws work by shearing past each other like the blades of a pair of scissors. Canines and pointed teeth are well adapted for a tearing action, while molars and premolars are effective at grinding food rather than cutting it.

Teeth form an even, oval-shaped arch with the incisors at the front and the canines, premolars and molars progressively placed further back. The dental arches normally fit together in such a way that, on biting, the teeth opposite interlock each other; this known as an *occlusion.*

Development of teeth

Around the age of six months, the first of the lower incisors begins to come through the gum, a process known as *dental eruption.* The age at which this occurs is variable: a very few babies have teeth at birth, while, in others, they may not emerge until the age of one.

After the lower incisors have emerged, the upper incisors begin to erupt, and these are followed by canines and molars, although the precise sequence may vary. Teething problems may be associated with any of the deciduous teeth.

By the age of two-and-a-half to three, the child will usually have a complete set of 20 'milk' (deciduous) teeth. Ideally they should be spaced in such a way that provides room for the larger permanent teeth.

Subsequently, after the age of six, the lower, then the upper deciduous incisors become loose and are replaced by the permanent teeth. The permanent molars develop not in the place of the deciduous molars but behind them. The first permanent molars come through at the age of 6, the second molars at the age of 12, and the third molars, or *wisdom teeth,* around the age of 18. There is, however, considerable variation in the timing of the emergence of all the teeth. About 25 per cent of people never develop one or more wisdom teeth. The reason for this may be an evolutionary one: as the jaw has got smaller, the number of teeth has lessened. Some wisdom teeth may never erupt through the gum, and if they become impacted (wedged closely together under the gum), they may need to be removed. This happens in 50 per cent of people.

Deciduous (baby) and permanent teeth

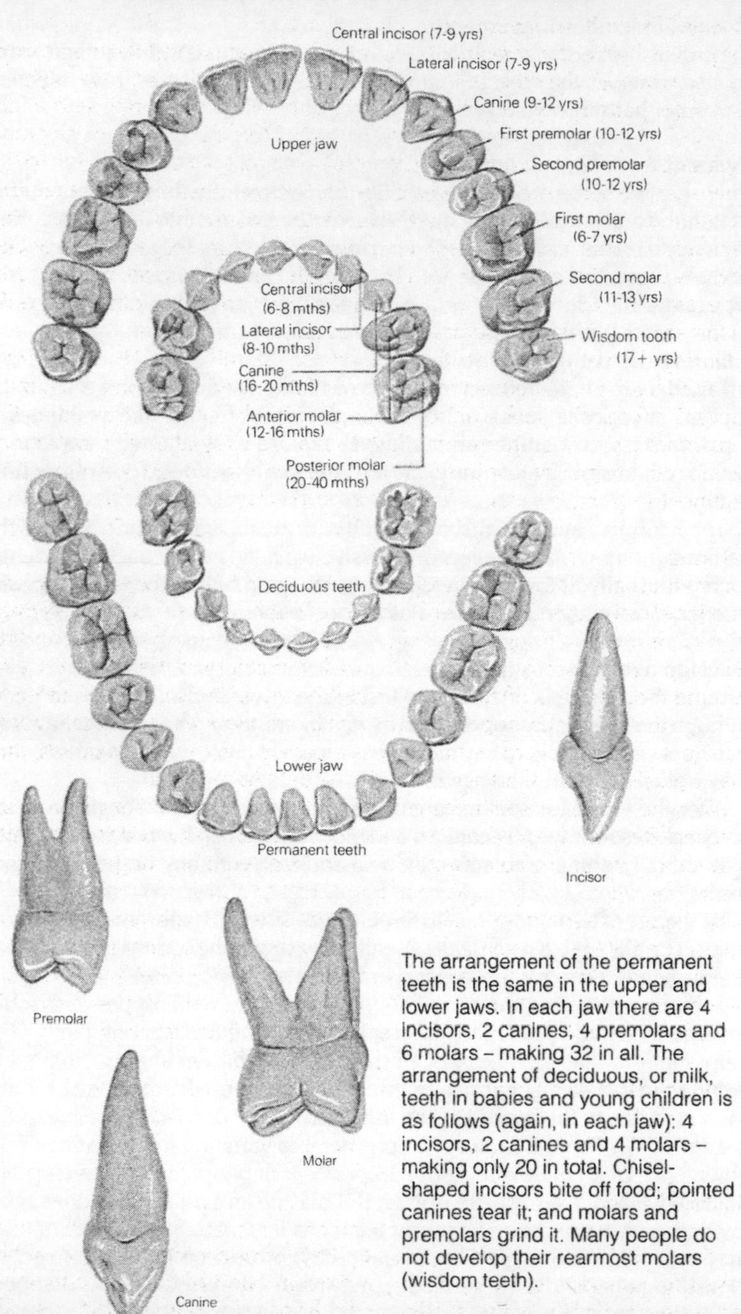

The arrangement of the permanent teeth is the same in the upper and lower jaws. In each jaw there are 4 incisors, 2 canines, 4 premolars and 6 molars – making 32 in all. The arrangement of deciduous, or milk, teeth in babies and young children is as follows (again, in each jaw): 4 incisors, 2 canines and 4 molars – making only 20 in total. Chisel-shaped incisors bite off food; pointed canines tear it; and molars and premolars grind it. Many people do not develop their rearmost molars (wisdom teeth).

Changes in teeth arrangement

The part of the jaw that supports the milk teeth increases very little in size from the age when all the milk teeth have erupted. Milk teeth tend to be smaller than their permanent replacements, and only when the large permanent incisors have erupted does the final form of the dental arches become apparent. The upper permanent incisors often appear out of proportion to the child's face when they first come through, but this naturally becomes less apparent as the face grows while the teeth remain the same size. Any tendency for the upper incisor teeth to protrude usually only becomes obvious when the milk teeth are replaced: the larger permanent teeth will exaggerate any discrepancy in their position. Similarly, crowding often only becomes clear when the permanent teeth erupt.

During the six years or so that it takes for the milk teeth to be entirely replaced by their 32 permanent successors, it is very common for a gap to appear between the upper incisors. This gap usually tends to close when the permanent canines erupt as they push the incisors together. Discrepancies either in the alignment or in the bite of the teeth may require orthodontic treatment to bring the teeth into the correct position. *See also* DENTAL CARE.

Teething

Tooth eruption is a normal developmental process, and can be quite painless, but many babies appear to suffer from a lot of discomfort, particularly as each new tooth breaks through. Sometimes a baby whose new tooth is hurting develops a red, inflamed patch on his or her cheek, and the gum may also become red. There is often excessive dribbling, rubbing of the mouth and crying; the cheeks may appear pinker than usual. Symptoms such as fever or diarrhoea are unlikely to be due to teething as is commonly supposed, and if they persist, medical advice should be sought immediately.

Where teething causes the baby some distress, a number of measures can be taken. Because the teething baby will occasionally suck or bite frantically on anything he or she can reach, then can be given a teething ring or hard dummy or, alternatively, a piece of raw carrot or a hard rusk. Never give a baby sweets to suck: they will not do much to relieve discomfort and will almost certainly be detrimental to the developing teeth. In some cases, it may be advisable to apply creams which have the effect of a local ANAESTHETIC on the child's sore gum, but bear in mind that these wear off rather quickly because the teething baby tends to salivate and dribble so much.

Temperature, *see* **Fever**

Tendons

Tendons, or sinews, play an important part in a wide variety of movements. Basically, a tendon is a very strong and tough band of fibrous connective tissue which joins the active section or 'body' of a MUSCLE to the part – usually a BONE – which it is intended to move. The force of the contracting muscle fibres is concentrated in and transmitted through the tendon, achieving traction on the part concerned and thus making it move.

Tendons are specialized extensions or prolongations of muscles, and they are formed by the connective tissue which binds the bundles of muscle fibres together, joining and extending beyond the muscle as a very tough, inelastic cord. They have very few nerve endings and, being essentially inactive tissues, little in the way of a blood supply. At one end, they are formed from the 'belly' of the muscle and at the other they are very firmly tethered to the 'target' bone, some of their fibres being actually embedded in the bone structure.

Location

Several tendons are located close to the surface of the body and can easily be felt. For instance, the 'hamstring' tendons, controlling knee bending, are at the back of the knee. Tendons are also often found where there are a large number of JOINTS to be moved in a relatively small space, since they take up much less room than 'meaty' muscles. Thus both the backs and the fronts of the hands and FEET contain a whole battery of different tendons. The muscles working these tendons are sited well back in the arms and legs.

An unusual tendon is found in connection with the muscle tissue that forms the wall of the HEART and brings about its pumping action. Here strips of thickened, fibrous connective tissue form tough strips within the heart muscle which both give it a firmer structure and form firm supporting rings at the points where the great blood vessels join the heart.

Tenosynovitis

In order that they can move smoothly and without friction or the danger of abrasion, tendons are enclosed in sheaths at the points where they cross or are in close contact with other structures. The tendon sheath is a double-walled sleeve designed to isolate, protect and lubricate the tendon so that the possibility of damage from pressure or friction is reduced to a minimum. The space between the two layers of the tendon sheath contains fluid, so that when the muscle is in action, the two layers slide over each other.

But the human machine cannot sustain repeated movements of the same sort without sustaining damage in the form of inflammation. This is because rest periods are necessary for the lubricating fluid to be replenished. If this does not happen, and the system is run without adequate lubrication, the two layers of the tendon sheath begin to rub against each other and chafe. Continued movement will then both be painful and cause a creaking sound called *crepitus*. This is the basis of the condition called *tenosynovitis* – inflammation of the tendon sheath. Any tendon sheath can be afflicted by this very annoying and painful condition which is particularly common in those such as typists, athletes, dancers and others who use one particular set of muscles repeatedly (*see also* REPETITIVE STRAIN INJURY).

Injury

Virtually all the disorders of tendons are due to injury of one sort or another.

A deep cut in the region of the foot, ankle, hand or wrist may sever one of the tendons which lie quite close to the surface. It is usually possible to sew the two ends together, though there is always the possibility of some weakness of the muscle or pain on use remaining. Extreme tension, 'over-stretching' or sudden forceful jerking strains on a tendon may damage it in a variety of ways of escalating severity.

What happens is that some of the fibres of the tendon anchoring it to the bone get torn away from their moorings. The tendon itself is not really stretched and only very rarely ruptured or snapped, since the force that would be required to do this would already have pulled it away from its attachment to the bone. Treatment of injuries is with ice packs and rest with the support of an elastic or crêpe bandage. In some cases, surgery may be needed: if permanent reinforcement of the tendon is required, the surgeon may implant carbon fibres into the tendon to strengthen it.

Tennis elbow, *see* **Tendons**

Tenosynovitis, *see* **Wrist**

Tension, *see* **Stress**

Termination of pregnancy, *see* **Abortion**

Testosterone, *see* **Hormones, Testes**

Test-tube babies

On 25 July 1978, at three minutes to midnight, a normal, healthy baby girl was delivered by Caesarean section at Oldham General Hospital in Lancashire. Louise Brown, weighing 5 lb 12 oz (2.6 kg) was the world's first test-tube baby.

It is estimated that about one in eight couples has a problem with INFERTILITY. Exact figures are hard to establish because not everyone chooses to try to have children nor seeks advice if there are difficulties. In perhaps just under a third of reported cases, however, the problem is the woman's Fallopian tubes, which are either blocked or damaged.

In the normal course of events, the ripened egg passes into one of the Fallopian tubes where it may meet and be fertilized by the SPERM. If the tubes are blocked and the passage of the egg is prevented, chances of pregnancy in the normal way are ruled out. In the majority of cases, it is pelvic infection which is responsible for blocked and damaged tubes, particularly infection with GONORRHOEA or CHLAMYDIA. Infections in users of the intra-uterine device (*see* CONTRACEPTION) have also been known to have this effect.

New developments in microsurgery – that is, fine surgery carried out under a microscope – have greatly increased the success rate in dealing with tubal problems. At present, it is only practised at certain centres to which women can ask to be referred. It should certainly be the first course of action – only if such surgery proves unsuccessful should test-tube fertilization be considered as a last resort.

In vitro fertilization

In the case of Louise Brown and other test-tube babies, fertilization took place outside the mother's body. In fact, a test-tube is not used at all, but a glass dish – hence the term *in vitro*, from the Latin meaning 'in a glass'.

One technique that has made a vital contribution to this form of fertilization is laparoscopy (*see* ENDOSCOPY). The patient is given a general anaesthetic and the abdominal wall is pierced with a slim needle through which gas is passed to distend the abdominal cavity. A small incision is then made just below the navel and the instrument known as the laparoscope is introduced. It works like a telescope and provides clear views of the UTERUS, OVARIES and the Fallopian tubes. The gynaecologist using a laparoscope can see exactly what he is doing and can carry out minor surgery if necessary.

To free the ovaries so that a ripened egg can be obtained without difficulty, a surgical procedure known as a *laparotomy* may first be needed to clear away any adhesions resulting from infection or previous unsuccessful surgery. The next stage is to recover one or more eggs from the patient's ovaries just before they are about to be shed. Fertility drugs are usually used to stimulate the woman's ovaries so that several eggs are produced at one time. The use of fertility drugs also means that procedures can be timed more conveniently for patients and doctors.

The eggs, removed via a hollow needle, are incubated for some hours in a special preparation. Then the husband's sperm, which has been freshly collected, is added. If fertilization takes place, it will be apparent after 18 hours. The fertilized egg is then transferred to another solution where it will start to divide. Now most embryos are transferred at the two-cell stage, with very few even reaching as many as eight cells.

The method for replacing the embryo is both simple and painless and done without anaesthetic. The embryo travels through in a cannula (a very fine tube) with an outlet at the side which is inserted through the vagina and cervix. Several days after insertion the woman is ready to return home. If pregnancy takes place, she will be carefully monitored.

Most teams report a success rate for recovering a suitable egg cell from laparoscopy of more than 90 per cent; fertilization is now also achieved in more than 90 per cent of cases. The problem then lies in implantation. Although the success rates of IVF are improving in most specialized centres, only about one attempt in four is successful. However, repeated attempts at IVF can be made for an individual couple. This can, nevertheless, be extremely stressful for them – *and* very expensive. IVF treatment is increasingly difficult to get on the NHS, and private treatment will cost approximately at least £3000 for each IVF attempt.

GIFT

Recently a somewhat simpler technique called gamete intrafallopian transfer (GIFT) has been developed. Eggs are removed from the woman's ovary in exactly the same way that is used for IVF, and then placed into the woman's Fallopian tube directly with a cannula. Some of the partner's sperm is inserted at the same time so that natural fertilization can proceed at the usual site within the tube. This technique does not need the services of a laboratory.

Testes

The normal human male has two testes (testicles) which develop in the embryo from a ridge of tissue at the back of the abdomen. When the testes have formed, they gradually move down inside the abdomen so that at the time of birth, each testis has usually arrived in its final position within the scrotum.

Function and structure

The function of the testes is twofold. First, they provide the site where SPERM is manufactured; each sperm contains all the genetic information for that particular male. Second, the testes contain cells which produce the male sex hormone *testosterone* and consequently the male characteristics such as the deep voice, male hair distribution and typical distribution of fat. These two functions are carried out by completely separate sets of cells within each of the testes: one function can fail without the other one necessarily doing so.

The testes are oval structures. Attached to the back of each one is a smaller structure which is shaped like a long comma and is called the *epididymis*. This consists of a series of microscopically tiny tubes which collect sperm from the testis. These tubes connect together to form one tube, called the *vas deferens*, which transfers the sperm towards the base of the bladder. All these structures, with the exception of the vas deferens, are microscopic in size.

Each testis is suspended in the scrotum by the *spermatic cord*, which contains the vas deferens, the *testicular artery* and the *testicular vein*. These three structures are surrounded by a tube of muscle called the *cremasteric muscle*. The spermatic cord, therefore, serves two purposes: first, to provide a blood supply to the testis and, second, to conduct the sperm away from the testis.

What can go wrong?

For the vast majority of males, the testes carry out their vital and complex role unaffected by problems. But sometimes structural or functional difficulties do occur which, fortunately, can usually be treated.

Undescended testes: For sperm to be manufactured, the testes have to be at a slightly lower temperature than the normal body temperature. And this is why the testes are suspended outside the abdominal cavity in the scrotum.

At birth, however, it may be noted that one or other testis is not in the scrotum. It may be in the groin, having got stuck on the way, or it may have failed to get as far as the groin. An undescended testis can have several effects: it will be unable to produce sperm; it may be damaged in the groin and be more liable to twisting, or torsion (*see below*); and there is an increased risk of a tumour occurring in an undescended testis.

It is important to distinguish between an undescended testis and one which is *retractile.* The latter means that the cremasteric muscle is over-active and has pulled the testis up into the groin. A retractile testis will probably descend into the scrotum at puberty; an undescended testis will not descend on its own, and will require surgery.

The operation for an undescended testis, an *orchidopexy,* is usually performed by the age of three or four years. It consists of a small incision in the groin to find the testis, followed by stitching it into place in the scrotum. There is some evidence that, if the operation is delayed beyond this age, irreversible damage to the testis may occur. However, even if a testis does not produce sperm because it has not descended, it still may be able to produce normal amounts of testosterone. And, in any event, one testis which is functioning normally should be perfectly adequate to produce sufficient sperm and testosterone.

Torsion: In some men, there is an abnormality in the way in which the testis hangs in the scrotum. This abnormality is present at birth, and usually affects both testes. The abnormality is such that one of the testes can twist on its spermatic cord, leading to a sudden cutting off of the blood supply to the testis. The most common age for this to occur is in the teens, but it can also happen in younger children or in young adults.

The usual symptom of a torsion of the testis is extreme tenderness and the sudden onset of severe pain on one side of the scrotum. Left untreated, the twisted testis swells up and becomes inflamed, and eventually becomes gangrenous. Irreversible gangrene can occur within hours of the onset of the pain. Because of the swelling and inflammation, there is a danger that a case of torsion could be mistaken for infection. Infection in the testis in a teenager is, in fact, quite rare, and so any case of inflammation of the testis in this age group should be treated as a torsion until proved otherwise.

Treatment involves surgical exploration, untwisting of the testis and fixing it with stitches so that it cannot twist again. If it is gangrenous, it will have to be removed. Because the abnormality is present on both sides, a small operation is usually done on the other side to prevent torsion from occurring.

Infection and inflammation: Sometimes infection can pass from the bladder along the vas deferens, and obtain access to the epididymis. This infection, called *epididymitis,* usually occurs in older men and may be related to PROSTATE disease. The symptoms are pain and swelling in one side of the scrotum.

Usually the urine is infected, and after treatment with the appropriate antibiotic, the infection clears up. There are usually no long-term effects, but the patient may be prone to repeated attacks.

Inflammation of the testis itself is known as *orchitis*. Infection with the MUMPS virus can cause orchitis, and, if both testes are affected, can lead to sterility. Fortunately, however, this complication is rare.

Cysts: There are several different types of CYST which can occur in the testes. They are usually associated with some congenital abnormality, but may not become apparent until the patient is quite old. The first type is known as an *epididymal cyst* and shows itself as a lump attached to the testis; the testis can still be felt as separate entity. Shining a strong light through the lump confirms that it is not solid, but is full of clear fluid.

The other type of cystic swelling is known as a *hydrocoele*. This may be larger and is different in that the fluid-filled cavity surrounds the testis, so that the testis cannot be felt separately. The former type of cyst is entirely harmless. The second type is usually harmless but occasionally may be associated with underlying inflammation in the testis, or, more rarely, a tumour.

The treatment of these various cysts is to remove them surgically, but only if they are causing symptoms.

Varicocoele: This is a condition where the veins in the spermatic cord become enlarged and twisted, like VARICOSE VEINS. The patient usually notices an aching sensation in the scrotum and may feel a lump just above the testis when he stands up. Because the lump is, in fact, the veins full of blood, it goes away when the patient lies down.

Apart from producing a dragging, aching sensation, varicocoeles are significant because they can cause a rise in the temperature of the tissues in the scrotum. This can eventually lead to impairment of sperm production and INFERTILITY.

Treatment involves surgical removal of the large veins and this sometimes leads to a rise in the sperm count.

Testicular cancer

Tumours of the testis are rare in comparison to the incidence of some other tumours. Many of them can be cured completely, even though they are technically speaking a form of CANCER. These tumours occur in young men, between the ages of 18 and 40 years, though they can occur in other age groups.

The commonest way in which they become apparent is by the patient noticing that one testis is bigger than the other one. There may be some pain.

Because malignant tumours of the testes can be cured by early treatment, all men should check their testes every month for any sign of abnormal swelling or tenderness. If an abnormality is found, medical advice should be sought.

Treatment involves removing the testis, followed by further investigations to see whether the tumour has spread. Even if there is spread, the results of treatment with X-rays and special drugs are good.

See also INFERTILITY, PENIS and VASECTOMY.

Tetanus

This is caused by a bacterium called *Clostridium tetani.* This organism is found freely in the soil, and is more likely to be encountered in manured and cultivated soil since it is very common in animal dung. However, it is not confined to the soil; street dust from the centre of a town certainly contains the spores of the bacteria, and they can even be found inside buildings in quite large amounts.

Any minor injury can implant tetanus spores into the skin. Since major injuries are usually treated in hospital, proper care is taken to prevent the disease. A minor injury – such as pricking your finger on a rose thorn – can set up a tetanus infection if you have not been immunized. About a third of all cases of tetanus in Britain occur as a result of an injury which was so trivial that the patient had not even noticed.

The bacterium has one very important characteristic that controls the way the disease behaves: it is killed off by oxygen and only grows in oxygen-free (anaerobic) surroundings. This is why the bacteria have to be introduced into the body via a wound of some sort, since the blood supply and therefore the oxygen supply are cut off as a result of the tissue damage. The deeper and more contaminated a wound is, the worse the risk of tetanus.

The toxin that the bacterium makes is a deadly substance, exceeded in potency only by the toxin responsible for botulism. A tenth of a milligram is the fatal dose for an adult. From its site of production in the wound contaminated by the bacteria, the toxin passes into the spinal cord and the brain. It is thought that it travels through the nerves, although spread via the blood could also be important. Once in the nervous system, the toxin cannot be neutralized by antibodies either produced by the body after immunization or given as antitoxin.

Symptoms

The incubation period is six to ten days as a rule, although in rare cases it may be several months. At the other extreme symptoms can occur within a day. There is a short vague illness with headache, general illness and fever, but the important first signs are due to the generalized muscle rigidity that is one of the two classical symptoms of the disease. This especially affects the jaw muscles (giving rise to 'lock jaw' by which name the disease is sometimes known), the muscles of the abdomen, which are found to be firm on examination, and the muscles of the back. Eventually the back may be arched right over and the neck bent right back.

Spasms develop later and can be brought on by any stimulus. Minor spasms may simply affect the face, with contraction of the facial muscles into a ghastly grin – known by the chilling Latin title *risus sardonicus,* meaning 'sardonic smile'. Breathing can be affected by these spasms, and when they become more generalized, they lead to even more exaggerated arching of the back and neck.

The difficulty in looking after tetanus patients really becomes marked when the disease interferes with the way that the brain controls vital functions. The heart may be affected, leading to abnormalities of rhythm and either very low, or very high blood pressure. Sometimes the temperature may shoot up rapidly. These changes are due to involvement of the autonomic nervous system.

Treatment

The aim of treatment is to tide the patient over the period of illness without any of the possible fatal problems occurring. These problems include exhaustion due to spasm, asphyxia (suffocation) during spasm, pneumonia due to stomach contents entering the lungs, and death due to disorders of the control of vital functions such as the heartbeat and blood pressure.

In milder cases, simple sedation and the avoidance of all types of disturbance will prevent spasms, but in the more severe cases, a tracheostomy (*see* STOMA CARE) is performed, and the patient is treated by total paralysis using *curare* (a paralysing drug), while breathing is taken over by a ventilator. Penicillin and antitoxin should be given to all patients in an attempt to neutralize any circulating toxin.

About half of all patients die from the disease, and without good medical care, fatality rates can be much higher.

Prevention

IMMUNIZATION with what is known as *tetanus toxoid* is given with a baby's first immunization, and boosters are given when starting school and again on leaving. After that, a booster should be given every ten years – or more often if you are at special risk – for example, if you work on the land. In people who have not been immunized, it is necessary to give an antitoxin after any serious wound.

Tetany, *see* **Calcium, Rickets**

Tetralogy of Fallot, *see* **Blue baby, Valves, heart**

Tetraplegia, *see* **Paralysis**

Thalassaemia

This is a form of ANAEMIA, and results from abnormalities in the structure of haemoglobin, an important component of BLOOD.

There are two basic forms of the disease: *thalassaemia major* and *thalassaemia minor.* In the minor form, there are usually no serious ill effects, but the major form can be fatal.

Thalassaemia tends to occur in the places where MALARIA is or has been common, but it is particularly prevalent on the Mediterranean coast and in the Middle and Far East. However, because the population of the world is now so mobile, thalassaemia can be found almost anywhere in the world.

It is thought that possessing one of the abnormal genes that give rise to thalassaemia gives some protection against the effects of malaria. Some doctors believe that this is because all the red cells in the body of a thalassaemic person are a bit fragile, so that when the malarial parasite gets inside a red cell, the cell breaks down and the parasite stops growing.

Causes

Haemoglobin is the substance that is responsible for carrying oxygen from the lungs to the tissues. It is made up of two substances which are chemically bound together: *haem* – the iron-containing central core of a haemoglobin molecule – and *globin,* the protein constituent of haemoglobin which exists as a chain.

The body produces a number of different chains, but it is the *alpha* and *beta* chains that are at the heart of the thalassaemic condition. Each molecule of haemoglobin has four globin chains attached to its central portion; normal haemoglobin in an adult – called haemoglobin A – is made of two alpha and two beta chains. The type of chain is determined by the genes inherited from our parents (*see* GENETICS and HEREDITY).

If the normal construction of the globin chain fails, the make-up of the haemoglobin is affected and thalassaemia is produced. The failure can be caused by both the presence of an abnormal gene, and an abnormality in what is called the *transcription process* – converting the genetic instructions into the production of new protein molecules.

Beta thalassaemia

We inherit two genes from our parents that control the production of beta chains. If one of the genes is faulty, the outcome is beta thalassaemia minor, a form of thalassaemia that gives no serious trouble. However, when both genes are defective, the very serious beta thalassaemia major is produced.

In this disease, the faulty haemoglobin – called haemoglobin F and normally only found in the foetus – is very slow to give up the oxygen to the tissues, and this leads to over-stimulation of the BONE MARROW. The marrow then expands and may deform the bones that contain it.

This long-standing and serious anaemic condition is particularly dangerous for children as it restricts growth and development.

Alpha thalassaemia

Alpha thalassaemia is slightly more complex – but not as serious – due to the fact that we inherit four genes which are responsible for the production of alpha globin chains. If one or two of these genes are defective in any way, the result is alpha thalassaemia minor which is not serious; the sufferer is only a little anaemic but will need treatment.

When there are three defective alpha genes, this produces a type of haemoglobin called haemoglobin H which turns into haemoglobin H disease. Here, the red blood cells break down very easily, and this leads to both anaemia and JAUNDICE. Although this condition cannot be cured, it can be successfully controlled through occasional blood transfusions, and the sufferer can lead a near-normal life.

However, when all four alpha chain genes are missing, this produces a type of blood which is not compatible with life and the foetus either aborts or is stillborn.

Treatment

The different types of thalassaemia are treated in much the same way; patients are provided with regular blood transfusions to keep the level of haemoglobin high, and so maintain the supply of oxygen to the tissues. The number of blood transfusions depends on the type and severity of the anaemia. As frequent blood transfusions can result in a dangerous build-up of IRON, some patients may need daily treatment with a special drug which allows the iron to be excreted safely in the urine. Treatment may also include antibiotics to counter infection, and in some cases, the SPLEEN is removed.

Prevention

Genetic counselling is the only preventive measure that can be taken. Using simple tests, it is possible to determine whether two people have the genes for beta thalassaemia. Where this is found one in four of the children are expected to have beta thalassaemia major.

It is also possible to examine the blood of the foetus at about 20 weeks into the pregnancy to see if there are any beta chains being produced. If there are not, a baby considered 'at risk' is likely to have the disease, and it may be thought wise to terminate the pregnancy.

See also SICKLE-CELL ANAEMIA.

Thirst, *see* Water

Threadworms, *see* Worms

Throat

This is the term popularly used to describe the area that leads into the respiratory and digestive tracts. It extends from the mouth and NOSE to the OESOPHAGUS and trachea (windpipe), and is composed of two main parts: the PHARYNX and the LARYNX.

Thrombosis

This describes a BLOOD clot in an ARTERY or a VEIN that blocks CIRCULATION. Although the smoker, the obese and the diabetic are more prone to thrombotic diseases, they can occur even among the healthy. But risks can be minimized and appropriate measures taken.

Thrombosis formation

The blood forms a clot (or *thrombus*) as a normal, healthy protective process, by which bleeding from a damaged blood vessel is stopped and the repair process begins. However, when blood circulation through the heart, limbs or brain is sluggish, or the blood contains an excess of clotting factors, or the blood vessels are affected by *atheroma* (*see below*), a clot may block a major artery or vein. The thrombosis may occur in different parts of the body.

When thrombosis occurs in one of the coronary arteries of the heart, a patient has a HEART ATTACK, or *myocardial* INFARCTION. In the brain, it results in a STROKE. Thrombosis in a leg vein causes PHLEBITIS; and if it occurs in the artery supplying a limb, gangrene may result.

An *embolism* occurs when a thrombus forming in a major blood vessel or on the lining of the heart breaks loose and is swept away by the bloodstream to become lodged in a narrow vessel, completely cutting off the blood supply to part of the lung or brain or to an arm or leg. Because of the anatomy of the circulatory system, thrombosis in a leg vein may break loose to form a pulmonary embolism in the lung. But if the clot originates from one of the neck arteries, it may be carried into the brain to produce a cerebral embolism.

Why does a thrombosis occur?

Thrombosis nearly always results from one or a combination of the following: CORONARY HEART DISEASE; artery disease; prolonged immobilization; the aftermath of major surgery; PREGNANCY; the CONTRACEPTIVE pill; or associated with cancer.

Apparently some individuals are more susceptible to thrombosis than others. In these, there is usually both an abnormality of blood vessels and a 'hypercoagulable' state in which blood has a tendency to clot more easily than normal. Any attempt to reduce the risk of thrombosis must either entail preventing or correcting the disease in the heart or blood vessels, or reducing the ease with which clotting occurs in the blood.

There tends to be a higher incidence of thrombosis in women who take a high-dosage oral contraceptive, particularly if they are over 35 and smoke. The modern low-dosage oestrogen pill, on the other hand, has only a very small risk of causing thrombosis – indeed a smaller chance than in pregnancy itself.

Disorders of the blood vessels

As we grow older, signs of degenerative disease become more marked in the major arteries. Pathologists describe the degenerative process as *atheroma* and the effect on the blood vessels as *arteriosclerosis*, or hardening of the arteries. Arteriosclerosis is most likely to occur first in the heart and the major arteries where the arteries are subjected to the most stress. Not surprisingly, when the BLOOD PRESSURE is abnormally raised, arteriosclerosis develops early in the blood vessels supplying the heart, brain and limbs. The arteries become narrower and more rigid, which has the effect of significantly reducing the flow of blood.

Atheroma in its earliest form can be detected in childhood. Tiny yellowish flecks develop in the linings of the major arteries, particularly where they branch or split into smaller tributaries. By middle age, the flecks have become distinct streaks, rich in cholesterol. The lining of the vessel may then become roughened and cracked. Platelets are attracted to the cracked surface and eventually a small clot may grow into the cavity of the artery. This may create a turbulence in blood flow, which may finally tear the clot loose, resulting in a dangerous embolism of the brain or the limbs.

Coronary thrombosis

Coronary thrombosis is the common cause of what the general public calls a heart attack and doctors usually refer to as myocardial infarction. One person in three will be affected by coronary artery disease, and it is still the commonest single cause of death in Britain. Until the age of 70, about four times as man men as women suffer a coronary thrombosis. Over 70, women are just as likely to be affected as men.

Those most at tisk of a heart attack are male, overweight, heave a diet rich in fats and lead a stressful life with minimal exercise. In addition, DIABETICS and people whose families have a history of heart attacks are prone to it. However, the biggest group of risk-takers are SMOKERS: a cigarette smoker is five times more likely to suffer a heart attack than a non-smoker, all other factors such as diet and lifestyle being equal.

Causes symptoms, treatment: The two coronary arteries, embedded in the muscular walls of the heart, divert oxygen-rich blood, fresh from the lungs, to small vessels feeding all parts of the heart muscle. It is vital that these arteries remain open; even a slight narrowing of the coronary arteries may cause symptoms during times of exertion.

Persons at risk from coronary disease have a tendency to form fatty deposits which roughen the lining of the arteries and narrow the central channel. If the blockage occurs gradually, the person may experience pain only on exertion. This is typical of the pain of *angina,* and usually is severe enough to make the sufferer stop what he or she is doing. The angina pain then subsides. Although frightening, it serves as a warning, making the sufferer rest long enough for blood flow to be restored to the oxygen-starved muscle before serious damage can be done, and allowing time for new circulatory channels to open up over the following weeks.

When a coronary thrombosis develops at a site of narrowing, it completely blocks the blood supply to part of the heart muscle. That part will be so severely damaged that it will cease to contract normally; the symptoms, then, will be sudden and severe. Patients experience crushing chest pain which is sometimes also felt in the arm and jaw; they may feel breathless and sweat profusely. These symptoms do not necessarily begin when patients are exerting themselves and do not usually improve even when they rest.

Coronary thrombosis almost always requires treatment in hospital, though patients will be allowed out of bed for short periods within the first fortnight and will emabark on a programme of graduated exercise. Drugs to dissolve clots, such as streptokinase, can now be given to disperse them. It is believed that once a firm scar has replaced the damaged heart muscle, exercise will encourage the formation of new channels to replace the thrombosed artery.

Cerebral thrombosis

Strokes resulting from cerebral thrombosis are one of the most common causes of death and disablement. Those most at risk are people who suffer from high blood pressure, or who are diabetics, have a high serum cholesterol, and who smoke. Strokes may run in families. Some people with heart disease are predisposed to strokes.

Causes, symptoms, treatment: A stroke can be caused by bleeding from a weakened artery into the brain (cerebral HAEMORRHAGE); a sudden blockage of an artery by a flake of material that has come adrift from a diseased artery or from the heart (embolism); or a more gradual blockage by clot formation within a diseased artery of the brain (thrombosis). The arterial disease that predisposes a person to all three types of stroke is arteriosclerosis.

The effect of a stroke depends entirely on the size and situation of the affected area of the brain. If the right side of the brain is damaged, there is usually weakness, paralysis of the facial muscles, with loss of sensation in the left arm and leg. If the left side of the brain is affected, the patient may lose total or partial control of speech and be paralysed on the right side of the body.

Cerebral thrombosis produces sudden paralysis or weakness which begins to improve within hours of the stroke occurring. Recovery is helped by early encouragement of the patient, and physiotherapy and/or speech therapy. A high proportion of stroke victims make a full recovery, but in the rest, the degree of recovery will depend on the severity of the initial damage to the brain.

See also PHLEBITIS and RHEUMATIC FEVER.

Thrush

This is caused by a fungus called *Candida albicans* (*see* FUNGAL INFECTIONS) and can affect many parts of the body, but is particularly likely to affect the VAGINA. It can also occur at any time of life, from the first few weeks to old age.

Causes

Compared with the number of bacteria that infect humans, there are very few fungi that cause problems. These fall into two groups: yeasts and filamentous fungi. *Candida* is one of the yeasts which are very similar in form to the type used to make bread rise. When examined under the microscope, they are seen as small round organisms, while the filamentous fungi produce long threads made up of a series of single-celled organisms joined together. But it may be difficult to identify a particular *Candida* organism.

A number of different types of *Candida* cause disease, the commonest being *Candida albicans* (meaning white). *Candida* is an organism which is often present on the skin or in the gut of most people. If it starts to cause symptoms, this is because some other problem has allowed the *Candida* organisms to multiply to a greater extent than usual. For example, elderly people often develop thrush in their mouths, and the precipitating factor is usually a cut or abrasion, perhaps where an ill-fitting denture rubs the gums or lips.

Vaginal thrush is the exception to this rule – it is very common for the *Candida* organism to breed in the vagina, even if the vaginal mucosa (lining) is quite normal and healthy.

It is very unusual for *Candida* to get into the body and cause systemic or deep infections (infections of the internal organs and tissues). This is most likely to happen in people who already have some illness that lowers their resistance to infection. Systemic infections may occur when patients are on drugs that suppress the IMMUNE SYSTEM, or when they have a disease – such as LEUKAEMIA or AIDS – which has this effect. Taking a course of ANTIBIOTICS can also allow this to happen, because the drug may kill off bacteria that were keeping the *Candida* in check.

Rarely, there may be a chronic infection of the mouth or the vagina, or elsewhere on the surface of the body. This is called *chronic mucocutaneous candidiasis*. The exact cause is not certain, but it is an inherited defect in the immune system's response to disease, and the problem starts in infancy and childhood.

Babies can also get thrush in their mouths any time after about the age of three weeks. This nearly always happens in those babies who are bottle-fed rather than breastfed, but it does not mean that there is anything wrong with the baby's immune system. Thrush may also cause a nasty rash in the baby's nappy area, with a white exudate lying on the skin (*see* NAPPY RASH).

Symptoms

The two commonest sites of *Candida* infection are the mouth and the vulva and vagina, where infection is called *vulvo-vaginitis*. Infection in the mouth is most often found in people who wear dentures, and takes the form of small white patches on the gums, lips and inside the cheeks. These may be very sore, particularly on eating and are usually worst in people who have a serious illness.

Vulvo-vaginitis as a result of thrush causes a white discharge with a lot of irritation. It affects women of almost any age, but it seems to be commoner in PREGNANCY and less common among children. DIABETICS are particularly prone to vaginal thrush, and it is often the reason why the disease initially comes to light before other symptoms develop.

Men also suffer from genital *Candida* infections. For example, inflammation of the tip of the PENIS (*balanitis*) is often caused by *Candida*. In men, it is even more common for genital infection to be associated with diabetes than in women, although candidal balanitis is overall less common than candidal vulvo-vaginitis.

Sometimes women get repeated vaginal thrush without some predisposing condition like diabetes. This problem seems to be occurring more frequently, and the conventional explanation is that these women are being repeatedly infected, perhaps by their sexual partners. This is, however, not a very satisfactory theory since *Candida* is an organism which nearly always exists in people but is only occasionally the cause of symptoms. It has also been suggested that the increase in the incidence of chronic vaginal thrush is due to the wider use of the CONTRACEPTIVE pill and there is some evidence to support this view.

Other parts of the skin may also be infected, including the nail-folds. Infection here is called *paronychia,* and *Candida paronychia* is common in people who constantly immerse their hands in water. Infection of damp sweaty skin folds also occurs.

Most attacks of thrush do not lead to complications, despite the intense itching and burning which may prove very troublesome, especially with vaginal thrush. Only deep-seated infections in people who are very ill are likely to prove dangerous.

Treatment

The treatment of simple thrush is effective and convenient, and differs greatly from that of the systemic disease. Drugs that work on surface infection – nystatin, amphotericin B and clotrimazole – are not absorbed when taken orally. The drugs are used in the form of pessaries and creams in the case of vaginal infection. Other drugs have become available which can be taken by mouth as a single dose to treat vaginal thrush if local treatment is ineffective. Treatment by mouth is used for people with recurrent mouth infections, or if it has spread into the gullet.

Once a systemic infection has been diagnosed, it is essential to use a treatment which reaches the bloodstream. The problem is that, when amphotericin B is given by injection, it becomes toxic and its effects have to be carefully monitored. Other new drugs are also effective and may ultimately prove more satisfactory.

Thymus

Over the last few decades, it has become clear that the thymus sits at the centre of the remarkable web of interconnected organs and tissues that make up the IMMUNE SYSTEM – defending us from attack by infection.

There is still considerable ignorance about exactly how the thymus does its job, but it is now known that it is essential for the proper running of the immune system, and that it carries out its major function during the first few years of life.

Where is it?

The thymus is found in the upper part of the chest, where it lies just behind the breastbone. In a young adult, it is a few centimetres long and weighs about ½ oz (15 g). However, this simple statement conceals the most remarkable thing about the twin-lobed thymus, and that is the way that, quite unlike any other organ, it is at its largest at about the time of puberty when it may weigh up to 1½ oz (45 g).

In a baby, the thymus is very large compared to the rest of the body, and it may extend quite a long way down the chest behind the breastbone. It grows quite quickly until about the age of seven, after which it grows more slowly until puberty.

After the age of puberty, the thymus starts to shrink in size – a process called *involution* – until, in an elderly person, there may be no more thymus tissue present apart from a bit of fat and associated connective tissue.

Structure and function

The thymus contains many of the small round cells, called *lymphocytes*, that are the basic unit of the immune system. These cells are found in the BLOOD, the BONE MARROW, the LYMPH glands and the SPLEEN, and they can be seen travelling into the tissues during an inflammatory reaction.

The outer layer of the thymus, called the *cortex*, has many lymphocytes. Inside this is an area called the *medulla* which contains lymphocytes and other sorts of thymus cells as well.

There seems to be little doubt that, in the early years of life, the thymus is concerned with 'programming' the way in which the immune system works, and in particular, it seems that the thymus is responsible for making sure that the system does not turn its activities against the body's own tissues.

It is now thought that the thymus is responsible for many of the most important aspects of the immune system. There are two main sorts of immune cells in the body and they are both different sorts of lymphocytes. The T or 'thymus' cell lymphocytes are under the control of the thymus and are responsible for the recognition of foreign substances and for many of the ways in which the body attacks them. The other sort – the B lymphocytes – are responsible for making antibodies to foreign substances.

The exact ways in which the thymus goes about controlling its T lymphocytes is not known, but one important mechanism has come to light. It seems that about 95 per cent of the new sorts of lymphocytes that are made in the thymus are, in fact, destroyed there, before they ever have an opportunity to get out into the rest of the body. The probable reason for this is that they would have the potential for turning against the body itself, and the only cells that the thymus allows to develop are those which will attack outside or foreign substances.

What can go wrong?

If the thymus is regarded as an isolated organ, it must be said that it is very rare for it to give rise to any trouble. However, it is important to remember that the T lymphocytes it controls are really the most central part of the body's immune system, and the activity of this system is extremely important in almost all serious diseases.

Still, in the thymus itself, as opposed to the wider aspects of its function, there are two important problems. Firstly, the thymus may fail to develop properly in babies, and as might be expected, this leads to a failure of the immune system and a failure to resist infection which may certainly prove fatal. Luckily, this is an uncommon problem. Second, TUMOURS can occur in the thymus. These are called *thymomas,* and they are treated by surgery followed by X-ray treatment.

Myasthenia is a nervous system disorder, and symptoms include weakness and tiredness of the muscles which gets worse during the course of the day. This disease is caused by the formation of antibodies to the junctions between nerves and muscles by the body's own immune system. These antibodies attack the junctions and the nerves cannot instruct the muscles to move. As the thymus is very much involved with the control of the immune system, it has been found that taking the thymus out can be effective in helping some sufferers.

In the United States, from the 1920s to the 1950s, a disease called *status lymphaticus* was supposed to be caused by an enlarged thymus in infants and very young children. Hundreds of thousands had their thymuses X-rayed to reduce the size. Later it was discovered that this disease did not exist at all, but in the meantime, a significant number of those who had been X-rayed developed thyroid and breast cancer from the treatment.

Thyroid

Problems associated with the thyroid gland cause the commonest type of hormonal disorders (*see* HORMONES), affecting large numbers of people. However, many of these problems can be completely cured, mainly because the hormone produced by the gland can be easily prepared and administered by mouth.

Of the wide range of thyroid disorders, by far the most important are those of over-activity – *thyrotoxicosis* or *hyperthyroidism* – and of under-activity: *myxoedema* or *hypothyroidism.* Both of these problems are a lot more common in women than in men, and up to 2 per cent of the adult female population may have difficulty from an over-active thyroid at some stage in their lives, with under-activity being only slightly less common than over-activity. One other disorder is worth noting here: *thyroiditis,* which is an inflammation of the thyroid as a result of a virus infection.

The thyroid gland

The thyroid gland is found in the neck, just below the level of the LARYNX, which can be seen or felt as the Adam's apple. There are two lobes to the gland, and these lie just in front and at either side of the windpipe, or trachea, as it passes down the front of the neck. The two lobes are connected by a small bridge of tissue, and there may be a smaller central lobe called the pyramidal lobe. In an adult, the gland will weigh about ⅔ oz (20 g).

The function of the gland is to make the thyroid hormone *thyroxine*. When the gland is looked at under a microscope, many small 'follicles' can be seen; these are islands of tissue containing collections of colloid, a protein substance to which thyroid hormone is bound.

It is not possible to tie the activity of thyroxine down to one specific thing. It is released from the gland and is then probably taken up from the blood into all the cells of the body. There appears to be a receptor on the surface of the cell nucleus that responds to the hormone. The overall effect of the hormone is to increase the amount of energy that the cell uses; it also increases the amount of protein that the cell manufactures. Although the exact role of the hormone in the cell is not known, it is essential for life.

The thyroid gland contains IODINE that is vital for its activity. This is the only part of the body that requires iodine and the thyroid is very efficient at trapping all the available iodine from the blood. An absence of iodine in the diet results in malfunction of the thyroid and the growth of the gland, a condition called *endemic goitre*.

The thyroid is one of the ENDOCRINE glands, and like so many of them it is under the control of the PITUITARY. The pituitary produces a hormone called *thyroid-stimulating hormone*, or TSH, which increases the amount of thyroxine that is released from the gland. The amount of TSH that the pituitary produces increases if the amount of thyroxine circulating in the system falls, and decreases if it rises – a system called 'negative feedback' – which results in a constant level of thyroid hormone in the blood.

The pituitary is itself under the influence of the HYPOTHALAMUS and the amount of TSH that is produced will be increased if there is a release of a substance called TRH (*TSH-releasing hormone*) from the hypothalamus.

This situation is further complicated by the fact that thyroid hormone comes in two versions, according to the number of iodine atoms that it contains. Most of the hormone released from the gland is in the form of *tetra-iodothyronine*, which contains four iodine atoms and is known as T4. However, the active hormone at the cell level is *tri-iodothyronine*, which contains three atoms and is known as T3. Although the gland releases some T3 into the blood, most of its output is T4, and this is converted into T3 in the tissues. Sometimes the tissues switch the way that they convert T4 to produce an ineffective compound called reverse T3. This means that there will be less thyroid hormone activity in the tissues even though the hormone level in the blood is adequate.

Goitre

Any enlargement of the thyroid gland is called a goitre. Small but still visible goitres are found in about 15 per cent of the population, with about four times as many in women as in men. Usually these are of no significance.

In the past, iodine deficiency would have been the main cause of goitre, but now most are caused by over-activity of the thyroid or are simple goitres that are not related to any abnormality of the thyroid's function. In a few cases, goitres are isolated lumps (nodules) in the substance of the thyroid, and these should be investigated using an isotope scan to see whether the lump is composed of functioning tissue. If it is not, and if an ULTRASOUND scan shows that it is solid, then it could be malignant and may need a surgical exploration.

Over-active thyroid glands

Most cases of thyroid over-activity are caused by *Graves' disease.* A goitre is usually present and the eyes become protruding and staring – a sign that many people associate with thyroid problems. It is the basic disease process that causes the symptoms and not the over-activity.

Graves' disease is caused by the presence of antibodies in the blood (*see* IMMUNE SYSTEM). Although these antibodies do not destroy thyroid tissue, they stimulate the gland to produce thyroxine. It is not known why some people are more prone to making these antibodies than others, although there is certainly GENETIC susceptibility. This can be demonstrated by the fact that many sufferers have a specific type of tissue group.

The effect of an over-active thyroid are weight loss, and increased appetite, anxiety and nervousness (sometimes with a tremor), palpitations of the heart, sweating with intolerance to heat and irritability. In addition to eye problems, there may be weakness of the muscles particularly at the shoulders and hips.

Once Graves' disease is suspected, the majority of cases can be diagnosed very simply by measuring the level of the thyroid hormone in the blood. Often the T3 level is measured as well as, or instead of, the T4 level, since T3 is always raised in Graves' disease, while it is possible to have the disease with a normal T4 level.

Treatment is given to suppress thyroid activity. This can be done with tablets for a year or more. If the gland is very large, it may be appropriate to operate to remove some of it. The alternative is to give a dose of radioactive iodine. This is, of course, taken up only by the thyroid so it presents no danger to other tissues. It will reduce the level of thyroid activity over the course of approximately six weeks.

While the hormone levels are being brought under control, the symptoms can be decreased by drugs which block the effects of adrenalin (*see* ADRENAL GLANDS), since high levels of thyroid seem to produce an increased response to adrenalin.

Under-active thyroid glands

This condition of the thyroid gland – myxoedema – is also caused by antibodies in the gland which seem to destroy it. *Hashimoto's disease* is very similar, except that the antibodies set up a long-term inflammation of the gland, causing goitre but leading to thyroid failure.

In many cases, weight gain results, together with a lack of energy, dry thick skin, hair loss, intolerance to cold, a slow heartbeat, hoarseness and deafness, and a typical puffy face. The presence of hypothyroidism makes elderly people much more susceptible to HYPOTHERMIA.

Under-activity of the thyroid is readily picked up by blood tests. The level of T4 is reduced, but this can occur on its own – in severe illness, for example. Much more important is the high level of TSH that is found in the blood, as the pituitary gland tries to drive the thyroid on to produce enough hormones.

Once a diagnosis is made, the thyroid hormone T4 can be given by mouth. The dose is built up fairly gradually since there is a risk of making patients with heart disease worse; myxoedema predisposes to CORONARY HEART DISEASE since it causes a very high level of CHOLESTEROL.

Patients with myxoedema must continue to take medication for the rest of their lives. Although Graves' disease is not quite as easy to treat as myxoedema, the results of treatment in both conditions are really very satisfactory, and the outlook is very good in both once the early difficulties have passed.

Tinea, *see* **Fungal infections, Ringworm**

Tinnitus

Commonly described as 'ringing in the ears', tinnitus – the sensation of noise in the EARS or head – is a symptom that affects more people than is generally realized. The sound is perceived by the sufferer even though it has no origin outside the body. In some, the noise is soft and barely noticeable, while in others, the noise is crashingly loud and can prevent the person sleeping. Although it is rarely the symptom of any serious disease, it can be extremely disturbing to the person who has it. The sound perceived can vary between a ringing, a hissing, a buzzing and a roaring noise, but the nature and quality of the sound has actually very little to do with the causes.

Outer ear causes

In the outer ear, there are two common causes. The first, and most common, is impacted wax, often caused by people trying to clean their ears out with cotton wool buds or the corner of a handkerchief. The quick and simple way to remove it is by syringing, where a doctor washes the wax away with water.

The other cause in the external ear is infection by a bacteria or a fungus. In this case the patient complains of both tinnitus and some kind of irritation, often accompanied by localized pain which is made worse by moving the outer ear. There is also some DEAFNESS and a scant, watery discharge. Fortunately, treatment is simple with antibiotic and steroid drops which quickly clear up the infection and the tinnitus abates.

Middle ear causes

Tinnitus also crops up in association with problems in the middle ear. The two main causes are infection and otosclerosis.

As with most types of infection, there are acute and chronic types. Acute infection of the middle ear – acute *otitis media* – as well as giving tinnitus, can also cause deafness, a mucous discharge from the ear and a raised temperature. Again, treatment for this is with antibiotics and also with decongestant nasal drops.

Chronic infection of the middle ear is usually rather more difficult to detect. The symptoms, although broadly similar to those of acute *otitis media,* are extremely variable and can be intermittent. Rarely, the patient suffers VERTIGO. If this happens, the patient must seek medical help rapidly to avoid severe and permanent hearing damage.

Tinnitus is an early symptom of the other type of problem in the middle ear. In this condition, *otosclerosis,* new bone is laid down round the stirrup bone (stapes) and it prevents it from moving freely and transmitting sound properly from the eardrum to the inner ear. The patient becomes progressively more deaf, but fortunately there is an operation in which the stapes is removed and a plastic replacement fitted. This restores the hearing and any remaining tinnitus is usually masked by the increased volume of external sound heard by the patient.

Inner ear causes

In the inner ear, there are the very delicate receptor cells in the cochlea. Damage to these cells is probably the most common cause of tinnitus. The damage can have several causes, the most usual of which is the simple degenerative ageing process that produces deafness. Although the degree of deafness and the age of onset vary greatly, there is almost always some tinnitus.

Another increasingly common cause of tinnitus is cochlear damage caused by sudden loud noises or prolonged exposure to noises of lesser intensity.

Some drugs, when given in high does, also cause cochlear damage, and thus tinnitus. There is a disease called MÉNIÈRE'S DISEASE which involves tinnitus, and a rare benign TUMOUR called an *acoustic neuroma* which gives tinnitus, usually only in one ear.

Tinnitus caused by problems in the inner ear can be difficult to treat. Certain drugs may help, such as betahistine or cinnarizine. They damp down excessive discharge from the damaged cells in the inner ear. However, the most effective treatment is usually a 'masking' device which is worn in the ear like a small hearing aid. It produces a constant noise which distracts attention from the tinnitus and makes life much more bearable for the sufferer.

Tissue typing, *see* **Heart transplants, Rejection of tissue, Transplants**

Tongue, *see* **Taste**

Tonsils

These are part of a ring of lymphoid tissue (*Waldeyer's ring*) which encircles the entrance to the food and air passages in the throat. Although they are present at birth, they are relatively small, but grow rapidly during the first few years of life, only to regress after puberty. However, they do not disappear completely.

The tonsils' exact function is not known but it has been suggested that they play a significant role in maintaining the body's IMMUNE SYSTEM. They are ideally situated to scrutinize ingested materials and to react to those which pose a threat to the body. This immunity is given by *lymphocytes* (*see* BLOOD) produced by the tonsils. In addition, the tonsils produce antibodies which deal with infections locally.

Tonsillitis

Almost everyone will have suffered an attack of tonsillitis at some time in life. The organism producing the infection is usually a *streptococcus* (a certain type of bacterium). Often, however, tonsillitis is caused by a viral infection.

The main difference between the ordinary sore throat – such as occurs at the beginning of a COLD – and tonsillitis is the presence of pus, or *exudate*, on the surface of the tonsils. This occurs only when the tonsils themselves have become infected. Often the illness starts quite suddenly, although symptoms do vary with the severity of the infection. There is always marked discomfort in the throat, making swallowing difficult. Pain from the throat may also be felt in the ear. Some patients even experience discomfort on turning their heads because of swelling of the lymph GLANDS in this region.

A raised temperature almost always accompanies the infection, but it varies in degree. Children, for example, tend to develop higher temperatures and consequently more symptoms – such as malaise and vomiting – than adults. And some children may have no symptoms in the throat but complain of abdominal pain instead. Many children with tonsillitis develop an unusual and unpleasant smell on their breath.

The tonsils become enlarged and inflamed. At first, pus may appear on the tonsils as a thin covering, but within a few hours, many specks of creamy pus can be seen all over the surface of the tonsils.

Symptoms can be alleviated by eating soft foods and drinking lots of liquids. PAINKILLERS such as aspirin or paracetamol both relieve the pain and reduce the temperature, although aspirin should not be given to children under 12 years of age. In most cases, the symptoms improve within 36 to 48 hours, although if antibiotics are prescribed, improvement usually occurs more quickly.

It is not uncommon for children to develop a slight RASH with tonsillitis. This tends to be a fine, red rash and occurs only when tonsillitis is caused by the streptococcus bacterium. The rash presents a mild form of the once-feared complication of tonsillitis, SCARLET FEVER or scarletina.

Tonsillitis tends to occur most frequently between the ages of four and six years and then again around puberty. The more often the tonsils are infected, the more prone they are to persistent and recurrent infection. A stage is therefore reached when removal of the tonsils is the only sensible way of controlling the disease.

Quinsy

In some cases, an infection is so sever that an ABSCESS forms in the tissue around the tonsils. This is known as *peritonsillar abscess*, or *quinsy*. Quinsy usually affects one side of the tonsils and is very rare in children. The affected tonsil swells to a considerable extent and may prevent swallowing altogether. Local inflammation contributes to this disability by limiting the opening of the jaw. Oral antibiotics are not only difficult to swallow but also are rarely effective. Higher doses of antibiotics are given by intramuscular injections for 24 to 36 hours, followed by oral antibiotics. If the quinsy is 'ripe' – that is, the abscess is 'pointing' – recovery may be accelerated by lancing the abscess and allowing the pus to drain.

In exceptional cases, an infection is not limited to the tonsils but spreads both down the neck to the chest and up towards the base of the skull – a *parapharyngeal abscess*. This is a life-threatening condition and requires urgent admission to hospital, where drainage and the administration of massive doses of powerful antibiotics can be undertaken. Patients who have had quinsy are thought to be more susceptible to this complication and are therefore advised to have their tonsil out even if they have not been troubled previously by recurrent tonsillitis.

Viral infections of the tonsils

Tonsillar tissue can be affected by viral infections which commonly lead to a sore throat. Symptoms are similar to those of tonsillitis, but are often milder and last for only 24 to 48 hours.

However, sometimes it may be very difficult if not impossible for a doctor to tell simply by examining the tonsils whether or not the tonsillitis is caused by the bacterium or by a virus. Only those cases caused by bacteria respond to antibiotics. There has been considerable controversy over whether or not it is right for doctors to use antibiotics routinely for tonsillitis. Most cases clear up within a few days whether or not antibiotics are given, and antibiotics do not help any of those cases caused by viruses. Because the risk of complications from tonsillitis is now so low, and the possibility of side-effects or reactions to the antibiotics always exists, some doctors prefer not to give antibiotics for tonsillitis unless there are complications. Other doctors take a throat swab first to be examined in a laboratory for the presence of bacteria, and give the patient antibiotics if streptococci are found on the swab.

The tonsils are also affected in GLANDULAR FEVER.

Tonsillectomy

In children, attacks of tonsillitis may precipitate attacks of *otitis media* (an infection of the middle EAR) or may prevent a complete recovery from secretory *otitis media*, a condition known more commonly as 'glue ear'. In these cases, the surgeon may advise tonsillectomy to prevent possible damage to the middle ear and avoid the DEAFNESS, which although temporary, is associated with these conditions.

A tonsillectomy is performed under general ANAESTHETIC. The tonsils are dissected away from the pharyngeal wall and the resulting bleeding is controlled by ligatures (tying off of blood vessels). On average about 1/5 pint (120 ml) of blood is lost during the operation, irrespective of the age of the patient. Surgeons are therefore very reluctant to operate on children who are very small or below the age of four; such an amount of blood loss is a significant proportion of their total blood volume. However, if an operation is necessary, the child will be given an intravenous drip for about 12 hours after the tonsillectomy.

The only serious complication that may arise after the operation is further haemorrhage. When this occurs, it is usually within the first few hours and requires a return to the theatre for further ligation.

Bleeding may also occur six to ten days after the operation if the tonsil bed becomes infected. Patients mostly affected are those who eat poorly post-operatively or have had an attack of tonsillitis immediately before admission to hospital. This late bleeding is treated with antibiotics, but if the patient has lost a lot of blood, a transfusion or a course of iron tablets may be necessary to stimulate rapid replacement of the lost blood.

Children tend to recover from the operation more quickly than adults and only require one to two days in hospital. Adults, however, may need four to five days' hospitalization before they are fit enough to be discharged, and they may need more than a week in bed afterwards.

See also ADENOIDS.

Toxaemia of pregnancy, *see* **Cerebral palsy, Eclampsia and pre-eclampsia**

Toxic shock syndrome

First described in the United States in 1978, this now appears to be a world-wide phenomenon. It is a potentially fatal illness that almost exclusively affects women during the course of their PERIODS. There is very good evidence to suggest that its occurrence is related to the use of tampons. In particular, it seems most likely to occur it a tampon is left in the vagina for too long. When new super-absorbency types were introduced, its incidence increased, probably because women were encouraged to believe that those tampons could be left in place much longer than previous types. However, it is very important to remember that millions of women use tampons, and the risks of toxic shock are extremely low. The super-absorbency tampons that were associated with an increased risk of the syndrome have now been withdrawn from sale, so there is no risk of unknowingly using one of this type.

Causes

The important ingredients in causing the syndrome seem to be the occurrence of a period, probably the use of a tampon and the presence of *staphylococci* bacteria in the vagina. Although staphylococci are not invariably found in the vagina, they are present in many more cases with the syndrome than not. It has been suggested that, when the staphylococci are present in the vagina, and a period starts, the presence of a blood-soaked tampon will provide an excellent culture medium for the organisms to grow on. It is thought that the symptoms result from the production of a toxin (poison) by the staphylococci, which is absorbed through the vaginal skin.

About 95 per cent of reported cases have happened in women who are having periods. The syndrome tends to occur in very young women, with the average age of 23, and 30 per cent of cases happen in girls aged between 15 and 21. In most cases, the woman tended not to have been changing her tampons very frequently. The longer the tampon is left in the vagina, the more likelihood there is of bacterial growth in the blood-soaked material of the tampon.

Toxic shock syndrome has been reported in a number of men, all of whom had a skin infection with staphylococci. One of these men was a plumber who had cleared a lavatory blocked with tampons.

Symptoms and dangers

Toxic shock syndrome is characterized by a high fever of over 102.2°F (39°C), a low blood pressure (SHOCK, in the emergency doctor's language); a flattish skin RASH that leads on to the loss of skin from the hands and feet after a week or two; and often a quite marked EYE infection.

Additionally, there will be involvement of at least four of the body's main systems. Failure of the KIDNEYS is very common, as is DIARRHOEA. There is nearly always *myalgia* – aching pains in the muscles – of the sort people get with flu. Headaches and disorientation occur, and there may be evidence of disturbance of the function of the LIVER.

Typically the illness develops suddenly on the fourth day of a menstrual period. The fever occurs first, and there may be abdominal pain. Watery diarrhoea develops during the first 24 hours in most cases. Then myalgia occurs: it is extremely painful in the muscles and the skin. The rash also appears during the first 24 hours, but it may not be noticed and may be mistaken for the first flush of fever. Later it becomes more marked, usually affecting the fingers, and sometimes the palms and the soles.

As the disease progresses, other problems such as pain in the joints and discomfort on looking towards a light (photobia) may occur. The kidneys often fail, and stop passing enough urine so that the level of waste products in the blood starts to rise. The kidney failure is probably related to the drop in blood pressure, as the kidneys are very sensitive to any changes in the amount of blood flowing to them.

Most patients recover after ten days, but at a rather late stage, the skin is lost from the palms and soles, and often from the face and even the tongue. The death rate from the disease is not easy to assess, but it is probably around 2 or 3 per cent.

Treatment and outlook

The most important aspect of the treatment is replacing fluid intravenously to correct the working of the circulation. The other problems that can happen have to be faced as they occur: a patient running into breathing difficulty might have to be put on a respirator, for example. There is no evidence that the infection with staphylococci involves the blood, but it is very worthwhile treating the patient with antibiotics to eradicate the organisms from the vagina. Not only may this hasten recovery from the illness, but it may also prevent repeated attacks.

Prevention
The best way to avoid the syndrome is to change tampons regularly and frequently during a period – at least four times a day, even if the tampon is hardly soiled – and to use the smallest tampons that will meet your needs. If possible, it may be wise to try to use external protection in the form of sanitary pads during the later stages of the period. Although there seems little doubt that the disease is directly related to the use of tampons, few women would be prepared to forgo their use completely to avoid such an uncommon condition.

Toxocariasis, *see* **Blindness, Worms**

Toxoplasmosis, *see* **Blindness**

Trace elements

A balanced diet includes PROTEIN, CARBOHYDRATES, FATS and also the VITAMINS and MINERALS that we need to keep us healthy. Some minerals are required in such tiny amounts that they are called the 'trace elements', because only a tiny trace of them is needed.

In terms of quantity, most of our needs are catered for by the three elements carbon, OXYGEN and hydrogen, and, to a lesser extent, nitrogen; we take in kilograms of these substances every day. Relatively large amounts of other elements such as sodium (*see* SALT), POTASSIUM, phosphorus and CALCIUM are also required, and we normally take in a few grams of these every day. However, trace elements such as copper, fluorine (*see* DENTAL CARE) and IODINE, which are just as essential for normal life, are needed only in minute quantities.

What they do
Most important trace elements have a role in bringing about the activity of the body's various ENZYMES. The function of enzymes is to assist in chemical reactions in the body, and although they set a process going, they remain unchanged at the end of the reaction. This means they act as *catalysts.*

All the enzymes are proteins, and what each one does depends on the shape into which the long string-like protein molecule winds itself. Trace elements play a role because it seems that a few of the body's enzymes require strong chemical forces – produced by atoms of certain metallic elements – to attain the correct shape for action. Therefore, most of the trace elements we need are metallic, and they either form part of the structure of an enzyme, or they take part in its chemical reaction in the body.

Also, a few trace elements seem to be part of the structure of other important substances in the body. Fluorine is associated with the structure of BONES and TEETH, and iodine is an essential constituent of the THYROID hormones.

Deficiencies of other trace elements cause problems: chromium deficiency causes glucose intolerance; cobalt deficiency causes anaemia; selenium deficiency causes growth retardation and manganese deficiency causes skeletal abnormalities and growth retardation.

Harmful trace elements

Traces of some substances, often present in food or air, are not only of no value, but can be positively dangerous. Metals such as lead, cadmium, mercury and arsenic are all poisonous in sufficient quantities and have absolutely no use within the body.

Apart from the purely poisonous metals, it is possible to accumulate high levels of normally beneficial, essential trace elements that can then cause illness. In *haemachromatosis,* an abnormality of the transport of IRON in the blood leads to an accumulation of iron in the liver and pancreas. This can cause CIRRHOSIS and DIABETES. A genetic-linked disease – called *Wilson's disease*– also occurs. The copper metabolism becomes disorganized and this leads to accumulations of copper in the heart and liver.

In other circumstances, accidental intake leads to poisoning by metals that are essential only in very small amounts. The most notorious example of accidental excess was in Quebec, Canada, where cobalt was added to beer to improve the froth and therefore get a better head. This led to an outbreak of heart failure in beer drinkers, as the cobalt slowly poisoned the heart.

Zinc

Zinc is an important trace metal and is found in comparatively high concentrations in the skin, eyes, liver, pancreas and bone.

One of the first discoveries about the importance of zinc was the realization that deficiency leads to disease. In some parts of both Egypt and Iran, there is a deficiency of zinc in the diet. In these areas, there is a tendency for boys not to mature properly, and not go through puberty. This leads to people over 20 having the appearance of 10-year-olds. Adding zinc to the diet brings about rapid maturation.

More relevant is the role that zinc plays in the healing of the skin. Zinc given in tablet form can help to speed up healing of various types of wounds. Also, in recent years, a disease called *acrodermatitis enteropathica* has been recognized. Here, the skin produces eczema-like symptoms; this happens particularly in the skin of infants at the time of weaning. The condition results from poor absorption of zinc and it responds well to zinc treatment.

Tracheostomy, *see* Larynx and laryngitis, Stoma care

Tracheotomy, *see* Stoma care

Trachoma, *see* Blindness, Chlamydia

Traction, *see* Fractures, Orthopaedics

Tranquillizers

All of us can cope with some STRESS in our lives – some even thrive on it. However, there are times when we feel particularly anxious for a definite reason – or indeed for no clear reason at all. There are several different types of drug which doctors can prescribe to relieve anxiety, but each has its own risk of possible side-effects. Although tranquillizers have been widely prescribed in the past for quite minor anxiety or worry, it is now known that dependence can arise quite quickly to certain types of tranquillizer – particularly the barbiturates and benzodiazepines (e.g. Valium and Librium). Doctors are therefore prescribing these drugs less often, and now often try to help the patient with other approaches, such as RELAXATION therapy or psychotherapy (*see* MENTAL THERAPIES).

Major tranquillizers

Drugs used to treat anxiety are divided into two major groups – the major and minor tranquillizers. The major tranquillizers are used for the treatment of psychotic states, where the working of the mind is disturbed (*see* PSYCHIATRY). They are of value in treating some of the major mental disorders such as SCHIZOPHRENIA, hallucinations and mania, as well as a number of other conditions, and they are sometimes used for treating anxiety. Among the best-known major tranquillizers are chlorpromazine (Largactil) and trifuoperazine (Stelazine). Most are given by mouth, but some can be given by 'depot' injections (an injection of a chemical which is stored in the body and remains effective for weeks).

An important advantage of the major tranquillizers is that they do not produce dependence. Their principal side-effect is muscle stiffness and shakiness but this stops when the drug is discontinued. This muscle stiffness can also sometimes affect the face and mouth or the eye muscles, which can be distressing, especially if the patient does not know the cause. Often another drug is prescribed to control those unwanted effects.

Another, more serious but rare side-effect of major tranquillizers is a condition called *tardive dyskinesia*. After some years of tranquillizer therapy – often at high dosages – the patient may develop curious writhing movements of the limbs. This condition does not improve much even if the drugs are stopped, and unfortunately there is no really successful treatment. Because side-effects of major tranquillizers occur more commonly with the higher doses, patients who need these drugs to control severe mental illnesses such as schizophrenia are always monitored very carefully by their doctors or by psychiatric nurses.

In low doses, side-effects are much less common so the major tranquillizers may be prescribed for severe anxiety in modest doses over a relatively short period of time without any serious risk of untoward effects.

Minor tranquillizers

All the most widely prescribed minor tranquillizers belong to a group called the *benzodiazepines*. The first drug of this type, chlordiazepoxide (Librium), was introduced in 1960, followed three years later by diazepam (Valium). Since there was already concern about abuse of barbiturates in the 1960s, the new drugs were hailed as a major advance in the treatment of a variety of psychological disorders because they were said to be relatively free from side-effects. There is no doubt that some of these claims were partly true. In particular, there is very little risk to any patient who overdoses on a benzodiazepine drug. Yet benzodiazepines were promoted as safe and effective treatment for conditions such as general tension or unhappiness, for the relief of all grades of anxiety, to help people over family worries or grief and as an aid in the management of psychosomatic disorders such as tension headaches. In short, they rapidly became an almost universal panacea for the stresses and worries of modern life.

By the early 1970s they were in widespread use. In 1975, 25 million prescriptions for minor tranquillizers were dispensed in Britain – more than for any other type of drug. The situation was much the same in the United States and many other countries, where minor tranquillizers were also the most widely prescribed single class of drugs.

Benzodiazepines proved not only to be effective in the relief of anxiety, but several different types became available which have been promoted and used as sleeping pills, although the effects of the different benzodiazepines are dissimilar.

In small doses benzodiazepines have a SEDATIVE or damping effect on the mind, with relief of anxiety and tension. In larger doses, they relieve muscular tension and also cause a feeling of drowsiness or sleepiness.

Some benzodiazepines have quite prolonged effects, lasting for well over 24 hours following a single dose. A small dose of a long-acting benzodiazepine may help anxiety, a larger dose can induce sleep, but there will be a considerable risk of a hangover effect when the person wakes. Other benzodiazepines have an intermediate effect (8–10 hours), while others have very short-lived effects (4–6 hours at most).

Regular tranquillizer use can often lead to patient's lives taking on a uniform 'grey' nature without any real emotions. While it is true that the emotions of sadness may be somewhat blunted, it is also the case that patients may not experience very much happiness either. In addition, it has been found that these sorts of tranquillizers are both physically and psychologically addicting when taken for a long time. Today they are recommended only for very short periods – two or three days, or a week at the most – to give patients short-term relief.

Coming off tranquillizers

A staged withdrawal programme is planned by the doctor with the help of the patient. At the very least, withdrawal after years of regular use will take a month, but it may take three months. Most doctors favour a very gradual reduction in dose over this period of time. However, some doctors suggest an initial switch to another drug and then a gradual withdrawal of this substitute. Although there may be minor symptoms during a withdrawal programme – for example, slight sleeping problems – these are usually very mild and easy to cope with.

Once the patients are off drugs, they will often feel not only much better physically, but emotionally as well. Often patients say that they had not realized what they had been missing in life while tied to the routine of tablet taking.

Beta-blocking drugs

When a person is really anxious, several things happen in the body as a result of over-activity of the sympathetic nervous system (*see* AUTONOMIC NERVOUS SYSTEM). The muscles tense, and may even tremble. The heart beats rapidly, the hands become sweaty, the mouth becomes dry and there is a feeling of 'butterflies' in the stomach. These feelings can arise from an acute stress, such as speaking or playing a musical instrument in public, or taking examinations, and if the stress is prolonged, the symptoms may sometimes also be prolonged. A person with a highly anxious personality can even focus on the very symptoms produced by anxiety, such as worrying about sweaty hands.

The *beta-blockers* are not strictly tranquillizers but a group of drugs which block these actions of the sympathetic nervous system, and are widely used in treating high BLOOD PRESSURE and HEART disorders. They do not affect psychological symptoms such as worry, tension and fear, but do reduce palpitations, tremor and sweating: therefore they are useful in patients in whom these symptoms dominate.

Other alternatives

For any sudden or severe mental stress, rest and RELAXATION is vital. Some people find regular EXERCISE a help, or MASSAGE. Daily sessions of MEDITATION or relaxation are a much more positive answer to such problems than taking tranquillizers.

For more severe anxiety, a PSYCHOLOGIST can help by relaxation training and by suggesting specific techniques to avoid developing the symptoms of anxiety or panic attacks.

Transplants

The idea of replacing diseased parts of the body with 'spares' is quite old, but it is only in relatively recent times that this has become a reality. There are considerable problems that must be overcome before transplants can be carried out, including locating suitable replacements, overcoming problems of REJECTION of the transplanted organ or tissue and resolving important ethical questions that might arise. Yet the field of transplant surgery is expanding, since it offers the hope of treating illnesses which must otherwise be disabling or fatal.

While we are concerned here with the replacement of organs, important and valuable work also takes place in the transplanting of other body tissue: skin grafts, corneal grafting and BONE MARROW transplants can be counted among the most successful procedures in this field.

In theory, any organ except the brain can be transplanted, but a consistent level of success has only been achieved in the case of the KIDNEYS, HEART, LUNGS (which are usually transplanted with the heart) and LIVER. Further research and development is taking place in the field of pancreas and small bowel transplantation.

Physical and ethical problems

Finding organs to transplant is one of the most difficult of the immediate problems that the surgeon has to face.

The organ should come from a person who was fit and preferably young at the time of death. The tragedy of modern living is that the most likely way for this to occur is through a road accident.

Great care must be taken to ensure that the organs are removed only after death has occurred, but at the same time, the organ to be used in a transplant will deteriorate quite quickly if it is no longer supplied with blood after death. Therefore it must be removed as soon as possible. It is this dilemma that has provoked most controversy in recent years, because it was rapidly discovered that the exact point of death was more difficult to define than to recognize.

The solution of this problem centred on whether the brain was alive in the sense of being capable of recovering independent life-support. After careful study of the survival of many victims of brain damage, there have now emerged clear-cut ways in which doctors can determine the point at which brain death has occurred.

If a person has expressed a positive wish to donate his or her organs – in a will, by carrying a Department of Health donor card or by stating the intention in the presence of two witnesses during the last illness – the relatives have no legal right to be consulted after the death. However, when death takes place in hospital and the coroner wants to perform a post-mortem, no part of the body can be removed without the coroner's permission.

Once brain death has been confirmed (and consent has been obtained), the organ for transplant can be removed immediately after the ventilator has been switched off. This may sound macabre, but the reality is no more unpleasant than the death of a victim in other circumstances.

Particularly where kidney and liver transplants are concerned, there is a crucial shortage of available organs. Much greater publicity is needed to encourage people to carry organ donation cards so that they can become potential donors.

When an organ has been taken from a dead donor, it must be preserved until it can be placed in the ill patient. The organ must be placed on ice and special fluid must be pumped through its blood vessel system to keep the system open and free of blood clots. The technology required during this crucial period is being constantly updated and, in the case of kidneys, is now quite advanced. The kidney is simply flushed through to remove the blood, and it is then put into a polythene bag which is surrounded by ice. It can be kept in this state for up to 24 hours before being used.

Living donor transplants
Organ transplants from living donors occur exclusively in kidney transplantation, since a normal person can easily survive in good health with only one kidney.

If a relative is prepared to give one of his or her kidneys, this is often the best match as it lessens the risk of rejection. A close relative such as a brother, sister or parent will share many genetic characteristics of the recipient; there is thus a chance that his or her IMMUNE SYSTEM will not recognize the graft as foreign and reject it violently. In addition, the kidney for transplantation can be removed calmly without the urgency that is called for in a recently dead donor, allowing more time to plan the operation.

Travel sickness

The main cause of travel sickness is the motion of the vehicle in which one is travelling – the rolling and tossing of a ship, the swaying of a car as it rounds a series of bends, the rhythmic movements of a train – so that travel sickness is sometimes called 'motion sickness'. However, psychological factors can also be important: the mere thought of a boat journey can make some people feel queasy, while fear of flying is a frequent cause of airsickness.

Why does it happen?
Travel sickness results from an imbalance of information reaching the brain from the various sense organs concerned with movement. One of the most important of these is the BALANCE organ in the inner ear, which contains three fluid-filled canals (the semicircular canals). These are like three spirit levels placed at right angles to each other: head movement in any direction causes movement of the fluid in one or more of the canals. A volley of nerve impulses is then sent to the brain via the vestibulo-cochlear nerve. At the same time, the brain receives information about movement from a number of other sources, particularly the eyes. If the brain's central computer can make sense of these various pieces of information, no harm will result. If, however, the information coming from the inner ear or the eyes is confusing or conflicting, signals are sent to a part of the brain called the VOMITING centre which triggers off both the feeling of NAUSEA and the physical act of vomiting. One way of understanding why this happens is to consider the difference between a cyclist travelling along a road, the driver of a following car and someone sitting in the back of the car reading a book. When the cyclist rounds a bend, both his eyes and inner ear send the same information about the movement to his brain, so no confusion results. The same applies to the driver of the car. The passenger in the back seat, however, senses the movement only with his inner ear; the car seat and the book in front of him do not move in relation to his eyes. The brain cannot make sense of this and sooner or later the passenger may feel nauseous and may want to vomit.

People who have been travel sick several times may develop a psychological association between a particular form of travel and the feeling of being unwell: they unconsciously expect to be sick even before the journey has started. Psychologists call this type of reaction a 'conditioned reflex'. It accounts for the fact that some people feel seasick before the boat has even left the dock.

Symptoms

The symptoms of travel sickness are different from person to person, although a particular individual always experiences the same symptoms and in the same order. Giddiness, nausea and vomiting are the most obvious, but other common ones include headaches, drowsiness, increased breathing efforts, yawning and pallid skin complexion.

Remedies

Fortunately there is a wide variety of travel sickness pills available under many brand names, and each contains a particular drug effective against motion sickness. Some of the drugs which are short-acting, being effective for only three or four hours, are more suitable for short journeys; others are longer acting and are more suitable for prolonged journeys. Most can be bought over the counter at the chemist's, but anyone with a recurrent problem with travel sickness should consult a doctor.

Different travel sickness pills have different effects on different people, so it may be necessary to try out two or three brands before one is found that is suitable and effective. Once this has been found, it is best to stick to it if possible.

Most of the drugs act on the central nervous system, damping down nerve activity either in the ear's balance organ or in the vomiting centre itself. Simply taking them probably also has a psychologically beneficial effect.

Most travel sickness pills have the side-effect of drowsiness, so are unsuitable for car drivers. It is a good idea to try the pills out in the safety of your own home some days before the journey; if drowsiness is a real problem, ask your doctor to prescribe or recommend an alternative drug. Drowsiness can also, of course, be a useful side-effect, especially for children during long car journeys.

Children do seem to be much more susceptible to travel sickness, the ages at which they are particularly vulnerable being between four and 12. By the time they reach their teens, most children have adapted to travel and know they should avoid such activities as reading in a moving car. Remember that children need a far smaller dose of travel pills than adults – if they don't work, do not be tempted to increase the dose. Ask your doctor to recommend some alternative drug suitable for children.

The doses and duration of action vary from drug to drug, and you should adhere strictly to the instructions supplied with the pills – take care not to exceed the maximum stated dose. Alcohol mixes very badly with these drugs and can produce a severe or dangerous degree of sedation.

Taking a pill when one already feels sick is usually of little use. The drug may be expelled immediately when one vomits, and in any case cannot reach its site of absorption into the body – the intestines – because the sphincter at the base of the stomach has sealed off. Sucking the pill may, however, have a useful effect if it does not taste too bad. In this case, the drug is absorbed into the bloodstream through the lining underneath the tongue.

One treatment which undoubtedly works for some people is to wear special elasticated wrist bands with a small plastic button which presses on an ACUPUNCTURE point on the inside of the wrist. This point is stimulated continually by the pressure from the band and sickness may be relieved.

Another simple remedy that has also been proved effective is to take some ginger an hour or so before travelling. A small teaspoonful of powdered ginger in water should be enough: or you could eat several pieces of crystallized root ginger. The advantage of both these treatments is their total lack of side-effects, although they may be less reliable than drug treatments.

Avoiding travel sickness

The chances of travel sickness can be minimized in a number of ways. On a ship, the best idea is to stay on deck and scan the horizon. In this way, the eyes receive a constant flow of information about the ship's movements which compensates for the information coming from the ear's balance organ. Leaning over the rails and looking at the sea itself is not such a good idea – the constant see-saw motion of the waves passing across one's visual field is likely to be just a bit more than the brain can cope with.

Similarly, as a car passenger, it is best to focus one's attention on objects in the far distance. Reading a book or watching a hedge whizz by through a side window are more likely to make one feel nauseous. Children in the back seat should be seated high enough for them have a good view. Having a window or two partly open to allow fresh air to circulate is also an extremely good idea, especially if one of the car's occupants is smoking.

Having some control over one's movements, such as driving a car or taking the tiller of a dinghy or motor boat, is another method of avoiding sickness. Occupying one's mind also seems to help: 'spotting' games are particularly useful for long car or coach journeys with children.

Travelling on either an empty of an overful stomach is best avoided. Frequent small snacks are a better idea and rich or fatty foods should be avoided. Alcohol should be avoided, particularly by anyone who has taken a travel pill. Heavy drinking the night before to take your mind off the impending journey is not to be recommended – in fact, a hangover will greatly increase the chances of experiencing travel sickness.

Trichinosis, ***see*** **Worms**

Trichology

This is the study of the hair and scalp, in healthy as well as diseased conditions. Hairdressers are nowadays trained in the basic elements of trichology and many will give their customers simple advice about keeping their hair healthy. Trichologists have received further training in a variety of non-medical treatments for hair and scalp disorders and are able to treat many minor disorders. However, more severe diseases of the scalp – which often affect the hair and hair growth – is a medical matter. Family practitioners treat conditions such as psoriasis of the scalp or seborrhoea; hospital specialists in skin disorders (dermatologists) may be consulted in difficult cases.

See also DANDRUFF.

Trichomoniasis

Trichomoniasis – or 'trich' – is a common condition, with at least one in five women likely to have it at some time during their lives. It can affect men, being responsible for about 4 per cent of cases of NON-SPECIFIC URETHRITIS (NSU), but more usually gives rise to disease in women, for whom it is among the common causes of vaginal discharge (*see* LEUCORRHOEA).

Causes

The trichomonas organism (*Trichomonas vaginalis*) responsible for the infection is rather unusual. It is neither a bacterium nor a virus, but a one-celled, pear-shaped protozoon or parasite. Its five whip-like tentacles enable it both to swim about in the vaginal secretion and to attract particles of material on which it lives.

Although trichomoniasis can often be caught as a result of having intercourse with somebody who already has the infection, it can be contracted in other ways. Indeed, the facts that the trichomonas infection occurs in a very much greater number of women than men, that it does not usually survive for long in males, and that the infection can develop in women who are not having intercourse confirm this. The answer to this apparent mystery lies in the ability of the trichomonas organism – unlike other sexually transmitted organisms such as the gonococcus (*see* GONORRHOEA) – to survive outside the human body for at least 30 minutes on objects with which the genital parts of an infected person have come in contact. It is, therefore, one of the few basically SEXUALLY TRANSMITTED DISEASES that can actually be caught from a lavatory seat as well as from contaminated towels, flannels or clothing.

Symptoms

Fortunately, almost all cases of trichomoniasis can be easily and completely cured. Usually, its only manifestation is vaginitis (inflammation of the vagina), the main symptom of which is a profuse vaginal discharge – this is generally quite runny, yellow to green in colour and has a strong odour. The discharge is often accompanied by soreness and irritation of the genital area. It is very unusual for any organ other than the vagina – either in the pelvis or elsewhere in the body – to be involved, and the infection has virtually no complications.

Diagnosis

The diagnosis of trichomoniasis can only be made by seeing the actual trichomonas organism under a microscope in a specimen of the vaginal discharge: there are no blood or other tests which will reveal it. There are, however, a large number of diseases that can give rise to vaginal discharge of one sort or another. And, even though the nature of the discharge may strongly suggest that it is trichomonas infection, this can only be proved and other possible causes ruled out by an internal examination and by looking at the discharge under the microscope.

Since trichomoniasis can only be cured completely by one particular type of drug (and there is no single treatment that is effective for all types of vaginal discharge), it is important that a positive identification is made of the trichomonas organism. Vaginal examination and tests are particularly advisable if the infection is likely to have been caught through sexual intercourse with a casual partner, since it is possible to have acquired other infections, such as gonorrhoea or THRUSH, at the same time. It is wise, therefore, to confirm or eliminate the presence of other infections so that appropriate additional treatment can be given if necessary. A full investigation can be carried out at a 'special clinic' – that is, a hospital clinic which specializes in sexually transmitted diseases.

Treatment

The treatment of trichomonas infection usually consists of taking oral doses of *metronidazole* (Flagyl) or another closely related drug. It is important that the effectiveness of the cure is checked after treatment, by the examination of vaginal secretion to make sure that no organism has survived. Until this has been done, the patient should refrain from intercourse to avoid the possibility of reinfection and of contaminating anybody else. The patient's partner is usually advised either to undergo the tests for trichomoniasis as well, or to take a course of metronidazole as a precautionary measure against the infection.

Metronidazole has few side-effects, although it makes some people feel slightly nauseated. It is also important that anyone taking the drug should avoid alcohol during the course of his or her treatment.

Trigeminal neuralgia, *see* Neuralgia

Trophoblastic disease, *see* Uterus

Tropical diseases

Now that air travel is so quick and convenient, both business travellers and holiday makers may be at risk of contracting tropical diseases during a trip to the tropics. Holiday destinations in India, Africa and the Far East are increasingly popular, but it is possible to contract a tropical disease in these areas even if the traveller stays within the confines of modern holiday resorts.

What are tropical diseases?

Tropical diseases include not only spectacular and bizarre parasitic disorders like *elephantiasis*, but also rare and deadly fevers like *Lassa fever* or *Marburg fever*. Relatively few diseases occur only within the tropics; and diseases such as leprosy and plague, which most people now think of as 'tropical', were once widespread in Europe. Likewise, diseases which are now familiar in Europe, such as MEASLES or TUBERCULOSIS, are of immense importance in the tropics; the mortality rate from measles is 400 times greater among malnourished African children than among European ones. Although most tropical diseases are due to VIRUSES, BACTERIA or PARASITES, malnutrition, RABIES and even snakebites must be considered too (*see also* FUNGAL INFECTIONS). There is no clear-cut definition of tropical diseases beyond the fact that they tend mainly to be associated with warm climates, poverty or poor hygiene.

Fighting tropical diseases

SMALLPOX is the only disease ever to have been totally eradicated. Unfortunately, it is not likely that we will be able to eradicate any more tropical diseases for many years to come – much more research is necessary, and the resources required will be enormous. However, the World Health Organization has determined that the following six tropical diseases be singled out for particular attention.

Malaria probably affects 200 million people each year and causes a million deaths. It is one of the world's greatest killers, and is still on the increase. (*See* MALARIA.)

Schistosomiasis (also known as *bilharzia*) is an unpleasant and sometimes fatal disease due to small worms which live in the liver, bowels and bladder. Eggs passed out in the urine and faeces hatch in water and produce organisms which infect certain kinds of snails. These produce other types of organisms which penetrate the intact human skin and then pass in the blood to the liver. It is usually caused by coming into contact with water polluted by faeces.

Sleeping sickness, spread by the tsetse fly, has made vast areas of Africa uninhabitable by humans and livestock. The disease is caused by a tiny, single-celled parasite which lives in the blood and the brain, and causes serious damage to the nervous system. Treatment is difficult, and there is no vaccine. The disease is a risk to visitors to African game parks, who should therefore take special precautions to avoid insect bites.

Leprosy still affects a large number of people around the world – there are probably 20 million sufferers, though no more than three million currently receive treatment.

Filariasis is caused by a variety of small worms which gain entry to the body through the bites of mosquitoes and flies. These are the worms that cause *elephantiasis* by blocking the lymph passages in the body. *African river blindness* is another form of filariasis – a disease that causes blindness by infestation with a worm that enters the body through a blackfly bite.

Leishmaniasis is spread by sandflies, and is caused by a parasite which attacks the skin, liver and spleen.

Immunization schemes

Measles, POLIO, TETANUS, tuberculosis, DIPHTHERIA and WHOOPING COUGH kill five million children in developing countries each year. And the World Health Organization has set itself an awesome task: immunization of all children in the world against these diseases. The practical problems are enormous as 80 per cent of the world's population lives in remote areas, and even when supplies of vaccine arrive, their effectiveness cannot always be guaranteed; unless refrigerated, vaccines are quickly inactivated by tropical heat. But the project is well under way, and considerable progress has already been achieved, with polio (now virtually unknown in developed countries) being on the verge of eradication.

See also HOLIDAY HEALTH.

Tuberculosis

Tuberculosis – or TB as it is more commonly known – remains one of the most important infectious diseases in the world. Although the improved standards of general living conditions have made it relatively uncommon in the West, it remains one of the great killers – especially of children – among Third World communities. In past centuries, it was known as 'consumption' because of the way it appeared to 'consume' the body.

TB is caused by a fungus-like bacterium called *Mycobacterium tuberculosis*. And there are two main strains of this particular organism that cause disease in humans: a human strain, which is the only important one in the UK; and a bovine strain, which primarily infects cattle, but which is also capable of causing human disease. Nowadays, all the cattle in the UK are tested for infection – so-called 'tuberculin-tested' herds – so that infection in cattle with the bovine strain of the disease is no longer a problem.

The incidence of this chronic infection and the problems it can cause vary from country to country. In the UK, there is no doubt that infection of the LUNGS – *pulmonary* TB – is the most usual form of the disease, whereas in Africa *abdominal* TB is very common.

How TB develops

At one time, most people growing up in a country like Britain would have been in contact with tuberculosis at an early age. Such early contact leads to an infection called *primary* TB which is often – but not always – without any significant symptoms. This first contact is picked up as a result of contact with someone who has a sufficiently severe disease in the lungs to cough up sputum (PHLEGM) containing TB bacteria. If the amount of bacteria inhaled is relatively small, the primary TB will be a minor infection which will help build up a partial immunity to the development of full-blown TB after exposure to the infection later on.

The more serious forms of the disease that occur in later life are called *post-primary* disease. It seems that the usual cause for these infections is that the immunity to the original infection has broken down and the TB bacteria have literally broken out of their original site. Although this is probably the usual mechanism of development of the disease, it is also likely that some people getting the disease later in life do so because they are exposed to a very high infective dose of bacteria.

The reasons why the immunity breaks down are not at all clear. In most cases, it seems that social rather than medical factors are of the greatest relevance. There is little doubt that TB these days is a disease that is increasingly frequently found among the homeless and alcoholics, although it may still occur in an apparently fit person who is well-fed and lives in good housing.

Complications of primary TB

Although primary TB is often a relatively minor infection with no symptoms at all, it can develop into a serious disease in very young children or in those who have some other debilitating disease.

The site of infection is nearly always the lungs, although in some parts of the world it may affect the ABDOMEN. The original infection causes a small area of inflammation in one of the lungs, and this goes on to produce a reaction in the LYMPH nodes that drain lymphatic fluids from the particular part of the lung. This patch of inflammation and enlargement of some of the nodes at the root of the lung is called the *primary complex*.

In the majority of cases, the living TB bacteria in the primary complex are contained by the lymph nodes and spread no further. But, in a few children and adolescents with primary TB, the defence mechanism breaks down soon after infection. This allows the organism to spread throughout the body, leading to a serious condition called *miliary* TB, which causes a lot of general illness, with loss of weight and a high fever. Diagnosis of miliary TB is made by X-ray examination of the chest which shows that both lungs are full of tiny nodules, each of which represents an area of tuberculous infection.

Sometimes the general spread of the disease soon after the primary infection leads to an infection in the nervous system, called TB MENINGITIS. Unlike the usual sort of meningitis that comes on within a day or so, TB meningitis may take some weeks to develop. The first symptoms are of general ill health, a slight fever, headaches – a relatively unusual complaint in a child – and, occasionally, fits. At a later stage, the fever rises and the signs of drowsiness and neck stiffness appear. Finally, the fever rises yet higher and obvious problems with individual nerves such as those controlling the eyes will occur. This is a very dangerous condition, and it is important to start treatment as soon as the diagnosis is made. This is done by performing a lumbar puncture which enables doctors to look at the cerebrospinal fluid that bathes the BRAIN and the SPINAL CORD. One of the findings that will indicate TB meningitis is that the level of sugar in the fluid is very much lower than that in the blood; this is almost unique to this condition.

Pulmonary TB

Although the primary focus occurs in the lungs, it is not until the post-primary stage of infection that the lungs give rise to any trouble. In a few cases of primary TB, the lymph nodes at the root of the lung may break down and liberate the bacteria into one of the main tubes (bronchi) supplying a particular lobe of the lung. This, in turn, will lead to a lobar pneumonia happening soon after the original infection.

Most cases of tuberculous lung disease, however, happen many years after the original infection with the disease. The primary focus actually has a tendency to attack the lower lobes of the lungs, while the post-primary infection is much more likely to occur in the highest segments of the upper lobes of the lungs. It seems that the large amounts of oxygen that are available there, together with the relatively poor supply of blood, are particularly suitable incubators for the lung disease.

When the disease has become established in the upper part of the lungs, it may cause cavities to form there. Once this has happened, large numbers of TB organisms may be produced in the sputum, and this means that the sufferer becomes a serious source of infection until he or she is treated. The sufferer is most likely to do damage to young children by giving them primary TB, TB meningitis and TB bronchopneumonia (*see* PNEUMONIA). And it may well be that someone excreting large numbers of TB organisms is able to rekindle the disease in people in older age groups who have already had the primary form.

Left untreated, pulmonary TB can lead to the formation of fluid in the pleural space which surrounds the lungs, to infection of the pleura (lining membrane) itself, and subsequently to pleural thickening and fibrosis. It is very characteristic of TB that the fibrosis it leaves behind is often full of calcium and is therefore very rigid. Obviously, a lung surrounded by a hard wrapping of bone-like fibrosis is not going to be able to move freely, and breathing will be seriously impaired.

Sometimes the same sequence of events will happen to the *pericardium* – the membranous bag that contains the heart. This has even more serious effects since tuberculous PERICARDITIS may effectively throttle the heart and therefore stop it pumping enough blood through to the rest of the body.

It is usually fairly easy to diagnose a case of pulmonary TB. In any well-developed infection, there will be quite marked changes on the chest X-ray, particularly in the upper parts of the two upper lobes. One of the difficulties on an X-ray, however, is to tell whether the changes represent new or old TB infection. The fibrosis caused by an early episode of TB will persist for life.

In a case of suspected TB, the first thing is to inspect the sputum that is produced under a microscope. When there is a heavy infection, there will be plenty of bacteria in the sputum. These will show up as thin red rods when stained with the special TB stain, called the Ziehl–Nielsen stain. The presence of bacteria on direct staining of the sputum is of very great importance since if there are no bacteria, the patient cannot be infectious, even if he or she does turn out to have TB at a later stage. For this reason, infection with the presence of bacteria on direct staining is called 'open' TB, and this is the only sort that can possibly be infectious.

Other forms of TB

Although TB in the lungs is the most common form of the disease, there are many other areas of the body that it may attack, such as the UTERUS (womb), GENITALS, KIDNEY, SKIN and spine (*see* BACK).

TB in the abdomen is a common problem, particularly in Africa and India. It can be quite difficult to make the diagnosis, since there is no convenient test, such as the chest X-ray, that picks up the disease. Sufferers simply appear to be rather unwell, and will have a temperature. One of the easiest ways of making the diagnosis is by performing a liver BIOPSY – that is, surgically removing a small piece of LIVER, and examining it under a microscope to see whether there are any TB bacteria present.

TB is also fairly likely to attack the glands in the neck, sometimes involving the overlying skin. This condition, known as *scrofula*, has a very long history. For many years, it was thought that the disease could be cured by the touch of a monarch. For this reason, it was called 'king's evil'.

Treatment

Prior to the 1950s, TB was frequently fatal. The cure for pulmonary TB, for instance, relied heavily on building up the patient's resistance with rest and nourishment. But, unfortunately, this care often came too late. The clarity of the air and the relative lack of oxygen at great heights was also thought to be helpful, and there were many sanatoriums in countries such as Switzerland for wealthy TB sufferers.

Patients were also operated on to remove the seriously infected parts of the lungs. The surgery reduced the volume of the lungs and obliterated the cavities, thereby halting the spread of the disease through the lungs. However, before antibiotics were introduced as a treatment for TB, attempts to achieve a cure were thwarted by the fact that the disease was often quite widespread before treatment was started. This often resulted in very intense fibrous scarring of the lung tissue, which prevented the organ from fulfilling the function of transferring oxygen from the air into the blood. Even today, if cases of TB are left untreated for too long, fibrosis will occur and cannot be helped by antibiotics.

With modern treatment, however, it is quite possible to stop the progress of TB within a few days of starting treatment, although it will take months to produce an actual cure. There are now a selection of drugs that can be used to treat the TB infection. The first of these was streptomycin, and although it is still used, it is somewhat limited by the fact that it has to be given by injection. The usual drugs used these days are rifampicin, isoniazid and ethambutol. To prevent the organism from becoming resistant to the use of any one drug, it is customary to use these drugs together during the early stages of the infection. Once the organism has grown, and this may take three months, it is possible to show that it is sensitive to at least two of the drugs and one is left out. Unfortunately, doctors in both the UK and the US are finding that, among homeless TB patients, drug resistance is an increasing problem.

The length of time it takes to cure TB varies depending on the particular type of infection. For instance, treatment has to continue for at least nine months in the case of pulmonary TB, but much longer in the case of abdominal TB.

Prevention

It is possible to test the population for immunity to TB by using a preparation of TB-derived protein called tuberculin. This is used in two tests – the Mantoux test and the Heaf test – usually performed on children by the age of 13. People with a partial immunity to the disease due to primary TB in the past will show a reaction when tuberculin is injected into the skin. In cases of established post-primary TB, the extent of the reaction will be greater.

If a child between the ages of 11 and 13 has not yet come into contact with the disease, it is well worth vaccinating him or her with BCG (Bacille Calmette-Guérin). This vaccine consists of a modified form of the TB bacterium and has the same effect as a minor primary infection, and gives some immunity. It is also worthwhile immunizing younger children (and doctors, nurses and medical students) where there is a risk of contact with the disease. However, because of the low incidence of tuberculosis now, some regions in the UK are following the American policy of not routinely giving BCGs.

Tumours

Strictly speaking, any type of abnormal growth should be called a tumour. This can cause some distressing misunderstandings, since medical staff tend to use the term accurately, while lay people often mistakenly think that all 'tumours' are malignant or cancerous growths (*see* CANCER).

The body's normal cells are subject to controls which ensure that, once we have stopped growing, new cells are made at the same rate as old cells are lost. For example, as skin cells are destroyed by friction and abrasion on the surface, equal numbers of new cells are formed. This means that the skin is roughly the same thickness throughout life.

No one understands the details of this control mechanism. But if it breaks down, cells are formed at an unchecked rate and a tumour is formed.

Types of tumour

There are two basic types of tumour, *benign* and *malignant*. Benign tumours are localized growths of tissue, which produce swellings. There is no tendency for these extra cells to spread or grow into other parts of the body. However, they can have serious consequences as a result of their location.

For example, a benign tumour of the nerve tissue in the spinal canal can put pressure on the spinal cord, causing loss of sensation and paralysis. Similarly, an organ may be damaged if pressure is put on one of the blood vessels that supply it.

The major identifying characteristic of malignant tumours is that they have a tendency to spread to other parts of the body. However, it can still be extremely difficult to identify a tumour as malignant, since some are, in fact, very slow-growing indeed.

Malignant tumours are separated into two further groups, *primary* and *secondary*. The original tumour is known as the primary one. As this grows, fragments of the tissue may break off and settle in other parts of the body either by lymphatics or bloodstream. These then multiply and the cells which make up the fragments form secondary tumours.

Secondary tumour cells can usually be identified under a microscope, because they consist of cells that are normally found in another part of the body. For instance, a primary tumour of the thyroid gland may spread to the bones, so that a secondary tumour formed of abnormal thyroid cells is found in a bone.

Turner's syndrome

Several different types of chromosome abnormality are known to affect the sex chromosomes of both males and females (*see* GENETICS). Turner's syndrome is one such abnormality which occurs only in females. It was first described in 1922 by a Dr Rossle, who noted that a number of INFERTILE women were also relatively short and had an unusual but characteristic appearance.

Causes

The genetic material in any human cell is composed of strands of DNA which are known as chromosomes. In a normal cell, there are 44 chromosomes arranged in pairs, and in addition, two more chromosomes which determine the sex of the individual. A normal male has two sex chromosomes, an 'X' and a 'Y'; the X-chromosome is inherited from the mother and the Y-chromosome from the father. Male sperm contain only 23 chromosomes (half the normal number) and each carries either an X or a Y chromosome. A normal female has two X-chromosomes, and so all her eggs (ova) carry a single X-chromosome. So if a Y-carrying sperm fertilizes the ovum, the baby will have one X-chromosome and one Y-chromosome and will be male. If an X-carrying sperm fertilizes the ovum, the baby's cells will carry two X-chromosomes (usually called 'XX') and will be female.

Babies born with Turner's syndrome have an abnormality of one of their X-chromosomes. In more than half of all cases of the syndrome, one X-chromosome is missing completely. This condition is called 'XO'. It seems that the likely cause of this situation is a loss of the X-chromosome from the father's side. The sperm which fertilizes the egg has no sex chromosome present at all, so the child just inherits one X-chromosome from the mother. In about 30 per cent of cases of Turner's syndrome, there are two X-chromosomes present, but one of them is faulty. An abnormality can be detected on one of the arms of one X-chromosome, and it may be so mis-shapen that it does not function. In other cases, there appears to be a mixture of different chromosomal abnormalities in different cells in the body; some cells have the XO condition whereas others have normal XX chromosomes, or even XY chromosomes. This situation is known as *mosaicism* because the cells in one individual are of two different types, rather like a mosaic pavement.

It seems that the genetic damage that affects the sperm is a purely chance event and there is no additional risk of it recurring in a later pregnancy.

Characteristic features

A baby born with Turner's syndrome is usually lighter than average – less than 6 lb 6 oz (2.9 kg) – and is also shorter than normal. The diagnosis may be suspected on the basis of fullness or 'webbing' of the tissues on either side of the neck.

As the child grows, other features may become more obvious. Many children develop a broad, rather flat chest or may have a deep depression in the middle of the chest. There may be prominent folds on the inner side of the eyes. The hair line at the back of the neck can be rather low. The elbows may be mildly deformed and the hands rather short, with brittle finger-nails.

Although not all the features of the syndrome may be present in any one individual, the major characteristic finding is of reduced height. Girls with Turner's syndrome fail to grow as fast as their peers. At the time of expected puberty, sexual development also fails to occur in most cases. The normal rounding out of the female figure does not occur, breast development is reduced or absent, and there is virtually no growth of pubic hair. Girls with Turner's syndrome very rarely start menstruating naturally. Ninety-nine per cent of them are infertile.

In addition to the external signs of Turner's syndrome, there may be internal abnormalities to various organs of the body. One in six women affected by the syndrome has a heart VALVE abnormality or a narrowing of the aorta, the major ARTERY which runs from the heart. A few have KIDNEY deformities, and about one in four develops high BLOOD PRESSURE. There may also be short-sightedness and DEAFNESS.

Most children with Turner's syndrome have average intelligence and ability, although they may not be quite so good at sports as other children of their age because of their short stature and minor skeletal abnormalities. However, a small percentage of children with the syndrome also have learning difficulties. This appears mostly to affect those children who have XO chromosomes, in whom the risk of this is about one in six.

Treatment

Once the syndrome has been diagnosed, there is nothing that can be done about the basic problem, because it is caused by a genetic defect. However, many paediatricians advise plastic surgery to remove webbing of the neck and to improve the appearance of the eyes if this is abnormal. If the child is deaf, a hearing aid will be provided. The child will be seen regularly by a specialist to check that there are no problems developing with the internal organs, such as the heart or kidneys.

When the child reaches the age of 11 or 12, she is usually started on a course of hormone treatment. The female sexual hormone, oestrogen, is given to the child for three weeks out of four and this is continued indefinitely into adult life. This treatment allows the child to develop a more normal adult female appearance; some children start to menstruate with this therapy but most still remain infertile. Many women with Turner's syndrome have a fairly unremarkable appearance, apart from their shortness, and live perfectly normal lives. Their life expectancy can also be quite normal, unless complications arise as a result of high blood pressure or kidney disease – but these are rare.

Typhoid and paratyphoid

The serious infectious fevers, TYPHUS and typhoid, have been recognized for centuries, but until the middle of the last century, there was no distinction between them and they were both called typhus.

In fact, the two diseases are quite distinct in their effects, and because typhoid particularly affects the INTESTINES, it came to be recognized as a separate disease. Its association with typhus remained, however, since the name typhoid simply means 'typhus-like'. Paratyphoid is a disease very like typhoid but is considerably less severe.

Causes

Typhoid is caused by one of the SALMONELLA organisms, which are spread by contaminated food and water and therefore give rise to FOOD POISONING. *Salmonella typhi* (the typhoid organism) has developed in such a way as to cause a generalized illness only in humans, without the severe intestinal symptoms that are characteristic of salmonella poisoning.

There are three types of paratyphoid caused by the organisms *Salmonella paratyphi* A, B and C. In the UK and Europe, paratyphoid B is the only one of any importance.

How infection is spread

Salmonella typhi has survived so successfully because some infected people continue to pass the organism in their faeces, yet remain quite fit and symptom-free. Such people are called 'carriers', and are obviously ideal hosts for the organism, which tends to settle in the GALL BLADDER, and can remain there for years while new organisms are excreted into the bowel via the BILE duct.

In the past, food and water became readily contaminated with human faeces, and this enabled typhoid to become very widespread. It is perhaps the disease more than any other that has largely been prevented by modern techniques of hygiene and sanitation. Another reason why the organism is so adapted to infect humans is that it survives well in fresh water – in fact, many of the serious epidemics have been water-borne. Organisms can, however, survive for any length of time in water only if there is decaying organic matter present for them to feed on – if water is simply stored in a clean reservoir, the number of organisms will be reduced.

Salmonella typhi do not survive well in sea water, so some coastal towns discharge untreated sewage straight into the sea. Nevertheless there is some risk of contracting typhoid by bathing in polluted coastal waters. Shellfish filter gallons of water to extract their food; sewage may contaminate seafood, giving a substantial risk of typhoid.

Dairy produce is a fairly common source of infection since it provides an excellent medium for the bacteria to grow in. Infected milk almost always occurs through a human carrier, and less often by contamination with sewage. Typhoid can, of course, be spread by any food, although the organism is destroyed by thorough cooking. Of course, a carrier who works with food is especially dangerous, since there is a very high risk of faecal contamination of the hands. The most famous carrier of all was an American cook who was known as 'Typhoid Mary'.

Symptoms

Typhoid has an incubation period of between 10 and 14 days. It begins as an illness resembling flu with a headache, muscle pains and abdominal discomfort. Initially, constipation is common and diarrhoea occurs occasionally.

The temperature rises slowly over the course of a week or so, in a classic 'step ladder' pattern. It is raised in the evening, but has fallen slightly by the following morning, until it finally reaches 104°F (40°C) by the end of a week.

By the end of the first week, the patient obviously has a serious disease and is in a poor general condition with a severe headache. At this stage, chest symptoms are very common, and sometimes pneumonia develops. The abdomen is distended, and two of the most significant symptoms will be present. The SPLEEN can be felt in the top left-hand corner of the abdomen, and a few pale pink patches appear on the skin.

The organisms may be grown in cultures of the blood during the course of the first week, and this is often how the diagnosis is made. The organisms are so widespread after about a week that they can also be grown in culture from a specimen of skin containing a rose-red spot – another method of diagnosis.

During the second week, patients become progressively more ill, with particular deterioration in their mental function and withdrawal from what is happening around them. Throughout the first two weeks, the organism is passing from the blood into various organs of the body, but it is in the intestines that serious complications can occur. At intervals down the length of the small intestine, there are collections of LYMPHATIC tissue called *Peyer's patches*. Typhoid particularly tends to infect these, and their surfaces may ulcerate to cause severe intestinal bleeding.

By the third week, an untreated patient is extremely ill with a swollen abdomen and a stupor that almost amounts to a coma. Diarrhoea occurs at this stage as the intestines become involved, but more serious than this is the risk that the walls of the intestine might perforate, particularly around the Peyer's patches. If this does not happen, the fever begins to settle after three or four weeks, although there is a high risk of a possibly serious relapse.

Treatment

The antibiotic *chloramphenicol* has made a great difference to the treatment of the disease, and once it is started, the illness should settle within about five days. Unfortunately, the drug can cause fatal depression of the BONE MARROW so that no blood cells are produced. Although this is very rare, it means that this antibiotic has to be reserved for potentially fatal illnesses such as typhoid. An alternative treatment is the drug *cotrimoxazole,* which is nearly as effective as chloramphenicol but without its side-effects.

Chloramphenicol is less effective in clearing up carrier states, and the antibiotic ampicillin is used quite successfully for this.

A useful and reliable vaccine against typhoid is available, and worth having if you are travelling to a country where the standards of hygiene are low. It is not 100 per cent effective, so it is still important to try to avoid food that could be contaminated.

Paratyphoid

Carriers of paratyphoid exist, but are not responsible for all outbreaks of the disease, as is the case with typhoid. The incubation period is shorter and it is not as infectious as typhoid. This means that you will not necessarily get the disease if you take in the organism.

Paratyphoid causes symptoms resembling both typhoid and salmonella poisoning. Thus there is an acute phase of GASTRO-ENTERITIS (as with salmonella) but no generalized disease develops, and only in very rare and isolated cases does paratyphoid prove to be fatal. Paratyphoid can be treated with cotrimoxazole tablets.

Typhus

There are actually a number of typhus illnesses, all caused by the same sort of organisms – the *rickettsiae.* Rickettsiae are spread from human to human by blood-sucking insects.

The most serious form of typhus is called *epidemic typhus,* and it often occurs in the social breakdown that can follow such disasters as war famine, floods and earthquakes. A less serious disease is *murine typhus.* This is basically a disease of rats and it spreads to humans via the rat flea. Finally, there is a disease of the Orient called *scrub typhus* or *tsutsugamushi fever.*

Causes of epidemic typhus

The organism of epidemic typhus is called *Rickettsia prowazekii* and the infection passes from human to human via infected body LICE; it cannot be caught directly from another human. A louse becomes infected by sucking an infected person's blood, but another human has to be very close for the louse to move on to him or her.

Once a louse is infected, the rickettsiae grow in its intestine and are passed out in the faeces. The invariable habit which the louse has of defecating as it eats leads to transfer of infection, since the human host will scratch the irritating bite and rub the faeces into the wound. Rickettsiae live for a long time in louse faeces and the dust from infected clothing can be very infectious.

Symptoms and treatment

The incubation period of epidemic typhus is about ten days. The disease starts very suddenly with a high fever and the patient feels ill, with muscular aches and pains; there is also a headache.

A rash appears after three or four days: it begins gradually and can simply be mistaken for the flush of a fever. It consists of small red flat spots, but after about a week or so, it gets darker, and the spots may start to look like little bruises.

The most serious stage of the disease occurs as the rash gets more obvious. The patient sinks into a stupor, and although he is awake, it is often impossible to communicate with him. At this point, the deterioration can be very alarming: the KIDNEYS start to fail; a cough develops; and the rash may actually progress to gangrene in the fingers, toes and genitals. In untreated infections, somewhere between 20 and 50 per cent of patients will die at this stage.

Those who are going to recover lose their fever in the third week and their brain starts working normally very quickly. However, they will need a very long period of convalescence.

The condition responds to treatment with certain antibiotics. The most likely drugs to be successful in controlling the infection are *tetracycline* and *chloramphenicol*.

Murine and scrub typhus

Murine typhus is less severe than epidemic typhus, and the death rate without treatment is probably around the 2 per cent mark. Murine typhus is a disease that is found in circumstances where humans are in quite close contact with rats. It is often endemic in rat-infested areas such as ports and food stores.

The characteristic feature of scrub typhus is that 60 per cent of infected people develop a hard scar at the site of the infecting bite within about five days. This scar is called an *eschar*. The disease then goes on in a very similar way to epidemic typhus. The illness exists in a large number of animals and is spread by a blood-sucking mite or 'chigger'. As the name suggests, this is a disease which happens in scrub land when the free-living chiggers leave the scrubby undergrowth to bite and infect.

Prevention

Vaccine against typhus does exist, and it provides quite good protection. It is also possible to take tetracycline when travelling in an infected area.

However, the most important means of prevention is to control the fleas and lice that carry the disease. In the case of epidemic typhus, this is not too difficult, since the louse is fairly easy to deal with. In areas with murine typhus, the thing to do is to try and eradicate the rats.

The most serious control problem is that of scrub typhus. This is found in rural areas, and the disease has many small animals in which it can survive; in fact, a human is probably an unusual host.

See also TYPHOID AND PARATYPHOID.

U

Ulcerative colitis, *see* **Colon and colitis**

Ulcers, peptic

'Ulcer' simply means a break or lesion in the lining, mucous membrane or skin in any part of the body. It is possible to get an ulcer almost anywhere: in your mouth, on your leg or in any part of the lining of your gut. A peptic ulcer is any sort of ulcer that results from the action of STOMACH acid – its name is derived from the enzyme *pepsin*, secreted by the stomach.

Peptic ulcers normally occur in the stomach itself, when they are called *gastric* ulcers, or in the DUODENUM – *dudodenal* ulcers. However, it is possible to get peptic ulcers in other places: for example, the effect of acid washing back from thc stomach into the oesophagus may cause an ulcer (*see* DIAPHRAGM). But the problem is mainly confined to the stomach and the duodenum.

When food is being broken down during DIGESTION, it churns round and round in acid produced by the stomach wall. So that the wall of the stomach is not digested as well, it is lined with a layer of tissue which is resistant to acid. Any break in this layer of acid-resistant tissue is an ulcer. Such a break in the tissue allows the acid gastric juices to attack the tissues underneath and gradually eat them away until a hole may develop.

Gastric or duodenal

Dudodenal ulcers are two or three times as common as gastric ulcers. In fact, gastric ulcers are becoming less common as time goes by, whereas at the end of the last century, they were more common than duodenal ulcers. No one knows why this change is taking place, but it suggests that people's way of life may influence the development of ulcers.

It also appears that people with BLOOD GROUP O have a higher chance of duodenal ulcers than people with other blood groups. It is also not known why this happens.

Causes and symptoms

It is not known why some people's stomach and duodenal linings are adversely affected by stomach acid. Diet and STRESS may well play a part and possibly drinking spirits on an empty stomach. Regular meals, with a high fibre content, and reduction of stress may help to prevent ulcers.

SMOKING certainly makes ulcers worse, and it may play a part in causing them, but it is not a sole cause.

The presence of a certain type of bacteria in the stomach called *Helicobacter pylori* has been associated with the development of peptic ulcers. Antibiotic treatment to eradicate the bacteria promotes healing of ulcers.

The pattern of pain in gastric and duodenal ulcers is usually different, although the pain is felt in the same are in the upper middle abdomen. Pain from a gastric ulcer occurs soon after eating (15–30 minutes) and is relieved by vomiting. In duodenal ulcer, the pain occurs 2–3 hours after meals and is relieved by eating. Patients often drink milk or eat biscuits in the middle of the night to help relieve the pain.

The pain is also similar to that caused by oesophagitis, which is an inflammation of the lower end of the OESOPHAGUS, caused by acid washing back into it from the stomach.

Ulcers can cause complications such as bleeding, when the patient may vomit blood or pass blood in the STOOLS. This can cause serious blood loss.

Dangers

Only a small percentage of people suffering from peptic ulcers are likely to need intensive medical attention. However, complications may occur which require hospital treatment.

The most important of the various complications is bleeding. Patients may start to vomit blood, which will come out as small, dark brown lumps called 'coffee-ground' vomit, or they may feel faint and then pass the black, tarry motions that are associated with altered blood passing through the colon. A lot of blood can be lost by bleeding from an ulcer, and the doctor's first priority is usually to treat the SHOCK associated with blood loss. The bleeding will often settle down if the patient rests in bed. If it does not settle, however, an operation may be necessary to stop the flow. In such operations, it can be difficult to work out where the bleeding is coming from, and the surgeon's job is made easier with the help of a gastroscope (*see* ENDOSCOPY), through which he or she can look down into the stomach and the duodenum.

Other complications may arise out of a peptic ulcer. The ulcer may *perforate,* causing inflammation – a condition called PERITONITIS. The signs of this complication are obvious, with collapse and severe abdominal pain. An operation at the earliest opportunity is usually vital as the consequences are serious.

The inflammation that surrounds a peptic ulcer may also cause problems by constricting part of the stomach that drains into the duodenum, resulting in a blockage called *pyloric stenosis* (*see* STOMACH). In minor cases anti-ulcer drugs may ease the inflammation and help reduce the blockage, but in established cases surgery is needed.

Another danger of gastric ulcers is that there is a small risk that they may become malignant (*see* CANCER). So all patients with gastric ulcers usually have an endoscopy to check for this possibility. There is virtually no risk of duodenal ulcers being malignant.

Diagnosis and treatment

Diagnosis is carried out either by X-RAY or fibre-optic endoscope. The X-ray diagnosis requires the patient to first eat a barium meal, a special preparation which makes the stomach show up on an X-ray. The fibre-optic endoscope is a flexible tube which can transmit images up its length, and is passed via the mouth into the stomach or duodenum so that the walls can be examined. The endoscope can be used to take samples from the stomach lining, which can then be examined in a laboratory to check if there is evidence of malignancy in the ulcer, for example.

If an ulcer is diagnosed, the initial treatment is with drugs. There are several which promote the healing of peptic ulcers by reducing the amount of acid secreted by the stomach. Antacid mixtures and tablets also help to bring relief by soaking up the acid, lessening the pain it causes in the stomach wall.

If drugs don't stop the pain, or if the ulcer causes additional problems, surgery may be necessary. But simply removing an ulcer by surgery does not necessarily cure the patient because another ulcer may well form somewhere else. So an ulcer operation usually aims to reduce the amount of acid produced by the stomach. This can be done by cutting some of the nerves that stimulate the stomach to produce acid (a vagotomy) or, occasionally, by removing part of the stomach altogether (a partial gastrectomy).

If any cancerous change is suspected in a gastric ulcer, the patient is likely to have a partial gastrectomy to remove the ulcer.

Ulcers, skin

Where an area of tissue loss occurs or erosion on the surface of the SKIN takes place, an ulcer is formed. It is often circular or oval in shape and sometimes irregular in outline. Ulcers on the surface of the body vary considerably in their depth, some involving skin loss only, but others extending deep into the muscle or bone.

The causes of ulcers are also numerous and range from the mild irritation or injury to a serious disease. The most common sites are inside the mouth, on the lips and face, in the groin region, on the legs and around the hips and lower back.

Mouth and lip ulcers

Mouth ulcers – also known as 'canker sores' – are a very common problem and can occur as a 'one-off' condition, or as a recurrent disease where the ulcers appear and disappear in periodic cycles.

Almost everyone has at some time or other suffered the discomfort of the non-recurrent type of mouth ulcer. They are brought on by a variety of factors, but are usually due to some identifiable physical, chemical or biological cause, or are a symptom of some underlying condition.

Physical causes of mouth ulceration include irritation from jagged teeth, compulsive cheek-chewing, too vigorous use of a toothbrush or burning from hot food or drink. Chemical causes include caustic drugs, tablets or sweets dissolved in the mouth, strong antiseptics and mouthwashes and chemicals used in dental treatment.

These two types of ulcers tend to clear up quickly on their own accord, but are extremely sensitive to salty and sour tastes like crisps or lemons.

Biological causes include the SYPHILIS bacterium, various FUNGI and the *Herpes simplex* virus. A syphilitic chancre in the mouth is rare, but very serious. It is sexually acquired, consisting of a single round, button-sized and painless ulcer on the lips or tongue. On the other hand, an acute herpes infection in the mouth consists of numerous, much smaller, painful ulcers on the gums, tongue and membranes which line the inside of the cheeks or the inside of the lips.

Non-recurrent, but persistent mouth ulcers may also be a symptom of DIABETES, various BLOOD diseases, TUBERCULOSIS, and inflammatory bowel disease such as Crohn's disease or ulcerative colitis. CANCER of the lip, though uncommon, often first appears as an ulcer.

Often, mouth ulcers are recurrent and indeed these are the commonest type of ulcer affecting about 1 in 5 adults. They are called *aphthous ulcers* and they are divided into major and minor types. In the minor form a single ulcer or small crop of ulcers appear in the mouth several times a year, lasting for about a week, and healing without scarring. Swallowing may be painful.

Major apthous ulceration affects 1 person in 10 of those who suffer from recurrent ulcers. It is characterized by more frequent attacks, often every 3–4 weeks, in which ulcers are multiple and may persist for years. This can be incapacitating. Both types of recurrent aphthous ulcers tend to improve after a few years.

It is still not clear what causes this problem. It does tend to run in families, and is more common in women, so there may be a link to hormonal changes, because the ulcers occur more often during menstrual PERIODS. Emotional STRESS also tends to trigger them off. Some researchers believe that they are caused by some disorder of the IMMUNE SYSTEM: it is known that this is affected both by stress and hormonal changes in the body. However, this type of ulcer may also be caused by VITAMIN deficiency, ANAEMIA or food ALLERGY.

Rarely, HERPES infections can cause recurrent ulceration in the mouth. This is a much more severe problem than aphthous ulcers. There may be as many as a hundred small painful ulcers, scattered all over the inside of the mouth, including the cheeks, tongue, gums and throat. The ulcers can take up to ten days to heal. Attacks may occur at intervals of three or four months.

The treatment of mouth ulcers depends greatly on the cause. Single mouth ulcers caused by jagged or decayed teeth stop occurring when appropriate dental treatment has been carried out. A single ulcer that persists for more than two weeks should always be investigated by a dentist or doctor. Although the cause may be quite simple, a cancerous ulcer is a possibility; surgery will then be required.

If you suffer from recurrent crops of mouth ulcers, it is also worth consulting your doctor. Although a variety of simple remedies such as anaesthetic gels or mouth washes are available from the chemist, your doctor will usually prescribe local STEROIDS. Either a steroid gel or a tablet containing hydrocortisone will probably be helpful. The gel is rubbed into the ulcers, and the tablet is sucked to provide a high concentration of hydrocortisone in the mouth.

In cases of severe herpes ulceration of the mouth, an anti-viral drug, acyclovir, may be prescribed.

Leg ulcers

Like mouth ulcers, leg ulcers are quite common and have a number of different causes: injury, infection, blood disease such as SICKLE-CELL ANAEMIA, and cancer. The most common cause, however, is disease of the blood vessels in the legs.

Blocked or narrow ARTERIES diminish the blood supply to the tissues, causing the tissues to die and break down and so produce an ulcer. Ulcers of this type tend to occur on the lower leg or foot and have a quite regular 'punched out' appearance. They may be several centimetres wide, quite deep and are very painful indeed.

Defective valves in the VEINS not only cause VARICOSE VEINS but can also bring about ulcers in the legs through the slow circulation of blood. In this case, the tissues break down to form large, shallow ulcers over the inside of the lower leg and ankle. The ulcers are not particularly painful, but may ache considerably.

The immediate treatment for leg ulcers is aimed at keeping the area as free from infection as possible. This includes frequent cleaning, the use of antiseptic ointments or soaks, the application of a sterile foam pad, and bandaging. Painkilling drugs may also be prescribed.

Longer-term treatment of leg ulcers must, however, be directed at the cause of the problem. If ulcers are caused by blocked or narrowed arteries, the arterial disease must be treated. The narrowing in the artery may be dilated with a balloon under X-ray control, or surgery can be undertaken to bypass the blocked artery, using a piece of vein (usually from the leg) or an artificial graft. In the last resort amputation may be necessary.

The commoner 'venous' ulcers are always associated with varicose veins, because the ulcers are caused by sluggish circulation of the blood in the skin around the ankle, which is in turn caused by back pressure from the enlarged veins. The ulcer will improve when this back pressure is relieved.

If there are superficial varicose veins with back pressure in the superficial veins of the leg, then surgery to those veins may improve ulceration. In other cases, bandaging the leg to provide increased pressure at the ankle and calf, or wearing a compression stocking, will promote healing of the ulcer. Elevation of the leg at rest during the day and at night, by raising the foot of the bed, will also help.

Other ulcers

Pressure sores – which are known medically as *decubitus ulcers* – commonly affect elderly, bed-ridden and long-term patients. These are caused by constant pressure impairing the blood circulation through an area of skin and underlying tissue, and commonly occur on the hips, heels and the base of the spine.

These sores are often referred to as 'bed sores' because they occur most commonly in people who are confined to bed, but they may also occur on the buttocks or over the sacrum in elderly people who sit still in hard chairs all day. The prevention of bed sores is essentially a matter of avoiding undue pressure on any one area of the skin for too long. Anybody who is bed-bound and unable to move around in bed must be turned regularly by a nurse or whoever is attending the patient. Sheepskin may be placed under pressure points to reduce the possibility of damage to the skin from hard surfaces. In the case of patients who are unconscious or comatose, special air-mattresses called 'ripple beds' may be used. Air-filled channels run through the mattresses which are automatically slowly inflated and deflated so that no area of the patient's skin is under pressure for more than a short time.

Once a bedsore has formed, professional nursing is essential. Care must be taken to avoid any further pressure to the area, and dressings are applied to encourage healing.

The *rodent ulcer* is a particularly nasty ulcer that occurs on the skin. This is actually a type of skin cancer, starting as a red lump which grows and breaks down to form a circular ulcer. Without treatment, this continues to grow and spread, but surgical removal or RADIATION THERAPY can result in a complete cure.

Ulcers in the groin region can occur for a variety of reasons including sexually acquired herpes or syphilis. Any ulcer in the groin area should be investigated immediately by your doctor as there is a chance that it may be due to syphilis – a very serious disease if left untreated.

Ultrasound

Ultrasound consists of sound waves which vibrate at frequencies beyond the range of human hearing. In medical ultrasonography (or echography), a beam of tiny bursts or pulses of ultrasound is generated by a small probe, which is moved over the surface of the body. What happens to each pulse of ultrasound depends entirely upon the structure and characteristics of the tissues and organs through which it passes – it may be transmitted, reflected or absorbed.

The probe produces 1000 pulses of ultrasound per second, and each pulse is so brief in duration – lasting a mere millionth of a second – that there is a relatively long interval between pulses. During these intervals, the probe picks up any echoes reflected back from the tissues within the body. Analysis of the echo pattern is a complex process which requires a computer, but the final result is usually an image on a kind of TV screen which represents a cross-section or 'slice' through the body along the path of the probe.

One further property of ultrasound is of vital importance: the doses of ultrasound needed to form images are so tiny that there is virtually no possibility of any harmful effect. This is one area where ultrasound 'scores' over X-RAYS.

Having an ultrasound scan

An ultrasound 'scan' is an entirely painless procedure performed by a doctor or technician with special training. After an initial explanation, the patient is asked to undress to expose the region to be examined. He or she then lies down on a couch. A thin layer of oil or gel is applied to the skin to facilitate contact with the probe and improve the quality of the image. The lights are dimmed during the procedure, so that the image on the screen may be viewed to best advantage, and the probe is passed gently to and fro over the area under examination.

There is no special preparation needed for an ultrasound scan, and the person to be scanned does not need to be kept in hospital either before or after the procedure, unless, of course, the scan reveals something that needs treatment.

Different types of ultrasound equipment produce different types of images such as moving pictures, or a sequence of 'still' pictures, both of which can be recorded for further analysis and review.

Ultrasound examinations in PREGNANCY are always performed with the bladder as full as possible, because this lifts the uterus into the most suitable position for a scan and pushes other organs out of the way. In addition, the urine in the bladder transmits ultrasound well, and greatly improves the quality of the image attained.

Ultrasound in pregnancy

Perhaps the most important use of this technique is in pregnancy. Here, ultrasound yields a wealth of information about the foetus at an early stage. The information gained can have a crucial bearing upon the outcome of the pregnancy for mother and foetus; and it may not be readily obtained by any other method of examination.

A pregnancy can be diagnosed by ultrasound about five or six weeks after the last menstrual period. At this stage, the sac holding the embryo can be identified. By the seventh or eighth week, the developing embryo – or more than one, if there is to be a MULTIPLE BIRTH – can be made out on the ultrasound picture.

Blood flowing through the foetal heart reflects ultrasound in a characteristic way, and a portable ultrasound device is often used by obstetricians to pick up the baby's heartbeat. An audible signal is produced by the machine.

Early in pregnancy ultrasound scans may be performed to diagnose the cause of unusual bleeding; this is often caused by a threatened MISCARRIAGE. If the foetal heartbeat can be seen on the scan, it is possible for the pregnancy to survive, and the patient will be rested in bed until the bleeding stops. If, on the other hand, there is no foetal heartbeat present, a miscarriage is inevitable; the obstetrician is likely to carry out a D & C to remove the remains of the pregnancy. Ultrasound scans can also detect other abnormalities in early pregnancy such as an ECTOPIC PREGNANCY, in which the embryo develops in one of the Fallopian tubes.

In a normal pregnancy, however, a routine ultrasound scan is often performed between the 7th and 14th week to assess the size of the foetus. By measuring the length (called the *crown–rump length*) on the scan, the duration of the pregnancy can be estimated with great accuracy. Later on in pregnancy, the diameter of the foetal head is measured with the scan to assess growth. This measurement is referred to as the *bi-parietal diameter* or BPD. (The parietal bones are the bones on each side of the skull.) If there is any concern about whether or not the baby is growing properly, a series of scans can be carried out at intervals right through the pregnancy. A scan is also able to detect certain abnormalities of the foetus itself, such as SPINA BIFIDA.

Apart from identifying a foetus, an ultrasound scan also shows up the size and position of the placenta. This is important if an amniocentesis is to be performed. In this procedure, a needle is inserted through the woman's abdomen into the uterus to draw off some liquid from around the baby for analysis in the laboratory. The technique is used to diagnose spina bifida and to detect GENETIC disorders. However, before it is carried out, an ultrascan is always performed to ensure that the needle will not damage the placenta as it passes through the wall of the uterus.

A scan is also very useful in all cases in which there is abnormal bleeding from the vagina later in pregnancy. Such bleeding may come from separation of the placenta from the wall of the uterus, or from a low-lying placenta which encroaches upon the opening of the uterus. This latter condition is known as a *placenta praevia*. A scan will reveal the cause of the bleeding and then the obstetrician can decide how to treat the patient. In certain cases, an emergency CAESAREAN operation may be needed if the scan shows severe problems with the placenta, which can be dangerous.

Its role in disease

Ultrasound is also used to investigate and diagnose diseases which change either the shape, or the sound-reflecting properties of organs accessible to the ultrasound beam. Air, bone and fat interfere with the ability of ultrasound to form satisfactory images which can be seen on the screen. Organs such as the lungs, the intestines and the brain are unsuitable for examination, but in other areas of the body, ultrasound scans have become routine diagnostic tests.

The heart: Ultrasound pictures and measurements of the HEART have brought about almost as great a revolution in cardiology as those of the foetus in obstetrics. Special types of ultrasound scans called echocardiograms are used which can not only show the structures inside the heart but also reveal the movements of the heart muscle and of the valves in the heart.

Kidneys and bladder: Ultrasound scans can show the size, shape and position of the KIDNEYS and reveal any major abnormality in their internal structure, such as scarring from infections. If there is blockage to the outflow of urine from the kidney, it shows up as a dilation of the collecting tubes within the kidney. Scans are often used as an initial diagnostic test for a wide range of kidney abnormalities, but are also used to detect internal abnormalities in the BLADDER such as small tumours.

Liver and gall bladder: An ultrasound scan of the LIVER may show up cysts or internal growths within the liver. It is now routine to use ultrasound scan to diagnose gallstones (*see* GALL BLADDER), which show up very clearly. This avoids the alternative investigation – a cholecystogram – which involves the patient taking a drug prior to special X-ray tests.

Blood vessels: Some blood vessels are prone to abnormal swellings called *aneurysms,* which occur particularly in the main blood vessels in the chest and abdomen (*see* ARTERIES). An ultrasound scan can easily detect such problems.

Glands: Both the THYROID gland and the PANCREAS may develop cysts which can be diagnosed with an ultrasound scan.

The eye: Specialized ultrasound equipment is available to detect abnormalities deep within the EYE. It is especially useful in cases of eye injury (for example, to locate foreign bodies within the eye) and in cases of retinal detachment.

Gynaecology: Ultrasound scans can be used in the diagnosis of FIBROIDS of the uterus or cysts in the OVARY. Cancers in the ovary may also be detected using scans, and some doctors have suggested that all women of middle age and beyond should have regular ultrasound scans to detect early cancers in the ovary. However, this screening test has not been proved conclusively to be of any really significant value.

Physiotherapy: Powerful ultrasound beams are used to provide 'deep heat', and to promote healing of inflamed tissues, especially around joints.

Unconsciousness

Normal consciousness may be defined as the state in which people are awake, alert and aware of their surroundings. Unconsciousness is a sleep-like state, but much deeper with people having no awareness of their surroundings and showing no response to any stimuli. This condition can vary in severity, ranging from a transient faint to a prolonged coma. Whatever its immediate cause, the condition only arises because of important changes in the BRAIN.

Mechanisms in the brain

Exactly how the brain functions in consciousness and unconsciousness is not yet fully understood. However, there are a number of critical areas in the brain that are deeply involved in maintaining consciousness: the cerebral cortex, the thalamus, the brain-stem and, in particular, a group of cells within the brain-stem called the reticular formation.

The cerebral cortex receives sensory inputs from the main sensory nerves and also from the reticular formation. Nerve routes from around the body branch out to the reticular formation and feed it a constant stream of electrical signals. This action, in turn, causes the reticular formation to fire off signals to targets all around the brain, to the appropriate centres where the signals are gathered, collated and acted upon. If this driving force slows down, or is prevented from occurring, the cerebral cortex becomes 'sleepy', and we become unconscious.

The brain-stem is also important in that it is responsible for keeping our essential body mechanisms – such as heartbeat, BLOOD PRESSURE and BREATHING – running smoothly without our even having to think about it.

It appears that when a person becomes unconscious – for whatever reason – the brain concentrates itself on keeping the body ticking over by using all available energy to keep the brain-stem functioning. Damage is thereby confined to what are regarded as 'non-essential' parts of the brain.

Degrees of unconsciousness

The brain's activity can be measured as electrical impulses on a machine called an ELECTROENCEPHALOGRAPH (EEG). The impulses of the brain are presented as a pattern of electrical waves. This pattern varies considerably according to the degree of alertness or unconsciousness, thus providing a clue to the severity of the unconscious state a person may be in. For instance, during unconsciousness, the pattern of waves is slow and large, about three waves per second. When someone is coming round from unconsciousness – or rousing from sleep – the waves come at about six to eight a second, and increase in frequency until, at full consciousness, the pattern of waves is rapid and jagged, showing increased electrical activity.

The machine is used to determine whether the brain has been severely damaged or even 'died'. If the EEG shows no electrical activity, then the person has almost certainly suffered brain death.

Causes

Unconsciousness can be caused by a variety of factors, ranging from shock to poisoning. The most likely cause that we are likely to come across is *syncope*, known as fainting.

Fainting can be brought on by anything from excessive heat to standing still for long periods, conditions which result in a temporary lack of blood supply to the brain. The resultant lack of oxygen forces the brain to 'shut down' for a brief spell until the oxygen supply is restored to normal levels. If, for some reason, the blood supply to the brain is not fully and quickly restored the person may enter a deeper state of unconsciousness.

Symptoms of fainting include dizziness, light-headedness and a lack of colour in the face. Someone who has fainted should remain lying down for a few minutes until a full recovery has been made. Allowing those who have fainted to get up too soon, or pulling them to their feet, could result in a more serious unconscious state.

Poisoning by fumes, chemicals or drugs can also cause unconsciousness, though by different means. For instance, barbiturates depress the central NERVOUS SYSTEM, in which case the brain-stem may be affected, necessitating emergency measures to ensure the maintenance of the life-support systems. Stimulants will be given to treat this form of poisoning when it has led to unconsciousness.

Carbon monoxide poisoning, however, replaces the oxygen in the blood which leads to an oxygen deficiency at the brain. Immediate treatment consists of removing the person from the source of the gas and artificial respiration.

Shock (*see* p. 782) can bring on unconsciousness through a collapse of the circulatory system. Once the circulatory system fails to maintain an adequate supply of blood to the brain, the collection of symptoms known as 'shock syndrome' becomes apparent. This will include sweating, blurring of vision, shallow, rapid breathing and faintness that can drift into unconsciousness.

Shock like this can be brought on by extensive internal or external bleeding, HEART ATTACKS and loss of body fluid due to various illnesses. In CHOLERA, for example, the body becomes so dehydrated that the sufferer actually dies of shock rather than the bacteria.

Treatment of shock varies according to the cause. Replacing lost fluid and raising the blood pressure are measures taken in hospital, but it is important to try to stop heavy bleeding as soon as possible. When individuals become unconscious, turn them on their side and make sure that they can breathe properly. If breathing stops, resuscitation should be started.

Head injuries (*see* p. 343) are a common cause of unconsciousness and they occur in many sports including rugby and boxing. Unconsciousness may be brought on either through direct injury to brain tissue or through a temporary contraction of blood vessels, which impairs brain function. This condition is known as *concussion*, and varies considerably in the degree of severity. A return to consciousness may be accompanied by a severe headache, nausea and difficulty in focusing the eyes. Loss of memory of what happened immediately prior to the injury also occurs, and is one of the main symptoms of concussion. Anyone who has been knocked out should see the doctor as soon as possible as there could be a chance of skull damage or internal bleeding.

Although a patient will often feel all right after concussion, the effects can last for up to two weeks. He or she may continue to have recurrent bouts of severe headaches and nausea, but these symptoms gradually disappear with time. However, it has been found that reading, bright lights and deep concentration delay recovery and often aggravate the situation.

Even a minor blow can have a serious, delayed effect in that unconsciousness follows some time later. This may often be preceded by vomiting and violent headaches, and indicates that there has been possible brain damage brought on by internal bleeding. Anyone who has had a blow on the head and starts to complain that he is feeling unwell should be taken to a hospital as soon as possible.

If you have had a number of knock-outs, or if you find that you lose consciousness easily, it is important that you are examined by your doctor. It could be that there is some lasting damage from an earlier concussion that may need treatment. Boxers have been known to suffer from their brain cells becoming permanently damaged – a condition known as 'punch-drunk' – but very few of us are likely to be subjected to the same sort of body punishment as boxers.

Epilepsy (*see* p. 282) can also cause unconsciousness and is usually accompanied by convulsions. Quite why the fit takes place is not fully understood, but it is known that it is brought on by an uncontrollable discharge of electricity in the brain.

'Breath-holding' can resemble an epileptic attack, but it usually only occurs in children between one and four years old and during a severe temper or crying fit. Usually they let out a cry before turning blue in the face and passing out; sometimes this is accompanied by small convulsions. Although these attacks can be frightening for parents, they are not serious, and a child will grow out of them. But it is important to inform your family doctor of what is happening, and have the condition properly diagnosed.

Coma

A coma is the most extreme form of unconsciousness, a state that is very serious and often long lasting. Unlike in sleep, the activity of the brain as a whole is depressed, and even reflex actions – such as coughing, corneal reflexes and tendon reflexes – may be absent. In the very deepest coma, the person may not respond even to the most painful stimuli.

The usual causes of coma are injury to the brain (such as bleeding or tumour), severe shock and blood poisoning. Damage to the thalamus may initiate a permanently comatose state.

Both DIABETES and hypoglycaemia are also common causes of a coma, but thankfully can be controlled.

Previously, any kind of coma that lasted for more than 24 hours usually resulted in permanent brain damage, but modern treatment and nursing has done much to change this. However, the longer a coma lasts, the less likelihood there is that a perfect recovery can be made.

In all cases of unconsciousness, treatment depends on the underlying cause, and may range from simple rest and recuperation to surgery. A comatose patient will require long-term and continual care in hospital.

Urethra

This is the duct (tube) which extends from the BLADDER to an opening on the outside of the body. In both sexes, its function is to discharge URINE. In men, the urethra is also the channel through which semen is ejaculated (*see* PENIS).

The male urethra

The mature male urethra averages 8 in (about 20 cm) in length and consists of three sections. The first, or *prostatic* section is about 1 in (2.5 cm) long and passes from the sphincter (valve) at the outlet of the bladder through the middle of the PROSTATE GLAND. The middle part of the urethra is only about ½ in (12 mm) long and is often called the *membranous* urethra. The final – and, at over 6 in (15 cm), the longest – section is called the *spongy or cavernous* urethra. This section is within the penis and opens to the outside at the urethral meatus (the slit in the tip).

The female urethra

In women, the urethra is very much shorter and its only function is to be a channel for the disposal of urine. It is about ½ in (1 cm) in diameter and is also surrounded with mucous glands. The fact that it is so short and opens into a relatively exposed area explains why women frequently get urinary infections.

Structural problems

Structural abnormalities in the female urethra are extremely rare. Occasionally small benign growths called *caruncles* occur at the opening of the urethra and cause some discomfort and soreness. They can easily be removed by a minor surgical operation.

Because the male urethra is longer and has a much more complicated path within the body structure, problems occur more commonly. The development of the urethra within the male foetus may be abnormal. Occasionally small valves form within the upper part of the urethra which cause an obstruction to the flow of the urine from the bladder. Unless they are removed, back pressure from urine accumulating in the bladder can ultimately damage the KIDNEYS.

Another development problem that occurs in boys is the condition of *hypospadias*. This results in the opening, or meatus, of the urethra being on the underside of the penis rather than at the tip. In most cases, there is no difficulty in passing urine. If the opening is near to the tip of the penis, then later there will be no problem in having intercourse or in fathering children. However, if the opening is towards the base of the penis, a small surgical operation can be performed when the child is older to place the meatus in approximately the right position. Occasionally hypospadias is associated with a minor deformity of the glans of the penis, which is abnormally bent downwards. This can also be corrected surgically.

Adult men may have a narrowing, or stricture, of the urethra. Such a narrowing can occur after infection of the urethra, or it may arise as a complication of surgery to it. The effect of the stricture is to reduce the flow of the urine to a trickle, and ultimately it may become almost impossible for the person to pass any urine at all. Treatment involves opening up (dilating) the stricture by passing smooth metal rods called bougies into the urethra and gradually increasing its diameter. This procedure is carried out under general or local anaesthetic and may need to be repeated at regular intervals. If this treatment fails, then an operation is required to remove the strictured part of the urethra.

Injuries to the urethra

A serious injury to the pelvis may result in injury to the urethra. In both men and women, the urethra lies just next to the pubic bone which forms the front of the pelvis. If this bone is fractured, the urethra may be torn or ruptured, which is much more likely to occur in men than in women. Urine can then pass from the urethra into other tissues around the pelvis. Such injury is serious and must be attended to by a specialist urological surgeon immediately. Usually a tube is passed into the bladder from the abdominal wall to divert the flow of urine away from the urethra. An operation to reduce the fracture of the pelvis and to repair the urethra many then be performed.

Urethritis

Inflammation of the urethra, called urethritis, is a common urethral disorder and can have several causes. The commonest are infections acquired as a result of sexual intercourse with an infected partner. NON-SPECIFIC URETHRITIS is the name given to one type of infection which may be caused by organisms such as CHLAMYDIA or ureaplasmas. Women may also get urethritis as a result of contamination from the anus.

Occasionally a urethral discharge in a man is caused by prostatitis – infection in the prostate gland. Although such infection may be acquired sexually, this is not always so. Prostatitis causes inflammation of the prostatic portion of the urethra, which gives rise to a discharge. There is also pain deep inside the pelvis, behind the scrotum.

The urethral syndrome

Many women experience repeated attacks of pain on urinating, which they have to do with increasing frequency. Often such symptoms are caused by CYSTITIS – infection in the bladder – but in as many as half the cases, no infection can be found when urine is examined in the laboratory. If no infection is present, then the symptoms are usually described as the 'urethral syndrome'. The causes remain obscure. Some cases undoubtedly occur as a result of bruising to the urethra during sexual intercourse, particularly if the woman's vagina is not well lubricated. Other cases seem to be associated with STRESS. In these instances, the muscles in the bladder may tighten up, causing discomfort and pain on urinating. Where symptoms persist, careful investigation by a urologist is necessary.

Treatment of urethral disorders

Most urethral disorders are treated by specialists. Urethritis may be investigated and treated by a general practitioner, but more often a specialist in genito-urinary medicine is involved. Usually antibiotics cure the condition, but follow-up treatment for several months may be necessary to ensure a complete cure.

Often, surgeons use special catheters when treating patients who have urethral problems. These catheters are tubes made of flexible rubber which have a small balloon attached around the upper end. The balloon can be inflated via a separate tube running up the side of the central, drainage tube. Once the catheter is inserted into the bladder, the doctor or nurse inflates the balloon to keep it in place. Urine can then flow through the catheter into a collecting bag.

Catheters are used when there is an obstruction to the urethra – for example, because of an enlarged prostate gland – or a stricture. They may also be used temporarily for patients who are unconscious or anaesthetized for long periods. After an operation to the urethra, the vagina or the prostate gland, a catheter may be left in place to act as a splint until the wound has fully healed. Rarely, some patients have to rely permanently on catheters to control the flow of urine. However, surgeons try to avoid this if at all possible because recurrent infections can easily occur if a catheter is left in place for a long time.

Urethritis, *see* **Gonorrhoea, Non-specific urethritis, Reiter's disease, Urethra**

Urine

This fluid, produced by the KIDNEYS, carries waste products out of the body. Disease often affects its composition, colour or volume, and thus it is also a valuable barometer for the detection of ill-health.

Throughout life – even inside the womb – the body is making and excreting urine. The composition is varied to keep the balance of chemicals in the body within very narrow limits. It is a process that we tend to take for granted, but its crucial nature is demonstrated when the mechanism breaks down. If failure is complete and the patient does not get regular treatment, death could result in a few days in some cases.

Why is urine manufactured?

The contents of the fluid inside cells are kept within very strict limits. Certain toxic substances such as urea and acids are constantly being formed, and these must be eliminated to keep their concentrations in the BLOOD acceptably low. Certain other substances such as salt and water must also be kept within strict limits, and this process, called HOMEOSTASIS, is a major function of the kidneys. Clearly a very flexible system is needed – particularly since fluid intake varies from zero to as much as 2½ gal (10 litres) in a single day.

How urine is made

Urine is made in the kidneys, which lie on either side of the spine. About a quarter of the blood leaving the heart passes through the kidneys – an enormous amount if you consider how small they are – and this blood is filtered through a specialized system of blood vessels. This filtrate (filtered liquid) is similar to blood but has had blood cells and larger molecules removed. It contains glucose, urea and salt (sodium). In the kidney, the filtrate passes into tubules where some constituents such as glucose are reabsorbed and others such as urea remain. The reabsorption of constituents such as salt and water is varied by the influence of HORMONES.

The composition of the urine finally excreted varies, depending on what toxic products the body is producing. Virtually everything found in urine is also present in the blood; only the concentrations differ, those in urine being enormously varied so as to keep those in the blood within narrow limits. The foul odour often associated with urine is due to its decomposition by bacteria from the air. The smell of fresh urine is not as disagreeable.

The whole picture is immensely subtle and complex, but the end result is that a fluid is formed within which waste products and variable amounts of other substances such as sodium can be removed from the body. About 250 gal (1200 litres) of blood pass through the kidneys daily, and about 25 gal (110 litres) of filtrate is formed. Nearly all of this is reabsorbed, leaving just 2 pints (1 litre) of urine. This passes continuously from the kidneys via the ureters to the BLADDER, and is the average amount of urine passed per day.

The effects of disease

Disease can alter many of the properties of urine, including its colour, its clearness and its smell. Thus disease can often be suspected from simply looking at the urine. This relationship between urine and disease was recognized a long time ago – for example, it was noticed that some people with extensive BOILS excreted sweet urine that attracted ants. It is likely that these people were suffering from DIABETES and, as a result, were excreting glucose (sugar) in their urine. Diabetes patients are also prone to many kinds of infection and this would explain the high incidence of boils.

The colour of urine is due mainly to substances produced by the metabolism of BILE. The amount of water excreted with this varies the colour accordingly, pale urine being very dilute and dark brown urine being concentrated. However, other substances can affect the colour. Many people have experienced momentary alarm when they have passed red urine after eating beetroot. Other foods have a similar effect. Certain drugs can colour urine, and it can be turned red by blood and in a rare disease called porphyria.

Probably the most common cause of colour change, however, is JAUNDICE. Certain types of jaundice cause increased secretion of the pigments which normally colour urine and therefore turn it a dark brown. The same pigment colours the FAECES (stools), and if the bile duct is obstructed the pigment cannot enter the bowel and the faeces become pale. The combination of pale faeces and dark urine is thus an important indication of jaundice.

The volume of urine passed in a day may also indicate disease. The rate of urine formation in a healthy adult can vary enormously – from an egg-cupful to 2 pints (1 litre) in one hour – depending on how much he or she has drunk.

Similarly, large amounts of fluid can be lost in sweat (PERSPIRATION) on a hot, humid day (or if the person has a fever), in VOMITING or in DIARRHOEA. So the excretion of small amounts of urine under these circumstances has a different significance than if it were excreted by an apparently healthy person.

It should be noted that measuring the volume of urine passed by somebody with diarrhoea or fever is a simple but important method of determining whether he or she is receiving enough fluid.

One of the manifestations of the disease *diabetes mellitus* – usually referred to simply as diabetes – is the excretion of large volumes of fluid by the patient. In this disease, the high level of glucose in the blood exceeds the capacity of the kidney to reabsorb it. The filtrate retains water and large amounts of urine are therefore excreted – this process is called *polyuria.* High levels of CALCIUM in the blood can have a similar effect. In another disease, the mechanisms in the tubules of the kidney for reabsorbing water are impaired and again large amounts of water are passed. This is called *diabetes insipidus,* which is completely different from diabetes mellitus.

On the other hand, conditions that cause a decreased excretion of urine are much rarer, but may occur in cases of kidney failure. Another common change that can be seen in urine is in its translucency. Usually urine is clear, but it can become slightly opaque, or cloudy. This does not necessarily indicate disease, but in some cases, cloudiness can be caused by infections of the bladder such as CYSTITIS because cells and bacteria are being excreted. Similarly, blood, even in tiny quantities, can make urine look smoky.

Urine tests

The commonest series of tests performed on urine are those which use specially impregnated strips that are dipped into the urine. These tests are used to detect blood, sugar and protein. The chemical reaction that takes place differs depending on the substance that is being tested for, but all involve a colour change in the strip if the substance is present. These tests are simple, but important: every patient who goes into hospital has his or her urine routinely 'screened'. Often an abnormality associated with a known illness is found; but more important are those cases of unsuspected disease – for example, glucose in the urine of an unrecognized diabetic or blood in that of a person with bladder or kidney cancer.

Microscopy is the basis for other tests. Any urine, if it is left standing, will develop a sediment, which can be examined. Distinguishing the various elements from each other requires a great deal of experience and may show, for example, whether blood detected in the urine is due to kidney disease or a disease lower down the urinary tract.

The detection of infections in the bladder and cystitis forms a major part of the work in any microbiology laboratory. The infecting bacteria are grown from the patient's urine on artificial media so that they can be identified and tested. The specimen used is called a 'mid-stream urine' or MSU. Essentially this involves ignoring the first part of the urine stream and collecting what comes after it. This is because the section of the urethra nearest the skin is normally contaminated with bacteria which are washed away by the first part of the stream. Otherwise the bacteria might contaminate the urine specimen and lead to a false result.

A standard measured amount of MSU is placed on growth media and incubated at body temperature; a preliminary identification of the infecting organism may be ready in as little as 24 hours.

Testing urine for PREGNANCY is common. The test is based on the detection of a HORMONE which is secreted by the developing foetus and placenta and is almost always specific to pregnancy, although other, very rare conditions can produce it. A variety of tests are available, including tests that can be carried out at home. They are all based on the reaction of the hormone with a particular antibody in the urine. The test becomes positive from about the sixth week of pregnancy.

Urticaria, *see* Allergy

Uterus

In the past, the uterus has been blamed for almost every mental and physical ailment from which women have suffered. Nowadays, we have a more rational, although still incomplete, understanding of this vital organ.

Function

The uterus is composed of two main parts – the *corpus* or body of the organ, and its CERVIX or neck – and it is capable of undergoing major changes during a woman's reproductive life. From puberty to the MENOPAUSE the lining of the womb (*endometrium*) develops each month to provide nutrition for a fertilized egg. If the egg is not fertilized, the endometrium is shed during menstruation (*see* PERIODS), and is slowly replaced in the course of the next menstrual cycle.

During PREGNANCY, the uterus expands to allow the foetus to grow, and provides it with protection and nutrition. At the same time, the large muscle fibres are prevented from contracting.

The uterus suddenly changes its role when the foetus is mature. It begins to contract in order to open the cervix and allow the baby and placenta to pass through (*see* CHILDBIRTH). The uterus then contracts tightly to close off the large blood vessels which have been supplying the placenta. After the birth, it rapidly returns to its pre-pregnant state, ready to accept another fertilized egg.

All these changes in the functioning of the uterus are orchestrated by HORMONES released from the PITUITARY gland and from the OVARIES, and by similar substances called prostaglandins which are released by the uterine tissue. The way in which these substances interact is still not fully understood.

Position

In an adult woman, the uterus is a hollow organ approximately the size and shape of a small pear, and lies inside the girdle of pelvic bones. The narrow end of the pear is equivalent to the cervix which protrudes into the vagina – the remainder forms the body of the uterus. This is connected to the two Fallopian tubes which carry the monthly egg from one or other of the ovaries. In this way, the uterus forms part of a channel between the abdominal cavity and the outside world.

Special mechanisms exist to prevent the spread of infection via this route into the abdominal cavity. The lining of the uterus is shed when a woman menstruates, the cervix secretes antibodies and the acidity of the vagina inhibits the growth of BACTERIA.

The front of the uterus sits on the BLADDER and the back lies near the RECTUM. The uterus is normally supported inside the PELVIS by muscles – called the *pelvic floor muscles* – and by bands of connective tissue and blood vessels from the side wall of the pelvis, which are attached to the cervix.

During pregnancy, the uterus enlarges so that, by the 12th week, it can just be felt inside the abdominal cavity above the pubic bone. At about 38 weeks it usually reaches the lower edge of the rib cage, but about two weeks after the baby is born, it can normally no longer be felt in the abdomen. After the menopause, the uterus shrinks in size.

The variations in size are controlled by the secretions of sex hormones, which also govern the nature of the glandular tissue lining the uterus – the endometrium. During the first half of a woman's menstrual cycle, the endometrium increases in thickness until the egg is released. It then stops growing but begins to secrete substances rich in nutrition to allow further growth of the egg if it is fertilized. If the egg is not fertilized, the endometrium is shed during menstruation.

Congenital variations

During the development of the female reproductive organs in the foetus, two tubes of tissue – called *Mullerian ducts* – grow from the side walls of the abdominal cavity and meet centrally. These tubes continue to grow downwards until they fuse with tissue which will later form the lower vagina. The upper portions of the tubes become the Fallopian tubes and the lower central portions fuse to form the uterus and upper vagina.

Very rarely, both the Mullerian ducts fail to form, with the result that the adult woman will have a short vagina but no uterus or Fallopian tubes. Nothing can be done to cure this condition, although sometimes plastic surgery is performed to lengthen the vagina. Such women are infertile and do not menstruate.

If only one of the Mullerian ducts develops, the woman will have a uterus and vagina but only one Fallopian tube. This does not cause any major problems.

Another rare occurrence during foetal development is incomplete fusion of the Mullerian ducts. This may result in any abnormality from a double uterus to a small dimple at the top of the uterus. Women with this problem seldom have difficulty in becoming pregnant, but they are slightly more likely to have miscarriages or go into premature labour. If such abnormalities create

Problems of the uterus

Part of the uterus affected	Name of condition	Possible symptoms	Treatment
Entire uterus	Absent uterus	No periods, infertile	None
	Congenital malformation (double uterus or abnormal division in the uterus cavity)	Often no symptoms (when pregnant, a woman may go into premature labour)	Very rarely it may be necessary to do plastic surgery to make the uterus a normal shape
	PROLAPSE of the uterus	No symptoms, or the sensation of 'a lump coming down into the vagina'	Special pelvic floor exercises, avoidance of constipation, weight loss if necessary. Sometimes surgery
Endometrium (lining of the cavity of the uterus)	Endometrial POLYPS	Bleeding from the vagina between periods or after the menopause	Dilatation and curettage (D & C)
	Endometrial hyperplasia (over-growth of the lining of the uterus)	Heavy irregular periods usually as a woman approaches the menopause	Diagnosis by D & C followed by a course of hormone tablets
	Endometritis (inflammation of the lining of the uterus)	Lower abdominal pain and heavy periods	Diagnosis by D & C followed by a course of antibiotics
	Endometrial carcinoma	Bleeding from the vagina after the menopause or between periods	HYSTERECTOMY and possible RADIOTHERAPY and/or hormones
	Trophoblastic disease (formation of placenta in the uterus with no foetus present)	A 'feeling' of pregnancy and irregular bleeding from the vagina	D & C, avoidance of pregnancy until the condition is cured, drugs if the placental tissue spreads outside the uterus

	Dysfunctional (abnormal) uterine bleeding	Heavy and/or frequent periods with no obvious physical abnormality of the uterus	Diagnosis by D & C, hormone treatment followed by hysterectomy if hormones unsuccessful
Myometrium (muscular wall of the uterus)	FIBROIDS	Often no symptoms – possibly heavy periods and enlarged uterus	If they cause a problem, fibroids may be surgically removed (myomectomy) or a hysterectomy may be performed
	SARCOMA (cancerous form of fibroid)	Often no symptoms – sometimes the uterus becomes enlarged	Hysterectomy and radiotherapy
	Adenomyosis (endometrial tissue deposited inside the muscular layers of the uterus)	Painful heavy periods	May be treated by hormonal therapy but only diagnosed by hysterectomy
CERVIX	Polyp	Often no symptoms – sometimes vaginal bleeding after sexual intercourse or between periods	D & C, and removal of polyp
	Erosion or ectropion (cells which normally line the cervix begin to grow on the outside)	Often no symptoms – sometimes a watery discharge	No treatment needed, but the area may be burnt (cautery) so that new cells form
	Cervical dysplasia (abnormal cells which may revert to normal or turn into cancer)	Abnormal cervical smear	Repeated cervical smears, and occasionally removal of the area of abnormal cells
	Cancer of the cervix	Bleeding from the vagina after sexual intercourse and between periods	Radiotherapy and sometimes hysterectomy

difficulties for the woman in carrying a pregnancy to term, plastic surgery can be done to re-form the uterus into a single cavity.

Problems with the uterus

Considering the complex mechanism that governs the normal functioning of the uterus, it is remarkable how few women have any problems.

Obviously, several different conditions can give rise to the same symptoms. For example, bleeding from the vagina between periods or after intercourse is often due to a minor condition such as a POLYP which can be easily cured. However, these symptoms may, very rarely, be caused by uterine CANCER. This can be completely cured if it is detected early enough, so it is very important for all women to have regular smear tests and for any woman who has these symptoms to seek her doctor's advice.

A *retroverted* uterus is one which tilts backwards from its attachment at the top of the vagina instead of forwards (an *anteverted* uterus). This is quite normal and occurs in about 20 per cent of women with no ill effect. Rarely, however, a disease process such as *endometriosis* or SALPINGITIS will cause a normally anteverted uterus to become stuck backwards, or retroverted. These diseases can cause a decrease in a woman's fertility and, as they are associated with a retroverted uterus, it is sometimes said that retroversion of the uterus causes infertility. A problem like endometriosis can be treated by surgery or hormone therapy – this does not always cure the retroversion but will improve the woman's chances of conceiving.

Treatment

It is difficult to diagnose problems that are due to an abnormality of the uterine cavity as this area cannot be examined directly. Therefore a woman may need to have a D & C (dilatation and curettage, when the lining of the uterus is scraped away) just to diagnose the cause of a menstrual problem or vaginal bleeding after the menopause. Once the correct diagnosis has been made, the doctor can then recommend appropriate treatment – for example, taking HORMONE REPLACEMENT THERAPY to regulate the menstrual cycle.

Unfortunately, doctors are not always able to control abnormal menstrual symptoms in this way. In such cases, both the patient and doctor may feel that the only way to cure the symptoms is by a HYSTERECTOMY. This will stop a woman having any more periods, and will also make her infertile, but should not otherwise alter her life. However, as modern medical therapies improve, this operation is being performed less frequently.

Uvula, *see* Cleft palate and hare lip

V

Vaccination, *see* **Immunization**

Vagina

This is the channel which leads from the vulva (external genitals) to the UTERUS. During a woman's life, the vagina undergoes several changes. The vagina of a child is obviously smaller than that of a mature woman. The lining of its wall is thinner in a child or post-menopausal woman than that of a woman during her reproductive years. These changes are largely influenced by a group of hormones released by the ovary: these are called *oestrogens.*

The vagina plays an important role during intercourse (*see* SEX AND SEXUAL INTERCOURSE) and CHILDBIRTH. The role during childbirth is relatively passive when the vagina forms the lower portion of the birth canal and is capable of opening sufficiently to allow the birth of the baby. We have only relatively recently begun to understand some of the changes which occur in the vagina during intercourse.

Structure

The vagina is a canal 2¾–3½ in (7–9 cm) long, surrounded by fibrous and muscular tissue, but lined with a layer of cells called *squamous epithelium.* The walls of the canal are normally collapsed on to one another and thrown into many folds. These properties make it easy for the vagina to be distended during intercourse or childbirth. The URETHRA lies on the front wall of the vagina and the RECTUM lies on the upper third of the back of the vagina. The anus is separated from the vagina by a fibro-muscular tissue called the *perineal body,* or *perineum.* The ducts from the two *Bartholin's glands* enter on either side of the outer end of the vagina, while the CERVIX protrudes into the top of the vagina.

During the reproductive years of a woman's life, the vaginal secretions are slightly acidic. This tends to inhibit the growth of harmful BACTERIA in the vagina, but during the pre-pubertal and post-menopausal years, the vagina becomes mildly alkaline. Under these circumstances, the bacteria can thrive and occasionally make the vagina rather sore.

The walls of the vagina are well lubricated with secretions from the cervical canal and Bartholin's glands. During intercourse, secretions also seep through the vaginal epithelium into the vaginal canal. A certain amount of discharge from the vagina is normal in all women (*see* LEUCORRHOEA). The amount increases during ovulation and sexual arousal.

The structure of the vagina

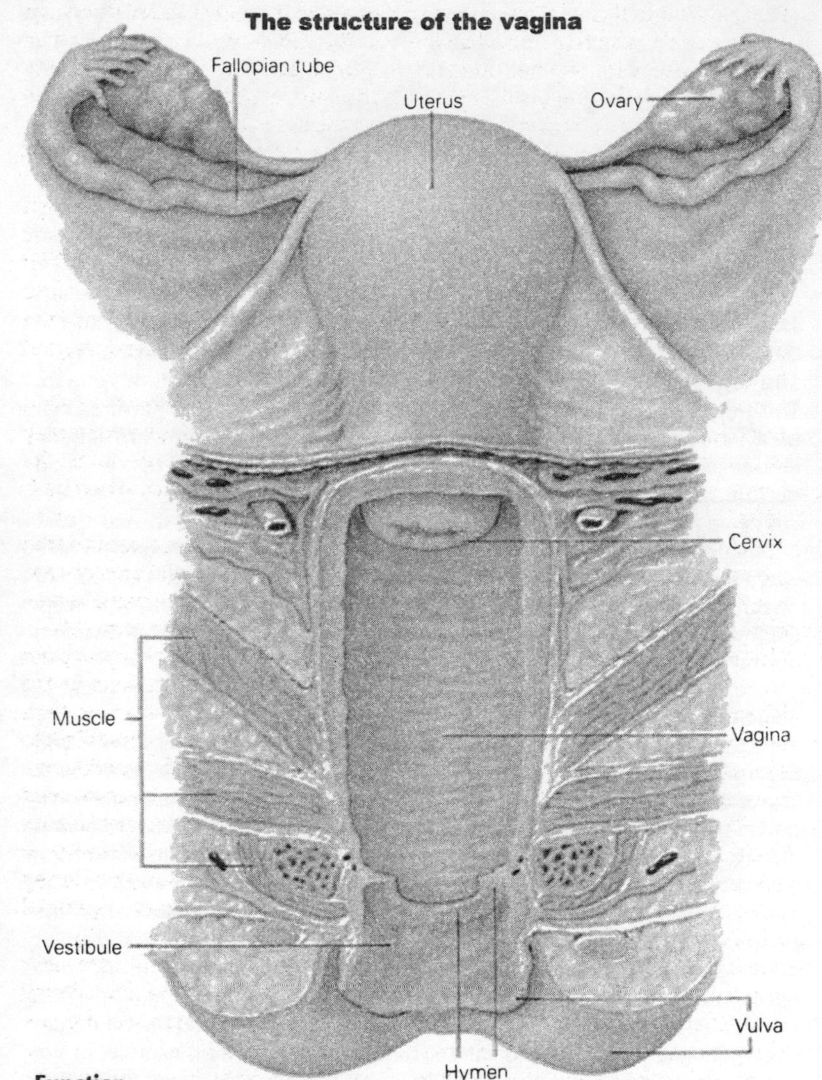

Function

During sexual arousal, the genital organs, especially the *labia minora* and lower vagina, become engorged with blood and the amount of vaginal secretion increases. During an orgasm, the muscles of the pelvis, including those surrounding the vagina, contract involuntarily.

If a woman is particularly tense during intercourse, the muscles surrounding the vagina will go into spasm. This condition, called *vaginismus*, makes the vagina narrower and makes sex painful. It can be cured by help from a psycho-sexual counsellor.

Disorders

Probably one of the most common problems is an irritating vaginal discharge called THRUSH, which is caused by the *Candida albicans* FUNGUS. This can be easily treated with vaginal pessaries. Unfortunately it is easy to become reinfected with this fungus. It is possible to guard against this by treating the woman's partner at the same time and warning her to be particularly careful about washing her towels and pants out thoroughly as the spores of this fungus can lodge in these articles.

There are several other infections which might also result in a vaginal discharge. During the past few years, doctors have discovered that many cases of vaginal soreness and discharge are caused by an organism called *Gardnerella vaginalis.* This bacterium was previously unsuspected as a cause of such problems. The condition can, however, be treated with tablets of the antibiotic metronidazole. *Trichomonas vaginalis* is another cause of vaginal discharge and irritation (*see* TRICHOMONIASIS).

GONORRHOEA seldom causes any abnormal symptoms in women unless it spreads to infect the Fallopian tubes, when it causes severe pain. SYPHILIS may also mature undetected as it initially causes small painless ulcers on the female genitalia. Most women learn they have these infections when their partners are diagnosed.

Although many SEXUALLY TRANSMITTED DISEASES produce little discharge from the vagina, it is important that any woman who has a discharge consults her doctor. She should be particularly careful to tell him or her if she has had a recent change in partner, because a sexually transmitted disease is then more likely. The only way that a doctor can reliably check for such a disease is to carry out an internal examination and take a number of swabs for analysis in the laboratory. Appropriate treatment can then be given. Any woman who feels embarrassed about seeing her own doctor for such problems can go straight to a hospital clinic for genito-urinary medicine, and be seen in strict confidence.

Soreness or discomfort in the vagina during intercourse may be associated with infection either in the vagina or in the uterus. Deep discomfort is more likely to be associated with uterine infection; a medical opinion would be advisable. Often, however, discomfort at the entrance to the vagina during intercourse is simply a result of tension, or lack of lubrication. Artificial lubrication (such as KY jelly) would help.

If a woman's partner uses condoms, and her vagina feels sore after intercourse and she later has extra discharge, this may be caused by allergy to the latex rubber which is used for manufacturing condoms. Special hypo-allergenic condoms, available from chemists, should be tried.

PROLAPSE of the vaginal wall tends to occur when women have experienced long or difficult labours during childbirth. This causes weakness of the supporting structures around the vagina, so that the vaginal walls collapse downwards, and are experienced by a woman as a lump coming down into the entrance of the vagina. There may be associated dragging pains and possibly INCONTINENCE of urine during laughing or coughing. A small operation can be undertaken to repair the prolapse. Alternatively, the patient may be fitted with a pessary which will keep the vaginal wall in place.

Another common problem is atrophic vaginitis, which affects women in their mid-60s, and tends to make the vagina sore and uncomfortable. This occurs because these women no longer have high enough levels of oestrogen in their circulation to stimulate the growth of the vaginal epithelium. The vagina then loses its acidity which favours the growth of the bacteria. The condition can be easily treated with oestrogen creams or a slightly acidic jelly which is inserted into the vagina.

Some women who use vaginal deodorants can develop a reaction to them, which tends to cause a heavier and more unpleasant vaginal discharge than normal. If a woman suffers from an unpleasant, foul-smelling vaginal discharge, she should consult her doctor, rather than using a deodorant.

Vaginismus, *see* **Sex and sexual intercourse, Vagina**

Vagotomy, *see* **Autonomic nervous system**

Valves, heart

The HEART is a muscular pump divided in two halves, whose function it is to maintain the CIRCULATION of BLOOD. Like so many pumps, it depends on a series of valves to work properly. On the right-hand side are the *pulmonary* and *tricuspid valves*; on the left-hand side are the *aortic* and *mitral valves*. The four valves open and close automatically to receive and discharge blood from and to the chambers, so that it can flow in only one direction.

The pulmonary and aortic valves are similar in structure. They have three leaf-like cusps, or leaflets, and are made of tough but thin fibrous tissue. The mitral and tricuspid valves are more complicated, though they, too, are similar in structure. The mitral valve has only two leaflets, whereas the tricuspid valve has three.

Each of these valves sits in a ring between the atrium and the ventricle. The bases of the leaflets are attached to the ring, while the free edges touch each other and close the passage between the ventricle and atrium when the valve is closed. These free edges are also attached to a series of fine strings – called the *chordae tendineae* – which pass down into the ventricle and stop the valve from springing back into the atrium when under pressure.

Problems

Only two things can go wrong with a valve. It can either become blocked so that blood can't pass through (*stenosis*), or it can allow blood to leak backwards in the opposite direction to the normal circulation (*incompetence* or *regurgitation*).

In the past, RHEUMATIC FEVER was the important cause of valve disease, with other causes being rather rare. In the case of rheumatic fever, the inflammation almost exclusively affected the valves on the left side (aortic and mitral), and could subsequently lead to stenosis or incompetence.

Today congenital abnormalities are probably the commonest forms of valve disease. Stenosis or incompetence can occur as a result of minor abnormalities of structure of any of the valves; however, the aortic and pulmonary valves are most likely to be affected. Problems may not come to light until late in life when the wear and tear starts to put strain on the valve. An abnormal valve may thicken and get deposits of calcium in it over the years, causing a reduction in efficiency. Abnormal valves also appear to be at risk of picking up germs from the bloodstream, which grow on the valve and start to destroy its substance. This gives rise to a disease called *infective endocarditis*, which can be very serious. This is why anyone who has valve disease should receive an antibiotic before dental treatment, which can release showers of bacteria into the bloodstream.

As well as isolated involvement of a single valve, there may be congenital problems that affect many parts of the heart and give rise to problems, sometimes as early as immediately after birth. One of the commonest is called *Fallot's tetralogy* (see BLUE BABY): this involves an obstruction to the pulmonary valve, together with a hole between the two ventricles (*ventricular septal defect*).

Another abnormality that can cause minor problems is *mitral valve prolapse*. This happens because there is some slack in the valve and its chordae tendineae, which allows it to balloon back into the atrium, resulting in a leakage of blood. The condition is extremely common, affecting 5 per cent of women and 0.5 to 1 per cent of men.

Valves that were normal at birth can also become stenosed as part of the ageing process, especially the aortic valve. The mitral valve is at risk following certain types of heart attack when the chordae tendinae rupture, causing mitral regurgitation.

Symptoms of valve disease

There are relatively few ways in which valve problems come to light. Murmurs are usually picked up by a doctor using a stethoscope. Aortic and mitral problems may cause a build-up of fluid in the lungs due to increased pressure, which results from an obstruction or leaking. This leads to breathlessness. Excessive thickening of the muscular wall of the heart, as a result of the extra strain that a blocked or leaky valve puts on it, may lead to heart pain (*angina*; *see* CORONARY HEART DISEASE). Finally, the heart's rhythm may be disturbed (*arhythmia*) as the orderly contraction of muscle breaks down. This may cause blackouts in aortic stenosis.

Investigation and treatment

Often the symptoms of minor valve problems can be controlled by tablets, but in some cases, an operation may be needed. To decide if this necessary, a cardiologist will make a number of tests, including an ordinary chest X-ray and an ELECTROCARDIOGRAM (ECG); these give a good idea of the level of strain that the heart is under. An echocardiogram, which uses ULTRASOUND to look at the heart, may be performed to build up a picture of the valves. Finally, a cardiac catheterization may be done; this will measure the pressure in the various chambers of the heart by inserting a narrow tube up a vein into the heart itself. Appropriate surgery can then be performed.

Varicella, *see* **Chickenpox**

Varicocoele, *see* **Infertility, Testes**

Varicose veins

VEINS are said to be 'varicose' when they become tortuous, thin-walled and widened and easily visible below the skin. The veins in the superficial (surface) tissues of the legs are the ones most commonly affected.

There is usually no clear-cut cause for varicose veins of the legs, but there are many factors which may lead to a worsening of varicose veins which are already present. Varicose veins do run in families, but there is no obvious reason for this. They are also much more common in women than in men.

The veins

Normally, the blood which supplies the tissues of the lower limbs flows down the ARTERIES to the feet and then back up the veins, and so to the HEART. In the lower limbs, there are two systems of veins: deep, and superficial.

The superficial system consists of veins in the tissues between the muscle and the skin. Both the superficial and deep veins contain valves every few centimetres. These consist of tiny folds of the lining of the vein, and they allow blood to flow up the limb, but not the other way.

In patients with varicose veins, these valves are found to be defective. It is not clear whether the defective valves cause the varicose veins, or whether it is the other way round. However, the final effect of having defective valves is that the blood in the vein can flow *down* the vein, leading to stretching of its wall. The superficial veins of the lower limb are divided into two main veins, the *long saphenous* and the *short saphenous*. The long saphenous vein carries blood from the front of the foot, up the inner side of the leg and goes deeply into the thigh just below the groin. The short saphenous vein carries blood from the outer side of the foot up to the back of the knee, where it also goes deeply to join the deep system of veins. The long saphenous vein and its many branches are the commonest sites of varicose veins.

Aggravating factors

Although there are no obvious causes of varicose veins, there are a number of factors that increase their possibility.

Constipation: In countries where a high-fibre diet is usual, varicose veins are almost unknown. It is therefore thought that anyone who regularly has to force out a hard constipated bowel motion may damage the valves in the leg veins as the pressure inside them increases considerably during such straining. Ultimately this may lead to distension of the veins and varicosities. *See* CONSTIPATION.

Pregnancy: Many women notice varicose veins after PREGNANCY. It is probable that the veins were abnormal before, but pregnancy made them worse. There are two theoretical reasons why this should happen. First, the presence of an enlarged uterus leads to pressure on the veins in the pelvis, causing increased pressure in those of the leg. This pressure may cause the veins to become swollen. Second, hormones which are produced during pregnancy lead to a general softening of supporting tissues to allow the baby's head to pass through the birth canal; the supporting tissues of the veins may also be similarly affected.

Obesity: Varicose veins can be brought on through obesity because of increased pressure inside the abdomen, together with general weakening of fibrous tissue in the wall of the vein.

Prolonged standing: Jobs which require prolonged standing may put an undue strain on the veins of the legs.

Injury: Sometimes, a large varicose vein develops at the site of an injury, such as where a cricket ball hits the leg. This may be the only varicose vein in an otherwise normal leg.

Deep-vein thrombosis: Occasionally, patients who have had a deep-vein THROMBOSIS may develop varicose veins in the lower leg, but these are usually of a different pattern compared with the more common varicose veins which start in the superficial veins.

Effects of varicose veins

Varicose veins do not look pleasant, and by far the commonest reason for people to seek medical help for their varicose veins is because of this. But varicose veins can cause complications, and these may necessitate surgical or other treatment.

Because these veins are thin-walled and near the surface, they are more susceptible to injury. This, coupled with the fact that the blood flow is much more sluggish in varicose veins, can lead to a THROMBOSIS (clot) in the vein. The resulting inflammation around the thrombosis – known as PHLEBITIS – causes pain and redness in the affected area.

Some patients with varicose veins develop quite bad ECZEMA on the lower leg because the presence of varicose veins reduces the flow of blood through the SKIN capillaries. This eczema can be treated with skin preparations, but if the varicose veins are treated, the eczema usually disappears.

Treatment

Several different forms of treatment are available.

Support hosiery: Mild varicose veins, such as those that develop during pregnancy, can often be controlled by wearing support tights or stockings. This can relieve the ache and may improve the appearance by flattening the veins.

Injections: A special substance is injected into different parts of the vein causing the lining of the vein to become inflamed. The leg is then tightly bandaged – and remains so for about a month – so that the vein is compressed. The object of the treatment is to get the opposite walls of the vein to stick together permanently, thus effectively closing it.

The main disadvantage of this form of treatment is that it is only effective on small varicose veins, and only if they are situated below the knee (it is virtually impossible to get a bandage to stay on the thigh for more than a few hours).

Surgery: The aim of surgery is principally to prevent back pressure occurring in the superficial veins of the leg so that the veins do not become so distended that they become varicose. Often the abnormal veins are removed, but unless all the veins feeding blood into the skin of the leg are removed or tied off, there is a risk that varicose veins could recur.

The surgeon therefore has to plan the operation very carefully. He or she first tests the flow of blood through the veins in the leg by lifting up the leg to empty all the veins of blood and then lowering it again, carefully observing how the blood flows back into the veins. 'Perforating' veins from deep tissues may be present which allow blood to flow into the varicose veins, and each of these can be identified by the surgeon.

When the operation is performed, the top of the varicose vein is tied off, as are any perforating veins. The abnormal vein can then be removed by stripping: after incisions are made in both the groin area and at the knee, a wire stripper is passed up the abnormal vein from knee to groin; this is then pulled out at the groin, taking the vein with it. Smaller veins may be removed simply by making an incision over the vein and taking it out a piece at a time.

After an operation for varicose veins, the patient is encouraged to get up and walk as soon as possible to re-establish blood flow in the normal veins of the leg. The hospital stay is unlikely to be more than a few days.

Vasectomy

This is a permanent form of sterilization or birth control (*see* CONTRACEPTION) for males. It is equivalent to the operation in a woman in which the Fallopian tubes, along which eggs pass from the OVARY to the uterus, are either cut, tied, clipped or sealed, so that she cannot become pregnant (*see* STERILIZATION, FEMALE). Both operations are intended to result in a permanent inability to have children.

How it works

SPERM are manufactured from cells that make up the walls of small tubes (*seminiferous tubules*) which form each TESTIS. When sperm have matured, they collect in larger tubes, the *vasa efferentia*. These join together and pass out of the testis as the *epididymis*, a long coiled tube almost wrapped around the outside of the testis. When the epididymis leaves the area of the testis, it becomes a long thin channel – the *vas deferens*. This is grouped together with the arteries, veins and lymphatics that supply the testis. Together they form a thick cord called the *spermatic cord*.

From the scrotum in which the testes lie, the two spermatic cords pass up into the lower part of the abdomen and loop over the lower end of each *ureter* (the tube carrying urine from the kidney to the bladder), before joining the URETHRA (the tube that takes urine away from the bladder) where it runs through the PROSTATE GLAND. Then during ejaculation, the sperm, now in a fluid called semen, are pushed forcefully down the urethra and out at the tip of the PENIS – and, during SEXUAL INTERCOURSE, deep into the vagina.

Sterilization in a male consists of removing a section of the *vas deferens*, which gives this method the name *vasectomy*. It works on the basis that, if a piece of the vas deferens is missing, it will be quite impossible for sperm to pass along it from the testes, to be released and bring about fertilization.

Pros and cons of vasectomy

Men who consider vasectomy are often in their late 30s and 40s or already have children, feel that their families are complete and prefer this method of birth control to any other.

Vasectomy has the great advantage of being absolutely reliable and permanent. However, its permanency is also, under certain circumstances, a disadvantage – a reversal of the surgical procedure is at the very least difficult and expensive and, in many cases, impossible.

The decision to have or not have a vasectomy is not one that men have to make entirely on their own, although it is, in the end, their decision and one for which they must take full responsibility. It is important that the decision is taken jointly by both partners. Although it is the man who will have the vasectomy, it will inevitably have some effect on the relationship. Therefore, before planning the operation a man should discuss the pros and cons with his partner and family doctor.

The operation

The operation is quite straightforward and minor. It does not require hospitalization but can be done in the doctor's surgery, a family planning clinic or the out-patient department of a hospital.

The vasectomy is done under local anaesthetic; two or three small injections are given into the site of the operation to deaden the area. The section of the vas deferens chosen for removal is that part which is most easily accessible and lies at the neck of the scrotum, just below where it joins the rest of the body. A small vertical cut is made through the anaesthetized skin and the vas deferens identified. It is then cut in two places 1 inch (2.5 cm) apart and the intervening section is removed. The ends are usually folded back on themselves before being securely tied with a material, such as silk, which will not dissolve or disintegrate. The wound is closed with a few stitches and the procedure is repeated on the other side. The whole operation takes only half an hour or less.

After surgery

The wound usually heals in a few days, after which the stitches are removed. There may be some soreness when the anaesthetic wears off, but this is normal. In a few patients, there may be some bleeding into the wound – *scrotal haematoma* – and this can cause pain, swelling and discoloration for a few days. Intercourse is likely to be painful for a day or two, and most men avoid it until the stitches are removed.

The main thing to understand about a vasectomy is that there is a time lag between the operation and the time when the patient is, in fact, infertile. Sperm have already passed up the vas deferens and 'escaped' before the vasectomy has been done. These sperm can remain capable of fertilization for several months after the operation. Usually, it is reckoned that, by the time three months have elapsed, they should all have been used up, but there are cases where pregnancy has occurred six months later. The exact time cannot be predicted, but is related to the number of times that the man ejaculates after the operation. If he has frequent sexual intercourse, then he will 'use up' the remaining sperm more quickly. To guard against unwanted pregnancy during this time, other forms of contraception, such as a condom, should be used. It is customary to examine two specimens of semen at eight and 12 weeks after the operation, and if these contain no sperm, it is considered safe to carry on with unprotected intercourse.

If seminal analysis after six months still shows the presence of live sperm in the man's ejaculate, the operation has not been successful and a re-operation may be necessary. Very rarely the two ends of the severed *vas deferens* manage to join up again – but this occurs in less than 0.5 per cent of cases. Where it does, it is usually within a few months of the operation. It has also been known for the *vas deferens* to join up again after a year or two, resulting in a return of fertility, but this is extremely rare.

Effects of vasectomy

It is important to realize that the operation of vasectomy is simply an interruption to the flow of sperm into the part where the semen is collected. Even though millions of sperm are released during normal intercourse, they are so small that their total volume will not make any appreciable difference to the volume of the semen. The other function of the testes – producing male hormones which are released directly into the bloodstream – is not affected in any way by a vasectomy, nor is a man's sexual drive or ability.

There is some evidence that tying off the *vas deferens* on each side can lead to the formation of antibodies against the patient's own sperm. This occurs in very few patients, and is of no relevance unless the patient wishes to have a reversal of his vasectomy.

Reversing the operation

Vasectomies have been successfully reversed, but this is a difficult procedure with no guarantee of success in the end. The operation – called *reanastomosis* – involves finding the cut ends of the *vas deferens* (usually only on one side) and meticulously sewing the various layers together again. Even if this is done, the internal tube may not remain open, and if it is open, sperm antibodies can prevent the development of satisfactory sperm. At present, the pregnancy rate in the partners of men who have had vasectomies reversed is no more than 60 per cent.

Veins

Veins are similar to ARTERIES in that they are similarly distributed – the arteries and veins associated with a particular organ or tissue often run together. However, there are major differences. For example, many veins have valves in them which the arteries do not, and the walls of an artery are always thicker than those of a vein of corresponding size, while the central channel, or *lumen*, will be much bigger in the vein than the artery.

Structure and function

Veins are tubes of muscular and fibrous tissue. The wall of a vein is divided into an outer layer (the *tunica adventitia*), a middle layer of muscular fibre (the *tunica intermedia*); and an inner lining (the *tunica intima*). Veins contain only a very thin layer of muscle.

After passing through the capillaries from the arteries, BLOOD enters the venous system (*see* CIRCULATION). It first passes into very small vessels called *venules* which are the venous equivalent of arterioles. It then makes its way into small veins and back towards the HEART along the veins which are large enough to be seen under the skin. Veins of this size contain valves which prevent blood from flowing back towards the tissues. The valves consist of little half-moon shaped cups that project into the lumen of the vein, and these make the blood flow in only one direction.

Eventually, blood flowing back to the heart enters one of two large veins: the *inferior vena cava* receives blood from the lower half of the body, and the *superior vena cava* receives blood from the head and arms. These vessels are about 1 in (2–3 cm) wide, and they enter the right atrium of the heart. Blood passes from here into the right ventricle, and then into the lungs via the pulmonary veins which enter the left atrium of the heart.

Special types of vein

There is one area where the veins are arranged in a very different way from the arteries, and this is in the INTESTINES. Here, instead of draining into a vein that passes straight into the heart, blood from the intestines is drained into what is known as the *hepatic portal system* of veins. This allows the blood, which may be rich in digested food, to be carried directly to the LIVER.

Once blood from the intestines reaches the liver, it passes in among the liver cells, in special capillaries which are called *sinusoids*, and then enters another system of veins called the *hepatic veins*. These eventually lead on to the inferior vena cava, and thus into the heart. This system ensures that food passed into the venous system from the intestines is brought to the liver for chemical processing in the most efficient way.

Other areas where there are special kinds of venous structure are in the extremities: the hands, feet, ears and nose. Here it is possible to find direct communications between the small arteries and veins, where blood may flow through from one to the other without having to go through a system of capillaries in the tissues. The main function of these arterio-venous connections is to do with control of body temperature (*see* FEVER). When they are open, heat loss increases and the body cools down.

There are similar connections between the arteries and veins in the genital areas. These allow for the engorgement of blood which occurs in the genitals as a result of sexual excitement (*see* SEX AND SEXUAL INTERCOURSE).

What can go wrong?

One serious problem that affects veins is the tendency of blood clots to form in them (*see* THROMBOSIS). This is likely to happen because of the slowness with which blood flows along the veins, in contrast with the rapid flow maintained in the arteries. SMOKING and the contraceptive pill increase the risk of clotting, although the low dose of oestrogen in modern contraceptive pills has much reduced this danger.

Another major trouble is caused by humans' upright stance – this leads to considerable pressure in the veins of the legs since they are supporting quite a high column of blood. This can result in VARICOSE VEINS – twisted engorged veins in the legs.

Venereal diseases, *see* Sexually transmitted diseases

Ventricular fibrillation (VF)

This is a form of TACHYCARDIA – disturbance of the orderly electrical activity of the HEART. Because the fibres that make the heart's pumping chambers start to relax and contract in a totally uncoordinated way, the heart is unable to pump blood. This means that, within seconds of an attack, a person will become unconscious, and death will follow in a minute or two. Obviously urgent treatment is needed – whether it be from a resuscitation team which can get quickly into the streets to reach the patient, or in a coronary CARE UNIT in hospital.

Causes of VF

The main cause of VF is a HEART ATTACK, which is responsible for many of the deaths from the condition. A heart attack usually arises from CORONARY HEART DISEASE, where the heart's own blood supply becomes obstructed.

Other heart problems can also cause VF, particularly those where there is an electrical disturbance of the heart. Sometimes the heart is affected by a disease that involves its own muscles – called *cardiomyopathy* (*see* HEART DISEASE) – and in a few cases, this may lead to VF.

Heart surgeons may deliberately put the heart into ventricular fibrillation. In the carefully controlled circumstances of heart surgery, where the work of the heart is taken over by the bypass machine, there is very little risk involved. The reason the heart is put into ventricular fibrillation is that it moves less and is therefore easier to operate on. It can be easily reversed by using a defibrillator (electrical shocking machine) which restarts the heart.

Mechanism of VF

The regular and automatic beating of the heart results from a very sophisticated timing system which conducts electrical impulses to the various parts of the heart. These impulses lead to the heart muscle contracting, and they are ordered so that the ventricles contract after the atria, and both sets of chambers have time to relax before the next heartbeat. In VF, the whole system breaks down so that individual muscle fibres contract and relax quite independently, with no overall contraction of the heart, and no pumping of blood.

In *atrial* fibrillation, the atria of the heart are beating in an uncoordinated way. This has little impact on the overall function of the heart since the two ventricles are still able to pump. In ventricular fibrillation, no blood is pumped through the heart, and death will follow unless the heart's electrical activity is restored to normal. Atrial fibrillation – a common and relatively minor heart problem – does not lead to ventricular fibrillation.

Treatment

The revolution in treatment of VF has been the introduction of *defibrillators*. These machines work by delivering a shock across the heart when two electrical pads are placed on the chest, one on the breastbone (sternum) and one at the apex of the heart, just below the left nipple. During heart surgery, two very much smaller pads are placed on the actual surface of the exposed heart, and a much lower current is used. For patients who go into ventricular fibrillation frequently outside hospital, implantable defibrillators are available which are sewn into the heart muscle. These are capable of delivering a shock when the patient has gone into ventricular fibrillation.

The basic principle of defibrillation is that an electric shock will cause the simultaneous electrical discharge of all the cells in the heart. This gives the normal conducting system what might be described as a clean slate on which to work, and enables it to reinstate normal orderly electrical activity.

Like any other effective form of treatment, defibrillation is not without its dangers. A shock can actually put a heart *into* VF, although this is only a risk when this form of treatment is being used for less serious forms of tachycardia; once the patient is in VF, there is obviously nothing to lose. Further, when defibrillation is performed, neither the patient not his or her bed must be touched. The electrical pads – or paddles – have insulated handles to protect the operator.

Prevention

Great efforts are made to identify patients who are at risk of getting VF, and then using drugs effectively to lessen that risk. One of the main indications that someone may be liable to suffer from VF is when they have already suffered an attack. Such patients will usually be given an intravenous infusion of the local anaesthetic lignocaine, which reduces the likelihood of extra electrical activity of the heart.

Much can also be done in coronary care units to reduce the risk of VF after a heart attack. Since the risk is greatest during the initial 24–48 hours after a heart attack, patients usually stay within these units until the critical period has passed. Even so, a number of patients still suffer attacks of VF after this.

VF outside hospital

Unfortunately, most heart attacks come out of the blue, with the result that patients are most likely to suffer from VF before they can reach the safety of a coronary care unit. The critical period is the first two hours, and hence it is imperative to get effective treatment to them immediately. Ideally there should be teams of resuscitation technicians available to rush to the spot when someone collapses with VF. Most large cities now have teams of ambulance crews trained as paramedics who can deal with VF on the spot.

Ventricular septal defect, *see* **Blue baby, Valves, heart**

Venules, *see* **Circulation, Veins**

Verruca

This is simply the Latin word for a WART, and has been adopted into the English language to refer to a wart on the sole of the foot. However, medically this is called a 'plantar wart'.

Cause

Warts are caused by a VIRUS that enters the skin through tiny injuries, especially if skin is wet and soggy. Most verrucae arise on the weight-bearing parts of the sole – that is, the heel and ball, not the instep.

A virus is a particle of living matter that can only reproduce itself inside a living cell, borrowing some of the cell's contents for this purpose. After the virus enters a cell in the SKIN's epidermis (outer layer), there is an incubation period of several months, while the virus multiplies and spreads, before enough skin cells are infected and deformed to produce a visible wart.

The epidermal cells deformed by the virus cause a hard, horny swelling – the wart – which on the sole of the foot is pressed inwards by standing and walking, irritating the sensitive nerve endings under the skin.

There are several strains of human wart virus. Verrucae are due to one strain, although the patient often has warts elsewhere. Another strain that affects only the soles of the feet causes a *mosaic wart*. This looks like a honeycomb and is actually a mass of closely packed polygonal warts, often at least 1 in (2.5 cm) across. Mosaic warts are extremely resistant to treatment and often last for several years, but fortunately they are not nearly as painful as verrucae.

Verrucae, like other common virus diseases, are unusual in infancy but begin to occur during the school years, reaching a peak at about the age of nine. They then decline in frequency becoming rarer after the middle 20s. Curiously, the sex incidence is equal up to the age of six but then they become commoner in girls.

Appearance

Like verrucae, CORNS AND CALLUSES are also painful and horny, and it may be very difficult to tell them apart. But if the horny cap of a verruca is carefully pared away, four distinguishing features will be clearly seen.

First, the verruca becomes wider the more skin is pared away. It is shaped like a pyramid with the point at the surface, and there is more hidden in the skin than is visible above it. It also has a horny collar which pushes aside the tiny lines on the skin of the sole. These never run across the verruca but encircle it and its horny collar. Finally, when the skin can no longer be pared without causing pain, pin-point bleeding spots appear. However, if the verruca has already been killed, the tiny blood vessels are clotted, showing as a few speckled black spots on the surface. This is therefore a sign that the verruca is healing.

Verrucae occur where the sole touches the ground but rarely at an exact point of pressure as is the case with corns and calluses. Therefore if the bit of hard painful skin has been present less than two years in a child or young adult, and is not exactly over a bony knot, it is probably a verruca. Occasionally, a verruca may arise in a callus, and will be revealed by careful paring.

Progress

The verruca wart virus – which is relatively harmless, and only affects a tiny area of the outer layer of skin – is often overlooked by the body's IMMUNE SYSTEM for many months. This is why warts last so long.

When the body finally notices the verrucae and mounts an offensive, they shrivel up and disappear leaving no scar – as if by magic. This accounts for the 'success' of many wart charms. About 20 per cent clear in six months and the majority within two years. Once this immunity is learned it is readily available to prevent re-infection. Sometimes, as a result of illness or the use of immune suppressive drugs, this immunity fades and warts recur, so that further treatment will be needed.

Treatment

There are no medicines or injections to kill the verruca virus in the way that antibiotics kill bacteria. The aims of local treatment are to destroy the skin cells containing the virus, and to stimulate the body's own defence mechanisms. Moreover, local treatment which kills the surface virus makes the verruca less infectious to others.

Local treatments that can be safely used in the home include paints, gels and soaks that contain salicylic acid, formaldehyde or related drugs. Rubbing down the horny cap of a verruca relieves the pain of walking on it. If this is not done, a layer of dead, hard tissue builds up over the verruca, shielding it from the paint you have to put on.

The simplest and one of the most effective treatments is a paint containing *salicyclic acid.* Some preparations contain *lactic acid* as well (e.g. Salactol, Duofilm, Cuplex and Salatic). These paints are all based on *collodion,* a substance that dries on the skin leaving a thin transparent film containing the active ingredients. It is very important, however, that these preparations are used properly.

In resistant cases, a doctor may prescribe an ointment or a paint containing the drug *podophyllin.* This is a substance that poisons dividing cells and can be very effective when used to treat warts. However, it may cause some pain when it is applied, and inflammation may occur with repeated use. It is used only under medical supervision.

If verrucae persist, there are other techniques for removing them surgically. A verruca may be scooped out under a local ANAESTHETIC using a special surgical instrument called a *curette.* Although the procedure itself is painless once the local anaesthetic has taken effect, there is inevitably some pain while the anaesthetic is injected into the sole of the foot. Because the tissues of the sole are so tightly bound together with connective tissue, any injection into this area tends to be painful. Once the verruca is removed, the resulting hole is covered with a sterile dressing.

An alternative technique is freezing the verruca with liquid nitrogen. This treatment causes a blister to form under the verruca and it then lifts off a few days after the treatment has been given. However, the blister can be quite painful and there is some risk of subsequent infection, so this technique is rarely used for verrucae, although it is widely used for warts on other parts of the body.

Prevention

Most verrucae are caught at swimming pools, since the skin barrier is weaker when it is wet. People with verrucae should therefore wear the thin rubber shoes that can be bought at swimming pools. In the home, a child can be prevented from spreading the virus by using his or her own towel and bath mat, and by covering the verruca with a waterproof plaster.

Vertigo

People often confuse vertigo with fear of heights. In fact, it can be a symptom of a variety of conditions – from the normal effects of spinning on a roundabout to the distressing results of some sorts of BRAIN damage.

Vertigo is a very common and often distressing symptom that occurs when the delicate BALANCE mechanisms in the inner part of the EAR or brain-stem are damaged or disturbed. Many of the causes of vertigo are not at all serious, but occasionally vertigo may indicate some quite worrying disease.

Problems in the inner ear

The part of the inner ear that contains the balance sensors is called the labyrinth because it curls into a spiral. The labyrinth can be the site of a viral infection and this can cause sudden and severe vertigo, called *labyrinthitis.* Sometimes the sensation of spinning is so strong that it causes VOMITING, and even slight head movements cause giddiness.

Labyrinthitis can also be caused as a result of other types of ear infection, such as *otitis media*. This type of ear infection is common among children, but fortunately vertigo is a rare complication.

MÉNIÈRE'S DISEASE can also be a cause of vertigo. It is caused by swelling in the fluid cavities of the inner ear, including the balance mechanisms themselves. No one knows quite why this happens, but it is usually characterized by severe vertigo with partial loss of hearing and a continuous buzzing in the affected ear. The latter symptom is called TINNITUS.

Again the vertigo can be treated with special drugs. Unfortunately, however, deafness ultimately develops and then the vertigo ceases. This is one of the causes of vertigo that makes prompt medical advice such a necessity.

A rare condition called *benign positional vertigo* causes brief spells of vertigo when the head is moved in a particular way. It is caused by hypersensitivity of cells in the inner ear.

Damage to the brain-stem

Nerve messages from the inner ear are analysed by a collection of cells in the brain-stem called the *vestibular nucleus*. Damage to this interpretative part of the system can also cause vertigo.

In older people, the ARTERIES that supply the brain-stem can become furred or even blocked up. Starved of sufficient oxygen, cells in the brain-stem stop working and messages from the inner ear are no longer properly analysed.

Sometimes the blood vessels get kinked in the neck as a result of arthritic neck joints. This may mean that the blood supply is momentarily blocked when the head is turned suddenly. This can produce vertigo. Occasionally, tumours or patches of inflammation (e.g. multiple sclerosis) may affect the vestibular nucleus, producing vertigo. Certain drugs, alcohol and migraine can also cause vertigo.

All these types of vertigo can be eased by drugs, but the root cause also has to be found and treated by your doctor.

Vesicles, *see* **Rash**

Vestibulitis, *see* **Balance**

Viruses

The basic structure of viruses is so simple that it is questionable whether they should be regarded as living matter at all. Essentially they consist of no more than a capsule of protein which contains their GENETIC material in the form of one of the nucleic acids, DNA or RNA – these are the substances which carry the genetic message from generation to generation in all living things. It is the DNA that is passed on in the process of reproduction and it ends up in the nucleus of living cells. The DNA then passes messages to the chemical 'factories' inside the cell instructing them to make various types of protein. These messages are carried by RNA.

Viruses work by invading the cells of the organism they are infecting. Once a virus is inside a cell, it liberates its DNA or RNA content. These substances interfere with the cell's own function and turn over the protein-producing apparatus of the cell to work for the virus instead of the cell itself. Having taken control of a cell, the virus manufactures more viruses, so that more cells and finally other individuals can be infected.

Thus viruses are very life-like in their ability to pass on their own characteristics from generation to generation by the use of genetic material. The two nucleic acids DNA and RNA are the basic stuff of life, and even if they are only contained in a thin capsule, they make up what is virtually a living organism.

Structure

The smallest viruses are 2–30 nanometres across (1 nanometre = one thousandth of a micrometre) and the largest are ten times that size. Nearly all of them are more or less round in shape, except the RABIES virus and its related viruses which are bullet-shaped, and the SMALLPOX virus and its related viruses which are shaped like bricks.

They are classified basically according to whether they carry the nucleic acid DNA or RNA. The nucleic acid core of a virus is called the *genome* and the protein capsule the *capsid*. The capsid is made up of many identical protein blocks called *capsomeres*. The way in which the capsomeres line up around the genome dictates the overall shape of the individual virus particle.

Different groups of viruses have different shapes, one of the commonest being the icosahedron, a structure with 20 flat sides of equal size, effectively forming a sphere. The capsid of other viruses forms a hollow cylinder. These differences in structure can only be determined by pictures taken with an electron microscope (electronmicrographs). Some viruses have another structure over their capsid, aptly called an *envelope*.

All these variations are taken together to classify a virus into a particular group. The viruses that cause human disease are now all classified.

Viruses and bacteria

There is a great difference in size between viruses and BACTERIA – for example, a streptococcus is 50 times greater in diameter than a POLIO virus.

An individual bacterium is able to reproduce itself by splitting in two, and it can live independently, having the apparatus to carry out many metabolic processes within its cell wall. All bacteria contain DNA and RNA. In contrast, although viruses can survive outside the cells of other organisms, they need these cells for any kind of metabolic activity. And individual viral particles (virons) also need the apparatus of host cells in order to multiply. They do this by making copies of themselves according to instructions from their DNA or RNA – a process known as replication. Finally, they only contain one kind of nucleic acid.

How are viruses spread?

Viral diseases can be very infectious. A disease like MEASLES is so infectious that, until immunization was introduced, it was certain that virtually every child in the UK would get it. The measles virus, like many others, is spread by droplet infection. A cough or sneeze from an infected person will carry the virus into the air to be inhaled by someone else.

The polio virus and *enteroviruses* (primarily infecting the intestines) enter the body via the digestive tract. Another group – the *togaviruses* which are carried by insects – make their way into the body through the skin as the result of an insect bite. And that most horrific of infections, rabies, also enters via a bite from an animal which has been driven to distraction by the disease. The HIV virus, which causes AIDS, is spread only by sexual contact or by inoculation of infected blood, for example on contaminated needles or syringes.

Once inside the body, the viruses invade the cells at the site of entry. Thus the *rhinoviruses* that are responsible for the common COLD, enter the cells of the mucous membrane lining the nose to create symptoms in upper airways.

Treatment of viral infections

A particular viral infection is usually diagnosed by studying the levels of particular antibodies in a patient's blood over a period of two weeks.

However, if there were any really effective method of treating a specific virus, a doctor would need a diagnosis earlier than two weeks after the onset of infection. But there are very few specific treatments for viral diseases.

Viruses cannot be treated with ANTIBIOTICS. Bacteria, which respond to antibiotics, are quite complicated organisms, although each consists of only one cell. On the other hand, viruses are very simple, consisting of nothing more than a core of nucleic acid (genetic material) surrounded by a protein capsule. Antibiotics work by finding a way of impeding the activity of the bacterial cell without harming the human cells. Since the virus has no metabolic activity to disrupt, the basic principle of antibiotics is of no value whatsoever.

Recently, however, there has been one important breakthrough in the search for treatment. This is the development of the drug *acyclovir* which has the property of killing cells infected with the herpes group of viruses while leaving normal cells untouched. The virus can therefore no longer replicate itself. This drug may prove useful against all kinds of herpes infections – from

COLD SORES to SHINGLES – and is already very valuable in treating the overwhelming kind of infection that people with deficient IMMUNE SYSTEMS suffer from. A related drug, gancyclovir, is particularly active against cytomegalovirus. Tribavirin inhibits a wide range of DNA and RNA viruses. It can be given by inhalation for the treatment of sever bronchiolitis in infants. Research continues on other similar drugs which may have anti-viral properties.

Prevention
Although viral infections cannot be satisfactorily treated yet, many of the serious ones can be successfully prevented. Smallpox, for example, has been totally eradicated through a combination of vaccination and isolation of cases. It is also possible to vaccinate against MEASLES, MUMPS, RUBELLA, YELLOW FEVER, polio and rabies.

There are some infections, however, against which it seems impossible to produce an effective vaccine. One of these is INFLUENZA. The influenza viruses have a remarkable ability to change their protein structure as they pass from person to person. These minor changes enable them to fool the body's immune system with each new infection. This explains why we get so many attacks of the same disease in a lifetime. A vaccine will be effective if it is made from the current strain of a virus, but for this to be possible, a manufacturer would have to predict accurately which strain this would be – a very difficult proposition. However, certain predictions can now be made and for certain groups of patients the flu vaccine is recommended. The problem is multiplied in the case of the common cold, for which there are many viral strains, so it is unlikely that vaccines for prevention or drugs for treatment of the cold will be available in the near future.

Viscera, *see* **Abdomen**

Vitamins

These are essential for the body to function efficiently, although they may only be required in very small amounts. Most cannot be made by the body, and instead have to be found in the diet. The vitamins – A, the B complex, C, D, E and K – are involved in the continual processes of repair and maintenance of the body's tissues. The lack of one or more vitamins can cause what are known as 'deficiency diseases'.

Such diseases are rare in the West, where even the poorest sections of the community seem to have a diet which provides adequate amounts (*see* NUTRITION); this is not the case in underdeveloped countries. For people to suffer a vitamin deficiency in a country such as Britain, there is more often some underlying reason such as a physical disease which might interfere with the way that the vitamin is absorbed from the intestines (*see* MALABSORPTION), or a mental illness which leads to an abnormal diet. The elderly, the infirm and ALCOHOLICS may also be at risk because of MALNUTRITION resulting from a poor diet.

Only very small amounts of vitamins are needed for health, and there is little convincing evidence that taking extra amounts is of any benefit at all. Some vitamins, especially vitamins D and A, can even cause a serious illness when taken in excessive amounts; this is called *hypervitaminosis.* A possible exception to this is vitamin C, and indeed some very respected scientists believe that large doses of this vitamin are beneficial to health and helpful at warding off infections. However, the evidence is not convincing and this idea is certainly not proven.

Alcohol and vitamin deficiency

Alcoholics often have very inadequate diets, even though the drink they consume may itself contain a reasonable number of calories. They are particularly likely to run short of B vitamins. Although it is possible to suffer from true beriberi as a result of alcoholism, there is an interesting condition known as *Wernicke's encephalopathy* which is very common in alcoholics. The disease involves unsteadiness, and nystagmus – regular jerking of the eyes and looking to one side. It may also involve memory loss – when the name *Korsakoff's syndrome* is used. Most of the symptoms respond to thiamin, although the memory loss is often permanent.

Vitamin A

This vitamin enables us to see in a dim light, keeps our skin healthy, ensures normal growth and renews the body tissue.

The vitamin A in our food comes in two different forms from two different sources. The pure form, called *retinol,* is found in foods such as fish liver oils, liver, kidney, cheese, eggs and butter, having already been manufactured by the animal concerned. The second form we make ourselves from *carotene,* which is found in such vegetables as carrots, spinach, cabbage, and tomatoes.

In fact, when a vegetable is orange, yellow or dark green in colour, what you are seeing is its carotene content, and the darker the green of the vegetable, the greater the carotene content. Spinach and watercress therefore contain more in each pound than cabbage, and dark green cabbage provides more than lighter types of vegetable.

Carotene is converted into retinol in the liver and the small intestine, and then some of the vitamin is absorbed into the bloodstream and circulated round the body to be used in its everyday function. The rest is stored in the liver.

Although vitamin A is not present in many foods, those which contain it are fortunately readily available. A fifth of our average intake comes from vegetables, mainly carrots. Milk and butter are other common sources, as is margarine, to which vitamin A is added.

Deficiency and excess

Probably the most widespread worldwide health problem is due to a deficiency of vitamin A. This deficiency is the cause of EYE problems, starting with night blindness, and leading on to *xerophthalmia*, a disease where the cornea becomes dull and hazy as a result of a thin skin forming over it. In the most severe cases, this disease leads to a thinning of the cornea, which eventually breaks down and perforates, causing BLINDNESS.

Vitamin A deficiency is not associated with any particular part of the world or with any staple food. Vitamin A is fat soluble – that is, it dissolves in fat or oil rather than water. This means that it is found in fat-containing foods, and it is these foods that are in such short supply in places where there is malnutrition.

Keratomalacia (the most severe form of vitamin A-deficient eye disease) is common wherever there is severe malnutrition. Thousands of children between the ages of two and five go blind permanently as a result of the deficiency every year.

There is danger in taking too much vitamin A. An excess can result in fragile bones, liver and spleen enlargement, and appetite loss. This is very unlikely to result from intake through food but can occur if large amounts are taken in concentrated forms such as halibut liver oil capsules.

Vitamin B complex

Vitamin B complex – a collection of eight separate vitamins – can be obtained in adequate supplies by eating a good balanced diet since B vitamins are present in a wide variety of foods. But they are easily affected by drugs or excessive alcohol and may not be absorbed properly during pregnancy or certain illnesses. If a deficiency occurs, disease can result.

Uses

The B vitamins have a number of uses in the body. They act with ENZYMES to maintain chemical actions, particularly to do with breaking down food.

Pyridoxine (B_6) assists in HORMONE production; *folic acid* and *B_{12}* are involved with red cell formation. *Riboflavin* (B_2) maintains the skin, liver and eyes, while other vitamins in this group, which include *thiamin* (B_1), *nicotinic acid* (niacin), *pantothenic acid* and *biotin*, play a part in growth and the repair of body tissues, the production of energy, food metabolism and other functions necessary to good health.

How the B vitamins are lost

The body does not store the B vitamins, making regular daily replenishment vital. Because they dissolve in water, much of their nutritive value can be lost in cooking. Thiamin is most affected and nicotinic acid the least.

Food processing also affects the B vitamins we get in our foods. Milling wheat to produce white flour results in a lowering of the thiamin and nicotinic acid content. Milling and the extraction of bran and germ from rice means that polished white rice contains less thiamin. Cereals which have been processed have fewer vitamins.

Canned meats contain fewer vitamins than home-cooked meats. Light affects riboflavin content in bottled milk.

Deficiency

The practice of eating white (polished) rice, which has been both washed and cooked in a large amount of water, considerably reduces the dietary supply of thiamin. For these reasons, *beriberi* is a disease of rice-eating countries, although improved health education has made it much less prevalent in South-East Asia, where it was once common.

Wet beriberi arises from a thiamin-deficient diet, and is characterized by OEDEMA: waterlogging and swelling of the body. Dry beriberi occurs through a thiamin deficiency, but the deterioration in health is slower and oedema may not appear. Both forms of beriberi affect the functioning of the nervous system, but the brain is usually unimpaired. Infantile beriberi is a disease which affects children breastfed by thiamin-deficient mothers: here brain malfunction exists, together with convulsions, uneasiness and loss of voice. In rare cases, beriberi might arise following fever, pregnancy or hard physical work. The cure for all types of beriberi is a diet containing thiamin, and bedrest.

Another deficiency disease is pellagra, caused by a deficiency of nicotinic acid (niacin). This disease is prevalent among those people whose staple diet is maize, and is found in large areas of Africa, and in parts of South America, India and Europe. In Africa, pellagra remains a big problem, while it seems to have been reasonably controlled in other parts of the world. Oddly enough, there is a great deal of nicotinic acid in maize, but unfortunately it is in a chemical form that cannot be separated out by the digestive system, so none is absorbed. It was found that people who had a satisfactory level of protein in their diet did not suffer from pellagra, even if the remainder of their diet consisted almost entirely of maize. This is because animal proteins contain a lot of tryptophan, a substance from which the body can make nicotinic acid. The protein in maize controls little or no tryptophan.

PERNICIOUS ANAEMIA is a disease which occurs mainly in people who lack the ability to absorb and utilize vitamin B_{12}, and vegans, who shun milk, eggs, meat and fish completely. B_{12} can be taken in tablet form or by injection, and eating raw liver is also a cure.

Sores on the skin, often at the corners of the mouth, are usually caused by a deficiency in riboflavin.

When a supplement is necessary

Pregnant women can benefit from taking folic acid, which is sometimes given along with iron supplements at ante-natal clinics to women who are found to be anaemic. It has also been shown to reduce the risk of neural tube defects if taken before contraception and for the first 12 weeks of pregnancy.

Folic acid is involved in the making of red blood cells: the body has to produce more of these cells in pregnancy to help with the nourishment and development of the foetus. Without folic acid, a pregnant woman will risk such complications as toxaemia (*see* ECLAMPSIA AND PRE-ECLAMPSIA), premature birth and haemorrhaging, all the result of a condition called megaloblastic ANAEMIA, which causes tiredness and weakness. There is also evidence that folic acid supplementation may prevent SPINA BIFIDA.

Great claims have been made for pyridoxine in a variety of conditions including premenstrual syndrome, but there is little sound evidence to support them and overdose can be dangerous.

Vitamin C

This is perhaps the most controversial of all the vitamins. Great claims have been made for its healing and protective qualities – not only in connection with the common COLD, but in ageing, HEART DISEASE, CANCER and many other conditions. And although scientists and doctors remain sceptical in regard to some or all of these claims, they agree that vitamin C is vital for the body to function properly. Nor do they deny that, even in affluent societies, we are more likely to be deficient in vitamin C than in any other nutrient.

Unfortunately, this vitamin does not occur in many foods, and in those that do contain it, the amount will vary according to season, freshness and cooking. Nor can the body store vitamin C, so it needs regular replenishment.

Vitamin C is vital for maintenance of the body's connective tissue – that is, the skin, fibres, membranes and so on – that literally hold it together. Collagen, a protein that is important for the formation of healthy skin, tendons and bones, depends partly on vitamin C for its manufacture, and the vitamin is also needed for the release of hormones and the production of other chemical substances which play a part in our survival and resistance to infection.

Even so, this vitamin is something of a mystery. Its complete function is unknown, but there are research scientists who look upon it as such an essential to life that it transcends all the other vitamins. For instance, it helps in the body's absorption of IRON.

Vitamin C deficiency

The extreme form of deficiency in vitamin C is a condition called SCURVY. When this occurs, the connective tissue disintegrates so that blood vessels break down and there is bleeding into the skin, joints and from the gums. Teeth are loosened, bruises appear and resistance to infection is lowered. Nowadays, this deficiency can be cured very quickly with high doses of vitamin C, but if the condition is neglected, there could be permanent damage.

Sources of vitamin C

If we were prepared to live on rose hips, we would be very well provided with vitamin C, as this is the richest source available – it may well be the reason that our ancestors thrived. Paprika is good, too, but since neither this nor rose hips are on everyone's daily menu, we have to rely on other sources.

Fortunately, vegetables such as potatoes, which do feature in most people's diets in the Western world, contain some vitamin C, as do Brussels sprouts, cauliflower and cabbage. Among fruits, blackcurrants are best, followed by strawberries. Further down on the list, but available all the year round, are citrus fruits – oranges, lemons and grapefruit.

There is not much vitamin C in apples or pears, virtually none in milk – with the exception of formula milks – and none in cereal grains, dried peas and beans, nuts or dried fruit. Although all green and root vegetables and fruit contain a certain amount, this does vary from season to season.

When extra is needed

Some distinguished experts maintain that we need far more than the normally recommended daily allowances. It is generally acknowledged that the body requires extra vitamin C after a severe illness or injury, and there have been experiments showing that burns heal faster when a vitamin C solution has been applied to the skin in conjunction with injections or doses taken by mouth.

High doses of vitamin C have also been used successfully in experiments to reduce cholesterol (fatty deposits) in the arteries, and it is thought that the vitamin might offer protection against gastric bleeding in those who have to take large regular amounts of aspirin for conditions such as arthritis.

This, of course, brings us to the vexed question of vitamin C and the common cold, over which many claims have been made and much research carried out. The current verdict is 'not proven' – with no conclusive evidence that points to vitamin C being effective protection against or treatment for colds.

The body excretes any surplus of this vitamin, and any massive dose of vitamin C that is not utilized by the body is simply flushed away in urine. This means that there is no possibility of an overdose, according to our present knowledge.

Vitamin D

This is sometimes called the 'sunshine vitamin' for the very good reason that we derive part of our essential supplies from exposure to the sun. We also obtain it from what we eat, but there is some danger of deficiency since it does not occur in many foods.

We need vitamin D so that it can work with CALCIUM to make healthy bones. Vitamin D helps the absorption of calcium and phosphorus from the intestinal wall and maintains correct levels in the blood.

Sources of vitamin D

There are two main types of vitamin D. When we derive it from sunshine, it is through ultraviolet rays hitting the skin and converting cholesterol in the skin into *cholecalciferol*, or vitamin D_3. This form is also directly available to us in fish liver oils: fish store surplus vitamin D in their livers. The other main kind of D is called *ergocalciferol*, or D_2, and it is manufactured from plant materials such as yeasts.

Comparatively few foods contain vitamin D. Besides cod liver oil, it is most richly available in herrings, kippers, canned salmon and sardines. If you think you are not taking a sufficient amount, you could increase your supplies with a daily spoonful of cod liver oil or a helping of canned fish one or twice a week. By law, margarine is required to have vitamin D added to it during production, and evaporated milk usually has extra, too. Butter and fresh milk have much smaller amounts, but because of their daily use, they are a good source. Eggs contain some as well.

Vitamin D deficiency

Perhaps the vitamin which is most affected by social habits and geography is vitamin D. It is lack of this important vitamin which leads to RICKETS in children and, in adults, *osteomalacia.* To be short of the vitamin you have to have an inadequate diet *and* be exposed to little sunlight.

In Britain, rickets and osteomalacia are found quite often in minor forms, although they don't often cause sever problems. The diseases most often occur in a number of social groups, including the relatively poor and the elderly, who not only have a diet which is lacking in the vitamins, but also lead a sedentary life which reduces the amount of sunlight that the skin is exposed to. Another group in Britain who are particularly at risk from vitamin D deficiency are Asian immigrants. This is partly because their diet tends to be low in vitamin D and also because social custom tends to restrict the time that women spend outside – and the deficiency is more common in women. However, another contributing factor is skin colour. The MELANIN in dark-skinned people is designed to protect the skin from the sun, but it will also have the effect of blocking the synthesis of vitamin D unless there is a great deal of sunlight about. Having dark skin in a country with low sunlight levels increases the risks of developing rickets and osteomalacia.

See also OSTEOPOROSIS.

Excessive vitamin D

Since vitamin D is stored in fat, any extra is not easily got rid of by the body. Instead it is stored in the liver and can lead to certain poisonous effects if the intake is too high. Early signs of vitamin D poisoning include loss of appetite, nausea, vomiting and general debility. There may be yellowish deposits beneath the finger nails, in the eyes and on the skin. Since vitamin D helps absorption of calcium, there may be unhealthily high concentrations of this in the blood, leading to brittle bones, hardening of the arteries, calcium deposits in the kidneys, and growth failure in children.

Vitamin E

Most orthodox nutritionists say that we probably get enough vitamin E in a balanced diet and that there is no reliable evidence to suggest that supplements will increase lifespan or produce cures or miracle improvements in virility or fertility. They point out that the vitamin is fat soluble (it dissolves in body fat), which means that it is not excreted in the urine; therefore we are able to store it and are unlikely to become deficient.

Vitamin E is the general name for a number of vitamin compounds called *tocopherols.* They are thought to play a part in the process concerned with the absorption of fats during digestion and the preservation of oxygen in the bloodstream. Beyond that, little clear knowledge exists about the function of this vitamin and it has not been proved to be essential to life.

Sources of vitamin E

The most potent source is in wheat germ oil, which is the oil present in every whole grain of wheat. When we eat wholewheat bread, we get the wheat germ intact, with its quota of oil, but when we eat white bread, the wheat germ along with other nutritious elements in the flour are no longer present. They have been removed by the processing involved in producing fine white flour. Some of the nutritious elements – calcium and iron, for instance – are put back artificially, but vitamin E is not usually replaced.

A similar loss occurs with white rice, any product made with white flour and most breakfast cereals that have been refined or processed, such as instant porridge or specially treated rice. However, biscuits and pastry contain fats which contribute vitamin E.

Other foods with vitamin E are peanuts, eggs and vegetable oils. Green leafy vegetables provide some, especially spinach. It is found in broccoli and cauliflower, too, but only in the leaves, not the florets.

Vitamin E deficiency

The standard medical view is that the main category of the population at risk from a deficiency are premature babies because they have low fat stores and cannot retain or utilize sufficient vitamin E for their needs. They may be given extra supplements at birth to counteract this. Others at risk are people suffering from a inability to absorb fats; they, too, may benefit from supplements. But since the function of the vitamins is not fully understood, these supplements are more a preventive measure than a treatment.

Despite the orthodox view, people have reported improvements in cases of HEART DISEASE, PHLEBITIS, SKIN conditions, burns, leg cramps, MISCARRIAGE and MENOPAUSE as a result of taking extra vitamin E. Unfortunately, these cases tend to be isolated, and controlled trials have not confirmed the favourable results.

However, as there are no known toxic (poisonous) effects if adults take large supplements of vitamin E, there is no danger in resorting to this treatment. The treatments often involve large doses of the vitamin, so large that the therapy is called megavitamin therapy, involving daily doses of anything from 800 to 1600 milligrams.

A high consumption of the polyunsaturated vegetable oils actually creates an increased need for the vitamin. This is because vitamin E has a complex biochemical effect on polyunsaturated fats which uses up supplies. Polyunsaturated fats are nowadays often recommended by doctors for patients with high cholesterol levels, as the fats help reduce these levels, but remember that more vitamin E is needed to maintain a balance.

To ensure a healthy intake of vitamin E without resorting to expensive megavitamin doses, a normal diet should include wholewheat bread, eggs and green vegetables. One or two teaspoons daily of wheat germ oil, available from health food shops, will make up for any deficiency in the diet of otherwise quite healthy people.

Vitamin K

This consists of vitamin K_1, a yellow oil found in a variety of vegetables, and vitamin K_2, a yellow waxy substance produced by bacteria. Although we get a supply of vitamin K_1 from leafy vegetables such as spinach and green cabbage, a normal diet will only provide us with a proportion of our needs. We get the remainder of vitamin K_2 from the bacteria which live in our intestines, and this ensures that we always have a steady supply. Thus in healthy people, a deficiency resulting from an inadequate diet seldom occurs.

Vitamin K deficiency

Vitamin K is used by the liver to produce 13 blood components known as the *clotting factors*. A deficiency results in the decreased production of three of these 13 factors, the most important of them being *prothrombin*. When an injury occurs, the ability of the blood to coagulate will be impaired. Small cuts will bleed vigorously, and large bruises will form under the skin in response to even minor injuries. In severe cases of vitamin K deficiency, serious and even fatal haemorrhaging may occur.

Because vitamins K_1 and K_2 are fat soluble (they are dissolved and stored in fat), a deficiency may occur in diseases which cause decreased digestion and absorption of fats and oils. These include a BILE duct obstruction and COELIAC DISEASE (where gluten in cereals suppresses normal food absorption). This deficiency can easily be treated with vitamin K injections or with tablets of synthetic vitamin K.

Some liver diseases, such as CIRRHOSIS and HEPATITIS, interfere with the utilization of vitamin K, and vitamin supplements in large doses may then be required. This deficiency is sometimes difficult to treat and can be dangerous in patients with liver failure, who may develop uncontrollable internal bleeding.

Finally, vitamin K deficiency is common in the newborn and may cause serious damage both from blood loss and from bleeding into the brain and other vital organs. Intestinal bacteria are not present at birth, milk contains very little vitamin K and the supply from the mother's bloodstream does not last very long. To make up this deficiency, babies are given vitamin K (either orally or intrasmuscularly) after birth and at intervals afterwards. This is especially important in premature babies and those who have had forceps delivery who are at greater risk of brain haemorrhage.

Excess vitamin K

Vitamin K is non-toxic (not poisonous) if taken in excessive amounts because the liver controls the rate of production of the clotting factors.

Some patients have an increased tendency to THROMBOSIS, or blood clot formation. These blood clots obstruct the healthy blood vessels in which they are first formed, and may also be carried around the body in the bloodstream to obstruct blood vessels elsewhere. The limbs, lungs, brain and heart may suffer serious damage. Thrombosis is not caused by excess vitamin K, but in such patients, further blood clot formation can be prevented by taking drugs such as warfarin, which prevent the liver from using vitamin K to produce clotting factors.

Volvulus, *see* Infarction, Intestines and intestinal disorders

Vomiting

This refers to the forceful ejection of the contents of the STOMACH through the mouth. Commonly known as 'being sick' or 'throwing up', this unpleasant and often exhausting experience, often preceded by NAUSEA, can be caused by a number of conditions.

Mechanism

The actual mechanism behind the ejection of food is quite straightforward. At the onset of vomiting, the *pylorus* – a muscular valve through which food normally passes from the stomach into the INTESTINES – closes. The waves of stomach contractions which normally push food downwards into the intestines go into reverse, causing pressure inside the stomach to build up until the contents burst out through the mouth.

There are three main areas of the body which, when stimulated, can bring about vomiting. Although the mechanism is the same in each case, the causes are very different.

Stomach irritation

Irritation of the stomach lining is the most common cause of vomiting. This can be brought on by a surprising variety of conditions, including gastritis, GASTRO-ENTERITIS, PERITONITIS, APPENDICITIS and ULCERS; TONSILLITIS can also cause vomiting in young children. These types of complaint are associated with viral infections and inflammation, and should be treated as soon as possible.

The commonest cause of stomach irritation is eating or drinking to excess, or taking in contaminated or impure food (*see* FOOD POISONING). The body actually protects itself against potentially harmful substances and does its best to expel what it has recognized as dangerous. The bout of vomiting is usually short-lived, lasting a day or two, and is rarely serious.

Putting fingers down the back of the throat will also cause vomiting, and use is made of this REFLEX action in trying to make people empty their stomach of certain poisonous substances that have been swallowed. The function of this reflex is to protect the body from swallowing anything that is unsuitable.

The ears and travel sickness

TRAVEL SICKNESS is another common cause of vomiting. This results from contrasting information reaching the brain from the various different organs of BALANCE. At the centre of this are the semicircular canals in the EAR. If what we see conflicts with the information from these canals, and the brain is not able to interpret the two, it triggers off impulses to the vomiting centre in the brain. This apparent 'warning' action results in nausea and vomiting.

Poor travellers are well aware of this problem, but it can also affect sufferers of MÉNIÈRE'S DISEASE, in which the organs of hearing and balance are affected.

The brain

A blow to the HEAD – it doesn't even have to be a hard blow – can be the cause of vomiting, and this usually indicates the likelihood of serious bleeding inside the skull. The desire to vomit usually occurs some time after the blow – often when one has completely forgotten about the injury, even a couple of days later – and indicates a damaged blood vessel that has allowed pressure to accumulate on the brain and around the vomiting centre. This must be treated as soon as possible, as there is a very real danger that the person can slip into a coma (*see* UNCONSCIOUSNESS).

Morning sickness

Vomiting also frequently occurs in PREGNANCY. Known as 'morning sickness', this form of vomiting is not fully understood, but it is believed that it is related to the changing level of hormones in the blood during early pregnancy. In a few women, the vomiting is persistent and severe and may even necessitate a spell in hospital.

Repeated vomiting

Repeated bouts of vomiting are often regarded as a symptom of a serious disorder and should be brought to your doctor's attention immediately.

What is brought up in the vomit is also important. It will usually consist of the last meal you have had or may be almost entirely yellow-green, bitter bile. However, if it contains any sign of blood, then the implications are very serious and you should get medical advice straight away. The blood may look like dark coffee beans, as it will have congealed in the stomach well before the vomiting started.

Treatment

Where vomiting has taken on a repetitive nature, or if it is accompanied by fever and general malaise, the condition must be diagnosed by the doctor, and the root cause treated.

When someone has been sick, avoid giving solid foods. Diluted milk, squashes and plenty of water are fine, but no fizzy or alcoholic drinks. If it is impossible to keep fluids down, ice cubes can be sucked. A level teaspoonful of bicarbonate of soda diluted in a teacup of water or milk can be helpful. As the person begins to feel better, he or she can take soups and custards, building up to a normal diet over three or four days.

If a baby, young child or elderly person vomits, it is imperative to give them enough fluids to avoid dehydration (*see* WATER).

W

Warts

These are a very common, usually harmless SKIN affliction which affects mainly children and, to a lesser extent, adults and teenagers. They consist of small rounded growths in the skin and can occur virtually anywhere on the skin surface, although they are most common on the hands, knees, face and genitals.

Rarely any cause for concern, warts are usually painless and can disappear without trace within a few months or years. A type of wart that appears on the sole of the foot – a *plantar* wart, commonly known as a VERRUCA – is often painful and requires treatment. Facial and genital warts may cause some embarrassment or discomfort, and these are best treated as they can persist for years.

Causes and transmission

Warts are caused by a VIRUS called *papavovirus*, which can infiltrate and multiply within the outermost layer of the skin cells. When the virus infects the skin, it causes the skin cells to proliferate in a disordered fashion, producing, in effect, a small, benign TUMOUR. This fact is of great interest to doctors as warts are the only type of growth found in humans that is definitely known to be caused by a virus.

The wart virus is contagious and can thus be transmitted from one person to another or from one part of the body to another, either by direct skin contact or indirectly via an intermediate object such as a towel. A break in the skin – such as a scratch – may facilitate entry of the virus. Hand warts are most probably transmitted by hand-holding and genital warts by sexual intercourse. The period between infection and appearance of the warts may be weeks or months.

Warts on children are rarely transmitted to adults, probably because adults have acquired some immunity to the virus through infection during their own childhood. However, the viruses that cause common hand warts and genital warts are slightly different, so a person who was afflicted with hand warts during childhood is not immune to genital warts during adulthood.

Appearance

The appearance of warts varies a little according to where they occur on the body. Warts on the palms of the hands are usually solitary growths consisting of a hard, dome-shaped, raised area of skin with hundreds of tiny conical projections which give the surface of the wart a 'velvety' appearance. Their colour also varies from pink to brown.

Warts on the hands, knees or face are often numerous and sometimes have a flat, plateau-like surface. Another variety, called *filiform warts,* consists of fine, elongated outgrowths from the face or neck.

GENITAL warts may be found in and around the folds of skin of the vulva in women or around the tip of the PENIS in men or anywhere in the surrounding genital area. They often grow and spread quite profusely, creating clusters of soft, cauliflower-like growths which may cause little discomfort despite their unsightly appearance. Their presence should always be reported to your doctor because they often accompany more serious SEXUALLY TRANSMITTED infections. Another risk for women is that certain types of genital warts may predispose to cancer of the CERVIX. Treatment is therefore important and should be followed up with regular smear tests.

People over the age of 50 are commonly afflicted with *seborrhoeic warts* on the covered parts of their skin (*see* SKIN AND SKIN DISEASES).

Treatment

Over the centuries, a wide variety of folk remedies have been used in the treatment of warts. Although these unconventional cures may sometimes appear to work, a visit to the doctor will probably be a more rewarding approach.

There are a number of different treatments for warts but no specific drugs for combating the wart virus. However, the growths can be attacked with corrosive ointments, or by freezing or electrically burning them off. All of these procedures are carried out by a doctor.

Common childhood warts on the hands and knees can either be left to disappear in their own time, or they can also be treated painlessly with an antiseptic-type acid paint. Applied twice a day, this usually causes the wart to disappear in two or three months.

Troublesome adult warts on the hands are sometimes treated by freezing with liquid nitrogen or solid carbon dioxide, which can be mildly painful but is very effective and causes little scarring. Electrically burning a wart off is more likely to cause a scar and is often followed by a recurrence of the infection, so this technique is less often used.

Genital warts are treated by painting with a corrosive substance called *podophyllum.* This must be applied by a doctor or nurse, as careless application can cause considerable soreness; the paint has to be washed off some four to six hours after application. The freezing and burning techniques outlined above are also sometimes used.

Water

Perhaps surprisingly, water is the largest single component of the human body – the average man contains about 10 gals (45 litres). To keep alive, we all need a regular intake of both food and water, but of the two we need water more regularly. The body has no method of storing water, and without it, death occurs in about three days since water is absolutely vital for all major bodily functions.

Importance of water

Water (chemically known as H_2O) is the simplest compound of hydrogen and oxygen, elements which are essential to living matter and to every life process.

The body is made up of approximately 70 per cent water, with certain tissues – such as the grey matter in the BRAIN – containing up to 85 per cent, and other tissues, such as fat layers, only 25 per cent. It is also the base for the body's major transport system: BLOOD is 80 per cent water, and this takes food (in the form of sugars) to the tissues and, on its return, takes waste to be excreted.

Luckily, the body has the necessary machinery to tell us when we need water. Thirst is a basic human drive; when we feel thirsty, the body is signalling its need for water. The volume of water we then drink in order to satisfy the body's needs is dependent on how much water the body has lost.

Water loss

The body is continuously losing water through cooling, lubrication and excretion. Most of this loss occurs through the KIDNEYS when we urinate. If our blood becomes too concentrated, special cells in the HYPOTHALAMUS signal this to the PITUITARY gland which then begins to secrete a HORMONE – called antidiuretic hormone – which acts on the kidneys. This hormone then makes the kidneys reabsorb more water from the renal tubules. If we take in too much fluid, the opposite happens; the KIDNEYS reabsorb less water and the URINE becomes more dilute and present in greater quantities.

In addition, up to 1¾ pints (1 litre) of water can be lost from the moist membranes of the lungs as we breathe out. This can be seen in the 'steaming breath' caused by water vapour condensing on a cold day. We also lose some in tears when we cry or when our eyes are irritated, in our saliva, in our faeces and mucous secretions – such as a streaming nose or even mucous lost during SEXUAL INTERCOURSE. In addition, we lose water in our sweat, not just when we are excessively hot, but during everyday activity (*see* PERSPIRATION). Only in extremely rare cases do we find ourselves short of water as we are continually taking in the amount we need through both drink (coffee, tea, milk, etc.) and food. In fact, up to 90 per cent of some vegetables are water.

Dehydration

If too much water is lost and not replaced, this will lead to dehydration, a condition that normally only occurs in hot climates where water is in short supply, and during illness. Severe dehydration can lead to both physical and mental changes. The physical symptoms include dry skin, weakening muscles, the loss of skin elasticity, and dark-coloured urine. Eventually the flow of urine ceases. If the person continues to be deprived of water, the kidneys fail and waste products, such as urea, accumulate in the bloodstream. If the situation is not remedied, the result is death.

Mentally, the sufferer can become disorientated and begin to hallucinate – hence the popular image of lost desert travellers seeing mirages of oases.

Water loss through illness

It is with illnesses such as CHOLERA and DYSENTERY, which produce fever, VOMITING and DIARRHOEA, that much water can be lost and severe dehydration result. During illness, water in the body is heavily involved in ridding the body of its poisons and wastes and in cooling the body during bouts of FEVER. So any cold or fever needs to be accompanied by an increase of fluid intake.

Severe diarrhoea in small children and babies can be extremely dangerous. When it leads to dehydration, their lips, tongue and mouth become dry, and they are continually thirsty. Their anterior fontanelle (the soft spot at the top of a baby's head where the bones of the skull have not yet fully fused) is depressed and the children may feel cold when you touch them; in its severest form, a child may begin to turn blue (*cyanosis*) as the circulation begins to falter.

Intravenous fluids may need to be administered to restore the water balance, although water and salts taken by mouth help the situation immensely. The cause of the diarrhoea and vomiting needs to be treated separately before water content in the body can be naturally restored.

See also HOMOEOSTASIS.

Waterbrash, *see* Indigestion

Water retention, *see* Oedema

Wax in the ear

Ear-wax, or cerumen, consists of a mixture of the oil secretions of the modified sweat glands situated in the outer third of the ear canal, scales from the skin and dust particles. It is sticky, water-resistant and forms a natural barrier against infection.

Although ear-wax is harmless, and is usually removed by the ear's self-cleaning mechanism, it may occasionally accumulate, causing temporary deafness. Medical treatment should be sought when this occurs.

Problems

In normal circumstances, wax does not accumulate in the EARS, as it is continually being moved outwards by the movement of the jaw-bones and the natural shedding of the skin.

However, some people do produce more ear-wax than others. An accumulation is more likely to occur in people employed in dusty occupations, or those who have excess hair in their ears, or those who have an inflammation of the skin or scalp.

Accumulated wax may cause a variety of symptoms, the chief one being temporary DEAFNESS. The wax may become impacted at the narrowest part of the ear canal by unskilled attempts to remove it with matches, hairpins, cotton wool buds or other implements. Accumulated wax may cause irritation and noises in the ear, but rarely pain.

Sudden deafness together with a feeling of pressure may occur after taking a swim or shower: this is due to water entering the ear and causing the wax to swell. Attempts to clear the ears will only push the wax deeper into the ear canal, and this will cause pain, noises in the ear or, more rarely, dizziness (*see* BALANCE).

Treatment

Impacted wax is one of the commonest conditions seen in a doctor's surgery. A doctor can remove the wax safely by picking it out with very fine forceps or by a blunt hook under direct vision.

Alternatively, the wax can be removed by syringeing the ears. This is a safe procedure in experienced hands. Before syringeing, the doctor may advise the patient to put drops such as bicarbonate of soda in solution, warm olive oil or a wax solvent in the ears to soften the wax and make it easier to syringe.

Syringeing is a painless procedure. A jet of warm water is forced into the ear canal without touching the skin with the syringe's metal tip. The ear is then carefully cleaned and dried. Relief from deafness is immediate and dramatic. Special care and gentleness is required when syringeing a child's ears. If the child is reluctant or uncooperative, it may be better to have the wax removed under anaesthesia.

If the patient has a previous history of ear trouble or has had an operation on his or her ears, there may be perforation of the eardrum. The normal drum is not easily ruptured, but where there has been a perforation which has healed, the scar tissue is vulnerable to injury and great care must be taken during syringeing.

Where wax has accumulated in large amounts and has become solid, it should be removed by a specialist in hospital.

Weals, *see* Rash

Weil's disease

Weil's disease or Leptospirosis is a disease caused by infection with an organism called *Leptospira icterohaemorrhagiae.* They are excreted in rodent urine (usually rats) to which humans are exposed. People who work in abattoirs and sewers are particularly at risk, but increasingly people who take part in water sports in infected rural waters are catching Weil's disease.

Symptoms

The incubation period is 10 days. Only 10–15 per cent of patients suffer from severe illness. The illness occurs in two phases: first, viral-type symptoms such as fever, headache and loss of appetite predominate; this is followed by the immune phase, in which 50 per cent of patients have meningism (irritation of the lining of the brain), and a small number go on to develop tender liver enlargement and jaundice. They may then progress to kidney and heart failure.

Diagnosis
Leptospires can be found in the blood when cultured and in the cerebrospinal fluid if a lumbar puncture is performed. A special antibody test may become positive at the end of the first week.

Treatment
Treatment is with penicillin. Liver and kidney failure may require more complex hospital treatment, e.g. dialysis.

Wernicke's encephalopathy, *see* **Vitamins**

Whiplash injury

This is a well-known term which conjures up images of a devastating injury to the neck. In fact, 'whiplash' refers to a single type of neck injury which is essentially a sprain. Like any sprain, it may vary greatly in severity, ranging from a few days of mild discomfort in the neck to many months of pain and restriction of movements, or even permanent disability. But in the majority of cases, although the condition may be irritating, recovery is complete within about a month.

Causes
Whiplash injury is nearly always caused by car accidents, usually when a stationary car is struck from behind by another car. When this happens, the occupants of the stationary car are suddenly accelerated forward, but their heads are momentarily 'left behind'. The effect is like suddenly looking upward: the neck is bent backward or 'extended'. The MUSCLES and ligaments at the front of the neck and throat are placed under a sudden strain. This results in minor haemorrhages into these muscles and ligaments which resolve within a short period of time. In more severe cases, there may be momentary dislocation of one or more small joints in the neck, or even FRACTURES of the neck bones.

Symptoms
Often there is little pain immediately after the accident. However, the following day there is pain in the neck which is difficult to pinpoint, and this may spread into the shoulders or upper arms. Neck movements may become restricted by muscle spasm. Those with more severe injuries may complain of blurred vision, headaches, dizziness, or difficulty in swallowing because of bruising around the nerves and blood vessels in the neck. X-rays are usually unhelpful since the injuries are located in the soft tissues, which don't show on ordinary X-rays.

In most cases, the symptoms settle down within a few days. However, people may develop persistent pain and stiffness which may last for many months. Some of these pains may be due to underlying ARTHRITIS in the joints of the neck which is triggered off by the injury. In other cases, there is a vicious circle of pain and stiffness giving rise to muscle spasm which in turn causes more pain and stiffness. In some cases, there is a psychological element which keeps the pain going – often while an insurance claim is awaiting settlement.

The main danger is that symptoms will become persistent. Serious injury to the neck is rare: fractures of the neck bones, SLIPPED DISC, dislocations of the joints, SPINAL CORD and nerve root injuries are more commonly caused by bending the neck forward, or by direct force applied to the top of the head. Other complications may include pain so acute as to be immobilizing. Constant headaches and dizziness may require medication heavy enough to impair routine activities.

Treatment

Initial treatment consists of resting the neck so that its muscles can relax and avoid going into spasm. This may be achieved by lying flat in bed so that the neck muscles do not have to work to hold the neck upright. A more convenient method is to apply a collar or neck brace to support the neck: this takes over the function of the muscles and allows the individual to remain fairly active. At this stage, PAINKILLERS are useful to prevent sore muscles from going into spasm and worsening the symptoms. If pain persists beyond one or two weeks, PHYSIOTHERAPY may be helpful. Gentle traction to the neck will relieve painful muscle spasm and lessen any pressure on the nerves that go into the shoulders and arms. Exercise to mobilize the neck, often combined with heat treatment, may also help to relax tense muscles. Some patients fail to respond to any form of treatment, and in such cases, only time seems to result in any improvement.

The associated symptoms of dizziness, blurred vision and headaches are often very difficult to treat. Again, drug treatment may be of some help, but often the patient simply has to learn to live with these irritating symptoms and wait patiently for them to subside.

In the rare cases where a dislocation or fracture occurs, it may be necessary to stabilize the neck bones by means of an operation which is designed to fuse several of the neck bones together.

'Whites', the, *see* **Leucorrhoea**

Whitlow

The area where the SKIN meets the nail is firmly covered by the cuticle or nail seal. But through damage to the cuticle, this seal can be broken, thereby allowing infectious agents to enter. *Paronychia* is the medical term for infections which result, but commonly they have acquired the distinctive name of *whitlow.*

WHITLOW

Causes

Wetness, soap and injury are the main causes of cuticle damage. Excessive immersion in water softens and weakens the cuticle, while prolonged contact with soaps and detergents removes oil from the skin, leaving it less supple and more liable to split.

Minor injuries may also damage cuticles – fingers are particularly prone to injury as they are used so much in work and play. A baby's whitlow may be caused by injury and by the wet environment produced by thumb-sucking. Careless manicuring may damage cuticles; but, equally, neglect may result in the cuticle, at the base of the nail, growing out over the half-moon and splitting and curling up so it is caught and damaged.

Whitlows are also more likely where the nails have been bitten regularly, because the nail fold is frequently damaged as well. Some people also have a nervous habit of chewing the nail fold at the side of the nail or picking off little loose pieces of skin around the nail. Again, this may also make whitlows more likely.

Lastly, a whitlow may be caused by infection with the *Herpes simplex* virus, when it is known as a 'herpetic whitlow'. This virus also causes the common COLD SORES that many people develop during a heavy cold, or with exposure to the sun or extreme cold. Someone who is suffering from a cold sore and then chews his or her fingernails may transfer the virus to the nail fold, setting up an infection.

Symptoms

The commonest type of whitlow is of sudden or 'acute' onset. This is known medically as an 'acute paronychia'. The nail fold becomes inflamed, hot and painful. Within less than 24 hours, the fingertip begins to throb. Pus may start to form internally and little beads of pus may escape at the side of the nail. If the infection is neglected, the pus begins to collect under the nail as well and the infection may even involve virtually the whole fingertip. The sufferer may feel unwell as a result of the general effects of the infection.

Chronic whitlows usually occur in fingertips damaged by excessive immersion in water. Often two or three fingertips are affected. The infection may develop over many days, or even weeks. The nail fold becomes thickened and is usually tender to touch, but may not be particularly painful. A little pus tends to ooze out of the nail fold from time to time. The nail itself may become ridged or furrowed due to infection having damaged it as it was forming, and it may become infected and discoloured at the edges.

A herpetic whitlow starts suddenly with one or more blisters appearing near the nail fold. The blisters enlarge and then multiply, filling first with clear fluid which after a day or two becomes cloudy, rather like thin pus. A herpetic whitlow can be extremely painful and, if untreated, may last for several weeks.

Treatment

Acute whitlows always need medical treatment. The infection is caused by a bacterium, and it can respond to antibiotics taken by mouth if the infection is at a very early stage. The doctor may also prescribe some antibiotic ointment or cream to be applied to the nail fold under a dressing.

Once an acute whitlow reaches the stage of pus formation, incision is usually required. A small cut is made by the doctor in the nail fold along the edge of the nail, to allow the pus to escape. Anaesthesia for this procedure may be provided by spraying the area with ethyl chloride, which literally freezes the tissues so that they are numbed. However, more often a procedure called a 'ring block' is used. Local anaesthetic is injected by the doctor into the base of the finger on either side (in a 'ring') to deaden the nerves to the fingertip. After a few minutes the whole finger becomes completely numb, allowing the incision to be carried out painlessly.

Once the whitlow has been incised, it is immediately much less painful and should heal within a few days. A neglected whitlow may not only require incision but also surgical removal of the nail itself.

A chronic whitlow is usually caused by a fungal infection, although occasionally a bacterial infection may be responsible. Before treating the whitlow, the doctor may take a swab for laboratory testing to find out the exact type of infection. If the infection is indeed fungal, an anti-fungal cream or paint will be prescribed, to be applied to the nail fold two or three times a day. At the same time, it is very important that the finger is kept dry, so rubber gloves (with cotton gloves worn underneath) must be worn during washing-up.

A chronic bacterial whitlow may respond to local antibiotic cream or antibiotics given by mouth, but surgical removal of the nail may be needed.

A herpetic whitlow is treated with local anti-viral paint or cream. Special anti-viral antibiotics such as idoxuridine or acyclovir are applied under a dressing, and are usually effective in curing the whitlow within a few days. Surgery is not indicated. If a herpetic whitlow is incised in error (for example, it could be mistaken for an acute whitlow), the infection may actually worsen because the virus can be spread further through the tissues. Hence an accurate diagnosis of herpetic whitlow is essential.

Whooping cough

Whooping cough, or *pertussis* as it is medically known, is a highly infectious bacterial disease caused by *Bordetella pertussis*. Anybody who has neither had, nor been immunized against, whooping cough, can catch it. The disease is spread by droplets of bacteria in the air. The bacteria settle in the mucous lining of the respiratory tract (lungs and throat), causing inflammation and production of a thick sticky mucus.

Incidence of whooping cough

Children between one and four years old are most susceptible, although since IMMUNIZATION, more adolescents and adults are the source of the disease. The death rate is highest in babies less than one year old, and particularly under four months. Epidemics tend to occur in three- or four-year cycles, starting in January and peaking in the spring, like many other respiratory infections of children and adults.

An attack of whooping cough confers life-long protection through acquired immunity. Unlike many other infectious diseases, protection does not seem to be transferred to babies from the mother, so they are susceptible from birth. Some immunity is transferred to a breastfed baby in the colostrum (the fluid secreted form the mother's breasts for the first few days after giving birth).

Since the introduction of immunization against whooping cough, there has been a fall in both incidence and deaths, but immunization is neither complete nor permanent, and some adults who were immunized as children do still catch whooping cough in later life, although it is usually a mild attack with very few if any complications.

Course of the illness

The incubation period lasts 6–20 days from contact, with 7 days as an average. The patient is infectious from the catarrhal phase for about three weeks, and should be isolated for this period or until the cough has subsided. In particular, children aged under one year should be kept away from those already suffering from the condition.

The illness can be divided into three distinct stages: the *catarrhal* phase, the *paroxysmal* phase and the *convalescent* phase. The catarrhal phase lasts one or two weeks. Initially the symptoms are rather like a cold: runny nose; red, runny eyes; a slight cough; and temperature.

The paroxysmal phase lasts from two to four or more weeks, and in this stage, there are episodes of coughing, becoming increasingly worse and more frequent – up to around 40 bouts a day. The bouts consist of 5–10 repetitive coughs while breathing out, followed by a sudden effort to breathe in, which in older children produces the characteristic 'whoop'. The face goes red or blue, the eyes bulge, the tongue sticks out, both eyes and nose run and the veins in the neck become more obvious. Episodes of this coughing occur until the patient manages to dislodge the plug of mucus. During this time, in severe attacks, young children may lack oxygen and stop breathing or have a convulsion. At the end of the coughing bout, the child will vomit. The vomiting is really more characteristic of whooping cough than the whoop. These episodes are extremely exhausting, and infants become tired and lose weight.

Attacks can be triggered by movement, yawning, sneezing, eating, drinking or even by thinking about them. In between attacks, the patient appears relatively well.

Very young infants, under three or four months of age, often do not have the characteristic whoop. They have spasms of coughing, and at the end of the spasm, they may stop breathing for a moment or two and go blue. They then recover and continue breathing normally. In severe cases, the spasm may be accompanied by a nose-bleed, or there may be little pin-point haemorrhages in the skin around the eyes. There may also be bleeding into the whites of the eyes.

During convalescence, the paroxysmal cough, whoop and vomiting gradually subside, although the cough and whoop may last for many weeks or months – and often recur if the child catches a cold or throat infection. Incidentally, the Chinese call it 'the hundred day cough' because it can drag on for so long.

Adults and teenage children who have whooping cough are rarely very ill with the infection, and it may be so mild that the person is unaware that he or she may be infectious. Nevertheless adults with whooping cough are just as infectious as children who have the disease and may be responsible for spreading the infection to the young ones. The symptoms are usually simply of a recurrent dry cough which may persist for two or three weeks.

Diagnosis

The diagnosis is usually made on the clinical symptoms, but in older children and adults with a milder attack, this can be difficult. The best method is to take a swab from the back of the nose and do a culture (inoculate the material into a special substance on which the bacteria can grow so that a diagnosis can be made). Blood tests are not very helpful, though the number of lymphocytes (a type of defensive BLOOD cell) may be very high, which aids diagnosis. Otherwise, two samples of blood are needed, at the beginning and end of the illness, to show a rise in pertussis antibodies during that time; if the sample is not taken early enough, it won't show a large enough rise to make the diagnosis.

More often than not, it is difficult for a doctor to carry out all the tests necessary for a precise diagnosis, and in some cases, the swabs fail to show the *Bordetella* organisms. So the doctor may make the diagnosis on the basis of a characteristic history and the symptoms. Because the early symptoms are very similar to an ordinary cold, it may be several days before the doctor can make a confident diagnosis of whooping cough. Unfortunately, by this time the infection may have already spread to other people in the household who have not been vaccinated.

Complications

Most of the deaths from whooping cough are caused by complications, such as PNEUMONIA. Usually pneumonia is not due to pertussis bacteria, but to other invading bacteria, which enter the affected LUNGS. Plugs of mucus may block off the bronchi (the tubes leading the air from the throat to the lungs) and cause the lung to collapse; then it may become infected by bacteria. Sometimes the lung collapse is permanent, leading to chronic scarring of the lungs.

EAR infections frequently occur at the same time. The lack of oxygen to the BRAIN during a severe coughing spell can cause convulsions or loss of consciousness. The pertussis bacteria can also affect the brain tissues, causing inflammation. Haemorrhage or bleeding can occur into the brain. There is a real risk of long-term damage in severe cases of whooping cough, particularly among very young babies. Sometimes the pressure of coughing can cause the RECTUM to come out of the patient's anus. Occasionally the force of coughing may even cause one or more ribs to fracture. This is more common in older children or adults, whose ribs are less pliable than those of a baby.

Often babies cannot keep down enough fluid and food and become dehydrated. About 10 per cent of children require hospital admission.

Treatment

Antibiotics are effective if given in the catarrhal phase when they will stop or decrease the severity of the infection. They are not effective in the paroxysmal phase. If the antibiotic is given to a child who has been in contact with the disease, *before* any symptoms appear, the severity of the illness may be reduced. The drug is given to children who have whooping cough as it makes these children less infectious to others. Other treatment is symptomatic: avoiding stimuli which cause coughing; a warm room, especially at night; small frequent drinks and meals, and no rushing about. Children who go blue during coughing bouts or cannot keep down fluid need hospital admission for oxygen, therapy, suction to remove mucous plugs, and replacement of fluids either by a tube through the nose into the stomach, or by injection into a vein. Some doctors give mild sedatives.

Prevention

Lifelong prevention only occurs after an attack of whooping cough, so that pertussis can only be prevented by active immunization with the pertussis vaccine.

The vaccine consists of a suspension of killed organisms of *Bordetella pertussis*. They stimulate the body to produce antibodies without actually giving rise to an attack of whooping cough.

The vaccine has to be given in three doses to give about 95 per cent protection against the disease. The vaccine is more effective if given at the same time as diphtheria and tetanus vaccine – hence the triple DPT vaccine given to most infants.

When not to vaccinate

If a child is suffering from a feverish illness or is generally unwell, the vaccination should be postponed until the child is better. However, if the baby just has the sniffles or a cold without any fever, there is no added risk and the vaccination can go ahead.

When a child is due to have the second or third dose of vaccine, the doctor always enquires if there were any reactions to the previous dose. If there was an extensive local reaction with swelling and redness around the injection site involving a wide area of skin, no further injections will be given, because the reaction to the vaccine could be even worse with subsequent doses. A high fever or other serious general reactions following a previous dose is also a contra-indication to proceeding with the course of injections.

There are some groups of children who may have a higher risk than others of complications from vaccination. These include children who have already had fits, or whose parents, brothers or sisters have EPILEPSY. Also children who have had any disorders of the nervous system may be at added risk of complications. In any of these circumstances, an individual decision should be made by the parents about the advisability of vaccination, after consultation with a paediatrician. Whooping cough infection in such children is likely to cause more complications anyway, so it may be preferable to accept the slightly higher risk of complications from the vaccine.

Contrary to former belief, hay fever, eczema and a history of other allergies in the family are not a contra-indication to having the vaccine. It is also possible for children to be vaccinated while they are taking a course of antibiotics, provided they are not feverish.

Side-effects of vaccination

Following vaccination either with pertussis alone or with the triple vaccine, there may be a mild feverish illness over the next 48 hours, or your baby may just be a bit miserable; older children may complain of a headache. There is often a small area of redness and swelling at the site of the injection which usually settles after a few days. A small firm lump may be felt for a couple of months afterwards.

Serious complications generally occur in the first week, usually in the first 72 hours; these may be convulsions, often associated with a high temperature or, extremely rarely, *encephalitis* (*see* BRAIN AND BRAIN DISEASE). Complications can be kept to a minimum by strictly keeping to the rules concerning which children should and should not have the vaccine.

Either your own doctor or the children's clinic doctor or nurse may give pertussis vaccine. They will know your medical history but, in addition, will ask you about any family history of convulsions or brain damage. They know the risks, both of catching whooping cough and of the complications of the vaccine, and will discuss any worries with you.

Wilson's disease, *see* Minerals, Trace elements

Wisdom teeth

These are the rearmost TEETH, and they are designed to grind food. They are the third molars and normally erupt from the age of about 17 onwards (the first molar teeth erupting around the age of six).

Why are they called 'wisdom teeth'? Normally these teeth erupt at a time when many people finish schooling. Combine this with the experiences of early adulthood, and one might reasonably say that, at this age, a person's wisdom is in the ascendant. Maybe this was the reason that early anatomists named these teeth *dentes sapientiae*, which translates as 'wisdom teeth'.

There are normally four wisdom teeth and they cut through at the back of the mouth, one on each side of the upper jaw (*maxilla*) and one on each side of the lower jaw (*mandible*). Their arrival completes the normal complement of 32 teeth in an adult: eight incisors (four top and bottom), four canines (two top and bottom), eight premolars (four top and bottom) and 12 molars (six top and bottom).

In our ancestors, the upper and lower jaws were more pronounced than modern ones. In effect, our jaws have become smaller as we have evolved, but the genetic material controlling the number of teeth that erupt remains the same. Because the wisdom teeth are the last to erupt and claim space in the jaw, they will 'impact' whenever the earlier teeth have occupied too much of the available space.

The upper wisdom teeth are able to erupt more easily than the lower ones, being slightly smaller. The eruption process is similar to that of all the other teeth in the mouth. The gum is pushed back and the calcified crown of the tooth pushes its way from the underlying bone. During this process, the gum can become very sore, but this can often be reduced by bathing the area with warm salty water. The tooth will push through in bursts of growth activity which usually last for about eight days at a time and may take up to a year to take up its final position.

Because teeth work in pairs, it is essential for both upper and lower wisdom teeth to erupt normally if they are to be of any use. A shortage of space may cause either tooth to compact or erupt at an unfavourable angle, causing them to rub the inside of the cheek. In such cases, it may be desirable to extract them. They are also extracted if there is a risk of them becoming infected. They are not usually removed if they remain deeply buried in the jaw bone and are unable to erupt while remaining symptomless. Nor are they extracted when they erupt normally and have a useful role as a molar tooth at the back of the mouth.

Extraction of wisdom teeth

X-rays not only tell the dentist how a tooth is going to erupt, they also show how easy it would be to remove it should this be necessary. The upper wisdom tooth lies beneath the maxillary sinus in the cheek bone. In the mandible, the lower wisdom tooth lies close to the nerve that supplies part of the tongue, and a second nerve that supplies the lower lip on that side. By looking at the root formation and the proximity of these structures, the dentist can assess the ease or difficulty of an extraction.

Simple extractions can be performed with local anaesthetic in the dental chair with little inconvenience and no need for time off work. More complicated or multiple extractions of wisdom teeth are often carried out under a general anaesthetic and may require a week's convalescence afterwards. Numbness (anaesthesia) of the lower lip or tongue tip is a possible consequence of difficult extractions, and patients may be warned of this risk by the surgeon performing the extraction. Any such numbness is usually temporary, and normal sensation returns after a few months, although in a few cases, a small area of permanent numbness persists.

Difficult extractions are sometimes followed by small particles of bone being rejected by the body through the wound, a process called *exfoliation*. This is quite normal, and the socket heals all the faster once these particles have been removed.

A rare finding on X-ray can be *cystic degeneration* of the area around the wisdom tooth. This is caused by a change in the nature of the layer of follicle cells that have surrounded the tooth ever since it first started to form. Cysts can expand quite rapidly and may weaken the jaw bone, and consequently should always be treated.

See also DENTAL CARE.

Withdrawal, *see* **Contraception, Penis**

Womb, *see* **Uterus**

Worms

Worms are referred to medically as *helminths*; they are many-celled animals as opposed to the single-celled bacteria and protozoa that are the other main parasites of humans. Of the parasitic worms, each species has a specific life-cycle that allows infestation to continue and to pass through another animal before infesting a human host – for example, schistosomes, which cause schistosomiasis (bilharzia), develop in the water snail before infesting humans (*see* TROPICAL DISEASES).

Some of the worms that cause trouble in humans actually have another animal as their 'primary host'. The host is the animal within which the worm reaches its adult form, and any animal that it infects during the egg or larva stage is called the 'intermediate host'.

Helminths that infect humans are divided into three major groups. The first are the *nematodes*; these are the roundworms producing such diseases as ascariasis and elephantiasis. Next are the *cestodes*, or tapeworms; and last the *trematodes*, or flatworms, which give rise to schistosomiasis and liver fluke infestation. The cestodes and trematodes have fairly similar life-cycles.

Nematodes – roundworms

The nematodes have a wide range of shapes and sizes and a great variability in the way their life-cycles work. Those of medical importance include the following types of roundworm.

Filariae are a very important group of worms which cause such diseases as elephantiasis, loa loa and river BLINDNESS. The adult worms are round, and both males and females need to be present in the primary host so that reproduction can take place. These worms are carried from person to person by a blood-sucking insect – with a different species for each species of worm.

Hookworms are very common throughout the tropics and sub-tropics. They all have a similar life-cycle where the adult worm lives in the DUODENUM, where it feeds on blood and lays its eggs, which then pass out in faeces. In warm soil, the eggs change into larvae; these make their way through human skin, should they come in contact with it. Once in the bloodstream, the larvae are carried to the lungs. They then travel up the windpipe to be swallowed, and pass to the intestine. There is often itching at the entry point.

Ascaris cause a large number of infestations; it has been estimated that up to a quarter of the world's population may be infected with ascaris to some degree. The worms live in the intestine, the eggs being ingested directly from food contaminated with faeces. Once the larva hatches in the duodenum, it works its way into the bloodstream and embeds itself in the lungs. From here it is coughed up the windpipe and swallowed, thus finding its way back to the intestine.

Ascaris causes few symptoms in most people, but there may be inflammation of the lungs as the larvae pass through. Large numbers of ascaris in the bowel can certainly cause abdominal symptoms and lead to blockage of the intestine.

Threadworms, common in children all over the world, also live in the intestines. The adult female worm emerges from the anus to lay eggs which then cause irritation. The infested person has probably picked up the eggs on his fingers when scratching and inadvertently swallowed them. This may lead to reinfection of the same person and to infection of others, a situation most common in children. The main symptom is anal itching.

Trematodes – flatworms or flukes

Schistosomiasis (bilharzia) is one of the diseases caused by a trematode. The Egyptian form affects the bladder because here the eggs of the organism hatch into adult worms and cause inflammation. The two other forms of the disease infect the bowel. Eggs are passed out in the faeces and develop in water snails before the larvae find their way back into the human body by burrowing into the skin.

The liver fluke is another trematode which causes problems, especially in South-East Asia where raw fish is a popular food.

Cestodes – tapeworms

Tapeworms affect only meat eaters. The typical tapeworm is the beef tapeworm, *Taenia saginata*. Humans are the primary hosts, and the worm anchors itself to the upper intestine, producing a great string of egg-bearing segments (the tape). Eggs pass out in the faeces; for the infestation to be passed on, they must be eaten by some suitable intermediate host such as a cow. Inside the intermediate host, they hatch into larvae which spread to invade all the muscles. The life-cycle continues if a person eats infested uncooked flesh. Despite the enormous size they may reach – up to 30 ft (9 m) – tapeworms usually produce few symptoms.

Treatment and control

The only really common problem in the UK is threadworm. A small percentage of the population is infested with trichinosis – a pork parasite – but there are often no symptoms of this. Perhaps the most serious problem arising from worms is infestation with the larvae of the dog worm *toxicara*, since this can lead to blindness. Tapeworms are very uncommon. It is possible to catch a liver fluke, however, by eating wild watercress.

Drugs are available to kill practically all the worms that infest humans, but some of these drugs are quite toxic in themselves (although this *not* true of the drug treatment used to eradicate threadworm). Worm infestation is a major public health problem, but it must be control rather than cure that is the answer.

Many sorts of infestation could be avoided by better sanitation and by reducing the risk of food and water being contaminated with human faeces. In other cases the intermediate host could be controlled, thus cutting down the risk of disease.

Hygiene is very important, since many roundworms are spread by taking in food or water contaminated with human faeces. Hookworm can be avoided by wearing shoes. Many of the filarial worms are spread by blood-sucking insects – so try to avoid insect bites, though obviously this can be difficult.

Some worms can be avoided by cooking food thoroughly. Both the common tapeworms are spread by undercooked beef and pork. The larvae die at 55°C (131°F), so very high temperatures are not necessary. A fish tapeworm (*Diphyllobothrium latum*) occurs in Scandinavia; it is acquired from uncooked fish. *Anisakis marina* is another parasite which can be ingested with raw fish; it is a parasite of herrings and infects humans in Holland and Japan, where raw herring is eaten as a delicacy. There are also two forms of liver fluke in the Far East which can only be caught by eating raw or undercooked fish.

Wrist

Each wrist is actually a complex of numerous JOINTS between lots of little BONES. This gives the joint great flexibility but makes it a potential weak spot. It is strengthened by a web of ligaments and TENDONS which link the bones and make lifting possible.

The structure of the wrist

The wrist is made up no fewer than eight separate bones called *carpals*. They are like small pebbles arranged in two rows and bound together by about 20 ligaments and tendons. The carpals sit between the *metacarpals* of the hand and the long bones of the arm. The wrist bones in the row nearest the arm, running from thumb to little finger, are called the *scaphoid, lunate, triquetral* and *pisiform*. The second row consists of the *trapezium, trapezoid, capitate* and *hamate*. The only one of these that is visible on the skin surface is the pisiform which can be seen as the bumpy wrist bone.

The tendons that almost completely surround the wrist joint are enclosed in a kind of tunnel called the *carpal tunnel* . This protects the tendons from rubbing against the moving wrist bones.

Movement of the wrist

The carpal joints are relatively immobile, although as a unit the wrist is very flexible indeed. The exception is the joint between the trapezium and the thumb bone. This type of joint makes it possible to grasp an object between the finger and thumb. An opposable thumb makes humans particularly adept at using tools.

Anatomically, the wrist joint is described as *ellipsoid.* This means that, although it enables up-and-down and side-to-side actions and some circular movement, it cannot rotate like the hip and shoulder joints. This limitation helps to ensure the stability of the joint. However, it is thought that the wrist joint is only properly stable when the tendons, ligaments and muscles act to keep all the components of the joint in the right place. This 'tension' is necessary, even when the body is completely at rest.

Such a fragile joint is clearly easy to damage; lots of people will have experienced a slight sprain or strain and noticed how much it affects manual manipulation – every tiny action hurts the damaged joints.

Fractures and dislocations

Of all the injuries that involve the wrist, the most common is a break, or FRACTURE, at the lower end of the radius – one of the two long bones in the forearm. This is called a *Colles fracture,* and is treated by manipulation to reset the bones and immobilization in a plaster of Paris cast.

The small carpal bones can also suffer hair-line cracks. Sometimes there is a swelling on the back of the hand, just below the thumb, but often there are no external signs, only pain and stiffness in the joint. Often even X-rays do not show up these small cracks, but they can still be a problem. A hair-line crack can separate a small portion of bone from its blood supply and this can result in bone death. If there is any suspicion that this is happening, the doctor will immediately immobilize the wrist joint to prevent any more damage.

The bones of the wrist can also become dislocated if banged or moved awkwardly, especially the lunate bone in the centre of the wrist and the triquetral below the little finger. The dislocation shows up as a bulge on the outside of the wrist and should be manipulated into position by a doctor as soon as possible.

Problems with the tendons

The most common problem to afflict the wrist is called *carpal tunnel syndrome.* The fibrous carpal tunnel encloses all the wrist tendons and one of the main nerves supplying the hand, the median nerve. If the fibres in the tunnel become swollen or squashed, they press the nerve against the wrist bones, causing considerable pain.

The syndrome can be caused by simple overuse of the thumb and fingers (*see* REPETITIVE STRAIN INJURY). It is also common in late PREGNANCY when OEDEMA (swelling) can put pressure on the median nerve. It is generally more common in women than men. Other conditions which cause carpal tunnel syndrome are diabetes, rheumatoid arthritis and hypothyroidism.

Whatever the cause, the syndrome begins with a sensation of PINS AND NEEDLES OR NUMBNESS, especially in the thumb and next two fingers. The part of the wrist near the thumb may swell up, and the forearm and thumb are often very painful.

Usually the symptoms will gradually ease as the swelling or pressure is reduced. But, occasionally the syndrome may be quite persistent or recurrent, and in this case, surgery may be required to effect a permanent cure. This involves removing some of the swollen or damaged tissue.

Another common problem is called *tenosynovitis.* The lubricated tendon sheaths become inflamed as a result of injury from overuse, or from RHEUMATOID ARTHRITIS. It becomes difficult and painful to uncurl the fingers, and sometimes movement may result in audible grating noises. The fingers and thumb may also feel numb as if they have permanent pins and needles. A doctor will usually prescribe an anti-inflammatory drug and suggest complete rest. A plaster cast may be needed to immobilize the tendons and allow healing.

X

X-rays

X-rays belong to the same 'family' as light waves and radio waves; like radio waves, they are invisible. They are produced artificially by bombarding a small tungsten 'target' with electricity in a device called an X-ray tube. X-rays travel in straight lines, and radiate outwards from a point on the target in all directions. In an X-ray machine, the X-ray tube is surrounded by lead casing, except for a small aperture through which the X-ray beam emerges.

Each of the body's tissues absorbs X-rays in a predictable way, and it is this particular property of X-rays which enables them to be used in medicine to form images of the body. Bones are dense, and contain calcium; they absorb X-rays well. Soft tissues – skin, fat, blood, and muscle – absorb X-rays much less efficiently. So when, for example, an arm is placed in the path of an X-ray beam, the X-rays pass readily through the soft tissues but penetrate the bones much less easily; the arm casts a shadow. X-rays blacken photographic film, so the shadow cast by the bones appears white, while the shadow of the soft tissues is a dark shade of grey.

The X-ray examination

The X-ray image, or *radiograph*, is really a demonstration of the anatomy of the part of the body under examination, and it is now possible to make a detailed inspection of almost any part of the body with X-rays. X-rays are therefore of greatest use in the diagnosis and follow-up of diseases and disorders which alter the structure of the body. Sometimes such changes in structure are so dramatic that they are immediately obvious even to the untrained observer; this is often the case with broken bones, for example. Frequently, however, the changes are more subtle and may only be apparent to the trained eye of a *radiologist* – a doctor who specializes in the interpretation of X-ray images. This is true of mammograms, special X-rays of the breast used to screen for breast cancer.

Prior to an X-ray examination, instructions about any special preparations which may be necessary are given to the patient when the appointment for the examination is made. In the case of examinations of the abdominal region, for example, it is often preferable for the patient to take laxatives and a special diet for two days beforehand, since empty bowels result in radiographs of much improved quality.

When the patient arrives at the X-ray department, the radiographer who will be 'taking' the X-rays explains the procedure. The patient undresses to expose the area concerned, and must remove all objects which might produce an image on the radiograph – such as jewellery, hair pins or dentures.

The position of the patient when the X-ray is taken is carefully and accurately chosen so as to provide the best possible demonstration of the part under examination, *and* expose the least amount of the body to the X-rays. This position may have to be modified if the patient is unwell or in severe pain. Positioning the patient is one of the radiographer's most important tasks.

Each X-ray film is usually carried in a flat cassette, and the patient lies, sits or stands with the region of interest in contact with the cassette. It is essential to avoid movement while the X-ray is taken, since this results in a blurred image. Every effort is made, therefore, to keep the patient comfortable and relaxed, to use the shortest feasible 'exposure' time (usually a mere fraction of a second) and, if necessary, to support or immobilize the region of interest with foam pads, sandbags or a cloth bandage.

When all is ready – the patient is in the correct position, the film is in place and the X-ray tube is ready for action – the radiographer leaves the room for a few moments, and presses the exposure button on the control panel to 'take' the X-ray. Although the control panel is situated behind a protective screen, the radiographer is still able to see and talk to the patient at all times. If, for any reason, it is necessary for someone to remain in the room while X-rays are taken, unnecessary exposure to X-rays is prevented by wearing a lead apron.

Special techniques

For most purposes, a standard X-ray examination is all that is required. Special techniques are available, however, which enable areas not adequately seen on standard radiographs to be studied in greater detail.

In general, these techniques necessitate the use of what are known as 'contrast media'. These are substances which cause the tissue concerned to become opaque – that is, to lose their transparency.

The use of contrast media – which are eliminated from the body by the kidneys – can be used to show the gall bladder and bile ducts, the urinary tract and the digestive tract. And when a contrast medium is injected directly into blood vessels, the arteries and veins are clearly outlined, and any abnormalities revealed. Likewise, using a contrast medium to highlight the fluid which surrounds the spinal cord is frequently useful in detecting a nerve compressed by a disc or a tumour.

By using a suspension of barium sulphate – an inert, chalky mixture which is opaque to X-rays – it is possible to visualize the ALIMENTARY CANAL throughout its length. During a 'barium meal' examination, the patient is given a glass of flavoured barium to drink. The patient's swallowing mechanism can be studied, abnormalities of the oesophagus (gullet) can be detected and the stomach is clearly outlined. The image is monitored continuously during the examination on a television screen, and the patient lies on a tilting table so that, with careful manoeuvring, each part of the stomach and duodenum can be studied in turn.

The lining of the stomach is seen more clearly when the stomach is distended with gas – the patient has to swallow fizzy tablets – because it then becomes coated with a thin film of barium. The examination is conducted by a radiologists, and usually takes around 20 minutes; a series of X-ray films are taken during the examination, to give a permanent record. This is one of the best methods of detecting peptic ulcers.

Barium can also be introduced into the large bowel by means of a rectal tube – in a 'barium enema' – and this has been one of the most important methods used to detect a cancer of the bowel. Nowadays, both barium meals and barium enemas have been largely superseded by ENDOSCOPY.

Opacification of the urinary tract is achieved by intravenous injection of a solution which contains iodine; this is rapidly eliminated by a the kidneys. Like barium, iodine is opaque to X-rays, and if X-ray films are taken at various intervals after the injection, the kidneys, ureters and bladder are clearly shown. The technique is called *intravenous urography* or *pyelography* (IVU or IVP) and is of great importance in the diagnosis of many types of kidney disease.

Dental X-rays

X-ray techniques simplify the diagnosis of a wide range of important dental problems, and are now in everyday use (*see* TEETH).

Tooth decay can sometimes be surprisingly difficult to detect, especially when it lurks in the space between the back teeth and in other inaccessible recesses. Decay, root disease, abscesses and infections can all be visibly demonstrated with X-rays, which will confirm the diagnosis at an early stage, document the extent of any disease and help determine the most suitable form of treatment. In fact, a basic X-ray examination has become a routine part of the dental check-up.

The equipment used is not normally very complicated. A low-powered X-ray unit is used and is often linked up to the dentist's chair. Small films – called 'bite-wing' films – are gripped in the patient's mouth next to the teeth to be examined.

More complex conditions – such as abnormalities of growth and development of teeth, jaw fractures, cysts and tumours – require a more detailed examination. One particularly valuable technique is *orthopantomography,* in which the X-ray machine moves around the jaw of the patient while the X-ray is taken, producing a 'panorama' of the teeth and jaws. This technique shows both upper and lower jaws, any unerupted teeth and the position and relationship of all the teeth on a single X-ray film.

When the two jaws do not fit together well, a side view of the face and jaws may be taken, showing the relationship of the teeth, jaws and soft tissue. The pictures help the orthodontist to plan treatment which may involve plates, braces or corrective surgery.

Hazards of X-rays

The early pioneers of radiology had no idea quite how dangerous excessive exposure to X-rays could be, so they took no precautions at all when working with X-rays. They discovered to their cost that large doses of radiation cause skin burns and dermatitis, cataract formation in the eyes, the appearance of various types of cancer, and damage to the reproductive organs resulting in genetic abnormalities in their children.

Today, we are in a rather more fortunate position, for we not only have a much more complete understanding of the nature of the hazards, but are better able to reduce them to an absolute minimum. Modern X-ray film, equipment and techniques are now designed specifically to produce high quality images at the lowest possible radiation dose to the patient.

The possible hazard of genetic damage is usually minimized by shielding the patient's reproductive organs from the X-ray beam whenever possible, with a sheet of lead. Furthermore, any non-urgent X-ray examinations of women of childbearing age are usually carried out only during the first 10 days of the menstrual cycle, (this is called the 'ten-day rule'), during which the possibility of pregnancy is exceptionally unlikely.

Recent advantages and the future

In 1972 came the first of a series of quite remarkable technological developments which have thrust radiology – or 'diagnostic imaging', as the speciality is better known – to the forefront of modern diagnostic medicine: this was the invention of *computerized tomography* (CT scanning; also known as computerized axial tomography – CAT – scanning).

The technique is based upon X-rays and the use of a computer to calculate precise tissue density at every point of a 'section' through the patient; the resulting images are in the form of series of dramatic 'slices' through the body. One crucial advantage of CT scanning is that it permits soft tissues, indistinguishable from each other by conventional techniques, to be clearly differentiated. In the brain, for instance, blood clots, tumours, grey matter and tissue swelling can be readily seen, and it would be no exaggeration to say that CT scanning has brought about a revolution in NEUROSURGERY. Digital radiology systems now use electronic sensors instead of X-ray film, and the final image is displayed on a TV screen. Computer processing of the image is possible and gives many new techniques – for example, the elimination of confusing bony shadows from an X-ray – at the touch of a button.

Imaging techniques which do not utilize X-rays have attracted much interest, as they eliminate radiation hazards. ULTRASOUND is increasingly used – especially in antenatal diagnosis – and ultrasound facilities are now widespread. In addition, there is the new technique, MRI (*magnetic resonance imaging*), which depends on the use of powerful magnetic fields to construct images.

One further trend in radiology is of particular interest, and this is the refinement of what are called 'interventional' techniques. It has now become possible for radiologists to perform a wide range of procedures under X-ray control, eliminating the need for major surgery. Examples include removal of stones in the bile ducts and dilation of blocked blood vessels.

See also RADIOTHERAPY.

Y

Yaws, *see* Ulcers, skin

Yeast infections, *see* Fungal infections

Yellow fever

This is one of the most important diseases caused by the family of viruses known as the *arboviruses*, which have in common the fact that they are transmitted by blood-sucking insects.

Yellow fever originated in West Africa but is now found in the whole of tropical Africa (*see* TROPICAL DISEASES). It also occurs in North and South America and the Caribbean, and it is thought that the infection was probably carried across the Atlantic on ships. Fortunately, it does not occur in tropical parts of Asia or in Europe, and there are strict controls to prevent the accidental spread of the infecting mosquito by aeroplane.

Yellow fever is slightly unusual in that LIVER failure – often associated with KIDNEY failure – is a common result, but bleeding problems are just as likely to be its chief characteristic.

The arboviruses typically infect animals as well as humans. In the case of yellow fever, monkeys and humans are the main host of the virus. The reservoir of infection in forest monkeys means that there is little likelihood of eliminating yellow fever. There will always be mosquitoes to carry the disease from monkey to monkey, and anyone bitten by such a mosquito might also get the disease. In fact, people who are raised in tropical forests have a considerable immunity to the disease, presumably because they are immune as babies and their resistance is built up by repeated exposure to the virus.

Apart from the cycle of infection which occurs high up in the canopy of a tropical rainforest, there is also the urban cycle of infection. Thus infection may be carried directly from person to person by the infecting mosquito outside the habitat of monkeys.

Symptoms

After the bite of an infecting mosquito, there is an incubation period of several days while the virus is multiplying in the body. Severe cases start characteristically with a sudden onset of fever, headache and pain in the abdomen, back and limbs. The patient may haemorrhage and vomit blood, and because the virus injures and destroys liver cells, JAUNDICE is common. The kidneys may start to produce blood and protein in the urine.